The Cleveland Clinic Foundation Intensive Review of Internal Medicine

FIFTH EDITION

The Cleveland Clinic Foundation Intensive Review of Internal Medicine

FIFTH EDITION

EDITORS

■ **JAMES K. STOLLER, MD, MS**

Jean Wall Bennett Chair
Head, Cleveland Clinic Respiratory Therapy
Executive Director, Leadership Development
The Cleveland Clinic Foundation
Cleveland, Ohio

■ **FRANKLIN A. MICHOTA, Jr., MD, FACP**

Director of Academic Affairs
Department of Hospital Medicine
The Cleveland Clinic Foundation
Cleveland, OH

■ **BRIAN F. MANDELL, MD, PhD**

Vice Chairman, Department of Academic Medicine
Department of Rheumatic and Immunologic Disease
Editor-in-Chief
The Cleveland Clinic Journal of Medicine
The Cleveland Clinic Foundation
Cleveland, Ohio

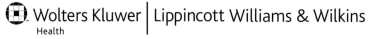

Wolters Kluwer | Lippincott Williams & Wilkins
Health

Philadelphia · Baltimore · New York · London
Buenos Aires · Hong Kong · Sydney · Tokyo

Acquisitions Editor: Sonya Seigafuse
Managing Editor: Kerry Barrett
Project Manager: Alicia Jackson
Senior Manufacturing Manager: Benjamin Rivera
Marketing Manager: Kimberly Schonberger
Designer: Holly McLaughlin
Cover Designer: Christine Jenny
Production Service: Aptara, Inc.

© 2009 LIPPINCOTT WILLIAMS & WILKINS, a WOLTERS KLUWER business
530 Walnut Street
Philadelphia, PA 19106 USA
LWW.com

Printed in China

Library of Congress Cataloging-in-Publication Data

The Cleveland Clinic intensive review of internal medicine / editors, James K. Stoller, Franklin A. Michota Jr., Brian F. Mandell. – 5th ed.
    p. ; cm.
  Includes bibliographical references and index.
  ISBN-13: 978-0-7817-9079-6
  ISBN-10: 0-7817-9079-4
  1. Internal medicine–Outlines, syllabi, etc.   2. Internal medicine–Study guides.
I. Stoller, James K.   II. Michota, Franklin A.   III. Mandell, Brian F., 1951-
IV. Cleveland Clinic Foundation.
  [DNLM: 1. Internal Medicine–Examination Questions.   WB 18.2 C635 2009]
  RC46.C548 2009
  616.0076–dc22

                                                    2008054709

Care has been taken to confirm the accuracy of the information presented and to describe generally accepted practices. However, the authors, editors, and publisher are not responsible for errors or omissions or for any consequences from application of the information in this book and make no warranty, expressed or implied, with respect to the currency, completeness, or accuracy of the contents of the publication. Application of the information in a particular situation remains the professional responsibility of the practitioner.

The authors, editors, and publisher have exerted every effort to ensure that drug selection and dosage set forth in this text are in accordance with current recommendations and practice at the time of publication. However, in view of ongoing research, changes in government regulations, and the constant flow of information relating to drug therapy and drug reactions, the reader is urged to check the package insert for each drug for any change in indications and dosage and for added warnings and precautions. This is particularly important when the recommended agent is a new or infrequently employed drug.

Some drugs and medical devices presented in the publication have Food and Drug Administration (FDA) clearance for limited use in restricted research settings. It is the responsibility of the health care provider to ascertain the FDA status of each drug or device planned for use in their clinical practice.

To purchase additional copies of this book, call our customer service department at (800) 638-3030 or fax orders to (301) 223-2320. International customers should call (301) 223-2300.

Visit Lippincott Williams & Wilkins on the Internet: at LWW.com. Lippincott Williams & Wilkins customer service representatives are available from 8:30 am to 6 pm, EST.

10 9 8 7 6 5 4 3 2 1

To my parents, for instilling the values that allowed this book to be, and to Terry and Jake, for inspiring and tolerating my passion to make it happen.

J.K.S.

To my wife and children for their ongoing support of a career that focuses my attention as much outside the home as it does inside.

F.A.M.

This textbook began several editions ago as a labor of love and commitment to lifelong professional education by Jamie Stoller and David Longworth, the first course directors. The annual Internal Medicine Review course, and this text's existence as a vibrant experience, would be impossible without the dedication and clinical expertise of the many Cleveland Clinic physician educators noted within these pages. On a personal note, I gratefully acknowledge the patience and support of my family during this enterprise of late night editing sessions.

B.F.M.

Contributors

ABBY ABELSON, MD Interim Chair, Department of Rheumatic and Immunologic Diseases; Vice Chair for Education, Orthopaedic and Rheumatology Institute; Rheumatology Education Program Director; Director of Education, Center for Osteoporosis and Metabolic Bone Disease, The Cleveland Clinic Foundation, Cleveland, Ohio

LOUTFI S. ABOUSSOUAN, MD Staff, Respiratory Institute, The Cleveland Clinic Foundation, Cleveland, Ohio

DAVID J. ADELSTEIN, MD Department of Hematology, The Cleveland Clinic Foundation, Cleveland, Ohio

GERALD B. APPEL, MD Professor of Clinical Medicine, Columbia University College of Physicians and Surgeons; Director, Department of Clinical Nephrology, Department of Medicine, Columbia Presbyterian Center of New York Presbyterian Hospital, New York, New York

WENDY S. ARMSTRONG, MD Department of Infectious Diseases, The Cleveland Clinic Foundation, Cleveland, Ohio

ALEJANDRO C. ARROLIGA, MD Head, Section of Critical Care Medicine, Department of Pulmonary, Allergy, and Critical Care Medicine, The Cleveland Clinic Foundation, Cleveland, Ohio

CHARLES J. BAE, MD Assistant Professor, Department of Medicine, Cleveland Clinic Lerner College of Medicine of Case Western University Staff, Neurological Institute, The Cleveland Clinic Foundation, Cleveland, Ohio

RACHID BAZ, MD Moffitt, Cancer Center, Tampa, Florida

PELIN BATUR, MD Staff, Medicine Institute, Women's Health Specialist, Independence Cleveland Clinic Foundation, Family Health Center, Independence, Ohio

GERALD J. BECK, MD Section Head, Clinical Trials Design and Analysis, Department of Quantitative Health Sciences, The Cleveland Clinic Foundation, Cleveland, Ohio

DAVID E. BLUMENTHAL, MD Department of Rheumatology, Metro Health Medical Center, Cleveland, Ohio

BRIAN BOLWELL, MD Chairman, Department of Hematologic Oncology and Blood Disorders; Vice Chief of Staff

JULIA BREYER-LEWIS, MD Professor, Department of Medicine, Division of Nephrology; Physician, Department of Medicine, Division of Nephrology, Vanderbilt University School of Medicine, Nashville, Tennessee

AARON BRZEZINSKI, MD Center for Inflammatory Bowel Disease, Department of Gastroenterology and Hepatology, The Cleveland Clinic Foundation, Cleveland, Ohio

MARIE M. BUDEV, MD Assistant Medical Director, Lung Transplant Program, Department of Pulmonary, Allergy, and Critical Care Medicine, The Cleveland Clinic Foundation, Cleveland, Ohio

CAROL A. BURKE, MD Director, Center for Colon, Polyp, and Cancer Prevention, Department of Gastroenterology and Hepatology, The Cleveland Clinic Foundation, Cleveland, Ohio

JEFFREY T. CHAPMAN, MD Staff Physician, Respiratory and Transplant Institute, The Cleveland Clinic Foundation, Cleveland, Ohio

LESLIE CHO, MD Section Head, Preventive Cardiology and Rehabilitation Director, Women's Vascular Center, Department of Cardiovascular Medicine, The Cleveland Clinic Foundation, Cleveland, Ohio

MINA K. CHUNG, MD Staff, Cardiac Electrophysiology and Pacing, Department of Cardiovascular Medicine, Heart and Vascular Institute, Molecular Cardiology, Lerner Research Institute, The Cleveland Clinic Foundation, Cleveland, Ohio

DANIEL A. CULVER, MD Staff, Respiratory Institute and Department of Pathology, The Cleveland Clinic Foundation, Cleveland, Ohio

ROSSANA D. DANESE, MD Division of Endocrinology, University Hospitals of Cleveland, Cleveland, Ohio

STEVEN R. DEITCHER, MD Vice President, Medical Affairs, Nuvelo, Sunnyvale, California

JOHN A. DUMOT, MD Staff, Department of Gastroenterology and Hepatology, The Cleveland Clinic Foundation, Cleveland, Ohio

RAED A. DWEIK, MD Director, Pulmonary Vascular Program, Respiratory Institute, The Cleveland Clinic Foundation, Cleveland, Ohio

CHARLES FAIMAN, MD Department of Endocrinology, Diabetes, and Metabolism, The Cleveland Clinic Foundation, Cleveland, Ohio

KRISTIN A. ENGLUND, MD Staff, Department of Infectious Diseases, The Cleveland Clinic Foundation, Cleveland, Ohio

KATHLEEN FRANCO-BRONSON, MD Staff Psychiatrist, Department of Psychiatry and Psychology; Associate Dean CCLCM, The Cleveland Clinic Foundation, Cleveland, Ohio

JORGE GARCIA, MD Assistant Professor, Department of Medicine, Cleveland Clinic Lerner College of Medicine of Case Western University Associate Staff, Department of Solid Tumor Oncology, The Cleveland Clinic Foundation, Cleveland, Ohio

BRIAN P. GRIFFIN, MD Director, Cardiovascular Disease Training Program, The John and Rosemary Brown Endowed Chair in Cardiovascular Medicine, US Associate Editor, Heart, The Cleveland Clinic Foundation Cleveland, Ohio

RICHARD GRIMM, MD Section of Cardiac Imaging, Department of Cardiovascular Medicine, The Cleveland Clinic Foundation, Cleveland, Ohio

CARMEL HALLEY, MD Advanced Fellow in Heart Failure, Department of Cardiovascular Medicine, The Cleveland Clinic Foundation, Cleveland, Ohio

AMIR H. HAMRAHIAN, MD Staff, Department of Endocrinology, The Cleveland Clinic Foundation, Cleveland, Ohio

CHRISTOPHER J. HEBERT, MD Staff Physician, Department of Nephrology and Hypertension, The Cleveland Clinic Foundation, Cleveland, Ohio

ROBERT E. HOBBS, MD Staff, Heart and Vascular Institute, The Cleveland Clinic Foundation, Cleveland, Ohio

EDWARD P. HORVATH, JR., MD Department of Veterans Affairs Medical Center, Cleveland, Ohio

CARLOS M. ISADA, MD Program Director, Fellowship Training, Vice Chairman, Department of Infectious Diseases, The Cleveland Clinic Foundation, Cleveland, Ohio

AMIR K. JAFFER, MD Associate Professor of Medicine, University of Miami Miller School of Medicine; Chief, Medicine Service; Division Chief, Department of Medicine, University of Miami Hospital, Miami, Florida

HANI JNEID, MD Assistant Professor of Medicine, Department of Cardiology, Baylor College of Medicine; Assistant Director of Interventional Cardiology, Department of Cardiology, The Michael E. DeBakey VA Medical Center, Houston, Texas

VIDYASAGAR KALAHASTI, MD Staff Cardiologist, Department of Cardiovascular Medicine, The Cleveland Clinic Foundation, Cleveland, Ohio

MATT KALAYCIO, MD Professor, Department of Medicine, Cleveland Clinic Lerner College of Medicine, Cleveland, Ohio

MATTHEW A. KAMINSKI, MD Cardiology Fellow, Department of Cardiovascular Medicine, The Cleveland Clinic Foundation, Cleveland, Ohio

SAMIR R. KAPADIA, MD Department of Cardiovascular Medicine, The Cleveland Clinic Foundation, Cleveland, Ohio

THOMAS F. KEYS, MD Consultant, Department of Post-Acute Medicine, The Cleveland Clinic Foundation, Cleveland, Ohio

OSSAM KHAN, MD Associate Staff, Department of Hospital Medicine, The Cleveland Clinic Foundation, Cleveland, Ohio

ALICE I. KIM, MD Staff, Department of Infectious Diseases, The Cleveland Clinic Foundation, Cleveland, Ohio

YULI Y. KIM, MD Senior Fellow, Boston Adult Congenital Service, Children's Hospital, Boston, Massachusetts

RICHARD A. KRASUSKI, MD Heart and Vascular Institute, The Cleveland Clinic Foundation, Cleveland, Ohio

RICHARD LANG, MD Chairman, Department of General Internal Medicine, The Cleveland Clinic Foundation, Cleveland, Ohio

CAROL A. LANGFORD, MD Director, Center for Vasculitis Care and Research, Department of Rheumatic and Immunologic Diseases, Orthopaedic and Rheumatologic Institute, The Cleveland Clinic Foundation, Cleveland, Ohio

JOYCE K. LEE, MD Chief Resident, Neurological Institute, Department of Neurology, The Cleveland Clinic Foundation, Cleveland, Ohio

SUSAN B. LEGRAND, MD Vice Chairman, Department of Cardiovascular Medicine, The Cleveland Clinic Foundation, Cleveland, Ohio

ANGELO A. LICATA, MD Director, Center for Space Medicine; Consultant, Department of Endocrinology, The Cleveland Clinic Foundation, Cleveland, Ohio

ALAN E. LICHTIN, MD Staff Hematologist-Oncologist, Department of Hematology/Oncology, The Cleveland Clinic Foundation, Cleveland, Ohio

MICHAEL LINCOFF, MD Director, Center for Clinical Research and Vice Chairman for Clinical Research, Lerner Research Institute; Director, Cleveland Clinic Coordinating Center for Clinical Research (C5 Research); Vice Chairman, Department of Cardiovascular Medicine, The Cleveland Clinic Foundation, Cleveland, Ohio

CAREEN Y. LOWDER, MD Division of Ophthalomology, Cole Eye Institute, The Cleveland Clinic Foundation, Cleveland, Ohio

JAMES M. LUTHER, MD, MSCI Instructor in Medicine, Division of Clinical Pharmacology, Vanderbilt University Medical Center, Knoxville, Tennessee

ANUJ MAHINDRA, MD Fellow, Department of Hematology and Medical Oncology, The Cleveland Clinic Foundation, Cleveland, Ohio

BRIAN F. MANDELL, MD Professor and Vice Chairman of Academic Medicine, Department of Rheumatic and Immunologic Disease, Center for Vasculitis Care and Research, Cleveland Clinic Lerner College of Medicine, Cleveland, Ohio

PETER J. MAZZONE, MD Department of Pulmonary, Allergy, and Critical Care Medicine, The Cleveland Clinic Foundation, Cleveland, Ohio

ATUL C. MEHTA, MD Vice Chairman, Department of Pulmonary, Allergy, and Critical Care Medicine, The Cleveland Clinic Foundation, Cleveland, Ohio

ADI E. MEHTA, MD Vice Chairman, Respiratory Institute, The Cleveland Clinic Foundation, Cleveland, Ohio

TAREK MEKHAIL, MD Director, Lung Cancer Medical Oncology Program, The Cleveland Clinic Taussig Cancer Center, The Cleveland Clinic Foundation, Cleveland, Ohio

CHAD MICHENER, MD Staff, Deaprtment of Obstetrics, Gynecology and Women's Health Institute, The Cleveland Clinic Foundation, Cleveland, Ohio

FRANKLIN A. MICHOTA, MD Head, Section of Hospital Medicine, Department of General Internal Medicine, The Cleveland Clinic Foundation, Cleveland, Ohio

HALLE C. F. MOORE, MD Staff, Solid Tumor Oncology, Taussig Cancer Institute, The Cleveland Clinic Foundation, Cleveland, Ohio

SHERIF B. MOSSAD, MD Staff Physician, Department of Infectious Diseases, Medicine Institute, The Cleveland Clinic Foundation, Cleveland, Ohio

JOSEPH V. NALLY, JR., MD Nephrologist, Department of Nephrology, The Cleveland Clinic Foundation, Cleveland, Ohio

CHRISTIAN NASR, MD Quality Control Officer, Department of Endocrinology and Metabolism Institute, The Cleveland Clinic Foundation, Cleveland, Ohio

CRAIG NIELSEN, MD Staff, Department of Internal Medicine, The Cleveland Clinic Foundation, Cleveland, Ohio

ROBERT M. PALMER, MD Head, Section of Geriatric Medicine, Department of General Internal Medicine, The Cleveland Clinic Foundation, Cleveland, Ohio

JOSEPH G. PARAMBIL, MD Staff, Department of Pulmonary and Critical Care, The Cleveland Clinic Foundation, Cleveland, Ohio

MANSOUR A. PARSI, MD Center for Endoscopy and Pancreatobiliary Disorders, Digestive Disease Institute, The Cleveland Clinic Foundation, Cleveland, Ohio

VICTOR L. PEREZ, MD Division of Ophthalmology, Cole Eye Institute, The Cleveland Clinic Foundation, Cleveland, Ohio

MELISSA PECK PILIANG, MD Associate Staff, Department of Dermatology and Anatomic Pathology, The Cleveland Clinic Foundation, Cleveland, Ohio

MARC A. POHL, MD Ray W. Gifford Jr. Endowed Chair in Hypertension, Department of Nephrology and Hypertension, Section Head, Clinical Hypertension and Nephrology, The Cleveland Clinic Foundation, Cleveland, Ohio

BRAD L. POHLMAN, MD Director, Lymphoma Program, Taussig Cancer Institute, The Cleveland Clinic Foundation, Cleveland, Ohio

LEOPOLD POZUELO, MD Section Head, Consultation-Liaison Psychiatry, The Cleveland Clinic Foundation, Cleveland, Ohio

SARINYA PUWANANT, MD Clinical Fellow, Advanced Cardiac Imaging, Department of Cardiovascular Medicine, The Cleveland Clinic Foundation, Cleveland, Ohio

YING QIAN, MD Ophthalmology Resident, Cole Eye Institute, The Cleveland Clinic Foundation, Cleveland, Ohio

ANITHA RAJAMANICKAM, MD Associate Staff, Department of Hospital Medicine, The Cleveland Clinic Foundation, Cleveland, Ohio

S. SETHU K. REDDY, MD Chairman and Program Director, Department of Endocrinology, Diabetes and Metabolism, The Cleveland Clinic Foundation, Cleveland, Ohio

JOEL E. RICHTER, MD Professor of Medicine and Chair, Department of Medicine, Temple University School of Medicine, Philadelphia, Pennsylvania

CURTIS M. RIMMERMAN, MD Staff Cardiologist, Department of Cardiovascular Medicine, The Cleveland Clinic Foundation, Cleveland, Ohio

STEVEN K. SCHMITT, MD Staff Physician, Department of Infectious Diseases, The Cleveland Clinic Foundation, Cleveland, Ohio

MARTIN J. SCHREIBER, JR., MD Chairman, Department of Nephrology and Hypertension, The Cleveland Clinic Foundation, Cleveland, Ohio

PRIYANKA SHARMA, MD Associate Staff, Department of Hospital Medicine, The Cleveland Clinic Foundation, Cleveland, Ohio

ROY L. SILVERSTEIN, MD　Staff, Department of Blood Disorders and Hematologic Malignancies, Taussig Cancer Center, The Cleveland Clinic Foundation, Cleveland, Ohio

EDY E. SOFFER, MD　Co-Director, GI Motility Laboratory, Division of Gastroenterology, Center for Digestive Diseases, Cedars Sinai Medical Center, Los Angeles, California

TYLER STEVENS, MD　Digestive Disease Institute, The Cleveland Clinic Foundation, Cleveland, Ohio

JAMES K. STOLLER, MD　Jean Wall Bennett Chair of Emphysema Research; Head, Cleveland Clinic Respiratory Therapy, Division of Medicine; Executive Director, Leadership Development, The Cleveland Clinic Foundation, Cleveland, Ohio

CHRISTY J. STOTLER, MD　Hematology Oncology Fellow, Taussig Cancer Institute, The Cleveland Clinic Foundation, Cleveland, Ohio

ALAN J. TAEGE, MD　Director, HIV Care, Department of Infectious Diseases, The Cleveland Clinic Foundation, Cleveland, Ohio

HOLLY L. THACKER, MD　Head, Section of Women's Health, Departments of General Internal Medicine and Obstetrics and Gynecology, The Cleveland Clinic Foundation, Cleveland, Ohio

KARL S. THEIL, MD　Staff Pathologist; Director, Pathology Residency Program, Department of Clinical Pathology, The Cleveland Clinic Foundation, Cleveland, Ohio

KENNETH J. TOMECKI, MD　Vice Chairman, Department of Dermatology, The Cleveland Clinic Foundation, Cleveland, Ohio

BENNIE R. UPCHURCH, MD　Staff Physician, Digestive Disease Institute, The Cleveland Clinic Foundation, Cleveland, Ohio

NIZAR ZEIN, MD　Digestive Disease Institute, The Cleveland Clinic Foundation, Cleveland, Ohio

ROBERT S. ZIMMERMAN, MD　Interim Chairman and Program Director, Department of Endocrinology, The Cleveland Clinic Foundation, Cleveland, Ohio

Preface

The fifth edition of the *Cleveland Clinic Foundation Intensive Review of Internal Medicine* reflects our ongoing fascination with how physicians learn best and our continued passion for clinical medicine, medical, education, and scholarship—values that define the culture of the Cleveland Clinic. This book has its origins in the Clinic's Intensive Review of Internal Medicine Symposium, a 6-day course offered annually since 1989, that is designed for physicians preparing for the certification and recertification examinations in internal medicine, and for those wishing for a comprehensive, state-of-the-art review of the field. The symposium celebrated its 20th offering in the United States in June 2008, and has been presented 4 times internationally.

We continue to be humbled and gratified by the success of the Symposium and of the first 4 editions of this book. Experience has taught us that practicing physicians learn best when using a case-driven format, and that factual knowledge and new developments in the field are best integrated into clinical practice through a discussion of case management. Never meant to be a comprehensive textbook of internal medicine, this fifth edition of the book builds on this concept and continues to use bulleted points, clinical vignettes, and review exercises to convey important "clinical pearls."

Each chapter in the fifth edition has been extensively reviewed and carefully updated where necessary, and many chapters have been substantially revised or completely rewritten. Several chapters are new since the fourth addition, reflecting input from our readers and attendees of the Intensive Review of Internal Medicine Symposium. Updated references have been provided in the suggested readings at the end of each chapter. New chapter features include call-out boxes with bulleted "Points to Remember" and the uniform inclusion of review exercises (with discussions) to test the reader's knowledge of key points.

This book continues to serve as the syllabus for both domestic and international offerings of the Cleveland Clinic Intensive Review of Internal Medicine Symposium. It also provides an independent study guide for those preparing for the certification and recertification examinations in internal medicine.

We remain extraordinarily grateful to our colleagues and contributors who have supported the Symposium and this book over the years. They represent the best and brightest among clinician-educators, adept at teaching the art and science of medicine, and facile in distilling their clinical wisdom into a concise and practical document. In addition, we are indebted to our many students, residents, fellows, and colleagues who have taught us so much over the years about clinical medicine and about how physicians learn best. Finally, there are several people without whom this book would not have come to fruition. We are indebted to David Longworth, M.D., our dear friend and former editor, now Chair of Medicine at Baystate Medical Center in Springfield, Massachusetts. As one of the founding editors of this book, his wisdom and organizational skills are still very evident in this fifth edition. We are grateful to Kerry Barrett and to Sonya Siegafuse of Lippincott Williams & Wilkins (LWW) for their ongoing support, both editorial and intellectual, in building on past editions. Lisa Consoli provided superb developmental editorial help in preparing and organizing the manuscript. We also offer our deep thanks to Sherri White, our administrative assistant, who contributed energy, and craftsmanship in shepherding each chapter through editorial revision, completion, and submission to the publisher. Finally, we are grateful for our families, who graciously tolerated and supported the many hours we devoted to preparing this book.

As editors, we take extreme pride in this book's content, and we accept sole responsibility for it shortcomings. We hope that this book deepens your own passion for clinical medicine and for medical education, just as it has continued to fuel our own.

James K. Stoller, M.D., M.S.
Franklin A. Michota, Jr., M.D.
Brian A. Mandell, M.D., Ph.D.

Contents

SECTION X: MOCK BOARD SIMULATION

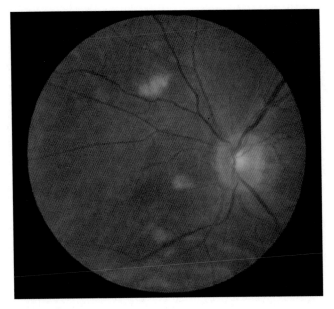

Color Plate 5.1 Cotton-wool spots.

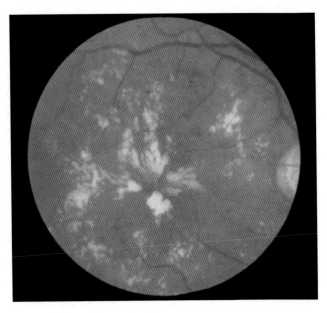

Color Plate 5.2 Hard exudates.

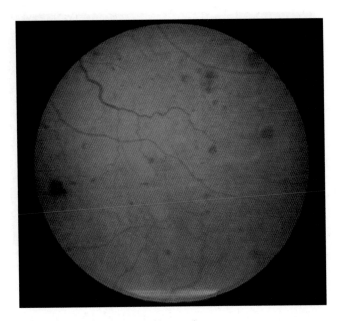

Color Plate 5.3 Intraretinal hemorrhages.

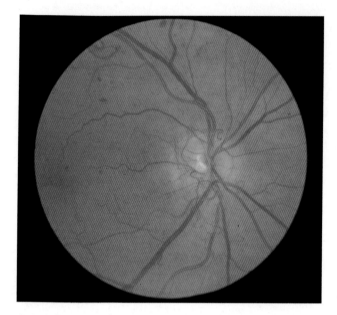

Color Plate 5.4   Neovascularization of the disc.

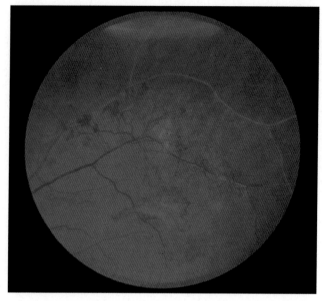

Color Plate 5.5   Neovascularization elsewhere.

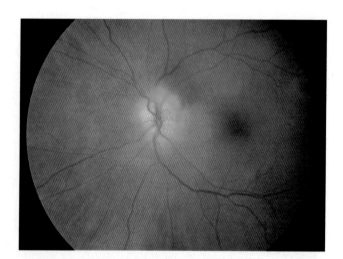

Color Plate 5.6   Pallid optic nerve edema in giant cell arteritis.

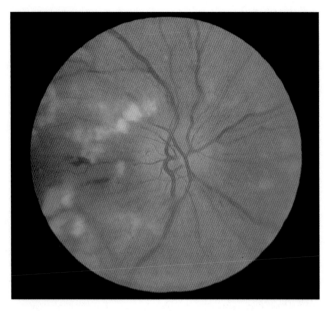

Color Plate 5.7 The edematous optic nerve is surrounded by cotton-wool spots and intraretinal hemorrhages in malignant hypertension.

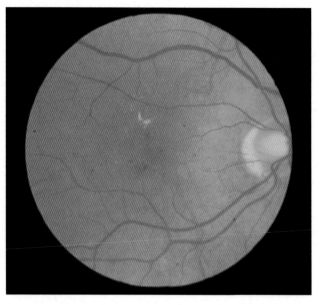

Color Plate 5.8 Background diabetic retinopathy consisting of dot hemorrhages and hard exudates.

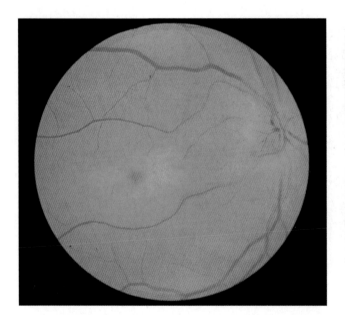

Color Plate 5.11 The retina is edematous, and there is a cherry-red spot in the macula of a patient with central retinal artery occlusion.

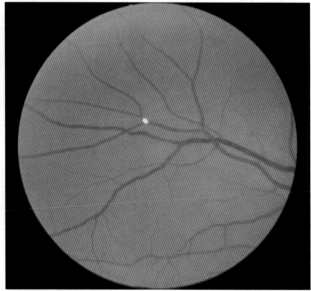

Color Plate 5.12 Hollenhorst's plaque.

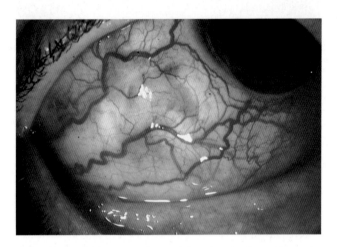

Color Plate 5.14   Avascularity of the sclera leads to scleromalacia in a patient with rheumatoid arthritis.

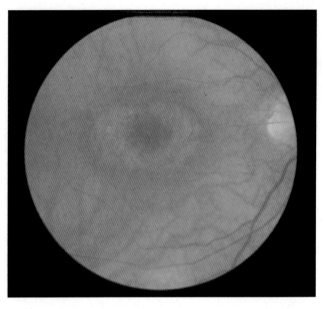

Color Plate 5.15   Bull's eye of hydroxychloroquine pigmentary maculopathy.

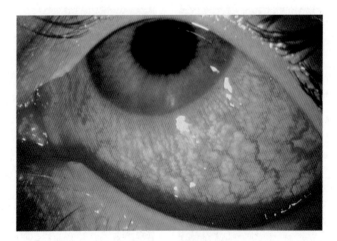

Color Plate 5.16   Marked conjunctival injection and ciliary flush in acute iritis.

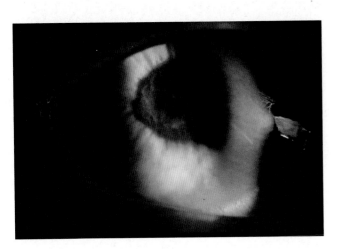

Color Plate 5.17 The anterior lens capsule is covered by a fibrinous exudate in a patient with HLA-B27–associated acute iritis.

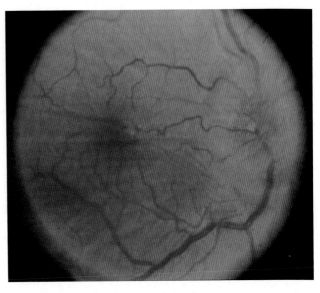

Color Plate 5.18 Fundus photograph show a swollen optic nerve and choroidal folds secondary to compression by enlarged muscles in a patient with thyroid optic neuropathy.

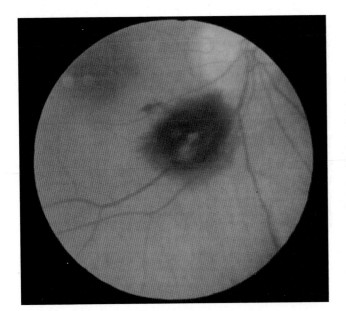

Color Plate 5.19 Leukemic retinopathy characterized by intraretinal and preretinal hemorrhages.

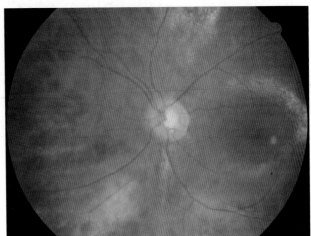

Color Plate 5.20 CMV retinitis in a patient with AIDS.

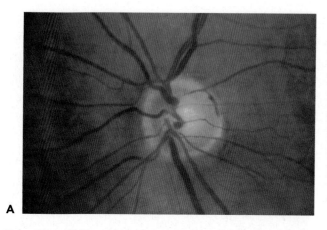 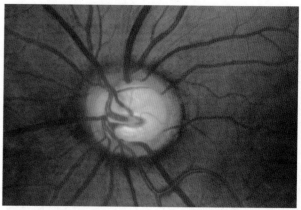

Color Plate 5.21   (A) Normal optic nerve. (B) Glaucomatous optic nerve.

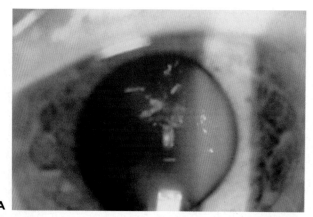 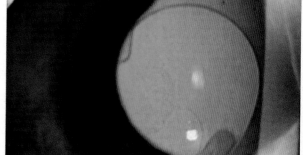

Color Plate 5.22   (A) Cataract. (B) Intraocular lens implant.

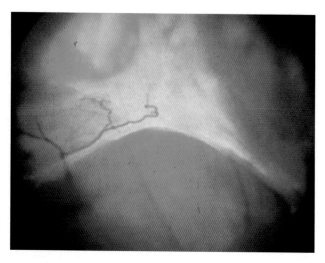

Color Plate 5.23 Retinal detachment.

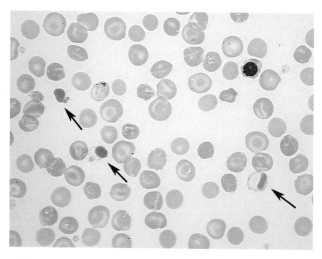

Color Plate 26.1 Peripheral blood smear: frequent target cells and hemoglobin C crystals (*arrows*).

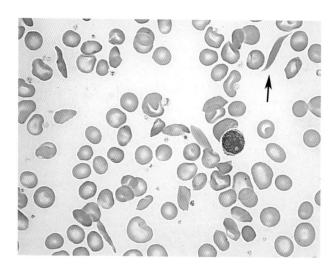

Color Plate 26.2 Peripheral blood smear in sickle cell disease showing polychromatophilic red blood cells and classic sickled cells (*arrow*).

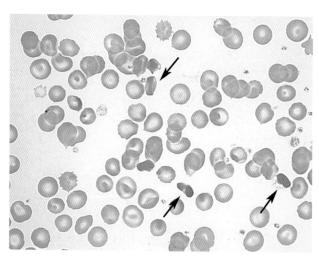

Color Plate 26.3 Peripheral blood smear: target cells and boat-shaped poikilocytes (*arrows*) in hemoglobin SC disease.

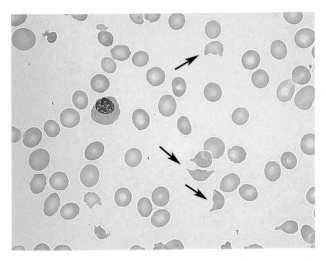

Color Plate 26.4 Peripheral blood smear: microangiopathic hemolytic anemias are characterized by the presence of red blood cell fragments (*arrows*).

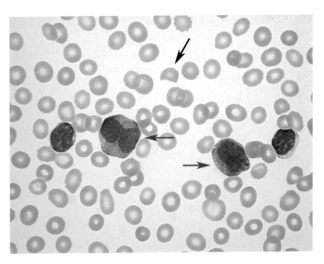

Color Plate 26.5 Peripheral blood smear in acute promyelocytic leukemia shows circulating blasts (*red arrows*). Severe thrombocytopenia and red cell fragments (*black arrow*) reflect a consumptive coagulopathy.

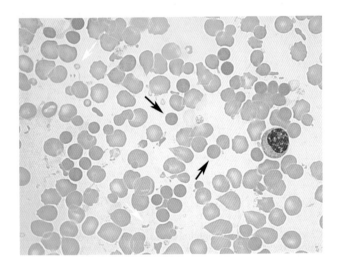

Color Plate 26.6 Peripheral blood smear: marked poikilocytosis with microspherocytes (*black arrows*) and red cell fragments (*white arrows*) following a severe burn.

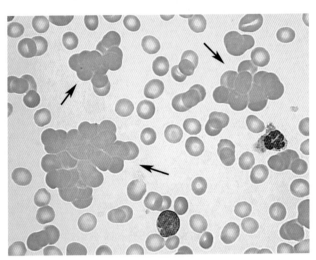

Color Plate 26.7 Peripheral blood smear: variably sized three-dimensional clumps of red blood cells (*arrows*) are the hallmark of a cold agglutinin.

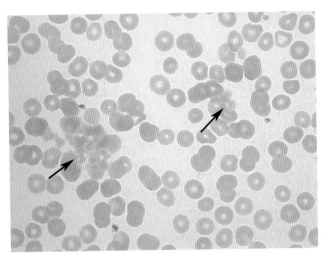

Color Plate 26.8 Peripheral blood smear shows amorphous extracellular light blue globules (*arrows*) in a patient with cryoglobulinemia.

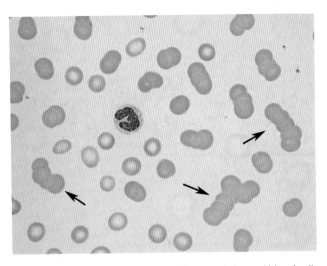

Color Plate 26.9 Peripheral blood smear shows red blood cells arranged as "stacks of coins" forming rouleaux (*arrows*).

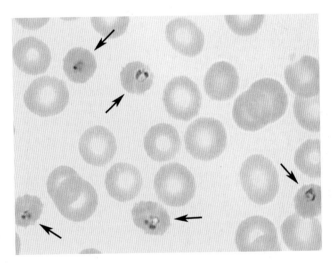

Color Plate 26.10 Peripheral blood smear shows several erythrocytes parasitized by ring trophozoites of malaria (*arrows*).

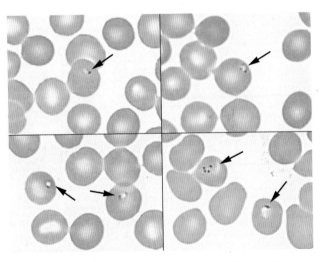

Color Plate 26.11 Peripheral blood smear in babesiosis shows small ring forms and characteristic tetrad form (*lower right*) within erythrocytes.

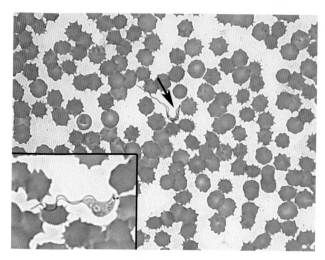

Color Plate 26.12 Trypanosomes (*arrow*) are extraerythrocytic parasites with an undulating membrane, central kinetoplast, and anterior flagellum.

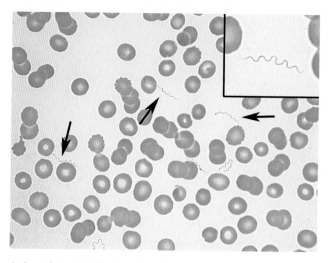

Color Plate 26.13 Peripheral blood smear in borreliosis shows extraerythrocytic spirochetes (*arrows*).

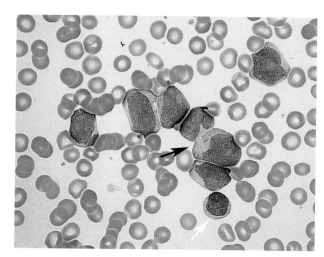

Color Plate 26.14 Peripheral blood smear with blasts and a lymphocyte (*white arrow*) from a case of acute myeloid leukemia. Auer rod (*black arrow*) within a blast is a distinctive feature associated with myeloid differentiation.

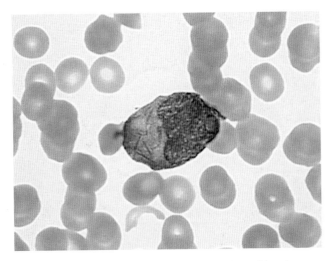

Color Plate 26.15 Multiple Auer rods within a blast in acute promyelocytic leukemia.

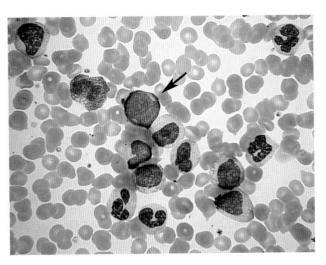

Color Plate 26.16 Peripheral blood smear in chronic myelogenous leukemia shows leukocytosis with left shift in granulocyte maturation, 1% to 2% circulating blasts (*arrow*), eosinophilia, and basophilia.

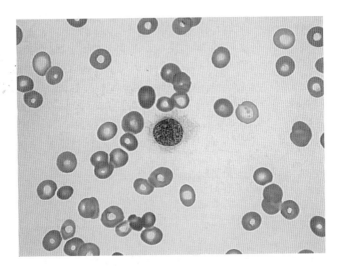

Color Plate 26.17 Peripheral blood smear in hairy cell leukemia shows a classic hairy cell with delicate cytoplasmic surface projections.

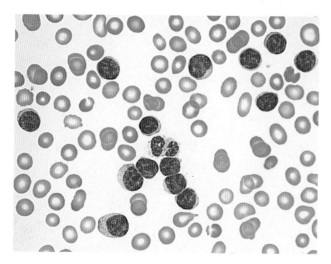

Color Plate 26.18 Peripheral blood smear in chronic lympho-cytic leukemia shows a mature lymphocytosis with clumped smudgy chromatin.

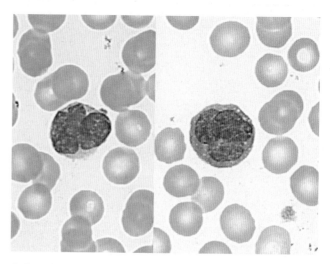

Color Plate 26.19 Sézary cells have characteristic convoluted nuclei.

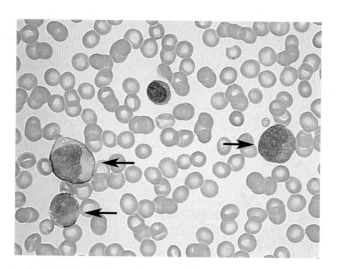

Color Plate 26.20 Reactive lymphocytes (*arrows*) as seen in infectious mononucleosis.

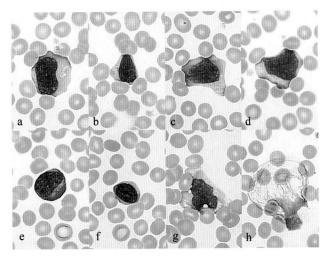

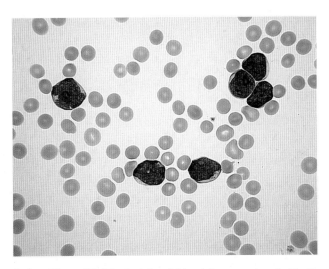

Color Plate 26.21 Reactive lymphocytes in infectious mononucleosis **(a–e)** contrasted with normal lymphocyte **(f)**, monocyte **(g)**, and smudge cell **(h)**.

Color Plate 26.22 Peripheral blood in acute lymphoblastic leukemia shows a uniform population of small blasts.

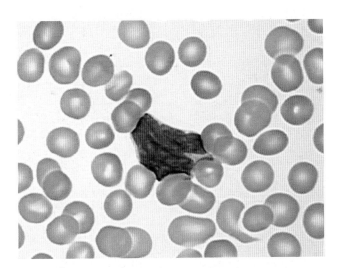

Color Plate 26.23 Follicular lymphoma cell in peripheral blood has clumped chromatin and indented nuclear outline with no visible nucleoli.

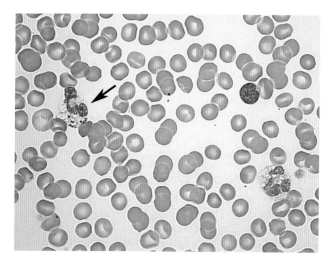

Color Plate 26.24 Peripheral blood smear with phagocytized bacteria (*arrow*) in a case of meningococcemia.

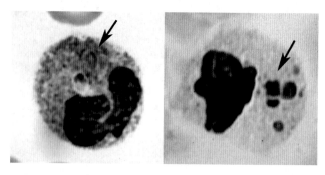

Color Plate 26.25 Peripheral blood smear with intracellular yeast in a case of disseminated histoplasmosis (*left*). Peripheral blood smear in anaplasmosis shows neutrophil with cytoplasmic morulae (*right*).

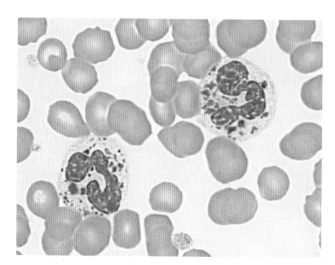

Color Plate 26.26 Peripheral blood smear in Chediak-Higashi syndrome shows abnormal cytoplasmic granulation.

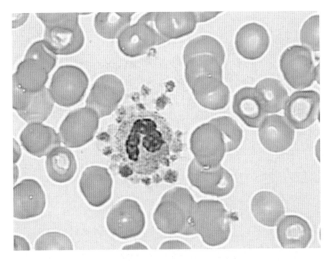

Color Plate 26.27 Peripheral blood smear showing platelet satellitosis.

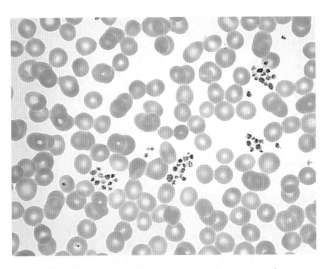

Color Plate 26.28 Platelet clumping can be a cause of spurious thrombocytopenia.

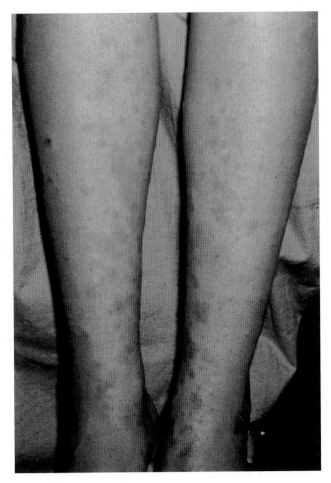

Color Plate 31.3 Rash.

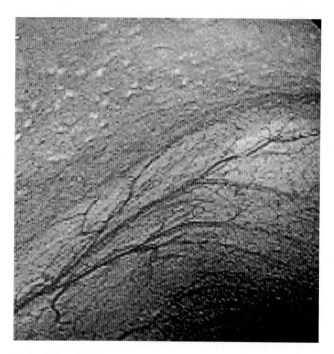

Color Plate 56.1   Line of demarcation in ulcerative colitis.

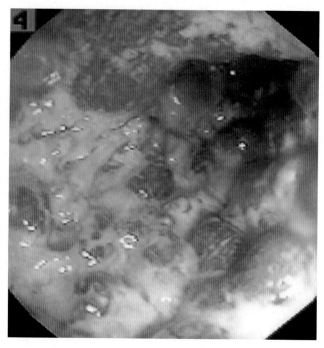

Color Plate 56.2   Severe Crohn's disease.

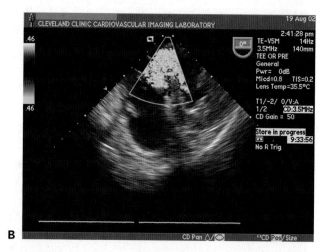

Color Plate 66.11B   Echocardiographic images of a ventricular septal defect in the inferior septum of the left ventricle with color Doppler depicting the blood flow from the left ventricle to the right ventricle (*arrow*).

Chapter 1

Health Screening and Adult Immunizations

Craig Nielsen   *Richard S. Lang*

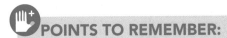

POINTS TO REMEMBER:

- Cardiovascular disease and cancer are the leading causes of mortality in the United States.

- Hypertension, diabetes, and hyperlipidemia are significant risk factors for cardiovascular disease and should be screened for in certain age groups.

- Abdominal aortic aneurysm screening is indicated in men ages 65 to 75 years who have ever smoked.

- Breast cancer screening with MRI is recommended in patients at very high risk for breast cancer.

- Human papillomavirus screening, along with Papanicolaou testing, is recommended in women ages 30 years or older.

- Colon cancer screening can be accomplished with fecal occult blood testing (yearly), sigmoidoscopy (every 5 years), or colonoscopy (every 10 years).

- Definitive evidence supporting prostate cancer screening is still lacking.

- In general, live attenuated viral vaccines should be avoided in immunocompromised and pregnant patients.

- Be familiar with recommended vaccines in certain patient populations (e.g., the patient with newly diagnosed HIV).

- Be familiar with recommended immunizations for healthy adults without chronic disease or special circumstances (e.g., pregnancy, immunocompromised state)

Conceptually, preventive medicine involves four tasks for the clinician: screening, counseling, immunization, and prophylaxis. Preventive interventions can be categorized as primary, secondary, and tertiary. *Primary prevention* is the reduction of risk factors before a disease or condition has occurred. Examples are immunization, use of safety equipment, dietary management, and smoking cessation. Primary prevention aims to reduce the incidence of a disease or condition. *Incidence* is the number of persons developing a condition or disease in a specific period of time (e.g., the number of new HIV cases this year). *Secondary prevention* is the detection of a condition or disease to reverse or slow the condition or disease and thereby improve prognosis. Examples of secondary prevention are mammography and Papanicolaou (Pap) smears. Secondary prevention ideally detects and intervenes in a condition before that condition is clinically apparent. Secondary prevention therefore aims to reduce the prevalence of a disease. *Prevalence* is the total number of individuals who have a condition or disease at a particular time (e.g., the total number of people currently diagnosed with HIV). *Tertiary prevention* is the minimizing of the future negative health effects of a disease or condition. An example of tertiary prevention is the aggressive treatment of cholesterol in a patient with a known history of coronary artery disease.

The considerations in screening for a disease or condition should include the following questions:

- Is the disease or condition an important problem? (What are the morbidity and mortality of the condition?)
- Is the disease or condition a common problem? (What are its prevalence and incidence?)
- Is the screening test accurate? (What are its sensitivity, specificity, and predictive value?)
- What is the cost of the screening procedure? (Consider both financial and health risks.)
- What are the available follow-up diagnostic procedures?
- What is the available treatment for the disease or condition?
- How acceptable to patients is the screening procedure?
- What are the circumstances for the screening? (What is the context—for example, health maintenance, occupational, preoperative screening?)

TABLE 1.1

PREDICTIVE VALUE OF TESTS

	Disease	No Disease	Total
Test positive	True (+)[a]	False (+)	All (+)
Test negative	False (−)	True (−)	All (−)
Total	All with disease	All without disease	Total patients

[a]Sensitivity = True (+) | [True (+) + False (−)] = how well the test correctly detects those with disease. Specificity = True (−) | [True (−) + False (+)] = how well the test identifies those without disease. Positive predictive value = True (+) | [True (+) + False (+)] = when a test is positive, the proportion of those with the disease. Negative predictive value = True (−) | [True (−) + False (−)] = when a test is negative, the proportion of those without the disease.

- What are the current recommendations for screening and the medical evidence to support these recommendations?

The ideal screening situation uses an inexpensive, noninvasive test with a high level of sensitivity and specificity to detect a common problem that can be treated but, if left untreated, leads to significant morbidity and mortality.

Sensitivity is the ability of a test to correctly identify those who have a condition or disease.

Specificity is the ability of a test to correctly identify those who do not have the disease or condition in question. The *predictive values* for a screening test are the proportions of people correctly labeled as having the condition or disease (positive predictive value) and those not having the condition or disease (negative predictive value). Table 1.1 illustrates these terms. This 2 × 2 table is a common method for viewing the application of a screening test in a population.

LEADING CAUSES OF MORTALITY

The optimal use of screening requires a basic understanding of the common causes of mortality. In the United States, the top two overall causes of mortality in adults are cardiovascular disease and cancer. Cardiovascular disease is the primary cause of mortality in the elderly. Accidents, homicide, and suicide are common causes of mortality in young adults. Motor vehicle injuries account for more than 25% of the deaths in persons 15 to 24 years of age. The use of seat belts, a form of primary prevention, can reduce crash mortality by as much as 50%. Homicide is the leading cause of death of black males in the 15- to 34-year-old age group. Therefore, counseling regarding handgun safety is an important intervention for this population. Suicide is another common cause of death in the younger age group; thus, surveillance and counseling for suicide in this patient population are important. HIV infection and other sexually transmitted diseases (STDs) continue to be an important cause of morbidity in the younger age groups. Preventive efforts related to sexual practices and to use of intravenous drugs are important interventions.

Heart disease and cancer are the leading causes of mortality in adults older than 45 years. Therefore, preventive efforts should be directed to these conditions. Projections indicate that cancer may become the leading cause of adult mortality in the future. The lifetime probability of developing cancer is estimated to be 45% in males and 38% in females. The lifetime probability of dying from cancer is estimated to be around 24% in males and 20% in females. Common cancer sites in women are the breast, lung, colon/rectum, uterus, and ovary. Leading cancer sites in men are the prostate, lung, colon/rectum, and bladder. Common causes of cancer death in women are lung, breast, and colon/rectum cancers, and in men are lung, prostate, and colon/rectum cancers. Screening and prevention efforts are thus targeted at the most common cancers as well as those most often leading to death—lung, colon/rectum, breast, and prostate cancers.

SCREENING TESTS BY ORGAN SYSTEM AND DISEASE

Cardiovascular System

For preventive purposes, atherosclerotic heart disease, stroke, and peripheral vascular disease are grouped together because of their similar risk factors:

- Previous atherosclerotic vascular disease
- Family history of premature vascular disease
- Smoking
- Hypertension
- Diabetes
- Hyperlipidemia
- Age older than 45 years in men and older than 55 years in women
- Premature menopause in women without estrogen replacement therapy

A high-density lipoprotein (HDL) cholesterol level >60 mg/dL is believed to be a negative risk factor, or "protective" factor, for the development of coronary vascular disease. Low-density lipoprotein cholesterol reduction has been proved to result in cardiovascular disease benefits in the setting of both primary and secondary prevention. The U.S. Preventive Services Task Force (USPSTF) recommends the measurement of total serum cholesterol level and HDL cholesterol level in a nonfasting state in "asymptomatic" adults, generally every 5 years beginning at age 35 years in men, at age 45 years in women, and at younger ages (20–35 years in men and 20–45 years in women) in those with additional cardiovascular risk factors. In persons of high risk, more frequent and earlier screening is suggested. The National Cholesterol Education Program recommends screening beginning at age 20 years with a fasting lipid profile, and it should be rechecked at least every 5 years. An age to stop screening is not established.

Most authorities advise measuring the blood pressure in normotensive persons at least every 2 years, particularly in those with prior diastolic readings of 85 to 89 mm Hg, prior systolic readings of 135 to 139 mm Hg, or those who are obese or who have a first-degree relative with hypertension. The current recommended classification of blood pressure, based on the Seventh Report of the Joint National Committee on Prevention, Detection, Evaluation, and Treatment of High Blood Pressure, is as follows:

- Normal blood pressure (BP) SBP <120 DBP <80
- Prehypertension SBP 120–139 DBP 80–89
- Stage 1 hypertension SBP 140–159 DBP 90–99
- Stage 2 hypertension SBP >160 DBP >100

Lifestyle modifications are appropriate for all stages of hypertension, including prehypertension. These modifications include optimizing weight; limiting alcohol; participating in regular aerobic exercise; reducing sodium intake; and maintaining an adequate intake of dietary potassium, calcium, and magnesium. Drug therapy is indicated for Stage 1 and Stage 2 hypertension.

Low-dose aspirin therapy should be considered for the primary prevention of ischemic heart disease in men older than 40 years who are at high risk. The optimal preventive aspirin dosage is not clearly established and ranges from 81 to 325 mg daily. The side effects and potential complications of chronic aspirin usage should be considered carefully.

The ECG is not a sensitive screening test for coronary artery disease in asymptomatic patients and therefore is not generally advised as a screening test. Considerations for obtaining a preoperative ECG include the patient's age, procedure planned, anesthesia to be used, cardiovascular risk factors, and presence of other systemic disease. Exercise treadmill testing has limited sensitivity (approximately 65%) and specificity (approximately 75%–85%) for detecting coronary artery disease. Stress testing is most useful when coronary artery disease is suspected or likely to be present. Therefore, treadmill testing is most effectively used for those with multiple risk factors. Stress testing should also be considered for those engaging in occupations that demand physical exertion or that may impact on public safety. Otherwise, exercise treadmill testing should not be used routinely in asymptomatic persons. This is consistent with USPSTF guidelines. The USPSTF recommends against screening with electrocardiography or exercise treadmill test in adults at low risk for congenital heart disease events. The USPSTF also does not recommend screening low-risk patients with new modalities such as the electron-beam CT.

Similarly, the use of noninvasive vascular evaluation of the carotid arteries should be reserved for patients in whom disease is suspected, based either on symptoms or the presence of carotid bruits. The prevalence of carotid bruits in the adult population is approximately 4% to 5%.

The USPSTF recommends a one-time screening for abdominal aortic aneurysms (AAAs) in all men between the ages of 65 and 75 years who have ever smoked at least the equivalent of 100 cigarettes. The recommended screening modality for an AAA is an abdominal ultrasound. If the aorta is of normal size, no additional screening is needed. The USPSTF does not make a specific recommendation for AAA screening in men who have never smoked. They recommend against AAA screening in women regardless of whether they have ever smoked.

In summary, risk factors for the development of vascular disease should be assessed in all patients, modifiable risk factors should be addressed, blood pressure and cholesterol should be monitored and treated appropriately, AAA screening should be performed in men ages 65 to 75 years who have ever smoked, and stress testing and assessment of carotid arteries are best undertaken in patients in whom coronary artery disease and carotid atherosclerosis are most likely to be present.

LUNG CANCER

Lung cancer is the most common cause of cancer death in the United States. Cigarette smoking is the most important risk factor for the development of lung cancer. Generally, smokers are 10 times more likely to die of lung cancer than nonsmokers. The risk for developing lung cancer depends on the number of cigarettes smoked, the age when smoking began, and the degree of inhalation. The risk for lung cancer decreases after smoking is stopped, particularly after 5 years or more. Therefore, the most important preventive interventions for lung cancer are avoidance and cessation of smoking. Other risk factors for the development of lung cancer are occupational exposures (asbestos, arsenic, chloromethyl ethers, chromium, polycyclic aromatic compounds, nickel, and vinyl chloride), chronic obstructive lung disease, previous lung cancer, previous head and neck cancer, and radon exposure.

Generally, screening for lung cancer in asymptomatic patients has not been advised because large-scale studies have not demonstrated a reduction in mortality when screening interventions such as serial chest x-rays and frequent sputum cytology were applied to high-risk populations. Therefore, routine screening chest radiography should be reserved for situations in which clinical evidence suggests the presence of disease. More recently, CT scanning techniques of the chest have shown promise as a screening modality in high-risk patients but are still not currently advocated as a general screening test by both the USPSTF and the American College of Chest Physicians.

BREAST CANCER

Risk factors for breast cancer are as follows:

- Family history of breast cancer
- *BRCA-1* and *BRCA-2* genes

- Previous breast cancer
- Menarche before age 13 years
- Late menopause (after age 50 years)
- Late first pregnancy (after age 35 years)
- Previous lobular carcinoma in situ of the breast
- Previous cancer of the uterus, ovary, or salivary gland

A family history of breast cancer is a particularly important risk factor when diagnosed in a premenopausal first-degree relative or bilaterally in any first-degree relative. A woman with a premenopausal first-degree relative who had breast cancer has a threefold risk of developing breast cancer herself. However, an estimated 80% of women diagnosed with breast cancer do not have a positive family history. High socioeconomic status, nulliparity, hormone replacement therapy, and prior exposure to high-dose radiation also convey modestly increased risk. A number of prediction tools are available to help determine breast cancer risk in women (e.g., the Gail and Claus breast cancer prediction models).

Screening for breast cancer includes breast self-examination, clinical breast examination by a physician or nurse, and mammography. A large number of breast cancers are found by palpation. Breast self-examination has low sensitivity and unknown specificity. Appropriate teaching is required for effective breast self-examination. Advisory groups now list breast self-examination as an optional test because of lack of evidence regarding its effectiveness. Annual clinical breast examination by a physician or health care professional is recommended by the major advisory panels for women older than 40 years. Mammography has a variable but good sensitivity for detecting breast cancer, in the range of 74% to 93%. Sensitivity is lower in patients with dense breast tissue or in patients younger than 50 years of age. Specificity is also relatively good, at approximately 90% to 95%. The positive predictive value of an abnormal mammogram is approximately 10% to 20%. A normal mammogram has a negative predictive value of approximately 99%. All major authoritative groups recommend routine mammography screening after age 50 years. Studies have shown that mammography screening in women 50 to 69 years of age leads to a reduction of approximately 30% in breast cancer mortality. The benefits of mammography for women of normal risk younger than 50 years have been uncertain, and much debate has taken place regarding screening for this age group. Some data suggest a positive benefit from screening in the age group of 40 to 50 years, leading most authorities to recommend mammography screening for women in this age group. Evidence is lacking as to the efficacy of screening mammography in women older than 70 years, but because of the high risk for breast cancer in this age group, many have recommended a continuation of screening. Life expectancy of the individual woman is a major factor to consider for screening in this age group. In general, clinical breast examinations should be instituted annually in women at around the age of 40, and annual mammography screening should be started between the ages of 40 and 50 years. Women with the greatest risk should be considered for screening at an earlier age. In 2007, the American Cancer Society recommended breast MRI screening in addition to mammography in high-risk individuals. High risk is defined by the following characteristics:

- *BRCA1* or *BRCA2* mutation
- A first-degree relative (parent, sibling, child) with a *BRCA1* or *BRCA2* mutation
- A lifetime risk of breast cancer of >20%
- A history of chest radiation between the ages of 10 and 30 years
- One of the following syndromes associated with an increased risk of breast cancer: Li-Fraumeni syndrome, Cowden's syndrome, or Bannayan-Riley-Ruvalcaba syndrome

COLON AND RECTAL CANCER

Risk factors for colon cancer are as follows:

- Prior colon cancer
- Familial polyposis
- Family history of hereditary nonpolyposis colorectal cancer
- Inflammatory bowel disease
- Family history of colorectal cancer
- History of endometrial, ovarian, or breast cancer
- History of adenomatous polyps of the colon
- Lifestyle factors: tobacco use, obesity, excessive alcohol use

The overall lifetime risk for colon cancer in the U.S. population is approximately 6%. The younger the age of a first-degree relative encountering colon cancer, and the more numerous the number of family members having had colon cancer, the greater the risk to the patient. Screening for colon cancer is best conducted by determining whether a patient has normal or high risk. The testing type and frequency can then be selected based on that risk stratification. Screening strategies for colon cancer vary somewhat between different advisory groups, but all agree that some form of screening is very important.

Fecal occult blood testing (FOBT) is a cheap screening test but often involves poor patient compliance, has a limited sensitivity of approximately 50% to 65% for colon cancer, and has a positive predictive value for cancer of approximately 10% to 15%. Rehydrating the stool sample increases the sensitivity of FOBT but lowers the specificity. Evidence supporting the use of FOBT in colon cancer screening comes from randomized controlled trials. It is estimated that yearly FOBT lowers colon cancer mortality in an individual by approximately 30%. In those of normal risk older than 50 years, most authoritative groups have advised yearly FOBT. This test can be falsely positive due to diet or medications and, for accuracy, should be combined with other screening tests.

Sigmoidoscopy has a relatively low sensitivity for detecting cancer of the colon, approximately 40% to 60%. Evidence supporting the use of sigmoidoscopy in colon cancer screening comes from case-control studies. Sigmoidoscopy is limited by examiner technique and the length of colon examined. In those of average risk, screening sigmoidoscopy is generally advised every 5 years beginning at approximately age 50 years.

Colonoscopy conveys a sensitivity for colon cancer of approximately 80% to 90%. Colonoscopy has the advantage of examining the whole colon and is believed by many to be the preferred method for screening (every 10 years). However, cost, bowel preparation, the potential need for sedation, the advanced training needed for the endoscopist, and limited data regarding its effect on colon cancer mortality must be factored in the screening decision-making process. In high-risk patients, most authoritative groups have advised screening starting at an earlier age, usually around age 40, or 10 years earlier than the earliest diagnosed colon cancer in the family, whichever number is lower. Most authoritative groups have suggested periodic colonoscopy at a frequency of approximately once every 5 years.

Both CT colonography (*virtual colonoscopy*) and fecal DNA mutation testing are promising new screening modalities. In their 2008 recommendations, the American Cancer Society now recommends that CT colonography every 5 years is an option for colon cancer screening. As technology advances, CT colonography has the potential to equal the sensitivity of a colonoscopy.

In summary, the risk for future development of colon cancer should be assessed in each patient. In those of low or average risk, screening should consist of FOBT yearly and sigmoidoscopy every 5 years after the age of 50 years or by colonoscopy every 10 years. In patients with a family history of colon cancer, the risk depends on the number of relatives affected. For patients with a family history that includes one first-degree relative or two second-degree relatives with colon cancer, colonoscopy screening can be initiated at around age 40 years. For patients with a family history that includes two or more first-degree relatives or one first-degree relative with cancer or adenomatous polyp before the age of 40, a colonoscopy should be performed every 5 years after the age of 40 years, or 10 years younger than the youngest affected family member. Those in a very high-risk group (e.g., familial polyposis, inflammatory bowel disease) should generally be referred to a specialty center for more aggressive screening and monitoring.

PROSTATE CANCER

Risk factors for prostate cancer are as follows:

- Advanced age
- African American race
- Family history of prostate cancer
- Smoking

With the advent of widespread screening for prostate cancer, the lifetime risk of a man being diagnosed with prostate cancer is approximately 15%, but the risk of death from prostate cancer is only around 3%. Digital rectal examination has a sensitivity of approximately 33% to 70% and a specificity of 50% to 95% for detecting prostate cancer. Digital rectal examination has not been shown to decrease mortality from prostate cancer. Prostate-specific antigen (PSA) has been used to screen for prostate cancer. A PSA level of >4 ng/mL has a sensitivity of approximately 71%, specificity of approximately 75%, positive predictive value of approximately 35% to 40%, and negative predictive value of approximately 90% for prostate cancer. PSA levels increase in both benign and malignant prostate disease. Variations on PSA testing, such as age-specific PSA, PSA density, PSA velocity, and free PSA levels, have sought to improve the sensitivity and specificity of the test but are currently not recommended by most advisory groups for routine screening. To date, no clear evidence has shown that the early detection and treatment of prostate cancer decreases mortality. Likewise, when prostate cancer is found at an early stage, no simple method currently exists for distinguishing clinically significant cancer from an indolent form. Screening for prostate cancer can lead to morbidity in those who may never have been affected by the disease and is costly when follow-up diagnostic studies are considered. Therefore, the use of digital rectal examination and PSA to screen for prostate cancer at this juncture is controversial and is not advocated by the USPSTF based on the current evidence. In fact, in the USPSTF 2008 guidelines, the task force recommends against screening for prostate cancer. The American Cancer Society has recommended offering annual digital rectal examination and PSA testing to men older than 50 years whose life expectancy is at least 10 years and screening men in a high-risk group yearly beginning at age 45 years. When considering prostate cancer screening, a discussion with the patient regarding the pros and cons of screening should take place.

CERVICAL CANCER

Risk factors for the development of cervical cancer are as follows:

- Multiple sexual partners
- History of STDs (especially human papillomavirus [HPV] and HIV)
- Previously abnormal Pap smear or cervical dysplasia
- First coitus at an early age
- Smoking
- Low socioeconomic status

The use of the cervical Pap smear has been shown to decrease mortality from invasive cervical cancer. The positive benefit of cervical Pap smear screening occurs because the natural history of the disease is known; the disease progresses relatively slowly; and screening via Pap smear is relatively accurate, inexpensive, and safe. A Pap smear has a low sensitivity of approximately 30% to 40%, but a high specificity greater than 90%. Liquid-based Pap smears have a higher sensitivity. Most advisory groups suggest Pap screening be initiated with the onset of sexual activity or at age 21 years, whichever occurs first. Thereafter, most advisory groups recommend annual Pap smears (or once every 2 years using liquid-based tests) in patients younger than 30 years of age. After age 30 years, Pap smears can be performed every 3 years if patients have undergone regular screening previously and are not considered high risk. Some advisory groups recommend HPV testing be combined with Pap smear screening every 3 years in patients older than 30 years. Beyond age 65 to 70 years, screening should be continued based on risk; in women who have been adequately screened at a younger age whose tests have been consistently negative, screening may be discontinued. Screening may also be discontinued in women who have undergone hysterectomy (with removal of the cervix) for benign gynecologic disease. Note that screening for the STD chlamydia, in women younger than 25 years, is also recommended at the time of their annual exams.

OTHER CANCERS

Insufficient evidence exists to recommend routine screening for testicular cancer by physician examination or patient self-examination. Similarly, the effectiveness of routine screening of women for ovarian cancer by pelvic examination, vaginal or abdominal ultrasound, or serologic testing (carcinoembryonic antigen CA-125) is not established. The screening of high-risk patients (for testicular cancer, those males ages 13–39 years with history of cryptorchidism, orchiopexy, or testicular atrophy; for ovarian cancer, those women with family history of ovarian cancer, familial breast-ovarian cancer syndrome, familial cancer syndrome, or *BRCA-1* mutation carriers) should be considered

An increase in melanoma incidence has occurred in the past few decades. Those with a high risk for melanoma (familial melanoma syndrome, or with first-degree relatives with melanoma) should be referred to and screened by a dermatologist. The benefit of screening average-risk patients for melanoma is currently not supported by medical evidence.

GENERAL PHYSICAL EXAMINATION

Over time, the use of the general physical examination as a screening tool has changed significantly. The general physical examination is now usually used to establish a baseline.

Thereafter, only blood pressure, weight, breast examination, and pelvic examination are advised by most advocacy groups for the screening of asymptomatic adults. The intervals to perform these examinations are not generally agreed on. Other components of the physical examination are not generally advised in truly asymptomatic persons. A more cost-effective approach for health care providers is to instead spend time and resources counseling patients about the following:

- Smoking
- Diet
- Exercise
- Mental health
- Sexual practices
- Alcohol use
- Drug abuse
- Use of seat belts

OTHER TESTS

Hearing testing is advised in all adults when hearing loss is suspected. In patients exposed to excess noise on a regular basis, audiograms should be performed periodically.

No general consensus exists for visual acuity testing. Some authorities have recommended screening in adults older than 65 years. Patients at high risk for glaucoma should instead be referred to an ophthalmologist for evaluation. Glaucoma prevalence is significantly higher in African Americans; the risk steadily increases with age.

Neither hematocrit/hemoglobin nor leukocyte determinations have been shown to be useful in screening asymptomatic patients. Chemistry profile panels are similarly not recommended for screening asymptomatic healthy adults. Fasting plasma glucose levels should be measured every 3 years in patients at a high risk for diabetes because of a family history of diabetes, in obese persons older than 40 years, and in women with a personal history of gestational diabetes. Native Americans, Hispanics, and African Americans have a higher risk for development of diabetes mellitus. The American Diabetes Association considers a fasting plasma glucose level of greater than 126 mg/dL on two separate occasions diagnostic of type II diabetes.

Urinalysis is also not advised for screening asymptomatic patients. Population-based studies have shown low rates for detecting serious and treatable urinary tract disorders in asymptomatic adults with either hemoglobin or protein present on dipstick urinalysis. All major authorities do recommend screening urinalysis in the prenatal care of pregnant women.

Generally, laboratory tests such as chemistry profiles, blood count, urinalysis, and other similar tests should be used for targeted select patients based on increased risk and likelihood of disease. Routine screening of asymptomatic healthy adults via these methods is not advised or supported by the current medical literature. Moreover, the

TABLE 1.2
SUMMARY—STANDARD IMMUNIZATIONS

HPV	Female patients ages 9–26	3 doses (0, 2, and 6 months)
Measles, mumps, rubella	Pts. born after 1957 (w/o immunity)	1–2 doses
Td	All adults	1 dose every 10 years
Tdap	Pts. <65 yo	1 dose (in place of Td)
Influenza	Pts. ≥ 50 yo	1 dose annually
Herpes zoster	Pts. ≥60 yo	1 dose
Pneumococcal	Pts. ≥65 yo	1 dose

Centers for Disease Control (CDC), does recommend routine HIV testing in adults.

ADULT IMMUNIZATIONS (TABLE 1.2)

Influenza

Influenza vaccine is made from an inactivated virus grown in eggs. It generally contains three viruses—two A-type and one B-type virus. The vaccine is given yearly in the fall, optimally in October or November. It is 65% to 80% effective. Side effects include local skin reaction, fever, myalgia, and malaise, which, if they occur, begin soon after the vaccination and last 1 to 2 days. Patients may mistake these side effects for influenza symptoms, which may create a barrier for their future use of the vaccine. The vaccine is made from an inactivated virus and does not cause influenza. Hypersensitivity reactions are rare. The vaccine should be avoided in those with a history of hypersensitivity reactions to eggs or to a previous dose of influenza vaccine and in those with an acute febrile illness. The vaccine should also be avoided in patients with a history of Guillain-Barré syndrome after a previous influenza vaccine. The vaccination can be given safely to pregnant women. Recommended recipients of the vaccine include the following:

- Those older than 50 years
- Those with chronic illness such as diabetes, chronic lung disease, asthma, congestive heart failure, kidney disease, cirrhosis, or hemoglobinopathy
- Nursing home patients
- Medical personnel
- Those with weakened immune systems, such as persons on long-term corticosteroid treatment or patients receiving cancer treatment with radiation or chemotherapy
- Those infected with HIV
- Those younger than 18 years on long-term aspirin therapy (to prevent Reye's syndrome)
- Persons frequently exposed to or living with persons at high risk
- Those who perform essential community service
- Women who will be pregnant during the influenza season

The vaccine, particularly in the elderly, is less protective for the recipient contracting the illness but does reduce the severity of the illness. The greatest percentage of deaths due to influenza occurs in those older than 65 years. Consequently, vaccination in this age group is particularly important. Also, the vaccine has been shown to be cost effective in healthy working adults between the ages of 18 to 64 years (through fewer missed work days).

A live attenuated influenza vaccine is also available. It is given intranasally and is currently indicated as an alternative to the regular flu vaccine in healthy nonpregnant patients ages 49 years or younger. Unlike the influenza vaccine, this is an intranasal live attenuated vaccine, and therefore it is contraindicated in the following:

- Pregnant patients
- Patients with chronic respiratory disorders (e.g., asthma, chronic obstructive pulmonary disease)
- Patients with chronic medical conditions such as diabetes, chronic kidney disease, and hemoglobinopathies
- Patients with immune deficiencies
- Patients with a history of Guillain-Barré syndrome

Pneumococcus

The current 23-valent vaccine was established in 1983. The vaccine is approximately 60% effective for establishing immunity and covers approximately 88% of bloodstream isolates of pneumococcal infections in the United States. High-risk patients include those 65 years and older and those younger than 65 years with chronic illness or other risk factors, such as the following:

- Chronic cardiac or pulmonary conditions
- Anatomical or functional asplenia
- Chronic liver disease
- Alcoholism
- Diabetes
- Immunocompromised state
- Chronic renal disease
- Residents of long-term care facilities

Patients with chronic renal disease, Hodgkin's disease, or multiple myeloma; those who have undergone organ transplantation; and those receiving hemodialysis or chemotherapy for cancer may have a diminished response to the vaccine. Adverse reactions to the vaccine are rare. Minor local side effects, such as pain and redness, are common. For those adults who are most at risk for serious pneumococcal infection, one-time revaccination after 5 years is recommended. This is particularly important in patients with functional or anatomical asplenia and in those who are likely to have diminishing antibody levels (e.g., patients on dialysis, those with nephrotic syndrome, those having had organ transplantation). Revaccination for healthy adults is advised for those who received the vaccine before age 65 years and more than 5 years have elapsed. Revaccination is generally safe and well tolerated. An Arthus-type reaction can occur. Pregnancy is not a contraindication to the use of this vaccine.

Hepatitis B

Hepatitis B vaccination is a three-part procedure presently given at 0, 1 to 2, and 4 to 6 months. The vaccination is 85% to 95% effective and is administered in the deltoid muscle. A decreased antibody response is seen in the presence of renal failure, diabetes, chronic liver disease, HIV infection, smoking, and advanced age. The vaccination series is advised for all patients through age 18 years and for adults at high risk, including the following:

- Health care workers
- Patients with HIV or a newly diagnosed STD
- Hemodialysis patients
- Intravenous drug users
- Institutionalized persons
- Homosexuals and bisexuals
- Public safety personnel
- International travelers to areas of high risk
- Immigrants from countries where hepatitis B is endemic

Vaccination is also recommended for contacts of hepatitis B virus carriers, those positive for anti–hepatitis C virus, and heterosexuals with multiple partners. The vaccine can also be given to all adults who want to be immunized against hepatitis B. The vaccine is contraindicated for those with yeast hypersensitivity (the vaccine is yeast recombinant). The vaccine is safe, producing in some patient's only mild soreness at the injection site that may last 1 to 2 days. Rarely, constitutional symptoms have been experienced. Postvaccination serologic testing to demonstrate immunity is advised in those with high occupational risk (e.g., health care workers) and in patients on hemodialysis. When antibodies to the hepatitis B surface antigen are not present, revaccination should use the three-dose series. After one dose, 20% of nonresponders will produce antibodies. Between 30% and 50% will respond after three additional doses. After six doses, further attempts to immunize the patient are not likely to be fruitful. The need for booster vaccinations to provide clinical protection is unproven. In patients receiving hemodialy-

sis, and whose immunity declines rapidly, annual serologic testing is recommended, and booster vaccination may be administered to those whose antibody level falls below 10 mIU/mL. The vaccine is safe to give to pregnant women.

Tetanus/Diphtheria

The primary tetanus/diphtheria (Td) toxoid vaccination should be given to all adults who have not received the primary series previously. The general recommendation for booster dosing has been every 10 years throughout life. One usually gets a last childhood booster at age 15 years. If a patient presents with a contaminated wound, a booster should be given if the last Td vaccine was given more than 5 years earlier. Local reactions of tenderness and erythema are common after Td injections. Severe reactions to the vaccine are rare. Hypersensitivity occurs most commonly in those receiving multiple booster vaccinations; therefore, those who have received the vaccination within 5 years should generally not be revaccinated. The vaccine is not contraindicated in pregnancy.

Tetanus/Diphtheria and Acellular Pertussis Vaccination

An increased incidence of pertussis infections in adults was seen during the 1980s and 1990s. One possible cause was believed to be the waning immunity in adults who were vaccinated against pertussis in childhood. The Advisory Committee on Immunization Practices (ACIP) recommends that tetanus/diphtheria and acellular pertussis (Tdap) vaccination should be given once, in place of Td, in all adults younger than 65 years. It is recommended to administer the Tdap to women in the postpartum period and not during pregnancy. It is also recommended that Tdap can be given as early as 2 years after the last Td vaccine in certain situations: health care workers, patients with close contact to infants younger than 12 months, and postpartum women.

Rubella

The rubella vaccine is a live attenuated virus vaccine and is therefore contraindicated in immunocompromised patients. It is available alone or in combination with measles and mumps. Rubella vaccine is recommended for all adults, particularly women. Infection in pregnant women during the first trimester usually results in congenital rubella syndrome, and vaccination attempts to prevent this disease. Susceptible women of childbearing age who do not have acceptable evidence of rubella immunity or vaccination should be vaccinated. Women of childbearing age should receive the vaccine only if they say they are not pregnant. They should be counseled not to become pregnant for at least 4 weeks after receiving the vaccination. If a pregnant woman is found to be rubella susceptible (no serologic evidence of immunity), she should be vaccinated as early in the postpartum period as possible. Adverse reactions occur only in susceptible persons. Those already immune to rubella who are receiving a second vaccination are not at risk for developing side effects. Side effects have included joint pain and inflammation, which have been persistent in some. Hospital workers who have the potential to transmit rubella to pregnant women should have their immunity checked and be vaccinated appropriately.

Measles

The measles vaccine is a live attenuated vaccine and is therefore contraindicated in immunocompromised patients. Those born before 1957 are likely to have had the virus and need not be vaccinated. Adults born after 1957, not previously vaccinated, and without demonstrated immunity to measles should receive the vaccine. A second dose is recommended in adults recently exposed to measles, health care workers, patients vaccinated between years 1963 and 1967 with an inactivated virus vaccine, students entering college, and persons who plan to travel internationally. Reactions to the vaccine are local redness, sometimes accompanied by a low-grade fever. Higher fevers developing 5 to 12 days after the vaccination and lasting 1 to 2 days occur in 5% to 15% of recipients.

Mumps

The mumps vaccine should be administered to adolescent boys who previously have not had mumps or who previously have not been given the vaccine because of the possibility of mumps orchitis complicating mumps infection. The vaccine should also be given to adults not previously immunized and without immunity to mumps. The vaccine should be avoided when hypersensitivity to eggs is present. The mumps vaccine is a live attenuated virus vaccine and contains trace amounts of neomycin. Therefore, contraindications include pregnancy, anaphylaxis to neomycin, and presence of immunosuppressive conditions. Asymptomatic HIV-positive patients can receive the vaccine. Side effects include fever and rash 5 to 14 days after the vaccination, arthralgia or arthritis when given with the rubella vaccine, and local pain.

Hepatitis A

All adults wanting to obtain immunity to hepatitis A can be vaccinated. Pre-exposure immunization with the hepatitis A vaccine is also advised for the following groups:

- Adults traveling to or working in countries in which hepatitis A is endemic
- Homosexual men
- Users of illicit drugs

- Those with chronic liver disease
- Those residing in an institutional setting where hepatitis A is an ongoing problem
- Those with an occupational risk for developing the disease
- Those with clotting factor disorders, such as hemophilia
- Food handlers, when health authorities determine the vaccination to be cost effective

The intramuscular injection is given as a primary vaccination followed in 6 to 12 months by a booster vaccination. Postexposure management of hepatitis A should employ immune globulin. Side effects of the vaccine include soreness at the injection site, headache, and malaise. Generally, the vaccine has a good safety profile.

Varicella

Those with a history of having varicella are assumed to be immune and need not be considered for vaccination. Many other adults without a reliable history of varicella infection often carry immunity to varicella. Therefore, serologic testing before vaccination should be considered. Persons for whom the varicella vaccination should be considered include the following groups:

- Health care workers
- Household contacts of immunocompromised patients
- Those living or working in high-risk environments for varicella transmission, such as schools and day care centers
- College students
- Military personnel
- Nonpregnant women of childbearing age
- International travelers
- Those without a history of the disease

The vaccine is given subcutaneously in two doses 4 to 8 weeks apart. The vaccine is a live attenuated virus and is, therefore, contraindicated in immunocompromised individuals. The vaccine is also contraindicated in those who have anaphylaxis to neomycin or untreated active tuberculosis, and in recent recipients of blood products or in pregnant women. Side effects may include pain and erythema at the injection site or a varicellalike rash.

Human Papillomavirus

Along with the increased use of HPV screening during a Pap smear in women older than 30 years, the introduction of the HPV vaccine should be another powerful tool in reducing the morbidity and mortality of cervical cancer. The HPV vaccine was recommend for use by the ACIP in 2007. The HPV vaccine is recommended in females ages 9 to 26 years. Ideally, it should be administered before one becomes sexually active. It consists of a series of three shots given at 0, 2, and 6 months. It is not a live virus vaccine.

Some have estimated that it may decrease the incidence of cervical cancer by up to 70%.

Herpes Zoster Vaccine

The herpes zoster vaccine is essentially a stronger version of the varicella vaccine. It was recommended by the ACIP for use in adults in 2007. The vaccine has been shown to reduce both the burden and incidence of herpes zoster infections in the elderly. It is recommended for adults 60 years or older and is given as a single dose. However, because it is a live virus vaccine, it has a same contraindication profile as the varicella vaccine.

Meningococcus

The meningococcal vaccine is recommended to all patients ages 11 to 18 years. College students, particularly freshmen living in dormitories, are at moderately increased risk for meningococcal disease and are advised to consider receiving the meningococcal vaccination to prevent meningococcal meningitis. Adults with functional or anatomical asplenia or terminal complement component deficiency should receive the meningococcal vaccination. Travelers to certain areas of the world (e.g., sub-Saharan Africa and Mecca, Saudi Arabia) should also be vaccinated. This single-dose polysaccharide vaccination has few side effects, principally localized erythema.

REVIEW EXERCISES

QUESTIONS

1. The optimal timing for the administration of the pneumococcal vaccination includes which of the following?
a) In the immediate postoperative period of a planned splenectomy
b) Every 10 years in a patient with chronic renal failure who received the vaccination previously
c) In a healthy 55-year-old patient
d) When a person is found to be HIV positive
e) After immunosuppressive therapy in a patient undergoing organ transplantation

Answer and Discussion
The answer is d. The pneumococcal vaccination is recommended in all patients age 65 years or older. Generally, it should also be given to immunosuppressed patients before their immunosuppression occurs or becomes advanced. Therefore, the vaccination should be given before a planned splenectomy, the administration of chemotherapy or immunosuppressant therapy, and when HIV infection is first detected. Because of waning immunity, the vaccination should be given after 5 years in a patient with chronic renal failure who received the vaccination previously. Therefore, the correct answer is d.

2. Which of the following statements regarding influenza vaccination is true?
a) It cannot be given at the same time as the pneumococcal vaccination.
b) It is 90% effective.
c) It often causes an influenzalike illness.
d) It is contraindicated in the presence of allergy to eggs.
e) It should not be postponed in the setting of a febrile illness.

Answer and Discussion
The answer is d. A common misconception among patients is that the influenza vaccination causes influenza infection. The vaccine may cause local skin reaction, fever, myalgia, and malaise, side effects that the patient may mistake for influenza symptoms. The vaccine does not cause influenza because the vaccine is made from an inactivated virus. The vaccine is contraindicated in those allergic to eggs because the vaccine is made from inactivated virus grown in eggs. It should be postponed in those with a febrile illness. It is 60% to 80% effective and can be given safely at the same time as the pneumococcal vaccination. Therefore, the correct answer is d.

3. A 35-year-old man presents to his physician's office for the first time requesting a "routine physical." He is on no medications and has no significant past medical or family history, and his review of systems is negative. In addition to checking blood pressure, which of the following screening tests would be considered to be most appropriate?
a) Lipid panel, urinalysis, complete blood count
b) Lipid panel, glucose
c) Glucose
d) Lipid panel
e) Lipid panel, ECG

Answer and Discussion
The answer is d. In asymptomatic patients, routine ECGs and screening lab tests, such as urinalysis, complete blood counts, chemistry panels, and liver function tests are generally not recommended. All major advisory groups recommend blood pressure screening and lipid panel testing by the age of 35 years. Therefore, d is the correct answer.

4. A 68-year-old wife and her husband are coming in for their annual evaluations. It is mid-November. They have many questions for you regarding prevention. As you begin to counsel them, you remember that which of the following statements is correct?
a) Herpes zoster vaccination is indicated in patients older than 55 years.

b) PSA and digital rectal exams are proven screening methods to reduce prostate cancer mortality.

c) Measles vaccine is recommended in individuals born before 1957.

d) Breast self-examination is a proven screening method to reduce breast cancer mortality.

e) The live attenuated influenza vaccine would not be recommended for this couple.

Answer and Discussion

The answer is e. Herpes zoster vaccine is recommended for patients age 60 years and older. Definitive evidence supporting prostate cancer screening is still lacking. Patients born before 1957 are likely to have had the measles virus and need not be vaccinated. Adults born after 1957 who are not previously vaccinated and without demonstrated immunity should receive the vaccine. Advisory groups now list breast self- examination as an optional test because of lack of evidence regarding its effectiveness. Answer e is a true statement—the live attenuated influenza vaccine is only approved for use in patients younger than 50 years.

5. A 35-year-old woman presents to you for a new patient evaluation and wants her "annual physical." Her current medications include an oral contraceptive and ibuprofen as needed. Her mother has a history of hypertension. She is married and works as a legal secretary. Her review of systems is negative. Her previous records report that she had a normal liquid-based Pap smear and an HPV screen 2 years ago. She does not remember any recent lab work and believes that her last immunizations were when she was a teenager. Which of the following screening tests are most appropriate for this patient?

a) Pap smear, lipid panel

b) Td vaccination, lipid panel

c) Pap smear, Td

d) Td

e) Pap smear, HPV testing, lipid panel, Td

Answer and Discussion

The answer is b. With both a normal Pap smear and negative HPV screen done 2 years ago, this patient does not need another Pap smear until next year (a 3-year interval). A Pap smear could be done sooner if this patient were considered to be at high risk for cervical cancer. A tetanus booster immunization should be administered every 10 years after the primary series is completed, and almost all major advisory groups recommend cholesterol screening in asymptomatic patients by the age of 3 years. Therefore, b is the correct answer.

SUGGESTED READINGS

Boulware LE, Marinopoulos S, Phillips KA, et al. Systemic review: the value of the periodic health evaluation. *Ann Intern Med* 2007;146:289–300.

Centers for Disease Control and Prevention, Advisory Committee on Immunization Practices (ACIP). Vaccines and Immunizations. ACIP Recommendations. Available at: www.cdc.gov/vaccines/pubs/ACIP-list.htm.

Chobanian AV, Bakris GL, Black HR, et al. The seventh report of the Joint National Committee on Prevention, Evaluation, and Treatment of High Blood Pressure. *JAMA* 2003;289:2560–2572.

Expert Panel on Detection, Evaluation, and Treatment of High Blood Cholesterol in Adults. Executive summary of the third report of the National Cholesterol Education Program (NCEP) Expert Panel on Detection, Evaluation, and Treatment of High Blood Cholesterol in Adults (Adult Treatment Panel III). *JAMA* 2001;285:2486–2497.

Guirguis-Blake J, Calonge N, Miller T, et al. Current processes of the U.S. Preventive Services Task Force: refining evidence-based recommendation development. *Ann Intern Med* 2007;147:117–122.

Immunization Action Coalition Web site: www.immunize.org.

Imperiale TF, Wagner DR, Lin CY, et al. Results of screening colonoscopy among persons 40 to 49 years of age. *N Engl J Med* 2002;346:1781–1785.

Jemal A, Siegel A, Ward E, et al. Cancer statistics, 2007. *CA Cancer J Clin* 2007;57:43–46.

Lang RS, Hensrud DD, eds. *Clinical Preventive Medicine*, 2nd ed. Chicago: AMA Press, 2004.

Lieberman D. Screening for colorectal cancer in average-risk populations. *Am J Med* 2006;119:728–735.

Mulshine JL, Sullivan DC. Lung cancer screening. *N Engl J Med* 2005;352:2714–2720.

Qasseem A, Snow V, Sherif V, et al. Screening mammography for women 40 to 49 years of age: a clinical practice guideline from the American College of Physicians. *Ann Intern Med* 2007;146:511–515.

The Seventh Report of the Joint National Committee on Prevention, Selection, Evaluation, and Treatment of High Blood Pressure. NIH Publication No. 98-4080. May 2003.

Smith RA, Cokkinides V, Eyre HJ. American Cancer Society guidelines for the early detection of cancer, 2006. *CA Cancer J Clin* 2006;56:11–25.

U.S. Department of Health and Human Services, Agency for Healthcare Research and Quality, Preventive Services Task Force Web site: www.ahrq.gov/clinic/uspstfix.htm.

World Health Organization. Immunization, Vaccines and Biologicals. Available at: www.who.int/immunization/en.

Chapter 2

Women's Hormonal Health Issues

Pelin Batur   Marie M. Budev   Holly L. Thacker

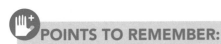

POINTS TO REMEMBER:

- The menstrual cycle is irregular at the extremes of reproductive life due to anovulatory cycles during the perimenarcheal and perimenopausal time frame.

- Bone mass declines starting in a woman's 30s and is accelerated during the menopausal transition period and early postmenopausal time.

- Increased exposure to estrogen modestly raises the risk of breast cancer.

- Pregnancy should be considered as the number one cause of secondary amenorrhea in all women.

- The benefits and risks of hormonal therapy should be discussed, and when prescribed, the lowest effective dose used.

With the increasing interest in women's health and gender-based biology, physicians are now more than ever being asked to have a greater understanding of gender-specific health care issues. In an effort to understand these issues effectively, it is helpful to divide a woman's life into the different hormonal phases—the reproductive phase, the menopausal phase, and the postmenopausal state. Understanding the changes in hormonal states during each phase depends on a keen understanding of the hypothalamic/pituitary/ovarian/endometrial axis. Any changes within this axis can lead to certain physiological and metabolic consequences. This chapter provides an overview of the three major hormonal phases in a woman's life, concentrating on the pathobiology, medical treatment, and management of these conditions.

ANATOMY AND HORMONES

Ovary

The ovary is composed of stroma and germ cells (oocytes). The greatest number of oocytes is present at the fifth month of gestation. Through atresia, a great number are reduced. At birth, 1 to 2 million oocytes exist, with only 400,000 existing by menarche; only a few hundred to a few thousand exist before menopause. The ovary is primarily responsible for synthesizing estrogen, progesterone, androgens, and peptides such as inhibin.

Estrogen

There are three human estrogens: estradiol (E_2), estrone (E_1), and estriol (E_3). More than 200 estrogenic substances (from plant, animal, and synthetic sources), however, interact with the estrogen receptors ($ER\alpha$ and $ER\beta$) and substances that affect estrogen metabolism. 17β-E_2 is the most potent human estrogen.

During reproductive years, the main source of estrogen, 17β-E_2, is produced by the dominant ovarian follicle (Fig. 2.1). E_1, the second major estrogen, is derived principally from the metabolism of E_2 and from the aromatization of androstenedione in peripheral adipose tissue. Only a small quantity of E_1 is secreted by the ovary and the adrenal glands.

In the postmenopausal state, estrogen production ceases, and the E_1 peripheral aromatization of androstenedione becomes the dominant form of estrogen. An increase in androstenedione conversion to E_1 occurs as a woman's weight increases, which results in increased overall estrogen levels.

The peripheral aromatization of testosterone to E_2 and E_1 has only a minimal contribution to overall E_1 and E_2 levels in the postmenopausal state. E_2 can also be converted to E_1 and vice versa through a reversible conversion that

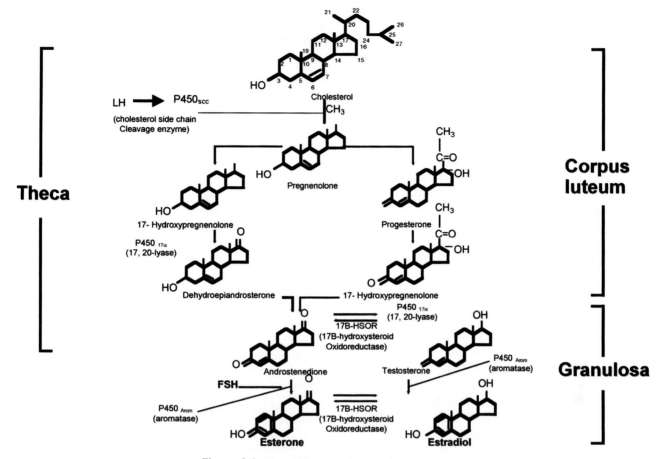

Figure 2.1 Steroid hormone biosynthesis in the ovary.

occurs in the liver. Another source of E_1 is from the reversible metabolism of E_1-3 sulfate.

The liver plays an important role in the metabolism and excretion of estrogens and is influenced directly by estrogen status. The first-pass effect of estrogens absorbed from the gastrointestinal tract and subsequent reabsorption of estrogens secreted in bile affect liver metabolism. The liver is also the primary conversion site of E_1 to E_2 as well as for the conjugation of estrogens.

All estrogens circulating in the body are either protein bound or free. Estrogen is bound tightly to sex hormone–binding globulin (SHBG) and more loosely bound to serum albumin. Alterations in SHBG change the concentration of unbound E_2, altering its bioavailability. Estrogen therapy (ET), pregnancy, and hyperthyroidism increase SHBG, whereas hypothyroidism, androgen excess, insulin, and obesity lower SHBG.

The biological activity of each estrogen depends on (a) its ability to cross the cell membrane, (b) its binding ability to a specific receptor protein and activation of the receptor, and (c) subsequent DNA synthesis. E_2 has the highest binding affinity of the estrogens. Two identified estrogen receptors (ERα and ERβ) are located throughout the body in different proportions.

Progesterone

Progestogens are divided into two classes: natural and synthetic. Progesterone is the sole naturally occurring progestogen. Synthetic progestins include 17-hydroxyprogesterone acetate, megestrol acetate, and compounds related to testosterone, including norethindrone and levonorgestrel and its derivatives. Naturally occurring progesterone is produced by the corpus luteum, and it prepares a secretory endometrium to accept a fertilized ovum. During anovulation, no corpus luteum develops; thus, estrogen is unopposed. This unopposed estrogen causes endometrial proliferation, leading to an endometrial lining that is unstable and subsequently sheds, leading to dysfunctional uterine bleeding. Therefore, progestins are prescribed to oppose the continuous effect of estrogen on the endometrium.

Androgen

In a premenopausal woman, androgens are produced by the adrenal gland and ovary. The ovarian androgens produced are androstenedione (which can be peripherally converted to E_1 in adipose tissue) and testosterone. Surgically induced menopause reduces not only a woman's level of estrogen and progesterone but also of total testosterone. Even with ET, many women may experience the effects of sexual dysfunction related to the relative androgen deficiency.

Inhibin

Inhibin is produced by the granulocytes of the ovary and inhibits pituitary gonadotropin production, specifically of follicle-stimulating hormone (FSH). When inhibin is at its highest level, FSH is suppressed. In the postmenopausal state, when inhibin is no longer produced, FSH levels remain elevated even in the face of ET.

MENSTRUAL CYCLE

The menstrual cycle begins with the onset of menarche, usually around 12 years of age, with a monthly cycle eventually occurring every 21 to 42 days. When menses occur at less than 21-day periods or more than 42-day periods, it is deemed to be irregular and likely anovulatory in etiology. It is important to note that the menstrual cycle is irregular usually at the extremes of reproductive life due to anovulatory cycles, during the perimenarcheal and perimenopausal time frame. Other common causes for a change in the usual menstrual cycle include changes in body mass index, changes in exercise patterns, parturition, and significant psychosocial distress (Tables 2.1 and 2.2). The menstrual cycle is divided into three phases: *follicular*, *ovulatory*, and *luteal*.

Follicular Phase

The first day of menstrual bleeding marks the beginning of the follicular phase (Fig. 2.2). During this time, one dominant follicle produces high levels of E_2. At this time, the other ovarian follicles become atretic. In response to the high levels of estrogen produced by the dominant follicle, the endometrium begins to proliferate. In response to high estrogen levels, the pituitary gland and hypothalamus decrease the production of FSH through negative feedback. An increase in luteinizing hormone (LH) release causes ovulation (the LH surge).

Ovulatory Phase

When LH reaches its peak, ovarian estrogen is temporarily inhibited and estrogen levels dip before ovulation, while progesterone levels continue to increase. Ovulation occurs due to the rupture of the dominant follicle and release of the mature oocyte into the peritoneal cavity. Often, with the release of the oocyte, women note symptoms of lower abdominal pain, termed *mittelschmerz*, which may be due to the release of follicular fluid and bleeding with the mature oocyte.

TABLE 2.1

CAUSES OF CHRONIC ANOVULATION

Chronic anovulation because of inappropriate pituitary feedback (e.g., in polycystic ovary syndrome)
Excessive extraglandular estrogen (as in obesity)
Functional androgen excess from adrenal or ovarian cause
Neoplasms that produce either androgens or estrogens
Neoplasms producing chorionic gonadotropin
Abnormal sex hormone–binding globulin (including liver disease)
Chronic anovulation because of endocrine or metabolic disorders
Thyroid dysfunction, either hyper- or hypothyroidism
Prolactin and/or growth hormone excess
Pituitary micro- or macroadenomas
Hypothalamic dysfunction
Drug-induced hyperprolactinemia
Malnutrition
Adrenal hyperfunction (Cushing's disease)
Congenital adrenal hyperplasia
Chronic anovulation of hypothalamic pituitary origin
Hypothalamic chronic anovulation
Psychogenic
Exercise induced
Associated malnutrition, weight loss, or systemic illness
Eating disorder (anorexia nervosa and/or bulimia)
Isolated gonadotropin deficiency (Kallmann's syndrome)
Hypothalamic pituitary damage
After surgery, trauma, radiation, or infection
Empty sella syndrome
After infarction (postdelivery Sheehan's syndrome)
Pituitary and parapituitary tumors
Idiopathic hypopituitarism

Luteal Phase

The luteal phase begins after the dominant follicle ruptures and then convolutes, forming the corpus luteum (Fig. 2.2). The term *corpus luteum* is used due to its yellow appearance as a result of the uptake of lipids and lutein pigment by the granulosa cells of the follicular walls. Once formed, the corpus luteum begins to secrete estrogen, progesterone, and androgens. The progesterone and the estrogens secreted by the corpus luteum begin the secretory phase, characterized by a coiling of the endometrial glands, resulting in a highly vascularized endothelium. If pregnancy does not occur, autolysis occurs, and the levels of progesterone and estrogen

TABLE 2.2

CAUSES OF SECONDARY AMENORRHEA

Pregnancy
Ovarian failure—menopause
Chronic anovulation
Endometrial atrophy (e.g., from continuous progestin use)
Traumatic amenorrhea (Asherman's syndrome)
Adrenal and/or thyroid dysfunction
Pituitary prolactinoma
Gestational trophic disease

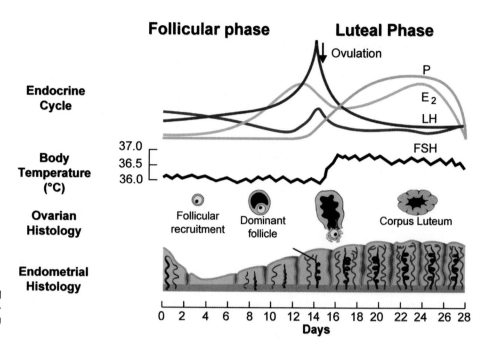

Figure 2.2 Follicular and luteal phases. E₂, estradiol; FSH, follicular-stimulating hormone; LH, luteinizing hormone; P, progesterone.

fall, owing to the absence of placenta human chorionic gonadotropin. With the fall in both estrogen and progesterone, the endometrium undergoes shedding.

PREMATURE MENOPAUSE/ PREMATURE OVARIAN INSUFFICIENCY

Premature menopause is better termed *premature ovarian insufficiency* (POI); this is said to occur before the age of 40 years and occurs in less than 1% of all women. POI before the age of 40 years usually occurs owing to premature cessation of ovarian function rather than depletion of the ovarian follicles. This is often termed *hypergonadotropic amenorrhea* (Table 2.3). The diseases associated with premature ovarian failure include sex chromosome abnormalities. POI has been linked to both familial and nonfamilial X chromosome abnormalities such as Turner's syndrome or XO chromosome and fragile X syndrome.

Women with POI should be offered testing for fragile X syndrome using *FMR-1* gene testing, particularly if any mental retardation exists in the family. Autoimmune disorders such as Addison's disease, myasthenia gravis, rheumatoid arthritis, systemic lupus erythematosus, and thyroid and parathyroid disease have been associated in women with POI. Physical insults to the ovary, including surgery, radiation, or chemotherapy (especially cyclophosphamide), or infection such as tuberculosis or mumps in utero can destroy ovarian follicles.

Other rare causes of premature ovarian failure and accelerated follicular atresia include isolated ovarian antibodies, interstitial diseases, and reduced follicular cell endowment. In rare cases, gonadotropic receptor defects leading to resistant ovarian syndrome can account for premature ovar-

ian failure. Hormonal contraceptives (HCs) (pills, patches, vaginal rings) do not suppress rare instances of ovulation in women with hypergonadotropic amenorrhea because contraceptive doses of hormones were developed to suppress ovulation in eugonadotropic women.

MENOPAUSE TRANSITION

Perimenopause or "menopause transition" is the time before and after the last period when hormone fluctuations occur, yielding some of the early symptoms of menopause.

TABLE 2.3
DIFFERENTIAL DIAGNOSIS OF HYPERGONADOTROPIC AMENORRHEA (FOLLICLE-STIMULATING HORMONE >20–40 IU/L)
Natural menopause (age range of 40–56 years, with mean of 51.3 years)
Physical causes
Surgical removal (castration)
Gonadal irradiation
Chemotherapy (especially alkylating agents)
Autoimmune disorders
Polyglandular failure involving the ovaries
Isolated ovarian failure associated with ovarian antibodies
Chromosomal abnormalities
Inherited tendencies producing premature ovarian failure
Genetically reduced cell endowment
Accelerated atresia
Gonadotropin receptor and/or postreceptor defects causing resistant ovary syndrome

TABLE 2.4

EFFECTS OF ESTROGEN LOSS

Symptoms (early onset)	Hot flashes/vasomotor symptoms
	Mood disturbances
	Sleep disturbances
	Irritability
	Urogenital symptoms
Physical signs (intermediate onset)	Vaginal atrophy
	Cervical atrophy
	Skin/dermal thinning
	Hair thinning
Diseases (later onset)	Osteoporosis

TABLE 2.5

DIFFERENTIAL DIAGNOSIS OF HOT FLASH/FLUSH

Psychiatric manifestations	Panic attacks
	Anxiety
Medications	Nitroglycerin
	Niacin
	Nifedipine
	Calcitonin
	Clomiphene citrate
	Danazol
	Gonadotropin-releasing hormone analogs
Endocrine	Thyrotoxicosis
	Carcinoid
	Diabetic insulin reaction
	Pheochromocytoma
	Insulinoma
	Autonomic dysfunction
Substances	Monosodium glutamate
Other	Lymphoma
	Tuberculosis

Symptoms during this time vary, depending on the production of E_2, androgens, and progesterone levels. Diagnosis is made clinically, and no method of serologic testing can predict the time of menopause. A persistent elevation in FSH (and LH) can signal that menopause is imminent.

MENOPAUSE

Menopause is defined as the permanent cessation of menses. This is diagnosed retrospectively after the absence of periods for 1 year. *Postmenopause* is the term used to refer to the time after menopause. The median age of menopause is 51 years of age. It has been noted that the average age of menopause is lowered in certain groups, such as smokers and women with chronic illness. Menopause occurs when the ovary no longer has active follicles producing E_2. The main symptoms of menopause are manifested by estrogen deficiency expressed by estrogen target tissues that are rich in estrogen receptors, including the urogenital system, breast, bone, the cardiovascular system (including the vascular endothelium), the central nervous system, and the gastrointestinal tract (Table 2.4).

Fluctuations in E_2 levels can trigger vasomotor symptoms such as hot flashes or flushes, the most commonly reported symptoms of menopausal transition and postmenopausal women. Other conditions can mimic vasomotor symptoms (Table 2.5).

MENOPAUSAL SYMPTOMS

Hot flashes are the sensation of warmth to extreme heat in the upper body, arms, and face. Usually, hot flashes are followed by a hot flush (visible erythema), which is characterized by the vasodilation of blood vessels and a noticeable blush to the skin. A prodromal aura may occur, consisting of head pressure, headache, and nausea, present with or without diaphoresis. The severity and resultant debilitating effects of these symptoms on each woman vary. This may be due to various hypothalamic receptors and dietary factors that are specific to an individual woman. Although the vasomotor phenomenon is not life threatening, it can frequently disrupt sleep and lead to chronic sleep deprivation, which can then lead to fatigue and mood changes, including depression. The pathobiology of hot flushes has yet to be clearly defined but is suggestive of a triggering response in the thermal regulatory centers in the hypothalamus. Hot flashes usually resolve with age, with a mean duration lasting 2 to 5 years after onset, although a small percentage of women continue to have these symptoms for more than 15 years.

Women who have induced menopause experience the most intense hot flash symptoms, but not all women with induced menopause experience vasomotor symptoms. Other vasomotor symptoms may include palpitations, dizziness, and, rarely, skin crawling sensations.

Psychiatric diseases such as major depression and panic disorder do not appear to occur at an increased rate in postmenopausal women. However, women who have suffered from affective disorders after a reproductive event (depression, premenstrual dysphoric disorder, and postpartum depression) are at an increased risk for recurrence related to changes in their reproductive hormonal status. Vasomotor symptoms can exacerbate panic disorders, depression, and anxiety. ET does have a role in ameliorating vasomotor symptoms, but standard psychiatric treatment and pharmacologic and psychological therapy should be recommended in these instances. In postmenopausal women without psychiatric disorders, mild mood changes can improve with ET.

Although epidemiologic data seem to indicate that ET reduces senile dementia of Alzheimer's type, recent placebo-controlled trials in patients with senile dementia of Alzheimer's type failed to show any delay in disease progression. Furthermore, the Women's Health Initiative (WHI), a large preventive trial, estrogen/progestin study in late postmenopausal women suggested an increased risk of dementia in older women. The timing of use of hormone therapy (HT) may explain the disparate findings between observation studies and randomized controlled trials in both dementia and cardiovascular disease. Subgroup analyses from the WHI study showed that women between the ages of 50 and 59 taking ET have a trend toward lower coronary disease risk compared to nonusers, although ET should not be used for the purpose of preventing heart disease. Similarly, women starting HT in their 60s seem to have an increased risk for dementia, whereas women using long-term HT starting in their 50s have decreased risk based on observational studies; however, larger randomized trials are not available to further confirm these findings.

Integument

Decrease or loss of E_2 decreases the mitotic activity of the dermis and epidermis and leads to a reduction in the synthesis of collagen and elastin fibers. Hair thinning may occur in an androgenic pattern in predisposed women. Also, excessive facial hair may occur with the change of the estrogen–androgen ratio. ET reverses some of these changes and may improve skin texture.

Genitourinary System

Multiple vulvar changes occur, including atrophy of the labia majora and the labia minora, atrophy of urethra, overall dryness, and sparser pubic hair owing to lack of estrogen and androgen. Reduced estrogen levels lead to a decrease in the vaginal rugae, with pale, dry vaginal mucosa noted on speculum examination. Atrophic vaginitis develops, which can lead to pain with routine pelvic examination and during intercourse. There may be an increase in urinary symptoms and urinary tract infections owing to a reduction in vaginal lactobacilli populations.

Cervical atrophy, which may cause the cervix to become flush with the vaginal wall, and uterine shrinkage may occur with decreased estrogen levels. Uterine fibroids generally shrink, and the ovaries also reduce in size and should not be palpable on routine examination within 1 to 2 years after menopause.

Urodynamic changes occur with the reduction in local estrogen levels as well, with changes in the epithelium of the urethra and a reduced closing pressure of the urethral sphincter. Frequently, urethral syndromes during menopause mimic symptoms of urinary tract infections, including urgency, frequency, dysuria, and suprapubic pain, which may occur without evidence of infection on routine dipstick examination.

Stress incontinence may develop during pelvic stress maneuvers such as coughing, sneezing, or lifting. Other types of incontinence include urge, overflow, function, and mixed (stress and urge), and can occur in combination in the postmenopausal period. Risk factors for stress incontinence include a history of obstetric trauma, weakness of pelvic floor muscles, and chronic cough. Kegel or pelvic floor exercises can be used for mild stress incontinence to strengthen the voluntary muscles of the pelvic floor and urethral sphincter. ET locally may help reconstitute the integrity of the vaginal and urethral mucosa. Bladder retraining and biofeedback may be helpful in treating mild cases of female incontinence.

Urge incontinence is associated with a strong urge to urinate but the inability to get to the bathroom before the onset of urination. The physiology of urge incontinence includes an uninhibited bladder contraction that is significant enough to overcome baseline urethral sphincter tone. Estrogen deficiency may further exacerbate bladder irritability owing to atrophy of the trigone of the bladder, thus worsening urge incontinence. Other substances that can worsen urge incontinence include caffeine, spices, and citrus products. Treatment for urge incontinence includes local estrogen treatment and medications such as tolterodine tartrate (Detrol) or oxybutynin chloride (Ditropan), along with bladder behavioral therapy.

The endopelvic fascia may also weaken with menopause, aging, weight gain, and trauma from childbirth, and this can lead to cystocele, rectocele, and cystourethrocele, or frank prolapse at the vaginal introitus, leading to irritation, incontinence, and frequent infections.

Bone Mass and Osteoporosis

Bone mass in a woman depends on multiple factors, including genetics, estrogen exposure, dietary calcium with vitamin D intake, and exercise. A rapid increase in bone mass occurs in puberty, with peak bone mass being reached by age 30. Bone mass declines starting in a woman's 30s and is accelerated during the menopausal transition period and early postmenopausal time. When menopause occurs and estrogen levels fall, the most rapid decline in bone mass is in the trabecular spine. Estrogen acts as an antiresorptive agent and inhibits bone loss. Evidence also suggests that progesterone plays a role in protecting bone mass, but overall it is primarily estrogen that preserves bone mass. The protection offered by estrogen/progestin therapy (named HT) is greatest if therapy is continuous. If therapy stops, typical menopausal bone loss will commence. Women who have used long-term HT for osteoporosis (OP) prophylaxis should have a bone density assessment periodically because a small percentage of these women on long-term therapy are considered bone nonresponders. Women using HT solely for bone benefits should consider other bone-specific options.

Alternatives to Hormone Therapy in Prevention and Treatment of Osteoporosis

Bisphosphonates that are approved for both treatment and prevention of OP include alendronate (Fosamax) and risedronate (Actonel), which can be taken daily or weekly, and ibandronate (Boniva), which can be taken daily or monthly. For many women, another alternative to HT is the use of selective estrogen receptor modulators (SERMs). Raloxifene (Evista) is the first SERM that was approved for both prevention and treatment of OP. The SERMs act similarly to estrogen on certain tissues. Raloxifene also has some positive lipid effects and effects on vascular reactivity, although overall these effects seem to be less potent than those of estrogen. The Raloxifene Use for the Heart trial, a large, randomized, prospective trial examining the use of raloxifene showed no increased risk of coronary events, and a 44% decreased risk of invasive breast cancer in raloxifene users compared to nonusers. The Study of Tamoxifen and Raloxifene (STAR) trial compared raloxifene and tamoxifen for breast cancer protection outcomes, and showed that both agents decreased invasive breast cancers and fractures similarly. Although tamoxifen is currently the only drug approved by the U.S. Food and Drug Administration (FDA) to reduce breast cancer diagnosis in high-risk women, the STAR study showed 38% lower endometrial cancer rates in the raloxifene group as compared to the tamoxifen group. This is related to the fact that tamoxifen has an estrogenic effect on the uterus, which can lead to endometrial hyperplasia, thus increasing the risk of endometrial cancer. The use of raloxifene and tamoxifen has been found to cause a slight increase in the risk of thromboembolism, similar to that of ET. Raloxifene does not treat any menopausal symptoms of hot flashes or vaginal atrophy and has not been shown to specifically reduce hip fracture, but it has been shown to reduce vertebral fractures.

Osteoprotegerin is a naturally occurring protein that is a regulator of osteoclast formation. A small, randomized, double-blinded study showed an 80% reduction in bone turnover markers in postmenopausal women who received daily injections of osteoprotegerin. Larger trials looking at these results are currently under way. Injectable Forteo (teriparatide) is FDA approved for the treatment of osteoporosis and has osteoblastic bone building effects. Women with Paget's disease or bone irradiation are not candidates due to the concern of osteosarcoma (seen in rats given very high doses).

Cardiovascular System

Despite significant advances in cardiovascular medicine over the decade, cardiovascular disease is still the leading killer of women in the United States and in the majority of developed countries. In the United States alone, more than half a million women die yearly due to cardiovascular disease, thus exceeding the number of deaths in men. Risk factors for cardiovascular disease in women are similar to those in men, including dyslipidemia, hypertension, diabetes mellitus, and smoking, but some gender-specific differences do exist. Selected studies have indicated that women are less likely than men to achieve risk factor goal therapies. Overall, the awareness of cardiovascular disease has increased in women, but a significant gap still exists in women's perceived and actual risk of cardiovascular disease.

Hypertension is more common in older women than older men. Early observational studies have suggested that ET can reduce the risk of coronary artery disease (CAD) up to 50% with estrogen alone and 34% with HT. The Heart and Estrogen/Progestin Replacement Study (HERS), the first large, randomized, placebo-controlled trial of estrogen for secondary prevention of CAD in postmenopausal women with established CAD showed no clinical benefit in HT users compared to placebo on overall cardiovascular events, despite favorable effects on the lipid profile. In fact, the HERS trial indicated a threefold hazard for venous thromboembolic events in HT users, particularly during early use. Based on the HERS findings, the American Heart Association (AHA) recommended that HT not be initiated solely for the purpose of secondary prevention of CAD. In 2002, the WHI Randomized Controlled Trial, the first primary prevention trial of HT in postmenopausal women, failed to demonstrate any benefit of estrogen plus progestin in the prevention of CAD or stroke after 5.2 years of follow-up. In addition, the WHI study demonstrated a twofold hazard of pulmonary embolism. It was concluded that HT should not be initiated or continued for the primary prevention of CAD.

Recently, the unopposed estrogen arm of the WHI, involving women without an intact uterus, showed no benefit and no risk of ET for the primary prevention of CAD. In the wake of the results from these major clinical trials, the AHA issued a set of collaborative evidence-based guidelines for the prevention of CAD in women, depending on clinical diagnosis and scenarios that group women into categories of high, intermediate, and lower risk.

In addition, the new guidelines show risk groups as defined by their absolute probability of having a coronary event in 10 years, according to the Framingham Risk Score for women. The new guidelines stress lifestyle interventions, including smoking cessation, encouraging physical activity every day of the week, cardiac rehabilitation after any recent cardiac event, heart-healthy diet including omega-3 fatty acids and folic acid, weight maintenance and reduction, and evaluation for depression. Major risk factor interventions include encouragement to achieve a new optimal blood pressure of <120/80 mm Hg through lifestyle approaches. In addition, optimal levels of lipoproteins in women including a low-density lipoprotein-cholesterol (LDL-C) of <100 mg/dL, high-density lipoprotein-cholesterol (HDL-C) of >50 mg/dL, and triglycerides of <150 mg/dL are described in the new guidelines. The guidelines stress the initiation of pharmacotherapy in high-risk women with an LDL-C of >100 mg/dL or in moderate-risk women with an LDL-C of >130 mg/dL to lower LDL-C with a statin simultaneously with lifestyle therapy. Statin agents, such as atorvastatin (Lipitor), lovastatin (Mevacor), pravastatin (Pravachol), rosuvastatin (Crestor), and simvastatin (Zocor), are recommended as initial first-line therapy. ET appears to have complementary effects on the lipid profile when combined with statin therapy, particularly in women with elevated levels of lipoprotein(a) (Lp[a]), although it is not used specifically for cardiovascular risk reduction, only for treatment of menopausal symptoms.

Preventative measures, including aspirin therapy, are recommended in high- and intermediate-risk women, but should probably not be used in low-risk women. In the sixth decade of life, aspirin appears to protect against stroke. Over the past several years, several large contrasting studies done by different methods cast controversy on when to start aspirin use in women; therefore, this is an area of active investigation. The AHA guidelines do not support the initiation or continuation of estrogen plus progestin HT to prevent cardiovascular disease in postmenopausal women. In addition, the guidelines do not support the use of antioxidant vitamin supplements in the prevention of cardiovascular disease, and the new guidelines recommend against the preventive use of aspirin in women at low risk for cardiovascular disease.

Breast Tissue

In the postmenopausal period, involution of the ductal and glandular breast tissue occurs with a reduction in estrogen and progesterone levels. For most women, the breast shrinks and becomes replaced with adipose tissue. The Gail Model Breast Cancer Risk Assessment Tool, a seven-question logistical mathematical regression model, computes an individual woman's 5-year risk and lifetime risk of breast cancer diagnosis. If a woman has a high Gail Model assessment percentage (lifetime risk of 30% or more), she should be further counseled regarding breast cancer risk assessment and be referred to a breast center for breast cancer chemoprevention study, tamoxifen therapy, or breast ductal lavage for further risk assessment.

Increased exposure to estrogen modestly raises the risk of breast cancer. Early menarche (before age 12 years) and/or late menopause (after age 55 years), both markers of increased estrogen exposure, confer some increased risk. The WHI showed a 26% increased risk of breast cancer at 5.2 years in women who use combination estrogen and progestin in the form of Prempro. When these same data are interpreted in the form of absolute risk, it is evident that the risk of breast cancer diagnosis to the individual woman is low. In the WHI, 38 cases of breast cancer occurred in HT users per year, compared with 30 cases in women not using HT—an absolute difference of 8 cases. In contrast, women in the estrogen-only arm of this trial, using Prem-

arin, had no increased risk of breast cancer. The Million Women Study in the United Kingdom is the largest nonrandomized study of hormone use. This study concluded that all types of hormone use, including estrogen-only forms, increased the risk of breast cancer compared with women receiving no hormone therapy.

DIAGNOSIS OF MENOPAUSE

The diagnosis of menopause is officially made retrospectively after the cessation of menses for 1 year. Pregnancy, however, should be considered as the number one cause of secondary amenorrhea in all women. If secondary amenorrhea remains suspected and pregnancy is ruled out, considerations in the differential diagnosis should include polycystic ovarian disease (most common ovarian cause), chronic anovulation, structural changes such as cervical stenosis or Asherman's syndrome (endometrial scarring), adrenal or thyroid dysfunction, endometrial atrophy (i.e., continuous progesterone use), pituitary prolactinoma, gestational trophoblastic disease, and nutritional disorders.

Clinical Diagnosis

The history and physical examination should focus on the skin, the bone, and the genitourinary structures, and the cardiovascular system. Key questions to ask about menopause include symptoms of estrogen deficiency, including hot flashes or hot flushes, sleep disturbances, palpitations, changes in skin texture, history of irritable bladder or incontinence, and history of painful intercourse. It is also pertinent to ask about symptoms of androgen deficiency, which may present as hypoactive sexual desire and a decreased ability to reach sexual climax, because this may represent a true female androgenic deficiency syndrome in a minority of postmenopausal women. Symptoms of progesterone deficiency in perimenopause present as heavy irregular menses (owing to unopposed estrogen).

The height, weight, and blood pressure should be recorded and compared with prior values. Thyroid examination; breast examination in sitting and supine position; skin examination; cardiovascular examination; and abdominal, pelvic, and rectal examinations should be performed. The clinician should note signs of genitourinary atrophy, including a thin, pale, atrophic vaginal mucosa, which may present with petechia or may be atrophic diffusely or in patches. The periurethral tissue is the most estrogen-sensitive tissue and usually shows initial signs of estrogen deficiency. Examples of severe vaginal estrogen deficiency include a stenotic introitus, varying degrees of urethral caruncle, and the presence of a small cervical os or possible stenotic os. In severe cases, the cervix may actually be flush with the vaginal walls and may be very difficult to distinguish from this surrounding vaginal tissue. A screening Papanicolaou (Pap) smear should be obtained of the ectocervix and the endocervix using a spatula and a cytobrush to screen for cervical cancer, with HPV testing in women older than 30 years or women with abnormal Paps. A Gail Model assessment of breast cancer risk should be considered to further define an individual woman's risk for breast cancer, and a Framingham Score should be used to assess for low, moderate, or high risk for cardiovascular disease.

Laboratory Studies

In most cases, FSH and E_2 levels are not needed to diagnose the menopausal state. In a woman who has had a simple hysterectomy (ovaries remaining), ovarian function may be present after the hysterectomy, and FSH and E_2 levels may aid the clinician in the decision to initiate ET. If a woman has been on HCs—pills, patch, ring, injection, or implants or hormonal intrauterine systems up to the time of menopause—measuring hormonal levels after several months of being off HCs (while a woman uses a barrier method) may also be helpful in determining whether menopause has occurred. Measuring these values in a menopausal transition female are not as clinically useful because these levels may fluctuate widely through the menopausal transition state. Again, this emphasizes that the diagnosis of menopause is always retrospective.

The American College of Physicians recommends screening of thyroid-stimulating hormone in all women older than 50 years, whereas the American College of Clinical Endocrinology recommends screening by age 35 years. Women receiving thyroxine, who may be clinically euthyroid, may actually be biochemically hyperthyroid and, therefore, at an increased risk for bone loss. Perimenopausal women who present with menopause-like symptoms and menstrual disorders may actually have hypo- or hyperthyroidism.

Standard screening mammograms and examinations of the breasts by a health care provider should be performed yearly, beginning at age 40 years for all women. Women with a strong family history of breast cancer (and/or those who have Gail Model–calculated lifetime risk of breast cancer of 30% or more) should be referred to a breast center. One randomized, double-blinded, placebo-controlled trial (Postmenopausal Estrogen/Progestin Interventions Trial) actually showed an increased breast density in some HT users, which in theory may make mammographic breast cancer detection more difficult. In women with dense breasts, the clinician may consider stopping hormonal therapy 2 to 3 weeks prior to annual mammography.

The National Osteoporosis Foundation (NOF) recommends that all women be screened for OP by the age of 65 years if one or more risk factors (including natural and surgically induced menopause, maternal or personal history of hip fracture, a weight of less than 128 lb, and smoking) are present. The NOF guidelines suggest that all women who have been on long-term HT have a bone density assessment because a small subset of women are bone nonresponders, even though they have been on long-term treatment. For a healthy postmenopausal woman who is contemplating initiating any therapy for bone protection reasons, a dual X-ray absorptiometry (DXA) scan may assist her in the decision to institute therapy. Any woman with a history of vertebral compression fractures or skeletal deformity should have a DXA performed initially at baseline. DXA scans also serve as screening for OP prevention in women with POI and for other persons with risk factors for OP (glucocorticoid use, eating disorders, anticonversant therapy, height loss, history of prolonged amenorrhea).

Along with body mass index calculations (weight in kilograms over height in meters), waist-to-hip ratios (waist circumference should be <35 inches in women and <40 inches in men), blood pressure, smoking history, diabetes, and lipids stratify a woman's cardiovascular risk. Several large studies indicate that ultrasensitive C-reactive protein (US CRP) screening, in addition to standard lipid screening, provided further information in identifying women who were at high risk for future cardiovascular events. These results may influence clinicians to more aggressively treat with statin agents in this subset of patients with elevated US CRP levels.

MANAGEMENT OF MENOPAUSE

The key to managing menopause and its associated symptoms is to tailor therapy to the individual woman. The minimum effective dose of replacement therapy should be used to treat the symptoms of menopause (vasomotor symptoms, genitourinary symptoms). The benefits and risks of hormonal therapy should be discussed with patients. Options should be provided regarding other bone therapy options with SERMs or bisphosphonates. Dietary, exercise, and lifestyle advice is paramount. A woman's individual medical history, family history, current menopausal symptoms, and response to HT should be reassessed periodically.

Risks and Benefits of Hormone Therapy

Benefits
- Relief of vasomotor symptoms
- Prevention of postmenopausal OP, fractures, and dental loss
- Curing of genitourinary atrophy
- Reduction in colon cancer and colon polyps in HT users
- Possible benefit in reducing age-related macular degeneration
- Probable improvement in mood and energy level and a sense of well-being in symptomatic women
- Possible reduction in cataract formation, knee osteoarthritis, and obstructive sleep apnea syndrome

TABLE 2.6

ORAL ESTROGEN DOSAGES

Trade Name	Ultra-Low Dose (mg)	Low Dose (mg)	Medium Dose (mg)	Intermediate Dose (mg)	Higher Dose (mg)	Highest Dose (mg)
Premarin (CEEs)	0.3	0.45	0.625	0.9	1.25	2.5
Estrace (micronized estradiol)	0.5		1.000		2.00	
Ogen (estrone)			0.625		1.25	2.5
Ortho-Est (estrone)			0.625		1.25	
Estratab (esterified estrogen preparation)	0.3		0.625		1.25	2.5
Menest (esterified estrogen preparation)	0.3		0.625		1.25	2.5
Cenestin (synthetic CEE)[a]			0.625		0.9	

[a]CEE, conjugated equine estrogen.

Risks
- Five- to 10-fold increase in endometrial cancer risk if ET is unopposed
- Slight increase in breast cancer diagnosis in women on estrogen/progestin HT for several years
- Increase in the relative risk of thromboembolic events of two- to threefold in HT users
- Increased stroke risk
- Increased incidence of gallbladder disease, which may necessitate cholecystectomy
- Premenstruallike side effects on a combination (estrogen/progestin) therapy
- Withdrawal menstrual bleeding on a cycled HT regimen
- Elevations of triglyceride levels on oral ET in susceptible women

If a woman has had a hysterectomy, ET alone is prescribed, but if a woman has an endometrium and uterus, *both* estrogen and progestin therapy should be given to avoid unopposed estrogen that can lead to endometrial hyperplasia and thus increase the risk of endometrial cancer.

If a woman is still using contraception before menopause, she should continue with contraception use 1 year after initiating HT therapy because the level of hormones in postmenopausal therapy is not high enough to inhibit the hypothalamic-pituitary-ovarian axis, which is needed for contraceptive protection.

Estrogen Therapy

Conjugated Equine Estrogens

A blend of multiple equine estrogens, Premarin, has been available the longest and studied the most extensively of all ET. Esterified estrogen preparations (Estratab and Menest) contain E_1 and equilin sulfate, but are not exact biochemical equivalents to conjugated equine estrogen (CEE). Cenestin is a synthetic conjugated estrogen formulation. Micronized 17β-E_2 (Estrace) can be given orally and is well absorbed by the gastrointestinal tract, but has a short half-life, necessitating a twice-daily dosage. E_1 is available as Ogen and Ortho-Est and is dosed daily. Dosages for oral ET are shown in Table 2.6.

The E_2 transdermal patch offers an alternative to women who prefer the convenience of dosing (most patches are changed every 3.5 days or once a week), who experienced nausea or drug-induced hypertension on oral preparations (Table 2.7), or who want to use "bioidentical" estradiol (although there is no evidence that bioidentical forms are any safer than standard regimens). In women who have elevated triglycerides, the patch preparation is also preferred.

TABLE 2.7

ESTRADIOL PATCH DOSAGES

Trade Name	Ultra-Low and Low Dose (mg)	Medium Dose (mg)	Intermediate Dose (mg)	Higher Dose (mg)	Change Patch
Estraderm		0.05		0.10	Every 3.5 days
Vivelle	0.025 0.0375	0.05	0.075	0.10	Every 3.5 days
Alora		0.05	0.075	0.10	Every 3.5 days
Climara	0.025	0.05	0.075	0.10	Weekly
CombiPatch	Contains 0.05 mg of estradiol with either 0.14 mg or 0.25 mg of norethindrone acetate (NA)				
Climara Pro	Contains 0.045 mg of estradiol with NA—weekly 0.015 of levonorgestrel				

The patch preparation avoids enterohepatic metabolism. The Estrogen and Thromboembolism Risk Study Group showed that in women with a history of deep venous thrombosis, use of transdermal ET resulted in no greater risk of thrombosis than the general population as compared to the oral ET formulations.

Overall, the side effects of estrogen include nausea, bloating, and breast tenderness, but they are lower with ET preparations in comparison with standard HCs because the overall estrogenic doses are four to five times lower in comparison with low-dose HCs. Lower doses of estrogen with CEE at 0.45 or 0.3 mg are recommended as starting doses, or patches may be used (0.025, 0.0375, or 0.045 mg). In general, women who have undergone surgical- or chemotherapy-induced menopause may need higher doses of estrogen to control vasomotor symptoms. Higher doses of CEE of 0.625, 0.9, or 1.25 mg daily, either by the oral route or the transdermal E_2 patches of 0.05, 0.075, or 0.100 mg, may be needed. Several weeks should elapse before dosages are increased. If women are on standard oral ET and continue to have genitourinary symptoms, vaginal preparations, in addition to systemic therapy, may be beneficial (Table 2.8). An example of this is Estrace or Premarin vaginal cream, 2 g daily for 2 weeks and then 1 g one to three times per week, given intravaginally. Some systemic absorption of estrogen cream in preparation occurs through the vaginal mucosa, but once the mucosal integrity is restored with local therapy, systemic absorption is minimal. If a woman prefers not to use vaginal cream preparations due to variability, absorbability, and application, other options have become available for urogenital symptoms of estrogen deficiency. A silicone vaginal ring (Estring) impregnated with E_2 can be inserted in the vagina by the woman every 3 months for relief of urogenital symptoms. Little systemic absorption of estrogen has been noted with the vaginal ring, thus making it a possible therapeutic option in women who want to avoid systemic estrogen treatment.

In addition, the Vagifem intravaginal tablet (17β-E_2) is another option for women who need local vaginal therapy and who have continued urogenital symptoms, or for women who are currently not on systemic therapy and continue to have urogenital symptoms. One tablet is inserted into the lower third of the vagina every night for 2 weeks, then twice a week thereafter for the relief of urogenital symptoms. An approximate 5% rate of systemic absorption of E_2 occurs using this treatment, unlike the vaginal ring, so endometrial stimulation is possible. Other kinds of estrogen systemic therapy include the Femring vaginal ring, changed every 3 weeks, which provides local and systemic estrogen, as well as estrogen lotions and gels, which are rubbed on the arms and legs and provide systemic estrogen to treat hot flashes.

Women who have low free testosterone levels may benefit from preparations containing esterified estrogen, 1.25 mg or 0.625 mg, combined with methyltestosterone, 2.5 mg or 1.25 mg (Estratest or Estratest HS). Side effects of androgen therapy include acne, hirsutism, and other virilization effects. It is important to note that any oral androgen may cause an elevation in transaminases and potential liver damage. Therefore, it is recommended that periodic monitoring of transaminases, lipid levels, and E_2-free testosterone levels be performed in women taking oral androgens. Compounded testosterone preparations are not routinely recommended because of variability in absorption and lack of standardization. Although testosterone patches are available (for male hypogonadism), the doses are generally too high for women.

Tibolone, available in Europe, is a synthetic steroid analog that has estrogenic, androgenic, and progestin activity without endometrial stimulation. After metabolism, the progestogenic metabolite predominates, producing an atrophic endometrium. Tibolone may prove to be a useful alternative in women wanting to avoid uterine bleeding or in women with endometriosis; however, in the Million Women Study, tibolone was shown to increase the risk of breast cancer. Tibolone may not only reduce bone reabsorption and decrease total cholesterol, Lp(a), and triglyceride levels, but it has also been noted to decrease high-density lipoprotein (HDL) levels as well.

Progestins

Combined estrogen/progestin therapy is mandatory in a woman with an endometrium to avoid stimulation of the endometrial lining, which may lead to the endometrial hyperplasia associated with unopposed estrogen use. In a hysterectomized patient, progestins are not recommended unless a residual endometriosis exists. The side effects of progestins include premenstruallike symptoms, which often cause women the discomfort that is associated initially with starting combined estrogen/progestin therapy. Progestins may have androgenic effects, depending on the type of agent used, dosage, and route of delivery. Also, the progestins seem to increase breast cancer and coronary event risks in comparison to the use of estrogen alone. Current epidemiologic studies do not recommend adding progestins to estrogen to prevent OP.

TABLE 2.8

OPTIONS FOR GENITOURINARY MENOPAUSAL SYMPTOMS

Premarin cream/Estrace cream/Ogen cream	2 g daily intravaginally for 2 weeks, then 1 g intravaginally one to three times weekly
Vagifem tablets (estradiol hemihydrate)	Insert 1 tablet in vagina each night for 2 weeks, then 1 tablet two times weekly for maintenance
Estring (estradiol ring)	Place ring intravaginally, change every 3 months

Cycled progestins are taken for the first 12 days of every calendar month. This *cyclic regimen* is associated with withdrawal bleeding in most women. If progestins are taken on a daily basis with estrogen, this is termed *continuous therapy*, and usually induces amenorrhea in most menopausal women within a 6- to 9-month period.

Provera, Cycrin, and Amen (medroxyprogesterone acetate, 5–10 mg) are examples of progestins that are given on days 1 through 12 of each calendar month for a cycled regimen (Table 2.9). Micronized progesterone (Prometrium, 100 mg continuous regimen or 200 mg cycled regimen, days 1–12) is centrally metabolized and may have sedative-hypnotic effects (Table 2.9). This may be an option for women who suffer from sleep disturbances secondary to menopause. Prometrium is micronized with peanut oil; therefore, women with peanut allergies must have progesterone compounded with another oil. Prochieve vaginal gel (4%–8%) is available for women intolerant of Prometrium use and is a vaginal progesterone.

A woman should expect mild to moderate bleeding during cycled therapy, usually occurring mid month between days 10 through 15. As long as the cervical os is not stenosed, the absence of withdrawal bleeding indicates the endometrial lining may simply be atrophic. Any abnormal bleeding occurring outside the day 10 to day 15 period should be further investigated with an endometrial biopsy, transvaginal ultrasound, hysteroscopy, or saline-infused sonogram to detect endometrial abnormalities.

If HT is given to relieve postmenopausal symptoms, therapy can be tapered off gradually while still monitoring for bone loss with periodic DXA scanning. The key to HT is to tailor the therapy based on an individual woman's risks and benefits and re-evaluate the need for HT periodically based on treatment goals using the lowest effective dose.

Contraindications to Hormone Therapy

Absolute contraindications to HT include pregnancy and undiagnosed vaginal bleeding. Any postmenopausal vaginal bleeding must be investigated with an endometrial biopsy, owing to a 5% to 10% incidence of simple or complex hyperplasia (with or without atypia), adenomatous endometrial hyperplasia, or frank endometrial cancers. The majority of women with postmenopausal bleeding have a proliferative endometrium (because of a lack of progesterone), endometrial polyps, cervical or vulvar lesions, submucosal fibroids, or simple bleeding from an atrophic vagina or atrophic endometrium.

Once uterine cancer is cured either by surgical excision of low-grade, early-stage cancer or by lack of occurrence after 5 years from initial surgical treatment, ET is an option. Ovarian cancers are not usually believed to be estrogen-dependent and therefore do not constitute a contraindication to HT.

A remote history of deep venous thrombosis (DVT) is not an absolute contraindication to HT. Any patient with a history of recurrent DVT or a family history of thromboembolic events, however, should be evaluated for the presence of a hypercoagulable state. Migraine headaches that have a hormonal pattern may improve or worsen at menopause. Postmenopausal women with a history of migraines usually benefit from continuous replacement therapy rather than cyclical therapy, thereby avoiding the variation in hormone levels that may actually exacerbate migraines.

TABLE 2.9

MEDROXYPROGESTERONE ACETATE (MPA) AND COMBINATION CONTINUOUS REGIMENS

Brand Name	Dosage
MPA regimens	
Provera	MPA 5–10 mg on days 1–12, or 2.5 mg daily
Cycrin	MPA 5–10 mg on days 1–12, or 2.5 mg daily
Amen	MPA 10 mg on days 1–12 (tablet is scored)
Combination continuous regimens	
Prempro (2.5 or 5.0)	MPA, 2.5 or 5.0 mg daily, and CEE[a] 0.625 mg daily (28-day pill pack), or new starting dose ultra-low-dose Premarin (CEE), 0.45 mg/1.5 mg of MPA or 0.3 mg/1.5 mg
Premphase	MPA, 5 mg/day for 14 days, with CEE, 0.625 mg daily (28-day pill pack)
Prometrium	Micronized progesterone, 200 mg for 14 days or 100 mg for 28 days in addition to ET, to be taken with food to improve absorption and in the evening due to sedative side effect
Femhrt	Norethindrone acetate, 1 mg with 5 μg EE daily (28-day pill pack)
Activella	Norethindrone acetate, 0.5 mg with 1 mg EE daily (28-day pill pack)
Prefest	Norgestimate, 0.09 mg with 1 mg estradiol daily (28-day pill pack); daily estrogen with *intermittent* norgestimate

[a]CEE, conjugated equine estrogens; EE, ethinyl estradiol; ET, estrogen therapy.

A rare side effect of HT is an idiosyncratic elevation of blood pressure in a small percentage of women. Also, women with hepatic disease or gallbladder disease may have worsening of the disease state on oral HT and may want to consider transdermal HT as an alternative (Climara Pro Patch or Novartis CombiPatch).

Alternative Options for Treatment of Menopausal Symptoms

Over-the-counter vaginal lubricants offer some temporary relief of symptoms of vaginal dryness but do not revive the atrophic vaginal mucosa. For the treatment of hot flashes, some of the selective serotonin reuptake inhibitors and the norepinephrine serotonin reuptake inhibitor venlafaxine have been shown to reduce hot flashes. Vitamin E, 400 IU per day, may also alleviate some vasomotor symptoms by reducing LH levels. In women with breast cancer, megestrol acetate (Megace) has also been used to treat vasomotor instability.

Alternative therapies such as black cohosh or red clover leaf have potential estrogenlike effects and may help in reducing vasomotor symptoms, but it is advisable to caution patients that these are not regulated substances in the United States; therefore, purity and strength can vary from product to product. Recently, soy products containing soy proteins and isoflavones (if ingested in amounts >25 mg/day) have been shown in studies to reduce total cholesterol levels. The resolution of vasomotor symptoms with soy has not been as consistent in studies. In a recent study, isoflavones in comparison with placebo were found to be no better in controlling vasomotor symptoms. In a recent placebo-controlled trial, dong quai was found to be no better than placebo in controlling hot flashes as well. In advising women regarding "natural remedies," it is important to stress that most herbal supplements have not been studied in large, controlled, prospective trials, and, therefore, the risk associated with these therapies remains questionable.

Diet and Exercise During Menopause

It is important to counsel patients that aging and menopause are risks for weight gain. During the menopausal transition period, women can gain on average 2 to 5 lbs or more. Also, a hormonally driven shift in fat distribution occurs, making central obesity more prevalent. A diet rich in fruits, vegetables, whole grains, nuts, and low-fat dairy products and low in saturated animal fats should be recommended. Trans fat ("partial hydrogenated oils") should be avoided, and essential fatty acids, such as omega-3 oils, should be consumed regularly.

Adequate calcium and vitamin D intake is important for OP prevention in women, as well as possibly reducing the risk of colon cancer and decreasing premenstrual symp-

toms. Three major sources for calcium exist: foods, calcium-fortified foods, and supplements. Dietary foods are the preferred means of obtaining adequate calcium intake. Dairy products have a high calcium content, have high calcium bioavailability, and are affordable. However, 25% of the U.S. population exhibits some degree of lactase nonpersistence (lactose intolerance) and have poor dairy intake. Calcium supplements should be considered if lactose intolerance or dietary preferences limit dietary dairy intake. The National Institutes of Health recommend the following daily elemental calcium intakes in women:

- Premenopausal women ages 25 to 50 years: 1,000 to 1,200 mg/day in divided doses
- Postmenopausal women younger than 65 years using ET: 1,200 mg/day total in divided doses
- Postmenopausal women not using ET: 1,500 mg/day total in divided doses
- All women older than 65 years: 1,500 mg/day total in divided doses

The use of higher calcium intakes produces no currently recognized health benefits and may expose the individual to further side effects. Vitamin D is essential for the intestinal absorption of calcium. The National Osteoporosis Foundation recommends 800 to 1,000 IU/day of vitamin D for women at risk of deficiency because of poor sunlight exposure, advanced age, chronic illness, being homebound, and living in northern latitudes. Daily requirements can usually be met with a multivitamin supplement (usually containing 400 IU of vitamin D) and with brief sun exposure of the skin.

Aerobic exercise and weight training are also beneficial for postmenopausal women and have been shown to increase bone mineral density, reduce OP fracture risks, and reduce the overall risk for fatal and nonfatal myocardial events, as well as to reduce breast and colon cancer risks.

Treatment of the Menopausal Transition State

Some women may experience only vasomotor symptoms while they are still menstruating regularly. Very low-dose ET may be a treatment option in this population. In the menopausal transition state, the failing ovary responds inconsistently to elevated levels of stimulating gonadotropins with estrogen surges. The endometrium may subsequently become thickened owing to this unopposed estrogen. Periodic monitoring (endometrial biopsy) of the endometrium is imperative to assess for hyperplasia if an unopposed estrogen state is suspected. Some women during the perimenopausal period may produce adequate amounts of estrogen from the ovaries and adrenal glands but may have evidence of progesterone deficiency due to a lack of production from the corpus luteum. These women may exhibit symptoms of mood irritability and menstrual disturbances, usually with heavy bleeding being the most common manifestation. The use of oral micronized progesterone in the form of Prometrium or the use of synthetic progestins may regulate menstrual flow in these women.

Hormonal Contraceptives

In the perimenopausal woman who is a *nonsmoker* and in general good health, HCs can be continued up to ages 50 to 55 years. HCs control the irregular cycles associated with the menopausal transition state and can control vasomotor symptoms and provide contraceptive protection as well. Once the woman becomes menopausal, if symptomatic, HCs can be converted to progestin/estrogen therapy (e.g., Femhrt, which is 5 μg ethinyl E_2 and 1.0 mg norethindrone acetate). Progestin/estrogen menopausal therapy *does not* provide contraceptive protection.

HCs provide four to five times more estrogenic activity than is needed during the menopausal state. Low-dose HCs (30–35 μg of ethinyl E_2) do not increase the risk of breast cancer or diabetes and have little effect on carbohydrate metabolism. For women who experience nausea, bloating, and other estrogenic side effects, very low-dose HCs, such as 20 μg of ethinyl E_2 (Loestrin, Mircette, Levlite), are options. These preparations should preserve bone mass, alleviate dysmenorrhea, and reduce menstrual blood flow (alleviating iron-deficiency anemia). In women with a history of ovarian cysts, higher doses of estrogen-containing HCs are needed to suppress ovulation. HCs are also beneficial in the treatment of acne and hirsutism by reducing absolute free testosterone levels via ovarian steroidogenesis suppression and reduced adrenal androgen production.

Newer Hormone Contraceptives: Yasmin, NuvaRing

Yasmin is a monophasic, low-dose oral contraceptive pill that contains E_2 and drospirenone, a progestin analog of spironolactone. Drospirenone is the only progestin with both antimineralocorticoid and antiandrogenic properties. Yasmin's 99% efficacy is similar to most other HCs. Yasmin helps improve acne, seborrhea, and hirsutism, while providing good weight stability due to its antiandrogenic, diuretic properties. As a result, it is a good choice in those with severe premenstrual symptoms such as bloating. Each Yasmin pill contains 3 mg of drospirenone, the equivalent to 25 mg of spironolactone, a potassium-sparing diuretic. Therefore, the serum potassium level should be monitored during the first month of therapy. Yasmin should be used with caution in women taking medications that predispose to hyperkalemia, such as other potassium-sparing diuretics, angiotensin-converting enzyme inhibitors, aldosterone antagonists, and nonsteroidal anti-inflammatory medications. Yasmin is contraindicated in women with renal, hepatic, or adrenal insufficiency. It is also available in a lower-dose formulation called Yaz, which is FDA approved for the treatment of significant premenstrual symptoms.

NuvaRing is a contraceptive vaginal ring that releases 120 μg of E_2 daily. The vaginal ring is colorless, odorless, 2 inches in diameter, and easily inserted vaginally by most women. The ring is left in place for 3 weeks, with withdrawal bleed occurring during the fourth, ringfree week. Although not recommended if a cystocele, rectocele, or uterine prolapse is present, NuvaRing is an excellent, convenient choice for most women.

A study comparing NuvaRing to standard HCs containing 30 μg of E_2 showed that NuvaRing users had less frequency of irregular bleeding and better cycle control. However, NuvaRing may cause a higher incidence of vaginal discomfort and vaginitis. Also, the ring may be accidentally expelled from the vagina, and if the ring is left out for more than 3 hours, efficacy is significantly reduced. To maintain the highest contraceptive efficacy, NuvaRing should be rinsed with warm water and reinserted in the vagina.

The other potential noncontraceptive health benefits of HCs include the following:

- Protection against endometrial and ovarian cancer (because of the suppression of chronic ovulation)
- Reduction of the risk of colon cancer (by induction of favorable changes in bile synthesis and reduction of bile acid in the colon)
- Reduction in incidence and severity of dysmenorrhea and *mittelschmerz* (ovulatory midcycle pain)
- Resolution of menstrual irregularity related to hormonal fluxes
- Stabilization of bone mineral density (which is advantageous in the female athlete with amenorrhea)
- Decrease in iron-deficiency anemia (because of the decrease in the length and flow of the menses)
- Reduction in ovarian cyst formation (higher doses of estrogen HCs may be needed for the suppression of large cysts)
- Lower incidence of endometriosis
- Reduction in the risk for developing uterine fibroids
- Reduced risk of benign breast disease
- Decrease in the risk of ectopic pregnancy
- Decreased risk of salpingitis/pelvic inflammatory disease
- Reduced risk of rheumatoid arthritis
- Possible improvement in menstrual exacerbations of porphyria and asthma

Since the introduction of HCs over the past 40 years, the overall dose of estrogen has been decreased by 90% and the dose of progestin by 80%. Third-generation progestins such as desogestrel (Desogen, Ortho-Cept) and norgestimate (Ortho Cyclen, Ortho Tri-Cyclen) have been developed to decrease some of the androgenic side effects that were present in higher-dose progestin-containing HCs. Studies from Europe, however, have indicated that the risk of nonfatal thromboembolic events associated with third-generation HCs (containing desogestrel or gestodene) seems to be higher than for the second-generation HCs (which contain levonorgestrel or norethindrone). In a woman with an increased risk of thromboembolic disease or with risk factors such as obesity or varicosities, these third-generation HCs should be generally avoided as first choice.

Data from the Nurses Health Study indicate no increased risk exists for CAD, stroke, or other cardiovascular complications in healthy HC users. A risk for cardiovascular complications does exist in women older than 35 years who *continue to smoke* while on HCs. In a woman who is generally healthy, is a nonsmoker, is without hypertension, and has well-controlled cholesterol levels, HCs can be continued well beyond the age of 40 years.

HCs have a mild favorable effect on lipid profiles, including a 5% to 10% increase in HDL-C levels and a mild decrease of 5% in LDL-C levels. Factor V Leiden mutation testing is *not* recommended before starting HCs in a patient who has no family history of thromboembolic events or no personal history of thromboembolic disease.

The first-generation oral HCs contain 50 μg or more of ethinyl E_2 and are indicated only for use in women with recurrent ovarian cysts needing ovarian suppression or in women with a seizure disorder on anticonvulsant therapy who may metabolize contraceptives at a faster rate.

Medroxyprogesterone acetate suspension (Depo-Provera) is an injectable hormone contraceptive that acts primarily by preventing ovulation by inhibiting the secretion of gonadotropins. The chief advantage of Depo-Provera is the avoidance of estrogenic side effects and the reduction of menstrual bleeding. By the end of the first year of use, approximately 50% of users will develop amenorrhea. The contraceptive protection of Depo-Provera lasts for approximately 12 to 14 weeks. The ideal time to initiate Depo-Provera is within 5 days after the onset of menses, and it is given by intramuscular injection (150 mg) in the upper outer quadrant of the gluteal region. The efficacy of Depo-Provera is high, with failure rates between 0.0% to 0.7%. Depo-Provera may be more desirable over HCs in certain disease states and in terms of compliance to therapy. Disease states, such as hypertension exacerbated by synthetic estrogens, renal hepatic disease, vascular disease, thromboembolic disease, hemoglobinopathies, and seizure disorders, and the postpartum lactating state are examples of medical conditions that make the use of Depo-Provera more desirable over HCs.

Contraindications to Depo-Provera use include pregnancy, undiagnosed bleeding, history of suspected malignancy or known malignancy of the breast, active thrombophlebitis, active liver disease, or known hypersensitivity to medroxyprogesterone acetate. The most common side effect of Depo-Provera is spotting bleeding (which makes it a poor choice of birth control in women in whom further investigation of vaginal spotting would be deemed appro-

priate, such as older women). Other side effects include weight gain (approximately 2-kg weight gain in the first year), exacerbation of headaches or migraines, abdominal pain, dizziness, and fatigue. The FDA has placed a black box warning to watch for osteopenia/low bone mass in patients on long-term use of this medication due to the possible deleterious effects of ovarian suppression on bone strength and attaining peak bone mass.

Implanon is a progestin-only contraceptive implant that is effective against pregnancy for 3 years. It consists of a single plastic rod measuring 40 mm in length and 2 mm in diameter (about the size of a matchstick). The rod is inserted just under the skin on the inside of the upper arm, is very flexible, and is not likely to be visible. The hormone etonogestrel is released slowly from the device into the bloodstream over 3 years. This is the active metabolite of desogestrel, one of the third-generation progestins commonly used in HCs. In clinical trials involving more than 2,300 women, no pregnancies have been reported after approximately 73,000 monthly cycles.

Postcoital contraception can be offered to women in the form of steroidal and nonsteroidal estrogens alone or in combination with progestin. Success rates are up to 75% if given within the first 72 hours after sexual exposure. Of note is that the earlier the administration of the first dose of postcoital contraception, the lower the failure rate. One example of postcoital contraception is the Yuzpe regimen, which consists of norgestrel and 100 μg ethinyl E_2 (Ovral, 2 pills, or Lo/Ovral, 4 pills), followed by a repeat dose 12 hours later. Major side effects with postcoital contraception include nausea (25%–66%) and vomiting (5%–24%). Preven Kit (estrogen and progestin) and Plan B (progestin only) are approved by the FDA for emergency contraception. Plan B is associated with less nausea compared with the Preven and is often the agent of first choice. It has FDA approval for over-the-counter availability.

Intrauterine contraceptive devices (IUDs) are an option still for parous, monogamous women. The copper IUD provides effective contraception for 7 to 10 years. Mirena-IUS (levonorgestrel-IUS) may be a treatment option to reduce bleeding in women with menorrhagia and can be a cost-effective alternative to hysterectomy to reduce heavy vaginal bleeding. The levonorgestrel IUS (Mirena) is therapeutic for 5 to 7 years. Women older than 35 years (particularly if they smoke, thus making HCs unacceptable) are excellent candidates for IUDs, assuming they have no history of pelvic inflammatory disease, ectopic pregnancy, leukemia, sickle cell disease, or valvular heart disease. IUDs are not the first choice for a young nulliparous woman due to the potential for dysmenorrhea and the high risk of sexually transmitted diseases.

Sterilization remains one of the most popular forms of contraception in the United States, either by tubal ligation or vasectomy, which are both considered irreversible procedures. Other options include *barrier methods*, such as latex condoms for men (or polyurethane condoms if either partner has a latex allergy). Several new female barriers have been developed in Europe, in addition to the Femdom (the female condom), including the Oves cap, Femcaps, and Lea's Shield (diaphragms), which require concomitant spermicidal use, as well as the contraceptive sponge, which is back on the market. The above caps come with user kits to promote correct and consistent use. Only a few clinical trials exist using these methods of contraception, thus limiting the availability of contraceptive efficacy data.

CONCLUSION

The various hormonal phases in a woman's life are periods of potential positive change that provide the patient and the physician a unique opportunity to address specific health care issues and health maintenance activities. Each life cycle hormonal phase requires the clinician to understand the physiology of gonadal hormones, pharmacology of the hormonal agent prescribed, and the importance of lifestyle modifications to individualize a woman's health regimen. The current approach to menstrual disorders management, contraceptive management, and menopausal care provides the potential for improved quality of life for women. Menopausal risk assessment and treatment provide the potential for improved quality of life for women and may include HT for symptoms, bone-specific agents for bone protection, and statin use for women at increased cardiovascular risk, with periodic re-evaluation.

REVIEW EXERCISES

QUESTIONS

1. A 54-year-old woman presents to your office with the chief complaint of vaginal dryness. She became postmenopausal spontaneously at 52 years of age and has had occasional nondescriptive hot flashes since then. She reports having at least two urinary tract infections in the past year, has noted that sexual intercourse has become more painful over the past year, and has experienced some stress urinary incontinence. Otherwise, she is healthy, has no history of breast or endometrial cancer, and has a normal Pap smear and screening mammogram. She is not interested in systemic HT at this time. Your best recommendations are which of the following?
a) Vaginal over-the-counter moisturizers and lubricants during intercourse
b) Estring vaginal ring
c) OCP therapy
d) Assessment of bone status
e) a, b, and d

Answer and Discussion
The answer is e. The use of the Estring vaginal ring would be an option for local ET in a patient with vaginal atrophy and genitourinary symptoms. The estrogen ring provides local estrogen to the vaginal mucosa to help alleviate symptoms of vaginal dryness. The use of nonhormonal over-the-counter vaginal moisturizers and lubricants, including Silk-E or K-Y Jelly, may provide some relief during sexual intercourse. In a woman *not* on systemic HT, it is important to establish her bone mineral density status because this might affect her decision to initiate HT, or select alternative therapy with a bisphosphonate (Actonel or Fosamax) or SERM such as raloxifene (Evista).

2. A 55-year-old Hispanic female who became menopausal 3 years ago presents to your office for routine physical examination. She is currently on CEEs and medroxyprogesterone acetate (Prempro), 0.625 mg/2.5 mg daily, and denies any vasomotor symptoms, sleep disturbances, or change in libido. She does report some "vaginal spotting" twice over the past 3 months. You would recommend which of the following?
a) Bleeding calendar to mark her days of bleeding
b) Hysterectomy
c) Increasing the progestin portion to Prempro, 0.625 mg/5 mg by mouth every day
d) Endometrial biopsy and consider low-dose Prempro

Answer and Discussion
The answer is d. The presence of abnormal vaginal bleeding or spotting in any postmenopausal woman on continuous combined HT should alert the physician to the possibility of endometrial hyperplasia or endometrial cancer. Other causes of spotting include endometrial polyps and uterine fibroids. The next step for therapy would be an endometrial biopsy to further evaluate the endometrial lining for changes. If the endometrial biopsy is benign, consideration should be given to a different hormonal therapy such as E_2/norgestimate (Prefest), E_2/norethindrone acetate (Activella), or Femhrt (ethinylestradiol/NA), or low-dose Prempro (0.45/1.5 or 0.3/1.5) (which may offer this patient a better chance of amenorrhea).

3. A 53-year-old white woman with a history of total abdominal hysterectomy, bilateral salpingo-oophorectomy for fibroids, and seizure disorder presents to your office with the chief complaint of having "hot flashes." She has been on CEEs (Premarin), 0.625 mg, since her hysterectomy. She is also taking phenytoin and folic acid. She has an isolated elevation of her triglyceride levels to 250 mg/dL. You would recommend which of the following?
a) Adding progestin, 5 mg daily
b) Increasing her oral Premarin dose to 1.25 mg daily

c) Adding isoflavones to her diet and then stopping Premarin

d) Changing her ET to a transdermal patch therapy such as weekly Climara

Answer and Discussion

The answer is d. Because of her history of using phenytoin for seizure disorder, this patient probably metabolizes estrogen at a faster rate than normal. By changing her ET to a transdermal patch, consistent estrogen levels can be maintained, which should alleviate her symptoms. Adding isoflavones and other plant-based estrogens in addition to her ET may or may not also help her symptoms. Other causes for her hot flashes should also be excluded, including checking for thyroid-stimulating hormone and a fasting blood sugar level. The patient will also benefit from transdermal patch therapy instead of oral ET due to her elevated triglyceride level. Fasting lipid levels should be periodically monitored.

4. A 48-year-old African American woman with a history of total abdominal hysterectomy and bilateral salpingo-oophorectomy 4 years ago for benign reasons comes to your office complaining of low sexual interest and an inability to reach sexual climax. She is currently on esterified estrogen (Menest), 0.625 mg every day, and denies other symptoms. You check her total serum E_2 level, which is 50 pg/mL. She has a normal vaginal and pelvic examination. You recommend which of the following?

a) Sertraline (Zoloft), 25 mg by mouth every day and sex therapy

b) Vaginal lubrication

c) Changing to esterified estrogens, 0.625 mg, plus methyltestosterone, 1.25 mg (Estratest HS) by mouth every day

d) Increasing her dose of Premarin to 1.25 mg by mouth every day

Answer and Discussion

The answer is c. This patient's symptoms seem to correlate with a female androgen deficiency (FAD) syndrome requiring therapy. Because she is already on adequate estrogen replacement, the only method currently available for androgen therapy is oral Estratest HS (1.25 methyltestosterone and 0.625 mg of esterified estrogen). At present, no agent is FDA approved for FAD. She should have periodic monitoring of her triglycerides, cholesterol profile, and free and total testosterone level before and after therapy is initiated.

5. A 56-year-old white woman who has been postmenopausal for 6 years comes to you for a routine examination. She has intermittent symptoms of gastroesophageal reflux disease and has a past medical history of esophagitis. She also had a recent DXA scan of her spine and hip that showed a T score of −2.5 standard

deviations below young normal. She states her mother was diagnosed with breast cancer, and she is not interested in HT. She has no personal or family history of DVT. You recommend which of the following?

a) Medroxyprogesterone acetate (Depo-Provera) injections every 3 months

b) Raloxifene, 60 mg by mouth every day

c) Alendronate, 70 mg by mouth every week

d) Calcium supplementation to a total of 1,500 mg daily with vitamin D, 400 IU to 800 IU daily

e) Both b and d

Answer and Discussion

The answer is e. This patient has OP on DXA, which is of concern and must be treated. Although calcium supplementation at 1.5 g plus vitamin D, 800 IU/day, is necessary but not sufficient to treat OP, she needs additional treatment to prevent further bone loss. The best option for treatment in this patient is a SERM such as raloxifene. Raloxifene will not only prevent further bone loss but will also offer her breast cancer reduction as well as a decrease in total cholesterol without an increase in US CRP. Because of this patient's past medical history of esophagitis and gastroesophageal reflux disease, Fosamax or Actonel can still be an option for treatment, but the gastrointestinal symptoms would have to be followed closely. Injectable Forteo, a bone building agent, could be considered.

SUGGESTED READINGS

Anderson GL, Limacher M, Assaf AR, et al. Effects of conjugated equine estrogen in postmenopausal women with hysterectomy: the Women's Health Initiative randomized controlled trial. *JAMA* 2004;291:1701–1712.

Batur P, Elder J, Mayer M. Update on contraception: benefits and risks of the new formulations. *Cleve Clin J Med* 2003;70:681–688.

Estrogen and progestogen use in peri- and postmenopausal women: September 2003 position statement of the North American Menopause Society. *Menopause* 2003;10:497–506.

Hulley S, Grady D, Bush T, et al. Randomized trial of estrogen plus progestin for secondary prevention of coronary heart disease in postmenopausal women. Heart and Estrogen/progestin Replacement Study (HERS) research group. *JAMA* 1998;280:605–613.

Kubba A, Guillebaud J, Anderson RA, et al. Contraception. *Lancet* 2000;356:1913–1919.

National Osteoporosis Foundation Web site: http://www.nof.org.

North American Menopause Society Web site: http://www.menopause.org.

Ridker PM, Hennekens CH, Buring JE, et al. C-reactive protein and other markers of inflammation in the prediction of cardiovascular disease in women. *N Engl J Med* 2000;342:836–843.

Treatment of menopause-associated vasomotor symptoms: position statement of the North American Menopause Society. *Menopause* 2004;11(1):11–33.

Utian W, Shoupe D, Bachmann G, et al. Relief of vasomotor symptoms and vaginal atrophy with lower doses of conjugated equine estrogens and medroxyprogesterone acetate. *Fertil Steril* 2001;75:1065–1075.

Writing Group for the WHI Investigators. Risks and benefits of estrogen plus progestin in healthy postmenopausal women: principal results from the Women's Health Initiative randomized controlled trial. *JAMA* 2002;288:321–333.

Chapter 3

Medical Disease in Pregnancy

Priyanka Sharma

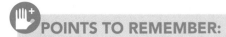

POINTS TO REMEMBER:

- Most medications used in pregnancy are category B or C.
- Pregnancy is associated with significant changes in cardiovascular physiology.
- The risk of thrombosis increases during pregnancy and postpartum.
- Glucose is difficult to control during pregnancy because the fetus is a constant energy sink, causing glucose values to dip when they otherwise would not.
- Pregnancy-induced hypertension is a multiorgan disease.

Chronic disease has an effect on pregnancy, and pregnancy has an effect on chronic disease. Table 3.1 describes basic maternal physiological changes during pregnancy. When considering the interactions of chronic medical disease and pregnancy, the general principles are as follows:

- The healthier the mother, the healthier the child.
- Although no drug is guaranteed to be absolutely safe in pregnancy, the risks of not treating a condition may outweigh the potential risks of treatment.
- The lowest effective dose should be used.
- Half of all pregnancies are unplanned.

PRECONCEPTION CARE

Primary care providers are in a unique position to practice preventive medicine for the not-yet-conceived patient (the fetus). Some women will consult with a provider before conception, but because up to half of all pregnancies are unplanned, and birth control methods are known to fail,

it is important to consider the following four points with all women of childbearing age, even those who "can't get pregnant":

- Recommend folic acid supplementation (0.4 mg/day) to prevent neural tube defects (NTDs). This amount is found in most multivitamins.
- Confirm immune status. A history of rubella vaccination is not predictive of rubella immunity. Planned pregnancy should be delayed 1 month after rubella vaccination. Check for varicella immunity; if no history of the disease is present, check blood titers. Vaccinations are available. Check for hepatitis B in susceptible patients because most vertical transmission (mother to fetus) occurs in chronic carriers.
- Consider family and genetic history, and offer consultation as needed.
- Consider medical history and the optimization of chronic disease—one-third of pregnancy complications are related to pre-existing conditions. "Tuning up" the treatment of chronic disease and a realistic risk assessment are helpful.

REVIEW OF U.S. FOOD AND DRUG ADMINISTRATION PREGNANCY CATEGORIES

Many medications are rated according to their potential risk to a developing fetus. These ratings are requested by the manufacturing companies themselves. For liability reasons, many manufacturers do not want their drugs used during pregnancy. To this end, some will provide no information concerning drug use during pregnancy, and some will stipulate contraindications not borne out in the literature (e.g., terbutaline, Pitocin). Other medications receive category B ratings even in their first year of general use. Because certain risk profiles may be acceptable to one patient

TABLE 3.1

BASIC MATERNAL PHYSIOLOGICAL CHANGES DURING PREGNANCY

Increased cardiac output
Decreased systemic vascular resistance
Increased intravascular volume and volume of distribution
Increased minute ventilation
Increased renal flow and excretion
Slowed gastrointestinal functioning
Hypercoagulability
Increased binding globulins affecting drug metabolism
Immune suppression

but not to another, the letter risk category designations of the U.S. Food and Drug Administration (FDA) do not tell the whole story, but rather give general guidance. See Table 3.2 for categories for drug use in pregnancy as suggested by the FDA.

Ninety-five percent of the 200 most-prescribed drugs appear to be safe for use during pregnancy. Currently, most medications used in pregnancy are category B or C. These categories may change soon to a descriptive system based on the strength of the evidence and the severity of the potential fetal effect.

Few drugs are rated category A because it is difficult to recruit pregnant patients for randomized, controlled, double-blind studies. A potential participant may be reluctant to forego a believed beneficial treatment or, conversely, may not be eager to expose her fetus to an unknown substance. Not all teratogens are category X. This applies only to those for which the indication for using the drug does not appear to outweigh the potential risk. Other known teratogens may be category C or D.

TABLE 3.2

CATEGORIES FOR DRUG USE IN PREGNANCY AS SUGGESTED BY THE U.S. FOOD AND DRUG ADMINISTRATION

Category	Description
A	Controlled human studies show no adverse effect.
B	Animal studies show no risk, and no anecdotal human evidence suggests otherwise; OR animal studies have shown risk, but human studies have not.
C	Animal studies have shown risk, and there are no human studies; OR no animal or human studies have been conducted.
D	Evidence exists for human fetal risk, but benefits may outweigh risk.
X	Evidence exists of human risk, and no benefit appears to outweigh it.

Most teratogens increase the relative rate of malformation from the background rate two- to threefold. Because the background rate of each particular malformation is usually less than 1%, the absolute incidence of any effect will be small, usually 2% to 3% at most. Even the most teratogenic substances known (e.g., thalidomide, isotretinoin) will affect only approximately 30% of exposed fetuses, leaving 70% unaffected. The factors involved are dose, timing of exposure, and cytogenetic makeup of the individual.

So, in the face of exposure to a teratogen, the mother must be counseled that it is more likely that her fetus will show no effect. It is nevertheless preferable to use the safest rated medications during pregnancy in all potentially fertile women.

Infection with measles or mumps during pregnancy causes fetal death or preterm birth rather than birth defects. Rubella increases the risk of miscarriage and causes congenital rubella syndrome. The risk with these infections appears to be highest in the first month of pregnancy. Vaccination with the measles, mumps, rubella vaccine, a live-attenuated vaccine, is recommended for non-pregnant females who do not have evidence of immunity to rubella. This vaccine is a category X drug and the Centers for Disease Control and Prevention advocates avoiding conception for 28 days after administration of this vaccine. However, this classification is based on scarce data, mostly retrospective. Bar-Oz et al. published a prospective study in the *American Journal of Medical Genetics* in 2004 in which they followed 94 women who received rubella vaccination 3 months pre- or postconception and a comparison group that were not exposed to known teratogens. No cases of congenital rubella syndrome were seen in the exposed group, and rates of major malformations, birth weights, and developmental milestones were similar in both groups. The Vaccine in Pregnancy Registry, which was active from 1971 to 1989, also did not report any evidence of congenital rubella syndrome in the offspring of 226 women who received the rubella vaccine and continued their pregnancy to term.

Vitamin A, even at doses of 800 to 10,000 IU/day, increases the risk of spontaneous abortions, and cardiac, renal, and facial anomalies in the child. Isotretinoin causes the isotretinoin syndrome; etretinate has been detected in maternal serum 7 years after the cessation of use, and conception is contraindicated for at least 3 years after discontinuation.

Ionizing radiation has an all-or-none effect in early gestation, causing miscarriage rather than birth defect, as well as fetal growth restriction and congenital malformations, particularly of the central nervous system during the period of organogenesis (approximately from week 3 to 10). There are no studies in humans on radiation risks, and most of the information is based on the data from survivors of the atomic bomb in Japan and the Chernobyl accident in the former Soviet Union. Most radiographic studies expose

TABLE 3.3

EXAMPLES OF CATEGORY X DRUGS AND THEIR POTENTIAL EFFECTS

Some Category X Drugs	Potential Effects
Live-attenuated vaccines for measles, mumps, rubella, and varicella	Congenital viral syndromes
Danazol	Ambiguous genitalia
Warfarin	Warfarin embryopathy: hypoplastic nose, epiphyseal stippling, optic atrophy, microcephaly, and growth restriction
Diethylstilbestrol	Vaginal adenosis and clear cell carcinoma in offspring
Vitamin A	Spontaneous abortions and fetal malformations
Isotretinoin	Isotretinoin syndrome
Triazolam	Cleft palate
Lovastatin	Bone malformation
Thalidomide	Limb-shortening defects
Ribavirin	Embryocidal
Lead, methyl mercury, polychlorinated biphenyls, polybrominated biphenyls, and organic solvents	Assorted mental, physical, and metabolic effects
Ionizing radiation	Miscarriage

TABLE 3.4

EXAMPLES OF CATEGORY D DRUGS WITH THEIR POTENTIAL EFFECTS

Some Category D Drugs	Potential Effects
Angiotensin-converting enzyme inhibitors	Unsafe after the first trimester; renal failure and death in neonate can occur
Anticholinergic drugs	Neonatal meconium ileus
Antithyroid drugs	Neonatal goiter and hypothyroidism, aplasia cutis (methimazole)
Carbamazepine	Neural tube defects (NTDs)
Lithium	Ebstein's anomaly
Nonsteroidal anti-inflammatory drugs	Constriction of the ductus arteriosus in third trimester
Phenytoin (Dilantin)	Fetal hydantoin syndrome
Psychoactive drugs	Fetal withdrawal syndrome
Tetracycline	Tooth discoloration, bone malformation
Valproic acid	NTDs

the mother to less than 1 rad, and the fetus to far less; 5 rads is considered acceptable fetal exposure. Patients who work near radiation should wear their detection badge near their pelvis to approximate the fetal exposure. When counseling a patient about the need for imaging, it is sometimes useful to remember that if the fetus was born, even prematurely, he or she would be radiographed as necessary for care.

Tables 3.3, 3.4, and 3.5 list a selection of drugs with their corresponding FDA pregnancy categories. Updated information may be found at www.motherisk.org, www.cdc.gov, or http://orpheus.ucsd.edu/ctis/.

MEDICAL DISEASES DURING PREGNANCY

A full review of all chronic disease and pregnancy is beyond the scope of this chapter. Common comorbidities and issues seen by the internist are reviewed in alphabetical order as follows. Additional diseases not mentioned in the text are included in Table 3.6.

Anemia

Anemia is a common finding in pregnancy due to a normal physiological response; on average, there is a 1,000-mL increase in plasma volume but only a 300-mL increase in red cell mass. Therefore, some dilutional decrease in hemoglobin and hematocrit is normal. Anemia in pregnancy is defined as a hematocrit level of less than 30% and a hemoglobin level of less than 10 g/dL. Besides dilutional factors, iron deficiency is the most common cause of anemia (90%). A trial of iron therapy is reasonable as a first step. Craving ice, starch, or dirt (pica) is a sign of iron deficiency. Folate deficiency is the second most common cause and is seen in multiple gestations; with drug therapy involving phenytoin, nitrofurantoin, pyrimethamine, or trimethoprim; or with large ethanol consumption. Thalassemias may present with microcytic, hypochromic anemia, and this has genetic implications for the offspring. Sickle cell disease may cause vaso-occlusive episodes (crises) that may lead to uteroplacental insufficiency, fetal growth restriction, and prematurity. Sickle trait carriers are at higher risk for urinary tract infections and should be screened regularly.

TABLE 3.5

SOME COMMONLY AVOIDED MEDICATIONS THAT HAVE BEEN SHOWN TO *NOT BE* TERATOGENIC

Bendectin (doxylamine and pyridoxine)
Diazepam (although some withdrawal syndrome occurs if used in third trimester)
Metronidazole
Oral contraceptives
Salicylates
Spermicides

TABLE 3.6

MEDICAL DISEASES DURING PREGNANCY

Disease	Considerations During Pregnancy
Headache	Pre-eclampsia must be ruled out. Acetaminophen and narcotics are first-line treatment choices. Ergot alkaloids are contraindicated, as are NSAIDs in the last trimester. Imitrex and propranolol can be used for refractory migraines (pregnancy category C).
Cerebrovascular accident	Occlusive disease is rare but increases fivefold during pregnancy, with the most common site being the middle cerebral artery. The potential benefit of making the diagnosis by imaging outweighs the minimal risk of fetal radiation exposure. Therapeutic heparin may be used if no evidence of intracranial bleeding is present. Subarachnoid hemorrhage, arteriovascular malformations (younger than 25 years), and berry aneurysms in the circle of Willis (older than 25 years) can also occur. Surgical repair is strongly recommended.
Epilepsy	Status epilepticus may be associated with a maternal mortality rate of 25% and a fetal mortality rate of 50%. Among the offspring of epileptics on medication, an increased risk (up to 10%) of congenital anomalies is present. Medication regimen should be changed to single-agent treatment (if possible), frequent dosing to avoid high peak concentrations, and increased doses of all medications based on monthly serum levels and clinical status. Seizure control is most important, regardless of how much and what medications are required. Carbamazepine (Tegretol) is the most widely used antiepileptic agent. Phenobarbital is next, despite a risk of cleft palate. Phenytoin is associated with fetal hydantoin syndrome: microcephaly, facial clefts and dysmorphism, limb defects, and distal phalangeal and nail hypoplasia. Valproic acid (Depakote) is associated with NTDs. Carbamazepine is also associated with NTDs, but to a lesser extent. Supplemental superdose folate (4 g/day) is added in early pregnancy and preconceptually to help neutralize the increased risk of NTDs. Maintenance folate during the rest of an epileptic's pregnancy is 1 g/day. Postpartum, the dose of antiepileptic medications should go back to the prepregnancy regimen. Breastfeeding is not contraindicated.
Depression	SSRIs and tricyclics are used in pregnancy. In severe cases, electroconvulsive therapy is considered safe. Postpartum exacerbation is common, affecting 10% of all mothers. SSRIs are safe for use during breastfeeding. For bipolar depression, valproic acid or lithium may be used, although both are associated with anomalies if used in the first trimester.
Rhinitis and upper respiratory infections	Sinusitis is reported to be six times more prevalent in pregnant women. Acetaminophen, guaifenesin with or without dextromethorphan, pseudoephedrine, diphenhydramine, loratadine, azithromycin, ampicillin-clavulanate, and ampicillin can be safely used. Oxymetazoline spray, pseudoephedrine, intranasal cromolyn, intranasal beclomethasone, oral tripelennamine, or chlorpheniramine may also be tried, in that order. A 3-week course is recommended because of difficulty with relapse and the increased chance of sepsis in treatment failure.
Substance abuse	Patients should be counseled against the use of smoking, alcohol, and other illicit drugs. Nicotine patches are preferable to smoking. Maternal methadone improves outcomes, but infants still withdraw.
Thrombocytopenia	In pregnancy, thrombocytopenia is defined as less than 100,000 platelets/μL. The various causes are similar to those in nonpregnant women, in addition to HELLP syndrome and DIC.
Von Willebrand's disease	It is diagnosed by measuring bleeding time at 36 weeks. Most patients do not bleed clinically despite abnormal tests. Desmopressin, von Willebrand's factor concentrate, or both may be needed to alleviate excess bleeding.
Carpal tunnel syndrome	Braces worn at night help, and symptoms usually resolve after delivery.
Tuberculosis	Inactive disease is often treated by oral isoniazid, 300 mg/day for 1 year. Active disease is treated with oral isoniazid, 5 mg/kg/day, plus rifampin, 10 mg/kg/day, plus pyridoxine.
Amniotic fluid embolism	It manifests as a sudden cardiovascular collapse, DIC, seizures, left ventricular dysfunction, and acute respiratory distress syndrome. It carries a 50% mortality rate. The best treatment is unknown, but it is usually supportive with inotropic medication and fresh-frozen plasma.
Pulmonary edema	It can be seen in association with tocolytic (terbutaline and magnesium sulfate) use. It is more likely in multiple gestations (twins, triplets). Careful diuresis and oxygen are used to treat edematous conditions.
Breast cancer	Chemotherapy can be given in the second and third trimesters, if necessary. Survivors (>5 years tumor free) need not be discouraged from conceiving if they are disease free for an additional 6 months or more.
Breast masses	These should be examined as usual, via unilateral shielded mammography or needle or open biopsy.
Hepatitis	Pregnancy does not affect the course of any type of hepatitis, except for occasional worsening of hepatitis E (up to 10% maternal mortality). Hepatitis A does not cross the placenta. Universal screening of mothers for hepatitis B is routine, and vertical transmission to the fetus at birth is the major risk. Infants receive hepatitis B immune globulin and vaccination if exposed.

(continued)

TABLE 3.6

MEDICAL DISEASES DURING PREGNANCY (*Continued*)

Disease	Considerations During Pregnancy
Intrahepatic cholestasis of pregnancy (pruritus gravidarum)	Bile acids are increased to 10 to 100 times normal, the alkaline phosphatase level is elevated, and the bilirubin level can be as high as 5 mg/mL, with a mild elevation of aminotransferases and cholestasis. The main symptom is intractable itching. Cholestasis of pregnancy is treated by delivery at term because an increase in fetal demise is reported if early induction is attempted. Diphenhydramine (Benadryl), hydroxyzine, calamine lotion, and cholestyramine are first-line therapy for symptomatic relief. Phenobarbital is used in severe cases. Pruritus gravidarum usually presents in late pregnancy, and recurrence in future pregnancies and with oral contraceptive use is likely.
HELLP syndrome	This is associated with pre-eclampsia and thus is usually found during the second half of pregnancy. Jaundice is mild, and aminotransferase levels are moderately elevated. HELLP syndrome is caused by a disruption in the vascular endothelium. Liver infarction and rupture can occur. DIC may follow. Delivery is the treatment of choice, even remote from term.
Acute fatty liver of pregnancy	It carries a mortality rate of 30%. It is usually seen during the last trimester in primigravidas. Symptoms include gastrointestinal dysfunction, epigastric pain, jaundice, confusion, coma, or coagulopathy. Bilirubin and transaminase levels are only moderately elevated, and biopsy shows small-droplet steatosis. A high index of suspicion and timely delivery decrease mortality.
Cholelithiasis	Symptomatic stones are treated with nasogastric suction, intravenous hydration, pain medication, and antibiotics as needed. Failure of these methods or the development of pancreatitis is an indication for cholecystectomy. Laparoscopic surgery is preferred in any trimester. All surgeries are safest in the second trimester.
Chronic renal disease	Pregnancy often has no adverse effect on those chronic renal disease patients with preconception creatinine levels of <1.4 mg/dL. Proteinuria occurs in half of all pregnancies and, in the absence of hypertension, is not a cause for concern. Patients with preconception serum creatinine levels of 1.5 to 2.5 mg/dL may have some worsening of renal function during and after the pregnancy. Poor fetal outcome is increased when creatinine levels are >2.5.
Renal transplantation	The prognosis for pregnancy after renal transplantation is fairly good if 2 years have passed since transplantation and no sign of impairment or rejection is present. Growth restriction, prematurity, and pre-eclampsia are more common in this group, but outcomes are generally good for mother and baby.
Urinary tract infections	Twenty-five percent of patients with asymptomatic bacteriuria will progress to symptomatic urinary tract infections or pyelonephritis if left untreated. Pyelonephritis is the most common medical complication of pregnancy requiring hospitalization. Twenty percent of pyelonephritis patients will have premature contractions; 10% will have positive blood cultures. Treatment of asymptomatic bacteriuria or urinary tract infection requires 3 days of antibiotics (oral ampicillin, 500 mg four times daily; oral amoxicillin, 500 mg three times daily; oral cephalexin, 500 mg four times daily; oral nitrofurantoin, 100 mg twice daily; and oral sulfisoxazole, 1 g four times daily). Sulfas and nitrofurantoin are avoided in the last month because they may theoretically displace bilirubin from the carrier proteins or cause hemolysis in a glucose-6-phosphate dehydrogenase–deficient neonate, respectively. The treatment for pyelonephritis is intravenous ampicillin and gentamicin, with prolonged oral therapy after resolution of pain. Gentamicin has been shown to be nephrotoxic in the neonate but not in the fetus. If intravenous therapy with appropriate antibiotics does not resolve pyelonephritis in 72 hours, obstruction needs to be ruled out using ultrasonography or a "single-shot" intravenous pyelogram.
Bacterial vaginosis	Bacterial vaginosis is associated with an increased incidence of preterm delivery, preterm rupture of membranes, amnionitis, postpartum endometritis, pelvic inflammatory disease, posthysterectomy cellulitis, and postabortal infection. No change in treatment is needed because of pregnancy. Typical treatments include oral metronidazole (Flagyl), 500 mg twice daily for 7 days; metronidazole vaginal gel 0.75%, one applicator daily for 5 days; or clindamycin cream 2%, one applicator daily for 5 days.
Group B β-hemolytic streptococcus	Group B β-hemolytic streptococcus colonizes 20% to 30% of women. The reservoir is the gastrointestinal tract, so the rectum is cultured in addition to the vagina. Approximately 0.1% of infants contract B streptococcus meningitis or sepsis. Currently, patients with risk factors are treated using intrapartum penicillin to decrease the colonization of the infant and subsequent infection. The risk factors for neonatal disease are prematurity, rupture of membranes for longer than 18 hours, maternal fever, previously affected infant, and B streptococcus urinary tract infection at any time during the pregnancy, which is believed to represent heavy colonization in the mother. Some practitioners culture all patients and treat the carriers during labor, even in the absence of risk factors. No regimen is 100% protective.
Chlamydia	Chlamydia in pregnancy is treated with 1 g of azithromycin or a 10-day course of erythromycin. Ampicillin may also be effective in a prolonged course. Tetracycline and doxycycline are not used because of tooth discoloration in the fetus.

(continued)

TABLE 3.6

MEDICAL DISEASES DURING PREGNANCY *(Continued)*

Disease	Considerations During Pregnancy
Cytomegalovirus	Ten percent of primary or recurrent infections in fetuses have anomalies such as hepatosplenomegaly, growth restriction, microcephaly, and intracranial calcifications that are worse with primary infections. No adequate screening method exists, and no treatment is available. Even asymptomatic infants can develop hearing loss, chorioretinitis, and neurologic or dental defects.
Gonorrhea	Screening for gonorrhea is routinely performed in pregnancy. Ceftriaxone or azithromycin are best practice for treatment and quinolones are avoided. Neonatal ophthalmia can be prevented at birth with the application opthalmalic erythromycin ointment. Presumed coincident chlamydia is always treated with azithromycin, erythromycin, ampicillin, or clindamycin. Tetracycline derivatives are avoided if possible.
Herpes simplex virus	Primary infection poses the greatest risk to the fetus because the IgG that forms with recurrent infection crosses the placenta and has a fetoprotective effect. Cesarean delivery is indicated if visible vulvar/vaginal lesions are present at labor. Cultures are not useful to predict shedding. Famciclovir and valacyclovir are pregnancy category B drugs and are used if clearly needed for symptomatic relief. These medications do not exert a definite effect on neonatal disease or on asymptomatic shedding.
Malaria	Mefloquine is an FDA pregnancy category C drug and should be used with caution. Chloroquine may be used, but it is not FDA rated.
Lyme disease	Early localized disease is treated with amoxicillin, 500 mg three times daily for 21 days. With asymptomatic seropositivity, no treatment is necessary.
Rubella (German or 3-day measles)	Fifteen percent of reproductive age women may lack immunity. A history of vaccination or infection is unreliable, so serum status is routinely checked during each pregnancy. Infection in the first trimester may lead to mental retardation, deafness, cataracts, and heart defects. The earlier the exposure, the worse outcome for the fetus. Immunoglobin M may be used to make the diagnosis, but immunoglobulin does not have a protective effect. Conception should be avoided for 3 months after infection or vaccination with the live virus on theoretical grounds.
Syphilis	Screening for syphilis is routinely performed once or twice during each pregnancy. Syphilis is caused by *Treponema pallidum*, which crosses the placenta. Abortion, stillbirth, and neonatal death are common. The classic stigmata of neonatal syphilitic syndrome are maculopapular rash, snuffles, mucous patches of the oral pharynx, hepatosplenomegaly, jaundice, lymphadenopathy, and chorioretinitis. Mulberry molars, Hutchinson's teeth, saddle nose, and saber shins may develop later. The diagnosis is made through blood screening tests. Because penicillin is the only effective antibiotic that crosses the placenta, treatment must use benzathine penicillin. In patients with penicillin allergies, desensitization may be needed before initiating treatment.
Toxoplasmosis	Toxoplasmosis develops as a result of exposure to undercooked meat from an infected animal or the infected feces of outdoor cats. Presently, in the United States, serial titers are not routinely determined in pregnant women. Infection is usually asymptomatic in the mother, but potential fetal effects are more severe the earlier in pregnancy the infection occurs. Maternal-fetal transmission rates, however, are increased later in pregnancy. Fetal effects include mental retardation, chorioretinitis, blindness, epilepsy, intracranial calcifications, and hydrocephalus. Treatment uses sulfadiazine and pyrimethamine.
Varicella	Varicella exposure during pregnancy rarely results in adverse neonatal outcomes, although a neonatal varicella syndrome that includes microcephaly and skin cicatrices has been described. Varicella pneumonia is more common in pregnant patients and is often fatal; acyclovir is used in this context. Presumed exposures are treated with varicella-zoster immune globulin if the patient is not immune. A history of disease is predictive of immunity. Half of those without a positive history are also immune. Conception should be delayed for 3 months after live-attenuated vaccination. No cases of neonatal syndrome from a fetus exposed to vaccine have been reported.
Abdominal surgery	Appendicitis is the most common surgical emergency during pregnancy. The maternal mortality rate in the first and second trimesters is 2%; mortality rises to almost 10% in the third trimester (compared with 0.25% for nonpregnant individuals). It is essential to thoroughly evaluate all pregnant women presenting with unusual abdominal pain for any potentially life-threatening conditions. Fetal risk from radiographic or invasive studies is low.
Abdominal trauma	The possibility of abruptio placentae must be kept in mind in all cases of direct abdominal trauma or sudden deceleration events (as occurs in automobile accidents). Serial hematocrits and coagulation studies will aid in the diagnosis, as will fetal hemoglobin titers (Kleihauer-Betke test) and ultrasonography. A normal ultrasonographic result, however, does not rule out abruption. In cases of penetrating trauma, surgical exploration is usually warranted.

(continued)

TABLE 3.6
MEDICAL DISEASES DURING PREGNANCY (*Continued*)

Disease	Considerations During Pregnancy
Inflammatory bowel disease	Ulcerative colitis is not exacerbated by pregnancy, but patients with ulcerative colitis have higher rates of miscarriage and preterm labor. Sulfasalazine, diphenoxylate, and steroids can be used safely during pregnancy. Regional enteritis is unaffected by pregnancy.
Pregnancy after gastro-intestinal bypass	Normal metabolism is found in most pregnant women who have undergone gastrointestinal bypass surgery. Screening for diabetes should be performed during pregnancy, and water-soluble emulsions of fat-soluble vitamins should be prescribed.
Spinal cord injury	Spinal cord–injured patients can complete a successful pregnancy, although in patients with lesions higher than T-10, self-palpation is needed to detect labor, and forceps delivery is required at the end of the birthing process because patients cannot push. If the lesion is above T-6, autonomic hyperreflexia can be life threatening during labor. Ironically, epidural anesthesia can help prevent this, even though it is not needed for pain management.
Multiple sclerosis	The severity of multiple sclerosis is often reduced during pregnancy, although postpartum relapses are common. No increase in fetal anomalies is reported. An increased incidence (up to a 5% lifetime risk vs. 0.1% in the general population) of multiple sclerosis in offspring is noted.
Myasthenia gravis	Pregnancy has no significant effect on the course of the disease. Labor and delivery are critical because of the increased work requirement and risk of anesthesia. Oral anticholinesterase drugs produce no fetal effects. A pyridostigmine parenteral preparation may be ordered during labor. Edrophonium also may be used safely during labor and delivery. Patients with myasthenia gravis are sensitive to narcotics; thus, their use must be carefully monitored. Magnesium should not be used. Neonatal myasthenia gravis occurs in 10% of neonates and is often transient.
Autoimmune-associated thrombosis	Lupus anticoagulant and anticardiolipin antibodies are collectively known as *antiphospholipid antibodies* and may be found in up to 50% of SLE patients and 4% of normal pregnant patients. Low-titer anticardiolipin antibodies in asymptomatic women are not worrisome because not all patients with antibodies have antiphospholipid antibody syndrome. Treatment is controversial, with minidose aspirin, heparin, or steroids used, depending on the seriousness of the history of thrombosis.
SLE	SLE is exacerbated in approximately half of all pregnancies. It is difficult to tell a lupus flare from pre-eclampsia (hypertension, proteinuria, thrombocytopenia, and edema). The flare, but not pre-eclampsia, will respond to steroids. The course of SLE in pregnancy usually mimics recent activity. The best time for pregnancy is when there are no recent flares, the disease is controlled on <10 mg/day of prednisone, and no renal compromise is present. Active SLE increases the risk to the fetus, with a 50% miscarriage rate. Neonatal lupus syndrome is associated with anti-Ro (SSa) and anti-La (SSb). Neonatal heart block, dermatitis, hemolytic anemia, thrombocytopenia, and hepatitis can be seen in severe cases. These resolve when the mother's IgG antibodies are cleared from the infant's circulation, usually within 3 to 6 months postpartum. The exception to this clearance time occurs with the heart block, which is often fatal, but otherwise requires a pacemaker. Common SLE medications used in pregnancy include aspirin, prednisone, azathioprine, and NSAIDs (first trimester only). Contraindicated medications include hydroxychloroquine sulfate, cyclophosphamide, warfarin, gold, and penicillamine.
Rheumatoid arthritis	Most arthritic conditions improve during pregnancy but flare during postpartum. Methotrexate is a known teratogen and must be avoided; NSAIDs in the third trimester can close the ductus arteriosus so should be used with extreme caution. Aspirin and steroids may be safely used throughout pregnancy.
Scleroderma	In patients with scleroderma, perinatal loss is increased, especially if the disease presents with renal involvement. Esophageal dysfunction is worsened during pregnancy.

DIC, disseminated intravascular coagulation; HELLP, **H**emolytic anemia, **E**levated **L**iver enzymes, **L**ow **P**latelets; NSAID, nonsteroidal anti-inflammatory drug; NTD, neural tube defect; SLE, systemic lupus erythematous; SSRI, selective serotonin uptake inhibitor.

Pregnant and postpartum women can tolerate much lower hemoglobin levels than others. No mortality or cardiac failure has been reported in patients with hemoglobin of >4.5 mg/dL as their only complicating factor. If transfusion is necessary for any pregnant patient, cytomegalovirus-negative blood is preferred to decrease the chance of devastating fetal infection. This precaution is not necessary postpartum.

Asthma

Asthma is seen in 1% of pregnant patients, of whom 15% have a severe attack. The course is unpredictable. One-third get better, one-third get worse, and one-third stay the same. Most pregnancies proceed uneventfully, but an increased risk of prematurity and growth restriction is present among asthmatics.

The general principles of management in asthma patients include continuing prepregnancy treatment and minimizing triggers. The routine use of a flow meter can detect onset before an attack becomes severe. Most asthma medications are safely used in pregnancy, including antibiotics and steroids, because minimizing the known risks of maternal hypoxia is preferred to minimizing the theoretical risk to the fetus from the medications. Inhaled medications minimize fetal exposure. Systemic theophylline levels must be reassessed every trimester and postpartum because binding globulins increase for two trimesters, and then clearance decreases. Allergy shots may be continued in pregnancy but are rarely initiated. Terbutaline is preferred to epinephrine, which may constrict uterine blood flow.

During a severe attack, fetal monitoring may be indicated. Oxygen pressure of less than 60 mm Hg correlates with fetal compromise. An aggressive attention to the patient's acid–base status, including early intubation, will optimize fetal health. Carbon dioxide pressure (P_{CO_2}) of >38 mm Hg or a pH level of <7.35 is highly abnormal for pregnancy and may represent retention and need for intubation.

Cardiac Diseases

Pregnancy is associated with significant changes in cardiovascular physiology (Tables 3.1 and 3.7), thus leading

---

TABLE 3.7

CARDIOVASCULAR "PEARLS" IN THE PREGNANT PATIENT

- Cardiac output increases 40% during pregnancy. Cardiac output peaks at 24 to 28 weeks' gestation, even during bed rest, and decreases somewhat during the last 10 weeks of pregnancy.
- Common signs of cardiovascular compromise, such as shortness of breath, palpitations, and tachycardia, are also found in normal pregnancies.
- Even in normal pregnancies, the chest radiograph shows cardiomegaly and venous congestion, and the ECG in normal pregnancy may include ST-T depression and flattening of T waves. Therefore, echocardiography is the preferred technique to evaluate cardiovascular disease in pregnancy.
- A 50% increase in intravascular volume and cardiac output occurs by the third trimester.
- Systemic vascular resistance decreases during pregnancy. This may worsen left-to-right shunts.
- Pregnancy is a hypercoagulable state, so dysfunctional valves and atrial fibrillation may need meticulous anticoagulation.
- Cardiac fluctuations occur during labor and delivery.
- Cardiac output increases by a further 50% during labor.
- Fluid shifts at delivery could go either way: blood loss or epidural-induced pooling can decrease effective volume, and redistribution from the contracted uterus or relief of caval obstruction may cause sudden increases in blood pooling. These fluid shifts affect both patients with preload-dependent cardiac output (pulmonary hypertension) and those with fixed cardiac output (stenosis).

TABLE 3.8

MATERNAL CARDIAC CONDITIONS ASSOCIATED WITH POOR AND GOOD OUTCOMES

Cardiac Conditions With Poor Outcomes	Cardiac Conditions With Good Outcomes
Eisenmenger's syndrome (pulmonary hypertension from shunting)	New York Heart Association functional classes I and II
Primary pulmonary hypertension	Mitral valve prolapse
Marfan's syndrome with aortic root dilation	Mild mitral and aortic disorders
Uncorrected tetralogy of Fallot	Septal defects
Dilated cardiomyopathy	Patent ductus arteriosus
Severe mitral or aortic stenosis	Repaired tetralogy of Fallot

---

to a potentially serious compromise of mother and fetus, depending on the nature of the maternal cardiac defect. Table 3.8 lists maternal cardiac conditions and their associated outcomes.

Endocarditis prophylaxis is of limited value for vaginal delivery or elective cesarean section because of the low risk of bacteremia in these situations. For low- or moderate-risk cardiac lesions, antibiotics are *not* recommended; they are considered optional for high-risk cardiac lesions. Nevertheless, most practitioners provide endocarditis prophylaxis because of possible intrapartum infection or the need for intrapartum cesarean section (Table 3.9). The standard antibiotic regimens for cardiac lesions are followed in the usual way in pregnancy.

A patient with a cesarean section after a long labor should be given prophylactic antibiotics. Aggressive antibiotics are used for gross infection. Patients with mitral valve prolapse without regurgitation are not given prophylactic antibiotics.

The offspring of patients with congenital heart disease are at increased risk over the general population for cardiac anomalies (up to 5%) but not necessarily the same ones present in their parents. If a sibling is also affected, then the risk increases to 10%. The fetus of a functionally impaired cardiac patient may exhibit growth restriction or premature delivery.

The careful management of preload and afterload is necessary for the severely affected patient. Most pregnancy-related cardiac deaths occur after delivery, probably exacerbated by the large fluid shifts that accompany delivery. Most cardioactive medications are safe for use during pregnancy with FDA categories B or C (e.g., digitalis, loop diuretics, thiazides, hydralazine, isosorbide, propranolol, metoprolol, nifedipine, verapamil).

Peripartum cardiomyopathy can occur in the last month of pregnancy or the first 6 months after delivery. It is treated similarly to other cardiomyopathies. Prognosis is related to

TABLE 3.9

ANTIBIOTIC USE IN PREGNANCY

Antibiotic	Comments on Use
Penicillins	All drugs in this class can be safely used during pregnancy.
Cephalosporins	All drugs in this class can be safely used during pregnancy.
Nitrofurantoin	Some question of fetal risk in the third trimester if glucose-6-phosphate dehydrogenase deficiency is present in fetus.
Erythromycin	Avoid estolate.
Clindamycin	Oral, intravenous, and topical forms can be used.
Metronidazole	Studies show no risk despite commonly held beliefs to the contrary.
Spectinomycin	Alternative gonorrhea treatment.
Azithromycin	Preferred agent because of long duration of action.
Gentamicin	No fetal effects despite causing neonatal renal failure.
Vancomycin	Only used if necessary.
Quinolones	Associated with cartilage problems in animals but no human evidence.
Trimethoprim-sulfamethoxazole	Not generally used in first trimester because trimethoprim is a folate antagonist; theoretical problems near delivery are suspected because the sulfa portion can displace bilirubin from binding proteins in the newborn and cause kernicterus.
Chloramphenicol	Contraindicated during pregnancy. Causes the "gray baby" syndrome.
Tetracycline and derivatives	Contraindicated during pregnancy. Causes tooth discoloration from second and third trimester use.
Kanamycin, streptomycin	Contraindicated during pregnancy. Causes eighth nerve deafness.

For current recommendations on antibiotic use, refer to www.cdc.gov.

cardiac size 6 months after delivery. Recurrence is likely, and death is a real possibility during the next pregnancy if the heart remains enlarged.

Maternal cardiac arrhythmias are treated as needed. Clinically significant arrhythmias are rare. Premature ventricular contractions and atrial contractions are common, as is paroxysmal supraventricular tachycardia. Wolff-Parkinson-White syndrome is managed with medication. Catheter ablation is not generally performed in pregnancy because of the fluoroscopy risk to the fetus. The most commonly used medications to treat Wolff-Parkinson-White syndrome are atenolol, quinidine, and procainamide. Larger doses than expected are often needed. Also used are the pregnancy category C drugs diltiazem, verapamil, disopyramide, flecainide, propafenone, sotalol, adenosine, and digoxin. Seldom used drugs include amiodarone, lidocaine, and mexiletine.

Rheumatic heart disease predisposes to congestive failure, pulmonary edema, subacute bacterial endocarditis, thromboembolic disease, and fetal loss. Symptomatic aortic or mitral valve stenosis can be treated with balloon commissurotomy or other procedures if necessary.

Women with mechanical valve prostheses need anticoagulation. Low-molecular weight heparin (LMWH) is preferred in the first trimester to avoid fetal anomalies (warfarin syndrome). A combination of LMWH and un-fractionated heparin is preferred in the third trimester because of easy reversibility. Warfarin is sometimes used in the middle trimester because unfractionated heparin can induce osteoporosis and thrombocytopenia in the mother. LMWH is used increasingly to avoid these side effects. Women with valvular bioprostheses do not need to be anticoagulated, but their chances of needing a replacement valve increase with each pregnancy.

Deep Vein Thrombosis

The risk of thrombosis increases during pregnancy and postpartum. Venous stasis, relaxed vasculature, occlusion by the gravid uterus, and hypercoagulability are contributing factors. Other factors, such as bed rest, pelvic surgery (cesarean section), obesity, increasing parity, and pre-existing coagulation disorders, can exacerbate the risk. Deep venous thrombosis (DVT) has an estimated incidence of up to 3%. The left leg is most often involved. Doppler testing of the symptomatic lower extremity is helpful, but because venography presents minimal risk to the fetus, it can be used to confirm the diagnosis of DVT if necessary. Treatment of DVT consists of LMWH anticoagulation. Coumadin is relatively contraindicated because of teratogenesis in the first trimester and risk of bleeding at delivery later in pregnancy.

Pulmonary embolism (PE) and DVT are more difficult to diagnose in pregnancy because many signs and symptoms of both are found in normal pregnancies. A false-positive Doppler result may be caused by the uterus interfering with venous return. An arterial oxygen pressure of <80 mm Hg may suggest PE. Diagnostic spiral CT and angiography present little radiation risk to the fetus. Ventilation-perfusion scans may also be used. Most of the radiation exposure to the fetus in this test is from collection of radiographic contrast agents in the bladder; therefore, hydration and a Foley catheter for drainage further decrease fetal exposure. Prompt anticoagulation reduces the mortality from PE. If PE is suspected, it is wise to begin heparin in the patient even before diagnostic tests are done. LMWH is the best choice in pregnancy, but a switch to regular heparin should occur before delivery for easy reversibility. Vena cava ligation or placement of a filter is acceptable during pregnancy if needed.

Sixty percent of women with venous thromboembolism in pregnancy also have activated protein C resistance. Others may have anticardiolipin antibody, lupus anticoagulant, or protein C, S, or antithrombin III deficiency. A diagnosis of protein S deficiency should not be made near term or postpartum because levels are normally low at that time.

Diabetes Mellitus

Both pre-existing and gestational onset diabetes affect 2% of pregnancies. Gestational diabetes mellitus is diagnosed during pregnancy and typically resolves after delivery. The proper preconception care of diabetics, types I and II, presents a unique opportunity for the internist to prevent birth defects. The incidence of malformations and miscarriages correlates with the quality of blood glucose level control. Even in well-controlled diabetes, a threefold increase in congenital anomalies is possible over the usual 2% baseline risk. Defects of the heart and neural tube are most common. The mermaid syndrome, or caudal regression (sacral agenesis), is seen only in diabetics.

Glucose is difficult to control during pregnancy because the fetus is a constant energy sink, causing glucose values to dip when they otherwise would not. Conversely, placental hormones, such as human placental lactogen, act as an anti-insulin agent and cause relative hyperglycemia. This effect intensifies as the pregnancy progresses and the placenta grows larger. The altered eating habits of early and late gestation further complicate the picture.

Incredibly tight control is desired of all diabetics (a fasting serum glucose level of <100 mg/dL and a 2-hour postprandial level of <120 mg/dL). Blood glucose is typically measured four times a day until a stable pattern emerges. Insulin is administered in two or three divided doses. Hemoglobin A1c is periodically measured for assessment of long-term control. Oral hypoglycemics are currently not used for fear of fetal effects, but this practice is currently under reconsideration. Glucose and oral hypoglycemic medication do cross the placenta; insulin does not.

Measurement of urine glucose has no value in the management of the pregnant diabetic because urine glucose does not correlate with serum levels during pregnancy. Glucosuria is common in any pregnancy and more so in patients with diabetes mellitus. Increased renal flow increases the diffusion of glucose into the urine beyond the capability of tubular reabsorption, thus resulting in the normal glucosuria of pregnancy of approximately 300 mg/day.

The pregnant woman with diabetes is at higher risk for pregnancy-induced hypertension, proliferative retinopathy, urinary tract infection, postpartum hemorrhage, and cesarean delivery. Diabetic ketoacidosis occurs more often as well. Retinopathy progresses in 15% of diabetic pregnant women, so an ophthalmologic examination is needed every 3 months.

The neonatal consequences seen with increased frequency in gestational and pre-existing diabetes include macrosomia, respiratory distress syndrome, polyhydramnios, hypoglycemia, hypocalcemia, hyperbilirubinemia, and shoulder dystocia with resultant Erb's palsy. Neonatal death and intrauterine growth restriction are seen in brittle diabetics or those with pre-existing end-organ compromise.

Gestational diabetes mellitus is diagnosed during pregnancy. Universal screening is done with a 50-g, 1-hour screening Glucola test during the second trimester. If the results of the 1-hour screen are abnormal, a diagnostic 3-hour test is indicated. The diagnosis is made with at least two abnormal values on a 100-g, 3-hour Glucola test. Earlier screening is recommended for higher-risk patients (obese, hypertensive, carrying multiple fetuses, glucosuria, history of a large baby, history of unexplained fetal death, strong family history of diabetes mellitus, or multiple miscarriages). The screen is repeated in the third trimester if the first result is negative. Fifteen percent of all gravidas will have an abnormal screen result, 15% of these will be diagnosed with gestational diabetes mellitus, and most of these patients will have diet-controlled diabetes.

Postpartum, the gestational diabetic rarely needs insulin; types I and II diabetics also experience a brief "honeymoon" period postpartum whereby less insulin needs are seen.

Glucose screening is advised 4 months after delivery and periodically thereafter (usually every 1 or 2 years) for any woman who had gestational diabetes because of an increased rate of regular diabetes later in life in these patients, particularly in women of Hispanic and Native American origin.

Oral hypoglycemic agents are now under investigation for use in pregnancy, and their continued use seems likely at this writing. Metformin is often used for women diagnosed prepregnancy as having metabolic syndrome or polycystic ovarian syndrome. Some studies have found metformin to help with weight loss, regulation of menstruation, and delaying the onset of type 2 diabetes. If a patient conceives while using metformin, current practice continues the metformin throughout the pregnancy. Metformin use confers a decreased chance of miscarriage and gestational diabetes.

The continuation of glyburide therapy during pregnancy for some diabetics, and the initiation of glyburide therapy for some gestational diabetics, is not yet the standard of care. Insulin therapy remains the safest approach.

HIV

The universal screening of all pregnant women for HIV is recommended. Reproductive age women represent an increasing percentage of the HIV-infected people in the United States. The majority of pediatric HIV infection occurs because of vertical transmission from mother to fetus. Up to 33% of infants born to untreated mothers are infected. With treatment, rates of transmission are decreased to less than 7%. Antiviral medication is given orally to the mother from 14 weeks' gestation to delivery, intravenously during labor, and orally to the infant for 6 weeks at least. If resources are tight, intrapartum zidovudine alone conveys most of the benefit. A triple-drug regimen is usually recommended, however, to reduce the development of resistance. Breastfeeding is discouraged when sterile formula is available.

The preferred route of delivery is an ongoing controversy; however, currently, planned cesarean section is favored to decrease the baby's exposure to maternal fluids.

Viral titers are correlated with transmission rates; thus, if the viral load is undetectable, perinatal transmission rates approach zero. Trimethoprim/sulfamethoxazole or aerosolized pentamidine are used for *Pneumocystis carinii* pneumonia (PCP) prophylaxis when indicated. HIV has no effect on the obstetric course when social factors are controlled. Pregnancy has no effect on the progression of HIV disease. If multiple drugs are used to control disease, they should be continued during the first trimester. If HIV is newly discovered, the start of medications should be delayed to the second trimester.

Hypertension

When hypertension occurs in pregnancy, four distinct syndromes may be in play: chronic hypertension, pre-eclampsia, pre-eclampsia superimposed on chronic hypertension, and gestational hypertension.

Chronic Hypertension

Chronic hypertension exists, by definition, before pregnancy or appears during the first 20 weeks of pregnancy. Consistent pressures of 140/90 mm Hg qualify as hypertension; medication use is not part of the definition. Chronic hypertension during pregnancy can be masked by the va-

sodilation that occurs in the first two trimesters. Methyldopa, hydralazine, and labetalol are antihypertensives with a long-term history of not adversely affecting fetal outcome. Nifedipine is a relative newcomer and has been used with good results.

Chronic hypertensives who are contemplating pregnancy are best started on medications that can be safely given during pregnancy. If a patient is stable on another medication, however, it is usual to wait until pregnancy actually occurs before changing medications. Diuretics should not be started during pregnancy because they may change fluid dynamics. They may be continued, however, if the patient has been stable while using them before pregnancy. Diuretics are most useful in left ventricular hypertrophy or salt-sensitive hypertension. They should be discontinued if fetal growth restriction or pre-eclampsia develops. Angiotensin-converting enzyme (ACE) inhibitors are contraindicated in pregnancy; these agents are associated with fetal growth restriction, neonatal renal failure, and death. Most of these effects are seen with ACE inhibitor exposure later in pregnancy; thus, it is prudent to change the medication on diagnosis of pregnancy. Atenolol has been associated with uteroplacental hemodynamic changes. If atenolol is used, fetal monitoring toward the end of term is recommended.

Poor maternal and fetal outcome is seen with diastolic pressures >110 mm Hg. Treatment of mild hypertension in pregnancy is not of proven benefit.

Pre-Eclampsia or Pregnancy-Induced Hypertension

Pregnancy-induced hypertension is a multiorgan disease that involves much more than elevated blood pressure. It is a disease of vascular endothelial cell damage (mechanism unknown) and volume contraction. Delivery of the placenta seems to remove the thus far unidentified precipitating agent, so delivery is the only "cure" for this condition. Maternal seizures are unpredictable but happen mostly within 24 hours before or after delivery. Magnesium is given intravenously as seizure prophylaxis. Neither phenobarbital nor phenytoin is as effective as magnesium in pre-eclamptic seizure control.

The subsets of pregnancy-induced hypertension are recognized, depending on end-organ effects:

- Pre-eclampsia (renal)
  - Proteinuria, edema, hypertension, decreased renal function
- Eclampsia (neurologic)
  - Convulsions
- HELLP syndrome (hepatic microvascular)
  - Hemolysis, Elevated Liver enzymes, Low Platelets, possible liver rupture

In the basic pathophysiology of pregnancy-induced hypertension, peripheral resistance is increased. Patients are volume constricted, not hypovolemic. Thus, they are not underfilled but rather constricted by the increased sensitivity of the arterioles to endogenous pressor substances, with a consequent increase in hematocrit in the early stages. Later, a decrease in hematocrit can occur from microangiopathic hemolytic anemia, a consequence of endothelial damage resulting from arteriolar spasm. Placental perfusion is decreased, as is perfusion of some end organs such as kidneys. Diuretics and antihypertensive agents do not improve uterine blood flow, but may decrease plasma volume even further and decrease uterine perfusion.

Mild pre-eclampsia is diagnosed by a sustained blood pressure of at least 140/90 mm Hg, 300 mg protein/24-hour urine, or nondependent edema. Some experts believe that an increase of 30 mm Hg systolic or 15 mm Hg diastolic over screening values represents significant hypertension, but this is currently a controversial point. The treatment of mild pre-eclampsia is to temporize with bed rest until fetal maturity or until the syndrome becomes severe. Delivery is the only "cure," and the syndrome resolves fairly promptly after delivery. Vaginal delivery is preferred, with cesarean section reserved for the usual obstetric indications. Intravenous magnesium is used during labor and 12 to 24 hours afterward to prevent seizures.

Severe pre-eclampsia is diagnosed with any of the following symptoms:

- Blood pressure greater than 160/110 mm Hg
- Nephrotic-range proteinuria (5 g protein/24 hours)
- Oliguria (<25 mL/hour)
- Eclampsia
- HELLP syndrome, disseminated intravascular coagulation
- Fetal distress

In these cases, prompt delivery is required, despite prematurity. Again, induction of labor is undertaken, hoping for a vaginal delivery. Magnesium is given intravenously during labor and for 24 hours after delivery to prevent seizures. Neither low-dose aspirin nor high-dose calcium has actually been proved to reduce the 30% risk of pre-eclampsia in subsequent pregnancies.

Pre-eclampsia superimposed on chronic hypertension carries the worst prognosis for both mother and child. Chronic hypertensives are at increased risk for pre-eclampsia. Proteinuria and increased serum uric acid are the first signs of pre-eclampsia in these patients, besides worsening hypertension.

Gestational hypertension that develops late in pregnancy with no signs of pre-eclampsia usually resolves after delivery.

Hyperthyroidism

The presence of increased binding proteins may confound the usual measurements of thyroid function, so determining the free thyroxine level is the best way to measure func-

tion. The level of thyroid-stimulating hormone remains the same during pregnancy.

Hyperthyroidism is found in 0.2% of pregnancies; 85% of these patients have Graves' disease. One must also consider acute and subacute thyroiditis, chronic lymphocytic (Hashimoto's disease) thyroiditis, toxic nodular goiter, hydatidiform mole, and choriocarcinoma.

Hyperthyroidism is treated with propylthiouracil in pregnancy, which has less placental transfer than methimazole. The patient need not be made completely euthyroid. Suppression adequate to allow satisfactory growth of the baby is sufficient. The neonate may be transiently hypothyroid after delivery. Propylthiouracil is not transferred to breast milk, but methimazole is transferred. Radioactive iodine is contraindicated in pregnancy.

The postpartum period is a time of relative increased risk for autoimmune thyroiditis. Two-thirds of cases are a reactivation of Graves' disease, in which the radioactive iodine uptake is normal or high, and one-third of cases are "silent" thyroiditis, in which radioactive iodine uptake is low. Spontaneous resolution usually occurs over months. Hypothyroidism follows in 25% of cases. Postpartum thyroiditis is histologically similar to Hashimoto's thyroiditis with lymphocytic infiltration. The rate is increased in patients who were previously type I diabetics (30%) or have had Hashimoto's thyroiditis previously (75%).

Thyroid storm can be precipitated by terbutaline (often used for preterm labor) if the hyperthyroidism is uncontrolled. Propranolol is used to counteract symptoms.

Hypothyroidism

Hypothyroidism is rarely diagnosed during pregnancy because it often disrupts fertility. Treated hypothyroidism is common, however, and there appears to be no adverse effects of medication use during pregnancy. In cases in which hypothyroidism is inadequately treated, one report finds a decrease in fetal intelligence may be possible. Free thyroxine or thyroid-stimulating hormone levels must be monitored every trimester as the binding protein concentration increases, and the dose of thyroxine may need to be adjusted.

Pneumonia

Pneumonia is uncommon but is a leading cause of nonobstetric death. The most common causes are *Streptococcus pneumoniae*, *Mycoplasma pneumoniae*, *Haemophilus influenzae*, fungi, varicella, and aspiration. Varicella can cause florid pneumonitis and death. Coccidioidomycosis can cause cavitary lesions and dissemination in pregnancy. Aspiration pneumonia is increased because of decreased esophageal sphincter tone and delayed gastric emptying.

LIFESTYLE ISSUES

For the pregnant or soon-to-become pregnant patient, here are the answers to a few common lifestyle questions ("Is it safe...?"):

- Hair dyeing—Yes
- Caffeine—Limit intake to 3 cups of coffee or tea per day
- Aspartame—Yes
- Exercise—Use perceived exertion as a guide and protect joints
- Scuba diving below 30 feet—No
- Sky diving or mountain climbing above 10,000 feet—No
- Physically hazardous job—If desired, the patient has a legal right to keep any job, although restricted duty is often appropriate. Time-honored restrictions are no lifting of more than 20 lb, no pushing of more than 50 lb, no standing for more than 4 hours without a break, and no exposure to known toxins, although these restrictions have not been proved to improve outcome in uncomplicated pregnancies.
- Flying—Flying in commercial airlines for less than 6 hours should be no problem at any gestational age, unless the cervix has started to dilate. Flights longer than 6 hours in duration have been associated with increased risk of DVT in nonpregnant individuals, and this would presumably further increase the risk in the pregnant patient.

REVIEW EXERCISES

QUESTIONS

1. A 32-year-old woman with no past medical problems is seen at her primary care physician's office. She is currently in her 12th week of gestation and was found to have HIV on routine screening. She is seeking further care for this. Which of the following is true?
a) The confirmatory Western blot test may be falsely positive in pregnancy.
b) Untreated, perinatal transmission approaches 60%.
c) Perinatal antiviral treatment will decrease the transmission rate to <7%.
d) PCP prophylaxis should be started.
e) Termination of the pregnancy will offer some protection against progression of her disease.

Answer and Discussion

The answer is c. Perinatal antiviral medication reduces transmission rates to near 7%. Up to 33% of infants born to untreated mothers are infected. Either trimethoprim/sulfamethoxazole or aerosolized pentamidine is used for PCP prophylaxis if indicated. Pregnancy does not affect the progression of disease.

2. A 28-year-old woman in her 20th week of gestation comes to the emergency department with shortness of breath. She has had asthma since childhood that was previously well controlled. She stopped all medications because of concerns for the fetus. On exam, she appears to be in severe respiratory distress with a respiratory rate of 28/minute. Her other vitals include a blood pressure of 102/56 mm Hg, pulse of 100/minute, and 97% saturation on room air. Her lung exam is significant for wheezing in all lung fields. The rest of the exam is unremarkable. You diagnose her as having an exacerbation of asthma. Appropriate therapy might include all *but*
a) Subcutaneous epinephrine
b) Inhaled metaproterenol
c) Oxygen by mask
d) Inhaled albuterol
e) Intravenous steroids

Answer and Discussion

The answer is a. Minimizing the known risks of maternal hypoxia to the fetus is preferred to minimizing the theoretical risks of medications. Therefore, encouraging compliance with medications is important. Almost all asthma medications are used safely during pregnancy. The exception is epinephrine, which can decrease uterine perfusion. A better choice is terbutaline, 0.25 mg subcutaneously, which is often used to treat preterm labor.

3. A 34-year-old female diabetic is in her 10th week of gestation. Her diabetes was previously well controlled, but she has had problems maintaining her blood sugar control with recent changes in diet. She is also concerned about her risk of hypoglycemia. Her exam is unremarkable. You advise her that all of the following have been associated with poor glycemic control in diabetic women who become pregnant, *except*
a) Increased first trimester miscarriages
b) Increased NTDs
c) Increased birth weight
d) Increased neonatal glucose levels
e) Increased neonatal respiratory distress syndrome

Answer and Discussion

The answer is e. Insulin does not cross the placenta, but glucose does. The fetus will make its own insulin to respond to high glucose levels. This leads to hypoglycemia after the umbilical cord is cut, as the glucose supply is interrupted. Both large-for-gestational-age and growth-restricted babies are born to diabetics, depending on the effect on the placenta, which is also an end organ like the kidneys and the eyes. Larger babies tend to have less mature lungs; the mechanism for this is unknown. Miscarriages and birth defects are more common in pre-existing diabetics, as opposed to gestational diabetics.

4. A 36-year-old woman with diabetes and hypertension has just found out that she is pregnant. Her blood pressure has been well controlled with enalapril 10 mg daily. She has come for her annual primary care visit and has not yet seen an obstetrician. Her blood pressure in your office is 136/78 mm Hg. Which of the following medications is contraindicated for the treatment of hypertension in pregnancy?

a) Propranolol
b) Methyldopa
c) Hydralazine
d) Enalapril
e) Labetalol

Answer and Discussion

The answer is d. Angiotensin-converting enzyme inhibitors are associated with fetal compromise and death when exposure occurs during the second and third trimesters. The other medications listed are commonly used.

5. A 26-year-old woman in her seventh month of pregnancy presents to the emergency department with increasing shortness of breath. She also complains of left leg swelling. She has no other medical problems and is not currently taking any prescription medications. On exam, she is in moderate respiratory distress. Her vital signs are respiratory rate of 28/minute, blood pressure of 108/64 mm Hg, pulse of 120/minute, and pulse oximetry shows 89% saturation on room air. Cardiac exam is significant for a regular, tachycardic rhythm; chest exam reveals no abnormalities; abdominal exam shows an enlarged uterus with palpable fetus; and extremities reveal left leg redness and swelling at the level of the calf. In addition to oxygen, what would be the most appropriate next step?

a) Doppler study of leg, then intravenous (IV) heparin if positive
b) Spiral CT, then weight-adjusted LMWH subcutaneously if indicated
c) V/Q scan, then IV heparin if positive
d) IV heparin while awaiting radiographic studies
e) Doppler leg study and vena cava filter to prevent PE if positive

Answer and Discussion

The answer is d. Early anticoagulation with heparin or LMWH decreases mortality. DVT and PE are increased during pregnancy. Heparin does not cross the placenta and is easily reversed, so immediate anticoagulation carries little risk. Once that is done, do not hesitate to make the definitive diagnosis. Fetal risk from radiation is minimal compared with the risk of untreated DVT or PE, or ongoing anticoagulation without a documented diagnosis. Ventilation-perfusion scanning, spiral CT, angiography, and venography are all worth the risk. Long-term full anticoagulation with heparin or LMWH is preferred to warfarin. A filter is indicated only if anticoagulation cannot be safely accomplished.

SUGGESTED READINGS

Coleman MT, Rund DA. Nonobstetric conditions causing hypoxia during pregnancy: asthma and epilepsy. *Am J Obstet Gynecol* 1997;177:1–7.

Coleman MT, Trianfo VA, Rund DA. Nonobstetric emergencies in pregnancy: trauma and surgical conditions. *Am J Obstet Gynecol* 1997;177:497–502.

Grubbs S, Brundage SC. Preconception management of chronic diseases. *J S C Med Assoc* 2002;98(6):270–276.

Kaaja RJ, Greer IA. Manifestations of chronic disease during pregnancy. *JAMA* 2005;294(21):2751–2757.

Koren G, Pastuszak A, Ito S. Drugs in pregnancy. *N Engl J Med* 1998;338:1128–1137.

Liccardi G, Cazzola M, Canonica GW, et al. General strategy for the management of bronchial asthma in pregnancy. *Respir Med* 2003;97(7):778–789.

Ramin SM, Vidaeff AC, Yeomans ER, et al. Chronic renal disease in pregnancy. *Obstet Gynecol* 2006;108(6):1531–1539.

Rayburn WF. Chronic medical disorders during pregnancy: guidelines for prescribing drugs. *J Reprod Med* 1997;42:1–24.

Roberts JM, Pearson G, Cutler J, et al. NHLBI Working Group on Research on Hypertension During Pregnancy. Summary of the NHLBI Working Group on Research on Hypertension During Pregnancy. *Hypertension* 2003;41(3):437–445.

Sibai BM. Chronic hypertension in pregnancy. *Obstet Gynecol* 2002;100(2):369–377.

Sookoian S. Effect of pregnancy on pre-existing liver disease: chronic viral hepatitis. *Ann Hepatol* 2006;5(3):190–197.

Wexler ID, Johannesson M, Edenborough FP, et al. Pregnancy and chronic progressive pulmonary disease. *Am J Respir Crit Care Med* 2002;175(4):300–305.

Chapter 4

Biostatistics in Clinical Medicine: Diagnostic Tests

Gerald J. Beck

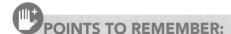

POINTS TO REMEMBER:

- The relationship between a dichotomous test result and the true diagnosis of disease can be summarized using a standard 2 × 2 table.

- The accuracy of the test is specific to a given cut-point value that distinguishes between a positive and negative test.

- A person's probability of having a disease is modified from the pretest probability to the posttest probability by incorporating information on the accuracy of the test.

- Positive and negative predictive values depend on the prevalence of the disease.

- The ratio of the sensitivity and the false-positive rate is called the *likelihood ratio*.

When determining the presence of a disease in a patient, physicians use the results of diagnostic tests (e.g., laboratory, radiologic, physical symptoms) to modify their pretest impression of the likelihood of the disease being present. Therefore, it is important that clinicians understand how diagnostic tests are used in reaching clinical decisions and how the accuracy of the diagnostic test can affect their conclusions. This chapter defines and illustrates the concepts of the sensitivity, specificity, and predictive value of a diagnostic test. A good general reference to the interpretation and use of diagnostic tests is given by Griner et al.

A diagnostic test is used as a decision-making tool in that the results of the test are used to predict whether a disease is present or absent. The relationship between a dichotomous test result (i.e., positive or negative) and the true diagnosis of disease can be summarized using a standard 2 × 2 ta-

ble with four cells (A–D, as in Table 4.1). This table shows that the test may provide the clinician with the correct answer (true positive [A] or true negative [D]) or may result in the wrong conclusion (false positive [B] or false negative [C]).

To quantify the accuracy of the test in making a correct decision, several diagnostic summary values can be calculated. To illustrate this, Table 4.2 gives some hypothetical data on the relationship of a screening test using prostate-specific antigen (PSA) in diagnosing prostate cancer. In this group of 400 men having both the PSA test and the definitive biopsy (gold standard test in this disease), 160 men were correctly identified as having prostate cancer, and 120 were correctly identified as not having prostate cancer. However, 120 men were misdiagnosed as either false positives ($n = 80$) or false negatives ($n = 40$). The accuracy of the PSA test can be summarized by (a) the proportion of truly diseased patients who test positive, called the *sensitivity of the test* (160 of 200, or 0.80, or 80% in the example), and (b) the proportion of truly nondiseased patients who test negative, called the *specificity of the test* (120 of 200, or 0.60, or 60% in the example). Similarly, the false-positive rate (1 − specificity) would be 80 of 200, or 40%, and the false-negative rate (1 − sensitivity) would be 40 of 200, or 20%.

The quantities of sensitivity and specificity can be determined for a diagnostic test, in general, when the result of the diagnostic test and the true disease status is known for a group of persons and tabulated, as shown in Table 4.1. Cells A, B, C, and D represent the frequencies of the various combinations of test and disease status. The sensitivity of the diagnostic test is $A/(A + C)$ and the specificity is $B/(B + D)$.

As in the PSA example, many diagnostic tests are based on a continuous measurement. The accuracy of the test is

TABLE 4.1

RELATIONSHIP BETWEEN A DICHOTOMOUS DIAGNOSTIC TEST RESULT AND THE OCCURRENCE OF DISEASE: THE 2 × 2 TABLE

Test Result	True Disease Status		
	Disease Present	Disease Absent	Total
Positive	True positive (A)	False positive (B)	A + B
Negative	False negative (C)	True negative (D)	C + D
Total	A + C	B + D	

TABLE 4.2

RELATIONSHIP BETWEEN PROSTATE-SPECIFIC ANTIGEN (PSA) TEST AND OCCURRENCE OF PROSTATE CANCER (HYPOTHETICAL DATA)

PSA Test	True Disease Status		
	Prostate Cancer	No Prostate Cancer	Total
Positive (≥4 μg/L)	160	80	240
Negative (<4 μg/L)	40	120	160
Total	200	200	400

then specific to a given cut-point value of the test that distinguishes between a positive and negative test. As shown in Figure 4.1, the choice of a cut-point will change the sensitivity, specificity, and false-positive and false-negative rates. The two curves in the figure represent the frequency distribution of the test value in the "disease absent" and "disease present" populations. Overlap usually occurs in these curves because no test perfectly discriminates between the "disease absent" and "disease present" groups. The different areas under the curves give the proportions of persons who are correctly or incorrectly classified in the "disease absent" and "disease present" groups. Therefore, moving the cut-point affects all the different areas. Moving the cut-point to the left (lower test value) increases the sensitivity but decreases the specificity (assuming a larger test value indicates the presence of disease). Hence, changing the cut-point cannot simultaneously increase both the sensitivity and the specificity or simultaneously decrease the false-positive and false-negative rates. The choice of an optimal cut-point is beyond the scope of this chapter, but it can be determined using receiver operating characteristic curves. The cut-point choice also depends on the purpose of the diagnostic test. For example, when screening donated blood for HIV, one should choose a cut-point that would reduce the false-negative rate as much as possible. If one uses the HIV blood test to identify infected individuals, however, one should reduce the false-positive rate as much as possible to avoid falsely alarming individuals about the presence of disease. Of course, in practice, repeating the test or using a second type of test to confirm the diagnosis is often done.

Of main interest to the physician (and patient) is the probability of having the disease given that the test was positive. This is easily seen in the PSA example in Table 4.2, in which out of the 240 men with a positive test, 160 actually have prostate cancer. That is, the test gave the correct diagnosis 0.667, or 66.7%, of the time (number of times the test was positive and the disease was present out of the total number of positive tests). This quantity is called the *positive predictive value* and is calculated by A/(A + B) using the general frequencies in Table 4.1. Similarly, the negative predictive value is the proportion of patients who have a negative test result and actually have no disease, out of the total number with a negative test result. In the example, this is 120 of 160 = 0.75, or 75%, or D/(C + D). In practice, the clinician only knows the result of the diagnostic test and is trying to determine the true disease status of the patient without having knowledge of the frequencies in Table 4.1.

The pretest probability of disease in a given individual is based on the physician's personal experience with patients who have characteristics similar to the patient being diagnosed and/or on the prevalence of disease in such patients, as reported in the published literature. The key point is that the person's probability of having a disease is modified from the pretest probability to the posttest probability (positive predictive value) by incorporating the information on the accuracy of the test. In the PSA example, the pretest probability of disease was .50 because 200 of the 400 men represented in Table 4.2 had prostate cancer, but this is not likely the case in practice.

Therefore, a general way of calculating the positive and negative predictive values is needed.

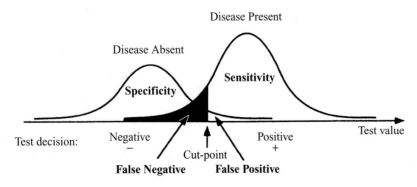

Figure 4.1 Diagnostic test terms when there is a continuous outcome for the test.

The positive and negative predictive values are calculated, in general, using the following two equations, which are derived from Bayes' theorem.

$$\text{Positive predictive value} = \frac{(\text{Prevalence})(\text{Sensitivity})}{(\text{Prevalence})(\text{Sensitivity}) + (1 - \text{Prevalence})(1 - \text{Specificity})}$$

$$\text{Negative predictive value} = \frac{(1 - \text{Prevalence})(\text{Specificity})}{(1 - \text{Prevalence})(\text{Specificity}) + (\text{Prevalence})(1 - \text{Sensitivity})}$$

In the PSA example, the sensitivity was 0.80, and the specificity was 0.60. So, if the prevalence is 0.5 (as assumed previously), the positive predictive value is $(0.5)(0.80)/[(0.5)(0.80) + (1 - 0.5)(1 - 0.60)]$, which equals 0.667, the same (160/240) as previously determined from Table 4.2. Likewise, the negative predictive value is $(1 - 0.5)(0.60)/[(1 - 0.5)(0.60) + (0.5)(1 - 0.80)]$, which equals 0.75, as before (120/160 in Table 4.2).

Suppose now that the prevalence (pretest probability) is 0.1 instead of 0.5. Applying the previous equations would give a positive predictive value of 0.182 and a negative predictive value of 0.964, quite a bit different from the previous values, in which the prevalence was 0.5. Table 4.3 shows these values and also gives the predictive values assuming other values of disease prevalence. This table dramatically shows that the positive and negative predictive values depend on the prevalence of the disease and that, as the prevalence increases, the positive predictive value increases while the negative predictive value decreases. This occurs even if the diagnostic test has very high sensitivity and specificity. Also, as can be seen from the previous equations, the positive predictive value can be increased by increasing the specificity of the test, and the negative predictive value can be increased by increasing the sensitivity of the test. It is important that the clinician understand these interrelationships when interpreting a diagnostic test or beginning a screening program. For example, if the general population, with low prevalence of HIV infection, is screened for HIV, the positive predictive value may be very low despite a very high sensitivity and specificity of the test. Also, this situation could lead to many more false-positive results than the number of true cases identified.

It is also important to understand how the diagnostic test result will modify the pretest probability (prevalence) values into the posttest probability. That is, a positive test will give a posttest probability (positive predictive value) larger than the pretest probability, whereas a negative test will give a posttest probability smaller (equal to 1 − the negative predictive probability) than the pretest probability. For example (as seen in Table 4.3), with a pretest probability of disease equal to 0.1, if the diagnostic test is positive, the posttest probability of disease is increased to .182, whereas, if the test is negative, the probability of disease is decreased to 1 − 0.964, or .036.

Without having to use the equations based on Bayes' theorem for determining the positive and negative predictive probabilities from the sensitivity, specificity, and prevalence of the disease (in the group setting of the individual being tested), one can use the simple nomogram of Fagan to go from the pretest to the posttest probability. This nomogram (Fig. 4.2) uses the ratio of the sensitivity and the false-positive rate (or 1 − specificity) as a way of incorporating both the sensitivity and specificity. This ratio is also called the *likelihood ratio*, and it is the ratio of obtaining a positive test result given the disease is present versus given

TABLE 4.3

INFLUENCE OF PREVALENCE OF DISEASE ON THE POSITIVE AND NEGATIVE PREDICTIVE PROBABILITIES (HYPOTHETICAL DATA, ASSUMING 80% SENSITIVITY AND 60% SPECIFICITY)

Prevalence	Positive Predictive Value	Negative Predictive Value
0.10	0.182	0.964
0.30	0.462	0.875
0.50	0.667	0.750
0.70	0.926	0.562
0.90	0.947	0.250

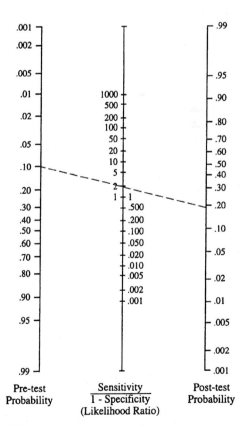

Figure 4.2 Fagan's nomogram to determine the posttest probability from the pretest probability, sensitivity, and specificity of a diagnostic test.

the disease is absent. As in the PSA example, if the sensitivity is 80% and the specificity is 60%, the likelihood ratio is $0.80/(1.0 - 0.60) = 2.0$. Then, if the pretest probability is .10, the posttest probability can be obtained using the nomogram in Figure 4.2 by drawing a straight line between the pretest value and the likelihood ratio and extending it to the posttest probability scale to reach a value. In this example, the posttest probability value read from Figure 4.2 is approximately .18 (very close to the exact value of .182 previously calculated). Selecting other pretest probabilities yields different posttest probabilities. Also, changing the sensitivity or specificity of the test gives different results. If the likelihood ratio is above (or below) 1, the posttest probability will be larger (or smaller) than the pretest probability.

In summary, diagnostic tests are commonplace in the practice of medicine. Understanding the interpretation of these tests is important and includes knowing the concepts of sensitivity, specificity, and positive and negative predictive value, the relationships among these, and the influence of the setting in which the test is applied—that is, the prevalence (or pretest probability) of the disease. Other biases can occur when using diagnostic tests; these have not been covered but should be considered to gain a better understanding of diagnostic testing. These biases include referral or verification bias, the use of an imperfect gold standard, the handling of uninterpretable results, and the influence of the case mix or spectrum of patients to which the test is being applied.

REVIEW EXERCISES

QUESTIONS

1. Assume that 20% of patients truly have disease X. Using a new test (X-ometry) to test 100 patients in your office for disease X, a total of 40 of these 100 patients are found to have positive X-ometry. The specificity of X-ometry is known to be 60%. What is the positive predictive value of positive X-ometry under these conditions?

a) 10%
b) 20%
c) 40%
d) 60%

Answer and Discussion
The answer is b. Tables 4.4, 4.5, and 4.6 use the partial information provided about a diagnostic test to complete the 2 × 2 table and then calculate the positive predictive value. The steps are as follows:

Step 1. The example specifies a population prevalence of disease X of 20%. Thus, of 100 patients who are tested, 20 are expected to have the condition disease X—that is, the frequencies A and C add to 20 (Table 4.4).

TABLE 4.4

DIAGNOSTIC VALUE OF X-OMETRY FOR DISEASE X: STEP 1

| X-ometry | Disease X | | |
	Present	Absent	Total
Positive			
Negative			
Total	20	80	100

Population prevalence = 20/100 (20%).

Step 2. The problem specifies that 40 of the 100 patients tested have a positive test, so A + B is 40, and the other marginal values of the table can be determined by subtracting the known values from 100, which is the total number of patients examined in this example (Table 4.5).

Step 3. The specificity of the test is designated to be 60%, so that 60% of the 80 patients without disease X in this example have a negative X-ometry test result. Frequency D is thus 60% of 80, or 48. The frequency in each of the other cells in this 2 × 2 table can then be specified (Table 4.6).

Step 4. Once the cells are all filled in, it is possible to calculate the value of the positive predictive value of X-ometry in this example by calculating cell A (= 8) divided by the sum of cells A + B (= 8 + 32, or 40). The correct answer for the positive predictive value is therefore 8 divided by 40, or 20%, in this example.

2. Suppose that a screening mammography test for breast cancer has both high sensitivity and specificity, say 95% and 90%, respectively. What are the positive and negative predictive values of the test when applied to women with a 1% prevalence of breast cancer?

Positive predictive value is
a) 0.514
b) 0.333
c) 0.154
d) 0.088

TABLE 4.5

DIAGNOSTIC VALUE OF X-OMETRY FOR DISEASE X: STEP 2

| X-ometry | Disease X | | |
	Present	Absent	Total
Positive			40
Negative			60
Total	20	80	100

Population prevalence = 20%.
Positive X-ometry in 40/100 (40%).

TABLE 4.6

DIAGNOSTIC VALUE OF X-OMETRY FOR DISEASE X: STEP 3

X-ometry	Disease X Present	Disease X Absent	Total
Positive	8	32	40
Negative	12	48	60
Total	20	80	100

Population prevalence = 20%.
Positive X-ometry = 40%.
Specificity X-ometry = 60%.

Negative predictive value is
a) 0.999
b) 0.994
c) 0.989
d) 0.950

Answer and Discussion

The answers are d and a. Apply Bayes' theorem to calculate the positive and negative predictive values given the specified values of sensitivity, specificity, and prevalence. The prevalence is 0.01, so the positive predictive value is $(0.01)(0.95)/[(0.01)(0.95) + (1 - 0.01)(1 - 0.90)]$, which equals $0.0095/(0.0095 + 0.099)$, or 0.088. Likewise, the negative predictive value is $(1 - 0.01)(0.90)/[(1 - 0.01)(0.90) + (0.01)(1 - 0.95)]$, which equals $0.891/(0.891 + 0.0005)$, or 0.999.

3. Using the same sensitivity and specificity as in question 2, what are the positive and negative predictive values of the test when applied to women with a 10% prevalence of breast cancer (e.g., those with a self-diagnosed lump in a breast)?

Positive predictive value is:
a) 0.667
b) 0.514
c) 0.333
d) 0.167

Negative predictive value is:
a) 0.994
b) 0.989
c) 0.950
d) 0.900

Answer and Discussion

The answers are b and a. The prevalence is 0.10, so the positive predictive value is $(0.10)(0.95)/[(0.10)(0.95) + (1 - 0.10)(1 - 0.90)]$, which equals $0.095/(0.095 + 0.09)$, or 0.514. Likewise, the negative predictive value is $(1 - 0.10)(0.90)/[(1 - 0.10)(0.90) + (0.10)(1 - 0.95)]$, which equals $0.810/(0.810 + 0.005)$, or 0.994.

Think about how the positive and negative predictive values changed when the prevalence increased from question 2 to question 3.

Using Fagan's nomogram (Fig. 4.2), the positive and negative predictive values can be approximated. Calculate the likelihood ratio, which is sensitivity/(1 − specificity). This equals $0.95/(1 - 0.90)$, or 9.5. Then, drawing a straight line from the pretest probability (prevalence) of 0.01 in part a, or 0.10 in part b, through the likelihood ratio of 9.5, one can read off the posttest probability (positive predictive value). These values are very close to those calculated previously by Bayes' theorem.

4. The positive predictive value of a diagnostic test can be increased (assuming other factors do not change) by
a) Increasing the sensitivity of the test
b) Increasing the specificity of the test
c) Decreasing the prevalence of the disease
d) Either a or b, or both

Answer and Discussion

The answer is d. Examining Bayes' theorem will show this, or it can be shown by calculating some examples.

5. In statistical hypothesis testing where the null hypothesis is like having no disease and the alternative hypothesis is like having disease, the statistical power of the hypothesis test is analogous to
a) Sensitivity
b) Specificity
c) 1 − sensitivity
d) 1 − specificity

Answer and Discussion

The answer is a. This has not been discussed in the chapter but is an important concept. Examining Figure 4.1 may be helpful. In a statistical test, rejecting the null hypothesis given that it is truly false is called the power of the test. This is equivalent to having a diagnostic test reject the presence of "no disease" to conclude that there is disease. Hence, this is analogous to sensitivity, the probability that the diagnostic test indicates there is disease when in fact there is disease present. Likewise, in hypothesis testing, the Type I error rate (i.e., significance level) of rejecting the null hypothesis when it is really true is analogous to 1 − specificity of a diagnostic test, the false-positive rate.

SUGGESTED READINGS

Begg CB. Biases in the assessment of diagnostic tests. *Stat Med* 1987;6:411–423.

Fagan TJ. Nomogram for Bayes' theorem [Letter]. *N Engl J Med* 1975;293:257.

Griner PF, Mayewski RJ, Mushlin AI, et al. Selection and interpretation of diagnostic tests and procedures: principles and applications. *Ann Intern Med* 1981;94:553–600.

Metz CE. Basic principles of ROC analysis. *Semin Nucl Med* 1978;8:283–298.

Meyer KB, Pauker SG. Screening for HIV: can we afford the false positive rate? *N Engl J Med* 1987;317:238–241.

Chapter 5

Ocular Manifestations of Systemic Disease

Ying Qian   Victor L. Perez   Careen Y. Lowder

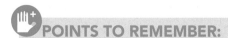

POINTS TO REMEMBER:

- Cotton-wool spots, hard exudates, and intraretinal hemorrhages are the most common nonspecific manifestations of retinopathy.

- Papilledema usually does not cause reduction in visual acuity unless it is long standing.

- If giant cell arteritis is suspected, the initiation of corticosteroids should be instituted immediately, even before the temporal artery biopsy.

- Patients with diabetes mellitus should be referred to an ophthalmologist for proper evaluation and care.

- Central retinal artery occlusion is a true ophthalmic emergency.

- Topical medications for glaucoma can have systemic side effects.

The ability of the physician to directly visualize ocular structures is unique to the eye as an organ system. The physician is able to make an immediate assessment of many systemic diseases, such as diabetes and hypertension, based on ocular findings. In systemic diseases with ocular manifestations, close collaboration between the ophthalmologist and the internist is required to provide the best medical care to the patient. The main goal of this chapter is to provide internists a comprehensive and simplified journey through the eye that will make for better communication between the specialties.

EYE EXAMINATION

The first step in the evaluation of any suspected ophthalmic disorder is a complete eight-part eye examination, which can be performed at the bedside in the following order:

1. Vision
2. Ocular motility
3. Pupil examination
4. Visual fields
5. External examination
6. Anterior segment examination (conjunctiva, sclera, cornea, anterior chamber, iris, and lens)
7. Intraocular pressure (IOP) examination
8. Dilated fundus examination

Vision, the vital sign of the eye, should always be documented, even if it means noting that the patient has light perception. The most common system is the Snellen notation, ranging from 20/20 (normal) to approximately 20/800. This is easily performed using a near card at the appropriate testing distance (check the card). Remember, the vision is checked for each eye separately while the fellow eye is occluded, and then with both eyes open. In the emergency room setting or at bedside, lower visual acuities are usually denoted as counting fingers at a specified distance (CF6′ is counting fingers at 6 feet), followed by the ability to see hand motions (HM12″ is hand motions at 12 inches), light perception, and no light perception. The most common error in vision testing is not completely occluding the fellow eye, leading to recording of better vision than is actually the case in an eye with poor vision.

Ocular motility testing is assessed by measuring versions and ductions. *Versions* are the movements of both eyes together while they are viewing the object of regard, whereas *ductions* are the movements of one eye while the other eye is occluded. These can be quickly evaluated by having the patient track the examiner's finger as it is moved through the 12 clock hours for both eyes together and then for each eye alone. Similarly, the patient is then asked to look in the six cardinal directions of gaze (up and right, right, down and right, up and left, left, and down and left), as well as up, down, and straight ahead for both eyes together and then for each eye alone. The evaluation of ocular movements may reveal cranial nerve palsies and mechanical restrictions of the muscles (thyroid eye disease, orbital inflammatory syndromes, and trauma).

Pupillary responses are a very important part of the ophthalmic exam. These responses should be tested by using a bright light source (muscle lamp or penlight). Pupillary testing may demonstrate a tonic pupil (Adie's syndrome, pharmacologic), relative afferent pupillary defect (asymmetric optic nerve damage; i.e., aneurysm), light-near dissociation (midbrain tumors), and Argyll-Robertson pupils (syphilis, chronic diabetes mellitus). Foremost, no drops should be placed in the patient's eyes before evaluation. The patient is then asked to focus on a distant object (at least 6 meters away) and maintain that focus throughout the examination. The light is shone into the right eye, and the pupillary response is noted. This is the direct response. A normal pupil should constrict immediately and briskly to a smaller circumference, followed by a small redilation to a level midway between the prelight stimulus and the maximal light stimulus. At this point (approximately 3 seconds), the light is swung to stimulate the left pupil (hence the name *swinging flashlight test*). The pupillary response of the left eye should be documented; this is called the *consensual response*. The normal consensual response is a pupil that may minimally dilate or stay constricted at the midlevel of the direct response. This is because the pupillary fibers cross in the optic chiasm, contributing approximately equal amounts of response to both sides. An abnormal pupillary response would be a redilation of the left eye to a size equal to or greater than the prelight stimulus. This would indicate that the left eye's optic nerve is not perceiving as much light stimulus. Another abnormal pupillary response would be a significant constriction of the left pupil, indicating that it is perceiving more light stimulus than the right eye. The light is then returned rapidly to the right eye after 3 seconds, and this process is repeated several times until the abnormality, if any, is determined. The patient is then allowed to recover, and the process is repeated starting with the left eye. Pupillary testing should be done in both dim and bright light conditions. One important point to remember is that if both optic nerves are equally damaged, no evidence of a relative afferent pupillary defect will be detected because there is no difference in the amount of light each optic nerve perceives it is receiving. Common errors to avoid are having the patient focus on the light source (this induces the near response with subsequent pupillary constriction) and not shining the light directly into the pupil (obliquely holding light in front of one pupil, but not the other, can simulate a relative afferent pupillary defect).

Confrontation visual field testing is easy, quickly performed, and reveals important information about the integrity of the visual system. Ask the patient to look directly and only at your nose while standing at approximately arm's length from the patient. Have the patient cover his or her left eye while you occlude your right eye so that you should both have similar fields of view (this only works if the examiner does not have a visual field defect). At this point, the examiner holds up the left hand at a distance midway between the examiner and the patient, extending fingers in the various fields of gaze (see previous discussion) so that the patient can also see them. Then the patient is asked to say how many fingers are present. Repeat the process for the other eye, reversing the eyes that are occluded for both the patient and the examiner and the hand that is being used to count fingers. Visual field testing can reveal the presence of pituitary masses, orbital masses, retinal detachments, advanced glaucoma, and intraocular lesions. Common errors of visual field testing include the patient not focusing on the examiner's nose (patient looks at the fingers), the examiner not occluding his or her own eye (could test outside the patient's field), and not having the patient wear his or her corrective lenses (the patient may not be able to see without them).

The external examination may reveal exophthalmos (anterior displacement of the globe), enophthalmos (posterior displacement of the globe), ptosis (lid droop), lid lesions, erythema, and edema. Palpation of the bony orbit may reveal discontinuities (orbital fractures) or masses (tumors, foreign body). Care should be taken to evaluate for the presence of a preauricular lymph node (common in viral conjunctivitis).

The anterior segment examination is best performed using a slit-lamp biomicroscope; however, a direct ophthalmoscope is just as useful at the bedside. A systematic approach is most useful: (a) lashes, lids, lacrimal system; (b) conjunctiva and sclera; (c) cornea; (d) iris; (e) anterior chamber; (f) lens; and (g) anterior vitreous. Conjunctival and scleral examination can demonstrate jaundice, paleness of the tarsal conjunctiva (anemia), subconjunctival hemorrhages (bleeding diatheses), or conjunctival edema (chemosis). Vascular congestion is common in conjunctivitis, and chemosis is typical of an allergic response. Ciliary flush or redness associated with severe iritis and light sensitivity (photophobia) should be taken seriously because these represent signs of severe inflammation of the anterior segment of the eye. The anterior chamber is assessed for depth, presence of cell (absent is normal), and flare (absent is normal).

The measurement of IOP is also very important. The normal range is 10 to 21 mm Hg, with a skewing toward the higher numbers. IOP should be assessed before dilation to minimize the possibility of worsening an attack of angle-closure glaucoma. Acute increases in IOP can mimic a systemic illness with the presence of headache, severe eye pain, nausea, vomiting, fatigue, loss of appetite, and abdominal pain.

The important structures of the posterior segment, such as the optic nerve, macula, and the major arcades and some of their branches, are easily visualized using the direct ophthalmoscope. The nerve is assessed for color (pale or pink), edema (sharp margins or blurred), hemorrhage, and the ratio of cup to disc. Symmetry between the nerves is noted. The presence of a foveal reflex should be noted. Narrowing and tortuosity of the arteries, arteriolar sclerosis, congestion, and tortuosity of the veins and arteriovenous (AV) crossing changes reflect disease processes such as hypertension, anemia, diabetes mellitus, and vasculopathies, among others. None of these findings is pathognomic of a specific disease; they only represent the limited number of ways that the retina can respond to injury.

RETINAL NONSPECIFIC SIGNS

Cotton-wool spots, hard exudates, and intraretinal hemorrhages are the most common nonspecific manifestations of retinopathy. These findings can be seen in disease processes such as diabetes mellitus, hypertension, hypotension, venous stasis, collagen vascular diseases, and radiation damage to the orbit.

Cotton-wool spots represent infarcts that result from the closure of the precapillary arterioles within the nerve fiber layer of the retina. The subsequent edema results in the classic appearance of small fluffy white lesions that may obscure the retinal blood vessels (Fig. 5.1). These lesions will characteristically disappear within 6 to 8 weeks.

Hard exudates are visualized as punctate yellowish spots that result from conditions that produce leaky blood vessels (Fig. 5.2).

Hemorrhages may be intraretinal or extraretinal extravasations of blood. Intraretinal hemorrhages may be flame shaped when present in the nerve fiber layer or dot shaped if in the outer plexiform layer (Fig. 5.3).

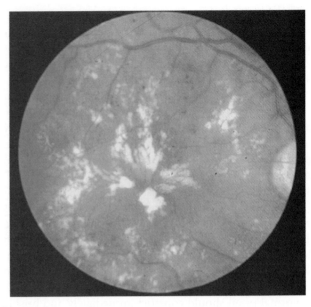

Figure 5.2 Hard exudates. (See Color Fig. 5.2.)

Neovascularization of the retina is characterized by the appearance of either loop or capillary structures that proliferate along the retinal surface and extend into the vitreous cavity. The new vessels demonstrate abnormal growth out of the retina, bleed easily, are prone to leaking exudates, and may involute. Retinal neovascularization is best associated with diabetes mellitus, but is also seen in numerous entities, including carotid artery disease, retinopathy of prematurity, inflammatory processes, and sickle cell disease. The vascular proliferation in diabetes mellitus typically appears on the optic nerve head (neovascularization of the disc, or NVD; Fig. 5.4) or may be

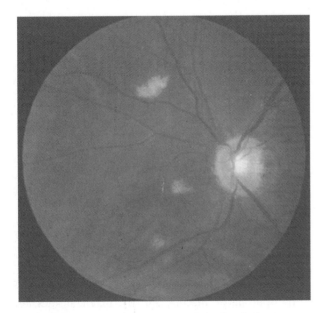

Figure 5.1 Cotton-wool spots. (See Color Fig. 5.1.)

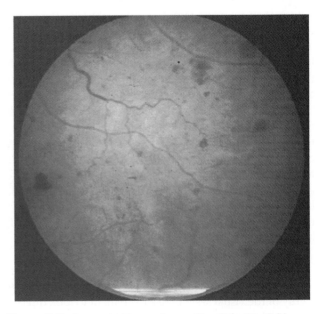

Figure 5.3 Intraretinal hemorrhages. (See Color Fig. 5.3.)

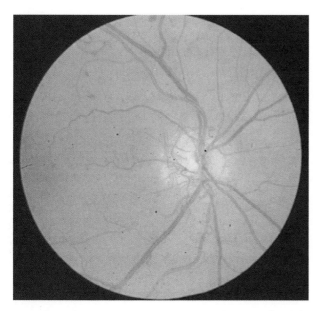

Figure 5.4   Neovascularization of the disc. (See Color Fig. 5.4.)

present elsewhere (neovascularization elsewhere; Fig. 5.5), but it is usually seen along blood vessels in the posterior pole.

Papilledema refers to swelling of the optic nerve head in patients with increased intracranial pressure. Disk edema refers to swelling of the optic nerve head from any other cause. These swellings are associated with stasis rather than inflammation. Swelling of the optic nerve associated with inflammation is called papillitis and is differentiated from papilledema by a reduction in vision. Papilledema usually does not cause reduction in visual acuity unless it is long standing.

OPHTHALMIC SIGNS OF SPECIFIC CONDITIONS

Giant Cell Arteritis and Temporal Arteritis

Giant cell arteritis is a systemic vasculitis that affects people older than 60 years with an increasing prevalence in each subsequent decade. No case has been documented histologically in a patient younger than 50 years. Histologically, the arteritis consists of cellular infiltration of the arterial wall by multinucleated giant cells and a breakdown of the internal elastic lamina.

Giant cell arteritis may present with sudden loss of vision in one or both eyes and diplopia. Patients may have systemic symptoms such as headache, arthralgias, myalgias, fever, weight loss, anemia, scalp tingling, jaw claudication, and depression prior to loss of vision. The diminished visual acuity is attributed to the occlusion of the posterior ciliary blood vessels that supply the optic nerve head. This results in an anterior ischemic optic neuropathy. Examination of the optic nerve head demonstrates typical pallid edema (Fig. 5.6). The diagnosis is based on a high degree of clinical suspicion in a patient population of the appropriate age having the symptoms outlined previously. Two useful tests are the erythrocyte sedimentation rate and the C-reactive protein level, which will generally be elevated in the presence of giant cell arteritis. These tests are nonspecific, however, and can be elevated normally in the typical age range of patients with this disease. Diagnosis can only be confirmed by a histologic demonstration of multinucleated giant cells within the muscular lining of the arterial wall and an accompanying breakdown of the internal elastic lamina, following biopsy of the superficial temporalis artery. In the appropriate clinical setting, if giant cell arteritis is suspected, the initiation of corticosteroids should be instituted immediately, even before the temporal artery biopsy. Patients can rapidly progress to no light perception vision in both eyes in the absence of treatment. A temporal

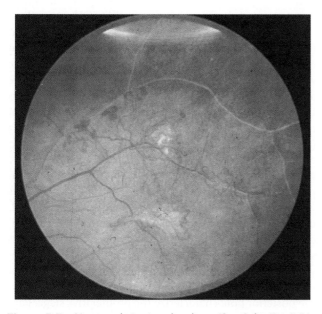

Figure 5.5   Neovascularization elsewhere. (See Color Fig. 5.5.)

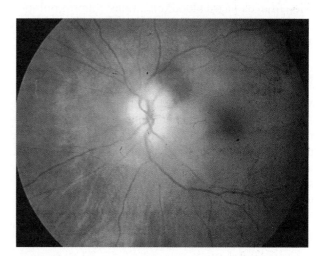

Figure 5.6   Pallid optic nerve edema in giant cell arteritis. (See Color Fig. 5.6.)

artery biopsy should be scheduled, but it should not delay treatment. Several studies have demonstrated that the biopsy remains positive for at least 3 weeks, even with intravenous (IV) corticosteroid treatment, and there have been anecdotal reports of positive biopsies several months after continuous corticosteroid use. The absence of a positive temporal artery biopsy does not ensure absence of disease. In the setting of high clinical suspicion and a negative biopsy, a biopsy of the uninvolved side is warranted. It has been reported that up to 10% of patients with giant cell arteritis have a negative temporal artery biopsy. Response to therapy and tapering of corticosteroids are guided by the erythrocyte sedimentation rate, which should be kept below 30 mm/hour. Therapy may need to be continued for more than a year.

Hypertension

Hypertensive retinopathy may develop through several stages, but in severe hypertension these stages may not be detected because of the accelerated nature of the hypertensive retinopathy. The stages of hypertensive retinopathy are:

■ Vasoconstrictive phase
■ Sclerotic phase
■ Exudative phase
■ Complications of the sclerotic phase

In the vasoconstrictive phase, elevated blood pressure causes the retinal arteries to increase their tone through autoregulation, resulting in arterial narrowing and tortuosity. The primary site of vasoconstriction is the precapillary arteriole, occurring most frequently in the second- and third-order arteries. A persistent elevation in blood pressure results in the hyalinization of the blood vessels, leading to a change in the light reflex of the vessel wall; AV crossing changes develop, and the arteries become more tortuous. In the exudative phase, flame-shaped hemorrhages develop from damaged blood vessel walls; cotton-wool spots or microinfarcts develop from closure of the precapillary arterioles.

Malignant Hypertension

Malignant hypertension is characterized ophthalmologically by papilledema and numerous flame-shaped hemorrhages and cotton-wool spots in the peripapillary area and posterior pole (Fig. 5.7). Malignant hypertension is a medical emergency, but care must be taken not to decrease the systemic blood pressure too rapidly because this may lead to infarction of the optic nerve.

Diabetic Retinopathy

In the Western Hemisphere, diabetic retinopathy is the leading cause of blindness in patients younger than

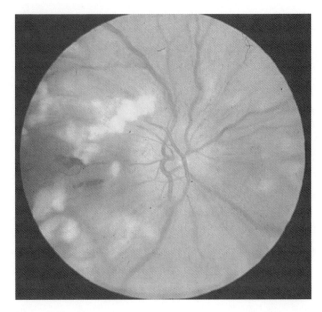

Figure 5.7   The edematous optic nerve is surrounded by cotton-wool spots and intraretinal hemorrhages in malignant hypertension. (See Color Fig. 5.7.)

65 years. The onset of diabetic retinopathy varies with the type of diabetes mellitus present. In type I diabetes (insulin-dependent diabetes mellitus), there is a delay of approximately 5 years between the diagnosis of diabetes and the onset of retinopathy. In type II diabetes (non–insulin-dependent diabetes mellitus), the retinopathy may be present at the time of diagnosis. Patients with diabetes mellitus should be referred to an ophthalmologist for proper evaluation and care.

Most patients with diabetes mellitus develop characteristic abnormalities of the retinal blood vessels. Retinal hemorrhages and hard exudates are not peculiar to diabetes mellitus, but their distribution and relative proportions lead to the highly characteristic and essentially pathognomonic appearance of the eye in patients with diabetes mellitus (Fig. 5.8). The hemorrhages and exudates are usually confined to the posterior pole, bounded by the superior and inferior temporal vessels. The leading cause of irreversible vision loss in patients with diabetes is macular edema. One test that is useful in the evaluation of diabetic retinopathy is IV fluorescein angiography. Fluorescein angiography is not needed to diagnose clinically significant macular edema (CSME) or proliferative diabetic retinopathy, but it is necessary to identify areas of precapillary closure and capillary nonperfusion (Fig. 5.9). Clinically, areas of capillary nonperfusion may have overlying cotton-wool spots. Patients with extensive capillary closure are at high risk for the development of proliferative diabetic retinopathy. Patients with diabetes mellitus who are noted to have cotton-wool spots should be monitored closely for the development of neovascularization or proliferative diabetic retinopathy. Neovascularization of the disc or of blood vessels elsewhere in the posterior pole characterize the proliferative stage. Pan-retinal laser photocoagulation is indicated in these patients.

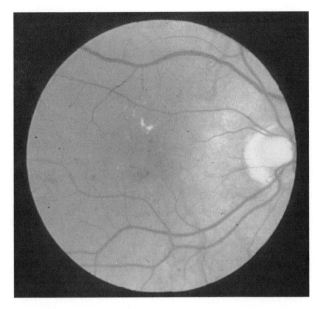

Figure 5.8 Background diabetic retinopathy consisting of dot hemorrhages and hard exudates. (See Color Fig. 5.8.)

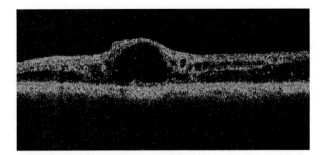

Figure 5.10 OCT image of diabetic macular edema showing large and small cystoid spaces and diffuse retinal thickening. The normal foveal contour is compact with a depression in the middle corresponding to the center of the fovea.

After the ophthalmologic examination, and according to the results from either the eye examinations or ancillary studies such as fluorescein angiography and optical coherence tomography (OCT), the patient is classified into one of nine different categories that will guide the treatment and follow-up care. OCT is a noninvasive scan that has revolutionized the way retinal pathology is diagnosed and treated. Using optical wave reflectivity (rather than sound echos in ultrasonography, for instance) to delineate interfaces, OCT provides a cross-sectional scan of retinal tissue architecture. In diabetic macular edema, for example, OCT is used to detect retinal thickening and to monitor the response to treatment (Fig. 5.10). Even newer OCT machines

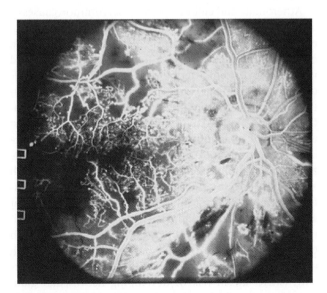

Figure 5.9 Fluorescein angiogram reveals areas of capillary nonperfusion.

and software are capable of generating three-dimensional images.

Depending on the presence or absence of retinopathy, the management of diabetic retinopathy will be as follows:

- *Normal or minimal nonproliferative retinopathy.* Fundus photographs, angiography, and laser treatment are not necessary. These patients should be examined once a year.
- *Nonproliferative retinopathy without macular edema.* These patients occasionally present with hard exudates and dot-and-blot hemorrhages, and fundus photographs may be taken to be used as baseline. Follow-up visits should be scheduled within 6 to 12 months.
- *Nonproliferative retinopathy with nonsignificant macular edema.* Nonsignificant macular edema does not involve the center of the fovea nor does it reduce visual acuity. Fluorescein angiography, OCT, and color fundus photography may occasionally be indicated for these patients. Follow-up visits should be scheduled within 4 to 6 months because these patients are at risk of developing CSME.
- *Nonproliferative retinopathy with CSME.* CSME has been defined as the presence of macular thickening, with 500 microns of the center of the fovea, hard exudates at or within 500 microns of the center of the fovea if associated with an area of adjacent retinal thickening, or an area of thickening one disc area or larger, any part of which is located within one disc diameter of the center of the fovea. These patients should be considered for fluorescein angiography, OCT, and focal laser photocoagulation. Referral to an endocrinologist should be considered. Follow-up visits should take place within 1 to 3 months.
- *Severe nonproliferative (preproliferative) retinopathy.* Nonproliferative retinopathy is characterized by the presence of four quadrants of hemorrhage and microaneurysms, two quadrants of venous beading, or one quadrant of intraretinal microvascular abnormalities. Depending on the extent of pathology, 10% to 50% of these patients will develop proliferative diabetic retinopathy within 1 year. Both color fundus photography and fluorescein

angiography are indicated. Follow-up visits should occur every 3 to 4 months.

■ *Non–high-risk proliferative retinopathy.* Non–high-risk proliferative retinopathy refers to patients who have not developed NVD and vitreous hemorrhage. Fluorescein angiography may help assess the extent of these areas of retinal nonperfusion and areas of retinal neovascularization. Laser surgery may occasionally be indicated for these patients, depending on their reliability to follow-up and the status of their fellow eye. Follow-up visits should occur within 3 to 4 months.

■ *Non–high-risk proliferative diabetic retinopathy with CSME.* Fluorescein angiography and OCT should be considered in these patients. Focal macular laser surgery is indicated for these patients. Follow-up visits should occur within 1 to 3 months.

■ *High-risk proliferative diabetic retinopathy.* High-risk proliferative retinopathy refers to patients who have developed NVD alone (greater than one-third to one-fourth of the surface disc area) or in association with vitreous hemorrhage. Panretinal photocoagulation is indicated for these patients. Some of them are candidates for early vitrectomy. Follow-up visits should occur every 3 to 4 months.

■ *High-risk proliferative diabetic retinopathy not amenable to photocoagulation.* High-risk proliferative retinopathy not amenable to photocoagulation refers to patients who have developed severe vitreous hemorrhage or to patients with active proliferative retinopathy despite laser treatment. Vitreous surgery may be indicated in these patients because it may be impossible to perform laser photocoagulation due to the vitreous hemorrhage. Follow-up visits should occur every 4 to 6 weeks.

The last two categories of patients are at high risk for developing neovascular glaucoma, a form of angle-closure glaucoma in which the trabecular meshwork is obstructed by neovascularization. Avastin (bevacizumab), an anti-vascular endothelial growth factor (anti-VEGF) antibody used to treat metastatic colon cancer, has been successfully injected intravitreally to treat neovascularization, although the antiangiogenetic effect is not long standing.

Retinal Artery Occlusion

Patients with central retinal artery occlusion have sudden loss of vision. Examination will reveal markedly narrow arteries with boxcar segmentation. The retina is opacified with a cherry-red spot in the macular area (Fig. 5.11). Central retinal artery occlusion (CRAO) is a true ophthalmic emergency. The usual site of obstruction is at the lamina cribrosa, the sievelike membrane at the optic nerve head. This is the location where the periarterial fibrous membrane becomes a mechanical barrier to the expansion of the artery. Digital massage over closed lids after instillation

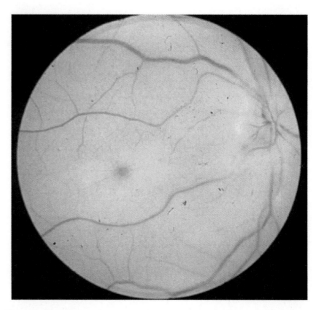

Figure 5.11 The retina is edematous, and there is a cherry-red spot in the macula of a patient with central retinal artery occlusion. (See Color Fig. 5.11.)

of antihypertensive drops such as a beta-blocker (timolol 0.5%) or an alpha-adrenergic agonist (Alphagan) can be performed immediately to decrease the IOP in the setting of acute CRAO. Systemic medications such as a carbonic anhydrase inhibitor may also be given to the patient. Alternatively, an anterior chamber paracentesis can be performed to acutely lower the IOP. Lowering the IOP may dislodge emboli and improve circulation. All reports of improvement following intervention are anecdotal in nature, and no intervention has ever been demonstrated to be effective over observation in restoring vision. Visual loss is permanent if the circulation is not restored within 90 minutes.

Atheromata and emboli are the most common causes of artery obstruction. The emboli may consist of calcific vegetations that originate from valvular disease of the heart, or they may be particles from atheromatous plaques found in the aorta, carotid artery, or more distal branches. Calcific emboli are matte white and nonscintillating, in contrast to lipid emboli, which appear yellowish and scintillating (Fig. 5.12). Lipid emboli usually originate in an atheroma of a stenotic carotid artery. Usually, multiple lipid emboli are seen clinically, and they tend to lodge at the bifurcations of the retinal arteries. These emboli are responsible for transient ischemic attacks. Platelet-fibrin emboli cause transient blindness and usually occur after myocardial infarction. Platelet-fibrin emboli are abolished with aspirin intake. Whenever a patient presents with CRAO, consider the possibility of giant cell arteritis, which can rapidly progress to involve the fellow eye. Patients with CRAO are at risk of developing neovascular glaucoma because of the elaboration of VEGF from ischemic retina.

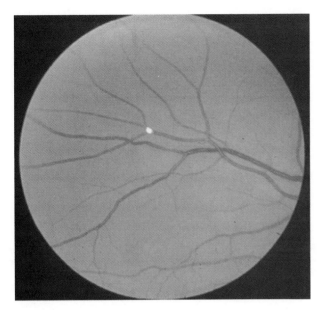

Figure 5.12 Hollenhorst's plaque. (See Color Fig. 5.12.)

Wegener's Granulomatosis

Wegener's granulomatosis is a necrotizing vasculitis of the small arteries and veins, and is associated with granuloma formation. About 95% of patients have respiratory tract disease; 85% may have renal disease. Eye, adnexal, and orbital involvement are present in 50% of patients. Virtually any vascularized part of the eye may be involved. Orbital disease is the most common ophthalmic manifestation of Wegener's granulomatosis and is usually secondary to nasal or paranasal sinus disease (Fig. 5.13). Orbital disease presents with pain, tenderness, limited extraocular movement, and proptosis. Optic nerve compression is the usual cause of blindness.

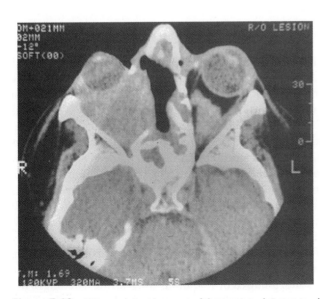

Figure 5.13 CT reveals involvement of the paranasal sinuses and orbits in a patient with Wegener's granulomatosis.

Rheumatoid Arthritis

The most common ocular problem in patients with rheumatoid arthritis is keratoconjunctivitis sicca or secondary Sjögren's syndrome associated with connective tissue disease. Dry eyes occur in 11% to 13% of patients. The lacrimal and salivary glands are infiltrated by lymphocytes, leading to glandular destruction with loss of tear and saliva production. Dry eyes should be treated with the frequent instillation of tears or bland ointment to prevent corneal opacification and melting.

Scleritis is the second most common ocular finding, occurring in 1% to 6% of patients with rheumatoid arthritis. The scleritis may be anterior, posterior, or necrotizing. Necrotizing scleritis has a poor prognosis because it is usually associated with systemic vasculitis (Fig. 5.14). Scleritis requires systemic treatment with nonsteroidal anti-inflammatory drugs (NSAIDs), in addition to topical corticosteroids. In severe cases, systemic corticosteroids and immunosuppressive drugs may be necessary.

Posterior segment lesions due to rheumatoid arthritis are rare. Probably the most common reason for a dilated eye examination in patients with rheumatoid arthritis is to screen for antimalarial drug toxicity. Hydroxychloroquine is accumulated in pigmented tissues, such as the retinal pigment epithelium and may cause a bull's-eye pigmentary maculopathy (Fig. 5.15). The retinopathy may be reversible if discovered early, but it is irreversible and even progressive despite discontinuation of the drug if not detected early. The frequency of retinopathy is less than 1% when dosages of <6.5 mg/kg/day of hydroxychloroquine are used (<400 mg/day) for a duration of less than 10 years.

HLA-B27–Associated Uveitis

More than 50% of acute anterior uveitis (iritis or iridocyclitis) is associated with the HLA-B27 antigen. In patients who have recurrent, unilateral, or acute attacks of iritis that alternate between the eyes, almost 90% of patients

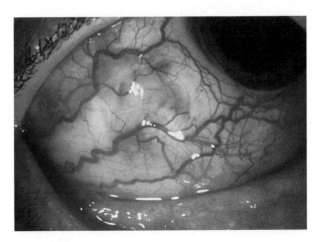

Figure 5.14 Avascularity of the sclera leads to scleromalacia in a patient with rheumatoid arthritis. (See Color Fig. 5.14.)

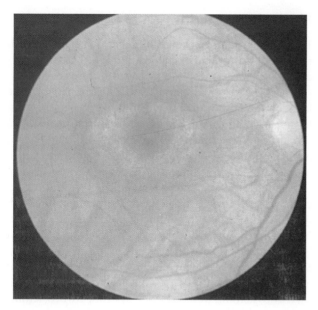

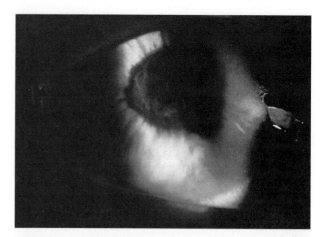

Figure 5.17 The anterior lens capsule is covered by a fibrinous exudate in a patient with HLA-B27–associated acute iritis. (See Color Fig. 5.17.)

Figure 5.15 Bull's eye of hydroxychloroquine pigmentary maculopathy. (See Color Fig. 5.15.)

have the HLA-B27 antigen. The iritis is characterized by severe pain, redness, and photophobia. Clinically, a marked conjunctival injection and ciliary flush are present (Fig. 5.16). The cornea may be hazy. Fibrinous exudates or a hypopyon may be present. The anterior lens surface may be obscured by fibrin (Fig. 5.17). These findings may be visualized using a direct ophthalmoscope. Both men and women may be affected, and approximately 50% of patients have an associated seronegative spondyloarthropathy. The most commonly associated systemic diseases are ankylosing spondylitis, Reiter's syndrome, psoriatic arthritis, and inflammatory bowel disease. In many instances, the patient may present first to the ophthalmologist with ocular complaints before any systemic diagnosis is made.

Approximately 10% of patients with inflammatory bowel disease (IBD) have ocular involvement, with the

highest incidence in those who are HLA-B27 positive. The most common ocular manifestations of IBD are episcleritis, scleritis, and uveitis. Episcleritis is reported to reflect systemic disease activity and subsides when systemic inflammation is brought under control. Scleritis is indicative of vasculitis and may result in scleral thinning.

Persistent and severe uveitis, scleritis, and vasculitis are manifestations of systemic inflammation and need systemic immunosuppression for disease control. Steroid-sparing agents such as methotrexate, mycophenolate, and azathioprine, as well as anti–tumor necrosis factor therapies, are often employed in conjunction with rheumatology consultation. Enbrel (etanercept) has also been reported to exacerbate intraocular inflammation or cause optic neuritis in patients with uveitis. A high clinical index of suspicion should be maintained when a patient presents with an atypical flare while taking etanercept.

Thyroid Eye Disease

Thyroid-related immune orbitopathy (Graves' orbitopathy, dysthyroid ophthalmopathy, thyroid eye disease) is the most common cause of unilateral and bilateral proptosis in adults. Thyroid eye disease usually occurs between the ages of 25 and 50 years. Findings include proptosis, eyelid retraction and lagophthalmos, and restriction of the extraocular muscles, resulting in diplopia. The signs may occur alone or at the same time. The compression of the optic nerve results from extraocular muscle enlargement and is sight threatening (Fig. 5.18). Formal visual field tests will reveal scotomas in patients with thyroid optic neuropathy. The clinical course of thyroid eye disease does not usually follow a linear progression in severity. Patients may have acute episodes characterized by edema and swelling of the tissues, followed by resolution and scarring. Swelling of the extraocular muscles causes diplopia. The patient, however, should not have corrective strabismus surgery until the

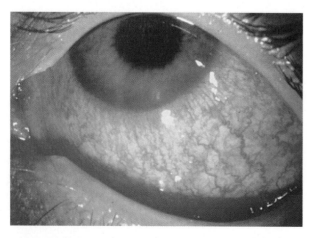

Figure 5.16 Marked conjunctival injection and ciliary flush in acute iritis. (See Color Fig. 5.16.)

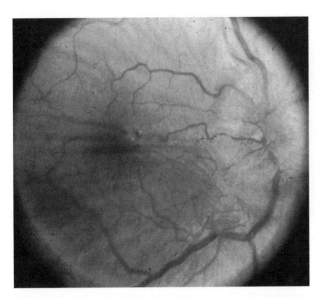

Figure 5.18 Fundus photograph show a swollen optic nerve and choroidal folds secondary to compression by enlarged muscles in a patient with thyroid optic neuropathy. (See Color Fig. 5.18.)

inflammatory process has subsided and stabilized, and scarring has developed.

Leukemia

The ocular involvement in leukemia varies in different series from a prevalence of 28% to 82%, the latter figure in an autopsy series. Leukemic infiltrates may be seen in the iris, retina, choroid, and optic nerve. Leukemic cells invading the anterior chamber mimic iritis and in the vitreous, vitritis.

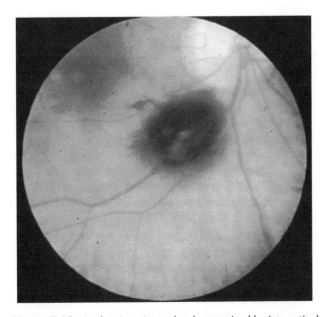

Figure 5.19 Leukemic retinopathy characterized by intraretinal and preretinal hemorrhages. (See Color Fig. 5.19.)

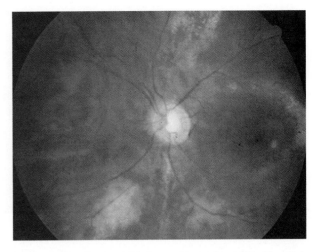

Figure 5.20 CMV retinitis in a patient with AIDS. (See Color Fig. 5.20.)

Leukemic retinopathy refers to the ocular findings in patients with leukemia who are suffering with anemia, thrombocytopenia, or increased blood viscosity. Hemorrhages may present as blots, dots, and flame shapes with or without white centers. The hemorrhage may spill into the vitreous. Cotton-wool spots are also commonly seen. Hyperviscosity of the blood may lead to vein occlusions, microaneurysms, retinal hemorrhages, and neovascularization (Fig. 5.19).

AIDS

The most common ocular manifestation in AIDS is the cotton-wool spot, a nonspecific finding seen in many other diseases. Infections of every ocular structure by unusual organisms have been reported in patients with AIDS. The most common and sight-threatening ocular infection is cytomegalovirus (CMV) retinitis (Fig. 5.20), which in the pre–highly active antiretroviral therapy era affected 20% to 35% of patients with AIDS and 30% to 40% of patients with a CD4$^+$ cell count $<50/\mu$L. The introduction of intravitreal sustained-release ganciclovir implants has greatly improved treatment of CMV retinitis because it avoids the need for prolonged IV treatment with ganciclovir or foscarnet.

OPHTHALMIC CONDITION OF RELEVANCE TO THE INTERNIST

Glaucoma

Glaucoma is a multifactorial disease process in which the end result is the characteristic optic neuropathy. Risk factors include elevated IOP, family history, age, race, long-term steroid use, and severe farsightedness. Because the only modifiable risk factor is IOP, all medical and surgical glaucoma treatments are aimed at lowering IOP. Elevated pressure within the eye can damage the cells of the retina (the lining of the eye) and the optic nerve (Fig. 5.21A and B).

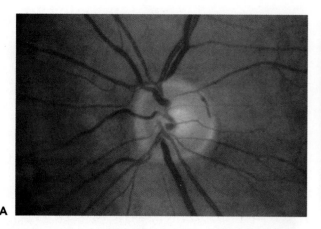
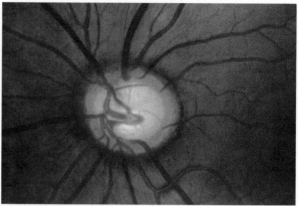

A   B

Figure 5.21   **(A)** Normal optic nerve. **(B)** Glaucomatous optic nerve. (See Color Fig. 5.21.)

The eye is like a ball that does not increase in size with more pressure. As the pressure increases, the walls of the ball become constricted, and damage occurs to the structures lining the ball (eye). Damage to the inner structures of the eye, because of eye pressure, leads to loss of visual field.

The risk of developing glaucoma increases with age. It usually occurs in people older than 45 years. According to the National Society for the Prevention of Blindness, 1 in 50 Americans older than 35 years and 3 of 100 older than 65 years have glaucoma.

People at greatest risk are those who have diabetes or who have relatives with glaucoma. There are different types of glaucoma:

- *Open-angle glaucoma*—This comprises about 90% of cases in the United States; it progresses slowly and is often unnoticed for months or years. Therapy usually consists of antiglaucomatous drops. This type of glaucoma is chronic and slowly progressive if untreated. Untreated open-angle glaucoma leads to loss of peripheral vision, which may be unnoticed by the patient because of its slow progression. Central visual acuity is preserved until late stages, but glaucoma ultimately leads to blindness.
- *Angle-closure glaucoma*—This is very different from open-angle glaucoma in that patients develop a sudden, drastic increase in pressure, severe pain, blurred vision, halos around light, and vomiting. Laser iridotomy is the treatment indicated. (See the Laser Surgery section.) Unlike open-angle glaucoma, an attack of angle closure is a medical emergency and must be treated immediately. If pressure is not relieved within several hours, the patient may develop permanent loss of vision.
- *Secondary glaucoma*—This increased IOP is caused by other conditions such as uveitis, corticosteroid treatment, trauma, and other factors. The increased IOP must be treated and monitored by an ophthalmologist.
- *Congenital glaucoma*—This is present at birth. The infant may have cloudy corneas, corneas that appear larger than normal, protruding eyes, tearing, and light sensitivity. The IOP must be relieved as soon as possible by means of a surgical procedure called goniotomy or trabeculotomy,

where the outflow or anterior chamber angle is incised to improve the flow of fluid out of the eye. Systemic conditions that predispose to glaucoma include Sturge-Weber syndrome, neurofibromatosis type 1, tuberous sclerosis, Axenfeld-Rieger syndrome, and oculodermal melanocytosis (nevus of Ota).

Diagnosis

The diagnosis of glaucoma is made by examination of the anterior chamber angle by gonioscopy, correlation between the optic nerve damage and visual field defect, and sometimes imaging of the nerve fiber layer with OCT. Patients at risk of developing glaucoma are called glaucoma suspects, and situations in which there is elevated IOP without any other risk or evidence of optic nerve damage are termed *ocular hypertension*. These patients are followed yearly with IOP checks and Humphrey visual fields. Patients with glaucomatous nerve damage are followed every 3 to 6 months, depending on severity of disease.

Treatment

Medical

Patients who have glaucoma need to have their IOPs monitored and medications (drops) prescribed according to the IOP. Medications decrease eye pressure by either slowing the production of fluid in the eye or improving drainage of fluid from the eye. For the medications to work, the patient must take them regularly and continuously. Even skipping one or two times can cause the pressure to go up. These topical medications for glaucoma can have systemic side effects that should be considered by internists in their assessment of patients with glaucoma (Table 5.1).

Laser Surgery

Laser surgery for glaucoma depends on the type of glaucoma. In *open-angle glaucoma*, the drain itself is treated. A laser is used to increase fluid flow through the drain in a procedure called laser trabeculoplasty. In *angle-closure glaucoma*, in which there is no room in the anterior chamber, the laser creates a hole in the iris (the colored portion of the

TABLE 5.1

SYSTEMIC SIDE EFFECTS OF TOPICAL GLAUCOMA MEDICATIONS[a]

Class Compound	Brand Name	Method of Action	Systemic Side Effects
Beta-adrenergic antagonists (beta-blockers)			
Timolol maleate	Timoptic XE Timoptic Ocudose Timolol gel	Decrease aqueous production	Bradycardia, heart block, bronchospasm, decreased libido, central nervous system depression, mood swings
Betaxolol	Betoptic (S)	Same as previous	Fewer pulmonary complications
Adrenergic agonists			
Epinephrine	Epifrin	Improve aqueous outflow	Hypertension, headaches, extra systoles
Alpha-adrenergic agonists			
Apraclonidine hydrochloride	Iopidine	Decrease aqueous production, decrease episcleral venous pressure	Hypotension, vasovagal attack, dry mouth and nose, fatigue
Brimonidine tartrate	Alphagan	Decrease aqueous production, increase uveoscleral outflow	Headache, fatigue, hypotension, insomnia, depression, syncope, dizziness, anxiety
Parasympathomimetic (miotic) agents			
Pilocarpine hydrochloride	Isopto carpine Pilocar	Increase trabecular outflow	Increased salivation, increased secretion (gastric), abdominal cramps
Echothiophate iodide	Phospholine iodide		Same as pilocarpine, more gastrointestinal difficulties
Prostaglandin analogs			
Lantanoprost	Xalatan	Increase uveoscleral outflow	Flulike symptoms, joint/muscle pain
Bimatoprost	Lumigan	Side effects and mode of action are the same as Latanoprost	
Travoprost	Travatan		
Hyperosmotic agents			
Mannitol (parenteral)	Osmitrol	Osmotic gradient dehydrates vitreous	Urinary retention, headache, congestive heart failure, expansion of blood volume, diabetic complications, nausea, vomiting, diarrhea, electrolyte disturbance, renal failure
Glycerin (oral)	Osmoglyn		Can cause problems in diabetic patients; similar to previous
Isosorbide (oral)	Ismotic		Similar to mannitol
Carbonic anhydrase inhibitors (CAI) ***ORAL***			
Acetazolamide	Diamox	Decrease aqueous production	Poor tolerance of carbonated beverages, acidosis, depression, malaise, hirsutism, flatulence, paresthesias, numbness, lethargy, blood dyscrasias, diarrhea, weight loss, renal stones, loss of libido, bone marrow depression, hypokalemia, cramps, anorexia, taste, increased serum urate, enuresis
Methazolamide	Neptazane		Same as previous
TOPICAL			
Dorzolamide	Trusopt		Less likely to induce systemic effects of CAI, but may occur; bitter taste

[a]Adapted from Basic and Clinical Science Course 2008–2009, American Academy of Ophthalmology.

eye). The procedure is called laser iridotomy, and the fluid behind the iris flows into the anterior chamber through the hole made by the laser and into the drain.

Surgery or Trabeculectomy

When a patient's IOPs cannot be controlled with medications and/or laser treatment, the surgeon must make an opening in the eye to allow the fluid to leave the eye. The fluid exits the eye through the opening and filters underneath a "bleb" or bubble covered by the conjunctiva, the covering of the sclera. *Untreated glaucoma or increased IOP can lead to blindness.*

CATARACT AND CATARACT SURGERY

A cataract is a clouding of the normal clear lens of the eye (Fig. 5.22A) that results in decreased vision, which may be described as:

- Blurred vision
- Fogged vision

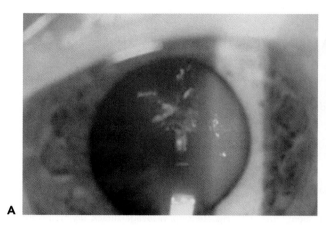
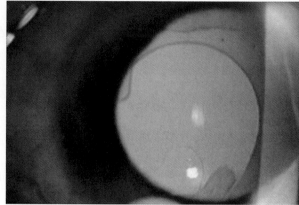

A　　　　　　　　　　　　　　　　　　　　　　　　　**B**

Figure 5.22　**(A)** Cataract. **(B)** Intraocular lens implant. (See Color Fig. 5.22.)

- Glare and halos around lights
- Double vision
- Requiring brighter light to read
- Frequent prescription changes
- Poor color perception

Cataracts are usually a result of aging, but may also develop because of medicines taken by the patient (e.g., steroids), ocular trauma, long-term exposure to bright lights, or medical conditions such as diabetes.

Treatment

Cataract surgery, or the removal of the cloudy lens, is the only way to clear the vision. An ophthalmologist must determine whether the patient's vision can be improved by examining the eye thoroughly to exclude any other causes of decreased vision. Cataract surgery, if recommended, is an elective procedure, meaning that a patient should only have surgery if the patient wants to have an improvement in vision because the decreased vision is interfering with normal daily activities.

Currently, the procedure is *phacoemulsification* (removal of the cataract by ultrasound to dissolve the cataract) and placement of a lens implant (a plastic lens, previously calculated to give good vision, to replace the biological lens; Fig. 5.22B). The surgery is performed as an outpatient procedure and under local anesthesia. Because sedation is used, patients must have someone to take them home after surgery; the eye is patched overnight, and the patch is removed on the first postoperative visit.

RETINAL DETACHMENT

The retina is the inner lining of the eye, and it is responsible for vision. The eye works in a way similar to that of a camera; that is, the light passes through the lens and is focused on the film (the retina is the film of the eye). The images on the film or retina are transmitted to the brain via nerve fibers.

Retinal detachment occurs when the lining of the eye comes off, thus causing loss of vision. Causes of retinal detachment include ocular trauma, posterior vitreous detachment, traction from an inflamed vitreous, long eyeballs (as in very nearsighted people), family predisposition, degenerative changes in the retina, complications from diabetes, and as a complication of intraocular surgery, including cataract surgery. A retinal detachment can be caused by a retinal tear or by scar tissue pulling the retina away from the wall of the eye. If the tear is not sealed (by laser), the liquid in the vitreous—the gellike substance in the eye—goes through the tear and gets under the retina, detaching it from the underlying tissues (Fig. 5.23). Vision is lost wherever the retina is detached.

Symptoms

The patient may notice loss of side and/or central vision, or a dark shadow, a veil, and—with total detachment—loss of vision. Frequently, patients describe seeing new floaters or flashes of light within the eye.

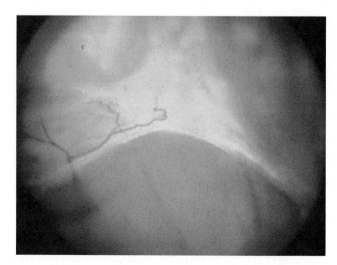

Figure 5.23　Retinal detachment. (See Color Fig. 5.23.)

Treatment

Retinal Tear

Laser treatment, cryotherapy, or both may be used to seal a retinal tear to prevent a retinal detachment from occurring. The laser beam is directed through a special contact lens. Cryotherapy freezes that part of the retina requiring treatment.

Retinal Detachment

If the retinal detachment is too large for laser treatment or cryotherapy alone, surgery becomes necessary to reattach the retina. The goal of surgery is anatomical reattachment of the retina. Successful reattachment of the retina does not always mean a return of good vision; vision depends on the length of time the macular area of the retina was detached prior to reattachment. Once the macula is detached, vision rarely returns to normal. An improvement in vision may require several months. Various procedures are available, and only the ophthalmologist can determine which procedure is most applicable after examining the patient and evaluating the type and extent of detachment.

OPHTHALMIC EMERGENCIES

There are some ophthalmic emergencies (Table 5.2) with which the internist should be familiar to better identify, treat, and triage patients, in order to protect the eye, to preserve vision, or both.

TABLE 5.2
OPHTHALMIC EMERGENCIES

Disease	Symptoms	Signs	Urgent in 12 (Ophthalmologist Hours)	Emergent (Immediate ER)	Treatment (Internist)
Trauma	Pain, photophobia, blurred vision or loss of vision	Laceration of the globe, redness, limitation of eye movements		×	Protective eye shield without underlying patch
Acute angle closure glaucoma	Pain, halos around lights, nausea, vomiting	Severe redness, corneal opacification		×	IV medication (mannitol)
Foreign body	Foreign body sensation, tearing, pain	Redness, discharge	×		Protective eye shield without underlying patch
Foreign body sensation in contact lens wearers	Tearing, severe pain	Redness, discharge, contact lens		×	Immediate removal of the contact lens, eye shield
Retinal detachment	Sudden loss of vision or field of vision, floaters, flashes of light	None or blunted red reflex	×		Bilateral eye patching, bed rest, "nothing by mouth" in anticipation of surgery
Sudden crossed eyes (adults)	Double vision	Crossed eyes		×	Glucose, head CT
Uveitis	Blurred vision, pain, tearing, floaters, photophobia	Hyperemia, anterior chamber cells, redness, vitritis, retinitis	×		
Scleritis	Severe pain with eye movement, photophobia	Diffuse or localized severe scleral injection, watery discharge	×		Oral nonsteroidal anti-inflammatory drugs, oral corticosteroid
Optic neuritis	Sudden loss of vision, severe pain with eye movement	Papillitis, afferent pupillary defect, change in color vision		×	IV (pulse) corticosteroid
Chemical burn	Severe pain, photophobia	Epithelial defect, chemosis, redness, whitening of cornea or conjunctiva		×	Copious irrigation with saline solution until pH of fornix neutralized, patch with antibiotic ointment

TABLE 5.3
OCULAR SIDE EFFECTS OF SYSTEMIC MEDICINES

Drug	Ocular Side Effect	Prevention and Monitoring	Therapy
Cidofovir	Uveitis and hypotony	Reduce dosage.	Topical corticosteroids and cycloplegics. If severe, discontinue cidofovir and switch to another agent.
Hydroxychloroquine (HC)/chloroquine (C)	Bull's-eye maculopathy	Baseline fundus exam, color plates, Amsler grid, ± visual field testing with red stimulus. Follow-up q6mo. Keep dose <6.5 mg/kg/day (HC) and <3 mg/kg/day (C).	Reduce dosage; discontinue.
Amiodarone	Corneal verticillata; green halos; ? optic neuropathy	Corneal changes usually visually insignificant. Association with optic neuropathy is weak.	Discontinue if cardiac risk is acceptable.
Tamoxifen	Maculopathy (edema and retinal crystals)	Baseline exam and q12mo follow-up. Keep dose <20 mg/day.	Reduce dosage; discontinue.
Sildenafil	Reversible ERG attenuation	Avoid high doses (>100 mg/day).	Reduce dosage; discontinue, especially with family history of retinitis pigmentosa.
Topiramate	Bilateral acute-angle closure glaucoma, acute myopia		Emergent referral to ophthalmology. Discontinue agent.
Anticholinergics	Pupillary dilation, may precipitate acute-angle closure glaucoma in pre-existing angle closure or narrow angles	Check with ophthalmologist before starting agent.	Discontinue if vision changes. Emergent referral if acute-angle closure.
Steroids	Cataract, glaucoma	Regular follow-up to check intraocular pressure.	Cataract surgery if necessary. Medical and surgical management of glaucoma.

ERG, electroretinography.
Adapted from Moorthy RS and Valluri S. Ocular toxicity associated with systemic drug therapy. *Current Opin Ophthalmol* 1999;10:438–446.

OCULAR SIDE EFFECTS OF SYSTEMIC DRUGS

See Table 5.3.

REVIEW EXERCISES

QUESTIONS

1. The most common cause of visual decline in a patient with diabetes mellitus is
a) Macular edema
b) Proliferative diabetic retinopathy
c) Diabetic papillopathy
d) Tractional retinal detachment

Answer and Discussion
The answer is a. In the Western Hemisphere, diabetic retinopathy is the leading cause of blindness in patients younger than 65 years. The leading cause of irreversible vision loss in patients with diabetes is macular edema.

2. The most appropriate initial intervention for a patient with a corneal ulcer is
a) No treatment
b) Corneal cultures and sensitivities
c) Eye patch
d) Broad-spectrum topical antibiotics four times a day

Answer and Discussion
The answer is b. Most corneal ulcers are caused by infections. People who wear contact lenses are at an increased risk of corneal ulcers. The risk of corneal ulcerations increases 10-fold when using extended-wear soft contact lenses. Patching is not indicated because it creates a warm, dark environment that allows bacterial growth. Antibiotic eye drops and oral pain medications are the mainstay of therapy.

3. The most common ocular manifestation in patients with rheumatoid arthritis is
a) Uveitis
b) Keratoconjunctivitis sicca
c) Conjunctivitis
d) Keratitis

Answer and Discussion

The answer is b. The most common ocular problem in patients with rheumatoid arthritis is keratoconjunctivitis sicca or secondary Sjögren's syndrome associated with connective tissue disease. Scleritis is the second most common ocular finding, occurring in 1% to 6% of patients with rheumatoid arthritis. Posterior segment lesions due to rheumatoid arthritis are rare.

4. In the Western Hemisphere, the leading cause of irreversible blindness in patients older than 65 years is
a) Cataract
b) Diabetic retinopathy
c) Glaucoma
d) Age-related macular degeneration

Answer and Discussion

The answer is d. In the Western Hemisphere, diabetic retinopathy is the leading cause of blindness in patients younger than 65 years; macular degeneration is the most common cause of irreversible blindness in patients older than 65 years.

5. Which of the following is a known cause of retinal detachment?
a) Diabetes
b) Cataract surgery
c) Ocular trauma
d) Severe nearsightedness (long eyeballs)
e) All of the above

Answer and Discussion

The answer is e. Retinal detachment occurs when the lining of the eye comes off, thus causing loss of vision. Causes of retinal detachment include ocular trauma, posterior vitreous detachment, traction from an inflamed vitreous, long eyeballs (as in very nearsighted people), family predisposition, degenerative changes in the retina, complications from diabetes, and complications of intraocular surgery, including cataract surgery.

SUGGESTED READINGS

Avery RL, Pearlman J, Pieramici DJ, et al. Intravitreal bevacizumab (Avastin) in the treatment of proliferative diabetic retinopathy. *Ophthalmology* 2006;113(10):1695–1705.

Bernstein HN. Ocular safety of hydroxychloroquine. *Ann Ophthalmol* 1991;23:292.

Digre KB. Principles and techniques of examination of the pupils, accommodation and lacrimation. In: Miller NR, Newman NJ, Biousse V, et al, eds. *Walsh and Hoyt Clinical Neuro-ophthalmology*, 6th ed. Baltimore: Williams & Wilkins, 2005:715.

Foroozan R, Deramo VA, Buono LM, et al. Recovery of visual function in patients with biopsy-proven giant cell arteritis. *Ophthalmology* 2003;110(3):539–542.

Frank RN. Diabetic retinopathy. *N Engl J Med* 2004;350(1):48–58.

Gillies MC, Sutter FK, Simpson JM, et al. Intravitreal triamcinolone for refractory diabetic macular edema: two-year results of a double-masked, placebo-controlled, randomized clinical trial. *Ophthalmology* 2006;113(9):1533–1538.

Kotoula MG, Koukoulis GN, Zintzaras E, et al. Metabolic control of diabetes is associated with an improved response of diabetic retinopathy to panretinal photocoagulation. *Diabetes Care* 2005;28(10):2454–2457.

Liozon E, Herrmann F, Ly K, et al. Risk factors for visual loss in giant cell (temporal) arteritis: a prospective study of 174 patients. *Am J Med* 2001;111(3):211–217.

Pepose J, Wilhelmus K, Holland GN, eds. *Ocular Infection and Immunity*. St. Louis, MO: Mosby–Yearbook, 1995.

Moorthy RS, Valluri S. Ocular toxicity associated with systemic drug therapy. *Curr Opin Ophthalmol* 1999;10:438–446.

Tay-Kearney ML, Schwam BL, Lowder C, et al. Clinical features and associated systemic diseases of HLA-B27 uveitis. *Am J Ophthalmol* 1996;121:47–56.

Wong T, Klein R, Islam FM, et al. Diabetic retinopathy in a multi-ethnic cohort in the United States. *Am J Ophthalmol* 2006;141(3):446–455.

Wong T, Mitchell P. The eye in hypertension. *Lancet* 2007;369(9559):425–435.

Chapter 6

Preoperative Evaluation and Management for Major Noncardiac Surgery

Amir K. Jaffer

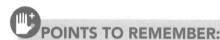

POINTS TO REMEMBER:

- The risk of a specific surgical procedure is proportional to the physiological stress associated with the procedure.

- Self-reported exercise tolerance is the key for cardiovascular risk stratification and is an independent predictor for postoperative cardiovascular complications.

- The frequency of pulmonary complications is higher than cardiovascular complications.

- The stress of anesthesia and surgery generally promotes hyperglycemia.

- Surgery increases the risk for the development of venous thromboembolism.

The primary aim of the preoperative evaluation is to assess and reduce perioperative risk through implementation of therapies that may help decrease perioperative morbidity and mortality, thereby improving patient outcomes and decreasing associated costs. Effective preoperative medical consultation depends on the internist's understanding of the issues faced by anesthesiologists and surgeons in planning and performing a surgical procedure and on communicating clear strategies to optimize the patient's medical status.

Perioperative risks fall into four major categories: *patient-specific, procedure-specific, anesthesia-specific,* and *provider-specific risks.* Patient-specific risks refer to patients' charac-

teristics (e.g., age, gender, race, level of fitness) and underlying medical conditions (e.g., diabetes, hypertension, coronary artery disease [CAD]). Optimization of these underlying conditions and identification of new risk factors or medical conditions that can be modified are some of the goals of the medical consultant.

The risk of a specific surgical procedure (procedure-specific risk) is proportional to the physiological stress associated with the procedure, as outlined in Table 6.1. Vascular procedures associated with major blood loss and/or that involve cross-clamping of the aorta cause the patient to experience the highest level of physiological stress and cardiac event risk of >5%. The intermediate level of risk is a cardiac event risk of 1% to 5% and is experienced by patients undergoing surgery (e.g., major joint replacement) where the blood loss is intermediate. The lowest level of risk occurs in minor procedures associated with minimal blood loss and physiological stress (e.g., breast biopsy) where the cardiac event risk is <1%.[1]

Modern anesthesia is generally safe, but there are anesthesia-specific risks that involve the direct and indirect effects of anesthetic agents in the context of the physiological responses to surgically induced hypotension, blood loss, anemia, and postoperative pain. During anesthesia induction, tachycardia and hypertension occur in response to anxiety and the mechanical effects of tracheal manipulation with intubation. Ten percent of cardiac events occur during this time. Later hypotension may occur as a result of vasodilation and myocardial depression associated with anesthetic agents, intermittent positive-pressure ventilation, hemorrhage, or infection. Balanced anesthetic

TABLE 6.1

CARDIAC RISK (NONFATAL MYOCARDIAL INFARCTION OR DEATH) STRATIFICATION FOR NONCARDIAC SURGICAL PROCEDURES

Vascular (reported cardiac risk often >5%)
- Emergent major operations, particularly in the elderly
- Aortic and other major vascular surgery
- Peripheral vascular surgery

Intermediate (reported cardiac risk generally 1%–5%)
- Carotid endarterectomy
- Head and neck surgery
- Intraperitoneal and intrathoracic surgery
- Orthopedic surgery
- Prostate surgery

Low (reported cardiac risk generally <1%)
- Endoscopic procedures
- Superficial procedure
- Cataract
- Breast

Adapted from Fleisher LA, Beckman JA, Brown KA, et al. ACC/AHA 2007 guidelines on perioperative cardiovascular evaluation and care for noncardiac surgery: a report of the American College of Cardiology/American Heart Association Task Force on Practice Guidelines (Writing Committee to Revise the 2002 Guidelines on Perioperative Cardiovascular Evaluation for Noncardiac Surgery): developed in collaboration with the American Society of Echocardiography, American Society of Nuclear Cardiology, Heart Rhythm Society, Society of Cardiovascular Anesthesiologists, Society for Cardiovascular Angiography and Interventions, Society for Vascular Medicine and Biology, and Society for Vascular Surgery. *Circulation* 2007;116(17):e418–e499.

techniques using opiates, sedative hypnotics, neuromuscular blockers, and inhalation agents cause fewer cardiovascular effects than with inhalation agents alone. Most anesthetic deaths are due to failure to ventilate adequately, unsuspected hypoxia, or anesthetic agent overdose. There is no single best anesthetic technique to reduce cardiac risk. One meta-analysis found that epidural or spinal anesthesia reduced the risk of mortality, thromboembolic complications, myocardial infarction (MI), transfusion requirements, pneumonia, and respiratory depression compared with general anesthesia.[2]

Provider-specific risk is related to the experience of the surgeon and/or the surgical team, and may vary according to their volume and expertise with that procedure. The medical consultant cannot modify this risk.

MANAGING CARDIOVASCULAR RISK

Overall risk of postoperative cardiac death or major cardiac complications is less than 6% in patients older than 40 years who are undergoing major noncardiac surgeries.[3] However, approximately 8 million individuals undergoing surgical procedures each year have known CAD or coronary risk factors,[4] and approximately 1 million individuals will have some perioperative cardiac complications.

The most common cardiovascular complications are the following:

- Perioperative acute ischemia and MI
- Congestive heart failure (CHF)
- Arrhythmias
- Hypotension
- Hypertension

In the early postoperative period, pain, hypotension, and increased catecholamines with associated tachycardia may lead to cardiovascular stress by increasing myocardial oxygen demand and coronary vascular tone. The catecholamine effects may also increase plaque instability and, with enhanced platelet aggregation and hypercoagulability owing to tissue injury, elevate the risk of coronary thrombosis. Limited cardiovascular reserve, particularly in elderly patients, increases the risk of a cardiac event. The incidence of MI peaks on the third postoperative day, and increased risk persists for up to 6 months after surgery. The greatest risk for acute pulmonary edema is in patients with known CHF; this risk occurs especially in the first few hours after anesthesia when anesthesia-induced hypotension abates and fluid resorption is most vigorous.

The critical first step in the cardiac evaluation of the patient having noncardiac surgery is identifying the need for surgery. Patients undergoing emergency surgery need to go to the operating room as soon as possible and receive perioperative surveillance and postoperative risk stratification and management. The second step is to evaluate the patient's clinical features, including the presence of unstable symptoms referred to as "active cardiac conditions" by the American College of Cardiology and American Heart Association (ACC/AHA) guidelines.[1] There is evidence that decompensated CHF, significant arrhythmias, severe valvular disease, or unstable coronary syndromes are associated with increased perioperative cardiac morbidity. A high index of suspicion may also identify individuals with occult symptoms. For example, dyspnea may be the only manifestation of underlying CAD. Identification and management of active cardiac conditions before elective surgery will greatly reduce postoperative cardiac morbidity.

In an attempt to quantify the preoperative risk in patients with known or suspected cardiac disease, several multivariate indices of risk have been developed. Some of the more well-known and studied indices include the Goldman Cardiac Risk Index (Table 6.2), Detsky Modified Risk Index (Table 6.3), and revised Goldman Cardiac Risk Index, also called the Lee Risk Index (Table 6.4). The role of the risk indices is to assist physicians in identifying low-, intermediate-, and high-risk patients for postoperative cardiac complications. Indices developed by Eagle et al.[5] (Table 6.5) and Vanzetto et al.[6] supported the usefulness of preoperative dipyridamole-thallium imaging (DTI) and clinical variables in predicting ischemic events after vascular surgery.

TABLE 6.2
CARDIAC RISK INDEX

Clinical Features	Points
Age older than 70 years	5
Myocardial infarction <6 months	10
S_3 gallop or jugular venous distension	11
Important valvular aortic stenosis	3
Non–sinus rhythm, premature atrial contractions or >5 premature ventricular contractions/minute	7
PO_2 <60 or PCO_2 >50 mm Hg, K <3.0 or HCO_3 <20 mEq/L, blood urea nitrogen >50 or creatinine >3.0 mg/dL, abnormal SGOT, signs of chronic liver disease, or patients bedridden from noncardiac cause	3
Intraperitoneal, intrathoracic, or aortic operation	3
Emergency operation	4

Risk Assessment

Class	Points	Risk
I	0–5	0.7% Complication 0.2% Death
II	6–12	5.0% Complication 2.0% Death
III	13–25	11% Complication 2.0% Death
IV	26+	22% Complication 56% Death

Adapted with permission from Goldman L, Caldera DL, Nussbaum SR, et al. Multifactorial index of cardiac risk in noncardiac surgical procedures. *N Engl J Med* 1977;297(16):845–850.

TABLE 6.3
MODIFIED MULTIFACTORIAL INDEX

Clinical Features	Points
Myocardial infarction (MI) <6 months	10
MI >6 months	5
Angina—class 3 unstable	10
Angina—class 4	20
Pulmonary edema	
■ Within 1 week	10
■ Ever	5
Critical aortic stenosis	20
Non–sinus rhythm, premature atrial contractions or >5 premature ventricular contractions	5
Age older than 70 years	5
Emergency operation	10
Poor general medical condition	5

Pretest Probabilities for Types of Surgeries

Major Surgery	Number of Severe Cardiac Complications (%)	95% Confidence Limits
Vascular	10/79 (13.2)	6.5–19.7
Orthopedic	9/66 (13.6)	6.0–21.2
Intrathoracic/ intraperitoneal	7/88 (8.0)	3.4–13.6
Head and neck	1/38 (2.6)	0.3–16.4
Minor surgery (e.g., transurethral, prostatectomies, cataracts)	3/187 (1.6)	0.5–1.6

Adapted with permission from Detsky AS, Abrams HB, Forbath N, et al. Cardiac assessment for patients undergoing noncardiac surgery: a multifactorial clinical risk index. *Arch Intern Med* 1986;146(11):2131–2134.

In 1977, Goldman et al. published a landmark study evaluating 1,001 patients undergoing noncardiac surgery.[3] Nine independent correlates of perioperative fatal or major nonfatal cardiac events were identified and assigned a certain number of points. Patients were then placed in four classes, depending on the total number of points. In class IV (highest risk category), 78% of patients had a major cardiac event compared to less than 1% of patients in class 1 (lowest risk category). The Cardiac Risk Index developed from this study (Table 6.3) divides patients into high- and low-risk categories, but a large group of patients are in the intermediate-risk category, where there is still a 9% chance of major cardiac event. Other limitations of this index include that relatively few vascular surgery patients were included in the study; it was developed in the mid-1970s and does not take into account advances in medical, anesthetic, or surgical care; and the data were only collected at one institution.

The Modified Multifactorial Index by Detsky et al.[7] (Table 6.3) modified the Goldman Cardiac Risk Index by assigning a higher score to emergency surgery and recent MI (<6 months) and including angina and pulmonary edema in the index. However, like the Goldman Cardiac Risk Index, Detsky et al. may also underestimate the cardiac risk in vascular patients.

The revised Goldman Cardiac Risk Index, also referred to as the Lee Risk Index[8] (Table 6.4), seeks to simplify the original criteria. In a prospective study of 4,315 patients at or older than 50 years undergoing elective major noncardiac surgeries, Lee et al.[8] identified six independent predictors of perioperative complications—namely, high-risk type of surgery, history of ischemic heart disease, history of CHF, history of stroke or transient ischemic attack, diabetes on insulin, and preoperative serum creatinine of >2 mg/dL—and assigned them 1 point each. Table 6.5 shows the rate of complication in each risk category during this study. This index appears to be more accurate than older indices in predicting major postoperative cardiac complications.[9]

The third step during the preoperative evaluation is to determine the patient's functional class. Self-reported exercise tolerance is the key for cardiovascular risk stratification and is an independent predictor for postoperative cardiovascular complications.[10] The Duke Activity Status Index[11] (Table 6.6) is one way of dividing patients into four functional classes (I–IV) based on their activity level that can help generate an estimate of their metabolic equivalents (METS). The ability to perform >4 METS of activity has been associated with a lower cardiovascular risk.[10]

TABLE 6.4

REVISED GOLDMAN CARDIAC RISK INDEX (LEE RISK INDEX)

High-risk type of surgery: intraperitoneal, intrathoracic, or suprainguinal vascular procedure

History of ischemic heart disease: history of myocardial infarction, positive exercise stress test, current complaint of ischemic chest pain or use of nitrate therapy, or ECG with Q waves. Patients with prior coronary artery bypass grafting or percutaneous transluminal coronary angioplasty were included only if they had current complaints of chest pain presumed due to ischemia

History of congestive heart failure: history of congestive heart failure, pulmonary edema, or paroxysmal nocturnal dyspnea, physical examination with bilateral rales or S_3, or chest radiograph showing pulmonary vascular redistribution

History of cerebrovascular disease

Diabetes mellitus treated with insulin

Preoperative serum creatinine >2 mg/dL

Revised Cardiac Risk Class	Number of Risk Factors	Major Cardiac Events	Rate (%)
I	0	5/1,071	0.5
II	1	14/1,106	1.3
III	2	18/506	3.6
IV	>3	19/210	9.1

From Lee TH, Marcantonio ER, Mangione CM, et al. Derivation and prospective validation of a simple index for prediction of cardiac risk of major noncardiac surgery. *Circulation* 2001;100:1043–1049.

TABLE 6.5

DIPYRIDAMOLE-THALLIUM IMAGING TO PREDICT POSTOPERATIVE CARDIAC ISCHEMIA

Clinical Group[a]	Postoperative	Event[b]
0 Factors	2/64	(3%)
1–2 Factors and − thallium	2/62	(3%)
1–2 Factors and + thallium	16/54	(30%)
3+ Factors	10/24	(50%)

[a]Factors including age older than 70 years, history of angina, history of VEA requiring treatment, diabetes mellitus on therapy, and Q wave on ECG.
[b]Cardiac death, myocardial infarction, ischemic pulmonary edema, unstable angina.
Adapted with permission from Eagle KA, Coley CM, Newell JB, et al. Combining clinical and thallium data optimizes preoperative assessment of cardiac risk before major vascular surgery. *Ann Intern Med* 1989;110(11):859.

The first three evaluation steps determine the need for noninvasive testing (step 4). Patients who are at low risk based on clinical features, good functional status (i.e., >4 METS), and proposed low-risk surgery do not generally require any further evaluation. However, patients who are deemed higher risk using clinical features developed by Lee et al.[8] (Table 6.4) (excluding high-risk surgery) and scheduled for vascular or intermediate-risk surgery would benefit from noninvasive testing if it will change management per the ACC/AHA guidelines (Fig. 6.1). In addition, patients with unreliable histories and poor functional status from vascular or orthopedic disease may make the assessment of angina difficult. In such patients, noninvasive cardiac testing may also be useful.

The fourth step is to determine the patient's surgery-specific risk, and Table 6.1 groups surgical procedures into three different categories labeled as vascular (reported cardiac risk >5%), intermediate (reported cardiac risk 1%–5%), and low (cardiac risk <1%).

TABLE 6.6

EVALUATION OF FUNCTIONAL STATUS USING SPECIFIC ACTIVITIES: THE DUKE ACTIVITY STATUS INDEX

Activity	Estimated Metabolic Cost of Each Activity (METS)
Can you...	
■ Walk indoors, such as around your house?	1.75
■ Do light work around the house, such as dusting or washing dishes?	2.70
■ Take care of yourself (i.e., eating, dressing, bathing, using the toilet)?	2.75
■ Walk a block or two on level ground?	2.75
■ Do moderate work around the house such as vacuuming, sweeping floors, or carrying in groceries?	3.50
■ Do yard work such as raking leaves, weeding, or pushing a power mower?	4.50
■ Have sexual relations?	5.25
■ Climb a flight of stairs or walk up a hill?	5.50
■ Participate in moderate recreational activities, such as golf, bowling, dancing, doubles tennis, or throwing a baseball or football?	6.00
	7.50
■ Participate in strenuous sports, such as swimming, singles tennis, football, basketball, or skiing?	8.00
■ Do heavy work around the house, such as scrubbing floors or lifting or moving heavy furniture?	8.00
■ Run a short distance?	

Reproduced with permission from Hlatky MA, Boineau RE, Higginbotham MB, et al. A brief self-administered questionnaire to determine functional capacity (the Duke Activity Status Index). *Am J Cardiol* 1989;64(10):651–654.

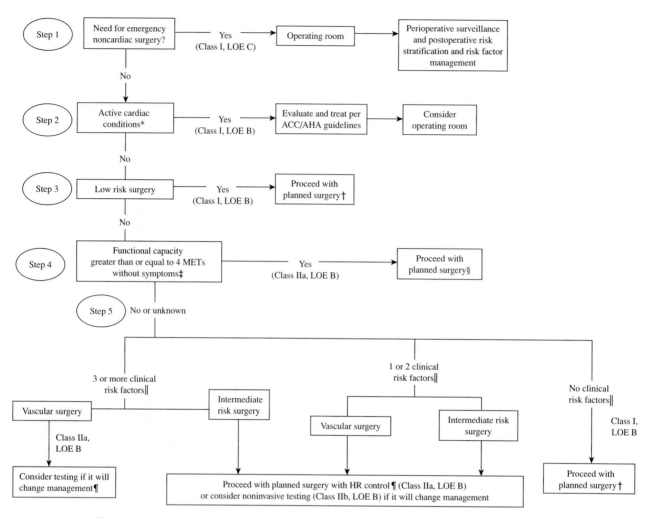

Figure 6.1 Stepwise approach to preoperative cardiac assessment. *Source:* Fleisher LA, Beckman JA, Brown KA, et al. ACC/AHA 2007 guidelines on perioperative cardiovascular evaluation and care for noncardiac surgery: a report of the American College of Cardiology/American Heart Association Task Force on Practice Guidelines (Writing Committee to Revise the 2002 Guidelines on Perioperative Cardiovascular Evaluation for Noncardiac Surgery): developed in collaboration with the American Society of Echocardiography, American Society of Nuclear Cardiology, Heart Rhythm Society, Society of Cardiovascular Anesthesiologists, Society for Cardiovascular Angiography and Interventions, Society for Vascular Medicine and Biology, and Society for Vascular Surgery. *Circulation* 2007;116(17): e418–e499.

In patients who can exercise, exercise stress testing can accurately stratify cardiovascular risk in patients undergoing major vascular surgery. Patients who achieve 75% of maximally predicted heart rate (HR) without ECG changes are low risk for cardiac complications.[4] DTI can accurately predict cardiac complications in selected patients undergoing vascular surgery. In patients with one or two risk factors (intermediate risk), a positive test is associated with a high cardiac complication rate, and a negative test is associated with a substantially lower rate (Table 6.5).[5] Data are limited in nonvascular surgery patients, but it is likely that DTI may be useful in the intermediate-risk patients as defined by the AHA/ACC guidelines.

Dobutamine stress echocardiography (DSE) may be useful in both intermediate- and high-risk patients, as defined by the AHA/ACC guidelines. In the largest study of

preoperative DSE undergoing vascular surgery, a normal test was associated with a very low cardiac complication rate.[12] In a meta-analysis of six noninvasive tests, DSE showed a positive trend toward better diagnostic performance than the other tests, but this was only significant in the comparison with myocardial perfusion scintigraph.[13] DSE should be avoided in patients with significant arrhythmias, very high or low blood pressures, and critical aortic stenosis.

The fifth step is to optimize medical therapy preoperatively, and this includes, but is not limited to, titrating medications to better control blood pressure and initiating beta-blocker therapy on those patients who would benefit from this therapy. Details regarding beta-blocker therapy are discussed in the section on this topic.

Management of Nonischemic Cardiac Disease

Hypertension

Patients with hypertension have a higher incidence of silent CAD and previous MI than the general population. Traditionally, surgery was delayed for patients presenting with diastolic blood pressure (DBP) >110 mm Hg, but review of the literature shows that these patients may be at increased risk for hemodynamic lability, not necessarily for MI. Chronic antihypertensive medications can be continued in the perioperative period with some exceptions for the morning of surgery, which are discussed as follows. Preoperatively, a systolic blood pressure >180 mm Hg and DBP >110 mm Hg are definite indications for preoperative intervention.

Heart Failure

Patients with clinically stable heart failure (HF) did not have high perioperative mortality rates in association with elective major noncardiac surgery, but they were more likely than patients without HF to have longer hospital stays and require hospital readmission, and had a substantial long-term mortality rate.[14] Therefore, it is important to stabilize HF prior to surgery and delay surgery if necessary. Optimizing medical management of patients with CHF is critical prior to elective surgeries, and if the surgery is emergent, invasive monitoring may be useful.

Cardiac Murmurs

When a murmur is detected on physical examination as part of the preoperative evaluation, one should try to ascertain the chronicity of the murmur and determine whether the murmur is functional or structural. If the murmur is believed to be functional, then a search for anemia, thyroid disorders, and other causes should be initiated. Evaluation by echocardiography is recommended for all diagnosed murmurs if none has been previously performed. Echocardiography can help determine the severity of the lesion and appropriate medical management as needed. Aortic stenosis increases the risk of perioperative mortality[15] and nonfatal MI by fivefold, regardless of the presence of the other revised cardiac risk index criteria.

Infective endocarditis prophylaxis for dental procedures is reasonable only for patients with underlying cardiac conditions associated with the highest risk of adverse outcome from infective endocarditis. This would include those with prosthetic valves or material, previous infective endocarditis, congenital heart disease, and cardiac transplant patients with valvular heart disease. For patients with these underlying cardiac conditions, prophylaxis is reasonable for all dental procedures that involve manipulation of gingival tissue or the periapical region of teeth, or perforation of the oral mucosa. Prophylaxis is not recommended based solely on an increased lifetime risk of acquisition of infective endocarditis. Administration of antibiotics solely to prevent endocarditis is not recommended for patients who undergo a genitourinary or gastrointestinal tract procedure.[16]

Beta-Blockers, Statins, and Reduction of Cardiac Events

Initial studies evaluating beta-blocker therapy during the perioperative period suggested that beta-blockers may be beneficial in reducing cardiac deaths and MIs. Later studies and recent meta-analyses, however, are less favorable, and suggest that beta-blockers may be associated with increased incidence of bradycardia and hypotension. Therefore, based on the available evidence and guidelines, patients currently taking beta-blockers should continue these agents. Patients undergoing vascular surgery who are at high cardiac risk should also take beta-blockers.[17] Current evidence would suggest that effective control of HR is associated with a reduced incidence of postoperative MI, suggesting that effective control of HR is important for achieving cardioprotection.[18]

One randomized trial and several cohort studies have found a significant reduction in cardiovascular complications with perioperative statin therapy. In addition, statin withdrawal is associated with increased postoperative cardiac risk. Statins should also be continued in patients already taking these agents prior to surgery. The optimal duration and time of initiation of statin therapy remains unclear.[17]

POSTOPERATIVE PULMONARY COMPLICATIONS

Postoperative pulmonary complications (PPC) may include atelectasis, infection (tracheobronchitis or pneumonia), acute respiratory failure requiring mechanical ventilation, acute exacerbation of underlying lung disease, and bronchospasm. The frequency of pulmonary complications is higher than cardiovascular complications. Risk factors for PPC include smoking, poor exercise tolerance, chronic obstructive pulmonary disease (COPD), surgical site (the risk of PPC increases as the incision approaches the diaphragm), surgery duration longer than 3 hours, general anesthesia, and use of intraoperative pancuronium.[19] Most pulmonary complications are the result of alteration of normal pulmonary physiology. Postoperative pain may cause splinting, and the residual effects of anesthesia and narcotics may impair cough and mucociliary clearance of respiratory secretions. In addition, altered pulmonary mechanics and altered pattern of breathing postoperatively may lead to a PPC.

Preoperative pulmonary risk reduction strategies[19] include the following:

- Encouraging patients to stop smoking for at least 8 weeks before surgery. Practically, this may never be possible because often the patients may not undergo a preoperative evaluation until a few weeks prior to surgery.
- Treating airflow obstruction with beta-agonists and steroids in patients with COPD or asthma.

■ Using antibiotics and delaying surgery for about 6 weeks if upper respiratory or pulmonary infection is present.

■ Educating patients preoperatively regarding lung expansion exercises and the techniques and use of incentive spirometry postoperatively.

PREOPERATIVE PULMONARY TESTING

In general, there is no single test or combination of tests that will reliably predict pulmonary complications. Preoperative history should focus on exercise tolerance, chronic cough, or unexplained dyspnea. Preoperative pulmonary function tests (PFTs) are not useful for noncardiothoracic surgery, except in cases where there is a significant smoking history, unexplained dyspnea, or uncharacterized lung disease, in which case preoperative PFTs may help provide a diagnosis or evaluate the degree of impairment. Forced expiratory volume in 1 second (FEV_1) remains a good indicator of surgical risk. If the FEV_1 is >2 L, the risk of complications is low. An FEV_1 <1 L is associated with a high risk of pulmonary complications or prolonged ventilation, whereas patients with an FEV_1 between 1 and 2 L have a moderately elevated risk that must be weighed against the need for the procedure.

These are the ACP guidelines for situations in which preoperative spirometry is indicated:[20]

■ Lung resection

■ Coronary artery bypass surgery and smoking history or dyspnea

■ Upper abdominal surgery and smoking history or dyspnea

■ Lower abdominal surgery and uncharacterized pulmonary disease, particularly if the surgery will be prolonged or extensive

■ Other surgery and uncharacterized pulmonary disease, particularly in those who might require strenuous postoperative rehabilitation programs

Arterial blood gases are generally not indicated preoperatively, except perhaps in patients planned for lung resection or in patients with underlying lung disease or risk for lung disease who have dyspnea. Small case series have asserted that $PaCO_2$ >45 mm Hg suggests limited pulmonary reserve and increased risk for PPC. However, clinicians should not use arterial blood gas analyses to delay surgery.[19]

Perhaps the most comprehensive risk index is the one developed by Arozullah et al.[21] This is a multifactorial risk index for postoperative respiratory failure that was derived and validated from a large Veterans Administration database. The factors in this index are listed in Table 6.7. The total points are added to develop a risk score, and patients are assigned in classes 1 to 5. Patients in Class 1 are at significantly lower risk for respiratory failure than patients in class 5. Type of surgery, emergency surgery, and

TABLE 6.7

RESPIRATORY FAILURE RISK INDEX

Preoperative Predictor	Point Value
Type of surgery	
Abdominal aortic aneurysm	27
Thoracic	21
Neurosurgery, upper abdominal, or peripheral vascular	14
Neck	11
Emergency surgery	11
Albumin 3 mg/dL	9
Blood urea nitrogen >30 mg/dL	8
Partially or fully dependent functional status	7
History of chronic obstructive pulmonary disease	6
Age	
Older than 70 years	6
60–69 years	4

Class	Points	N (%)	Rate of Respiratory Failure (%)
1	≤10	48	0.5
2	11–19	23	2.1
3	20–27	17	5.3
4	28–40	10	11.9
5	>40	2	30.9

Adapted with permission from Arozullah et al. *Am Surg* 2000; 232:242.

metabolic factors play large roles in predicting postoperative respiratory failure. In addition to developing an index to assess risk of postoperative respiratory failure, Arozullah et al. have also developed a similar index to assess the risk for postoperative pneumonia. Type of surgery, age, and functional status appear to be the most predictive factors for postoperative pneumonia.

In general, a careful history and physical exam are key in identifying potential PPC. Lung expansion maneuvers, including deep breathing and incentive spirometry, are the mainstays in postoperative prevention of pulmonary complications. Medical optimization of COPD and asthma will reduce the risk of postoperative complications significantly.

DIABETES MELLITUS

Advances in surgical management now mean patients have shorter preoperative and postoperative hospital stays, increasing the challenge of perioperative management of patients with diabetes mellitus. The patient with diabetes carries a cardiac event risk that is equivalent to the nondiabetic patient with known ischemic heart disease. Evaluation of the patient with diabetes must include the careful assessment of long-term complications, particularly renal, cardiovascular, and neuropathic complications that add to overall risk. A key factor in planning the pre- and intraoperative care of patients with diabetes is careful coordination of the management with the anesthesiologist. The stress of anesthesia and surgery generally promotes hyperglycemia by increasing the counterregulatory hormones epinephrine, cortisol, glucagon, and growth hormone. It is desirable to maintain intraoperative glucoses in the range of 150 to 200 mg/dL, to avoid both hypoglycemia and hyperglycemia. Hyperglycemia above 250 to 300 mg/dL is associated with osmotic diuresis and increased vascular instability. Preoperative glucose levels >300 mg/dL cause an osmotic diuresis, complicating volume management. Therefore, surgery should usually be delayed until the fasting glucose is <200 mg/dL. In type 2 diabetes mellitus treated with diet alone, supplemental short-acting insulin is used to maintain glucoses in the therapeutic range if needed. For patients with type 2 diabetes mellitus treated with oral agents, these medications are taken the day before surgery, but held on the morning of surgery. Short-acting intravenous (IV) insulin may be used intraoperatively and in the postoperative period, especially with major surgery or in poorly controlled diabetics on oral therapy. Renal function should be monitored in those patients receiving contrast media or having borderline renal insufficiency before restarting metformin after surgery. In those patients with type 1 or type 2 diabetes mellitus using insulin, the timing and expected duration of the procedure and the usual insulin regimen must be considered when planning therapy. For early morning minor procedures, just delaying the usual daily therapy until after surgery may be appropriate. If the patient uses insulin, then one-third to one-half of the usual dose is given before the planned surgery for minor procedures. For patients undergoing major surgery, the anesthesiologist monitors glucose control intraoperatively and uses IV insulin.[22] There is increasing evidence of the benefit of tight blood sugar control in the postoperative period in reducing complications.

THYROID DISORDERS

Patients with pre-existing hypothyroidism should be questioned as to recent changes in therapy, symptoms of hypo- or hyperthyroidism, and results of any recent thyroid tests. Newly diagnosed hypothyroid patients do not need to be treated before surgery unless signs of severe hypothyroidism or myxedema are present. It is not essential for patients to take their thyroid replacement on the morning of surgery.

Patients currently under treatment for hyperthyroidism should take their antithyroid drugs on the day of surgery and resume therapy as soon as possible because these drugs have a short half-life. Elective surgery should be postponed until hyperthyroid patients become euthyroid because of

TABLE 6.8

RECOMMENDED PERIOPERATIVE HYDROCORTISONE DOSAGE FOR PATIENTS ON LONG-TERM STEROID THERAPY

Surgery Type	Stress Dose (mg/day)	Duration[a] (days)
Minor (e.g., inguinal herniorrhaphy)	25	1
Moderate (e.g., total joint replacement)	50–75	1–2
Major (e.g., cardiopulmonary bypass)	100–150	2–3

[a]In the absence of complications.
Reproduced with permission from Shaw M. *Cleve Clin J Med* 2002;69(1):9–11.

the mortality associated with "thyroid storm." Patients with hyperthyroidism or severe hypothyroidism should be managed in conjunction with an endocrinologist preoperatively and perhaps perioperatively.

CHRONIC STEROID USAGE

Patients receiving ≥5 mg of prednisone or its equivalent daily for more than 2 weeks over the past year are at risk for adrenal insufficiency during stress after cessation of steroid therapy. Given the degree of morbidity and mortality associated with adrenal insufficiency, prophylactic glucocorticoids are outlined in Table 6.8.

DELIRIUM RISK

The incidence of postoperative delirium is in the range of 10% to 15% and is associated with higher mortality and poor functional recovery. The costs of care increase substantially when an acute confusional state complicates postoperative recovery. Marcantonio et al.[23] developed and validated a clinical prediction rule for the postoperative development of delirium. The findings were confirmed and slightly modified by Litaker et al.[24] Independent correlates of delirium risk included age older than 70 years; pre-existing cognitive impairment; previous episodes of delirium; self-reported alcohol use; poor functional status; markedly abnormal serum sodium, potassium, or glucose level; noncardiac chest surgery; and aortic abdominal surgery. Assessing risk allows for potential interventions to reduce delirium incidence. In addition to correcting preoperative metabolic abnormalities, the best preventive intervention is to avoid psychotropic drug use and hypoxia perioperatively, and pay careful attention to managing perioperative metabolic abnormalities, particularly in those patients identified as high risk.

TABLE 6.9

RECOMMENDATIONS FOR LABORATORY TESTING BEFORE ELECTIVE SURGERY

Test	Incidence of Abnormalities That Influence Management (%)	Indications
Hemoglobin	0.1	Anticipated major blood loss or symptoms of anemia
White blood cell count	0.0	Symptoms suggest infection, myeloproliferative disorder, or myelotoxic medications
Platelet count	0.0	History of bleeding diathesis, myeloproliferative disorder, or myelotoxic medications
Prothrombin time	0.0	History of bleeding diathesis, chronic liver disease, malnutrition, recent or long-term antibiotic use
Partial thromboplastin time	0.1	History of bleeding diathesis
Electrolytes	1.8	Known renal insufficiency, congestive heart failure, medications that affect electrolytes
Renal function	2.6	Age older than 50 years, hypertension, cardiac disease, major surgery, medications that may affect renal function
Glucose	0.5	Obesity or known diabetes
Liver function tests	0.1	No indication; consider albumin measurement for major surgery or chronic illness
Urinalysis	1.4	No indication
ECG	2.6	Men older than 40 years, women older than 50 years; known coronary artery disease, diabetes, or hypertension
Chest radiograph	3.0	Age older than 50 years, known cardiac or pulmonary disease, symptoms or exam suggest cardiac or pulmonary disease

Adapted with permission from Smetana GW and Macpherson DS. The case against routine testing. *Med Clin North Am* 2003;87(1):7–40.

PREOPERATIVE LABORATORY STUDIES

The goals of preoperative testing are to identify and minimize the risk factors for surgery. Potential reasons for ordering preoperative laboratory tests are (a) to detect unsuspected abnormalities that might influence the risk of perioperative morbidity or mortality, and (b) to establish a baseline value for a test that will be monitored or altered after the surgery is complete. Existing literature suggests that 30% to 60% of abnormalities discovered on routine preoperative tests are ignored.[25] Given this fact, routine preoperative testing without documentation of abnormalities may actually lead to more medicolegal risk. In general, it is safe to use test results that were performed and were normal within the past 4 months given that no change has occurred in the patient's clinical status. Macpherson and Litaker reported that only 0.4% of such tests repeated at the time of surgery were abnormal and could have been predicted by the patient's history.[26] Table 6.9 provides some evidence-based recommendations for laboratory testing before elective surgery.

MANAGEMENT OF MEDICATIONS

There are few controlled trials on the safety of drugs in the perioperative period. Therefore, the recommendations on which medications to stop or continue during this time are based on expert consensus, case reports, in vitro studies, manufacturer's recommendations in the package insert, and, finally, on known information such as the drug's pharmacokinetics, known effects, perioperative risks, and possible interactions with anesthetic agents.[27] In addition, it is key to take a detailed history to include not only prescribed medications, but also over-the-counter medications, vitamins, and herbal supplements. A recent review found that one-third of the presurgical population was taking an herbal medication; it concluded that physicians should explicitly elicit and document a history of herbal medication, and be aware of the potentially serious perioperative problems associated with their continued use.[28] Potentially harmful perioperative effects of some herbs include excessive bleeding, sedation, and even hypoglycemia. As a general rule, we recommend all herbal remedies and vitamins be stopped 14 days prior to surgery.

Aspirin irreversibly inhibits platelet cyclo-oxygenase and should be discontinued 7 to 10 days before surgery to allow replacement of the circulating platelet pool. In patients undergoing coronary artery bypass surgery, a prospective study showed that continuing aspirin leads to increased postoperative bleeding.[29]

Nonsteroidal anti-inflammatory drugs (NSAIDs) reversibly inhibit the platelet cyclo-oxygenase. Most NSAIDs can be stopped 3 to 5 days before surgery, except some long-acting drugs such as piroxicam and oxaprozin, which must be stopped 14 days prior to surgery. In vitro studies show no increased risk of bleeding with cyclo-oxygenase-2

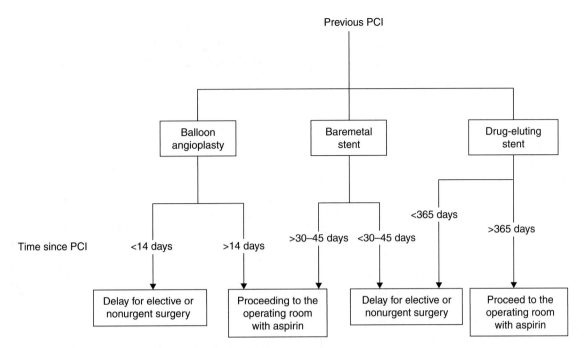

Figure 6.2 Proposed approach to patients with previous percutaneous coronary intervention. *Source:* Fleisher LA, Beckman JA, Brown KA, et al. ACC/AHA 2007 guidelines on perioperative cardiovascular evaluation and care for noncardiac surgery: a report of the American College of Cardiology/American Heart Association Task Force on Practice Guidelines (Writing Committee to Revise the 2002 Guidelines on Perioperative Cardiovascular Evaluation for Noncardiac Surgery): developed in collaboration with the American Society of Echocardiography, American Society of Nuclear Cardiology, Heart Rhythm Society, Society of Cardiovascular Anesthesiologists, Society for Cardiovascular Angiography and Interventions, Society for Vascular Medicine and Biology, and Society for Vascular Surgery. *Circulation* 2007;116(17):e418–e499.

inhibitors; therefore, theoretically, these can be continued perioperatively. However, because all NSAIDs can inhibit renal prostaglandin synthesis, they can induce renal failure in combination with other drugs and hypotension. Therefore, it may be best to stop all NSAIDs in patients with underlying renal insufficiency.

Clopidogrel causes irreversible antiplatelet effect by inhibiting adenosine diphosphate–induced stimulation of platelets. Therefore, it should be discontinued at least 7 days before surgery. However, with increasingly more patients on this drug because of drug-eluting stents, and due to the fact that premature cessation of this drug in these patients can increase the risk for catastrophic stent thrombosis, death, and MI, it has been recommended that patients undergoing elective surgery with this type of surgery have their procedure delayed unless the procedure can be done on dual antiplatelet therapy. A proposed approach to the management of patients with previous PCI who require noncardiac surgery is outlined in **Figure 6.2**.

Hormone replacement therapy (HRT) use is associated with a 2.7-fold increased risk of venous thromboembolism (VTE) compared to nonusers.[30] However, the perioperative management of HRT is still controversial. Some still recommend stopping HRT about 4 weeks before surgery; however, we recently completed a case-control study that found no association between perioperative HRT use and postoperative VTE in patients undergoing major orthopedic surgery as long as they were receiving pharma-

cologic prophylaxis with either enoxaparin or warfarin postoperatively.[31]

Among cardiovascular medications, all forms of nitrates, digoxin, beta-blockers, calcium channel blockers, statins, and antiarrhythmic can be safely continued, including on the morning of surgery. However, diuretics, angiotensin-converting enzyme inhibitors, and angiotensin receptor antagonists should be held on the morning of surgery[32,33] due to reports of refractory hypotension.

Pulmonary medications such as theophylline, inhaled beta-agonists, ipratropium, and corticosteroids can be safely continued perioperatively. In addition, all antiseizure medications, H_2-blockers, and proton pump inhibitors should also be continued perioperatively.

Among the antidepressants, selective serotonin reuptake inhibitors are safe perioperatively. Monoamine oxidase inhibitors have a large number of drug interactions and potential for hypertensive crisis. Tricyclic antidepressants may enhance the action of sympathomimetics. Patients on these last two classes of medications usually have more severe depression, and there is the potential for these patients to have a severe recurrence of depressive symptoms postoperatively with increased risk for suicide. Therefore, in our own practice, we tend to continue all antidepressants but alert anesthesiologists to these medications so that potentially interacting sedatives and/or anesthetics can be avoided.

Warfarin is a commonly used anticoagulant. Most patients needing major surgery or invasive procedures will require discontinuation of warfarin. It takes approximately 5 days for the antithrombotic effect of warfarin to wear off.[34] Therefore, in many patients with preoperative international normalized ratios (INRs) between 2 and 3, warfarin can be discontinued 5 days before surgery. During this time, patients may be at increased risk of thromboembolism. In addition, discontinuation of oral anticoagulation may be associated with a rebound hypercoagulable state, which has been described but not validated in clinical practice. Surgery increases the risk for the development of VTE. To minimize the risk of thromboembolism, some higher-risk patients may require treatment with IV unfractionated heparin in the hospital, or as outpatients with subcutaneous low molecular weight heparin as a bridge to surgery. Patients undergoing minor surgery can be managed using a nomogram that adjusts the perioperative dose of warfarin and minimizes the time the patient has a subtherapeutic INR.[35] Certain procedures such as cataract surgery and minor dermatologic and dental procedures can be performed without stopping or adjusting warfarin dosing. For further reading on the topic of perioperative management of anticoagulation, we refer you to a recent comprehensive review.[36]

VENOUS THROMBOEMBOLISM PREVENTION

The risk of VTE is determined by several factors: the type of surgery, the patient's clinical risk factors for VTE, and the period of perioperative immobilization.[37] The clinical risk factors for VTE include increasing age, prior VTE, obesity, stroke, immobility, paralysis, CHF, cancer, trauma, varicose veins, pregnancy, estrogen use, and a hypercoagulable state (e.g., protein C deficiency, factor V Leiden). Table 6.10 outlines a risk stratification scheme put forth for surgical patients by the American College of Chest Physicians. The risk categories range from low risk to highest risk.

TABLE 6.10

CATEGORIES OF RISK FOR VENOUS THROMBOEMBOLISM IN SURGICAL PATIENTS

Low Risk
- Minor surgery in patients younger than 40 years with no additional risk factors present[a]

Moderate Risk
- Minor surgery in patients with additional risk factor present,[a] or nonmajor surgery in patients ages 40–60 years with no additional risk factor, or major surgery in patients younger than 40 years with no additional risk factors

High Risk
- Nonmajor surgery in patients older than 60 years or with additional risk factor present,[a] or major surgery in patients older than 40 years or with additional risk factor

Highest Risk
- Major surgery in patients older than 40 years with additional risk factor present,[a] or hip or knee arthroplasty, hip fracture surgery, or major trama such as spinal cord injury

---

[a]Additional risk factors include one or more of the following: advanced age, prior venous thromboembolism, obesity, heart failure, paralysis, or presence of a molecular hypercoagulable state (e.g., protein C deficiency, factor V Leiden).
Adapted from Geerts WH, Pineo GF, Heit JA, et al. Prevention of venous thromboembolism: the seventh ACCP conference on antithrombotic and thrombolytic therapy. *Chest* 2004;126(3 Suppl):338S–400S.

The approximate prevalence of calf deep vein thrombosis (DVT), proximal DVT, and clinical pulmonary embolism in the absence of prophylaxis is listed for each category of risk in Table 6.11, along with suggested prevention strategies.

CONCLUSION

There are many medical considerations in the preoperative evaluation and perioperative management of patients undergoing major noncardiac surgery. Careful attention to

---

TABLE 6.11

LEVELS OF VENOUS THROMBOEMBOLISM RISK AND RECOMMENDATIONS FOR PROPHYLAXIS

Level of Risk	Calf DVT (%)	Proximal DVT (%)	Clinical PE (%)	Fatal PE (%)	Prevention Strategies
Low risk	2	0.4	0.2	0.002	No specific measures Aggressive mobilization
Moderate risk	10–20	2–4	1–2	0.1–0.4	LDUH q12hr or LMWH, or ES or IPC
High risk	20–40	4–8	2–4	0.4–1.0	LDUH q8hr or LMWH or IPC
Very high risk	40–80	10–20	4–10	0.2–5	LMWH or OA IPC/ES + LDUH/LMWH, or ADH; consider pharmacologic prophylaxis for extended duration (i.e., up to 30 days)

ADH, adjusted-dose heparin; DVT, deep vein thrombosis; ES, elastic stocking; IPC, intermittent pneumatic compression; LDUH, low-dose unfractionated heparin (e.g., unfractionated heparin 5,000 U SQ q12); LMWH, low molecular weight heparin (e.g., enoxaparin 40 mg SQ qd, dalteparin 5,000 IV/day); OA, oral anticoagulant (e.g., warfarin with target international normalized ration = 2–3); PE, pulmonary embolism.
Adapted from Geerts WH, Pineo GF, Heit JA, et al. Prevention of venous thromboembolism: the seventh ACCP conference on antithrombotic and thrombolytic therapy. *Chest* 2004;126(3 Suppl):338S–400S.

risk assessment during the history and exam, optimization of the preoperative medical conditions, institution of evidence-based risk reduction therapies, and excellent communication with other members of the team can assist the anesthesiologist and surgeon in delivering the best care to the patient.

REVIEW EXERCISES

QUESTIONS

1. You are asked to see a 54-year-old man for a preoperative evaluation prior to total hip arthroplasty. He has a 15-year history of non–insulin-dependent diabetes mellitus, chronic renal insufficiency, and hypertension. His medications include glyburide, metformin, and lisinopril. He has mild retinopathy and 300 mg/day of proteinuria. His last laboratory studies 2 weeks ago showed a creatinine of 2.1 mg%, total cholesterol of 256 mg%, high-density lipoprotein cholesterol 39 mg%, low-density lipoprotein cholesterol of 152 mg%, triglycerides of 210 mg%, and glycosylated hemoglobin of 7.2%. He has no past history of cardiovascular disease and denies current chest pain, palpitations, or dyspnea of exertion. For the past year, he has had limited physical activity due to progressive osteoarthritis of the hip. On examination, his weight is 220 lb with a body mass index of 32, his blood pressure is 132/84 mm Hg, and his pulse is 84/minute. His funduscopic examination shows mild background retinopathy. His cardiac and pulmonary examinations are normal, whereas the remainder of his examination is otherwise unremarkable except for mildly diminished dorsalis pedis pulses and decreased position sense in his toes. His ECG shows nonspecific ST-T-wave changes. Which of the following is the most appropriate preoperative recommendation at this time?

a) Ultrasound vascular evaluation of the lower extremities
b) DTI or DSE
c) No further cardiac testing and proceed with surgery
d) Cardiac catheterization

Answer and Discussion

The answer is b. Using the ACC/AHA guidelines, this patient has several clinical risk predictors (h/o type 2 diabetes mellitus and chronic renal insufficiency) and is scheduled for an intermediate risk surgery. Because his functional class is poor with activity <4 METS, he should undergo further risk stratification with noninvasive testing.

2. You are asked to evaluate a 73-year-old man with stable class II angina treated with nitrates and atenolol, and no previous myocardial infarction or coronary heart failure. He has mild hypertension controlled on lisinopril and no history of diabetes. He had excellent exercise capacity (7 METS) until he injured his ankle 2 weeks ago. At that time, he was found to have a 5.2-cm abdominal aortic aneurysm. His examination is unremarkable, his blood pressure is 144/86 mm Hg, and his heart rate is 65/minute. His ECG is normal. He is scheduled to undergo abdominal aortic aneurysm repair. Which of the following is the most appropriate recommendation at this time?

a) Exercise stress test
b) DSE or DTI
c) No further cardiac testing and proceed with surgery
d) Cardiac catheterization

Answer and Discussion

The answer is c. Applying the ACC/AHA guidelines to this case of a patient with chronic stable class II angina with excellent functional class would suggest that he not undergo any further risk stratification with a stress test unless there would be change in management.

3. A 48-year-old woman is referred for preoperative evaluation before planned elective laparoscopic cholecystectomy. She has no prior cardiac history but has had asthma since age 16 years. Her current medications are oral theophylline and inhaled albuterol. She does not smoke and notes no dyspnea on moderate exertion. On examination, her weight is 97 kg (213.4 lb), her height is 163 cm (5 ft, 4 in.), her blood pressure is 144/78 mm Hg, and her pulse is 76/minute and regular. Her lungs reveal moderate wheezing that does not clear with cough. Her heart is normal, and, other than obesity, the remainder of her examination is normal. Which of the following is the most appropriate next step?

a) Add inhaled salbutamol before surgery.
b) Add inhaled betamethasone before surgery.
c) Reassure her that her risk is low because of the planned laparoscopic approach.
d) Cancel the surgery and optimize antiasthma treatment regimen before rescheduling.

Answer and Discussion

The answer is d. The presence of active wheezing places this patient at greater risk for postoperative pulmonary complications and increased bronchospasm during anesthesia induction. The patient's surgery should be delayed until her asthma treatment is optimized. The laparoscopic approach may reduce the risk of pulmonary complications compared with open cholecystectomy, but a level of risk remains because of gaseous peritoneal distention and postoperative pain.

4. A 35-year-old man is referred to you for a preoperative evaluation prior to inguinal hernia repair. He has no prior cardiac history and does not smoke or drink. On exam, he weighs 80 kg (176 lb), and his blood pressure is 140/80 mm Hg and a pulse of 80/minute. His heart and lungs, as well as the remainder of his exam, are normal. You recommend which of the following?

a) Complete metabolic profile
b) Complete blood count
c) Urine analysis
d) All of the above
e) None of the above

Answer and Discussion

The answer is e. This patient is completely healthy, and evidence would suggest that ordering routine preoperative blood work would be both unnecessary and costly, and not indicated in this patient's case. Table 6.9 reviews in detail indications for various tests. A screening urine analysis is never indicated unless symptoms suggest that the patient may have an underlying infection.

5. A 50-year-old woman with a 20-year history of rheumatoid arthritis is scheduled for spine surgery. Her medications include prednisone 10 mg/day orally for the past year, vitamin E, gingko biloba, garlic, and aspirin. Her functional class is limited, but she can still climb a flight of stairs with her groceries (>4 METS). She denies history of chest pain, shortness of breath, and prior cardiac problems. Her exam reveals weight of 60 kg and height of 5 ft, 5 in., blood pressure of 120/70 mm Hg, and heart rate of 80/minute. Heart and lung exam are normal. Her neck exam reveals decreased range of motion, and her extremities reveal deformities consistent with rheumatoid arthritis. Which of the following is the most appropriate recommendation?

a) Discontinue vitamin E, gingko biloba, and garlic.
b) Discontinue aspirin 10 days before surgery.
c) Obtain cervical spine films.
d) Stress dose steroids.
e) All of the above.

Answer and Discussion

The answer is e. Current evidence and consensus would support discontinuing vitamin E, ginkgo, and garlic about 2 weeks prior to surgery because they may all increase the risk of bleeding. Aspirin irreversibly inhibits platelet cyclo-oxygenase and should be stopped 7 to 10 days before surgery. Cervical spine films are indicated in patients with rheumatoid arthritis before they undergo general anesthesia because the presence of severe atlantoaxial disease can cause compromise of the cervical cord during manipulation of the neck during intubation; however, there is no role for further spine imaging. Stress-dose steroids would be recommended in this patient to prevent iatrogenic adrenal insufficiency.

REFERENCES

1. Fleisher LA, Beckman JA, Brown KA, et al. ACC/AHA 2007 guidelines on perioperative cardiovascular evaluation and care for noncardiac surgery: a report of the American College of Cardiology/American Heart Association Task Force on Practice Guidelines (Writing Committee to Revise the 2002 Guidelines on Perioperative Cardiovascular Evaluation for Noncardiac Surgery): developed in collaboration with the American Society of Echocardiography, American Society of Nuclear Cardiology, Heart Rhythm Society, Society of Cardiovascular Anesthesiologists, Society for Cardiovascular Angiography and Interventions, Society for Vascular Medicine and Biology, and Society for Vascular Surgery. *Circulation* 2007;116(17):e418–e499.
2. Rodgers A, Walker N, Schug S, et al. Reduction of postoperative mortality and morbidity with epidural or spinal anaesthesia: results from overview of randomised trials. *BMJ* 2000;321(7275):1493.
3. Goldman L, Caldera DL, Nussbaum SR, et al. Multifactorial index of cardiac risk in noncardiac surgical procedures. *N Engl J Med* 1977;297(16):845–850.
4. Mangano DT, Goldman L. Preoperative assessment of patients with known or suspected coronary disease. *N Engl J Med* 1995;333(26):1750–1756.
5. Eagle KA, Coley CM, Newell JB, et al. Combining clinical and thallium data optimizes preoperative assessment of cardiac risk before major vascular surgery. *Ann Intern Med* 1989;110(11):859–866.
6. Vanzetto G, Machecourt J, Blendea D, et al. Additive value of thallium single-photon emission computed tomography myocardial imaging for prediction of perioperative events in clinically selected high cardiac risk patients having abdominal aortic surgery. *Am J Cardiol* 1996;77(2):143–148.
7. Detsky AS, Abrams HB, Forbath N, et al. Cardiac assessment for patients undergoing noncardiac surgery: a multifactorial clinical risk index. *Arch Intern Med* 1986;146(11):2131–2134.
8. Lee TH, Marcantonio ER, Mangione CM, et al. Derivation and prospective validation of a simple index for prediction of cardiac risk of major noncardiac surgery. *Circulation* 1999;100(10):1043–1049.
9. Devereaux PJ, Goldman L, Cook DJ, et al. Perioperative cardiac events in patients undergoing noncardiac surgery: a review of the magnitude of the problem, the pathophysiology of the events and methods to estimate and communicate risk. *Can Med Assoc J* 2005;173(6):627–634.
10. Reilly DF, McNeely MJ, Doerner D, et al. Self-reported exercise tolerance and the risk of serious perioperative complications. *Arch Intern Med* 1999;159(18):2185–2192.
11. Hlatky MA, Boineau RE, Higginbotham MB, et al. A brief self-administered questionnaire to determine functional capacity (the Duke Activity Status Index). *Am J Cardiol* 1989;64(10):651–654.
12. Poldermans D, Arnese M, Fioretti PM, et al. Improved cardiac risk stratification in major vascular surgery with dobutamine-atropine stress echocardiography. *J Am Coll Cardiol* 1995;26(3):648–653.
13. Kertai MD, Boersma E, Bax JJ, et al. A meta-analysis comparing the prognostic accuracy of six diagnostic tests for predicting perioperative cardiac risk in patients undergoing major vascular surgery. *Heart* 2003;89(11):1327–1334.
14. Xu-Cai YO, Brotman DJ, Phillips CO, et al. Outcomes of patients with stable heart failure undergoing elective noncardiac surgery. *Mayo Clin Proc* 2008;83(3):280–288.
15. Kertai MD, Bountioukos M, Boersma E, et al. Aortic stenosis: an underestimated risk factor for perioperative complications in patients undergoing noncardiac surgery. *Am J Med* 2004;116(1):8–13.
16. Wilson W, Taubert KA, Gewitz M, et al. Prevention of infective endocarditis: guidelines from the American Heart Association: a guideline from the American Heart Association Rheumatic Fever, Endocarditis, and Kawasaki Disease Committee, Council on Cardiovascular Disease in the Young, and the Council on Clinical Cardiology, Council on Cardiovascular Surgery and Anesthesia, and the Quality of Care and Outcomes Research Interdisciplinary Working Group. *Circulation* 2007;116(15):1736–1754.
17. Daumerie G, Fleisher LA. Perioperative beta-blocker and statin therapy. *Curr Opin Anaesthesiol* 2008;21(1):60–65.

18. Beattie WS, Wijeysundera DN, Karkouti K, et al. Does tight heart rate control improve beta-blocker efficacy? An updated analysis of the noncardiac surgical randomized trials. *Anesth Analg* 2008;106(4):1039–1048, table of contents.
19. Smetana GW. Preoperative pulmonary evaluation. *N Engl J Med* 1999;340(12):937–944.
20. Preoperative pulmonary function testing. American College of Physicians. *Ann Intern Med* 1990;112(10):793–794.
21. Arozullah AM. Multifactorial risk index for predicting postoperative respiratory failure in men after major noncardiac surgery. The National Veterans Administration Surgical Quality Improvement Program.
22. Schiff RL, Welsh GA. Perioperative evaluation and management of the patient with endocrine dysfunction. *Med Clin North Am* 2003;87(1):175–192.
23. Marcantonio ER, Goldman L, Mangione CM, et al. A clinical prediction rule for delirium after elective noncardiac surgery. *JAMA* 1994;271(2):134–139.
24. Litaker D, Locala J, Franco K, et al. Preoperative risk factors for postoperative delirium. *Gen Hosp Psychiatry* 2001;23(2):84–89.
25. Roizen MF. More preoperative assessment by physicians and less by laboratory tests. *N Engl J Med* 2000;342(3):204–205.
26. Macpherson DS, Litaker D. Preoperative screening. *Med Clin North Am* 2003;87(1):7–40.
27. Spell NO III. Stopping and restarting medications in the perioperative period. *Med Clin North Am* 2001;85(5):1117–1128.
28. Ang-Lee MK, Moss J, Yuan CS. Herbal medicines and perioperative care. *JAMA* 2001;286(2):208–216.
29. Taggart DP, Siddiqui A, Wheatley DJ. Low-dose preoperative aspirin therapy, postoperative blood loss, and transfusion requirements. *Ann Thorac Surg* 1990;50(3):424–428.
30. Grady D, Wenger NK, Herrington D, et al. Postmenopausal hormone therapy increases risk for venous thromboembolic disease. The Heart and Estrogen/progestin Replacement Study. *Ann Intern Med* 2000;132(9):689–696.
31. Brotman DJ, Hurbanek J, Jaffer A, Morra N. Postmenopausal Hormone Replacement Therapy and Venous Thromboembolism Following Orthopedic Surgery. Paper presented at Society of General Internal Medicine; May 2004.
32. Brabant SM, Bertrand M, Eyraud D, et al. The hemodynamic effects of anesthetic induction in vascular surgical patients chronically treated with angiotensin II receptor antagonists. *Anesth Analg* 1999;89(6):1388–1392.
33. Coriat P, Richer C, Douraki T, et al. Influence of chronic angiotensin-converting enzyme inhibition on anesthetic induction. *Anesthesiology* 1994;81(2):299–307.
34. White RH, McKittrick T, Hutchinson R, et al. Temporary discontinuation of warfarin therapy: changes in the international normalized ratio. *Ann Intern Med* 1995;122(1):40–42.
35. Marietta M, Bertesi M, Simoni L, et al. A simple and safe nomogram for the management of oral anticoagulation prior to minor surgery. *Clin Lab Haematol* 2003;25(2):127–130.
36. Jaffer AK, Brotman DJ, Chukwumerije N. When patients on warfarin need surgery. *Cleve Clin J Med* 2003;70(11):973–984.
37. Geerts WH, Pineo GF, Heit JA, et al. Prevention of venous thromboembolism: the seventh ACCP conference on antithrombotic and thrombolytic therapy. *Chest* 2004;126(3 Suppl):338S–400S.

SUGGESTED READINGS

Fleisher LA, Beckman JA, Brown KA, et al. ACC/AHA 2007 guidelines on perioperative cardiovascular evaluation and care for noncardiac surgery: a report of the American College of Cardiology/American Heart Association Task Force on Practice Guidelines (Writing Committee to Revise the 2002 Guidelines on Perioperative Cardiovascular Evaluation for Noncardiac Surgery): developed in collaboration with the American Society of Echocardiography, American Society of Nuclear Cardiology, Heart Rhythm Society, Society of Cardiovascular Anesthesiologists, Society for Cardiovascular Angiography and Interventions, Society for Vascular Medicine and Biology, and Society for Vascular Surgery. *Circulation* 2007;116(17): e418–e499.

Geerts WH, Pineo GF, Heit JA, et al. Prevention of venous thromboembolism: the seventh ACCP conference on antithrombotic and thrombolytic therapy. *Chest* 2004;126(3 Suppl):338S–400S.

Jaffer AK, Brotman DJ, Chukwumerije N. When patients on warfarin need surgery. *Cleve Clin J Med* 2003;70(11):973–984.

Lee TH, Marcantonio ER, Mangione CM, et al. Derivation and prospective validation of a simple index for prediction of cardiac risk of major noncardiac surgery. *Circulation* 1999;100(10):1043–1049.

Chapter 7

Geriatric Medicine

Robert M. Palmer

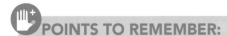

POINTS TO REMEMBER:

- Delirium is potentially preventable during hospitalization of elderly patients by maintaining their hydration, optimizing their cognitive function, keeping them mobile, enabling them to achieve satisfactory sleep, and providing hearing and vision aids as required.

- The incidence of delirium in a hospitalized patient is a sign of a serious underlying illness and should be evaluated and managed promptly with attention to contributing factors.

- Accidental falls are common in older patients, but high-risk patients can usually be identified rapidly in the office by asking them if they have fallen in the previous year or have a balance or gait problem.

- Resistive exercises to strengthen leg and hip muscles, and balance exercises such as tai chi, are effective in reducing the risk of subsequent falls in cognitively normal older patients at high risk of falling.

- Treating contributing conditions (shared risk factors, such as generalized weakness, impaired mobility, and use of psychotropic medications) can reduce the incidence of falls, delirium, and urinary incontinence.

- Nonpharmacologic therapies including behavioral therapies (e.g., patient continence logs, biofeedback, habit training) reduce the number of incontinence episodes in cognitively intact women with mixed (stress/urge) types of incontinence, often obviating the need for medications.

The aging process predisposes elderly patients to homeostatic failure, chronic disease, and functional decline (i.e., a loss of independence in performing daily activities). Illness often manifests as a *geriatric syndrome*, a clinical problem with a wide array of etiologies and complex pathophysiology. Included among these geriatric syndromes are cognitive dysfunction (altered mental status), falls, and urinary incontinence.

These syndromes, which increase in frequency and importance as patients age, are frequently encountered by internists in ambulatory, hospital, and long-term care settings. These common problems are often left undiagnosed or untreated, resulting in a loss of quality of life for older patients. Importantly, these syndromes share common risk factors that are amenable to preventive strategies, and there are effective interventions for their management.

COGNITIVE DYSFUNCTION: DELIRIUM

The common causes of cognitive dysfunction in elderly patients are dementia, delirium, and depression. (Dementia and depression are discussed in Chapter 10.) Delirium (acute confusion, altered mental status) is an organic mental syndrome characterized by:

- A reduced ability to maintain or shift attention
- Disorganized thinking
- An altered level of consciousness
- Perceptual disturbances
- Increased or decreased psychomotor activity
- Disturbances of the sleep–wake cycle
- Disorientation to time, place, or person
- Memory impairments

Typically, the disturbance in cognition develops over a short period (hours to days) and fluctuates throughout the day. Delirium occurring in hospitalized elderly patients often goes undetected or is misdiagnosed as dementia, depression, functional psychosis, or personality disorder. The sequelae of delirium is associated with a prolonged length of hospitalization, higher costs of care, and a greater risk of institutionalization and mortality: all underscoring the importance of early detection, a search for likely etiologies, and appropriate therapeutic interventions designed to prevent or rapidly resolve the syndrome of delirium.

TABLE 7.1

MEDICATIONS TO AVOID IN ELDERLY PATIENTS: REASONS, EXAMPLES, AND ALTERNATIVES

Antihistamines
Reasons: Confusion (delirium), oversedation, orthostatic hypotension, falls, constipation, and urinary retention due to anticholinergic effects
Examples: Diphenhydramine, hydroxyzine
Alternatives: *Hypnotics*: temazepam 7.5 mg HS, zolpidem 5 mg HS, trazodone 50 mg HS; *Nonsedating antihistamines*: loratadine 10 mg daily, fexofenadine 60 mg daily or BID

Benzodiazepines
Reasons: Confusion, sedation, and falls
Examples: Diazepam, chlordiazepoxide
Alternatives: *Alcohol or benzodiazepine withdrawal*: lorazepam 0.5–1 mg q4–6hr PRN, oxazepam 10 mg q4–6hr PRN
Agitation/psychosis: haloperidol 0.5–1.0 mg BID or TID, risperidone 0.5 mg BID

Tricyclic Antidepressants (First Generation)
Reasons: Confusion, oversedation, orthostatic hypotension, falls, constipation, and urinary retention due to anticholinergic effects
Examples: Amitriptyline, imipramine
Alternatives: *Neuropathic pain*: second-generation tricyclics: desipramine 10–20 mg daily, nortriptyline 10–25 mg daily

Antiemetics
Reasons: Confusion, oversedation, orthostatic hypotension, falls, constipation, and urinary retention due to anticholinergic effects
Examples: Trimethobenzamide (a low-potency antiemetic, highly anticholinergic)
Alternatives: Promethazine 12.5 mg q6hr PRN, prochlorperazine 5 mg q6hr PRN

Narcotic Analgesics
Reasons: Meperidine—confusion, oversedation, orthostatic hypotension, falls, constipation, and urinary retention due to anticholinergic effects; metabolite may produce agitation and seizures; short duration of analgesia. Propoxyphene—poor analgesic effect with usual opioid anticholinergic effects
Examples: Meperidine, propoxyphene
Alternatives: Acetaminophen—provides analgesia equivalent to propoxyphene, add codeine or oxycodone if pain relief is inadequate, oxycodone 2.5 mg q4–6hr; morphine—initially low doses (e.g., 4–6 mg for robust patients [2–4 mg for frail patients] q3–4hr) suffice, titrate dose response

BID, twice a day; HS, at bedtime; PRN, as needed; TID, three times a day.

Etiology

Virtually any acute physical stress can precipitate delirium in vulnerable patients. Delirium is most commonly associated with:

- Infection (e.g., urosepsis or pneumonia)
- Hypoxemia
- Hypotension
- Psychoactive medications (e.g., benzodiazepines)
- Anticholinergic medications

Other causes of delirium include:

- Alcohol withdrawal or intoxication
- Partial complex seizures
- Stroke
- Uremia
- Electrolyte disorders (e.g., hyponatremia)

Drugs are common preventable causes of delirium. Many antiarrhythmics, tricyclic antidepressants, neuroleptics, analgesics, and gastrointestinal medications can induce delirium in elderly patients. One common characteristic of many of these agents is their central anticholinergic effect. Some medications to avoid prescribing to elderly patients, and their alternatives, are shown in Table 7.1.

Epidemiology

Delirium occurs primarily in patients who are acutely ill or hospitalized. Among medically ill hospitalized elderly patients, the prevalence of delirium at admission is 10% to 15%; the incidence is 10% to 15% during hospitalization. The incidence of postoperative delirium is 10% to 15% in general surgical patients and 30% to 50% of patients admitted to the hospital with hip fractures or to undergo knee surgery.

The independent risk factors for incident delirium in medically ill hospitalized elderly patients include:

- Dementia
- Fever
- Use of psychoactive drugs
- Azotemia
- Fracture
- Abnormal serum sodium (dehydration)

In older patients admitted to a medical intensive care unit, where the incidence of delirium is 70% or higher, risk factors for delirium present at admission include baseline dementia, receipt of benzodiazepines before unit admission, elevated creatinine, and low arterial pH. In both medical and surgical older patients, dementia is the major risk factor for delirium, increasing the risk nearly threefold. Other medical conditions that are often associated with delirium include prolonged sleep deprivation, sensory impairments (vision and hearing), and changes in environment.

Delirium that occurs in the hospital in high-risk patients is precipitated by factors that are potentially amenable to medical interventions or change in therapies. These include:

- Use of physical restraints
- Malnutrition
- More than three added medications
- Use of a bladder catheter
- Any iatrogenic event (e.g., unintentional injury or pressure ulcer)

Pathophysiology

The pathophysiology of delirium remains poorly understood. Patients with risk factors for delirium are regarded as vulnerable or high risk, based on the assumption of limited homeostatic (brain) reserves. For a high-risk patient, even a minor insult such as fever can precipitate delirium. A metabolic derangement with disturbances in neurotransmitter activity likely accounts for the cognitive features of delirium. For example, delirium can be induced by centrally acting anticholinergic drugs. In hepatic encephalopathy, the presence of delirium correlates with the accumulation of toxic metabolites (e.g., ammonia). In other patients, dopaminergic excess, lymphokines, interleukin (IL)-1, IL-2, IL-6, tumor necrosis factor-alpha, and interferon are associated with delirium.

Clinical Presentation

An acute change in mental status with disturbed consciousness, impaired cognition, and fluctuating course is characteristic of delirium. A reduced ability to focus, sustain, or shift attention is evident and accounts for the behavioral manifestations of incoherent or tangential speech and disorganized or erratic thought processes. Perceptual disturbances (misperceptions), illusions, or delusions and hallucinations are common, particularly in patients with increased psychomotor activity. Most often, delirium presents as a "quiet confusion" in acutely ill patients, although extremes in behavior and cognition may occur throughout the day.

Diagnostic Evaluation

The diagnostic evaluation of a patient with detected delirium is driven by a search for the most probable etiologies,

and delirium may represent a life-threatening disease. In many cases, the etiology seems obvious (e.g., urosepsis), but vigilance is needed to exclude other possible concurrent causes (e.g., hypoxemia) that may contribute to the delirium. For example, a patient with delirium associated with pneumonia might also have hypoxemia, dehydration, fever, an adverse drug reaction, or sleep deprivation as contributing causes. In high-risk patients, delirium is often a nonspecific but common initial presentation of an acute infection, cardiovascular, or pulmonary event.

Rarely is an extensive laboratory evaluation of delirium needed. Because infection is so frequently the cause of delirium, a complete blood count, blood chemistry panel, and urinalysis are recommended. In select cases (e.g., fever, hypotension), blood and urine cultures are warranted. Likewise, chest films, electrocardiography, and arterial blood gases may be useful to identify the likely etiology of delirium or contributing factors and precipitants. Lumbar puncture, head neuroimaging, and electroencephalography are recommended in select cases when the delirious patient has focal neurologic deficits, a history of head trauma, or unclear etiology of the delirium.

Screening and Diagnosis of Delirium

Even subtle cases of delirium can be detected through careful observation of the patient (e.g., change in cognition, reasoning, or alertness) and the use of instruments, such as the digit span test for measuring attention and the confusion assessment method for confirming the diagnosis of delirium. With the digit span test, patients are asked to repeat a random list of numbers that are stated in a monotone at 1-second intervals. Typically, healthy patients can correctly repeat five or more of these numbers in correct order, whereas delirious patients repeat fewer than five numbers. With the confusion assessment method, a diagnosis of delirium can be achieved with >90% sensitivity and specificity by documenting a change in mental status characterized by inattention, an acute onset and fluctuating course, and either or both disorganized thinking and an altered level of consciousness. Instruments to measure cognitive function (e.g., Mini-Mental State Examination) are often used to quantify the degree of dysfunction or to monitor the patient's response to treatment.

Differential Diagnoses

Delirium should be distinguished from functional psychosis, depression, and dementia as follows:

- Functional psychosis (e.g., late-onset schizophrenia) is not characterized by impaired attention or fluctuating mental status.
- Depression is suspected in patients who give variable responses or many "I don't know" answers to questions during a mental status examination. A dysphoric mood, irritability, and a withdrawn appearance further suggest

TABLE 7.2
DELIRIUM VERSUS DEMENTIA

Feature	Delirium	Dementia
Onset	Rapid, often at night	Usually insidious, as in Alzheimer's disease
Duration	Hours to weeks (usually transient)	Months to years (persistent)
Consciousness	Depressed	Normal
Awareness	Always impaired	Usually normal
Alertness	Reduced or increased (fluctuates)	Usually normal
Attention span	Decreased (less than four digits)	Usually normal (in mild to moderate states) (five or more digits)

the diagnosis. Depressed patients are alert and attentive, although their ability to concentrate may be limited, especially if they are anxious or agitated.

■ Delirium occurs more often in demented patients, but clinical features help distinguish these conditions (Table 7.2).

Treatment

Prevention

Although evidence from randomized controlled trials is sparse, delirium can be prevented in both medical and surgical elderly patients. The incidence of delirium is decreased by reducing modifiable risk factors in patients. A clinical trial of intervention protocols targeted at risk factors for delirium resulted in a 40% reduction in the incidence of delirium. The protocols served to optimize cognitive function (reorientation, therapeutic activities), prevent sleep deprivation (relaxation, noise reduction), avoid immobility (ambulation, exercises), improve vision (visual aids, illumination), improve hearing (hearing devices), and treat dehydration (volume repletion). In elderly patients admitted to the hospital for acute or elective hip surgery, the incidence of postoperative delirium was not reduced by an intervention of haloperidol 1.5 mg/day given 1 day before and up to 6 days after surgery; yet, there was a reduction in the severity and duration of delirium. However, based on the limited data from clinical trials, routine pretreatment with an antipsychotic agent is not recommended.

Management

The management of delirium begins with the treatment of the underlying etiologies. Effective nursing and environmental interventions include:

■ Continuity of nursing care
■ Alternatives to physical restraints (restraints can paradoxically increase patient agitation)
■ Correction of sensory impairments (visual and hearing)
■ Placement of the patient in a room near the nurses' station for closer observation and greater socialization
■ Social visits with a family member, caregiver, or hired sitter

■ Promotion of normal sleep cycles through noise control, dim lighting at night, and reality orientation

Pharmacologic Treatment

No medication has an indication for treating delirium. Medications are considered for treatment of symptoms (e.g., frightening hallucinations) that are highly disturbing to the patient or for behaviors (e.g., severe agitation) that threaten to disrupt life-maintaining therapies. Antipsychotic agents (neuroleptics) are considered for the treatment of hallucinations, delusions, or frightening illusions. Haloperidol, 0.5 to 1.0 mg, can be given orally or intramuscularly every 6 to 8 hours as necessary. Doses of more than 3 mg daily are to be avoided to reduce risks of harm to patients. Higher doses of haloperidol, or more frequent intervals, are often used in critically ill patients whose heart rhythm and vital signs are continuously monitored, but the long-term safety of high doses of haloperidol and other neuroleptics is uncertain. Patients with anxiety or agitation associated with benzodiazepine or alcohol withdrawal should be considered for treatment with lorazepam 0.5 to 1.0 mg given orally or parenterally every 4 to 6 hours as necessary. Delirious patients in severe pain can be treated with morphine sulfate 4 to 6 mg parenterally as needed (but begin with lower doses in very old or frail patients). Repeated doses of meperidine should be avoided because of the neurotoxic effect of its metabolite. Psychotropic medications, however, should be used judiciously and for the shortest time necessary because they can cause paradoxic confusion and increase the risk of falls. Neuroleptics can be tapered and discontinued over a few days once the delirium or behavioral symptom has resolved. Physical restraints should be avoided in most cases because they can increase patient agitation and the risks of pressure ulcer and physical deconditioning.

Prognosis

Most episodes of delirium improve rapidly, usually within days of appropriate therapy. However, functional and cognitive deficits often persist after discharge from the hospital, probably related to the underlying etiology or risk factors for delirium, especially dementia. The patient's mental status should be re-evaluated after hospital discharge, and the patient should be monitored for possible dementia.

FALLS

Accidental falls, defined as "unintentionally coming to rest on the ground, floor, or other lower level," are common and potentially preventable causes of morbidity and mortality in the elderly. Falls account for many serious injuries, including hip fractures and soft tissue trauma. A loss of mobility and fear of falling again are common consequences of a fall and contribute to the patient's inability to live independently. Falls are often attributed to either host (intrinsic) or environmental (extrinsic) predisposing or situational risk factors.

Etiology

Epidemiology

The incidence of falls and related injuries increases with advancing age. Falls occur in approximately one-third of community-residing persons 65 years of age and older and in approximately 50% of persons 80 years of age and older. Approximately 5% to 10% of falls by community-residing elderly persons result in a fracture or head trauma, or soft tissue injury. Approximately 90% of hip fractures in elderly people result from falls. Accidental injurious falls increase the probability of hospitalization, nursing home placement, and death.

In prospective studies, the independent intrinsic risk factors for accidental falls are weakness, prior history of fall, balance deficit, gait deficit, vision impairment, dependence in activities of daily living, depression, and cognitive impairment. Among extrinsic factors for falls are psychotropic drug use (especially benzodiazepines, antipsychotics, and antidepressants) and environmental hazards such as uneven walking surfaces, throw rugs, cluttered floors, poor lighting, and lack of handrails. Hip fractures are more common in women with multiple risk factors ("high risk") for falling, a prior history of falls, poor performance on tests of neuromuscular function (e.g., gait speed), and low bone mineral density.

Clinical Causes

Accidental falls stem from the combination of environmental hazards and the increased susceptibility to falls related to aging or diseases. Accidents, simple slips or trips, are the most common cause of falls occurring in the community-dwelling elderly population, and these occur more often in the presence of environmental hazards. Other common causes are disorders of gait and balance, dizziness and vertigo, drop attack, and confusion. Lower extremity weakness from deconditioning, stroke, and chronic diseases cause gait impairment leading to falls. Syncope accounts for less than 3% of falls. Postural hypotension and visual disorders are less frequent causes of falls.

Pathophysiology

The maintenance of normal balance and gait requires the successful integration of sensory (afferent), central (brain and spinal cord), and musculoskeletal systems. A disturbance in sensory input (e.g., peripheral neuropathy), central nervous system functioning (e.g., dementia), or motor function (e.g., arthritis, muscle weakness) predisposes elderly patients to falls. Weakness of the lower extremity muscles, which is often associated with deconditioning, impairs gait and predisposes the patient to falling in the face of a minor perturbation. The aging process may also predispose patients to falls by increasing postural sway and reducing adaptive reflexes.

Screening and Diagnosis

Patients at risk for accidental falls can be identified with a medical history, brief physical examination, and basic laboratory studies. For patients new to an internist's practice, the falls screen begins with a question, "Have you had any falls in the past year?" If the answer is "No," then ask, "Do you have any problems with gait (walking) or balance (steadiness)?" Patients screening positive for either question are at a significantly increased risk of falling (at least 50%) in the next year. Observation of the patient's balance and gait identifies patients at risk of falling. The Timed Up and Go (TUG) test is quickly performed and predictive of falling. This test requires a patient to stand up from a chair, walk 10 feet, turn, walk back, return to the chair, and sit down. Older adults at high risk of falls require longer than 20 seconds to complete this task. As the patient performs this task, postural instability, lower extremity weakness, reduced step height, increased lateral sway, stride variability, and ataxia can be readily identified, and further diagnostic evaluation can be pursued. A review of risk factors, medications (e.g., vasodilators, adrenergic blockers, psychotropic agents), and screening instruments (e.g., vision, mental status, balance, gait) will further help identify patients at high risk for future falls. Further diagnostic assessment is invaluable for patients who have a prolonged TUG or risk factors for recurrent falls. For high-risk patients, a detailed examination of their vision, gait and balance, lower extremity strength and function, and mental status, as well as a basic neurologic examination, is recommended. Often, this assessment is completed with the assistance of other health professionals, such as physical therapists.

On routine annual examinations, all elderly patients should be asked about the occurrence of falls and balance or gait problems since their last office visit. For high-risk patients, these questions are asked at each office visit.

TABLE 7.3

INTERVENTION TO DECREASE THE RISK OF FALLS

Risk Factor	Intervention
Polypharmacy medication review	Reduce or discontinue doses of psychotropic agents (antidepressants, benzodiazepines), vasodilators, and adrenergic blockers
Lower-extremity weakness, deconditioning	Low-intensity resistive exercises, high-intensity resistance exercises under therapist supervision, tai chi exercises, water-walking exercises, and assistive devices (e.g., cane, walker)
Hearing and visual impairment	Hearing aid and corrective lenses
Postural hypotension	Reconditioning exercises, graded compression stockings, salt repletion, and medication changes (reduce doses of diuretics, vasodilators)
Environmental hazards	Home safety evaluation (rugs, lighting, stairs, handrails, assistive devices)

Diagnostic Evaluation

The diagnostic evaluation of a patient who has fallen is based on the circumstances surrounding the fall. Syncopal falls are evaluated differently from nonsyncopal falls. An ambulatory cardiac monitor is indicated for the patient with syncope, unexplained lightheadedness, or palpitations preceding the fall. With an acute fall, an acute illness should be suspected because a fall is often the sentinel symptom of underlying disease. For example, a basic chemistry panel could reveal evidence of dehydration or electrolyte disorders, and a complete blood count might indicate anemia or an elevated white blood count, implying the presence of an infection. A head CT scan is indicated if there is evidence from the history or physical examination of head trauma or an acute change in mental status associated with the fall.

Treatment

Although treatment of specific causes of falls can be easily treated (e.g., syncope owing to complete heart block), more often a multifactorial intervention is needed to reduce the risk of falls by optimizing the patient's sensory, central, and musculoskeletal systems (Table 7.3), and removing environmental risks. Clinical trials support the effectiveness of multifactorial interventions. In a trial of community-residing persons 70 years of age and older at risk for falling, an adjustment of medications, behavioral instructions, and an exercise program (balance exercises, gait training, low-intensity resistive exercises) reduced the numbers of falls in the subsequent year among patients receiving the intervention compared with control patients. An exercise program conducted in home visits by a physiotherapist led to a nearly 50% reduction in the 1-year incidence of falls in women 80 years of age and older. Systematic reviews suggest that the risk for future falls can be reduced in high-risk patients by reducing or stopping psychotropic medications, by introducing home visits by occupational therapists, and by performing exercises.

The most effective exercises to prevent falls in high-risk patients are tai chi and resistive exercises. Tai chi exercises appear to enhance balance and body awareness to reduce the fear of falling and the rate of falls in healthy elderly people. In a 6-month randomized controlled trial, nondemented elders who practice tai chi three times per week were significantly less likely to fall or to experience injurious falls compared to control patients performing just stretching exercises. Low-intensity and progressive high-intensity resistive exercises improve lower extremity strength and are effective as single interventions or as part of a multifactorial intervention to prevent falls. Bands, tubes, pulleys, and weight machines have been used under therapist supervision in various studies. For these reasons, nondemented patients at high risk for falling should be advised to participate in community-based exercise programs or referred to physical therapists for strengthening, balance, and gait exercises.

Fractures occur more commonly in older people with osteoporosis who fall. The treatment of osteoporosis (e.g., calcium and vitamin D supplementation, bisphosphonates) reduces the risk of hip fractures. Many older people have low body stores of vitamin D. Systematic reviews and controlled clinical trials support the efficacy of vitamin D supplementation alone to reduce the risk of falls in high-risk patients, perhaps by enhancing neuromuscular function. In addition, vitamin D supplementation with 800 international units (IU) daily reduces the incidence of both hip and vertebral fractures in frail older people. Benefits are seen with all analogs of vitamin D. For these reasons, vitamin D supplementation with 800 IU daily is advised for all high-risk older patients. The effectiveness of hip protectors to prevent hip fractures is unclear and may depend on the type of protector used, the duration of compliance with the device, and the setting in which it is used (e.g., being less effective with nursing home patients).

URINARY INCONTINENCE

Urinary incontinence (UI) is the involuntary loss of urine of sufficient severity to be a social or health problem. Incontinence impairs the quality of life of older patients, is costly to treat, and is a risk factor for institutionalization. Never a consequence of normal aging, UI is always treatable and often curable.

Epidemiology

The prevalence of UI in community-residing elderly people increases with advancing age from 5% to 15% in women 65 years of age to more than 25% in men and women 85 years of age and older, and nearly 50% in nursing home residents. In community studies, UI often goes unreported by patients to physicians. However, UI is strongly associated with impaired cognition and physical function, and a lower quality of life, underscoring the need to identify and treat these patients. Medications, fecal impaction, environmental barriers (e.g., lack of bathrooms in close reach), estrogen depletion in women, and pelvic muscle weakness increase the risk of incontinence. The adverse consequences of UI include the placement of indwelling urinary catheters with risks of infection, impaired healing of perineal pressure ulcers, and rashes.

Pathophysiology

UI results from neurologic or anatomical defects that interfere with normal urinary micturition. The urinary bladder is responsible for the storage and emptying of urine. Lesions that interfere with bladder contraction and emptying (e.g., sensory neuropathy) predispose patients to incontinence. Parasympathetic stimulation by the sacral nerves (S2–S4) produces detrusor muscle contractions; disruption of these nerves results in an acontractile bladder. As the bladder fills, the parasympathetic system is inhibited. When intravesical pressure increases (typically with bladder volumes of >250 mL), inhibitory pathways from the frontal lobe are overcome, and detrusor contraction is able to exceed urethral resistance to enable urinary flow from the bladder.

The contraction of the detrusor muscle at low bladder-filling volumes (detrusor instability or overactive bladder) occurs in patients with central nervous system disease (e.g., stroke) or increased sensory stimulation from the bladder (e.g., urinary tract infection, prostatic hyperplasia). Loss of detrusor contractility or bladder outlet obstruction results in a distended bladder; intravesical pressure exceeds urethral resistance and results in incontinence. Incompetence of the internal urethral sphincter (e.g., secondary to pelvic relaxation) allows urine to leak from the bladder during increases in intra-abdominal pressure. A common cause of UI in frail older patients (up to two-thirds of nursing home patients) is detrusor underactivity, a contraction of reduced strength and/or duration, resulting in prolonged bladder emptying and/or a failure to achieve complete bladder emptying within a normal time span. It is commonly associated with impaired contractility of the bladder (detrusor hyperactivity with impaired contractility [DHIC]).

Clinical Presentations

Four basic types of UI occur in elderly patients (Table 7.4):

- Stress incontinence
- Urge incontinence
- Overflow incontinence
- Functional incontinence

TABLE 7.4

TYPES, CHARACTERISTICS, AND TREATMENT OF URINARY INCONTINENCE

Type	Characteristics	Cause	Treatment
Stress	Urinary leakage with an increase in intra-abdominal pressure (cough, sneeze, physical exertion)	Sphincteric weakness of pelvic floor muscle or urethral sphincter weakness	Medical: pelvic floor muscle exercises, scheduled toileting Surgical: bladder neck suspension or vaginal sling and periurethral injections for intrinsic sphincter deficiency
Urge	Urinary urgency and frequency, usually with small to moderate volume of urine	Detrusor overactivity (overactive bladder)	Bladder retraining (scheduled or prompted voiding, biofeedback, urinary diary) and antimuscarinic bladder relaxants
Mixed	Combination of stress and urge	Overactive bladder/pelvic floor muscle weakness	Bladder retraining/antimuscarinic bladder relaxants
Overflow	Incomplete or unsuccessful voiding or continuous dribbling	Bladder outlet obstruction (e.g., stricture, prostate enlargement, or large cystocele)	Acontractile bladder: intermittent or chronic catheter drainage Obstructed outlet: surgical relief of obstruction
Functional	Inability or unwillingness to get to toilet	Physical or cognitive disability, inability to toilet	Change treatments (e.g., discontinue loop diuretics and restraints), bedside commode or urinal, prompted voiding, and absorbent pads and garments for incurable incontinence

Stress incontinence is the most common type in women younger than 75 years, whereas urge incontinence is the most common type in patients older than 75 years. Stress incontinence results from sphincteric incompetence, and urge incontinence results from detrusor overactivity (overactive bladder). Intrinsic sphincter deficiency (ISD) is commonly associated with multiple incontinence surgical procedures or hypoestrogenism.

Overflow incontinence is seen in patients with an acontractile bladder or bladder outlet obstruction. Functional incontinence occurs as a consequence of cognitive, physical, psychological, or environmental barriers to urination (e.g., delirious patient in physical restraint). Often two or more clinical types, commonly stress and urge, are present in elderly patients. A functional component is also common with the oldest and most frail patients. For example, patients with polyuric states (e.g., uncontrolled diabetes), gait impairments, or cognitive impairments are particularly likely to have a functional component to their incontinence. Patients with DHIC have symptoms that overlap with urge and overflow incontinence.

Diagnosis

Screening patients for UI is recommended when they are seen for the first time and at least annually. A simple question, "Do you have difficulty (trouble) holding your urine?", if answered positively by the patient, should lead to further questioning for lower urinary tract symptoms and leakage. Urinary incontinence may present as either an acute (*transient*) or a chronic (*established*) condition. Acute incontinence typically has a sudden onset and is associated with an acute illness (e.g., infection, delirium) or iatrogenic event (e.g., polypharmacy, restricted mobility). Incontinence may occur in hospitalized patients as a result of delirium (cognitive dysfunction), excessive infusions of intravenous (IV) fluids, fecal impaction, and metabolic disorders such as hyperglycemia with glucosuria.

The clinical types and most likely causes of established urinary incontinence are often determined by a careful medical history, a brief physical examination, and a few laboratory studies (e.g., urinalysis, blood chemistries). The medical history is key to the diagnosis (Table 7.4). Elderly patients should be asked about symptoms of incontinence (e.g., "How often do you lose urine when you don't want to?"). The physical examination identifies pelvic conditions such as vaginal prolapse, genital atrophy, or urethral leakage in women and abnormal prostate glands in men, and rectal or abdominal masses due to bladder distention or fecal impaction in both men and women. A postvoid residual urine obtained by straight catheterization of the bladder or estimated by a bladder scan can exclude urinary retention resulting from either an acontractile bladder or bladder outlet obstruction. A residual of >150 mL is abnormal and might indicate the need for further urologic evaluation or medical treatment.

Surgical referral should be considered for patients with complicated urinary tract infections (e.g., when upper urinary tract obstruction or stones are suspected), severe pelvic prolapse (prominent cystocele with observed leakage of urine), severe symptoms of prostatism, hematuria, and poor response to behavioral and medical treatments. When the pathophysiological mechanism of incontinence is unclear, office cystometry is useful to determine bladder filling capacity, detrusor compliance and contractility, and postvoid residual urine. A detailed urodynamic evaluation is needed in cases of incontinence refractory to medical treatments, particularly before surgical treatments. These studies can identify a definitive cause of overflow incontinence due to an acontractile bladder or outlet obstruction, secure the diagnosis of DHIC, and determine whether stress incontinence is due to urethral hypermobility or ISD.

Treatment

Therapeutic strategies for the management of urinary incontinence include behavioral techniques, medications, patient and caregiver education, surgical procedures, and catheters and incontinence supplies. Behavioral interventions, including bladder training, biofeedback, and pelvic muscle exercises, are recommended as a first line of treatment in the management of stress and urge incontinence in motivated women. Pelvic muscle exercise is assumed to enhance urethral resistance by increasing the strength and endurance of the periurethral and perivaginal muscles and by improving the anatomical support to the bladder neck and proximal urethra.

Intravaginal, oral, or transdermal estrogen replacement therapies have modest effects on stress incontinence in elderly patients and are not often prescribed due to concerns of long-term adverse effects. Surgical options for stress incontinence include bladder neck suspension for women with urethral hypermobility that fails to respond to conservative measures, a vaginal sling for women with findings of both urethral hypermobility and sphincteric incompetence, and periurethral injections of collagen for women with ISD.

Urge incontinence resulting from overactive bladder often responds to scheduled toileting and bladder retraining, scheduled toileting (e.g., every 2 hours), or prompted voiding. Bladder relaxant medications with anticholinergic properties are the most effective drug therapies for urge incontinence (Table 7.5). Oxybutynin and tolterodine are the most commonly prescribed agents. These medications are moderately effective, but can produce significant side effects of constipation, dry mouth, blurred vision, and, occasionally, confusion in vulnerable patients. Long-acting preparations of oxybutynin (XL) and tolterodine (LA) are available, are similar in efficacy, and may enhance compliance compared to the shorter-acting preparations. Newer medications, trospium, darifenacin, and solifenacin also

TABLE 7.5

ANTIMUSCARINIC MEDICATIONS FOR OVERACTIVE BLADDER

Medication	Dosages

Potential Adverse Effects. *All antimuscarinic medications:* dry mouth, constipation, blurring of vision, increased intraocular pressure. In select patients: cognitive impairment, delirium. Use lower doses in patients age 75 years and older and those with renal or liver impairment.

Darifenacin	Initial: 7.5 mg daily
	Maximum: 15 mg daily
Oxybutynin	
Short acting	Initial 2.5 mg up to three times daily
	Maximum: 5 mg three times daily
Long acting	Initial: 5 mg daily
	Maximum 15 mg daily
Transdermal	3.9-mg patch every 4 days
Solifenacin	Initial: 5 mg daily
	Maximum: 10 mg daily
Tolterodine	
Short acting	Initial: 1 mg twice daily
	Maximum: 2 mg twice daily
Long acting	2–4 mg daily
Trospium	20 mg once daily for age 75 years and older (or renal impairment) or twice daily for other patients

appear to be efficacious in older people. Although significant differences in side effects or in adverse drug–drug interactions (e.g., with cholinesterase inhibitors for treatment of Alzheimer's disease) might exist, there is no clear evidence of significant differences in the effectiveness of these agents.

Acute overflow incontinence, which may have been precipitated by medications (e.g., anticholinergic drugs causing underactivity of the bladder) (Table 7.5), anesthesia, or urethral manipulation may be treated with intermittent urethral catheterization until the acute precipitating event subsides. Overflow incontinence resulting from bladder outlet obstruction (e.g., urethral stricture, prostatic hyperplasia) needs either surgical correction or intermittent catheterization. Some patients with urge symptoms and outlet obstruction resulting from prostatic hyperplasia may respond to α-adrenergic antagonists (e.g., terazosin, tamsulosin, doxazosin) that reduce internal sphincter tone. Intermittent self-catheterization is warranted for patients with atonic (acontractile) or bladders. Chronic indwelling urinary catheterization is usually reserved for patients who cannot be catheterized intermittently because of discomfort or terminal illness. External (condom) catheters for men often fail and can lead to local skin infection. The condom catheter is most useful in mobility-impaired patients with either functional or urge incontinence at night.

Functional incontinence responds to improved caregiving, frequent toileting, and treatment of underlying causes. When incontinence is incurable, incontinence aids such as absorbent pads or external catheters are helpful.

REVIEW EXERCISES

QUESTIONS

1. A previously well 78-year-old man is admitted to the hospital for treatment of community-acquired pneumonia. The nurses report that he is sometimes hard to arouse, quiet, and withdrawn, while at other times he is agitated, disoriented, and accusatory, and behaves inappropriately. Physical examination is unremarkable except for findings of pneumonia. Which of the following is the most accurate statement about his mental status?
a) He has dementia with "sundowning."
b) The symptoms are potentially preventable.
c) A head CT scan is needed.
d) He has the "pseudodementia" of depression.

Answer and Discussion
The answer is b. The acute onset of change in mental status, the fluctuating course, and the altered level of consciousness are diagnostic of delirium. Although cognitive dysfunction at night in a new environment (sundowning) can occur in patients with either dementia or delirium, the patient does not have a history of dementia, in which symptoms usually progress over a duration of months to years, and attention and level of consciousness are normal. A head CT scan is rarely useful in the diagnostic evaluation of a patient with delirium and is reserved for patients with new or focal neurologic signs or suspected head trauma. Patients with major depressive disorder often have cognitive dysfunction ("pseudodementia"), but are alert and attentive and do not have a fluctuating course. A clinical trial of hospitalized elderly patients demonstrated a 40% decrease in the incidence of delirium with an intervention that targeted risk factors for delirium (cognitive impairment, sleep deprivation, immobility, visual and hearing impairment, dehydration); total days of delirium were also reduced by the intervention.

2. A 77-year-old man has a 6-month history of frequent falling. Because he loses his balance while walking, he is walking less and has a fear of falling. He takes a diuretic for hypertension and a nitrate for angina pectoris. On physical examination, he takes small, short steps, and has postural instability and decreased steppage. Routine blood test results are normal. The treatment most likely to reduce this patient's risk of falling is
a) Change in medications
b) Gait training
c) Low-intensity resistive exercises
d) All of the above
e) None of the above

Answer and Discussion

The answer is d. Recurrent falls occur in patients with disorders of balance and gait, lower extremity weakness (often from muscular deconditioning or atrophy), polypharmacy, and a fear of falling. Drugs with cardiovascular (e.g., α-adrenergic blockers, vasodilators) or central nervous system (e.g., benzodiazepines) effects may worsen postural stability or balance, increasing the risk of a fall. Clinical trials provide strong evidence that balance and gait training, low-intensity resistive exercise (e.g., with weights, bands, or tubes), walking, or tai chi exercises can reduce the incidence of falls.

3. A 68-year-old man presents in the office with a 3-day history of urinary urgency, dysuria, two episodes of large-volume urinary incontinence, and difficulty initiating urination. His examination is unremarkable. A urinalysis is positive for pyuria, nitrite, and trace protein, but no glucose. A postvoid residual urine (by bladder scan) = 40 mL. His past medical history is only significant for benign prostatic hyperplasia, mild hypertension controlled with diet, and osteoarthritis of the knees. The treatment most likely to relieve his urinary incontinence is

a) Transurethral resection of the prostate
b) Antibiotics
c) Alpha-blocker (e.g., doxazosin)
d) Bladder relaxant (e.g., tolterodine)
e) Cholinergic agent (e.g., bethanechol)

Answer and Discussion

The answer is b. The patient has a urinary tract infection and is likely to respond to an antibiotic that will reduce his lower urinary tract symptoms as well. Acute causes of urinary incontinence can be recalled by the pneumonic DRIP: Delirium, Restricted mobility, Impaction or Iatrogenic (physical restraints, excessive IV fluids) or Infection, Polyuria (glucosuria, loop diuretics, anticholinergics) or Pharmaceuticals. Transurethral resection of prostate is indicated for men with severe lower urinary tract symptoms and/or bladder outlet obstruction unrelieved by medications, but his symptoms are acute and not associated with large postvoid residual urine. An α-adrenergic blocker is often effective in reducing the irritative and obstructive symptoms of benign prostatic hyperplasia, but he did not have a history of chronic symptoms and an improvement with these medications might not be seen for several days or weeks. A bladder relaxant might reduce the intensity of his urinary urgency but would not eliminate the infection. A cholinergic agent would not eradicate the infection and might exacerbate his urge symptoms because it increases the detrusor muscle contractions.

4. An 84-year-old man is recovering from abdominal surgery in the hospital. Four days after surgery, he attempts to get out of bed for the first time. He feels lightheaded and unsteady and falls without an injury. He is now afraid to walk. Before the operation, he walked normally. He is taking a cardioselective beta-blocker, a statin, and acetaminophen. Physical examination reveals normal cognition and vital signs and generalized weakness. He appears worried. Laboratory studies are unremarkable. Which of the following is most likely to improve his symptoms?

a) A beta-blocker with intrinsic sympathomimetic activity rather than the cardioselective agent
b) Low-intensity resistive exercises for his lower extremities
c) A low dose of a psychostimulant (e.g., methylphenidate)
d) A four-prong cane
e) A benzodiazepine (e.g., lorazepam) to treat anxiety

Answer and Discussion

The answer is b. The patient probably has deconditioning associated with major surgery and prolonged immobility. With prolonged bed rest, generalized weakness of the extensor and flexor muscles of the knees and hip muscles is common. Low-intensity exercises, active resistance against flexion or extension, and therapeutic bands or tubes increase muscle strength and lessen the chance of a fall. A beta-blocker with intrinsic sympathomimetic activity could cause orthostatic hypotension and more lightheadedness. A psychostimulant might be considered for a patient with depression and delayed recovery from surgery but will not increase muscle strength. A four-prong cane is helpful when patients have weakness in one extremity, but is not indicated for a patient with generalized weakness due to deconditioning. An anxiolytic could cause gait impairment and increase the risk of a fall.

5. A 71-year-old woman presents with an 8-month history of urinary urgency, frequency, and nocturia, and daily urinary incontinence. Her past medical history is significant for occasional "stress incontinence" (with sneezing, coughing, and straining) for 12 years. She takes no daily medications. Physical examination reveals slight anterior vaginal prolapse and no visible leakage or pelvic mass. A screening urinalysis and basic metabolic panel are normal. Which of the following is most likely to relieve her urinary incontinence?

a) Bladder relaxant (oxybutynin)
b) Topical (vaginal) estrogen
c) α-Agonist (pseudoephedrine)
d) Behavioral therapies
e) Periurethral injections (collagen)

Answer and Discussion

The answer is d. The patient has mixed stress and urge incontinence. The stress incontinence is most likely a result of urethral hypermobility, whereas the urge incontinence likely represents an overactive bladder. Although bladder relaxants alone reduce the frequency of incontinent episodes due to urge incontinence, they have little or no effect on stress incontinence. Behavioral therapies (training), including pelvic floor exercise, pelvic floor stimulation, and biofeedback, are more effective than placebo or bladder muscle relaxants for mixed forms of incontinence. In one study, biofeedback to teach pelvic floor muscle control, verbal feedback based on vaginal palpation, and a self-help booklet in a first-line behavioral training program all achieved comparable improvements in urge incontinence in community-dwelling older women. Periurethral injections with bulking agents (collagen) are indicated for intrinsic sphincter deficiency (ISD) and have no effect on urge incontinence. The α-agonists and vaginal estrogen are of questionable value in the treatment of stress incontinence and have no proven effect in women with ISD.

SUGGESTED READINGS

Agostini JV, Leo-Summers L, Inouye SK. Cognitive and other adverse effects of diphenhydramine use in hospitalized older patients. *Arch Intern Med* 2001;161:2091–2097.

American Geriatrics Society, British Geriatrics Society, American Academy of Orthopaedic Surgeons Panel on Falls Prevention. Guideline for the prevention of falls in older persons. *J Am Geriatr Soc* 2001;49:664–672.

Bischoff-Ferrari HA, Dawson-Hughes B, Willett WC, et al. Effect of vitamin D on falls: a meta-analysis. *JAMA* 2004;291:1999–2006.

Bischoff-Ferrari HA, Willett WC, Wong JB, et al. Fracture prevention with vitamin D supplementation: a meta-analysis of randomized controlled trials. *JAMA* 2005;293:2257–2264.

Broe KE, Chen TC, Weinberg J, et al. A higher dose of vitamin D reduces the risk of falls in nursing home residents: a randomized multiple-dose study. *J Am Geriatr Soc* 2007;55:234–239.

Burgio KL, Goode PS, Locher JL, et al. Behavioral training with and without biofeedback in the treatment of urge incontinence in older women: a controlled trial. *JAMA* 2002;288:2293–2299.

Burgio KL, Locher JL, Goode PS, et al. Behavioral vs. drug treatment for urge incontinence in older women: a randomized controlled trial. *JAMA* 1998;280:1995–2000.

DuBeau CE. Beyond the bladder: management of urinary incontinence in older women. *Clin Obstet Gynecol* 2007;50:720–734.

Fick DM, Cooper J, Wade WE, et al. Updating the Beers criteria for potentially inappropriate medication use in older adults. *Arch Intern Med* 2003;163:2716–2724.

Ganz DA, Bao Y, Shekelle PG, et al. Will my patient fall? *JAMA* 2007;297:77–86.

Gill SS, Mamdani M, Naglie G, et al. A prescribing cascade involving cholinesterase inhibitors and anticholinergic drugs. *Arch Intern Med* 2005;165:808–813.

Gillespie LD, Gillespie WJ, Robertson MC, et al. Interventions for preventing falls in elderly people. *Cochrane Database Syst Rev* 2003;4:CD000340.

Hartikainen S, Lonnroos E, Louhivuori K. Medication as a risk factor for falls: critical systematic review. *J Gerontol A Biol Sci Med Sci* 2007;62A:1172–1181.

Hay-Smith J, Herbison P, Ellis G, et al. Which anticholinergic for overactive bladder symptoms in adults. *Cochrane Database Syst Rev* 2005;3:CD005429.

Inouye SK. Delirium in older persons. *N Engl J Med* 2006;354:1157–1165.

Inouye SK, Bogardus ST, Charpentier PA, et al. Multicomponent intervention to prevent delirium in hospitalized older patients. *N Engl J Med* 1999;340:669–676.

Inouye SK, Studenski S, Tinetti ME, et al. Geriatric syndromes: clinical, research, and policy implications of a core geriatric concept. *J Am Geriatr Soc* 2007;55:780–791.

Kalisvaart KJ, deJonge JF, Bogaards MJ, et al. Haloperidol prophylaxis for elderly hip-surgery patients at risk for delirium: a randomized, placebo-controlled study. *J Am Geriatr Soc* 2005;53:1658–1666.

Kannus P, Sievanen M, Palvanen M, et al. Prevention of falls and consequent injuries in elderly people. *Lancet* 2005;366:1885–1893.

Kiel DP, Magaziner J, Zimmerman S, et al. Efficacy of a hip protector to prevent hip fracture in nursing home residents: the HIP PRO randomized controlled trial. *JAMA* 2007;298:413–422.

Leslie DL, Zhang Y, Holford TR, et al. Premature death associated with delirium at 1-year follow-up. *Arch Intern Med* 2005;165:1657–1662.

Li F, Harmer P, Fisher KJ, et al. Tai chi and fall reductions in older adults: a randomized controlled trial. *J Gerontol A Biol Sci Med Sci* 2005;60:187–194.

Marcantonio ER, Flacker JM, Wright RJ, et al. Reducing delirium after hip fracture: a randomized trial. *J Am Geriatr Soc* 2001;49:516–522.

Mardon RE, Halim S, Pawlson G, et al. Management of urinary incontinence in medicare managed care beneficiaries. *Arch Intern Med* 2006;166:1128–1133.

Pisani MA, Murphy TE, VanNess PH, et al. Characteristics associated with delirium in older patients in a medical intensive care unit. *Arch Intern Med* 2007;167:1629–1634.

Pitkala KH, Laurila JV, Strandberg TE, et al. Multicomponent geriatric intervention for elderly inpatients with delirium: a controlled trial. *J Gerontol A Biol Sci Med Sci* 2006;61:176–181.

Prince RL, Austin N, Devine A, et al. Effects of ergocalciferol added to calcium on the risk of falls in elderly high-risk women. *Arch Intern Med* 2008;168:103–108.

Siddiqi N, Stockdale R, Britton AM, et al. Interventions for preventing delirium in hospitalized patients. *Cochrane Database Syst Rev* 2007;(2):CD005563.

Taylor JA III, Kuchel GA. Detrusor underactivity: clinical features and pathogenesis of an underdiagnosed geriatric condition. *J Am Geriatr Soc* 2006;54:1920–1932.

Tinetti ME. Clinical practice: preventing falls in elderly persons. *N Engl J Med* 2003;348:42–49.

Tinetti ME, Baker DI, McAvay G, et al. A multifactorial intervention to reduce the risk of falling among elderly people living in the community. *N Engl J Med* 1994;331:821–827.

Van Schoor NM, Smit JH, Twisk JW, et al. Prevention of hip fractures by external hip protectors: a randomized controlled trial. *JAMA* 2003;289:1957–1962.

Chapter 8

Dermatology

Melissa Peck Piliang   Kenneth J. Tomecki

POINTS TO REMEMBER:

- An awareness and appreciation of the cutaneous manifestations of systemic diseases help guide the internist in determining the diagnosis, therapy, or need for referral to a dermatologist.

- Drug eruptions occur in approximately 2% of all hospitalized patients.

- Basal cell carcinoma (BCC) and squamous cell carcinoma (SCC) are the most common types of skin cancer. Together, they account for more than 1 million skin cancers each year in the United States.

- Melanoma affects approximately 60,000 people each year in the United States. The lifetime risk in fair-skinned individuals is 1 in 75 (approximately 1%).

- Sarcoidosis is a chronic, often multisystem, granulomatous disease. Approximately one-third of patients have skin disease, which has a variety of presentations, including nasal edema, midfacial papules, annular or scaly plaques, or nodules.

- Approximately one-half of all patients with diabetes have skin disease, most commonly diabetic dermopathy (shin spots), thickened skin, acanthosis nigricans, yellowed nails and skin, or cutaneous infections (fungal or yeast, or bacterial most commonly).

The skin is often a window to systemic disease. An awareness and appreciation of the cutaneous manifestations of systemic diseases help guide the internist in determining the diagnosis, therapy, or need for referral to a dermatologist. This chapter provides a broad overview of skin diseases that are clinically germane and relevant to internists and medical subspecialists.

GENERAL DERMATOLOGY

Common Benign Cutaneous Disorders

Acne vulgaris is an inflammatory disorder of the pilosebaceous follicle, characterized by comedones, papules, pustules, and nodules, occasionally with scars, on the face, neck, chest, and back. Acne typically affects teenagers and young adults. Concomitant hyperandrogenism may occur in women with acne, hirsutism, and irregular menses.

Rosacea, or adult acne, is an inflammatory disease of the midface, characterized by erythema, telangiectasia, papules, and pustules. Rhinophyma is an uncommon complication.

Seborrheic dermatitis is a common inflammatory disease that favors hair-bearing areas of the scalp, face, ears, and central chest. Seborrheic dermatitis is characterized by erythematous plaques with greasy, yellow scale. Scalp pruritus is a common symptom. Disease can affect infants and adults, and tends to be common and extensive in adults with neurologic disorders such as Parkinson's disease and HIV infection.

Seborrheic keratoses are warty, age-related plaques. Although common and benign, they may indicate an underlying adenocarcinoma of the gastrointestinal tract if they appear suddenly in great numbers (sign of Leser-Trélat).

Urticaria, or hives, is often caused by medication (antibiotics, aspirin), food (shellfish, nuts, strawberries), or infection (chronic sinusitis). Affected patients have pruritic, edematous, evanescent wheals that usually resolve within 24 hours. Acute urticaria is usually self-limited, but may last 4 to 6 weeks.

Pruritus may be a symptom of a primary dermatosis, eczema, internal disease (e.g., hepatic or renal disease), hematologic malignancy (especially lymphoma), iron deficiency, psychiatric disease, or endocrinologic disorders. Aquagenic pruritus is unique to polycythemia vera.

Drug eruptions (Fig. 8.1) occur in approximately 2% of all hospitalized patients. The most common type of reaction is *exanthematous* or *morbilliform*, which can resemble a viral exanthem; common causes are penicillin, sulfonamides,

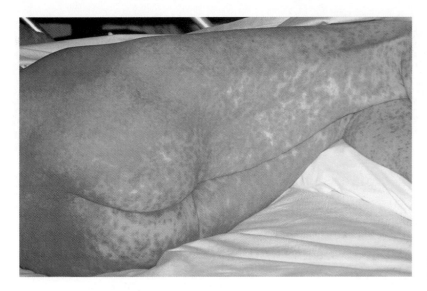

Figure 8.1 Drug eruption: exanthematous type caused by vancomycin.

and blood products. *Urticarial reactions*, characterized by transient wheals and edematous plaques, may occur with systemic anaphylaxis; the most common causes are aspirin, penicillin, and blood products. Phototoxic and photoallergic reactions are two types of drug-induced photosensitivity. *Phototoxic reactions*, essentially exaggerated sunburn responses, may occur in anyone; tetracycline is a common cause. In contrast, *photoallergic reactions* are immunologic responses that occur only in previously sensitized individuals; they occur on sun-exposed areas and may spread to unexposed areas. Drugs that cause photoallergic reactions include sulfonamides, thiazides, griseofulvin, and phenothiazines.

Erythema multiforme (Fig. 8.2) is a hypersensitivity reaction of the skin and mucosa, characterized by macules, papules, plaques, vesicles, or bullae, often with a targetoid appearance. The most common cause of erythema multiforme is recurrent herpes simplex virus infection; less common causes are other infections such as *Mycoplasma pneumonia* and hypersensitivity to medications such as sulfonamides, barbiturates, and antibiotics.

Psoriasis (Fig. 8.3) is a common disease that affects 1% to 2% of the population. The characteristic silvery-white scaly papules and plaques commonly occur on the scalp, elbows, and knees. Nail dystrophy, such as onycholysis, pitting, and oil spots, occur often. Disease typically begins in the third decade, and approximately 50% of patients have an affected family member. Approximately 5% to 10% of patients develop psoriatic arthritis (see Psoriasis and Psoriatic Arthritis section later in this chapter).

Vitiligo, characterized by depigmented macules, affects approximately 1% of the population. The disease can be localized, usually to bony prominences or orifices, or generalized. Some patients have an associated autoimmune disease such as thyroid disease (30% of all patients), alopecia areata, type I diabetes mellitus, pernicious anemia, or Addison's disease.

Erythema nodosum (Fig. 8.4) is a hypersensitivity panniculitis characterized by painful reddened nodules on the shins, less so on the thighs and forearms. The most common cause of erythema nodosum is streptococcal pharyngitis, closely followed by drug sensitivity (sulfonamides, oral contraceptives), and a variety of illnesses, primarily inflammatory bowel disease and sarcoidosis.

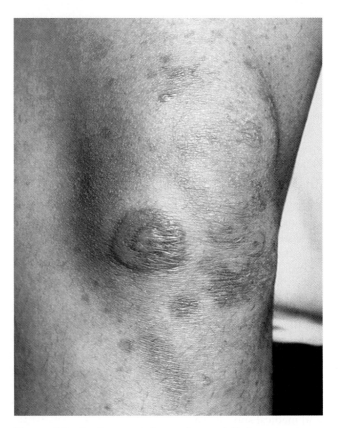

Figure 8.2 Erythema multiforme: "targetoid" plaques.

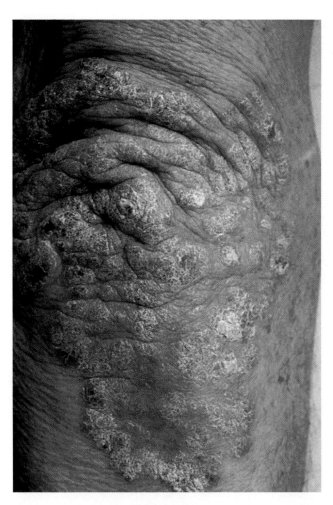

Figure 8.3 Psoriasis: scaly plaques.

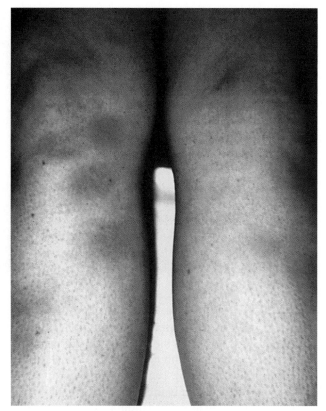

Figure 8.4 Erythema nodosum: reddened nodules on the shins.

Autoimmune Bullous Diseases

Autoimmune bullous diseases are characterized by the deposition of immunoglobulin within the epidermis (pemphigus) or at the dermal–epidermal junction (dermatitis herpetiformis, bullous pemphigoid, epidermolysis bullosa). *Pemphigus vulgaris* is a chronic, debilitating, blistering disease characterized by painful mucosal erosions and flaccid, often eroded blisters. Immunologically, deposition of immunoglobulin G (IgG) occurs within the epidermis. Despite treatment with systemic corticosteroids and/or systemic immunosuppressives, morbidity and mortality are appreciable. *Bullous pemphigoid* is the most common autoimmune bullous disease. It almost invariably affects the elderly, usually with large, tense blisters and urticarial plaques. Pruritus is common and may be severe. Mucosal disease is rare. Immunologically, deposition of IgG at the dermal–epidermal junction occurs. With treatment, usually systemic immunosuppressives, affected patients have a good prognosis.

Dermatitis herpetiformis (**Fig. 8.5**) is a chronic, intensely pruritic disease characterized by the deposition of immunoglobin A at the dermal–epidermal junction. Affected patients have symmetric groups of vesicles, papules, and wheals that appear on the elbows, knees, scalp, and buttocks. Most patients have an asymptomatic gluten-sensitive enteropathy, and approximately 35% have thyroid disease.

Epidermolysis bullosa acquisita is a blistering disease characterized by skin fragility, milia, scarring alopecia, and nail dystrophy. Skin disease typically follows trauma. Immunologically, IgG deposition occurs at the dermal–epidermal junction (similar to bullous pemphigoid).

Exfoliative Dermatitis

Exfoliative dermatitis (**Fig. 8.6**) is an uncommon itchy eczematous disease that is usually generalized and insidious in nature. The most common causes are a pre-existing skin disease (e.g., psoriasis, atopic eczema) and drug hypersensitivity (drug rash). A less common but important etiology is cutaneous T-cell lymphoma (mycosis fungoides).

PRIMARY SKIN CANCER

Basal cell carcinoma (BCC) (**Fig. 8.7**) and *squamous cell carcinoma* (SCC) (**Fig. 8.8**) are the most common types of skin cancer. Together, they account for more than 1 million skin cancers each year in the United States. BCC outnumbers

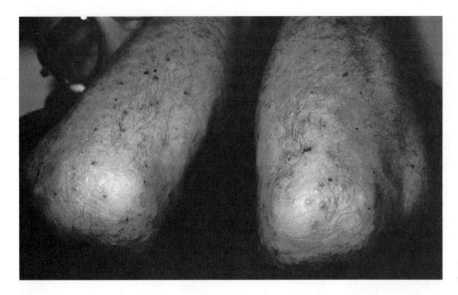

Figure 8.5 Dermatitis herpetiformis: excoriated papules and vesicles.

SCC at a 5:1 ratio. BCC is usually a "pearly" papule, plaque, or nodule with a telangiectatic surface and a rolled border. The vast majority occur on the head and neck. The tumor can be locally aggressive, although its ability to metastasize is limited (less than 0.1%). Tumors near the nose, eye, or ear may invade the eye or brain.

SCC is typically an ill-defined indurated papule, plaque, or nodule with central ulceration and a hyperkeratotic edge, most commonly found on the face, ears, dorsal hands, and forearms. Metastatic potential is 3% to 4%, especially for tumors on the head and neck, which require more aggressive treatment.

Melanoma (Fig. 8.9) affects approximately 60,000 people each year in the United States. The lifetime risk in fair-skinned individuals is 1 in 75 (approximately 1%). Approximately 30% of melanomas arise in a pre-existing melanocytic nevus; the remainder arise de novo. Most

melanomas have *a*symmetry, an irregular *b*order, uneven *c*olor, and a large *d*iameter (greater than 6 mm), all of which constitute the "ABCD" signs of melanoma. Most occur on the head, neck, upper extremities, back, chest, and legs. Common sites for metastases are regional

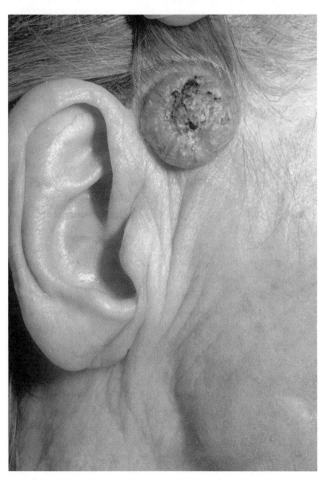

Figure 8.7 Basal cell carcinoma: erythematous plaque with rolled border.

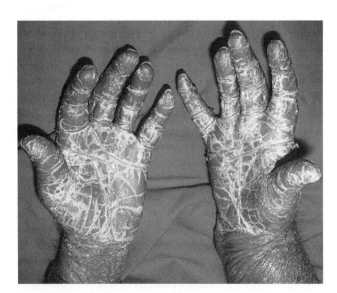

Figure 8.6 Exfoliative dermatitis: eczematous, scaly plaques.

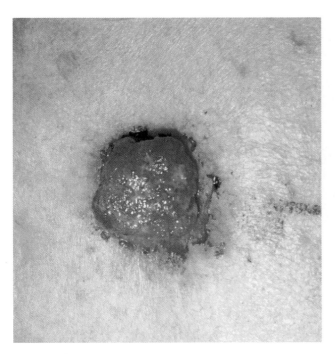

Figure 8.8 Squamous cell carcinoma: indurated, erythematous papule.

lymph nodes, skin, lungs, liver, bone, and brain. The most important prognostic indicator is the histologic depth of invasion (Breslow depth). Thin melanomas (<0.75 mm) have an excellent prognosis (greater than 95% 5-year survival), but thick melanomas (>3.5 mm) carry a much graver prognosis (35%–40% 5-year survival).

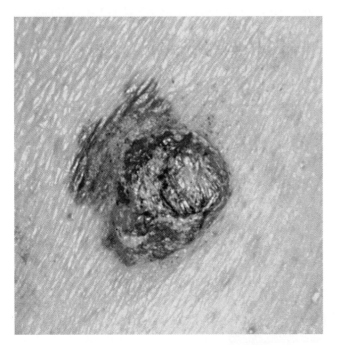

Figure 8.9 Melanoma: asymmetric plaque with an irregular border, uneven brown-black color, and large diameter (greater than 6 mm)—the "ABCD" signs of melanoma.

SKIN DISEASE AND INTERNAL CANCER

Cutaneous Metastases

Cutaneous metastases (Fig. 8.10) occur in 3% to 5% of patients with cancer, and most metastases occur on the head, neck, and trunk, or in close proximity to the underlying tumor. Metastases typically reflect the more common types of cancer in the general population (e.g., cancers of the breast, lung, or gastrointestinal tract). Clinically, cutaneous metastases may be nondescript, but are often juicy red to violaceous nodules.

Paget's Disease of the Breast

Paget's disease of the breast (Fig. 8.11), a unilateral, eczematous plaque of the nipple and areola, invariably implies an underlying intraductal carcinoma of the breast. *Extramammary Paget's disease* (Fig. 8.12), typically a persistent, eczematous plaque on the perineum, often indicates the presence of an underlying adnexal (apocrine) carcinoma or an underlying cancer of the genitourinary tract or distal gastrointestinal tract. Approximately 50% of affected patients have an underlying malignancy.

Acanthosis Nigricans

Acanthosis nigricans (Fig. 8.13), smooth, velvetlike, hyperkeratotic plaques on the neck and intertriginous areas, may indicate an underlying adenocarcinoma of the gastrointestinal tract, usually the stomach. The most common causes of acanthosis nigricans are obesity and type II diabetes. Occasionally, disease occurs with certain medications, such as systemic corticosteroids, nicotinic acid, diethylstilbestrol, and isoniazid.

Acquired Ichthyosis

Acquired ichthyosis (Fig. 8.14), a scaly, platelike thickening of the skin, is a relatively specific marker for lymphoma when it appears de novo in an adult.

Glucagonoma Syndrome

The *glucagonoma syndrome* (Fig. 8.15), characterized by a distinctive necrolytic migratory erythema (erosive, crusted plaques usually on periorificial, acral, and intertriginous areas), implies the presence of an islet cell (glucagon-secreting) tumor of the pancreas. Dermatitis without glucagonoma occasionally occurs with malabsorption or poor nutrition (e.g., zinc deficiency). Patients with necrolytic migratory erythema are usually ill, with weight loss, diarrhea, stomatitis, glossitis, and anemia. An elevated serum glucagon level confirms the diagnosis.

Carcinoid Syndrome

The triad of flushing, secretory diarrhea, and valvular heart disease characterizes *carcinoid tumor*. Other

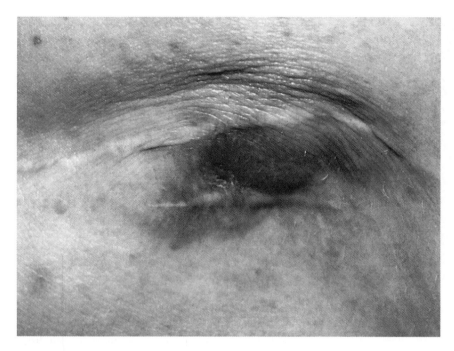

Figure 8.10 Metastatic breast cancer: thoracic nodule.

manifestations include telangiectasia, wheezing, and paroxysmal hypotension. Carcinoid tumors most commonly secrete serotonin. Affected patients have elevated levels of urinary 5-hydroxyindolacetic acid, a by-product of serotonin metabolism.

Gardner's Syndrome

Gardner's syndrome (Fig. 8.16) is an autosomal dominant cancer syndrome characterized by colonic polyposis; osteomas of the maxilla, mandible, and skull; scoliosis;

epidermoid cysts; and soft tissue tumors such as fibromas, desmoids, and lipomas. Approximately 60% of affected patients will develop adenocarcinoma of the colon by age 40 years, secondary to a malignant transformation of the gastrointestinal polyps.

Muir-Torre Syndrome

Muir-Torre syndrome (MTS) is an uncommon autosomal dominant cancer syndrome characterized by at least one sebaceous gland tumor (sebaceous adenoma, epithelioma,

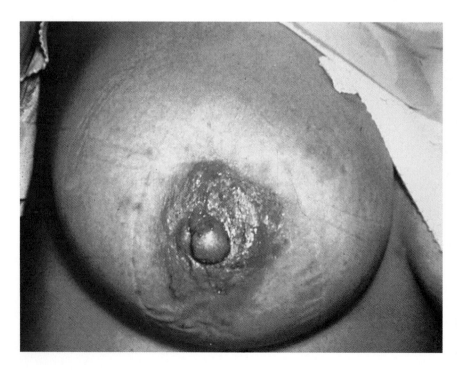

Figure 8.11 Paget's disease of the breast: unilateral eczematous plaque on areola.

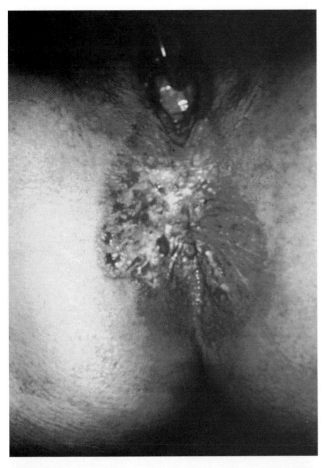

Figure 8.12 Extramammary Paget's disease: eczematous plaque on perineum.

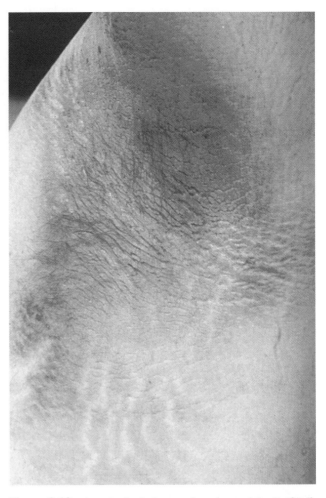

Figure 8.13 Acanthosis nigricans: velvety hyperpigmented axillary plaques.

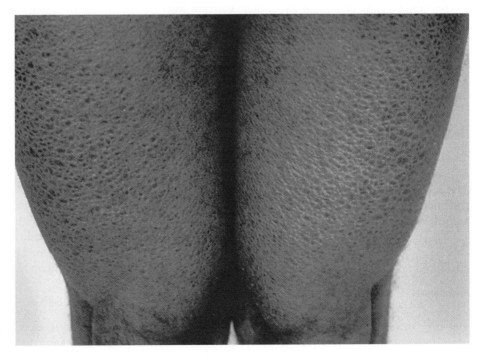

Figure 8.14 Acquired ichthyosis: platelike, scaly plaques.

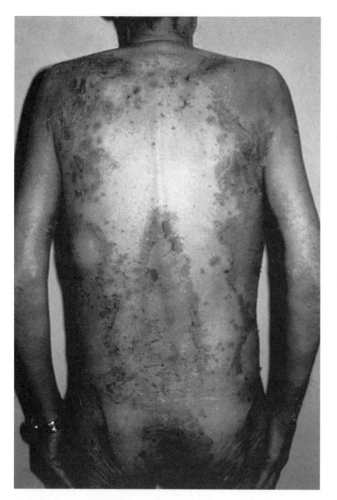

Figure 8.15 Necrolytic migratory erythema (glucagonoma syndrome): erosive, necrolytic plaques.

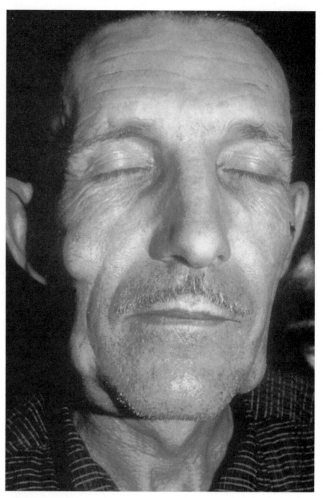

Figure 8.16 Gardner's syndrome: facial cysts.

carcinoma) and one or more internal malignancies, usually colorectal, genitourinary, or lymphoma. The sebaceous gland tumors generally appear on the face and trunk. MTS is a variant of hereditary nonpolyposis colon cancer syndrome (Lynch syndrome) with defects in the same genes.

Cowden's Syndrome

Cowden's syndrome (aka multiple hamartoma syndrome) is a rare autosomal dominant cancer syndrome characterized by multiple tricholemmomas (wartlike papules) on the nose, ears, and periorally. A high incidence of breast and thyroid cancer occurs in affected individuals.

Hirsutism

Hirsutism (Fig. 8.17) is the presence of coarse male-type hair in the beard area, chest or abdomen of a woman, which may indicate androgen excess, with or without an adrenal or ovarian tumor.

Sweet's Syndrome

Sweet's syndrome (Fig. 8.18), or acute febrile neutrophilic dermatosis, is characterized by the presence of painful, reddened plaques on the face, extremities, and trunk. The syndrome is associated with acute leukemia in about 20% of patients, either myelocytic or myelomonocytic. Sweet's syndrome may be induced by medications that stimulate neutrophil production, such as granulocyte colony-stimulating factor. Fever, a flulike illness, and arthralgias often accompany Sweet's syndrome, which primarily affects women.

Multiple Mucosal Neuroma Syndrome

Multiple mucosal neuroma syndrome, characterized by numerous fibromas of the skin and mucosa, is associated with the cancer syndrome, multiple endocrine neoplasia II, which includes medullary thyroid carcinoma, pheochromocytoma, and parathyroid adenoma.

Dermatomyositis

Dermatomyositis (Fig. 8.19) is a connective tissue disease characterized by symmetric proximal muscle weakness

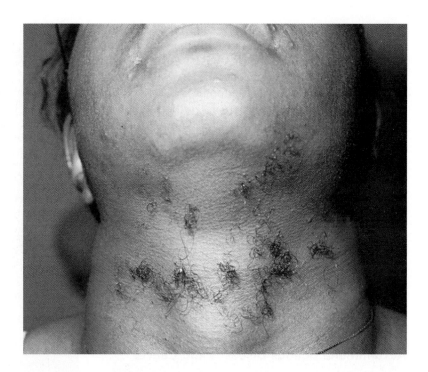

Figure 8.17   Hirsutism: coarse, male-type hair.

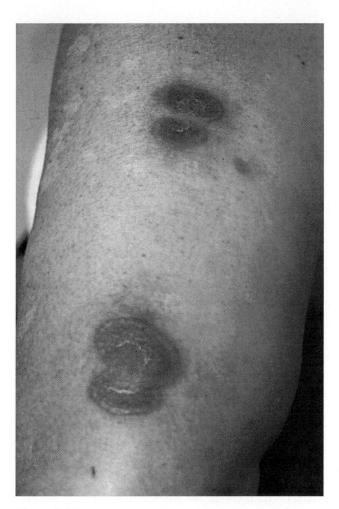

Figure 8.18   Sweet's syndrome: juicy, reddened plaques.

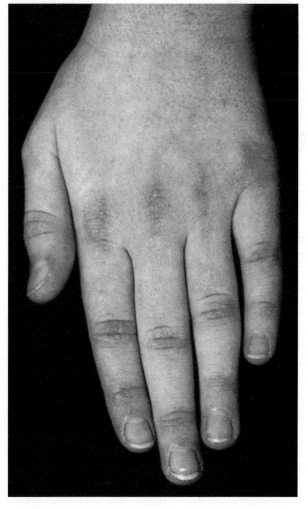

Figure 8.19   Dermatomyositis: Gottron's papules and plaques.

(myositis); pathognomonic papules and plaques on the hands, elbows, and knees (Gottron's papules); and periorbital edema with a violaceous hue (heliotrope). Other features include poikiloderma (hypopigmented/hyperpigmented, telangiectatic, atrophic macules) on the face, neck, trunk, and extremities; malar erythema; and nail abnormalities (periungual telangiectasia and cuticular hypertrophy). Accurate diagnosis requires a muscle biopsy, electromyelogram, and muscle enzyme tests. Adult dermatomyositis has a strong association with malignancy, usually adenocarcinoma of the breast, ovary, gastrointestinal tract, or lung.

Amyloidosis of the Skin

Amyloidosis of the skin, typically expressed as waxy papules of the orbits and midface that become purpuric with pressure or rubbing, may be a sign of multiple myeloma. Other features include macroglossia, "pinch purpura" after trauma, and alopecia.

Autoimmune Bullous Diseases and Cancer

Some autoimmune bullous diseases (see the preceding section on Autoimmune Bullous Diseases) may occur as a paraneoplastic phenomenon. *Paraneoplastic pemphigus*, which clinically and histologically resembles pemphigus vulgaris, bullous pemphigoid, and erythema multiforme, has a strong association with leukemia and lymphoma. Dermatitis herpetiformis is occasionally associated with an intestinal lymphoma, and epidermolysis bullosa acquisita has a weak association with multiple myeloma.

Erythema Gyratum Repens

Erythema gyratum repens is a rare but distinctive skin disease characterized by reddened concentric bands in a whorled pattern; it has a strong association with breast cancer.

SKIN DISEASE AND CARDIOVASCULAR DISEASE

Multiple Lentigines

Multiple lentigines and cardiac abnormalities occur with *LEOPARD syndrome* (Moynahan syndrome), which includes *l*entigines *e*lectrocardiographic changes, *o*cular hypertelorism, *p*ulmonary stenosis, *a*bnormal genitalia, *r*etarded growth, and *d*eafness. Variants of LEOPARD syndrome include Carney complex, which encompasses *LAMB syndrome* (*l*entigines, *a*trial myxoma, *m*ucocutaneous myxomas, and *b*lue nevi) and *NAME syndrome* (*n*evi, *a*trial myxoma, *m*yxoid neurofibromas, and *e*phelides).

Pseudoxanthoma Elasticum

Pseudoxanthoma elasticum (**Fig. 8.20**) is an inherited disease (either autosomal dominant or autosomal recessive)

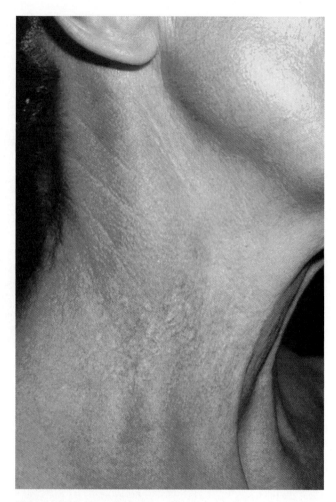

Figure 8.20   Pseudoxanthoma elasticum: pebbled skin on the neck.

characterized by yellow, pebbled skin on the neck, abdomen, and intertriginous areas, giving the appearance of "plucked chicken skin." The disease represents a defect in elastic fibers, which become brittle and calcified. Associated internal manifestations include hypertension, peripheral vascular and coronary artery disease, and retinal and gastrointestinal hemorrhage. Funduscopic examination reveals angioid streaks in Bruch's membrane.

Ehlers-Danlos Syndrome

Ehlers-Danlos syndrome, characterized by hyperextensible and hypermobile joints, fragile skin, and "fish-mouth" scars, represents an abnormality in collagen biosynthesis. Several variants exist, and associated features include angina, gastrointestinal bleeding (perforation), poor wound healing, hernias, and peripheral vascular disease.

Marfan's Syndrome

Marfan's syndrome is an autosomal dominant connective tissue disease affecting the skin and cardiovascular, musculoskeletal, and ocular systems. Patients are generally thin, with long, spindly extremities. Complications include striae distensae, elastosis perforans serpiginosa, aortic aneurysms, mitral valve prolapse, and displacement of the lens.

Fabry's Disease

Fabry's disease is an X-linked abnormality of glycosphingolipid metabolism caused by a deficiency of α-galactosidase A, characterized by angiokeratoma corporis diffusum (blue-black nonblanchable papules in a bathing trunk distribution). Associated cardiovascular abnormalities include mitral valve prolapse, angina, myocardial infarction, congestive heart failure, and hypertension. Other features are painful neuropathy, renal failure, and stroke.

SKIN DISEASE AND PULMONARY DISEASE

Sarcoidosis

Sarcoidosis (Fig. 8.21) is a chronic, often multisystem, granulomatous disease. Approximately one-third of patients have skin disease, which has a variety of presentations, including nasal edema, midfacial papules, annular or scaly plaques, or nodules. Lupus pernio is cutaneous sarcoidosis of the central face with involvement of the upper respiratory tract. Erythema nodosum, an acute painful panniculitis that commonly affects the shins, may accompany acute sarcoidosis; if so, it portends a good prognosis.

SKIN DISEASE AND RHEUMATIC DISEASE

Psoriasis and Psoriatic Arthritis

Psoriatic arthritis (PSA) (Fig. 8.22) is an uncommon, asymmetric, seronegative spondyloarthropathy characterized by fusiform swelling of the distal and proximal interphalangeal joints. PSA affects approximately 10% of psoriatic patients. The most common presentation is asymmetric oligoarthritis, characterized by "sausage" digits and the involvement of a few large joints.

Reiter's Syndrome

Reiter's syndrome (Fig. 8.23) is an inflammatory disorder with three features: urethritis, conjunctivitis, and arthritis. Reiter's syndrome invariably affects young men, and most patients have skin disease that resembles psoriasis—erythematous scaly plaques on the penis (circinate balanitis) and palms and soles (keratoderma blenorrhagicum). Most patients have the HLA-B27 antigen.

Acrosclerosis

Acrosclerosis (Fig. 8.24), a thickened tapering of the skin, often with secondary ulceration, may occur with angiitis, chilblains, cryopathies, and scleroderma, or may follow exposure to polyvinyl chlorides.

Erythema Chronicum Migrans

Erythema chronicum migrans (Fig. 8.25), the cutaneous expression of Lyme disease, is an annular erythematous

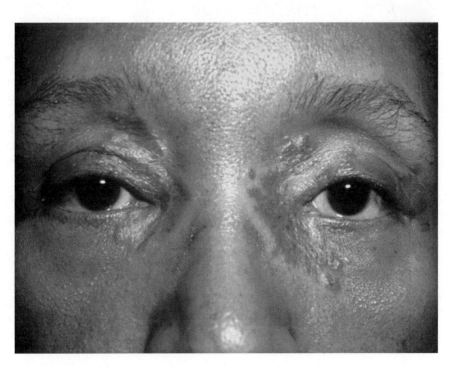

Figure 8.21 Cutaneous sarcoidosis: annular facial plaques.

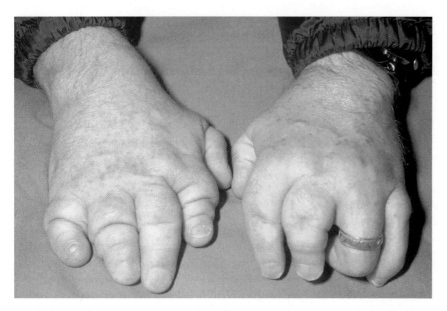

Figure 8.22 Psoriatic arthritis: "sausage" digits.

plaque that follows and surrounds the site of a tick bite. Lyme disease is a multisystem illness that includes fever, arthralgias, and myalgias, and may also include meningoencephalitis, myocarditis, and peripheral neuropathy. The causative agent in the United States is usually the spirochete *Borrelia burgdorferi*, transmitted by the bite of a tick, either *Ixodes scapularis* or *Ixodes pacificus*. Primary endemic areas are New England, the upper Midwest, and the Pacific Northwest.

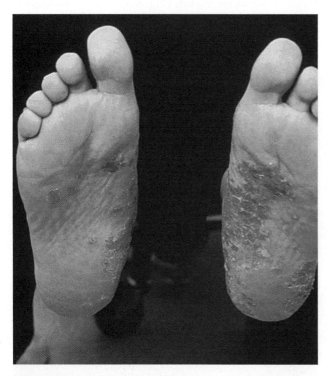

Figure 8.23 Reiter's syndrome: psoriasiform plaques on the feet (keratoderma blenorrhagicum).

SKIN DISEASE AND GASTROINTESTINAL DISEASE

Aphthae

Aphthae are common painful superficial ulcerations of the mucosa. They occur with Crohn's disease, gluten-sensitive enteropathy, and HIV infection.

Acrodermatitis Enteropathica

Acrodermatitis enteropathica is an inflammatory disease, either inherited or acquired, characterized by diarrhea, alopecia, and erosive plaques in the perineum and on the face, hands, and feet. Affected individuals have a zinc deficiency either due to malnutrition or malabsorption.

Hepatitis C Infection

Hepatitis C infection is a common cause of chronic liver disease and hepatoma. Infection can induce cryoglobulinemia with vasculitis, porphyria cutanea tarda, chronic arthropathy, and lichen planus (an itchy papulosquamous skin disease characterized by flat-topped polygonal purple papules, usually on flexural sites).

Hereditary Hemorrhagic Telangiectasia

Hereditary hemorrhagic telangiectasia (Osler-Weber-Rendu syndrome) (Fig. 8.26) is an autosomal dominant disease characterized by cutaneous (typically acral) and mucosal (lips, nose, and tongue) telangiectasia that may bleed. Affected patients typically have frequent nosebleeds (epistaxis) and occasionally gastrointestinal bleeding. Pulmonary arteriovenous fistulae and vascular malformations of the central nervous system may occur; aortic aneurysms are rare.

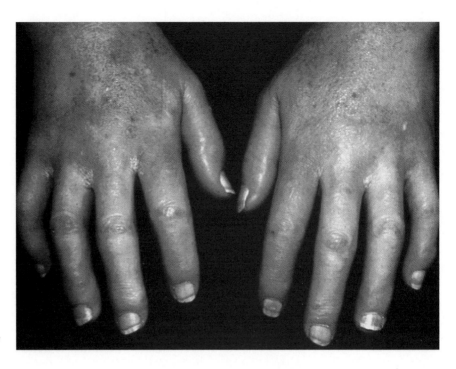

Figure 8.24 Acrosclerosis: thickened, sclerotic digits.

Peutz-Jeghers Syndrome

Peutz-Jeghers syndrome (Fig. 8.27) is an autosomal dominant disease characterized by perioral, mucosal, and acral lentigines and gastrointestinal polyps, usually hamar-

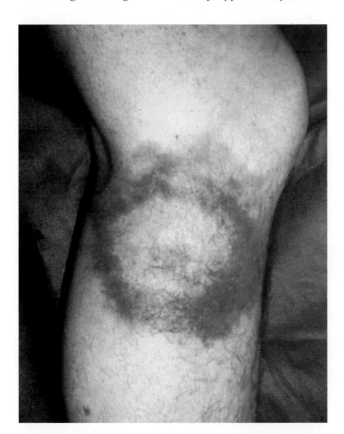

Figure 8.25 Erythema chronicum migrans (Lyme disease): annular, reddened plaque.

tomas, in the small intestine. The malignant potential of the polyps is low, but affected patients do have a higher risk of colon cancer than the general population.

Pyoderma Gangrenosum

Pyoderma gangrenosum (Fig. 8.28) is an inflammatory ulcerative skin disease with a distinctive morphology: inflammatory ulcers with undermined edges and a border of gray or purple pigmentation. The legs are most commonly affected, and the ulcers typically start as a pustule and may follow trauma. Most patients have either inflammatory bowel disease (usually ulcerative colitis) or rheumatoid arthritis. Some patients may have paraproteinemia, usually an IgA gammopathy. Bullous pyoderma gangrenosum occurs with leukemia.

SKIN DISEASE AND ENDOCRINE OR METABOLIC DISEASE

Skin Disease With Diabetes

Approximately one-third to one-half of all patients with diabetes have skin disease, most commonly, diabetic dermopathy (shin spots), thickened skin, acanthosis nigricans, yellowed nails and skin, or cutaneous infections (fungal or yeast, or bacterial most commonly).

Shin spots (diabetic dermopathy) are small, discrete, scar-like plaques on the legs. They are a common, although nonspecific, occurrence in diabetic patients.

Thickened skin, which may vary from pebbling to scleroderma-like changes, is another common finding.

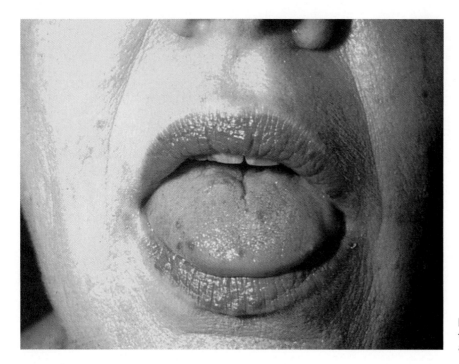

Figure 8.26 Hereditary hemorrhagic telangiectasia: telangiectasiae of the skin and mucosa.

Scleredema, a chronic thickening of the skin on the upper back and shoulders, usually affects men with long-standing, uncontrolled diabetes. *Stiff hand syndrome*, a waxy thickening of the skin combined with restricted mobility, occurs in young patients with insulin-dependent juvenile diabetes; renal and retinal vascular disease often follows the syndrome.

Acanthosis nigricans (see earlier section) commonly occurs with obesity and other insulin-resistant disorders, primarily diabetes.

Yellowed nails and skin occur in approximately 50% of patients with diabetes, primarily on the palms and soles, probably secondary to either carotenemia or protein glycosylation. The significance is unknown.

Granuloma annulare, characterized by reddened annular papules and plaques, usually on the hands and feet, may occur with or without diabetes.

Uncommon but specific conditions include necrobiosis lipoidica diabeticorum, diabetic bullae (bullous diabeticorum), and eruptive xanthoma.

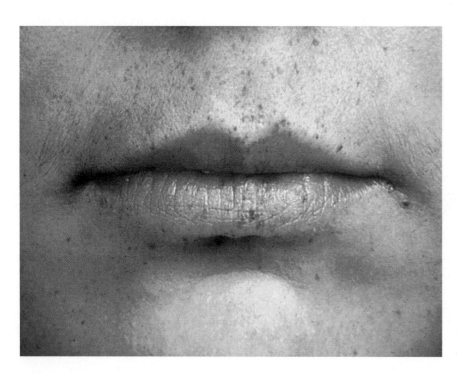

Figure 8.27 Peutz-Jeghers syndrome: hyperpigmented macules (lentigines) on the skin and mucosa.

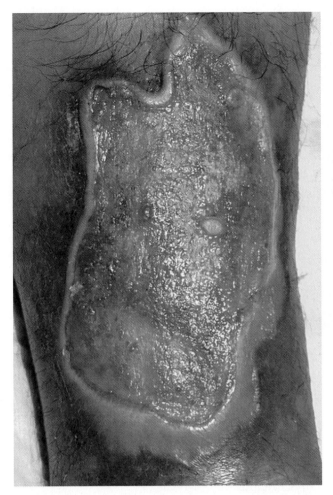

Figure 8.28 Pyoderma gangrenosum: inflammatory, undermined ulcer.

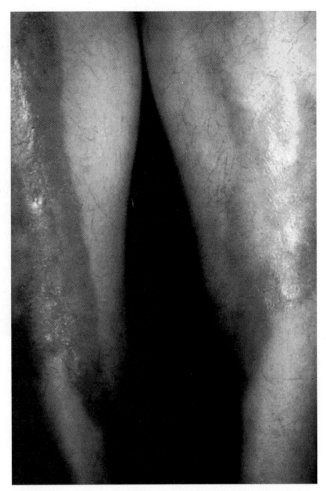

Figure 8.29 Necrobiosis lipoidica diabeticorum: shiny atrophic plaques.

Necrobiosis lipoidica diabeticorum (**Fig. 8.29**)—yellowed, atrophic plaques usually on the shins that may ulcerate—is uncommon but highly specific for diabetes.

Diabetic bullae are also very uncommon. Bullae erupt and resolve spontaneously and heal without scarring. They occur mainly in male patients with type II diabetes mellitus.

Eruptive xanthomas, characterized by discrete yellow papules on the extremities and buttocks, occur in patients with diabetes and hyperlipidemia (markedly elevated triglycerides). Pruritus can be significant. Xanthomas resolve with treatment of the hyperlipidemia.

Skin Disease and Renal Disease

Acquired perforating disorders primarily affect patients with diabetes mellitus and renal failure, especially those on hemodialysis. Patients have pruritic hyperkeratotic papules in a generalized distribution, especially on the legs.

Calciphylaxis is characterized by painful, inflammatory necrotic plaques that primarily affect adults with end-stage renal disease, diabetes mellitus, and secondary hyperparathyroidism. Calciphylaxis is caused by calcium deposits within the cutaneous vasculature, which lead to necrosis.

Nephrogenic systemic fibrosis (also known as nephrogenic fibrosing dermopathy) is a recently described entity characterized by fibrosis of the skin, viscera (heart, liver, and lungs), and muscle that occurs in patients with renal failure and gadolinium contrast exposure.

Porphyria cutanea tarda (see next section) is characterized by acral bullae, hypertrichosis, and scarring, and occurs in dialysis patients with iron overload.

Porphyrias

Porphyrias are a group of disorders related to abnormalities in heme biosynthesis that may be erythropoietic, hepatic, or mixed; each type, whether inherited or acquired, has a specific enzyme defect. Porphyria cutanea tarda (PCT) (**Fig. 8.30**), the most common porphyria, is a hepatic porphyria that may be inherited or acquired. Affected patients lack uroporphyrinogen decarboxylase, which converts uroporphyrin to coproporphyrin; as such, uroporphyrins accumulate in the urine. Precipitating factors

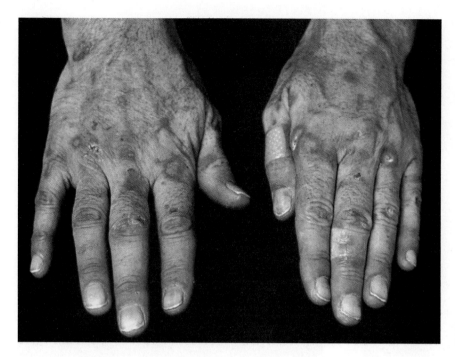

Figure 8.30 Porphyria cutanea tarda: vesicles and erosions.

include hepatitis C infection, alcohol ingestion, estrogen use, iron overload, dialysis, and exposure to toxins such as hexachlorobenzene. Skin disease typically includes photosensitivity, skin fragility, vesicles, bullae, and erosions, usually on the hands (dorsum), forearms, and face. Hyperpigmentation and hypertrichosis (excess hair growth) may occur, usually on the face.

Pseudoporphyria resembles PCT but without the enzyme defect; plasma and urinary porphyrins are normal. Common causes are hemodialysis and certain medications, such as nonsteroidal anti-inflammatory drugs, furosemide, nalidixic acid, and tetracycline.

REVIEW EXERCISES

QUESTIONS

1. Acute urticaria in a healthy young woman commonly follows all *except*
a) Crash dieting
b) Chocolate ingestion
c) Pregnancy
d) Alcohol ingestion
e) Stress

Answer and Discussion
The answer is c. The most common causes of acute urticaria are medications, food, and infection.

2. A 35-year-old woman developed several painful, reddened plaques on the face, arms, legs, and trunk associated with fever, arthralgia, and myalgia. The most likely diagnosis is
a) Lyme disease
b) Sweet's syndrome
c) Dermatomyositis
d) Sarcoidosis
e) Erythema multiforme

Answer and Discussion
The answer is b. Sweet's syndrome, characterized by painful, reddened plaques on the face, extremities, and trunk, typically affects women, often in association with a flu-like illness.

3. Sweet's syndrome is often associated with which of the following?
a) Adenocarcinoma of the breast
b) Adenocarcinoma of the gastrointestinal tract
c) Pulmonary disease
d) Myocarditis
e) Leukemia

Answer and Discussion
The answer is e. Sweet's syndrome is strongly associated with myelocytic or myelomonocytic leukemia.

4. Which is the most common type of drug eruption?
a) Exanthematous or morbilliform
b) Urticarial
c) Phototoxic
d) Photoallergic
e) None of the above

Answer and Discussion
The answer is a. The most common type of drug eruption is the exanthematous reaction.

5. Which is the most important prognostic indicator for melanoma?
a) Lymph node involvement
b) Site of the tumor
c) Histologic depth of invasion (Breslow depth)
d) Age and gender of the patient
e) Tumor size

Answer and Discussion
The answer is c. The histologic depth of invasion is the most important prognostic indicator for melanoma.

6. A 30-year-old man with ulcerative colitis developed an inflammatory undermined ulcer on his left leg. The most likely diagnosis is
a) Necrobiosis lipoidica diabeticorum
b) Stasis ulcer
c) Gangrene
d) Pyoderma gangrenosum
e) Kaposi's sarcoma

Answer and Discussion
The answer is d. Pyoderma gangrenosum is an inflammatory ulcerative disease of the legs. Ulcers have undermined edges and gray or purple borders. Approximately 50% of affected patients have inflammatory bowel disease, usually ulcerative colitis, or rheumatoid arthritis.

7. An elderly woman with tense bullae on the extremities most likely has
a) Bullous pemphigoid
b) Pemphigus vulgaris
c) Dermatitis herpetiformis
d) Erythema multiforme
e) Epidermolysis bullosa

Answer and Discussion
The answer is a. Bullous pemphigoid is an uncommon blistering disease of the elderly, characterized by tense bullae, most commonly on the extremities. Mucosal involvement is rare.

8. Dermatitis herpetiformis is strongly associated with
a) Recurrent herpes virus infection
b) Atopic dermatitis
c) Gluten-sensitive enteropathy
d) Nonsteroidal anti-inflammatory drug use
e) Colon carcinoma

Answer and Discussion
The answer is c. Most patients with dermatitis herpetiformis have an asymptomatic gluten-sensitive enteropathy; some have thyroid disease.

9. A 35-year-old woman has tender targetoid plaques on her hands and oral erosions. What is the most likely cause?
a) Toxic shock syndrome
b) Herpes simplex virus infection
c) Diabetes mellitus
d) Pemphigus vulgaris
e) Syphilis

Answer and Discussion
The answer is b. Patient most likely has erythema multiforme, which is most commonly associated with recurrent oral herpes simplex virus infection.

10. Lupus pernio describes central facial inflammation (plagues) and airway involvement of
a) Tuberculosis
b) Systemic lupus erythematosus
c) Psoriasis
d) Sarcoidosis
e) Granuloma annulare

Answer and Discussion
The answer is d. Sarcoidal involvement of the central face and upper respiratory tract characterizes lupus pernio.

SUGGESTED READINGS

Callen JP. Neutrophillic dermatoses. *Dermatol Clin* 2002;20:409.
Callen JP. Pyoderma gangrenosum. *Lancet* 1998;351:581.
Giuffrida TJ, Kerdel FA. Sarcoidosis. *Dermatol Clin* 2002;20:435.
Kahn LE, Russo G, Millikan LE. Genetic and acquired cutaneous disorders associated with internal malignancy. *Int J Dermatol* 1995;34:749.
McDonnell JK. Cardiac disease and the skin. *Dermatol Clin* 2002;20:503.
Perez MI, Kohn SR. Cutaneous manifestations of diabetes mellitus. *J Am Acad Dermatol* 1994;30:519.
Poole S, Fenske NF. Cutaneous markers of internal malignancy. I, II. *J Am Acad Dermatol* 1993;28:147.
Rivers JK. Melanoma. *Lancet* 1996;347:803.
Robson KJ, Piette WW. Cutaneous manifestations of systemic disease. *Med Clin North Am* 1998;82:1359.
Scott JE, Ahmed AR. The blistering diseases. *Med Clin North Am* 1998;82:1239.

Chapter 9

Occupational Medicine

Peter J. Mazzone   *Edward P. Horvath, Jr.*

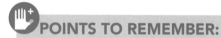
POINTS TO REMEMBER:

- Organophosphate compounds are readily absorbed through intact skin.
- Asbestosis may appear and progress long after exposure has ceased.
- Individuals with chronic silicosis have an incidence of mycobacterial tuberculosis that is three times greater than that of age-matched controls.
- To diagnose occupational asthma, we need to confirm the presence of asthma, confirm an exposure, and confirm a work-related pattern.

General internists are called on to manage many occupational health–related issues. Services commonly provided include preplacement examinations, injury care, and return-to-work evaluations. In addition, the internist needs to be knowledgeable about the evaluation and management of toxicity related to exposures in the environment and the workplace.

This chapter provides information that will help the reader recognize and manage three common chemical exposures, three common pneumoconioses, and occupational asthma. The Suggested Readings expand on these and other topics.

CHEMICAL EXPOSURES

Chemical exposures can result from occupational exposure, industrial accidents, natural disasters, recreational contact, chemical warfare, or acts of terrorism. Here, we discuss three common exposures: the asphyxiant carbon monoxide, cholinesterase inhibitors such as organophosphate insecticides, and heavy metal exposure to lead.

Asphyxiants—Carbon Monoxide

Asphyxiants are chemicals that lead to tissue hypoxia after exposure. Cardiovascular and neurologic symptoms predominate. Simple asphyxiants (e.g., methane, propane, nitrogen, carbon dioxide) cause tissue hypoxia by displacing oxygen in inspired air. Chemical asphyxiants (e.g., carbon monoxide, cyanide, hydrogen sulfide) cause tissue hypoxia by interfering with oxygen transport and/or cellular respiration in the body. We focus on carbon monoxide, the most commonly encountered asphyxiant.

Carbon monoxide poisoning is one of the most common forms of poisoning in both occupational and nonoccupational settings. As a by-product of incomplete combustion, it is present in virtually every workplace and home environment, particularly during the heating season. As an odorless, colorless, and tasteless gas, it gives no warning of its presence. In addition, its typical early symptoms of nausea, headache, and dizziness occur frequently with common disorders, such as viral illness. Practicing physicians must be aware of the possibility of carbon monoxide poisoning, particularly among certain workers and during the heating season. Measurement of blood carboxyhemoglobin always should be obtained in such circumstances.

Occupational Exposure

Certain employees are recognized as being at particular risk for carbon monoxide poisoning, including firefighters, coal miners, coke oven and smelter workers, mechanics, and drivers. Exhaust from the operation of vehicles indoors, such as propane-powered forklift trucks, is a frequently overlooked source of exposure. Overexposure is particularly likely to occur during winter months, when ventilation of the work environment may be decreased to lower the costs of heating. Methylene chloride, a solvent widely used as a paint stripper, produces a unique form of carbon monoxide poisoning by being metabolized to carbon monoxide in the body.

Environmental Exposure

Carbon monoxide is also a significant cause of poisoning in nonoccupational environments. Despite widespread recognition of this hazard, fatalities occur each year from prolonged exposure to automobile exhaust in enclosed spaces. Deaths of entire families from carbon monoxide poisoning caused by malfunctioning furnaces or space heaters are disturbingly common. Deliberate personal exposure from cigarette or cigar smoke can produce blood carboxyhemoglobin levels from 2% to 10% and sometimes as high as 18%. Nonexposed persons have an average level of 1% or less from endogenous hemoglobin metabolism.

Clinical Effects

Carbon monoxide has an affinity for hemoglobin approximately 200 to 300 times that of oxygen; however, the formation of carboxyhemoglobin is not the only way in which carbon monoxide exerts adverse physiological effects. It also shifts the oxygen-hemoglobin dissociation curve and binds to both myoglobin and cytochrome oxidase. The central nervous system and myocardium are sensitive to tissue hypoxia produced by carbon monoxide. Clinical effects in a given patient depend on the intensity and duration of clinical exposure and the presence of any pre-existing conditions, such as atherosclerosis. Blood carboxyhemoglobin levels of 10% or less rarely produce symptoms. At levels of 10% to 30%, patients may complain of headache, nausea, weakness, and dizziness. Mentation begins to be impaired at 30% to 35%, and levels of 35% to 40% may result in coma. Death can occur with levels exceeding 50%. As with many chemical exposures, there is considerable individual variation. Death has occurred from blood levels of 36% to 38% in circumstances of prolonged exposure, presumably from the longer time available for the cytochromes to be inhibited. Although many patients with carbon monoxide poisoning recover completely, others exhibit delayed neurologic and neuropsychiatric manifestations believed to be due to diffuse demyelination. These complications can include a parkinsonian movement disorder, cranial nerve dysfunction, peripheral motor or sensory loss, and disorders of cognition and affect.

Laboratory Studies

A person who has been overcome by carbon monoxide and brought to the emergency room from a typical exposure environment (e.g., a running vehicle in a closed garage) seldom poses a diagnostic problem. In some instances, however, exposure to carbon monoxide may not be readily apparent, and the patient's symptoms may be nonspecific. A key diagnostic clue is the presence of discordance between the oxygen saturation as measured by pulse oximetry and that measured by an arterial blood gas (by co-oximetry). The oxygen saturation measured by pulse oximetry is usually falsely normal. Arterial blood gases show a normal partial pressure of oxygen, but the oxygen saturation is decreased. Electrolytes may show hypokalemia. In the presence of tissue damage, creatine kinase and lactate dehydrogenase are elevated. The ECG may show ischemic

changes. Measurement of the carboxyhemoglobin level confirms the diagnosis of carbon monoxide poisoning.

Treatment

The objectives of treatment are to increase tissue oxygenation and speed the elimination of carbon monoxide. Administration of 100% oxygen by a tightly fitting face mask reduces the half-life from 5.5 hours to approximately 1.5 hours. Hospitalization should be considered if there is evidence of end-organ dysfunction (e.g., an abnormal ECG or neurologic findings) or carbon monoxide levels >25%. Assisted ventilation is required for patients in respiratory distress. Treatment with hyperbaric oxygen at 2 to 3 atm should be considered for severely affected patients with coma or seizures or for those in whom neurologic and cardiovascular dysfunction does not resolve with other forms of oxygen therapy. Oxygen at 3 atm not only reduces the half-life for carbon monoxide elimination to 23 minutes, but it also results in enough available oxygen dissolved in the plasma to support metabolism, even in the absence of functioning hemoglobin. The prompt use of hyperbaric oxygen may also reduce the risk of delayed neurologic symptoms.

Cholinesterase Inhibitors—Organophosphate Insecticides

Chemicals that inhibit the enzyme acetylcholinesterase include organic phosphorus pesticides, carbamate pesticides, and organophosphorus "nerve agents" (e.g., sarin, VX). The result of exposure is overstimulation of the cholinergic system with both muscarinic and nicotinic effects. Exposure may result from inhalation, ingestion, or absorption through the skin. Antidotes include atropine, pralidoxime, and benzodiazepines (for seizure control). Here, we focus the discussion on organophosphate insecticides.

Internists occasionally encounter patients either acutely poisoned by pesticides or fearful of potential long-term effects from past exposure. Although a large number of different pesticides are in commercial use, physicians are most likely to encounter clinical problems caused by the organophosphate insecticides. The toxicity of organophosphate insecticides varies widely. One of the least toxic, malathion, commonly results in home-use exposures. Poisoning from more toxic agents, such as parathion, is rare except in agricultural regions or in a pesticide manufacturing or formulating facility.

Occupational Exposure

In occupational settings, exposures occur during the manufacturing, formulation, transportation, and application of pesticides. Firefighters and hazardous waste workers may encounter these substances in their work. Organophosphate insecticides are readily absorbed by inhalation, through intact skin, and by ingestion.

Environmental Exposure

Exposures may occur among families of field workers or farmers who come in contact with contaminated clothing. Haphazard aerial spraying can also result in exposure in rural families. The general public often expresses concern about pesticide contamination of food or water, although actual clinical toxicity in such circumstances is rare. Organophosphate poisoning from accidental ingestion by children remains regrettably common, particularly when unused pesticide is stored in an inappropriate container, such as a soda bottle or can.

Clinical Effects

Anticholinesterase compounds produce their clinical effects through phosphorylation of acetylcholinesterase enzyme at nerve endings. The resultant accumulation of the neurotransmitter acetylcholine at these nerve endings produces overstimulation and then paralysis of nerve transmission. Both nicotinic (ganglionic and neuromuscular) and muscarinic (parasympathetic) effects are observed. Various mnemonics have been devised to assist clinicians in remembering the clinical signs and symptoms of cholinesterase inhibition. A common one, STUMBLED, stands for Salivation, Tremors, Urination, Miosis, Bradycardia, Lacrimation, Emesis, and Diarrhea. The developmental sequence of systemic effects and the time of onset after exposure can vary. Acute toxicity is usually rapid in onset, although symptoms may be delayed up to 12 hours after exposure. In cases of inhalation, respiratory and ocular symptoms may appear first. In cases of ingestion, gastrointestinal effects may be the initial manifestations. Occupational exposures insufficient to produce symptoms following a single event can result in symptoms after continued daily exposure. Depending on treatment, complete symptomatic recovery usually occurs within a week; however, increased susceptibility to the effects of anticholinesterase agents may persist for several weeks after a single exposure.

A delayed peripheral neuropathy has been reported after poisoning by some organophosphates. This condition, organophosphate-induced delayed neuropathy, is believed to be due to phosphorylation and inhibition of the enzyme neurotoxic esterase, followed by degradation of the phosphoryl-enzyme complex. This predominantly motor polyneuropathy occurs 2 to 3 weeks after acute poisoning, usually by intentional ingestion. An "intermediate syndrome" after acute poisoning has also been reported. It consists of a paralytic syndrome involving primarily proximal limb muscles, neck flexors, certain cranial motor nerves, and the muscles of respiration, which occurs 24 to 96 hours after heavy exposure. Neuropsychiatric or cognitive complaints, such as irritability, depression, anxiety, fatigue, difficulty in concentration, and short-term memory impairment, are commonly reported after acute exposures. In the assessment of individual cases, however, it is often difficult to distinguish organically based neurobehavioral symptoms from the psychological reactions likely to occur after exposure events.

Laboratory Studies

The diagnosis of organophosphate poisoning depends on a history of exposure, the presence of typical signs and symptoms, and laboratory documentation of cholinesterase inhibition. Two types of cholinesterase levels can be measured: plasma cholinesterase (pseudocholinesterase) and red cell cholinesterase (true acetylcholinesterase). Plasma cholinesterase, which is synthesized by the liver, declines sooner but regenerates faster than red cell cholinesterase. Typical regeneration time is days to a few weeks. Depressed plasma cholinesterase levels are also seen in genetic pseudocholinesterase deficiency and in chronic liver disease. Red cell cholinesterase more accurately reflects the degree of actual enzyme inactivation at neuroeffector sites; however, it is depressed more slowly and for longer periods than plasma cholinesterase. Typical regeneration time is 1 to 3 months. Cholinesterase levels are of greater clinical utility when they can be compared with a pre-exposure baseline. Unfortunately, such data are rarely available, except in pesticide-exposed workers in whom prior medical surveillance testing has been conducted. A cholinesterase depression of 25% or more, compared with the pre-exposure baseline, is regarded as evidence of excessive absorption. A reduction of more than 50% is usually seen with frank poisoning.

Treatment

For relatively mild cases, treatment may consist only of removal from further exposure and decontamination of clothing and skin. Health care personnel need to avoid direct cutaneous contact with obviously contaminated clothing inasmuch as organophosphate compounds are readily absorbed through intact skin. Gastric lavage is indicated in cases of pesticide ingestion. Anticonvulsant medication may be necessary (benzodiazepines are the agents of choice). In severe cases, a patent airway needs to be established, both for removal of excess secretions and to institute ventilatory support. In the absence of cyanosis, atropine sulphate should be administered intravenously in high doses, typically 1 to 4 mg. This is repeated every 15 minutes until signs of atropinization appear: dry, flushed skin, tachycardia as high as 140 beats/minute, and pupillary dilatation. A mild degree of atropinization should be maintained for at least 24 hours. Pralidoxime chloride (Protopam) reactivates the enzyme cholinesterase by breaking the acetylcholinesterase-phosphate complex. One to 2 g are given as an intravenous infusion and can be repeated 1 to 2 hours later if muscle weakness has not improved. Additional doses can be given at 10- to 12-hour intervals. Treatment with pralidoxime chloride is most effective if initiated within 24 hours after exposure. In addition to assessment of clinical response, red cell cholinesterase levels should be monitored.

Heavy Metals—Lead Intoxication

Lead has been used extensively since antiquity. Considerable information regarding the cause, clinical effects, prevention, and treatment of lead poisoning has been compiled. Despite a reduction in clinical cases arising in industrialized settings, lead poisoning continues to occur in both occupational and nonoccupational environments, providing a challenge to both internists and pediatricians.

Occupational Exposure

Although many industrial workers still regularly come in contact with lead-containing compounds, modern control measures, such as those found in the lead standard of the Occupational Safety and Health Administration (OSHA), have reduced the incidence of overt cases of clinical poisoning in high-risk operations, such as battery manufacturing, brass and bronze foundry work, and lead smelting and refining. However, cases continue to be reported in occupations in which lead exposure is less well appreciated. Bridge reconstruction workers are exposed to airborne lead arising from lead-painted surfaces that are subjected to abrasive blasting or oxyacetylene torch cutting or welding. Avid marksmen, particularly those frequently engaged in shooting competitions, may develop symptoms from exposures in inadequately ventilated indoor firing ranges. The risk of clinical toxicity is generally low in occupations such as soldering and lead glass manufacturing.

Environmental Exposure

Exposure to lead paint continues to be a serious hazard to both children and adults. Youngsters, particularly those in inner cities, regularly ingest paint chips from deteriorating interior surfaces. Adults are exposed to lead-containing dust generated by the abrasion of painted surfaces during building renovation. Although lead water pipes and storage tanks are no longer used in homes, some pipes still contain lead solder. Lead can enter domestic water supplies under certain conditions, particularly if the water is slightly acidic and has been in contact with a leaded surface for a prolonged time.

The declining use of alkyl lead compounds as antiknock agents in gasoline has decreased the risk from this source of exposure. Improperly manufactured lead-glazed earthenware can be an unusual source of lead poisoning, particularly with acidic foods and beverages, which may dissolve lead from the glaze. The risk is low with commercially manufactured stoneware, which is fired at a sufficiently high temperature. Although improvements in canning technology have decreased the lead content of canned foods substantially, folk remedies and "health foods" are generally unregulated and may be a source of unsuspected exposure.

Clinical Effects

Inorganic lead can enter the body by inhalation or ingestion. The former is more common in occupational exposures and the latter in environmental settings. After absorption, it is distributed to the erythrocytes, liver, and kidneys. Over time, lead is redistributed to the bones, following a metabolic pathway similar to that of calcium. Through its ability to interact with sulfhydryl groups, lead exerts toxic effects on a number of organ systems, resulting in a wide range of clinical effects.

Classic lead colic, which is due to spasmodic contraction of intestinal smooth muscle, is now encountered only rarely. More common are insidious gastrointestinal symptoms, including vague abdominal discomfort, anorexia, and constipation. Because lead interferes with hemoglobin synthesis, anemia is a frequent clinical finding. This condition has been described as microcytic, hypochromic, normocytic, and normochromic. Lead also shortens erythrocyte life span by a poorly understood mechanism. The resulting increased erythropoiesis in the bone marrow leads to the additional findings of reticulocytosis and basophilic stippling of red cells. Heavy persistent exposure lasting 10 years or longer may result in lead nephropathy characterized by progressive renal impairment and hypertension. Tubular dysfunction may be sufficiently severe as to result in a Fanconilike syndrome with aminoaciduria, glucosuria, and hyperphosphaturia. Lead interferes with the excretion of urates. The resulting hyperuricemia can lead to a form of gout referred to as *saturnine*, an old term for lead poisoning.

Severe involvement of the peripheral nervous system, leading to paralysis of the extensor muscles of the wrist (wrist drop) or ankles (foot drop), is now uncommon. Likewise, occupationally induced lead encephalopathy is rare; however, acute encephalopathy remains a regrettably frequent and serious complication of childhood lead poisoning. Although chelation treatment has reduced the mortality substantially, approximately 25% of survivors exhibit permanent brain damage. Some cases of mild poisoning in adults may present with vague neuropsychiatric complaints such as headache, poor concentration, and memory loss. Because these symptoms are relatively common nonspecific complaints in clinical practice, the diagnosis of lead poisoning may not be suspected without obtaining a thorough occupational history. Reproductive effects in both men and women have been described, including increased rates of miscarriages and stillbirths, prematurity, reduced birth weights, and decreased sperm counts and motility.

Laboratory Studies

The diagnosis of lead poisoning, like that of all occupational and environmental disorders, is an exercise in clinical judgment requiring full consideration of the medical and occupational history, the physical examination, and the relevant laboratory studies. Measurement of blood lead is the single most useful diagnostic test. It is also the preferred test for biological monitoring of exposed workers. It reflects recent exposure and is less variable than urinary lead measurements; however, the mere elevation of blood lead slightly above the upper limits of laboratory "normal" should not necessarily lead to a diagnosis of lead poisoning. Clinical symptoms (e.g., abdominal complaints) or organ system effects (e.g., anemia) should be present before the diagnosis is made. Concentrations $>40 \, \mu g/dL$, but $<60 \, \mu g/dL$, indicate increased absorption, but they may or may not be accompanied by clinical symptoms. Patients with blood lead levels $>80 \, \mu g/dL$ usually have clinical manifestations of lead toxicity and detectable anemia. Although an approximate dose–response relationship exists between blood lead levels and clinical effects, there are differences in individual susceptibility and in interpretation of test results.

Measurement of free erythrocyte protoporphyrin or zinc protoporphyrin relate to lead's effect on heme synthetase. Free erythrocyte protoporphyrin and zinc protoporphyrin levels begin to increase when the blood lead level exceeds $40 \, \mu g/dL$. They stay elevated longer than blood lead and are therefore better indicators of chronic intoxication; however, they are less specific than blood lead and may also be elevated in patients with iron-deficiency anemia. Other laboratory studies that should be ordered in the initial assessment of any lead-exposed patient include a complete blood count with peripheral smear, blood urea nitrogen, creatinine, and urinalysis.

The assessment of a causal role for remote lead exposure in a chronic disorder, such as nephropathy, can be difficult. The usual measures of recent exposure, such as the blood lead level, are generally normal. Over time, most of the body burden is redistributed to the kidneys, liver, and especially bone. A lead mobilization test using calcium disodium edetate (CaEDTA) has been advocated. A newer technique using radiographic fluorescence and bone densitometry can also measure accumulated lead.

Treatment

The initial treatment of lead poisoning is removal from further exposure. In adults with mild symptoms and only slight anemia, this may be all that is necessary. In patients with higher blood levels, more striking clinical symptoms, and significant anemia, chelation therapy is indicated. CaEDTA is the parenteral agent of choice and is usually given in cases of acute or severe poisoning. An orally administered agent, 2,3-dimercaptosuccinic acid (Succimer), has gained acceptance for lead poisoning in both children and adults. The prophylactic use of chelating agents to prevent elevated blood lead levels in workers who have been occupationally exposed is expressly prohibited by OSHA's lead standard.

PNEUMOCONIOSES

The term "pneumoconiosis" is derived from Greek and simply means "dusty lungs." The term is used today to describe the permanent alteration of lung structure caused by inhalation of a mineral dust and the reaction of the lung tissue to this dust. The reactions that occur within the lungs vary with the size of the dust particle and its biological activity. Some dusts (e.g., barium, tin, iron) do not result in a fibrogenic reaction in the lungs. Others can evoke a variety of tissue responses. Nodular fibrosis may occur with exposure to crystalline silica, diffuse fibrosis with exposure to asbestos, and macule formation with focal emphysema after exposure to coal. Still others, such as beryllium, can evoke a systemic response and induce a granulomatous reaction in the lungs. Treatment is supportive because specific therapies do not exist. The next section contains a discussion of the traditional dust exposures (asbestos, silica, coal) and the illnesses they produce.

Asbestos

Exposure to asbestos can lead to a variety of manifestations in the lungs. Pleural disease, parenchymal disease (asbestosis), and asbestos as a carcinogen are discussed.

Exposure

Exposure to asbestos occurs during its mining, milling, and transporting, as well as during the manufacture and application of asbestos-containing products. Plumbers, pipe fitters, insulators, and electricians working in the construction and shipbuilding industries are most commonly exposed. Manifestations of the various associated lung diseases typically occur many years after the initial exposure. A careful occupational history is often needed to identify the exposure.

Clinical Manifestations

Pleural Diseases

Four forms of pleural disease related to asbestos exposure have been described: pleural plaques, benign asbestos pleural effusions, pleural fibrosis, and malignant mesotheliomas.

Pleural Plaques

Pleural plaques are the most common manifestation of asbestos exposure. They are smooth, white, raised, irregular lesions found on the parietal pleura. Most commonly located in the lateral and posterior midzones or over the diaphragms, the plaques are typically asymptomatic, recognized only on chest imaging. Macroscopic calcification is common. Plaques are not associated with the development of a malignant mesothelioma. They are, however, markers of asbestos exposure, and thus, individuals with pleural plaques are at risk of developing parenchymal disease, mesothelioma, and lung cancer.

Benign Asbestos Pleural Effusions

Benign asbestos pleural effusions may be silent or present with pain, fever, and shortness of breath. They are an early manifestation of asbestos exposure, occurring within 15 years after initial exposure. The diagnosis of this condition is one of exclusion. It requires known asbestos exposure; the finding of an exudative, blood-stained, lymphocyte-predominant effusion; the lack of tumor development over a 3-year follow-up; and no evidence of another cause of the effusion. Frequently, a thoracoscopy with biopsy is performed to exclude other causes. A benign asbestos pleural effusion is usually transient but requires close follow-up. There is no specific therapy required. Benign asbestos pleural effusions are not associated with the development of a malignant mesothelioma.

Pleural Fibrosis

Pleural fibrosis typically occurs in individuals who have had a remote exposure to asbestos (more than 20 years before) that was short lived and heavy in intensity. Individuals may be asymptomatic or present with progressive shortness of breath and restriction on pulmonary function testing, depending on the degree of fibrosis. The fibrosis can occur as a focal or diffuse process. The fibrosed pleura may surround the lung, leading to a trapped lung, or fold in on itself, encasing a portion of the parenchyma. The masslike lesion that results is known as rounded atelectasis. All degrees of pleural fibrosis are difficult to distinguish from malignancy, and frequently require biopsies to ensure benignity. Pleural stripping ("decortication") is a treatment option for those who are symptomatic with a trapped lung and otherwise well enough to tolerate the procedure. The presence of pleural fibrosis indicates an increased risk of parenchymal disease.

Malignant Mesothelioma

Asbestos exposure is responsible for most cases of malignant mesothelioma. The presentation is typically the insidious onset of nonpleuritic chest wall pain, 20 to 40 years after the initial exposure. The pain can radiate to the upper abdomen or shoulder and is often associated with dyspnea and systemic symptoms. The mass typically involves both parietal and visceral pleura. Local invasion is common, with symptoms stemming from the organs invaded. Chest imaging frequently reveals an effusion ipsilateral to the pleural disease and may show pleural plaques in the contralateral hemithorax. Open biopsy is required for the diagnosis. Treatment options are unsatisfactory. For local disease in an otherwise healthy individual, extrapleural

pneumonectomy with adjuvant chemotherapy ± local radiation therapy is recommended. For unresectable disease, a platinum-containing chemotherapy regimen is used. There is no synergy between smoking and asbestos exposure for the development of a malignant mesothelioma.

Asbestosis

The term "asbestosis" refers to pulmonary fibrosis secondary to asbestos exposure. Risk factors for the development of asbestosis include increased levels and duration of exposure, younger age at initial exposure, and exposure to the amphibole fiber type. It is not associated with smoking.

Common symptoms include progressive shortness of breath and a nonproductive cough. Chest pain may be reported. On examination, inspiratory crackles on lung auscultation and digital clubbing are present with variable frequency.

The parenchymal fibrotic changes are most prominent in the lower lobes and subpleural areas. Pulmonary function testing reveals restrictive lung disease with a decreased diffusing capacity for carbon monoxide. These radiographic and physiological findings can be indistinguishable from those of other causes of pulmonary fibrosis. The presence of concomitant pleural disease and the finding of asbestos or ferruginous bodies in pathological samples help support the diagnosis.

Asbestosis may appear and progress long after exposure has ceased. It may remain static or advance over time. There is no known effective therapy. The number of reported deaths from asbestosis has increased over time, related to the use of asbestos in a time-delayed manner. The age-adjusted mortality rate from asbestosis is 5.0 per million population from 1985 to 1999.

Asbestos as a Carcinogen

Asbestos is classified as a class I carcinogen (carcinogenic to humans) by the International Agency for Research on Cancer (IARC). Lung cancer and mesothelioma have been consistently linked, whereas the evidence for laryngeal and gastrointestinal malignancies is more variable. The risk of developing lung cancer in an individual exposed to asbestos is enhanced in a multiplicative fashion by concomitant cigarette smoking. Lung cancer more commonly occurs in individuals who also have asbestosis. All cell types are associated with exposure. The lag time to the development of lung cancer is usually more than 20 years. Treatment follows the principles of lung cancer therapy in individuals without prior asbestos exposure (see Chapter 34). Comorbid lung disease may limit the treatment options.

Silica

Exposure

Exposure to crystalline silica occurs when silica-containing rock and sand are encountered. This most commonly occurs in occupations associated with construction, mining, quarrying, drilling, and foundry work. A variety of conditions have been associated with the inhalation of crystalline silica, including silicosis, tuberculosis, obstructive lung disease, and lung cancer.

Clinical Manifestations

Silicosis

Inhalation of crystalline silica can lead to a fibronodular parenchymal lung disease known as silicosis. This most commonly occurs in a form known as chronic or simple silicosis. Individuals with chronic silicosis typically have had more than 20 years of silica exposure. They are frequently without symptoms, although shortness of breath and cough can develop. Their disease is thus recognized radiographically as multiple small nodules with upper lobe predominance. Hilar adenopathy with "eggshell" calcification can be seen. Pulmonary function abnormalities do not invariably occur. Pathologically, the nodules are recognized as silicotic nodules.

The pulmonary nodules seen with chronic silicosis can become progressive. They may be seen to conglomerate and be accompanied by fibrosis, which has been termed "conglomerate silicosis and progressive massive fibrosis." Shortness of breath and cough can become debilitating. Pulmonary function testing often shows a mixed obstructive and restrictive defect with a reduction in the diffusing capacity. Death due to silicosis continues to occur. The age-adjusted mortality rate was 1.4 per million population from 1985 to 1999.

Acute and accelerated forms of silicosis are more rapidly progressive, typically associated with intense exposure to silica. Acute silicosis can develop within months of exposure. The exposed individual may develop progressive shortness of breath and coughing. The radiographic picture is compatible with acute airspace disease. Pathology mimics alveolar proteinosis with proteinaceous material in the alveoli, but interstitial involvement and early nodule formation can be seen. Rapid progression to acute respiratory failure is common. Accelerated silicosis occurs after 5 to 15 years of exposure. Patients are usually symptomatic and often progress to respiratory failure and death. They are recognized by the development of upper zone nodules and fibrosis on radiographs, and numerous nodules with interstitial fibrosis on pathology.

Mycobacterial Disease

Mycobacterial disease is known to occur with increased frequency in individuals with silicosis. Individuals with chronic silicosis have an incidence of mycobacterial tuberculosis that is three times greater than that of age-matched controls. Those with acute and accelerated silicosis have the highest incidence of mycobacterial disease. Others exposed to silica but without silicosis may have an excess risk of developing tuberculosis. It is recommended that individuals with silicosis (or long-term exposure to crystalline silica) should receive a tuberculin skin test. If the reaction is ≥ 10 mm and there is no evidence of active tuberculosis, standard treatment for latent tuberculosis should be administered. If symptoms or radiographic changes suggest the possibility of active mycobacterial disease, routine or induced sputum should be obtained. If active tuberculosis is confirmed, standard tuberculosis therapy, with a regimen containing rifampin, should be administered. Similarly, if a nontuberculous mycobacterium is identified, standard therapy for that organism should be administered.

Obstructive Lung Disease and Lung Cancer

Exposure to crystalline silica has been associated with the development of obstructive lung disease, chronic bronchitis, and emphysema. These associations are more prominent in those with silicosis. The intensity of dust exposure appears to affect the development of obstructive lung diseases. Tobacco smoking may cause an additive effect.

According to the IARC, there is sufficient evidence to classify silica as carcinogenic in humans. Available studies are complicated by multiple confounders and selection biases. Despite this, the bulk of the evidence supports an increased risk for lung cancer in tobacco smokers with silicosis. The relationship is less clear for never-smokers and for individuals exposed to silica who do not have silicosis.

Other Associations

Evidence suggests a relation between appreciable silica exposure and the development of scleroderma. Less evidence is available to support an association with rheumatoid arthritis or systemic lupus erythematosus. Similarly, reports of renal disease associated with silica exposure require further evidence to confirm a link.

Coal Dust

The deposition of coal dust in the lungs can lead to lung disease. In addition to coal worker's pneumoconiosis (CWP), coal dust exposure is also related to the development of airflow limitation, chronic bronchitis, and emphysema. Silica exposure frequently occurs in combination with coal dust exposure; thus, the previously described silica-related illnesses may also be seen.

Exposure

Coal mining is the major source of exposure. The tissue reaction to coal dust inhalation is the development of a coal macule. Over the course of years to decades, focal emphysema may form around the macule. This combination is termed a "coal nodule" and is the characteristic lesion of simple CWP.

Clinical Manifestations

Coal Worker's Pneumoconiosis

Most individuals with CWP are asymptomatic. This presentation is termed "simple CWP." Given the frequent absence of symptoms, simple CWP is often a radiographic diagnosis. Chest imaging reveals small nodules with upper and posterior zone predominance. Hilar lymph node enlargement is not uncommon, although eggshell calcification does not generally occur. Simple CWP tends to have little effect on lung function.

The presence of shortness of breath or a productive cough in an individual with simple CWP is often related to the coexistence of chronic bronchitis or airflow obstruction. Progressive massive fibrosis (PMF) can occur, more frequently when there has also been exposure to silica. Symptoms advance as the PMF worsens. When PMF occurs, the small nodules seen in simple CWP coalesce, forming opacities >1 cm. These lesions are odd shaped, usually bilateral, and progressive, and may cavitate or become calcified. Care must be taken because lesions diagnosed radiographically as PMF are often shown later to have been tumors, tuberculosis scars, or Caplan's nodules. Airflow limitation, restriction, and reduction in diffusing capacity can all be seen when PMF develops. Pulmonary hypertension may develop in advanced disease.

Deaths from CWP continue to occur.

Complications

Complications of CWP include a higher incidence of mycobacterial disease (although not as high as with silicosis), scleroderma, and increased risk of stomach cancer. Tuberculin skin testing, chemoprophylaxis, and treatment of active tuberculosis are as recommended in silicosis. Caplan's syndrome is a nodular form of CWP seen in individuals with rheumatoid arthritis. The nodules are multiple, tend to be larger than typical coal nodules, develop over short periods of time, and more frequently cavitate. These findings usually occur concomitantly with the joint manifestations, active arthritis, and presence of circulating rheumatoid factor.

OCCUPATIONAL ASTHMA

Occupational asthma now represents 5% to 15% of new asthma in working adults.

Exposures

More than 250 exposures are known to cause occupational asthma. Individuals may be exposed to sensitizing agents in a repeated fashion or have had a single exposure to a potent respiratory irritant. Latex exposure is the leading cause in health care workers. Isocyanates found in auto body shops or spray painters are also common. Many others exist, including wood products, textiles, and grains as sensitizing exposures, and chlorine gas, bleach, and strong acids as respiratory irritants.

Clinical Manifestations

The symptoms of occupational asthma are the same as those for nonoccupational asthma (see Chapter 35). The additional feature is that there is a work-related pattern to these symptoms. The work-related pattern of illness can mean that the asthma symptoms began after a new workplace exposure or that pre-existing asthma was made worse by the exposure. The asthma can be "work aggravated"—exacerbation of asthma that was previously subclinical or in remission, "asthma with latency"—new-onset asthma caused by a sensitizing exposure, or "asthma without latency"—asthma resulting from a single heavy exposure to a potent respiratory irritant. Symptoms are made worse by continuing exposure. This is manifest by increased asthma symptoms in the workplace that diminish when away from work.

To diagnose occupational asthma, we need to confirm the presence of asthma, an exposure, and a work-related pattern. Asthma may be confirmed by the classic symptoms and signs—shortness of breath, cough, and wheeze. An exposure can be confirmed from a detailed history, including review of Material Safety Data Sheets from the workplace. When the diagnosis is not clear, further testing is necessary.

Diagnostic Testing

Testing to confirm the presence of asthma includes spirometry looking for obstruction with a bronchodilator response. If this is not present, then a methacholine challenge test may be useful. Testing to confirm a sensitizing exposure may include skin or radioallergosorbent (RAST) testing by demonstrating antigen-specific antibodies. Testing to confirm a work-related pattern of the asthma manifestations may include peak flow recordings at work and away from work. Peak flows that fall while the exposure is occurring can objectify the work-related pattern of illness. This is complicated in that some substances (e.g., isocyanates) produce a delayed onset of symptoms (6–8 hours).

Treatment

Treatment follows the principles of asthma management for nonoccupational asthma. This includes a patient-centered approach with education about the illness and active monitoring of symptoms and peak flows. Inhaled corticosteroids and bronchodilators are the mainstays of medical therapy (see Chapter 35). Avoidance of the incriminated exposure must be highlighted.

REVIEW EXERCISES

QUESTIONS

1. During a preplacement examination for a bridge reconstruction job, a 32-year-old woman was found to have a blood lead level of 4.0 μg/dL (normal, 0.0–11.0 μg/dL) and a zinc protoporphyrin of 104 μg/dL (normal, 0.0–70.0 μg/dL). She is asymptomatic, and her physical examination is normal. Her medical history is unremarkable except for four pregnancies. The most likely explanation for these laboratory results is
a) Unrecognized environmental lead exposure
b) Iron-deficiency anemia
c) Erythropoietic protoporphyria
d) Laboratory error
e) Thalassemia minor

Answer and Discussion

The answer is b. An elevated zinc protoporphyrin with a normal blood lead level is most often due to iron-deficiency anemia, particularly in a woman of reproductive age. Because these studies were obtained during the preplacement evaluation, the patient has not yet encountered lead exposure in the workplace. The physician should always inquire about possible environmental or household exposures, such as the use of glazed ceramic ware, folk remedies, or lead-soldered water pipes. A completely normal lead level excludes recent or ongoing lead exposure from any source.

Erythropoietic protoporphyria is a rare disorder that results in significant symptoms, including photosensitivity. Thalassemia minor and laboratory error are theoretically possible, but highly unlikely explanations for these results.

2. In the proper medical management of lead toxicity, all the following are true, except
a) Removal from exposure is mandatory
b) Symptomatic patients with high lead levels should undergo chelation therapy
c) All patients with elevated blood lead levels should be chelated, even if asymptomatic
d) Calcium disodium edetate is the preferred parenteral agent
e) 2,3-Dimercaptosuccinic acid (Succimer) is the oral agent of choice

Answer and Discussion

The answer is c. The first step in the management of lead toxicity is removal from exposure, and, in some cases, this may be all that is necessary. Chelation therapy in adults should be reserved for patients with significant signs or symptoms (e.g., encephalopathy or renal injury). Commonly used chelators have potential side effects (e.g., calcium disodium edetate [CaEDTA] can cause acute tubular necrosis) and should not be

used routinely in asymptomatic patients. The indications for chelation therapy in children are more liberal. The Centers for Disease Control and Prevention recommend that children with blood levels of 45 μg/dL be referred for therapy, and some practitioners routinely treat children with levels between 25 and 44 μg/dL.

Although several chelators have been used in the treatment of lead poisoning, CaEDTA is the drug of choice when a parenteral agent is needed. When an oral agent is preferred (e.g., in children), Succimer is used.

3. The appropriate management of a patient poisoned by organophosphate cholinesterase-inhibiting agents includes all of the following, except
a) Atropine
b) Sodium nitrite
c) Pralidoxime chloride (Protopam)
d) Maintenance of airway
e) Decontamination

Answer and Discussion

The answer is b. Atropine blocks the muscarinic effects of organophosphates and should be administered promptly. Pralidoxime chloride (Protopam) reactivates the enzyme cholinesterase by breaking the acetylcholinesterase-phosphate complex. Its advantages over atropine include its ability to reverse muscle paralysis and possibly central nervous system depression.

Decontamination procedures may include removal of contaminated clothing, washing of skin and hair, and, if indicated by route of exposure, emptying the stomach. In severe cases, a patent airway needs to be established for removal of excess secretions and institution of ventilatory support.

Sodium nitrite is used in cyanide poisoning. It has no role in the management of organophosphate toxicity.

4. Acute poisoning from organophosphate insecticides can result in which delayed neurologic effect?
a) Cerebellar degeneration
b) Dementia
c) Bell's palsy
d) Motor polyneuropathy
e) Seizure disorder

Answer and Discussion

The answer is d. Acute poisoning with organophosphate insecticides can result in a variety of central nervous system manifestations. A small percentage of patients may exhibit neuropsychiatric or cognitive complaints, such as irritability, depression, anxiety, and short-term memory impairment, weeks to months after initial intoxication. It is often difficult, however, to distinguish organically based neurobehavioral symptoms from the psychological or emotional responses likely to occur after acute chemical exposures.

A delayed peripheral neuropathy has been reported after poisoning by some organophosphates. This condition, organophosphate-induced delayed neuropathy, is a predominantly motor polyneuropathy that occurs 2 to 3 weeks after acute poisoning.

5. A 52-year-old male employee of a local warehouse operation is seen at an urgent care center complaining of gradual onset of headache, nausea, and dizziness. He relates experiencing similar symptoms over the past few days, which tend to occur near the end of his workshift and resolve overnight. During this time, all windows in his warehouse have remained closed to reduce heating costs. None of his family members is ill, but he claims that other employees in his work area are experiencing similar complaints. He has been in good health, despite having smoked one-half pack of cigarettes daily for the past 30 years. Physical examination is unremarkable. A blood carboxyhemoglobin level is 20%. An ECG and cardiac enzymes are normal. Proper medical management of this patient would entail the following:
a) Nothing, except removal from exposure
b) Administration of 100% oxygen by face mask
c) Assisted ventilation
d) Hospitalization overnight for observation
e) Hyperbaric oxygen at 2 to 3 atm

Answer and Discussion

The answer is b. Removal from further exposure is usually the first step in the management of any toxic event. This has already been accomplished in this case, at least for the time being. However, the treating physician does have an obligation to promptly report the diagnosis of work-related carbon monoxide poisoning to the employer to ensure appropriate corrective measures are undertaken to lower further employee exposure below permissible limits.

Although this patient would ultimately recover without specific therapy, administration of 100% oxygen by face mask would reduce the half-life from 5.5 to 1.5 hours and hasten the patient's symptomatic improvement.

Assisted ventilation, hospitalization, or hyperbaric oxygen are indicated only for those more severely affected than this patient.

SUGGESTED READINGS

American Thoracic Society. American Thoracic Society Documents. Diagnosis and initial management of nonmalignant diseases related to asbestos. *Am J Respir Crit Care Med* 2004;170(6):691–715.

American Thoracic Society. American Thoracic Society Documents. Guidelines for assessing and managing asthma risk at work, school, and recreation. *Am J Respir Crit Care Med* 2007;169:873–881.

Bardana EJ. Occupational asthma. *J Allergy Clin Immunol* 2008;121: S408–S411.

Beckett W, Abraham J, Becklake M, et al. Adverse effects of crystalline silica exposure. Official statement of the American Thoracic Society Committee of the Scientific Assembly on Environmental and Occupational Health. *Am J Respir Crit Care Med* 1997;155:761–768.

Beckett WS. Occupational respiratory diseases. *N Engl J Med* 2000; 342:406–413.

Chong S, Lee KS, Chung MJ, et al. Pneumoconiosis: comparison of imaging and pathologic findings. *Radiographics* 2006;26:59–77.

Eddleston M, Buckley NA, Eyer P, et al. Management of acute organophosphorus pesticide poisoning. *Lancet* 2008;371:597–607.

Ernst A, Zibrak JD. Carbon monoxide poisoning. *N Engl J Med* 1998;339:1603–1608.

Hessel PA, Gamble JF, McDonald JC. Asbestos, asbestosis, and lung cancer: a critical assessment of the epidemiological evidence. *Thorax* 2005;60:433–436.

Hu H, Shih R, Rothenberg S, et al. The epidemiology of lead toxicity in adults: measuring dose and consideration of other methodologic issues. *Environ Health Perspect* 2007;115:455–462.

Kales SN, Christiani DC. Acute chemical emergencies. *N Engl J Med* 2004;350:800–808.

Kosnett MJ, Wedeen RP, Rothenberg SJ, et al. Recommendations for medical management of adult lead exposure. *Environ Health Perspect* 2007;115:463–471.

National Institute for Occupational Safety and Health (NIOSH). NIOSH Hazard Review. Health Effects of Occupational Exposure to Respirable Crystalline Silica. DHHS (NIOSH) Publication No. 2002-129, April 2002.

O'Reilly KMA, McLaughlin AM, Beckett WS, et al. Asbestos-related lung disease. *Am Fam Physician* 2007;75:683–688, 690.

Pelucchi C, Pira E, Piolatto G, et al. Occupational silica exposure and lung cancer risk: a review of epidemiological studies 1996–2005. *Ann Oncol* 2006;17:1039–1050.

Procop LD, Chichkova RI. Carbon monoxide intoxication: an updated review. *J Neurol Sci* 2007;262:122–130.

U.S. Department of Health and Human Services (DHHS), Centers for Disease Control and Prevention, Division of Respiratory Disease Studies. Work-Related Lung Disease Surveillance Report, 1999. DHHS (NIOSH) Publication No. 2003-111.

Wagner GR. Asbestosis and silicosis. *Lancet* 1997;349:1311–1315.

Weaver LK, Valentine KJ, Hopkins RO. Carbon monoxide poisoning: risk factors for cognitive sequelae and the role of hyperbaric oxygen. *Am J Respir Crit Care Med* 2007;176:491–497.

Chapter 10

Psychiatric Disorders in Medical Practice

Kathleen Franco-Bronson   Leopold Pozuelo

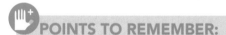

POINTS TO REMEMBER:

- Patients with a diagnosis of major depression can often present with physical symptoms.

- Depressed patients have a two- to fourfold greater risk for a recurrent cardiovascular event.

- Somatoform disorders respond better when intervention is early, without reinforcement by the excessive ordering of tests and evaluations.

- Low-dose antidepressants are generally first-line therapy for long-term management of panic disorder patients.

- White blood count must be closely monitored while on clozapine to avoid agranulocytosis.

Primary care physicians can find almost any psychiatric presentation in their practices, but some are more frequent and require that diagnostic and treatment skills be kept up to date. Most depressed patients present to their primary care physician rather than to a psychiatrist and have physical complaints rather than opening with emotional concerns. Major depression can be a life-threatening illness requiring a rapid assessment of suicide risk and expedient, safe therapy. Somatoform disorders can lead to expensive, unnecessary testing or risky procedures if medical mimics have not been considered. The same can be said for panic disorders, which if accompanied by depression, can carry the highest suicide risk. Patients with generalized anxiety disorder frequently seek medical attention and pharmacologic relief. Hospitalized patients, particularly elderly patients, are at risk for delirium or acute confusional states. As a greater number of people survive into later years, primary care physicians find themselves providing for not only the physical needs, but also the cognitive and emotional needs of patients with dementia.

This chapter explores the initial assessment and treatment for commonly seen psychiatric disorders and provides selected case vignettes for more in-depth exploration.

DEPRESSION

Case Vignette 1

A 76-year-old woman complained of epigastric pain, constipation, and loss of appetite for longer than 1 month. The pain awakens her at night, which she believes is the cause of daytime fatigue. Various gastrointestinal medications have been tried without success. The results of the upper and lower gastrointestinal series ordered by your colleague for this patient were normal. Although the chart indicates that her husband died 3 months ago, the patient states that she does not believe that his death is holding her back and would not describe herself as depressed. She has been devoted to her church throughout her life, but her physical symptoms have kept her from going to services the past few months. She moved out of her home a month ago and into a senior's apartment to live near a female friend. Her friend was admitted to the hospital 2 weeks earlier and has been diagnosed with cancer. The patient has never been treated for a psychiatric disorder, and there is no family history. The patient has a 10-lb weight loss since her last visit 6 weeks ago. She has a history of partially controlled hypertension. On an ECG, her heart rate is 82, PR 0.120 seconds, QRS 0.100 seconds, and QT/QTc 0.430/0.465 seconds. She has a 15-mm Hg orthostatic blood pressure drop, but she does not complain of dizziness. Her electrolytes, blood urea nitrogen, creatinine, and physical examination indicate dehydration. Her total protein is slightly low, as are her hemoglobin and hematocrit. Her liver function tests and urine analysis are normal. Her physical examination and chest x-ray do not reveal any additional information.

The patient has some features of depression, including weight loss, insomnia, fatigue, and discontinuation of normal activities. Bereavement generally occurs within the first 2 to 3 months after the death of a loved one. Subjects with persistent depression at 2 months are much more likely to be depressed at 2 years, are less likely to engage in new relationships, and are more likely to experience worse generalized health than before their loss. Basic laboratory studies, including a thyroid-stimulating hormone (TSH) test, would be helpful in this case to exclude underlying medical disorders.

As you talk to the patient longer, you learn that she believes she must have done something wrong for her husband to die, and now she is losing her best friend. She talks about her daughters, one who is a nun and has much responsibility and the other who lives in a distant state with her husband and the patient's only grandchildren.

She admits to withdrawal from others. She says, "I should be stronger. My daughters have important things to do. As for other friends, if I get close, they'll just be taken away from me." The patient acknowledges that she thinks about these things a great deal and also wonders whether her body is developing cancer. She does not drink alcohol or smoke cigarettes, and she has no suicidal thoughts.

The patient has many of the criteria for major depressive disorder (see criteria for major depressive episode in *Diagnostic and Statistical Manual of Mental Disorders*, 4th Edition, Text Revision [DSM-IV-TR]). Prior to her husband's death, the patient had no history of free-floating or pervasive anxiety. She did not have a "track record" for believing she had serious, life-threatening illness in the absence of any findings. No hallucinations, delusions, or evidence that she is out of touch with reality are present.

The mnemonic SIGECAPS is helpful in remembering the common signs and symptoms of depression. To meet criteria for major depression, the patient should have been depressed or dysphoric most of the day for 2 or more weeks, with difficulties in social interactions or at work and problems with at least four of the following:

S   Sleep is poor with early morning awakening and a fragmented pattern or excessive.
I   Interest in normal activities is diminished.
G   Guilt is excessive or inappropriate.
E   Energy is lower than normal.
C   Concentration is poor.
A   Appetite is reduced or increased, with a consistent weight change.
P   Psychomotor retardation, slowed speech, and physical involvement or agitation are present.
S   Suicidal thoughts or thoughts of death are reported.

Because patients who have physical illness alone may have disturbances of sleep, appetite, and energy, it is wise to further explore psychological symptoms.

In the medically ill patient with depression, we also consider the mnemonic WART; H/H:

W   Withdrawal from others
A   Anhedonia
R   Ruminating thoughts
T   Tearfulness
H/H   Helplessness/Hopelessness

Listen for the emotional aspects. Patients may not identify themselves as depressed and may continue stoically despite their losses. It may take some additional questions to find the psychological aspects of their condition. Ruminating on negative thoughts, excessive guilt, or belief of punishment, as well as a lack of interest and pleasure in former activities, are key symptoms. Physical symptoms of weight loss and insomnia may be associated with a variety of conditions and can be explored further, but depression should be treated when the criteria exist. One should treat patients who meet the criteria for major depression regardless of whether a comorbid physical illness or any "good physical reason to be depressed" exists.

A rapid, safe, first-line choice for treatment would be a selective serotonin reuptake inhibitor (SSRI) such as escitalopram. Avoiding additional orthostasis, cardiac conduction delays (quinidinelike), and anticholinergic effects would recommend and thus avoid tricyclic antidepressants (TCAs). Psychoanalytic psychotherapy is a lengthy procedure and would not be recommended as a stand-alone treatment in this case. Electroconvulsive therapy would be a later option if two or more antidepressants were not effective or if the patient were acutely suicidal with extreme psychomotor retardation.

During any given week, approximately 60% to 80% of the general public has a physical complaint, and physicians may be unable to identify an organic cause in 20% to 80% of patients bringing these symptoms to the office visit. Patients with a diagnosis of major depression can often present with physical symptoms to their primary care physician.

Case Vignette 2

A 52-year-old woman reports that she "just doesn't feel well." You also hear in her history that she has had poor appetite, with an 8-lb weight loss over the past 2 months. She has gradually withdrawn from her family and friends because she is just "too tired." Her interest in her church and grandchildren has deteriorated. She feels guilty about this but cannot seem to energize herself. Although she sometimes wishes she were dead, she convinces you that she would never do anything to hurt herself and has no plan or intent to commit suicide. Your patient is significantly overweight, demonstrates psychomotor retardation, and has marked orthostasis (170/90 mm Hg sitting, pulse 85/minute, 140/80 mm Hg standing, pulse 115/minute). Her evaluation includes a TSH testing of 5.5 and cholesterol of 240. On her ECG, she has a normal sinus rhythm and ventricular rate of 85, PR of 0.150 seconds, QRS of 0.100 seconds, and QT/QTc of 0.420/0.468 seconds. She had one earlier episode of depression at age 25 years and responded to amitriptyline.

There are many options of antidepressants to use in patients, which include the TCAs such as amitriptyline, serotonin norepinephrine reuptake inhibitors (SNRIs) such as venlafaxine or duloxetine, another dual-acting antidepressant such as mirtazapine, or an SSRI such as citalopram. Although she responded to amitriptyline in the past, her current QTc, orthostasis, and weight would advise against that. With her pre-existing hypertension, venlafaxine would not be the first choice. Weight gain, orthostasis, and hypercholesterolemia could be more problematic with mirtazapine. Of these choices, citalopram would be the best.

After 4 weeks of 20 mg of citalopram and a partial response, you increase the dose to 40 mg. She has tried an exercise program to promote wellness and increase activity, and her blood pressure is under better control. However, after 8 weeks of being on the citalopram, even though her mood is partially better, she still complains of low motivation, interest, and energy. Her repeat TSH is normal. The patient is wondering if this is the right antidepressant.

Switching to sertraline (another SSRI) or to another class of antidepressant such as venlafaxine or bupropion are all treatment possibilities. According to the landmark Sequenced Treatment Alternatives to Relieve Depression (STAR*D) study, if patients have not achieved remission of their depressive symptoms on citalopram, switching to another SSRI (sertraline) or another class of antidepressant (venlafaxine or bupropion) produced the same rates of remission.

Another possibility for this patient is staying on citalopram and augmenting with either bupropion or buspirone. Buspirone augments diverse serotonin receptor sites and has been used to improve response to various SSRIs with or without anxiety being present. Bupropion tends to be a little more activating antidepressant than the SSRIs. According to the STAR*D trial, augmenting with either of these agents (buspirone or bupropion) would also be effective. Perhaps due to our patient's low energy status, bupropion would be the better initial augmentation strategy. However, more research is needed to determine whether adding another medication (augmentation) is better than changing to another medication (switching).

Case Vignette 3

A 76-year-old man presents with a poor appetite, weight loss, and sleep disturbance, and is generally apathetic. He is not tearful or suicidal. The patient does not report any significant loss during the past year but is aware that his interest in nearby family, friends, neighbors, and hobbies (gardening, local community groups) has diminished. He has little energy and finds concentrating on the newspaper too great a challenge. He has a distant

history of "hepatitis" in his 20s. You have ordered baseline laboratory tests, including liver function studies, and are ready to order an antidepressant when you notice that his TSH is undetectable and his T$_4$ is elevated. You treat his hyperthyroidism first. Although he makes some physical improvements, symptoms of depression continue. He feels more hopeless and withdrawn from others. He ruminates on the time he has lost and wonders whether life is worthwhile at his age. He also has a history of coronary artery disease and acute myocardial infarction (MI) 5 years ago, for which he takes one aspirin a day. Today his vitals are temperature 37.1°C, pulse 105/minute, blood pressure 130/85 mm Hg, respiration rate 16/minute, and O$_2$ saturation 95%.

When reviewing treatment options, including observation, the risk of not treating a major depression in this patient can have more serious consequences than the risk of treatment side effects. Current research confirms that when all else is held constant, depressed patients have a two- to fourfold greater risk for a recurrent cardiovascular event. Many choices are safe for this patient, such as an SSRI (e.g., sertraline or citalopram). This class of medications is considered a first-line option. Clinical research has shown that depression can increase platelet aggregation and that SSRIs reduce platelet aggregation, with or without depression being present. SSRIs can also compete with warfarin through the P450 cytochrome 2C9. Although generally not a problem clinically, if acute bleeding occurs, the SSRI should be stopped. Trazodone is an antidepressant that could improve his sleep; however, it is unlikely to be an adequate antidepressant alone and can increase the risk of orthostasis. Methylphenidate is used for some medically ill and depressed patients, but the potential for tachycardia in this case makes it a less preferable choice.

Case Vignette 4

In the next examination room, you encounter another elderly man who had an MI 2 weeks ago and is back for follow-up as an outpatient. His hypertension has been treated with the same beta-blocker for 5 years. You find that he meets criteria now for his first major depression and recommend an antidepressant. His daughter says, "Isn't this a normal reaction, and can't we just wait it out?"

Treatment considerations are as follows. The risk of recurrent cardiovascular morbidity in a depressed cardiac patient is high, and the benefit of treatment for depression is potentially significant. The patient should be started on antidepressant medication, such as an SSRI. If he has been on the same beta-blocker for 5 years, it is unlikely to contribute to new-onset apathy. Evidenced-based medicine has *not* proven that for patients like this treatment with antidepressants will increase survival. However, there is ample evidence the treatment of the depressed cardiac patient can increase medication adherence, rehabilitation effort, as well as increase in mood, and quality of life.

Case Vignette 5

A 32-year-old woman reports frequent headaches extending from both temples to the back of her head and down her neck. As you explore her history further and complete your physical examination, you find adequate criteria to merit diagnosis of a recurrent major depressive disorder. Although she is willing to try an antidepressant medication because her symptoms responded in the past, she admits that she discontinued the antidepressant early because she experienced side effects. She wants to discuss the pros and cons of various medication options.

Sexual dysfunction is a common side effect. Patients taking SSRIs (fluoxetine, sertraline, paroxetine, citalopram, and escitalopram) are more likely to report sexual dysfunction than those taking other agents such as bupropion or mirtazapine. Weight gain will be more pronounced in medications such as mirtazapine and the TCAs. Although only a minority of patients will report insomnia with antidepressants, this side effect is more prominent in patients taking traditional activating SSRIs (e.g., sertraline more than paroxetine) and with bupropion. Mirtazapine and the TCA can be more sedating. Mirtazapine is unique in that lower doses are sedating, but above 30 mg, it is more activating.

Case Vignette 6

The patient's younger sister, age 21 years, is endorsing classic symptoms of depression. The sister appropriately discusses this with her primary care physician. She meets criteria for depression via SIGECAPS, and her quality of life is suffering. She does not endorse thoughts of suicide.

In exploring pharmacologic treatment options, all antidepressants need to be administered with caution in younger patients. The U.S. Food and Drug Administration (FDA) requires that *all* antidepressant medications carry a black box warning about increased suicidal behavior and ideation in children, adolescents, and young adults ages 18 to 24 years. This warning was placed due to concerns of increased suicidal behavior and ideation, which are more pronounced in younger patients who are receiving antidepressants. The clinician must weigh this concern with increased monitoring of the younger patient when starting an antidepressant, especially in the first 4 to 6 weeks of treatment. Psychotherapy should also be considered. The risk–benefit determination for any antidepressant prescription must include the potential higher risk of suicide in the untreated patient.

Patient Health Questionnaire and Treatment Phases for Depression

An easy screening and assessment tool for depression is the Patient Health Questionnaire (PHQ-9), which can be self-administered to the patient and used for monitoring of progress (Fig. 10.1). The nine-item symptom questions are scored on a Likert scale of 0 for "not at all," 1 for "several days," 2 for "more than half the days," and 3 for "nearly every day." A total score of ≥ 10 correlates with clinical depression. The PHQ-2, which consists of the first two questions of the PHQ-9, can be effectively used as a screening tool for depression, with a cut-off of ≥ 3 indicative of depression.

Finally, Figure 10.2 outlines treatment guidelines of antidepressant therapy, which includes the acute phase (1–3 months), the continuation phase (3–9 months), and the maintenance phase (≥ 9 months) of antidepressant therapy. Targeting depressive symptoms to achieve not only response, but also remission, should be the standard of care in depression treatment. The continuation phase is managed with the full antidepressant dose used in the acute phase, and after the continuation phase is complete, the antidepressant can be slowly tapered off. For those patients with two or more recurrent depressions in their lifetime, or for those who elect to stay on antidepressant medication due to the severity of the experienced depression, maintenance therapy is recommended. Psychotherapy for all treatment phases should also be considered.

SOMATOFORM DISORDERS

Case Vignette 1

A 45-year-old woman presents to your office complaining of intermittent chest pain for the past month. She initially noticed it walking up the stairs from her basement with a basket of laundry. Since then, she has been aware of the pain on several occasions: once at the office while working on a complex project for her boss, another time when rushing to the school performance of her youngest child, and, most recently, during a phone call with her mother. She believes the pain is growing in intensity and is taking longer before it passes.

The information provided suggests that some or all episodes occur when the patient is fatigued or potentially under duress. Rather than jumping in to order costly tests or prescribe unnecessarily, gathering additional past and family history is a valuable first step.

The patient confirms that her demands at work are increasing and that it is difficult to get everything done on time, both at work and at home. Past history from the patient includes irregular menses, double vision, pelvic pain, fatigue, headaches, nausea and vomiting, joint symptoms, insomnia, bouts of diarrhea, and frequent upper respiratory infections and urinary tract infections, among a variety of other symptoms. As you peruse the archival record, you notice your predecessor has done extensive workup on this patient on a variety of occasions and found little. She has had a dobutamine stress test in the past year that was normal.

Talking to her further, she tells you that her 75-year-old father died of an MI several months ago. She describes her mother as one who frequently requests others to take her to the doctor for a variety of concerns. Her mother is now quite distraught and needs or requests more visits with her doctors and more time from

PATIENT HEALTH QUESTIONNAIRE-9				72883

THIS SECTION FOR USE BY STUDY PERSONNEL ONLY.

Were data collected? **No** ☐ *(provide reason in comments)*

   If **Yes**, data collected on visit date ☐ **or** specify date:_____
                                                    DD-Mon-YYYY

Comments:

Only the patient (subject) should enter information onto this questionnaire.

Over the last 2 weeks, how often have you been bothered by any of the following problems?	Not at all	Several days	More than half the days	Nearly every day
1. Little interest or pleasure in doing things	0	1	2	3
2. Feeling down, depressed, or hopeless	0	1	2	3
3. Trouble falling or staying asleep, or sleeping too much	0	1	2	3
4. Feeling tired or having little energy	0	1	2	3
5. Poor appetite or overeating	0	1	2	3
6. Feeling bad about yourself – or that you are a failure or have let yourself or your family down	0	1	2	3
7. Trouble concentrating on things, such as reading the newspaper or watching television	0	1	2	3
8. Moving or speaking so slowly that other people could have noticed? Or the opposite – being so fidgety or restless that you have been moving around a lot more than usual	0	1	2	3
9. Thoughts that you would be better off dead or of hurting yourself in some way	0	1	2	3

SCORING FOR USE BY STUDY PERSONNEL ONLY

  *0*___ + _____ + _____ + _____

=Total Score: _____

If you checked off any problems, how difficult have these problems made it for you to do your work, take care of things at home, or get along with other people?

Not difficult at all	**Somewhat difficult**	**Very difficult**	**Extremely difficult**
☐	☐	☐	☐

I confirm this information is accurate.	Patient's/Subject's initials:	Date:

Figure 10.1 Patient Health Questionnaire-9. *Source:* Developed by Drs. Robert L. Spitzer, Janet B.W. Williams, Kurt Kroenke and colleagues, with an educational grant from Pfizer Inc. Copyright © 2005 Pfizer, Inc. All rights reserved. Reproduced with permission.

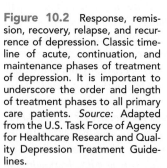
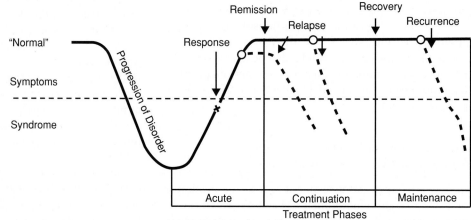

Figure 10.2 Response, remission, recovery, relapse, and recurrence of depression. Classic timeline of acute, continuation, and maintenance phases of treatment of depression. It is important to underscore the order and length of treatment phases to all primary care patients. *Source:* Adapted from the U.S. Task Force of Agency for Healthcare Research and Quality Depression Treatment Guidelines.

her daughter. The rest of the family history is unremarkable. Sleeping and eating patterns, concentration, and general interest level are all good at this time. The physical examination on the patient is completely normal.

The patient meets criteria for somatoform disorder, which is reviewed in the next section.

Diagnostic Criteria for Somatoform Disorder (from DSM-IV-TR)

The DSM criteria include finding a history of many physical complaints beginning before age 30 years that occur over a period of several years and result in treatment being sought or significant impairment in social, occupational, or other area of functioning. These criteria include:

- Four pain symptoms at different sites or functions
- Two gastrointestinal symptoms other than pain
- One sexual symptom
- One pseudoneurologic symptom
- After appropriate investigation, symptoms not fully explained by a known medical condition or effects of a substance
- When a related general medical condition exists, physical complaints or resulting social or occupational impairment are in excess of what would be expected

Watch the patient's affect and behavior closely while questioning about how easy or difficult daily life has been and how upsetting recent social changes have been. These responses can add clues to a psychosocial connection when there is a lack of support from physical findings. Reviewing medical records and emergency room visits are also a must.

Evaluating for Somatoform Disorders

In evaluating patients for somatoform disorders, key questions to ask include the following:

- In general, how stressful or difficult is this patient's daily life?
- Have there been newer or recent changes in the life of the patient or his or her loved ones, moves, job loss or switch, financial problems, disagreements with family members, or other concerns?
- Are there anniversary responses to past loss around this time of year?
- Is there a time connection with physical symptom(s)?
- Could symptom(s) serve to distract the patient from emotional conflict?
- Are there any potential gains or benefits from others having the symptom(s)?

Treating the patient with short but regularly scheduled visits; reassurance; referral to a psychoeducational group, if available, to enhance optimal health; ordering only "necessary" testing; and treating comorbid psychiatric disorders, such as depression if it arises, are the cornerstones of managing these cases.

Somatoform disorders respond better when intervention is early, without reinforcement by the excessive ordering of tests and evaluations and when patients are told that the symptoms are "real" but not life threatening and that you want to see them again for a scheduled return visit.

Case Vignette 2

A 24-year-old female student in allied health is admitted to the hospital 1 month after a motor vehicle accident. She complains of severe pain, edema, and skin temperature and coloration changes. Your anesthesiology colleagues performed three separate nerve blocks to reduce symptoms of a complex regional pain syndrome. The pain was relieved for only a few hours each time. They have discovered that she had two earlier admissions to your hospital 3 years ago. The patient was admitted at that time for red cells in her urine in close proximity to the appearance of a "butterfly" rash on her cheeks. The workup for systemic lupus and other autoimmune disorders was negative, as well as negative for urinary tract conditions. Your colleagues want to know whether the current symptoms have anything to do with those identified during the two prior hospitalizations.

As you talk to the patient, you realize there are many stressors and concerns in her life in addition to the physical symptoms limiting her ability to work part time and do her studies. It is important to be certain that all appropriate, but now excessive testing has been ordered and reviewed while requesting a psychiatric consultation. It is critical to listen closely, while being open with her about concerns that stress, depression, and anxiety can greatly affect both emotional and physical well-being. Patients can be directly or indirectly causing harm to themselves without their physician being aware.

This patient meets criteria for both major depressive disorder recurrent and factitious disorder. Included in the criteria for factitious disorder is the intentional production or feigning of physical or psychological symptoms. Symptoms of factitious disorder are motivated by psychological gain, as when a person wants to be in a sick role, either physically or emotionally. Alternatively, malingering would have been diagnosed if the patient was attempting to avoid financial or legal responsibility, or otherwise "better" her current situation. Working closely with mental health professionals, the internist in this case was able to treat the patient successfully. After the depression was treated and adequate individual and group psychotherapy provided, the self-destructive behavior ended (rubber band tourniquets, scratching with razor blades), and the patient returned to regular activities. Although patients like this are at risk during periods of great stress, re-entry into therapy as early as possible is of great advantage.

PANIC DISORDER

Case Vignette 1

A 20-year-old man presents to the office and states that last week, during his examination at the university, he had two episodes of choking. They came on unexpectedly and made it difficult for him to finish the test. On another occasion, he was watching television in his room. The patient is concerned that these episodes will return and is fearful of going anywhere alone that would make it difficult for him to obtain medical care. As you begin to question him further, he answers that he does feel short of breath, as though he might pass out for some minutes. The patient remembers feeling dizzy and sweaty toward the end of each of these episodes. He does not recall chest pain, headache, or abdominal pain.

Past history indicates some complaints of dizziness 2 years earlier that did not occur on more than a few occasions and then disappeared. He stated that he was told once that he might have mitral valve prolapse. Although he states that he never visited a mental health professional, his parents had planned to take him during elementary school because he did not want to leave home to attend class. A 35-year-old aunt had a history of chest pain and a rapid heart rate off and on; she has been taking fluoxetine for several years.

Criteria for Panic Attack (from DSM-IV-TR)

The criteria include a discrete period of intense fear or discomfort in which four (or more) of the following symptoms develop abruptly and reach a peak within 10 minutes:

- Palpitations, pounding heart, or accelerated heart rate
- Sweating
- Trembling or shaking
- Sensations of shortness of breath or smothering
- Feeling of choking
- Chest pain or discomfort
- Nausea or abdominal distress
- Feeling dizzy, unsteady, lightheaded, or faint
- Derealization (feelings of unreality) or depersonalization (being detached from oneself)
- Fear of losing control or going crazy
- Fear of dying
- Paresthesias (numbness or tingling sensation)
- Chills or hot flashes

Panic Disorder (from DSM-IV-TR)

To establish a diagnosis of panic disorder, both 1 and 2 must be present:

1. Recurrent unexpected panic attacks
2. At least one of the attacks has been followed by 1 month (or longer) of one (or more) of the following:
   a) Persistent concern about having additional attacks
   b) Worry about the implications of the attack or its consequences
   c) Significant change in behavior related to attacks

In addition, one should determine if comorbid agoraphobia is present.

A frequently chosen treatment option is low-dose antidepressants are generally first-line therapy for long-term management of panic disorder patients. To avoid precipi-

tating an attack, patients with panic disorder require tiny increments of antidepressant until they are able to tolerate a therapeutic amount with good control of symptoms. A small amount of benzodiazepine can be added for any breakthrough panic attacks occurring during the first 2 to 3 weeks.

This patient meets criteria for panic disorder and requires further assessment. He is also at risk for agoraphobia, considering that he is starting to alter where he will go for fear of an attack. Any medical concerns (e.g., thyroid, cardiac, or respiratory, and substance issues) should be explored. It is reported that patients with panic disorder often have six medical visits or more before the diagnosis is entertained. Past history of separation anxiety or school phobia during childhood may be an important clue, as is a positive family history. After basic laboratory studies, a chest x-ray, and the ECG are determined to be normal, the patient can be reassured and educated about panic disorder. A stress test may be recommended for some because reports indicate reduced heart rate variability in some patients with panic disorder as well as those with depression and schizophrenia.

A wide range of therapeutic options for panic disorder is available, including antidepressants, anxiolytics, and cognitive or other behavioral therapies. Often low-dose antidepressants are prescribed to avoid the frequent side effects that these patients experience. A small amount of benzodiazepine can be prescribed for the first 2 to 3 weeks while the antidepressant is slowly increased. An appropriate rate of increase for the antidepressant would be, for example, 12.5 mg of sertraline, 5 mg of paroxetine, or 10 mg of citalopram added every 4 to 5 days until the typical therapeutic dosage is reached.

Case Vignette 2

On your rounds at the extended-care facility, you are asked to see a new resident. She is 60 years old and suffers from late-stage Huntington's disease. During her 20s and 30s, she suffered from recurrent major depression and obsessive-compulsive disorder. Her daughter took care of her at home until a few years ago, at which time her son took her to live in a facility near his home. Over the past few years, her medication was changed from haloperidol to risperidone. In addition, she was "out of control" at times. The onset of these episodes was sudden, with loud vocalizations and pounding on her chest. They were infrequent 1 year ago, and the 0.5 mg of lorazepam twice daily seemed to control them well. Later, the dose was increased to three times a day, but eventually the symptoms recurred and led to 1.0 mg three times daily dosing.

On the new ward, her nurse tells you she thinks the patient awakens with these attacks, but once they get "medication into her she begins to calm down." Although the patient has limited detail in her spontaneous communication, she is able to indicate "yes" and "no" appropriately. She acknowledges her heart beating rapidly and feeling short of breath when the events occur.

MOOD DISORDER QUESTIONNAIRE (MDQ)

INSTRUCTIONS:

Please answer each question as best you can.   Yes   No

1   Has there ever been a period of time when you were not your usual self and...

    – you felt so good or so hyper that other people thought you were not your normal   □   □
self or you were so hyper that you got into trouble?

    – you were so irritable that you shouted at people or started fights or arguments?   □   □

    – you felt much more self-confident than usual?   □   □

    – you got much less sleep than usual and found that you didn't really miss it?   □   □

    – you were more talkative or spoke much faster than usual?   □   □

    – thoughts raced through your head or you couldn't slow your mind down?   □   □

    – you were so easily distracted by things around you that you had trouble   □   □
concentrating or staying on track?

    – you had much more energy than usual?   □   □

    – you were much more active or did many more things than usual?   □   □

    – you were much more social or outgoing than usual, for example, you telephoned   □   □
friends in the middle of the night?

    – you were much more interested in sex than usual?   □   □

    – you did things that were unusual for you or that other people might have thought   □   □
were excessive, foolish, or risky?

    – spending money got you or your family in trouble?   □   □

2   If you checked YES to more than one of the above, have several of these ever   □   □
happened during the same period of time?

3   How much of a problem did any of these cause you—like being unable to work;
having family, money or legal trouble; getting into arguments or fights?

□ No problem   □ Minor problem   □ Moderate problem   □ Serious problem

Figure 10.3 Mood Disorder Questionnaire (MDQ). *Source:* Modified from Hirschfeld RM, Williams JB, Spitzer RL. Development and validation of a screening instrument for bipolar spectrum depression: the mood disorder questionnaire. *Am J Psychiatry* 2000;157:1873–1875. Copyright © 2000–2007, James R. Phelps, MD.

During the day, the patient does not fall asleep while taking lorazepam. She communicates great distress when her chest pain begins, and she worries that the episodes are coming more often. You order a dipyridamole thallium stress test, and it returns normal. Although the patient never drank alcohol, her father and brother were alcoholics. Her mother and aunts were treated for depression.

It is difficult for her to communicate, but the symptoms seem likely to be those of panic disorder. Her "yes" and "no" responses are consistent and indicate no hallucinations or delusions. She does not have fluctuations in her attention span indicative of delirium, and she does not have a long history of somatic complaints without physical findings. As she became tolerant of lorazepam, breakthrough panic occurred nearly every morning, when blood level was lowest. Before discounting other conditions, it is important to rule out hypoxia and various endocrinopathies.

When comorbid psychiatric disorders exist, medication adjustments are most important. For example, if panic disorder exists with depression, doses must start low, with gentle titration upward (e.g., fluoxetine, 5 mg, taken orally each day for several days before increasing by another 5 mg daily). It may take 2 to 3 weeks to titrate up to the maintenance level (e.g., 20 mg fluoxetine). If obsessive-compulsive disorder exists along with major depression, it is not unusual for the patient to eventually need higher doses of SSRI (e.g., paroxetine, 40–80 mg daily).

DELIRIUM

Case Vignette 1

A 51-year-old male patient in the intensive care unit presents with acute onset of confusion 36 hours postoperatively, after a successful coronary artery bypass graft. The patient is taking several medications, including insulin, atenolol, promethazine, metoclopramide, levothyroxine, and others. The patient has no respiratory distress and has good arterial blood gases. His electrolytes,

TABLE 10.1

ANTIDEPRESSANT THERAPY

Drug	Starting Single Dose (mg) for Elderly or Frail Medically Ill Patients	Average Total Daily Dose (mg) for Many Patients	Important Considerations
Amitriptyline (Elavil)	10–25	75–150	Highly sedating; anticholinergic, orthostasis, ECG changes
Amoxapine	25	75–150	Antipsychotic properties with EPS
Bupropion[a] (Wellbutrin)	75–150	300	Less weight gain, watch BP ↑, less sexual side effects
Citalopram[a] (Celexa)	10–20	20–40	Less drug interaction
Clomipramine (Anafranil)	25	75–150	For obsessive-compulsive disorder; ↑ orthostasis and anticholinergic
Desipramine (Norpramin)	25	75–150	More overdoses associated with death
Doxepin (Sinequan)	25	75–150	Weight gain, sedating
Duloxetine (Cymbalta)	20–30	60	Nausea (take with food); helpful in diabetic neuropathy, pain syndromes
Escitalopram[a] (Lexapro)	5–10	10–20	Less drug interactions
Fluvoxamine (Luvox)	25–50	100–150	For obsessive-compulsive disorder, need BID dosing
Fluoxetine[a] (Prozac)	10–20	20–40	Longest half-life, self-tapers
Imipramine (Tofranil)	10–25	75–150	Orthostasis, ↑ ECG changes, anticholinergic
Maprotiline	25	75	Side effects similar to other TCAs
Mirtazapine[a] (Remeron)	7.5–15.0	15–30	Less sexual side effects; sedating at low doses activating at higher doses, weight gain; oral dissolvable tablet (SolTab) available
Nortriptyline[a] (Pamelor)	10–25	50–100	Less orthostasis, some ECG changes
Paroxetine[a] (Paxil)	10–20	20–40	Constipation on higher doses and more sedation; must taper; more withdrawal symptoms
Protriptyline (Vivactil)	5–10 (am)	20 (10 mg, am and noon)	Activating, but very anticholinergic
Selegiline (Emsam)	6 mg/24 hr patch	6–9 mg/24 hr patch	Selective MAO-B inhibitor; at >6 mg/24 hr patch, loses selectivity, must observe tyramine diet; requires 2-week wash out before changing to another antidepressant
Sertraline[a] (Zoloft)	25–50	50–100 (am)	Loose stools, less drug interaction at lowest levels
Trazodone[a] (Desyrel)	50	150–300	Sedating, orthostasis, priapism with rapid increase
Trimipramine (Surmontil)	10–25	50–100 (am)	Very anticholinergic, sedating and increased ECG cardiac changes
Venlafaxine[a] (Effexor XR)	37.5	75–150	Reduces pain, ↑ BP at higher doses

BID, twice a day; BP, blood pressure; EPS, extrapyramidal symptoms; MOA-B, monoamine oxidase type B; TCA, tricyclic antidepressants.
[a]Used in elderly patients.

blood sugar, ECG, creatinine, and liver function tests are within normal range at present. A TSH is ordered, and oral haloperidol (5 mg) is given to reduce symptoms of delirium. The patient does not improve; in fact, the nurses report his behavior has further deteriorated, and his arms and legs have become somewhat rigid.

Drug–drug interactions are frequent causes of delirium. It is wise to avoid multiple anticholinergic drugs that may cause delirium, including antipsychotic agents, antiemetic agents, antiparkinsonian agents, TCAs, and antihistamines such as diphenhydramine. Using multiple

agents that block dopamine (e.g., haloperidol, promethazine, metoclopramide) may affect multiple dopamine receptors, producing a paradoxical response and severe hypotension. If this occurs, a nondopaminergic pressor agent can be used. Vitals should be monitored, and the presence of rigidity or cogwheeling should be observed.

If the patient's QTc had been long, it would have been quite important to avoid medications that might further lengthen that interval: TCAs; carbamazepine; antipsychotics, including pimozide; and antiarrhythmics,

TABLE 10.2

ANTIPSYCHOTIC MEDICATIONS: DOSAGE FOR MEDICALLY ILL PATIENTS WITH PROMINENT CHARACTERISTICS

Agent	Starting Oral Dose (mg)[a]	Comments and Characteristics
Phenothiazines		
Chlorpromazine (Thorazine)	10–25	Significant hypotension risk, lowers seizure threshold, highly sedating, anticholinergic
Thioridazine (Mellaril)	10–25	Similar to chlorpromazine but more likely to alter ECG (prolongs QT more than others), not available IM
Mesoridazine (Serentil)	10–25	Similar to chlorpromazine and thioridazine
Perphenazine (Trilafon)	4	More sedation and hypotension than haloperidol, but less than chlorpromazine
Trifluoperazine (Stelazine)	2	High frequency of EPS (acute dystonias, akathesias, pseudoparkinsonian syndrome, tardive dyskinesia)
Fluphenazine (Prolixin)	2	High frequency of EPS similar to trifluoperazine
Prochlorperazine (Compazine)	5–10	Weak antipsychotic, used more as an antiemetic, but can produce EPS
Pimozide (Orap)	2	Has been used for monodelusional disorder, Tourette's syndrome
Other Typical Antipsychotics		
Haloperidol (Haldol)	0.5–2.0	High frequency of EPS, except when given IV (twice as potent when given IV); ECG monitoring when using IV
Thiothixene (Navane)	1–2	High frequency of EPS similar to trifluoperazine
Loxapine (Loxitane)	10	Moderate in most side effects noted previously
Molindone (Moban)	5–10	Less weight gain, but blurring of vision frequently
Atypical Antipsychotics		
Aripiprazole (Abilify)	10 QD	Nausea, akathisia can occur at first; partial antagonist of 5-HT and dopamine
Clozapine (Clozaril)	25 QHS	Recommended for patients who have treatment-resistant or chronic schizophrenia or evidence of tardive dyskinesia; very low EPS profile. However, has the most weight gain, orthostasis, and tachycardia. Agranulocytosis risk requires CBC monitoring
Quetiapine (Seroquel)	25–50 QHS	Very low incidence of EPS, preferred agent in Parkinson's disease. Can cause sedation, weight gain
Risperidone (Risperdal)	0.5–1.0 QD or BID	At low dose, few EPS, but at higher dosages (>4 mg) can cause EPS; increases prolactin levels. Risperdal Consta IM maintenance bimonthly injections
Olanzapine (Zyprexa)	2.5–5.0 QHS	Sedation, orthostasis, weight gain, increased diabetes mellitus reported, very few EPS, available IM for acute use. Oral (Zydis) dissolvable form also available
Ziprasidone (Geodon)	20 BID	Few EPS, less sedating, less weight gain, do not use if ↑ QTc on ECG, take with food to increase absorption, available IM for acute use

5-HT, 5-hydroxytryptamine (serotonin); BID, twice a day; CBC, complete blood cell; EPS, extrapyramidal symptoms (akathisia, pseudoparkinsonian syndrome, acute dystonias, tardive dyskinesthesia); IM, intramuscularly; IV, intravenously; QD, every day; QHS, at bedtime.
All atypical antipsychotics may increase risk for diabetes mellitus. Little is known about the additional risk of diabetes mellitus when combining with antidepressants.

including lidocaine, propafenone, and quinidine. Other QT-prolonging conditions include electrolyte imbalance, underlying cardiac abnormalities, hypothyroidism, and familial long QT syndrome. Haloperidol (Haldol) carries a risk of arrhythmias (QT prolongation) and sudden death (torsades de pointes) when administered intravenously or at higher than recommended dosages. Due to this risk, the FDA issued a safety alert and recommends ECG monitoring when haloperidol is given intravenously. The prolonged metabolism of some QTc-increasing drugs can also occur with fluoxetine, grapefruit juice, and ketoconazole, via inhibition of the P450 3A4 isoenzyme.

Numerous reasons may exist for this patient's acute confusional state. Medication-induced delirium (anticholinergic), thyroid disease, alcohol or benzodiazepine withdrawal, and other conditions should be ruled out. Neuroleptic malignant syndrome, a serious clinical condition consisting of hyperthermia, rigidity, change in mental status, and hemodynamic instability, must always be monitored for when exposed to dopamine blocking agents. It is more likely that the metoclopramide and oral haloperidol may have increased his extrapyramidal side effects. Discontinuation of offending agents, supportive therapy with close monitoring of vital signs, laboratory studies, and patient responses will further direct treatment.

MANIA

Case Vignette 1

A 50-year-old female who is followed by your colleague drops in to ask if she can start a medicine she heard can help stop smoking. She is leery of trying varenicline, has tried the nicotine patch and gum, and had a friend that did well in smoking cessation with Zyban. The two of you determine that bupropion (Zyban or Wellbutrin) may be helpful.

As you assess her smoking dependency, you also consider contraindications to the medication. Patients who have epilepsy or who have brain pathology may have an increased risk for seizures while using this medication. Being overweight alone is not a contraindication, and in fact, this antidepressant is more effective in allowing patients who follow a healthy diet and exercise to lose weight. However, patients with either anorexia or bulimia nervosa are at higher risk for seizures when taking bupropion. Patients with cardiac disease can be treated safely, unless their blood pressure increases, which can sometimes occur at higher doses.

After 5 days, the patient's husband calls you on the phone, stating that "there's something wrong with her." He says she hasn't been able to sleep, and he wants you to prescribe a sleeping pill. Because you are in a hurry, you start to ask where he wants you to call in the prescription, but then reconsider and ask to speak with his wife, the patient. When you ask her how she is doing, she responds "terrific" and goes on to tell you all the many activities she's planning.

Patients with bipolar disorder exhibit depression and manic symptoms in their lifetime. The depressed phase of a bipolar patient may look very similar to the depressed phase of a depressed (unipolar) patient. The symptoms of a classic hypomanic/manic phase include pressured speech, racing thoughts, little to no sleep, boundless energy, euphoric mood, grandiose plans, and inappropriate judgment. Exposure to antidepressants can precipitate mania as occurred in our patient.

TABLE 10.3

ANTIANXIETY AGENTS AND NIGHTTIME SEDATIVES[a]

Agent	Half-Life (hr)	Onset	Starting Dose (mg)	Comments
Benzodiazepines				
Triazolam (Halcion)	1.5–3.5	Rapid	0.125 QHS	More frequent amnesia and hallucinations, rarely used
Oxazepam (Serax)[a]	8–20	Moderate	10 TID	More gradual onset
Lorazepam (Ativan)[a]	10–20	Rapid	0.5 TID	IV, IM, or PO preferably short-term use
Temazepam (Restoril)[a]	12–24	Rapid	15 QHS	Bedtime only
Alprazolam (Xanax)	12–24	Moderate	0.25 TID	Higher risk for dependency, short half-life
Chlordiazepoxide (Librium)	12–48	Moderate	10 BID or TID	Taper, used for benzodiazepine or alcohol withdrawal at higher doses
Clonazepam (Klonopin)	20–30	Rapid	0.5 BID	Long half-life, may be used for withdrawal taper
Diazepam (Valium)	20–90	Rapid	2–5 BID	Rapid onset, increased dependency may be used for withdrawal taper, IV, PO, or IM
Clorazepate (Tranxene)	20–100	Rapid	7.5 BID	Significant dependency risk, rarely used
Flurazepam (Dalmane)	20–100	Rapid	15 QHS	Rebound insomnia when stopped, long half-life, rarely used
Nonbenzodiazepines				
Zolpidem (Ambien)	2.6	Rapid	5 QHS	Hypnotic, short half-life
Zaleplon (Sonata)	1.0	Rapid	5 QHS	Hypnotic, similar to zolpidem
Eszopiclone (Lunesta)	6.0	Rapid	1–2 QHS	Hypnotic

Elderly or extremely debilitated patients should be given lower doses. Caution should be used when prescribing long-acting sedating medications because they have been associated with a high incidence of falls and hip fractures.

BID, twice a day; IM, intramuscularly; IV, intravenously; PO, orally; QHS, at bedtime; TID, three times a day.
For generalized anxiety disorder, buspirone (BuSpar). Slow onset of action; take 2 weeks 5 mg TID and increase; may need 45 or even 60 mg/24 hr.
[a]Preferred for elderly patients, one pass through liver. Glucuronidation only in lorazepam, oxazepam, and temazepam. (All others also require oxidation and should be given in lower doses to avoid accumulation, and increasing risk for falls and fractures.)
i) Antidepressants (for panic disorder): May use lower doses than for depression.
ii) Beta-blockers (for autonomic symptom control): Performance anxiety but not panic disorder. Propranolol (Inderal) 10–20 mg TID.
iii) Antihistamines: May be safer in some cases when dependency is a concern, but not advisable in the elderly or anyone prone to delirium. Diphenhydramine (Benadryl), 25 mg; starting doses BID; hydroxyzine (Vistaril), 25–50 mg; starting doses TID.

TABLE 10.4
ANTIPSYCHOTICS—THERAPEUTIC AND SIDE EFFECT PROFILE

	Aripiprazole (Abilify)	Haloperidol (Haldol)	Thioridazine (Mellaril)	Clozapine (Clozaril)	Risperidone (Risperdal)	Olanzapine (Zyprexa)	Quetiapine (Seroquel)	Ziprasidone (Geodon)
Reduces apathy, other negative symptoms	+			+	+	+	+	+
Intravenous use		+						
Intramuscular use	+	+			+ q2wk	+		+
Sedating			++	+++	+	++	++	
Anticholinergic		+	++	++		+	+	
Extrapyramidal		++	+		++	+		
Orthostatic hypotension	+		++	++	+	+	+	
Weight gain	+		++	+++	++	+++	++	+
Weekly CBC required (agranulocytosis)				+				
Can prolong cardiac conduction		+	++					+
CBC monitoring		QTc (IV)	PR, QRS, QTc	+ weekly biweekly, monthly				QTc

CBC, complete blood count.

TABLE 10.5

SELECTIVE SEROTONIN REUPTAKE INHIBITORS—SIDE EFFECTS

- Anticholinergic: very few side effects (paroxetine has some; still lower than tricyclic antidepressant)
- Arrhythmias: very few side effects; occasional bradycardia
- Sedation: very little, but some patients respond in paradoxical fashion; can increase with dose. Paroxetine most, fluoxetine least
- Seizure threshold is of very little concern
- Gastrointestinal side effects: sertraline provokes more diarrhea; paroxetine provokes constipation at higher doses
- Sexual dysfunction
- Toxicity in overdose: little to none
- Extrapyramidal symptoms: tremor and akathisia
- Headache
- Hyponatremia occasional
- Reduced platelet aggregation; prolongs bleeding time, especially with higher doses of antidepressant, presence of warfarin, and pre-existing bleeding

On further history, the patient states that she has a history of postpartum depression that was never treated, but quickly bounced back. You decide to stop the bupropion and have your psychiatrist colleague see her the next day.

The psychiatrist confirms bipolar disorder and wants to begin lithium carbonate and asks you to order lab tests. Considerations for the internists are that lithium has renal clearance and is not hepatically metabolized. More than 10% of patients on lithium develop hypothyroidism, so you want to know her TSH level before starting lithium. Likewise, her white blood count may rise with lithium, and ST elevation can occur. If we have baseline values before initiating the drug, we can better assess possible side effects. If her creatinine is elevated, she is unlikely to clear lithium adequately and would be at greater risk for toxicity.

Drug interactions with certain common medications can increase lithium levels. These include lisinopril and

TABLE 10.6

SELECTED SSRI DRUG INTERACTIONS

- Antiarrhythmic (propafenone, flecainide); increased plasma level of antiarrhythmic due to inhibited metabolism
- Beta-blockers (propranolol, metoprolol); decreased heart rate (addictive effect) reported with fluoxetine. Beta-blockers are metabolized by cytochrome P450 2D6. Fluoxetine and paroxetine is an inhibitor or 2D6. Therefore, fluoxetine will increase the side effects of lethargy, hypotension, and bradycardia of propranolol when administered together. Monitor blood pressure, heart rate, and sedation
- Calcium channel blockers (nifedipine, verapamil); increased side effects (headache, flushing, edema) resulting from inhibited clearance of blocker with fluoxetine
- Digoxin; decreased level (area under curve) of digoxin by 18% reported with paroxetine
- Warfarin can displace warfarin through p450 2C9/19 and secondarily increase risk of bleeding

TABLE 10.7

CYCLIC ANTIDEPRESSANTS

Anticholinergics
   Most: amitriptyline, imipramine
   Less: desipramine
Quinidine-like
   Most: amitriptyline, imipramine
   Less: protriptyline
Sedation
   Most: amitriptyline, doxepin
   Less: desipramine, nortriptyline
Seizures
   Most: clomipramine (TCA/SSRI), maprotiline (tetracyclic), amoxapine (TCA/antipsychotic)
   Less: desipramine
Weight gain
   Most: doxepin, amitriptyline
   Less: desipramine
Orthostatic
   Most: amitriptyline, imipramine
   Less: nortriptyline
Gastrointestinal
   Most: clomipramine (TCA/SSRI)
   Less: desipramine
Sexual dysfunction
   Most: "toss up" may be slightly better than SSRIs
Toxicity in overdose
   Most: "toss up" (more deaths reported with desipramine)

SSRI, selective serotonin reuptake inhibitor; TCA, tricyclic antidepressant.

other angiotensin-converting enzyme inhibitors, nonsteroidal anti-inflammatory drugs (NSAIDs), and hydrochlorothiazide. All drugs are able to significantly *increase* lithium levels to the point of toxicity in only several days. Theophylline, osmotic diuretics, and steroids can reduce lithium levels, and the patient's mood may switch into depression or mania.

Mood Disorder Questionnaire

Differentiating depressive symptoms in bipolar disorder versus depression from major depressive disorder can be very difficult due to similarities in presenting symptoms while clinically depressed, and bipolar patients are often prescribed antidepressants when seen as "just depressed." Screening for mania symptoms in depressed patients with a family history of bipolar depression, personal history of mania, or poor response to antidepressants can be pivotal to making the correct diagnosis and ensuring that the patient receives the correct treatment. Bipolar disorder patients who require mood stabilizers (lithium, anticonvulsants, or atypical antipsychotics) will not likely receive them if they are diagnosed as "just depressed." In **Figure 10.3**, the Mood Disorder Questionnaire is provided as a screening instrument to better identify bipolar disorder. Seven out of 13 positive ("yes") responses on question 1, coupled with a "yes" answer to question 2, and a response of "moderate"

TABLE 10.8

COMORBIDITY TABLE: PSYCHOTROPICS EFFECTIVE WITH AFFECTIVE AND RELATED DISORDERS

Psychotropic	MDD	PMDD	ADD	OCD	Panic	Eating Disorder	GAD	Bipolar	Pain Syndrome
Clomipramine (Anafranil)	T	T		T	T		T	a	?
Fluoxetine (Prozac)	T	T	T	T	T	T	T	a	T
Sertraline (Zoloft)	T	T	T	T	T	T	T	a	T
Paroxetine (Paxil)	T	T	T	T	T	T	T	a	T
Fluvoxamine (Luvox)	T	T	T	T	T	T	T	a	?
Citalopram (Celexa)	T	T	T	T	T	T	T	a	?
Mirtazapine (Remeron)	T	?			?	T	?	a	?
Trazodone (Desyrel)	T						T	a	?
Venlafaxine (Effexor)	T	?	?		?		T	a	T
Duloxetine (Cymbalta)	T	?			?		?	a	T
Amitriptyline (Elavil)	T				T		T	a	T
Imipramine (Tofranil)	T				T		T	a	T
Bupropion (Wellbutrin)	T	?						a	
Alprazolam (Xanax)					T		T		
Buspirone (BuSpar)	M	?					T		
Methylphenidate (Ritalin)[b]	c		T						
Lithium (Eskalith)	M							T	
Atomoxetine (Strattera)			T						
Carbamazepine (Tegretol)	M?							T	
Valproate (Depakote)	M?							T	
Gabapentin (Neurontin)							?	?	T
Topiramate (Topamax)								?	
Lamotrigine (Lamictal)	T?							T	
Oxcarbazepine (Trileptal)								?	
Atypical antipsychotics	M								?
T3	M								

ADD, attention deficit disorder; GAD, generalized anxiety disorder; MDD, major depressive disorder; OCD, obsessive-compulsive disorder; PMDD, premenstrual dysphoric disorder.
M, may be used to augment an antidepressant; T, effective treatment; ?, possibly effective or partially effective due to mechanism of action, but currently inadequate evidence-based data.
[a]Only administer in depressed phase and while on a mood stabilizer.
[b]Used in psychomotor retarded, medically ill patients, with quick response in 2 to 3 days.
[c]Alternative for medically ill patient with depression.

TABLE 10.9

MOOD STABILIZERS

Medication	Starting Dose	Usual Dose (mg)	Common Drug Interactions or Concerns
Lithium	300 mg	900–1,200	ACE inhibitors, NSAIDs, thiazide diuretics (will ↑ Li level), check TSH
Carbamazepine	100–200 mg	600–800	Autoinduction of compound, will lower other medications; SIADH (can ↓ sodium)
Divalproate	125–250 mg	750–1,000	Carbamazepine, lamotrigine, and many others
Gabapentin	100 mg	600–900	↓ level if creatinine is ↑, helpful for pain; limited data as mood stabilizer
Lamotrigine	25 mg (slow-dose titration to avoid Stevens-Johnson syndrome rash)	200–300	Valproate can ↑ lamotrigine; effective in depressed phase of bipolar depression
Oxcarbazepine	300 mg, increase q3days	600–1,200	Like carbamazepine, can ↓ sodium, but no autoinduction of compound; limited data as mood stabilizer
Topiramate	25 mg, increase every week	100–150	Can ↓ new learning; limited data as mood stabilizer

ACE, angiotensin-converting enzyme; NSAIDs, nonsteroidal anti-inflammatory drugs; SIADH, syndrome of inappropriate antidiuretic hormone; TSH, thyroid-stimulating hormone.
It is recommended that all patients on anticonvulsants be frequently monitored for suicidal ideation.

or "serious" to question 3 all indicate a positive screen for bipolar spectrum disorder.

DEMENTIA

Case Vignette 1

A 72-year-old man is brought to see you for "agitation" secondary to dementia. He has diabetes mellitus, is significantly overweight, and has hyperlipidemia. His ECG was read as normal with a QTc 400. The family wants to avoid placing him in a nursing home. They say he has tantrums when he cannot find his wallet, glasses, or other personal possessions. Lists, color coding possessions, reminder signs, and other behavioral techniques have been tried, but to little avail. The family asks if a medicine could help.

Although antianxiety, antidepressants, antipsychotics, and anticonvulsants have all been used for agitation in dementia, the etiology of the symptom, the intensity or nature of the behavior, and the side effects of these medications should be considered. In this case, the patient is likely forgetting where he placed his possessions, and if a cholinesterase inhibitor helps improve his recall, it would be an optimal pharmacologic choice with which to start.

Donepezil is started and successful for a few years until paranoid delusions about his neighbors stealing from him are heard. He insists that they send criminals into his home to remove his favorite shoes and gloves. He even saw them in his living room, although when the family arrived, they found no evidence that anyone had been there.

At this point in his care, memantine could help curb some of the agitation due to memory loss, but because he has visual hallucinations and paranoid delusions, an antipsychotic should be considered. Thioridazine is extremely anticholinergic and hypotensive; thus, it is not well indicated in the elderly and can prolong the QTc significantly. A newer agent (atypical antipsychotic) with less risk for tardive dyskinesia and orthostatic and anticholinergic effects is preferable. If visual hallucinations are prominent and Lewy body disease is suspected, quetiapine, due to its low extrapyramidal syndrome profile, may be a preferred agent. However, all atypical antipsychotics carry a risk of increased cardiovascular events when treating psychosis or behavioral disturbances in patients with dementia, and this should be factored in the risk–benefit analysis.

PSYCHOTROPICS IN THE MEDICALLY ILL

It is important to evaluate for underlying medical problems before prescribing any psychotropic medication. Several psychotropic medications have been implicated in association with the onset of diabetes mellitus. Insulin resistance has been reported as mechanistic underpinning. Hyperinsulinemia, increased leptin, and weight gain are also described. Weight gain is not believed to be the sole reason for the development of diabetes.

Before starting various psychiatric medications in a patient with multisystem disease, it is wise to assess blood pressure with venlafaxine, duloxetine, bupropion, and TCAs; assess renal clearance with lithium, Neurontin, and mirtazapine; and lipid profile with all atypical antipsychotics and antidepressants such as mirtazapine. Due to the risk of increased cardiovascular events, TCAs should not be prescribed to established cardiac patients.

Of the atypical antipsychotics, white blood count must be closely monitored while on clozapine to avoid agranulocytosis. Blood is drawn weekly for the first 6 months and biweekly for the following 6 months, and then monthly thereafter for the duration of treatment with this medication.

Finally, board review questions about patients with psychiatric disorders in the medically ill draw on your knowledge of psychopharmacology. To assist with learning how medications differ, review tables are included in this chapter. The pharmacologic profile for common psychiatric medications is summarized in Tables 10.1 to 10.3; side effects are reviewed in Tables 10.4, 10.5; and drug interactions are listed in Table 10.6. Table 10.7 reviews TCA profile. The relative use of different compounds is summarized in Table 10.8. Mood stabilizers are listed in Table 10.9.

REVIEW EXERCISES

QUESTIONS

1. Which of the following side effects is most commonly seen with selective serotonin reuptake inhibitors?
a) Weight gain
b) Sexual dysfunction
c) Sedation
d) QTc prolongation
e) None of the above

Answer and Discussion
The answer is b. Sexual dysfunction is a common side effect. patients taking selective serotonin reuptake inhibitors (fluoxetine, sertraline, paroxetine, citalopram, and escitalopram) are more likely to report sexual dysfunction than those taking other agents such as bupropion or mirtazapine.

2. Which of the following statements about somatoform disorders is correct?
a) There is a history of many physical complaints beginning before age 30 years.
b) When a related general medical condition exists, physical complaints are in excess of what would be expected.
c) These disorders respond better when intervention is early, without reinforcement by the excessive ordering of tests and evaluations.

d) Patients should be told that the symptoms are "real" but not life threatening.

e) All of the above.

Answer and Discussion

The answer is e. The DSM Criteria include finding a history of many physical complaints beginning before age 30 years that occur over a period of several years and result in treatment being sought or significant impairment in social, occupational, or other area of functioning. Treating the patient with short but regularly scheduled visits; reassurance; referral to a psychoeducational group, if available, to enhance optimal health; ordering only "necessary" testing; and treating comorbid psychiatric disorders, such as depression, are the cornerstones of managing these cases.

3. Which of the following is not a characteristic feature of a panic attack?

a) Chest pain

b) Feeling dizzy

c) Diarrhea

d) Paresthesias

e) Sweating

Answer and Discussion

The answer is c. Diarrhea is not a characteristic feature of panic attack. Nausea and abdominal distress may be seen.

4. Which of the following medications increases the risk for lithium toxicity?

a) Enalapril

b) Hydrochlorothiazide

c) Ibuprofen

d) Losartan

e) All the above

Answer and Discussion

The answer is e. Lithium has renal clearance and is not hepatically metabolized. Medications that can alter sodium excretion should be used with caution (e.g., diuretics, angiotensin-converting enzyme inhibitors, nonsteroidal anti-inflammatory drugs) because lithium levels may increase to the point of toxicity in only several days.

5. Which of the following should be obtained before initiating haloperidol?

a) Thyroid-stimulating hormone

b) Hematocrit

c) ECG

d) Liver function tests

e) All of the above

Answer and Discussion

The answer is c. Haloperidol may alter cardiac conduction and prolong QT Interval; life-threatening arrhythmias have occurred with therapeutic doses of antipsychotics, but risk may be increased with doses exceeding recommendations and/or intravenous administration (unlabeled route). Haloperidol should be used with caution or avoided in patients with electrolyte abnormalities (e.g., hypokalemia, hypomagnesemia), hypothyroidism, familial long QT syndrome, concomitant medications that may augment QT prolongation, or any underlying cardiac abnormality that may also potentiate risk.

SUGGESTED READINGS

Belmaker RH, Galila A. Major depressive disorder. *N Engl J Med* 2008;358:55–68.

Brown LC, Majumdar SR, Johnson JA. Type of antidepressant therapy and risk of type 2 diabetes in people with depression. *Diabetes Res Clin Prac* 2008;79:61–67.

Drugs for Psychiatric Disorders. Treatment Guidelines from the Medical Letter [online]. *The Medical Letter* 2006;4(46):35–46. Available at: http://medicalletter.org/html/archivesTG.htm.

Franco-Bronson K, Williams K. Emotional and psychiatric problems in patients with cancer. In: Skeel R, ed. *Handbook of Cancer Chemotherapy*, 7th ed. New York: Lippincott Williams & Wilkins, 2007.

Freeman R. Drug therapy: Schizophrenia. *N Engl J Med* 2003;349:1738–1749.

Friedman RA, Leon AC. Expanding the black box: Depression, antidepressants, and the risk of suicide. *N Engl J Med* 2007;356:2343–2346.

Gaynes BN, Rush AJ, Trivedi MH, et al. The STAR*D study: treating depression in the real world. *Cleve Clin J Med* 2008;75:57–66.

Iosifescu DV. Treating depression in the medically ill. *Psychiatry Clin N Am* 2007;30:77–90.

Katon WJ. Panic disorder. *N Engl J Med* 2006;354:2360-2367.

Kessler RC. Prevalence, severity, and comorbidity of 12-month DSM-IV disorders in the National Comorbidity Survey Replication. *Arch Gen Psychiatry* 2005;62:617–627.

Lee HB, Lyketsos CG. Depression in Alzheimer's disease: heterogeneity and related issues. *Biol Psychiatry* 2003;54:353–362.

Muzina DJ, Colangelo E, Sloan Manning J, et al. Differentiating bipolar disorder from depression in primary care. *Cleve Clin J Med* 2007;74:89–105.

Schneider LS, Tariot PN, Dagerman KS, et al. Effectiveness of atypical antipsychotics drugs in patients with Alzheimer's disease. *N Engl J Med* 2006;355:1525–1538.

Stunkard AJ, Faith MS, Allison KC. Depression and obesity. *Biol Psychiatry* 2003;54:330–337.

Whinney CM, Pozuelo L, Locala J. Evaluation and management of medical patients with psychiatric disorders. In: Williams, MV ed. *Textbook of Comprehensive Hospital Medicine*. Philadelphia: Saunders Elsevier, 2007:851–862.

Chapter 11

Genetic Disease

Franklin A. Michota

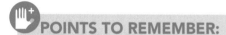

POINTS TO REMEMBER:

- Most diseases encountered in the practice of medicine have genetic components in both cause and pathogenesis.

- Down syndrome is associated with maternal age older than 35 years.

- The functional consequence and clinical implications of single gene disorders may be extremely variable.

- Virtually all males with an X-linked recessive mutation are affected clinically.

- The process of considering, ordering, and interpreting a genetic test is not straightforward.

Genetic disease is not as rare as once believed. Most diseases encountered in the practice of medicine have genetic components in both cause and pathogenesis. It is unlikely that any disease is entirely nongenetic because the interaction of both genetic and environmental factors influences the development of an individual. Many conditions previously believed to be nongenetic are now understood to be multifactorial diseases with the contribution of various genetic and environmental determinants. Medical genetics has broad relevance in adult clinical medicine. More adult patients with genetic conditions are being recognized, genetic testing for adult-onset genetic conditions is expanding, and children with genetic conditions are now more likely to survive into adulthood. This chapter summarizes the principles and methods in molecular genetics relevant to clinical practice, and discusses important disease entities that illustrate genetic disorders.

THE GENOME

The nucleus of every human cell contains the full complement of the human genome, which consists of approximately 30,000 to 70,000 named and unnamed genes and many intergenic DNA sequences. A gene is defined as a contiguous region of DNA that includes a defined set of exons (protein-coding regions) and introns (DNA interspersed between exons). The basic unit of DNA is made up of one of four nitrogenous bases (adenine [A], guanine [G], thymine [T], cytosine [C]). The double-helical DNA molecule in a human cell, associated with special proteins (histones and regulatory proteins), is highly compacted into 22 pairs of autosomal chromosomes and an additional pair of sex chromosomes (46 total chromosomes). The entire cellular DNA consists of approximately 3 billion base pairs, of which only 1% is believed to encode a functional protein or a polypeptide. The information contained in a given gene is expressed if the DNA sequence of the gene is first transcribed into an RNA molecule (transcription) that, after being processed in the nucleus, will carry the information (messenger RNA or mRNA) into the cytoplasm for translation into a protein. Many newly synthesized proteins are further modified after or during polypeptide synthesis. Posttranslational or cotranslational modifications of proteins ensure proper protein folding, targeting, activation, and stability. The specific processes include proteolysis, glycosylation, phosphorylation, acylation, metal binding, and assumption of secondary and tertiary structures.

GENETIC DISORDERS

Genetically determined disorders may be subdivided into three major groups: chromosome, single gene, and multifactorial (polygenic) diseases. The different types of genetic disease may manifest clinically at different prenatal and postnatal ages (Fig. 11.1).

Chromosome Disorders

As a group, chromosome disorders are common. However, most conceptions with chromosome anomalies abort early, and thus, the observed frequency of chromosome defects is much lower. Some chromosome anomalies are "balanced" and include the full complement of genetic material in a rearranged form. Most people with balanced chromosome rearrangements are healthy. In contrast, most

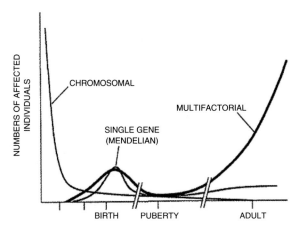

Figure 11.1 Age at manifestation of the different types of genetic disorders. *Source:* Reprinted from Geleherter TD, et al. *Principles of Medical Genetics*, 2nd ed. Baltimore: Williams & Wilkins, 1998:1–42.

individuals with a clinically important chromosome disorder have a net loss or gain of chromosome material and consequently of genes. This can occur when an individual has a chromosome number other than the expected 46 (aneuploidy or polyploidy) or when a portion of a chromosome is altered (via a deletion or duplication). Aneuploidy occurs when there is other than a multiple of the typical 46 chromosomes. Trisomy 21 (Down syndrome), 18 (Edward syndrome), and 13 (Patau syndrome) (Table 11.1) are seen at considerable frequencies in newborns, and Down syndrome is associated with increased maternal age older than 35 years. Turner syndrome (45,X) is most often caused by loss of the paternal X chromosome and is present in 1% of all conceptions (Table 11.1). Chromosome polyploidy occurs when the number of chromosome sets is other than two. The most common type of polyploidy is triploidy

TABLE 11.1

CHROMOSOME DISORDERS

Disorder	Abnormality	Clinical Features
Down syndrome	Trisomy 21 47,XX,+21	Oblique eye fissures with epicanthic skin folds on the inner corner of the eyes, muscle hypotonia (poor muscle tone), a flat nasal bridge, a single palmar fold, a protruding tongue (due to small oral cavity and and enlarged tongue near the tonsils), a short neck, white spots on the iris known as Brushfield spots, excessive joint laxity including atlantoaxial instability, congenital heart defects (typically ventricular septal defects), excessive space between large toe and second toe, a single flexion furrow of the fifth finger, and a higher number of ulnar loop dermatoglyphs can be seen. Most individuals with Down syndrome have mental retardation in the mild (IQ 50–70) to moderate (IQ 35–50) range. Hearing deficits (possibly due to sensorineural factors or chronic serous otitis media, also known as glue ear), thyroid disorders, and Alzheimer's disease are common. Other less common serious illnesses include leukemia, immune deficiencies, and epilepsy. Average life span is 49 years.
Edward syndrome	Trisomy 18 47,XX,+18	The survival rate of Edward syndrome is very low. About half die in utero. Of liveborn infants, only 50% live to 2 months, and only 5%–10% will survive their first year of life. Major causes of death include apnea and heart abnormalities.
Patausyndrome	Trisomy 13 47,XX,+13	Most embryos with trisomy 13 do not survive gestation and are spontaneously aborted. Of those surviving to term gestation, approximately 82%–85% do not survive past 1 month of age, and 85% do not survive past 1 year of age [2]. Certain malformations, especially holoprosencephaly and other central nervous system malformations, yield a more grave prognosis. Of those infants that survive past 1 year, most have few major malformations, but the prognosis remains poor, owing to multiple factors, including long-term neurologic disability, feeding difficulty, and frequent pneumonia and other respiratory infections. Presently, there are reports of more than 70 children around the world living with Trisomy 13.
Turner syndrome	Monosomy X 46,X	Common symptoms of Turner syndrome include short stature, lymphoedema (swelling) of the hands and feet, broad chest (shield chest) and widely spaced nipples, low hairline, low-set ears, reproductive sterility, amenorrhea, increased weight (obesity), small fingernails, webbing of the neck, bicuspid aortic valve (increased risk for dissection), coarctation of the aorta, horseshoe kidney, visual impairments (glaucoma), ear infections, and hearing loss.
Klinefelter's syndrome	47,XXY	Development of small testicles and reduced fertility. Some degree of language learning impairment may be present, and neuropsychological testing often reveals deficits in executive functions. In adults, possible characteristics vary widely and include little to no signs of affectedness; a lanky, youthful build and facial appearance; or a rounded body type with some degree of gynecomastia (increased breast tissue). The more severe end of the spectrum of symptom expression is also associated with an increased risk of germ cell tumors, breast cancer, and osteoporosis.

(69 chromosomes). Chromosome translocations, deletions, and duplications represent another unbalanced chromosome anomaly despite retention of 46 chromosomes. Although certain "hot spots" exist for chromosome alteration, virtually any chromosome could be affected in any position.

Single Gene Disorders

Single gene (monogenic) disorders are caused by alterations (mutations) in one or both alleles of a gene, involving changes at the nucleotide level that disrupt the normal function of a single gene product. Approximately 14,000 single gene disorders have been classified to date, and this number is expected to increase over time as the human genome is explored further. Single gene mutations are classified into three basic categories: single nucleotide substitutions, deletions, and insertions. Single nucleotide substitutions, transitions, and transversions are the most common types of single gene mutation. Transitions are substitutions of a pyrimidine for pyrimidine ([C] or [T]) or purine for purine ([A] or [G]). Transversions are substitutions of a pyrimidine for a purine or vice versa. Further classification of a single nucleotide substitution can be made on the basis of how the nucleotide change affects the resulting protein structure. An exon (coding region) mutation that still specifies the same amino acid is considered a silent or synonymous mutation. A missense or nonsynonymous mutation alters the codon and leads to a single different amino acid. A nonsense mutation terminates further protein assembly by introducing a premature stop codon. Base substitutions occurring in an intron can also result in an altered gene product because the intron/exon boundaries play an important role in splicing mRNA from transcribed RNA (excision of intronic sequences). The functional consequence and clinical implications of single gene disorders may be extremely variable. Deletions are subtractions of nucleotides from the normal DNA sequence, and insertions are additions of nucleotides to the normal sequence. Both deletions and insertions may involve a single nucleotide or many nucleotides. Exonic deletions and insertions may alter the "reading frame" of RNA translation at the point of the deletion/insertion and give rise to a new sequence of amino acids in the finished product resulting in a frameshift mutation. In-frame deletions and insertions can occur when the number of nucleotides affected is a multiple of three. Not all nucleotide changes create a new gene product that causes or modifies a clinical disease state. A DNA sequence variation that may or may not alter the encoded protein is called a common polymorphism if present in at least 1% of the population. Variation that occurs in <1% of a population is considered a mutation. Although polymorphisms may not necessarily be pathogenic or disease causing, they can be functional and exert important effects by influencing responses to endogenous and exogenous stimuli.

Inheritance Patterns

Single gene disorders may be inherited in a simple Mendelian fashion with autosomal dominant, autosomal recessive, X-linked dominant, or X-linked recessive inheritance patterns. Examples of disorders with Mendelian inheritance are shown in Table 11.2. The inheritance pattern is based on which type of chromosome (autosome or sex) the altered gene loci is found and whether the phenotype is expressed only when both chromosomes of a pair carry the abnormal allele (recessive) or whether the phenotype can be expressed when just one chromosome carries the mutant allele (dominant). Typical features of an autosomal dominant inheritance pattern (Fig. 11.2) include multigenerational presence of symptoms (vertical transmission) and equal involvement of sexes. Only one copy of a gene pair needs to be altered for clinical symptoms (heterozygous). Dominant conditions are often caused by aberrant structural or developmental processes, and only a minority result from enzymatic defects. Autosomal recessive disorders require two altered gene copies (homozygous). Heterozygotes are unaffected, and the inheritance pattern shows equal involvement of both sexes, affected individuals in the same single generation, and absence of disease appearing in multiple generations (Fig. 11.3). Virtually all males with an X-linked recessive mutation are affected clinically, with rare symptomatic females (Fig. 11.4). All daughters of an affected male are carriers of the mutated allele, and the risk for any of the daughters' sons to inherit the gene responsible for the condition is 50%. X-linked dominant conditions affect both male and female heterozygotes (Fig. 11.5). Random X inactivation would result in less severely affected females, unless they are homozygous for the disease allele. In some X-linked dominant conditions, affected males are rarely seen because of a lethal effect of the mutant allele in the hemizygous male. X-linked dominant inheritance pattern features include multigenerational involvement, presence of symptoms in all daughters and none of the sons of an affected male, and equal involvement of both sexes when transmitted by females.

Single gene mutations may also demonstrate non-Mendelian inheritance patterns, including genomic imprinting, mosaicism, mitochondrial disorders, and triple repeat disorders. Differential expression of genes, depending on whether the mutant allele is of maternal or paternal origin, results from genomic imprinting. Normally, the fetus receives one maternal and one paternal chromosome for each chromosome pair. Two intact chromosomes from one parent is a meiosis error called uniparental disomy (UPD). When UPD for specific imprinted chromosome regions is present, clinical symptoms may manifest. The underlying mechanism of genomic imprinting is an alteration in chromatin affecting gene expression without changing its sequence. The gene is not necessarily mutated but reversibly inactivated, generally by a process of methylation. A classic example of genomic imprinting is Prader-Willi syndrome (hyperphagia, obesity, small hands and

TABLE 11.2

MENDELIAN DISORDERS

Disorder	Inheritance	Frequency	Ethnicity	Gene	Diagnosis	Genetic Testing
Polycystic Kidney Disease	AD	1/1,000	None	PCK1/PKD2 Chromosome 16/4	Renal Ultrasound	Linkage analysis DNA sequencing

Clinical Features

Most common hereditary renal disease. Represents 10% of all cases of renal failure that reach end-stage disease. There is wide phenotypic variability. From birth, thin-walled spherical cysts develop in the cortex and medulla of both kidneys. The cysts range from millimeters to centimeters in diameter and are usually visible on ultrasonography or CT by 25 years of age. Other cysts can be found in the liver, spleen, pancreas, and brain (arachnoid cysts), and occasionally, in the esophagus, ovaries, uterus, and seminal vesicles. Liver cysts are common, with a higher prevalence in women. Pregnancy is a risk factor for massive hepatic cystic involvement. Symptoms typically develop in the third to fourth decades, with flank pain and hematuria. Urinary tract infections are common and must be treated using lipophilic antibiotics (fluoroquinolones, sulfonamides) that penetrate the cysts. Other manifestations include nocturia, kidney stones, and hypertension. Left ventricular hypertrophy is a common early complication of adult polycystic kidney disease (PKD), with cardiovascular disease representing the leading cause of death. PKD is also associated with cardiac valve myxomatous degeneration, diverticulosis, and intracranial aneurysms. Subarachnoid hemorrhage from an intracranial aneurysm causes death or neurologic injury in approximately 10% of patients. Hematocrit may be increased secondary to elevated erythropoietin levels or decreased from excessive hematuria and blood loss.

Disorder	Inheritance	Frequency	Ethnicity	Gene	Diagnosis	Genetic Testing
Hereditary Hemochromatosis	AR	1/500	Northern European	HFE/SLC11A3 Chromosome 6	Liver biopsy/ Genetic testing	Mutation analysis

Clinical Features

Hereditary hemochromatosis (HHC) is a disorder of iron storage, whereby an inappropriate increase in intestinal iron absorption results in deposition of excessive quantities of iron in parenchymal cells, with eventual tissue damage and functional impairment. The most commonly affected organs include the liver, pancreas, heart, and pituitary gland. Clinical expression of HHC is modified by several factors, including blood loss in menstruating women. HHC is expressed five to ten times more frequently in men. Symptoms develop in most untreated patients between the fourth and sixth decades. HHC is rarely clinically evident before age 20 years. Early symptoms include weakness, weight loss, change in skin color, abdominal pain, loss of libido, and symptoms related to the onset of diabetes mellitus. More established disease presents with hepatomegaly, skin pigmentation, spider angiomas, palmar erythema, splenomegaly, ascites, loss of body hair, testicular atrophy, arthropathy, cardiac arrhythmias, congestive heart failure, and jaundice.

Disorder	Inheritance	Frequency	Ethnicity	Gene	Diagnosis	Genetic Testing
Sickle Cell Anemia	AR	1/500	African	HBB gene Chromosome 11	Hemoglobin Electrophoresis	Mutation analysis DNA sequencing

Clinical Features

The most common heritable hematologic disease affecting humans. Patients have an electrophoretically abnormal hemoglobin (HgbS) that differs from HgbA by substitution of valine for glutamic acid at the sixth position of the β chain. On deoxygenation, HgbS begins to polymerize and changes the red blood cell (RBC) from a biconcave disk to an elongated sickle shape. Patients with SSA have a selective advantage against *Plasmodium falciparum* malaria. The rate of polymerization depends on the concentration of HgbS and the extent of deoxygenation. The sickling may be irreversible if enough cell damage occurs. Fetal hemoglobin (HgbF) is protective against polymerization and varies in its distribution among RBCs in patients with SSA. Signs and symptoms of the disease do not usually appear until the sixth month of life, at which time most HgbF has been replaced by HgbS. The elongated sickle shape of RBCs is responsible for the vaso-occlusive phenomena seen in patients with SSA. Microinfarcts develop, leading to painful bone crises, and macroinfarcts cause chronic organ damage. SSA leads to impaired growth and development, and recurrent splenic infarction results in an increased susceptibility to serious infections, particularly pneumococcal infections. Patients with SSA typically have severe hemolytic anemia, with an RBC life span of only 2 weeks. Infection or folate deficiency may suppress erythropoiesis enough to cause aplastic crisis. Chronic anemia often causes congestive heart failure, and progressive renal insufficiency typically develops, with most patients suffering from hyposthenuria. Other clinical findings include chronic skin ulcers, retinal infarcts and ocular disease, seizures, neurologic thrombosis with an increased risk for subarachnoid hemorrhage, avascular necrosis of bone, and increased risk of gallstones. The most common cause of death in adult patients with SSA is from acute chest syndrome. In a multicenter study, 45% of all acute chest syndrome cases had an unknown etiology. Its cardinal features are fever, pleuritic chest pain, referred abdominal pain, cough, lung infiltrates, and hypoxia. Approximately 30% were due to infections with atypical organisms and 9% from fat embolism secondary to long-bone infarction.

Disorder	Inheritance	Frequency	Ethnicity	Gene	Diagnosis	Genetic Testing
Cystic Fibrosis	AR	1/2,500	Northern European	CFTR Chromosome 7	Clinical+ Sweat chloride/ Genetic testing	Mutation analysis DNA sequencing

Clinical Features

Cystic fibrosis (CF) is a monogenetic disorder with clinical manifestations due primarily to the dysfunction of exocrine glands, producing viscid dehydrated secretions. Approximately 3% to 4% of patients with CF are diagnosed as adults. This group usually presents with chronic respiratory problems, and in contrast to CF patients diagnosed as children, they have milder lung disease, less pseudomonal infection, and are more likely to be pancreatic sufficient. Clinically, CF is characterized by chronic airway infection leading to bronchiectasis and bronchiolectasis, exocrine pancreatic deficiency, abnormal sweat glands, and urogenital dysfunction. Patients typically have chronic sinusitis as children, with eventual lower respiratory tract involvement represented by cough. The cough is progressive and productive, *(continued)*

TABLE 11.2

MENDELIAN DISORDERS (*Continued*)

Disorder	Inheritance	Frequency	Ethnicity	Gene	Diagnosis	Genetic Testing

ultimately leading to frequent exacerbations with decrements in pulmonary function. Advanced lung disease ensues, leading to digital clubbing, respiratory failure, and cor pulmonale. Other respiratory complications include pneumothorax and hemoptysis, both of which are poor prognostic indicators. After multiple clinical exacerbations and antibiotic exposures, *Pseudomonas aeruginosa* becomes the predominant organism recovered from sputum. Almost 50% of patients have *Aspergillus fumigatus* in their sputum, with up to 10% exhibiting the syndrome of allergic bronchopulmonary aspergillosis. Infection with *Burkholderia cepacia* species is pathogenic and causes rapid clinical deterioration, often with fulminating pneumonia, bacteremia, and death (cepacia syndrome). More than 85% of patients with CF demonstrate some degree of exocrine pancreas deficiency, but most adults remain asymptomatic. Insufficient pancreatic enzyme release, however, yields the typical pattern of protein and fat malabsorption with frequent, bulky, and foul-smelling stools. Young adults may present with distal intestinal instruction, which may be confused with appendicitis. Late onset of puberty in CF is common in both sexes, with almost all men being azoospermic.

Marfan Syndrome	AD	1/10,000	None	FBN1 Chromosome 15	Clinical + Genetic testing	Linkage analysis Mutation analysis DNA sequencing

Clinical Features

Severe Marfan syndrome is characterized by a triad of features: (a) long, thin extremities frequently associated with other skeletal changes; (b) reduced vision as the result of dislocations of the lenses (ectopia lentis); and (c) aortic aneurysm that typically begins at the base of the aorta. Other skeletal abnormalities include severe chest deformities, scoliosis, kyphosis, and pes planus. Joint hypermobility may be seen, although not commonly. Cardiovascular abnormalities are the major source of morbidity and mortality. The rate of aortic dilatation is unpredictable, but dilatation can cause aortic regurgitation, dissection, and rupture. Dilatation is probably accelerated by physical and emotional stress, particularly pregnancy. Mitral valve prolapse is common and progresses to regurgitation in 25% of patients. Other clinical manifestations include spontaneous pneumothorax and inguinal and incisional hernias. Approximately 25% to 30% of patients do not have affected parents and most likely represent spontaneous mutations.

Fabry Disease	X-linked Recessive	Rare	None	α-Gal A gene X chromosome	Biochemical Testing	Mutation analysis DNA sequencing

Clinical Features

Fabry disease is a lysosomal storage disease resulting from a deficiency of α-galactosidase A. The inheritance pattern is X-linked recessive. Onset is usually in childhood or adolescence. Clinical signs include telangiectatic angiokeratomas of skin and mucous membranes; acroparesthesia; corneal opacities and cataracts; infiltrative cardiac disease with left ventricular hypertrophy, arrhythmias, and, occasionally, a short PR interval on ECG; and renal disease with hypertension. The most frequent cause of death is renal failure, followed by cardiac or cerebrovascular disease.

Neurofibromatosis	AD	1/4,000 (NF1) 1/40,000 (NF2)	None	Unknown Chromosome 17/22		

Clinical Features

Von Recklinghausen disease, or neurofibromatosis type 1 (NF1), is the first of two genetically distinct types of neurofibromatosis, both AD disorders. NF1 is associated with café-au-lait macules, axillary and inguinal freckling, Lisch nodules of the iris, neurofibromas, and, occasionally, pheochromocytomas and scoliosis. As many as 30% to 50% of patients do not have affected parents and most likely represent spontaneous mutations. Type 2 (NF2) is characterized by bilateral vestibular schwannomas with associated symptoms of tinnitus; hearing loss; and balance dysfunction, other nervous system gliomas, and cataracts.

Kartagener Syndrome	AR	Rare	None	DNAI1/DNAH5/DNAH11 Chromosome 5,7,9		

Clinical Features

Disorder of ciliary ultrastructure with absent or reduced ciliary motility. Patients have recurrent pneumonia, sinusitis, bronchitis, and bronchiectasis. Kartagener syndrome is clinically distinct from other ciliary dyskinesias by the presence of situs inversus and dextrocardia. Female patients are fertile. Male patients have immotile spermatozoa, and in the absence of micromanipulation, they are functionally infertile.

Gaucher Disease	AR	1/1,000	Ashkenazi Jews	β-glucocerebrosidase Chromosome 1		

Clinical Features

Lysosomal storage disorder caused by a deficiency of the enzyme β-glucocerebrosidase. Lipid storage is found in the spleen, liver, bone marrow, and other organs. Gaucher disease encompasses a continuum of clinical findings from a perinatal lethal form to an asymptomatic form or one that is initially diagnosed in the elderly. Five clinical subtypes have been identified. Type 1 is the most common and is characterized by the absence of central nervous system disease; it occurs most frequently in Ashkenazi Jews and responds well to enzyme replacement treatment. Hepatomegaly, splenomegaly, anemia, thrombocytopenia, and degenerative bone disease (osteopenia, focal or sclerotic lesions, osteonecrosis) may develop in untreated patients. Types 2 and 3 are characterized by the presence of primary neurologic disease, with expected life spans ranging from childhood to the third and fourth decades.

(continued)

TABLE 11.2

MENDELIAN DISORDERS (*Continued*)

Disorder	Inheritance	Frequency	Ethnicity	Gene	Diagnosis	Genetic Testing
von Hippel-Lindau Syndrome	AD	Rare	None	VHL gene Chromosome 3		

Clinical Features
Disorder characterized by retinal, spinal cord, and cerebellar hemangioblastomas; cysts of the kidneys, pancreas, and epididymis; pheochromocytoma and renal cell cancers; and endolymphatic sac tumors. Cerebellar hemangioblastomas may be associated with headache, vomiting, gait disturbances, or ataxia. Retinal hemangioblastomas may be the initial manifestation of von Hippel-Lindau syndrome and can cause vision loss. Renal cell carcinoma occurs in 40% of patients and is the most common cause of death. If renal cell carcinoma occurs, hematuria and anemia are typical, but erythrocytosis may be seen in up to 5% of patients. Endolymphatic sac tumors can cause hearing loss of varying severity, which can be a presenting symptom.

Disorder	Inheritance	Frequency	Ethnicity	Gene	Diagnosis	Genetic Testing
Osler-Weber-Rendu Disease	AD	1/50,000	None/Danish	Unknown Chromosome 9		

Clinical Features
Osler-Weber-Rendu disease, or hereditary hemorrhagic telangiectasia, is an autosomal dominant condition in which occult or overt gastrointestinal bleeding is often present. Telangiectases of the skin and mucous membranes are seen (recurrent epistaxis occurs in 50%–80%), and approximately 20% of patients have pulmonary arteriovenous malformations. Patients are also at risk for high-output cardiac failure, ischemic stroke, migraines, and paradoxical emboli. Less than 10% of patients die of complications of the disease.

Disorder	Inheritance	Frequency	Ethnicity	Gene	Diagnosis	Genetic Testing
Friedreich Ataxia	AR	1/50,000	None	FXN gene Chromosome 9		

Clinical Features
Disorder characterized by slowly progressive ataxia with onset usually before age 25 years, typically associated with depressed tendon reflexes, dysarthria, Babinski responses, loss of position and vibration senses, and cardiomyopathy. Approximately 25% of cases have an atypical presentation with later onset (after age 25 years), retained tendon reflexes, or unusually gradual progression of disease. Other clinical associations include diabetes mellitus (10%), optic atrophy (25%), dementia, and respiratory dysfunction due to kyphoscoliosis. Death is often related to cardiomyopathy and diabetes. The mean age of loss of ambulation is 25 years.

Disorder	Inheritance	Frequency	Ethnicity	Gene	Diagnosis	Genetic Testing
Fragile X	X-linked Dominant	1/400	None	FMR1		

Clinical Features
Leading hereditary cause of developmental and learning disabilities. Methylation of the FMR1 locus in chromosome band Xq27.3 is believed to result in constriction of the X chromosome, which appears "fragile" under the microscope at that point, a phenomenon that gives the syndrome its name. Characteristics of the syndrome include an elongated face, large or protruding ears, flat feet, larger testicles in men (macro-orchidism), and low muscle tone. Speech may include cluttered or nervous speech. Behavioral characteristics may include stereotypic movements (e.g., hand-flapping) and atypical social development, particularly shyness and limited eye contact. Some individuals with fragile X syndrome also meet the diagnostic criteria for autism. Most females experience symptoms to a lesser degree because of their second X chromosome; however, they can develop just as severe symptoms. Most boys have mental retardation, and one-half to two-thirds of girls have normal IQ or learning disabilities. Emotional and behavioral problems are common in both sexes.

Disorder	Inheritance	Frequency	Ethnicity	Gene	Diagnosis	Genetic Testing
Huntington's Disease	AD	1/30,000	Western European	Huntington gene Chromosome 4		

Clinical Features
Onset of symptoms is gradual; patients eventually exhibit jerky, random, and uncontrollable movements called chorea, although some exhibit very slow movement and stiffness (bradykinesia, dystonia). These abnormal movements are initially exhibited as general lack of coordination and an unsteady gait, and gradually increase as the disease progresses. This eventually causes problems with loss of facial expression (called "masks in movement") or exaggerated facial gestures; inability to walk, sit, or stand stably; problems with speech (slurring of words); and some uncontrollable movement of the lips and problems with chewing and swallowing (dysphagia), which commonly causes weight loss. In the later stages of the disease, speaking is impaired with slurred words and uncontrollable movements of the mouth; continence, eating, and mobility are extremely difficult, if not impossible. Selective cognitive abilities are also progressively impaired, including abstract thought and other executive functions. Psychopathological symptoms vary more than cognitive and physical symptoms, and include depression, impulsivity, egotism, and aggressive behavior.

Disorder	Inheritance	Frequency	Ethnicity	Gene	Diagnosis	Genetic Testing
Duchenne's/Becker's Muscular Dystrophy	X-linked Recessive	1/30,000 (B) 14,000 (D)	None	Dystrophin gene X-chromosome		

Clinical Features
Progressive skeletal weakness occurs, with the clinical diagnosis being supported by markedly increased creatine kinase levels. Duchenne's muscular dystrophy is rapidly progressive, with affected children being wheelchair bound by age 12 years. Cardiomyopathy occurs in all patients after age 18 years, and few survive beyond the third decade. Becker's muscular dystrophy has later-onset muscular weakness, with patients remaining ambulatory into their 20s. Despite the milder skeletal muscle involvement, heart failure from dilated cardiomyopathy is a common cause of morbidity and the most common cause of death. Mean age of death for Becker's muscular dystrophy is in the fifth decade, but some patients will survive beyond the sixth or seventh decade.

(continued)

Disorder	Inheritance	Frequency	Ethnicity	Gene	Diagnosis	Genetic Testing
Charcot-Marie-Tooth Disease	AD	1/3,000	None Chromosome 1	MFN2		

TABLE 11.2

MENDELIAN DISORDERS (Continued)

Clinical Features
Charcot-Marie-Tooth (CMT) disease is a hereditary neuropathy categorized by mode of inheritance and causative gene or chromosomal locus. CMT disease is the most common genetic cause of neuropathy and is characterized by chronic motor and sensory nerve symptoms. The typical patient has distal muscle weakness and atrophy often associated with mild to moderate sensory loss, depressed tendon reflexes, and high-arched feet. CMT disease is genetically heterogeneous and may be inherited through autosomal dominant, autosomal recessive, and X-linked patterns. CMT1 is autosomal dominant, represents the most common of the subtypes, and is associated with hearing loss.

AD, autosomal dominant; AR, autosomal recessive; CT, computed tomography; ECG, electrocardiogram; SSA, sickle cell anemia.

feet, short stature, and variable mental retardation); 70% of cases are caused by a deletion on an allele on chromosome 15 inherited from the father.

Mosaicism is the presence of at least two cell lines within an individual or a specific tissue that differ genetically but are derived from a single fertilized egg. In other words, a person may have some of the cells in their body with 46 chromosomes, whereas other cells in their body have 47, XY+21 chromosomes. This is an example of chromosomal mosaicism (mosaic Down syndrome). The clinical consequences of single gene mosaicism depend on the type of the mutation and the extent of tissue involvement. Either somatic or germline mosaicism for single gene mutations may be the underlying etiology in families with unusual clinical pictures and/or pedigrees.

Mitochondrial disorders are clinically heterogenous and associated with mutations of either nuclear DNA or mitochondrial DNA. Nuclear gene defects are primarily inherited in an autosomal recessive manner. However, in contrast to chromosomes in the nuclear genome, there is no tightly controlled segregation of the mitochondrial DNA. At cell division, the mitochondrial DNA replicates and sorts randomly among mitochondria, which are also distributed randomly among the two resultant daughter cells.

Therefore, parent point mutations in mitochondrial DNA are variably transmitted to children, which may lead to pronounced intrafamilial phenotypic variability. The percentage of altered mitochondrial DNA may influence the variability of the condition expressed. Ultimately, the recurrence risk for offspring is difficult to predict in mitochondrial disorders.

Triple repeat disorders are the most common group of diseases that are caused by unstable dynamic mutations in a gene. In these disorders, a segment of DNA containing a repeat of three nucleotides increases in number when passed from generation to generation, undergoing expansion. Once a critical degree of expansion occurs, a change in gene expression and function ensues leading to a disease phenotype. Examples of this include fragile X syndrome, Friedreich ataxia, and Huntington disease.

Multifactorial Disorders

Many genetic disorders appear familial but do not follow a single gene pattern of inheritance. These disorders are the result of a combination of alterations in multiple genes with varying degrees of effect working together with environmental factors. The genetic heterogeneity seen in

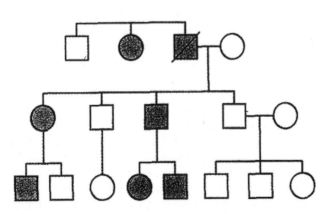

Figure 11.2   Autosomal dominant inheritance pattern.

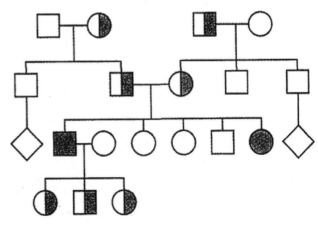

Figure 11.3   Autosomal recessive inheritance pattern.

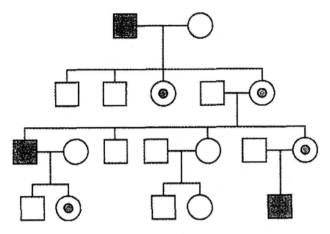

Figure 11.4 X-linked recessive inheritance pattern.

complex disorders may result from different mutations at the same gene locus or as a result of mutations at different loci or both.

DIAGNOSIS OF GENETIC DISEASE

With our increased understanding of the hereditary basis of common adult conditions, genetic disorders may be suspected by clinical presentation (e.g., idiopathic venous thromboembolism and factor V Leiden) or a routine physical examination that demonstrates dysmorphic features. All patients with a suspected genetic disorder should undergo a comprehensive history, including a family history with detailed information on relatives' ages, current and past medical health, and birth defects. Specific questions regarding miscarriage, stillbirth, infant deaths, and infertility should be sought. Racial and ethnic background is of importance in identifying higher-risk groups. The possibility of consanguinity in the family history should be explored when clinically relevant. Drawing a family pedigree that symbolically represents the family and demon-

strates relationships between affected family members is helpful.

Genetic Testing

Genetic testing refers to cytogenetic, molecular genetic, and biochemical analyses. The process of considering, ordering, and interpreting a genetic test is not straightforward. Genetic tests for a variety of disorders may use different methodologies, may have different detection rates, and are often used differently in various situations. Genetic tests typically have less than a 100% detection rate, and some genetic conditions include genetic heterogeneity. Genetic tests are often most informative if a clinically affected family member is tested first to determine whether a specific genetic test is informative within a family before using the test to predict genetic status for a clinically unaffected family member. The presence of a certain genotype does not always result in a specific phenotype but instead predicts risk for a phenotype. Some gene mutations have different effects on phenotype, depending on the presence or absence of certain genetic backgrounds and/or modifier genes. A specific mutation may have no effect with some genetic backgrounds but a severe effect with others. Many genetic variants will have uncertain clinical significance.

Cytogenetics

Clinical cytogenetic testing primarily includes chromosome analysis. Condensed chromosomes can be visualized by light microscopy as cells enter the metaphase of division. With staining methods, chromosomes are divided into individual bands, each with a characteristic location, size, and staining intensity. G-banding (treating with trypsin and staining with Giemsa solution) is the most common chromosome staining procedure. With high-resolution banding methods, chromosomes of early metaphase and late prophase have more than 850 bands per haploid set of chromosomes. This allows for more precise localization of genes and detection of subtle chromosome anomalies. A karyotype is an individual's or cell's chromosomal constitution (number, size, morphology) determined by examination of chromosomes with light microscopy and use of stains. An additional technique to visualize chromosomes includes fluorescence in situ hybridization (FISH). Radioactive (fluor-colored) DNA probes for highly repetitive sequences are used to bath metaphase or interphase cells that have had their genomic DNA denatured by using heat and formamide. Probe DNA anneals with complementary DNA sequences in the chromosome, and the fluorescent signal is observed with a fluorescence microscope. FISH probes are generally classified by where they hybridize in the genome or by the type of chromosome anomaly they detect. Many microdeletion and microduplication syndromes of individual genes (see Single Gene Disorders section) have been identified with FISH probes (Fig. 11.6).

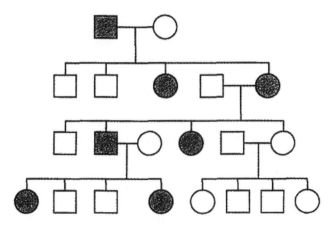

Figure 11.5 X-linked dominant inheritance pattern.

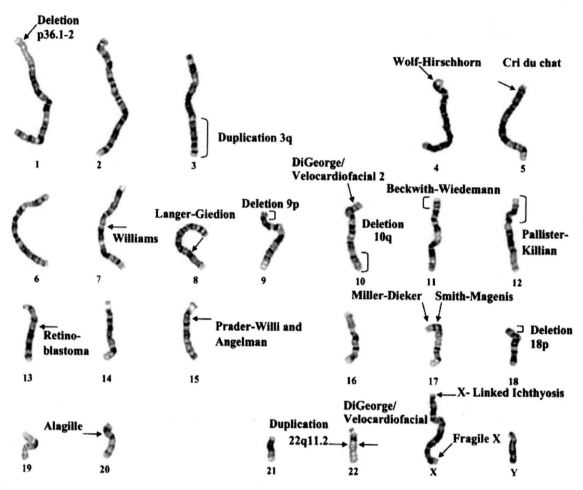

Figure 11.6   Haploid karyotype indicating the loci of selected congenital cytogenetic disorders. *Source:* Reprinted from Spurbeck. *Mayo Clin Proc* 2004;79(1):58–75.

Molecular Genetic Testing

DNA testing investigates alterations in a gene that is believed to result in disease. The finding of a disease-causing mutation may confirm the suspected clinical diagnosis, identify a disease carrier, or show a pronounced genetic predisposition to disease. There are several techniques available to identify genetic mutations, including polymerase chain reaction (PCR), southern blot analysis, restriction enzyme analysis, sequencing, and linkage analysis. Most molecular genetic tests are labor intensive and time consuming. Depending on the rarity of the disease, results might become available after a few weeks to months.

PCR is a technique of in vitro cloning or replicating relatively small DNA sequences into millions of copies over a short period. One has to know the nucleotide sequence of the DNA fragment of interest (target) to use PCR technology. Single-strand PCR is often used in embryo preimplantation diagnosis of genetic disease. For adults, PCR assays can be performed directly on genomic DNA samples to detect clinical disorders (e.g., leukemia, lymphomas) that involve translocation-specific malignant cells with very high sensitivity. In southern blotting, DNA is cut into pieces using restriction endonucleases (enzymes that digest DNA at specific sites that are marked by a four- to eight-member specific nucleotide sequence), and then the restriction fragments are subjected to agarose gel electrophoresis (DNA separation by size and topology). A DNA sequence of interest is then visualized by a radiolabeled reporter probe after a hybridization step followed by autoradiography. In addition to target identification and quantification, southern blotting may allow detection of mutations that result in alterations of restriction fragment lengths (e.g., restriction fragment length polymorphisms). Linkage analysis is a form of indirect DNA testing used when only the location of a gene is known but not the gene itself or when currently available direct gene testing has been unable to detect a mutation, although the gene location has been identified. Linkage testing investigates polymorphism around or within a gene and their transmission through the family, thereby identifying with a high degree of certainty who has and who has not inherited the "disease allele." Linkage analysis is most informative for patients and families who have a highly affected family (multigenerational involvement) with multiple relatives available to test.

Biochemical and protein testing refers to analyses of affected proteins or metabolites that are either the substrates or the products of a deficient enzyme. If abnormal metabolites are identified, the disease may then be confirmed by enzyme analysis when available.

GENETIC COUNSELING

Genetic counseling is a communication process that deals with human problems associated with the occurrence or risk of occurrence of a genetic disorder in a family. Testing results are explained completely, and education is provided about the particular genetic disease and its implications. Assessment of risk for the patient and family members, including reproductive implications and risk for offspring is discussed. The psychosocial implications of the diagnostic evaluation and risk assessment are also explored with the patient and family.

REVIEW EXERCISES

QUESTIONS

1. A 44-year-old man reports intermittent gross hematuria. He is very concerned about his health following the recent death of his younger brother from a subarachnoid hemorrhage. Family history is remarkable for kidney disease. On examination, he is hypertensive with a mitral regurgitation murmur. No rash or skin lesions are found. Urinalysis shows more than 25 red blood cells but no white blood cells, casts, protein, or stones. Blood urea nitrogen is 31 mg/dL, and creatinine is 2 mg/dL. Of the following tests, which is most likely to be helpful in diagnosis?
a) 24-Hour urine collection for protein
b) Plasma immunoglobulin A levels
c) Renal ultrasound
d) Total and C3 complement levels
e) Renal biopsy

Answer and Discussion

The answer is c. This patient has adult polycystic kidney disease (PKD). In PKD, thin-walled spherical cysts develop in the cortex and medulla of both kidneys from birth. The cysts range from millimeters to centimeters in diameter and are usually visible on ultrasonography or CT by 25 years of age. Renal ultrasound is the diagnostic method of choice for screening individuals at risk. Sensitivity is >85% in those from 20 to 30 years of age. Although proteinuria is common in PKD, it rarely exceeds 2 g/day. Immunoglobulin A nephropathy may present with hematuria but is usually associated with erythrocyte casts and glomerulonephritis. Complement levels are normal in PKD and have no role in the diagnosis of this disorder. Renal biopsy is not necessary for the diagnosis.

2. A 56-year-old white man with a history of pseudogout and diabetes mellitus type II complains of fatigue and weight loss. His family history is significant for diabetes, liver cancer, and arthritis. On examination, a mildly enlarged liver is noted, together with palmar erythema and bilateral knee effusions. Blood chemistry reveals mildly elevated alanine transaminase and aspartate transaminase values; total bilirubin is 2.0 mg/dL, international normalized ratio is 1.95, and ferritin is 2,500 ng/mL (normal, 10–200 ng/mL). The treatment most likely to decrease this patient's risk for hepatocellular carcinoma is which of the following?
a) Ursodeoxycholic acid (ursodiol)
b) Repeated phlebotomy
c) Penicillamine
d) Deferoxamine
e) None of the above

Answer and Discussion

The answer is e. This case illustrates the clinical presentation of symptomatic hereditary hemochromatosis (HHC), one of the most common autosomal recessive disorders. HHC is a disorder of iron storage, whereby an inappropriate increase in intestinal iron absorption results in deposition of excessive quantities of iron in parenchymal cells, with eventual tissue damage and functional impairment. The liver is usually the first affected organ. Hepatomegaly develops and, when hepatic iron concentration reaches a threshold of 400 μmol/g dry weight, cirrhosis is common. The iron threshold is lower in patients with other risk factors for liver diseases, such as heavy alcohol consumption or chronic hepatitis. Splenomegaly develops in 50% of symptomatic patients. Manifestations of portal hypertension and esophageal varices occur less commonly than in alcoholic cirrhosis. Hepatocellular carcinoma develops in 30% of those with cirrhosis and is the most common cause of death among treated patients. Clinical HHC is only present in the setting of iron overload. The serum ferritin level defines the point at which hemochromatosis is expressing iron overload and treatment should be initiated. Treatment involves removal of mobilizable iron stores. Weekly phlebotomy is usually required for 2 to 3 years. When the transferrin saturation and ferritin level become normal, phlebotomy is performed at the time intervals required to maintain levels in the normal range. Chelating agents, such as deferoxamine, are more expensive and less effective than phlebotomy, but may play a role in HHC when anemia or hypoproteinemia are severe enough to preclude further blood removal. When treatment is initiated before the development of hepatic cirrhosis or diabetes, patients with HHC appear to have a normal life expectancy. In the case example, elevations in INR, bilirubin, and transaminases suggest that liver damage and cirrhosis have already occurred. Once hepatic cirrhosis develops, no treatment is available to alter the risk of hepatocellular carcinoma.

3. A 19-year-old African American man presents to the emergency department with severe abdominal pain and jaundice. His past medical history is unremarkable, although his mother reports "growing pains" as a child. Further questioning reveals that the patient is adopted. He is febrile and tachycardic. The abdomen is diffusely tender. No rebound is present, and bowel sounds are present throughout. A small skin ulcer is noted on his left lower extremity. Complete blood cell count shows white blood cells at 17 K/μL, hemoglobin at 6.3 g/dL, and mean corpuscular volume at 89 μm^3. Aspartate transaminase and alanine transaminase values are normal. Indirect bilirubin is 3.6 mg/dL. A peripheral smear was performed and displays crescent-shaped RBCs. Which of the following statements regarding this patient's condition is true?

a) Sepsis is the most common cause of death in adults.
b) In the United States, few patients survive beyond the fifth decade.
c) A selective advantage against *Plasmodium vivax* malaria is present.
d) Transmission is autosomal dominant with variable penetrance.
e) Symptoms do not develop until the patient is older than 6 months.

Answer and Discussion

The answer is e. This patient has sickle cell anemia (SSA), the most common heritable hematologic disease affecting humans. Inheritance is autosomal recessive, and among African American adults, SSA has a prevalence of 1 in 500, with 10% being carriers of the sickle trait. Patients have an electrophoretically abnormal hemoglobin (HgbS) that differs from HgbA by substitution of valine for glutamic acid at the sixth position of the β chain. On deoxygenation, HgbS begins to polymerize and changes the RBC from a biconcave disk to an elongated sickle shape. Patients with SSA have a selective advantage against *Plasmodium falciparum* malaria, with preferential sickling of parasitized cells. The rate of polymerization depends on the concentration of HgbS and the extent of deoxygenation. The sickling may be irreversible if enough cell damage occurs. Fetal hemoglobin (HgbF) is protective against polymerization and varies in its distribution among red blood cells in patients with SSA. Signs and symptoms of the disease do not usually appear until the sixth month of life, at which time most HgbF has been replaced by HgbS. The most common cause of death in adult patients with SSA is from acute chest syndrome. Worldwide, approximately 120,000 babies with SSA are born each year, but <2% survive to the age of 5 years. In the United States and other developed countries, SSA patients often survive into their fifth or sixth decade.

4. A thin, 21-year-old white woman presents to the emergency department with acute-onset shortness of breath. Examination is consistent with pneumothorax. Chest radiography confirms this finding, along with evidence of mild hyperinflation and ring shadows in the upper lobes. She states that she was adopted and grew up in foster homes, noting that she was a "sickly" child with many episodes of sinusitis and bronchitis, and that lately she cannot get rid of a productive cough. Genetic testing reveals a mutation in the *CFTR* gene on chromosome 7. Which of the following statements regarding this patient's condition is false?

a) Adults make up approximately 40% of patients with this disease.
b) Pneumothorax and female sex are poor prognostic indicators.
c) *Pseudomonas aeruginosa* is associated with rapid deterioration in lung function.
d) Two-year survival for lung transplantation patients exceeds 50%.
e) Allergic bronchopulmonary aspergillosis has been noted in 10% of patients.

Answer and Discussion

The answer is c. This patient has cystic fibrosis (CF). In white populations, CF, which occurs in approximately 1 in 2,500 live births, is the most common lethal autosomal recessive genetic disorder, with a carrier frequency of 1 in 25 persons. During the past three decades, however, the number of adults with CF has increased dramatically, attributable in large part to a significant improvement in survival. For patients born in the 1990s, the median survival is now predicted to be longer than 40 years. More than one-third of the patients in the Cystic Fibrosis Foundation Registry are now older than 30 years. CF is a monogenetic disorder caused by mutation in the CF transmembrane conductance regulator (*CFTR*) gene on chromosome 7. The clinical manifestations are due primarily to the dysfunction of exocrine glands, producing viscid dehydrated secretions. Clinically, CF is characterized by chronic airway infection leading to bronchiectasis and bronchiolectasis, exocrine pancreatic deficiency, abnormal sweat glands, and urogenital dysfunction. Patients with CF exhibit characteristic sputum microbiology, with *Haemophilus influenzae* and *Staphylococcus aureus* often being the first organisms recovered from lung samples in patients newly diagnosed with CF. After multiple clinical exacerbations and antibiotic exposures, *P. aeruginosa* becomes the predominant organism recovered. Almost 50% of patients have *Aspergillus fumigatus* in their sputum, with up to 10% exhibiting the syndrome of allergic bronchopulmonary aspergillosis. Infection with *Burkholderia cepacia* species is pathogenic and causes rapid clinical deterioration, often with fulminating pneumonia, bacteremia, and death (cepacia syndrome). Female sex and pneumothorax are poor prognostic indicators in CF.

5. A 43-year-old man undergoes a preoperative evaluation for inguinal hernia repair. He is a tall, thin man without previous medical problems. Examination reveals normal vital signs, pectus excavatum, mild kyphoscoliosis, and a mitral regurgitation murmur. Subsequent echocardiography demonstrates normal left ventricular function, 2+ mitral regurgitation, and mild ascending aortic aneurysm. Further workup reveals a negative urine cyanide-nitroprusside test result and a slit-lamp examination consistent with ectopia lentis. Which of the following is the most likely diagnosis?

a) Ehlers-Danlos syndrome type IV
b) Homocystinuria
c) Marfan syndrome
d) Familial aortic aneurysm
e) Ehlers-Danlos syndrome type VI

Answer and Discussion
The answer is c. This case illustrates the clinical presentation of Marfan syndrome. Marfan syndrome is inherited as an autosomal dominant disorder with a wide phenotypic range both within affected families and between families. Severe Marfan syndrome is characterized by a triad of features: (a) long, thin extremities frequently associated with other skeletal changes; (b) reduced vision as the result of dislocations of the lenses (ectopia lentis); and (c) aortic aneurysm that typically begins at the base of the aorta. Other skeletal abnormalities include severe chest deformities, scoliosis, kyphosis, and pes planus. Joint hypermobility may be seen, although not commonly. Other clinical manifestations include spontaneous pneumothorax and inguinal and incisional hernias. Marfan syndrome shares clinical characteristics with other syndromes, and in the absence of classic features, diagnosis may be difficult. Patients with homocystinuria may have tall stature, pectus deformities, scoliosis, pes planus, and progressive lens dislocation. Homocystinuria may be detected by a positive urinary nitroprusside test result or elevated urinary homocystine by amino acid chromatography. Ehlers-Danlos syndrome type IV (vascular type) presents with aortic aneurysms and rupture, joint hypermobility, mitral valve prolapse, and spontaneous pneumothorax. Ehlers-Danlos syndrome type VI (ocular type) may exhibit characteristics similar to those of type IV, with the addition of retinal detachment and ocular symptoms. Ectopia lentis is not a feature of Ehlers-Danlos syndrome.

SUGGESTED READINGS

Claster S, Vichinsky EP. Managing sickle cell disease. *BMJ* 2003;327:1151–1155.

Ensenauer RE, Michels VV, Reinke SS, et al. Genetic testing: practical, ethical, and counseling considerations. *Mayo Clinic Proc* 2005;80(1):63–73.

GeneClinics Web site: www.geneclinics.org.

McCarthy GM, McCarthy CJ, Kenny D, et al. Hereditary hemochromatosis: a common, often unrecognized genetic disease. *Clev Clin J Med* 2002;69:224–242.

OMIM (Online Mendelian Inheritance in Man): www.ncbi.nlm.nih.gov/Omim.

Pietrangelo A. Hemachromatosis. *Gut* 2003;52(Suppl):23–30.

Steinberg MH. Drug therapy: management of sickle cell disease. *N Engl J Med* 1999;340:1021–1030.

Tefferi A, Wieben E, Dewald G, et al. Primer on medical genomics: part II: background principles and methods in molecular genetics. *Mayo Clinic Proc* 2002;77(8):785–808.

Wilson PD. Mechanisms of disease: polycystic kidney disease. *N Engl J Med* 2004;350:151–164.

Yankaskas JR, Marshall, BC, Sufian BJD, et al. Cystic fibrosis adult care: consensus conference statement. *Chest* 2004;125(Suppl):1S–39S.

Chapter 12

Neurology

Joyce K. Lee   Charles J. Bae

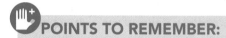

POINTS TO REMEMBER:

- Tension-type headaches or muscle contraction headaches are the most common type of primary headache.

- Centrally acting anticholinesterase drugs are indicated for use in mild to moderate Alzheimer's disease.

- Based on the results of the diagnostic studies and the time window, the stroke patient may be a candidate for intravenous or intra-aortic thrombolytic therapy.

- Antiplatelet therapy is a mainstay of treatment for stroke unless a high-risk condition such as atrial fibrillation is present.

- A resting tremor that is relieved by action is most likely due to Parkinson's disease.

Neurology is an enormous field that contains its own core information and, in addition, borders on a number of other fields of medicine, including internal medicine, pediatrics, neurosurgery, neuroimaging, neurophysiology, psychiatry, geriatrics, and neuropathology. This chapter focuses on the major areas within clinical neurology.

DISORDERS OF CONSCIOUSNESS

Consciousness is difficult to define, but in neurologic terms it consists of two components: arousal (wakefulness) and awareness. Each component has a separate functional neuroanatomical basis. Arousal is predominantly a function of the ascending reticular activating system (ARAS). ARAS cell bodies are located in the pons and midbrain, and have projections to the thalamus and hypothalamus. Awareness is a direct function of the cerebral hemispheres, which receive input from the thalamus, hypothalamus, and brainstem. Disorders of consciousness can occur when three specific anatomical areas are damaged: the reticular formation (upper midbrain), bilateral diencephalon (thalamus,) and bilateral cerebral hemispheres.

Disorders of consciousness are divided into two categories: those caused by an abnormality in arousal and those attributable to a loss of awareness. Disorders of arousal lie on a spectrum that ranges from alertness to deep coma. Four degrees of disordered arousal are described for clinical utility: confusion, drowsiness, stupor, and coma. Refer to Table 12.1a for a description of these disorders. Disorders of awareness refer to states during which there is an abnormal interaction with the environment when the patient is apparently awake. Refer to Table 12.1b for a description of these disorders.

The examination of a patient with disorder of consciousness must include a thorough general medical examination and complete neurologic examination. As with all medical emergencies, the ABCs (airway, breathing, circulation) should be assessed. Endotracheal intubation, mechanical ventilation, or pressure support may be required. The head should be inspected for any signs of trauma. Periorbital ecchymoses ("raccoon eyes"), ecchymoses behind the ear ("Battle's sign"), and cerebrospinal rhinorrhea or otorrhea are signs of a basilar skull fracture. Examination of the optic discs with an ophthalmoscope may demonstrate papilledema due to increased intracranial pressure or subhyaloid hemorrhages in the setting of a subarachnoid hemorrhage. Abnormal breathing patterns such as central neurogenic hyperventilation, apneustic breathing, or ataxic breathing indicate brainstem dysfunction.

The neurologic examination is critical and should be used to help localize the problem to cerebral hemispheric dysfunction versus brainstem pathology. The initial state of responsiveness can be estimated by observing responses to verbal stimuli or noxious stimuli if needed. Examining the pupils for size, reactivity to light, and symmetry is imperative. Pupils that are normal (3–5 mm in diameter), reactive to light, and symmetric suggest bihemispheric disease. Pupils that are very large or very small in diameter, not reactive to light, and asymmetric indicate brainstem disease. A unilateral enlarged, nonreactive pupil (>5 mm diameter) is a localizing sign for

TABLE 12.1a

DISORDERS OF AROUSAL

Disorder	Description	Associated Findings
Confusion or delirium	Inability to maintain a coherent stream of thought or action due to a diffuse abnormality of the nervous system caused by metabolic or toxic encephalopathy. Other causes include sedative drug withdrawal, alcohol withdrawal, high fever, and use of stimulant medications	Eyes open but unable to perform tasks that require attention (i.e., serial 7s, digit span) Hyperactivity of the sympathetic nervous system (dilated pupils, diaphoretic, tachycardic, tremulous)
Drowsiness	State of apparent sleep	Overcome by simple verbal command or physical stimulus
Stupor	State of deeper sleep	Overcome by noxious stimulus
Coma	State of unresponsiveness to the external environment	Not overcome by noxious stimulus

brainstem herniation and requires immediate neurosurgical consultation.

Eye movements are tested by observing spontaneous eye movements and by testing the oculocephalic reflex (OCR) or the vestibulo-ocular reflex (VOR). If the eyes are moving, the portion of the brainstem (from the vestibular nuclei in the upper medulla/lower pons to the oculomotor nucleus in the midbrain) that controls eye movements is intact. Eyes that are fixed or dysconjugate indicate brainstem pathology. Eyes that spontaneously move back and forth ("roving") suggest bihemispheric disease. Conjugate deviation of the eyes away from the paralyzed or paretic side can be seen with large hemispheric lesions. The converse is seen with seizures, which can cause a conjugate gaze deviation toward the convulsing side.

If the eyes are not moving spontaneously, the OCR can be tested with the "doll's-eyes maneuver." This maneuver is performed by quickly turning the head from side to side while observing the eye movements. In cases of cervical fractures or indeterminate OCR testing, the VOR should be tested with cold calorics. After making sure that the tympanic membrane is intact, 10 cc of ice water are infused into the external auditory canal, and the eye movements are observed over the next 30 to 60 seconds. In the normal person, the eyes will slowly move conjugately toward the side of the ice water infusion, followed by a fast, compensatory phase away from the irrigated ear. In the setting of coma due to bihemispheric disease, the fast "corrective phase" is absent, and the eyes remain deviated toward the side of the cold water infusion. In the setting of brainstem disease, there are no eye movements. In addition to these reflexes, special attention should be made to test the corneal reflex. An absent corneal reflex may be due to brainstem injury.

The first part of a motor examination consists of observing the patient, looking for purposeful or involuntary movements. Noxious stimulation of the stuporous or

TABLE 12.1b

DISORDERS OF AWARENESS

Disorder	Description	Associated Conditions
Abulia	State of reduced will or motivation	Bilateral prefrontal disease (i.e., dementia) Hydrocephalus Anterior cerebral artery Distribution strokes Frontal lobe malignancies Basal ganglia lesions Psychiatric illness
Catatonia	Condition marked by changes in muscle tone or activity, consisting of either a frozen, motionless state or a violent, excitable state	Neuroleptic malignant syndrome Head trauma Stroke Encephalitis Metabolic disorders Psychiatric illness
Conversion disorder	Condition in which one unconsciously converts psychological stress into physical manifestations	Psychological stress Psychiatric illness
Dissociative state	Hypnotic condition in which the patient dissociates various components of the personality	Psychological stress Psychiatric illness

comatose patient may result in movements that can indicate patterns of weakness such as hemiparesis, paraparesis, tetraparesis, or monoparesis. Spontaneous movements or normal withdrawal to noxious stimuli suggest an intact brainstem. Conversely, a lack of spontaneous movements, in addition to abnormal posturing of the extremities, suggests brainstem pathology. Lesions in the bilateral midbrain or pontine areas result in decerebrate posturing, characterized by opisthotonus and extension with internal rotation of all four extremities. Hemispheric disease or upper midbrain lesions (classically above the red nucleus) can result in decorticate posturing, characterized by extension with internal rotation of the lower extremities and flexion with adduction of the upper extremities.

Brain death is defined as the "irreversible cessation of all functions of the entire brain, including the brainstem." Refer to Table 12.2 for current brain death criteria guidelines.

The vegetative state is a state of complete unawareness of the self and environment despite preservation of some brain functions, often those involving brainstem centers for cardiovascular and autonomic control. A persistent vegetative state is present when the comatose state lasts for at least 1 month after initial injury, and a permanent vegetative state is present after 6 months of unresponsiveness with no signs of improvement. An algorithm for the management of an unconscious patient is shown in Figure 12.1.

TABLE 12.2
AMERICAN ACADEMY OF NEUROLOGY BRAIN DEATH CRITERIA

- Unresponsiveness
- Absent brainstem reflexes (e.g., pupillary, caloric, corneal, pharyngeal reflexes)
- Absence of effective respiratory movements in the presence of adequate oxygenation and arterial pCO_2 of 60 mm Hg
- Clinical or neuroradiologic evidence of an etiology adequate to explain the clinical findings
- Adequate observation period to guarantee irreversibility
- Exclusion of reversible factors that can confound assessment (drug intoxication or body core temperature <90°F)
- Use of serial exams or confirmatory tests (e.g., electroencephalogram, transcranial Doppler ultrasonography, somatosensory-evoked potentials)

HEADACHE

Headache is one of the most common complaints for which people seek medical attention. It is important to note that not all structures within the head are pain sensitive. Nociceptors are only present in the dura mater and closely related structures, in proximal portions of the cerebral arteries, and in the scalp and its vessels. The brain is therefore not pain sensitive. Headaches are caused by traction, displacement, inflammation, or distention of the

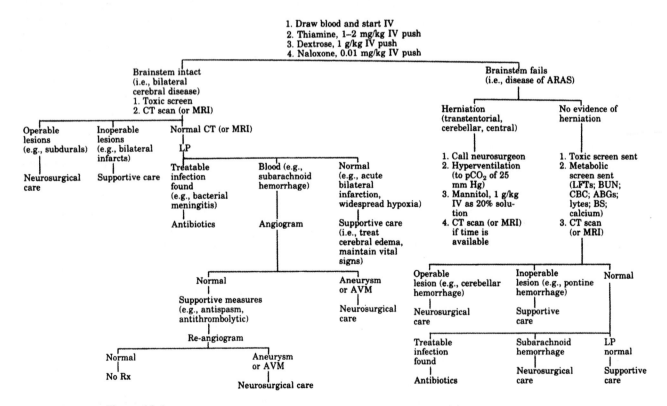

Figure 12.1 Diagnosis and treatment protocol in the comatose patient. ABGs, arterial blood gases; AVM, arteriovenous malformation; BS, blood sugar; LFT, liver function test; LP, lumbar puncture. *Source:* Reprinted with permission from Samuels MA, ed. *Manual of Neurologic Therapeutics*, 6th ed. Philadelphia: Lippincott Williams & Wilkins, 1999.

pain-sensitive structures within the head and neck. The trigeminal and cervical nerves are a common pathway for pain signals, and the impulses are carried to way stations in the brainstem known as the trigeminocervical complex.

Historically, three major theories exist for head pain. The vascular theory of head pain is based on the concept that the pain is related primarily to vasodilatation and the stimulation of nociceptive fibers by this process. Supporting this theory is the fact that serotonin receptors are known to exist on blood vessels, and medications that affect serotonin receptors, such as the triptans (5-hydroxytryptamine [5-HT1d] agonists), are known to improve head pain. An older theory that migraine is due to a biphasic phenomenon of vasoconstriction followed by vasodilatation is probably incorrect. The neurologic theory argues that head pain is an entirely neurologic phenomenon caused by abnormalities in the way the brain handles nociception. The effect of drugs that act on catecholamines (i.e., tricyclic antidepressants) in pain syndromes supports the neurologic theory of head pain. The current leading theory for the cause of head pain is the neurovascular theory, which provides a unifying hypothesis that some aspects of head pain are generated from peripheral mechanisms involving blood vessels, while other aspects are mediated by the central nervous system (CNS) processing of these signals. The neurovascular theory also argues that head pain may actually be related to neurogenic inflammation caused by the release of inflammatory substances from synaptic terminals into blood vessels and related tissues in the periphery.

Regardless of the cause, several major headache syndromes are recognizable clinically and can be managed by syndrome recognition. The 1988 International Headache Society (IHS) classification of headache system is almost universally accepted and has become the basis for headache classification in the International Classification of Diseases (ICD-10b). It is used to aid the physician in diagnosing and treating headaches appropriately.

Tension-type headaches (TTHs) are the most common type of primary headache. TTH is also known as muscle contraction headache or cervicogenic headache. Patients with TTH report having a constant pressurelike pain across the forehead as if it was being squeezed in a vise. The pain is typically bilateral and mild to moderate in severity. In contrast to migraines, the pain does not increase with exertion.

Migraine headaches are the second most common primary headache syndrome. There is often a positive family history, and women tend to have more migraines than men. Pertinent historical findings include colic in infancy, motion sickness in childhood, episodic abdominal pain in childhood, catamenial headaches at the time of menarche, and food-induced headaches, particularly for such foods as red wine, aged cheeses, peanuts, and chocolate. For migraine without aura, five attacks are needed, each lasting 4 to 72 hours and having two of the following four characteristics: unilateral location, pulsating quality, moderate to severe intensity, and aggravation by routine physical activity. In addition, the attacks must have at least one of the following: nausea (and/or vomiting,) photophobia, or phonophobia.

There are four phases of a migraine: prodrome, aura, headache and postdrome. The prodrome consists of premonitory phenomena occurring hours to days prior to headache onset and include mental and mood changes, stiff neck, fatigue, yawning, food cravings, fluid retention, and increase in urination. The aura is characterized by focal neurologic symptoms, usually lasting less than 60 minutes. Visual auras are the most common type (i.e., zigzag or scintillating figures, scotomata), followed by motor, sensory or brainstem disturbances. The headache phase is typically characterized by unilateral, throbbing pain, moderate to severe intensity, and aggravated by exertion. Other common features include nausea (occurs in 90% of patients), vomiting, sensory excitability (photophobia, phonophobia, osmophobia) and other systemic symptoms (i.e., anorexia, diarrhea, abdominal cramps, diaphoresis, lightheadedness, irritability). In the postdrome phase, the head pain wanes, and the patient often reports feeling tired, washed out, or depressed.

It is important to recognize comorbidities associated with migraines. These include psychiatric illnesses (anxiety, depression, mania), epilepsy, and stroke. The proportion of strokes attributed to migraine varies from 1% to 17% in clinical series and is believed to be related to vasospasm or hypercoagulable states. The prevalence of epilepsy in migraine patients is 5.9%, greatly exceeding the population prevalence of 0.5%.

Cluster headaches are the most severe type of primary headaches, but are relatively uncommon. Patients report having severe unilateral "ice pick" headaches that are maximal at onset and occur in clusters. The IHS classification for diagnosis requires that the patient have at least five attacks of severe, unilateral, orbital, supraorbital, and/or temporal pain that last 15 to 180 minutes and are associated with at least one of the following: ipsilateral lacrimation, conjunctival injection, rhinorrhea, nasal congestion, forehead and facial sweating, miosis, ptosis, or eyelid edema. Unlike migraine patients, these patients do not sit still; they pace the floor or even bang their heads against the wall to try to alleviate the pain. Cluster headaches are also much shorter in duration than migraines, with an average duration of 45 minutes to 1 hour. Men tend to have this type headache more than women, and there is a circadian pattern to the headaches.

Chronic daily headaches refer to headaches that occur more than 5 days a week. Most chronic daily headaches are related to analgesic withdrawal, also known as "rebound headaches." This syndrome is the final common pathway for any chronic headache problem that is characterized by excessive analgesic use.

Thunderclap headache refers to a headache that is maximal at onset. In such circumstances, a subarachnoid hemorrhage should be ruled out by using noncontrast CT, and a lumbar puncture if the CT scan is normal. Most thunderclap headaches are benign headaches seen in people with migraines.

Refer to Table 12.3 for an overview of the different types of headache syndromes.

Headaches in elderly persons can represent a special problem. If there is no prior history of headache, temporal arteritis, also termed giant cell arteritis, should be excluded. These patients typically complain of headaches involving the temples, profound scalp tenderness, jaw claudication while talking or eating, and visual disturbances. They may report systemic symptoms, such as fever, anorexia, and night sweats. If the syndrome is quite suggestive of temporal arteritis, these patients should be treated with steroids urgently to prevent vision loss. A temporal artery biopsy is the only way to definitively diagnose this condition. The American College of Rheumatology's criteria for diagnosing temporal arteritis include age older than 50 years, new-onset headache, abnormalities of the temporal arteries, erythrocyte sedimentation rate (ESR) >50 mm/hour, and positive temporal artery biopsy. The presence of three or more criteria has a sensitivity of 97% and specificity of 79%. An association has been recognized between temporal arteritis and polymyalgia rheumatica. It is considered standard of care to initiate treatment if there is a strong clinical suspicion for temporal arteritis, rather than delaying treatment while awaiting temporal biopsy results.

The treatment of the common primary headache disorders is based on a clear understanding of the anatomy and neuropharmacology of head pain. The goals of headache management are to relieve or prevent the pain and associated symptoms of the headache in order to restore the ability to function normally. The current view of managing migraines is to use abortive treatments unless the headaches are so frequent that they interfere with daily life, in which case prophylactic treatments can be used. Examples of acute migraine treatments include triptans (5-HT1d), analgesics, antiemetics, anxiolytics, anti-inflammatory drugs, and steroids. For refractory headaches, dihydroergotamine administered intravenously after an antiemetic usually provides excellent headache relief.

Preventive medications for migraines include antidepressants, anticonvulsants, beta-blockers, and calcium channel blockers. Among the beta-blockers, propranolol appears to be the most effective, probably because it penetrates the blood–brain barrier most effectively. Among the antiepileptic drugs, valproic acid is probably the most effective, but the side effects of hair loss and lack of safety in pregnancy make it difficult to use in the patient population that is more likely to have migraines—young women. Gabapentin is another useful anticonvulsant that is not metabolized by the liver and has a minimal side effect profile. Among the tricyclic antidepressants, amitriptyline has been shown to be most effective, but it also has the most side effects: dry mouth, constipation, blurred vision, and some degree of confusion and drowsiness. Botulinum toxin type A is a promising alternative therapy, but it is still undergoing clinical trials for efficacy.

Treating migraines during pregnancy is a particular problem. In general, no medication is completely safe for the fetus.

It is generally believed, however, that acetaminophen is relatively safe. Short courses of steroids can be used. Opiates are probably safe if given occasionally, and promethazine may also be useful for occasional use, when administered per rectum.

The treatment of acute cluster headache is 100% oxygen by face mask to abort the attacks. Prophylactic treatment involves the use of lithium carbonate or verapamil, a calcium channel blocker.

Hemicrania continua is responsive to indomethacin, which can be given per rectum to abort attacks and orally for prophylaxis. Calcium channel blockers, such as verapamil, sometimes work prophylactically.

TTH is generally treated using nonpharmacologic techniques such as exercise, biofeedback, and relaxation techniques. If possible, the underlying cause (i.e., depression, anxiety, neck pain) should be treated. Recently, clinicians have used the spasticity drug tizanidine (Zanaflex) for its muscle relaxant properties. Botulinum toxin injections of the frontalis muscle are also used for muscle contraction headaches.

Chronic daily headache is best avoided by not using analgesics more than 3 days a week, either prescription or over-the-counter analgesics. Treatment requires withdrawing the analgesics and often giving the patient steroids if necessary during this period.

DEMENTIA

Dementia is a group of disorders characterized by intellectual dysfunction. It is important when evaluating dementia to consider three major types of abnormalities in intellectual dysfunction. Dementia is a progressive loss of previously acquired intellectual ability. Mental retardation is a subnormal intellectual capacity. Pseudodementia consists of intellectual problems caused by disorders in affect, mood, or thought. When a patient, or more often a family member, complains of an abnormality in intellectual function, there are ten published warning signs to look for (American Academy of Neurology clinical practice guidelines). Refer to Table 12.4.

If the patient does have any of these symptoms, any one of a number of abbreviated screening examinations may be carried out, including the Folstein mini-mental status examination and the Solomon 7-minute mental status battery to assess the severity of the dementia. The neurologic examination itself involves a careful evaluation of

TABLE 12.3

OVERVIEW OF DIFFERENT TYPES OF HEADACHES

Headache Type	Typical Age of Onset (years)	Usual Location	Duration	Frequency/ Timing	Severity	Quality	Associated Features
Migraine	5–40	Hemicranial	Several hours to 3 days	Variable	Moderate to severe	Throbbing	Nausea, vomiting, photo/phono/osmophobia, scotomata, neurologic deficits; F > M
Tension type	10–50	Bilateral	30 minutes to 7+ days	Dull ache, may wax/wane	Viselike, bandlike pressure	None
Cluster	15–40	Unilateral, peri/ retro-orbital	30–120 minutes	1–8 times per day, nocturnal attacks	Excruciating	Stabbing, piercing	Ipsilateral conjunctival injection, lacrimation, nasal congestion, rhinorrhea, miosis, facial sweating; M > F
Hemicrania continua	Any	Unilateral	Constant	Daily	Mild to moderate	Stabbing	Has a mixture of cluster and migrainous features, but distinguished based on good response to indomethacin; F > M
Mass lesion	Any	Any	Variable	Intermittent, nocturnal, upon awaking	Moderate	Dull steady, throbbing	Vomiting, nuchal rigidity, neurologic deficits, seizures
Subarachnoid hemorrhage	Adult	Global, occipitonuchal	Variable	N/A	Excruciating, "worst headache of my life"	Explosive	Nausea, vomiting, nuchal rigidity, loss of consciousness, neurologic deficits
Trigeminal neuralgia	50–70	Second to third > first division of CN V	Seconds, occur in volleys	Paroxysmal	Excruciating	Electric, shocklike	Facial triggers, spasms of muscles ipsilaterally (tics)
Giant cell arteritis	>55	Temporal	Intermittent, then continuous	Constant	Variable	Variable	Tender scalp arteries, jaw claudication, visual changes; associated with PMR
Pseudotumor cerebri	20–45, young obese females	Diffuse, usually nonspecific	Variable	Variable, increased with Valsalva maneuvers and postural changes	Moderate to severe	Variable	Nausea, visual blurriness, horizontal diplopia, pulsatile tinnitus; papilledema on funduscopic; persistent optic atrophy can lead to blindness

Adapted from Silberstein SD, Lipton RB, Goadsby PJ. *Headache in Clinical Practice*, 2nd ed. UK: Taylor & Francis, 2002.

149

TABLE 12.4

WARNING SIGNS OF DEMENTIA

- Memory loss that affects job skills
- Difficulty performing familiar tasks
- Problems with language
- Disorientation to time and place
- Poor or decreased judgment
- Problems with abstract thinking
- Misplacing things
- Changes in mood or behavior
- Changes in personality
- Loss of initiative

TABLE 12.5

CAUSES OF DEMENTIA

Primary Causes of Dementia
- Alzheimer's disease
- Vascular (multi-infarct) dementia
- Pick's disease (frontotemporal dementia)
- Lewy body disease
- Normal pressure hydrocephalus
- Huntington's disease
- Parkinson's disease
- Parkinsonian-plus syndromes (corticobasal ganglionic degeneration, progressive supranuclear palsy, multisystem atrophy)
- Multiple sclerosis
- Head injury

Secondary Causes of Dementia
- Medication effects (antidiarrheals, antiepileptics, antihistamines, lithium, tricyclics)
- Chronic alcohol or drug abuse and dependence
- Vitamin deficiency (vitamin E, B_{12}, folic acid, thiamine)
- Infections (HIV, syphilis, meningitis, encephalitis)
- Creutzfeldt-Jakob disease (prion disease)
- Metabolic disorders (cortisol derangements, diabetes, calcium and sodium imbalance, kidney and liver failure, thyroid disease)
- Pseudodementia (depression)
- Brain tumors

the mental status by testing four major spheres of mental functioning: level of consciousness, memory, language, and visual-spatial skills. The level of consciousness is tested using specific tests of attention, such as the digit span test or serial 7s. If the patient is confused or delirious, a careful search should be done for a metabolic or toxic cause or a right hemisphere problem, such as a stroke or tumor. Short-term memory can be tested by discussing current events of which the patient should have some knowledge, including questions relating to current events, sports, hobbies, politics, and music. Long-term memory is quite difficult to test in the office and is best relegated to a formal neuropsychological evaluation, if necessary. Language is assessed by analyzing fluency, comprehension, and repetition. Visual-spatial skills are evaluated by having the patient write his or her name and address and a sentence, followed by a large rendition of a clock face with the hands put on the clock at an arbitrary location. This four-part mental status examination should be kept in the record for future reference. The rest of the neurologic examination is done with the aim of uncovering visual field defects, weakness, sensory loss, or incoordination.

The diagnostic evaluation for a demented patient will vary, depending on the history and physical examination findings, but some form of brain imaging, preferably MRI, should be considered at some point in the course of the evaluation. Ancillary testing, depending on the history, would include metabolic and toxic screens (basic metabolic profile, liver function tests, complete blood count [CBC]); serological test for syphilis and HIV; thyroid function tests; vitamin B_{12} and folate level tests; homocysteine and methylmalonic acid level tests; an electroencephalogram (EEG) to assess brain wave activity; a lumbar puncture for measurements of pressure, cellularity, opportunistic infection, and the clinical response to lowering the spinal fluid pressure; and formal psychological tests performed by a neuropsychologist. Recently, genetic testing for dementia with Lewy bodies, Creutzfeldt-Jacob disease, and APOE genotyping for Alzheimer's disease (AD) has become more widely available and is considered to be part of the routine evaluation of the demented patient.

Multiple causes of dementia, both primary and secondary, are listed in Table 12.5. Details about specific primary demential syndromes can be seen in Table 12.6a.

The most important dementing illness in terms of prevalence and conceptual importance is AD. AD is believed to be a cerebral amyloidosis caused by an accumulation of a neurotoxic amyloid β-protein (A-β), which is cleaved from a normally occurring amyloid precursor protein (APP) by a γ-secretase enzyme. The neurotoxicity may be mediated in part by an inflammatory reaction to the amyloid and preferentially may affect cholinergic systems that are important for memory. Oxidative stress and excitotoxicity may also contribute to neuronal death.

Many routes to this final common pathway exist; these include (a) having a third copy of chromosome 21 (Down syndrome) that contains the gene for APP, thus having 50% too much APP; (b) having a mutation in the genes that code for the γ-secretase enzyme, such as occurs in the two known presenilin mutations on chromosomes 1 and 14; (c) having an abnormal isotype of the transport protein apoprotein E (APO E4) coded on chromosome 19, which may lead to increased amounts of the neurotoxic form of A-β in neurons; and (d) having a reduced amount of estrogen (as in men and postmenopausal women), which normally partially protects neurons against the neurotoxic effects of A-β.

There is no cure for AD, but there have been many advances in the treatment of this disease. Many treatments involving centrally acting anticholinesterase drugs are indicated for use in mild to moderate AD. Donepezil (Aricept), rivastigmine (Exelon), and galantamine (Reminyl)

TABLE 12.6a

PROMINENT FEATURES OF DIFFERENT TYPES OF PRIMARY DEMENTIA SYNDROMES

Syndrome	Genes Implicated	Pathophysiology	Prominent Clinical Features
Alzheimer's disease	Chr 21 (amyloid precursor protein) Chr 14, 1 (presenilin 1,2) Chr 19 (APOE4)	Deposition of β-amyloid protein, neurofibrillary tangles and senile plaques, mainly in the cerebral cortex and hippocampus	Memory loss, disorientation, visuospatial problems, depression, anxiety, delusions
Pick's disease (frontotemporal dementia)	Chr 17	Deposition of tau (microtubule-associated protein) in the neurons and glia; atrophy of the frontal and anterior temporal lobes; presence of Pick cells on pathology	Apathy, disinhibition, anosognosia, echolalia; earlier onset and more prominent cognitive dysfunction at presentation than Alzheimer's
Dementia with Lewy bodies		Deposition of Lewy bodies (round, eosinophilic intracytoplasmic neuronal inclusions) in the cerebral cortex and brainstem; these contain α-synuclein and tau proteins	Cognitive decline without prominent early memory impairment (different from Alzheimer's), visual hallucinations, Parkinson features (rigidity, bradykinesia)
Huntington's disease	Chr 4 (Huntington gene)	Expanded CAG trinucleotide repeat coding	Dementia with chorea and dramatic personality changes

are available, and have been demonstrated to have a modest beneficial effect on the natural history of AD. Memantine (Namenda), an N-methyl-D-aspartate receptor antagonist, has recently been approved by the U.S. Food and Drug Administration (FDA) for use in patients with moderate to severe dementia. Gingko biloba, an over-the-counter complementary medication, may contain a weak anticholinesterase drug. Estrogen replacement therapy may also delay and/or slow the progression of the disease, as do nonsteroidal anti-inflammatory drugs (NSAIDs). Antioxidants such as vitamin E (1,000 IU PO BID) may also delay the onset or slow the progression of the disease in susceptible persons and is being clinically used in conjunction with the anticholinesterase therapies. Currently, most therapies involve the use of symptomatic therapy for behavioral problems, and include the use of benzodiazepines and phenothiazine drugs when necessary. γ-Secretase-inhibiting drugs and drugs that interfere with the amyloid fibril self-assembly are presently under development but are not currently available.

Vascular dementia refers to patients who become demented because of multiple cerebral infarcts or because of chronic cerebral ischemia causing white matter injury (Binswanger's disease). No specific treatment for the disorder is available, but stroke prevention and maintaining reasonable blood pressure goals throughout life may decrease the incidence. Hydrocephalus is divided into two types, noncommunicating and communicating, depending on whether the ventricles of the brain are openly communicating with each other. Most dementias caused by hydrocephalus are of the communicating type. Normal-pressure hydrocephalus is a disorder in which patients present with the triad of dementia, gait abnormalities, and urinary incontinence. Imaging studies often suggest the diagnosis because the ventricles are large and the cerebral

sulci are not particularly deep. The clinical response to a lumbar puncture or subarachnoid drain is the best predictive test as to whether a permanent shunt procedure would be beneficial.

Many multisystem neurodegenerative diseases have dementia as a feature of a larger syndrome. The most common of these diseases are Parkinson's disease, diffuse Lewy body disease, progressive supranuclear palsy, cortical basal ganglionic degeneration, multisystem atrophy (Shy-Drager syndrome), frontotemporal dementia (Pick's disease), and olivopontocerebellar atrophy. There are other conditions that are associated with dementia. Refer to Table 12.6b for details.

DIZZINESS

Dizziness is an extremely common problem that generally refers to one or more of four common sensations: vertigo, near syncope, disequilibrium, and ill-defined lightheadedness.

Vertigo is defined as an illusion of movement and always reflects a disorder of the vestibular system. Vertigo originating from the CNS tends to spare hearing, produce less torsional vertigo, and is associated with other brainstem symptoms and signs, such as double vision, dysarthria, and ataxia. A common cause of peripheral vertigo is benign paroxysmal positional vertigo (BPPV) resulting from the escape of otoliths from the utricle and saccule into the posterior semicircular duct, thereby producing violent spinning vertigo when the affected ear is turned down in the supine position. This vertigo is transient (i.e., lasting less than 60 seconds), fatigues with repeated movements into the "bad" position, reverses direction on sitting up, spares hearing, and is associated with rotatory nystagmus.

TABLE 12.6b
OTHER CONDITIONS WITH ASSOCIATED DEMENTIA

Endocrine disorders	Thyroid disorders: adult hypothyroidism, cretinism in children, Hashimoto's encephalopathy
Infectious diseases	Syphilis, HIV, toxoplasmosis (most commonly seen in immunocompromised persons), prion disease (i.e., Creutzfeldt-Jacob disease, fatal familial insomnia, Gerstmann-Straüssler disease)
Nutritional diseases	Cobalamin (vitamin B_{12}) deficiency, thiamine deficiency (Wernicke-Korsakoff), nicotinamide (niacin deficiency) otherwise known as pellagra
Demyelinating disease	Multiple sclerosis, progressive multifocal leukoencephalopathy, osmotic demyelination (formerly central pontine myelinolysis)
Chronic metabolic insults	Hypoglycemia, hypoxemia, uremia, hepatic failure with portosystemic shunting
Intracranial space-occupying lesions	Gliomas, metastases, abscesses (after oral surgery or ear infections)
Brain trauma	Trauma with two copies of APO E4 genotype increases risk of dementia

Refer to Table 12.7 to differentiate central versus peripheral vertigo.

Treatment of vertigo depends on the cause. For BPPV, the best treatment is to reposition the otoliths by moving them from the posterior semicircular duct back into the utricle and saccule. This treatment can be done using a physical therapy maneuver called the Epley maneuver (Fig. 12.2).

If the Epley maneuver fails, the labyrinth can be reconditioned by placing the head in the "bad" position

TABLE 12.7
DISTINGUISHING CENTRAL VERSUS PERIPHERAL CAUSES OF VERTIGO

Central Causes		Peripheral Causes	
Features:		**Features:**	
▪ Usually gradual onset of vertigo with progressive worsening		▪ Associated with hearing loss and tinnitus	
▪ Associated nystagmus is often nonfatigable and vertical rather than horizontal		▪ Vertigo typically episodic and transient	
▪ Other brainstem signs (dysarthria, dysphagia, diplopia, focal weakness, or sensory loss)		**Common Causes:**	
▪ Usually no hearing loss or tinnitus		**Cause**	**Description**
Common Causes:		Acute labyrinthitis	Inflammation of the labyrinth in organs caused by viral or bacterial infection
Cause	**Description**	Acute vestibular neuronitis (vestibular neuritis)[a]	Inflammation of the vestibular nerve, usually caused by viral infection
Cerebellopontine angle tumor	Vestibular schwannoma (i.e., acoustic neuroma) as well as infratentorial ependymoma, brainstem glioma, medulloblastoma, or neuro-fibromatosis	Benign positional paroxysmal vertigo (benign positional vertigo)	Transient episodes of vertigo caused by stimulation of vestibular sense organs by canalith; affects middle-age and older patients; affects twice as many women as men
Cerebrovascular disease such as transient ischemic attack or stroke, vertebrobasilar insufficiency	Arterial occlusion causing cerebral ischemia or infarction, especially if affecting the vertebrobasilar system	Cholesteatoma	Cystlike lesion filled with keratin debris, most often involving the middle ear and mastoid
Migraine	Episodic headaches, usually unilateral and throbbing accompanied by other symptoms such as nausea, vomiting, photophobia, or phonophobia; may be preceded by aura	Herpes zoster oticus (Ramsay Hunt syndrome)	Vesicular eruption affecting the ear; caused by reactivation of the varicella zoster virus
Multiple sclerosis	Demyelinization of white matter in the central nervous system	Ménière's disease (Ménière's syndrome, endolymphatic hydrops)	Recurrent episodes of vertigo, hearing loss, tinnitus, or aural fullness caused by increased volume of endolymph in the semicircular canals
		Otosclerosis	Abnormal growth of bone in the middle ear, leading to immobilization of the bones of conduction and a conductive hearing loss
		Perilymphatic fistula	Breach between middle and inner ear often caused by trauma or excessive straining

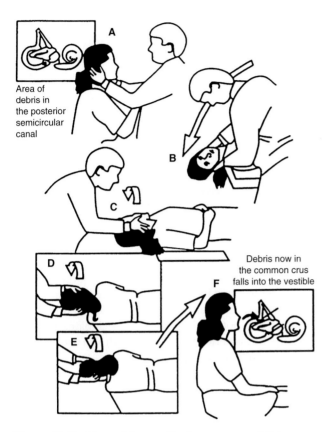

Area of
debris in
the posterior
semicircular
canal

Debris now in
the common crus
falls into the vestible

Figure 12.2   The otolith repositioning maneuver of Epley.

repeatedly each day. This treatment is unpleasant and less than satisfactory. Vestibular sedatives, which are anticholinergic and act primarily on the CNS, can also be used. Many are available over the counter, including meclizine (Bonine, Antivert), diphenhydrinate (Dramamine), and diphenhydramine (Benadryl). Promethazine (Phenergan) and scopolamine (Scope Trans-Derm) are prescription drugs. An acoustic or vestibular schwannoma can usually be removed by neurosurgeons and otolaryngologists often working as a team. In patients with vertebrobasilar insufficiency, the blood pressure should be raised slightly, and aspirin or other antiplatelet drugs should be implemented. Recently, more innovative treatments, including both surgical and endovascular revascularization techniques of the basilar and vertebral arteries have been tried with varied results. All known vestibulotoxic drugs should be discontinued, if possible.

Near syncope refers to a sensation of almost fainting caused by inadequate cerebral perfusion pressure. This usually occurs in the upright position and represents a failure of the nervous system's autonomic response to the upright posture. In clinical practice, it is often associated with the use of medications that cause vasodilation, volume depletion, or both. Drugs that interfere with the ability of the heart to respond to low blood pressure, such as beta-blockers, which prevent tachycardia, can also aggravate the symptoms of this type of dizziness. A careful cardiac evaluation should be performed to ensure that the patient is

not suffering from a serious cardiac condition, such as left ventricular outflow obstruction, as seen in aortic stenosis; asymmetric septal hypertrophy; or coronary artery disease. Most causes of near syncope are benign and are often related to volume depletion and vasodilation; these problems can be managed by reducing the medications that cause these adverse effects.

Disequilibrium refers to a sensation of dizziness caused by gait disorder. In clinical practice, the common gait disorders that cause dizziness include cerebellar ataxia, spasticity, and proprioceptive difficulties, such as those commonly seen in cervical spondylosis. Vitamin B_{12} deficiency has the tendency to produce stiff, weak legs and poor proprioception. An extrapyramidal disorder such as Parkinson's disease may also cause a gait disorder that patients refer to as dizziness. Treatment of the gait disorder often improves the sensation of dizziness.

Ill-defined lightheadedness refers to a sensation caused by anxiety, which many patients call dizziness. In some of these patients, episodes of severe dizziness are caused by hyperventilation attacks, but in many others the sensation is simply a chronic feeling of dysphoria in which the word dizziness is used metaphorically to mean anxious or depressed. Such patients are best treated without medications or, if necessary, with medications aimed specifically at the anxiety and depression.

BACK AND NECK PAIN

Back and neck pains are among the most common complaints for which people seek medical attention. For clinical purposes, it is useful to divide these patients into two major categories: those suffering from low back and leg pain and those suffering from neck and arm pain. Most lower back and leg pain is due to degenerative disease of the lumbar spine or intervertebral disc disease. Nondiscogenic pain should be suspected when the pain is worse at night or at rest, when severe local tenderness is present, or when systemic symptoms or signs of an underlying disease are present. For many patients, the pain is localized to the lower back without much local tenderness or radiation to one or the other leg. Using proprioceptive reflexes, it is usually possible to ascertain the level of the greatest nerve root compression. Table 12.8 demonstrates how it is possible to do this using the reflexes and the sensory and motor examination. Conservative therapy consists of bed rest for 72 hours, NSAIDs, and muscle relaxants. Patients with pain that is refractory to conservative measures may benefit from epidural steroid injections into the affected lumbar roots. Surgical therapy is reserved for patients who fail medical and pain management therapies.

Most neck and arm pain is due to degenerative changes in the cervical spine or intervertebral disk disease. Cervical spondylosis refers to degenerative change in the cervical spine resulting from degeneration of the intervertebral discs

TABLE 12.8

SYMPTOMS AND SIGNS OF LATERAL RUPTURE OF LUMBAR DISK

Disk	Root	Pain and Paresthesias	Sensory Loss	Motor Loss	Reflex Loss
L3–4	L4	Anterior surface of thigh, inner surface of shin	Anteromedial surface of thigh, extending down along shin to inner side of foot	Quadriceps	Knee jerk
L4–5	L5	Radiating down outer side of back of thigh and outer side of calf, and across dorsum of foot to great toe	Usually involves outer side of calf and the great toe	Extensor hallucis longus; less commonly, muscles of dorsiflexion and eversion of foot	None
L5–1	S1	Radiating down back of thigh and outer side and back of calf, to foot and the lesser toes	Almost always involves outer side of calf, outer border of foot, and the lesser toes; less commonly, the back of the thigh	Gastrocnemius and occasionally muscles of eversion of foot	Ankle jerk

and their intermittent protrusions and calcifications, which can lead to nerve root or spinal cord compression. Unlike intervertebral disc disease in the lumbosacral spine, disk disease in the neck can be dangerous in that it can compress the spinal cord, resulting in a myelopathy.

Most cervical spondylosis produces radiculopathy, with its consequent pain in the shoulder, arm, and hand. This disease has a natural history that is characterized by waxing and waning symptoms without significant long-term disability. The vast majority of patients can be treated medically with episodic use of a collar, anti-inflammatory and antispasmodic drugs, and time. Table 12.9 demonstrates how it is possible using proprioceptive reflexes and motor and sensory examination to determine the level of the intervertebral disc that is most likely to be responsible. Patients who fail medical treatment using immobilization and analgesia may benefit from epidural steroid injections into the affected cervical roots. For patients who fail conservative and epidural therapies, surgical approaches are available using both anterior and posterior approaches, depending on the specific location of the disk protrusion.

It is important to note that current guidelines dissuade physicians from ordering imaging test (x-rays, CT, MRI) for every patient presenting with back pain unless the patient has severe or progressive neurologic deficits. Other reasons to consider imaging include a history and physical examination suggestive of cancer, infection, or other underlying condition as a potential cause of the back pain. When an imaging study is performed, an MRI with and without contrast is the preferred imaging modality.

SEIZURES AND EPILEPSY

A seizure is any stereotypical experience or activity arising from hypersynchronous discharges in the cerebral cortex and perhaps some subcortical structures. Epilepsy is a disorder characterized by recurrent seizures that are not due to a demonstrable metabolic insult. Status epilepticus is the term used to describe seizures lasting for longer than 30 minutes or repeated seizures lasting a total of 30 minutes from which the patient does not recover awareness between episodes. Status epilepticus is a neurologic emergency and requires prompt treatment. Please refer to Figure 12.4 for management of status epilepticus. A nonepileptic seizure (pseudoseizure) refers to episodic neuropsychiatric phenomena that cannot be demonstrated to be due to hypersynchronous discharges. Epileptic seizures are divided

TABLE 12.9

SYMPTOMS AND SIGNS OF LATERAL RUPTURE OF CERVICAL DISK

Disk	Root	Pain and Paresthesias	Sensory Loss	Motor Loss
C4–5	C5	Neck, shoulder, upper arm	Shoulder	Deltoid, biceps
C5–6	C6	Neck, shoulder, lateral aspect of arm, radial aspect of forearm to thumb and forefinger	Thumb, forefinger, radial aspect of forearm, lateral aspect of arm	Biceps
C6–7	C7	Neck, lateral aspect of arm, ring and index fingers	Forefinger, middle finger, radial aspect of forearm	Triceps, extensor carpi ulnaris
C7–T1	C8	Ulnar aspect of forearm and hand	Ulnar half of ring finger, little finger	Intrinsic muscles of the hand, wrist extensors

Reproduced with permission from Samuels MA, ed. *Manual of Neurologic Therapeutics*, 6th ed. Philadelphia: Lippincott Williams & Wilkins, 1999:89.

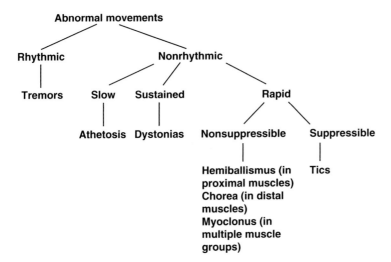

Figure 12.3 Classification of hyperkinesias.

into four major categories: primary generalized (centrencephalic seizures), secondary generalized (beginning partial), partial (formerly called focal), and neonatal (occurring in the first 30 days of life). Primary generalized seizures are subdivided further into tonic or clonic seizures (formerly known as grand mal seizures) and absence seizures (formally known as petit mal seizures). Partial seizures are subdivided on the basis of consciousness: complex partial seizures (consciousness is affected) and simple partial seizures (consciousness is not affected).

In evaluating a presumed seizure, it is important to obtain a history that includes a birth and developmental history and any history of remote neurotrauma or neurologic infectious disease. On physical examination, in addition to a standard neurologic examination, a careful evaluation of the head and the skin should be performed, giving particular attention to body asymmetries because these may reflect early life brain insults. In the emergent setting, stroke and blood (intraparenchymal or subarachnoid) must be ruled out. Ancillary tests include the use of imaging and an EEG to aid in determining the nature of the seizure and its localization. If a hemorrhage, any type of brain swelling, or mass effect is suspected, a noncontrast CT is indicated. Otherwise, an MRI with and without gadolinium should be performed. A spinal fluid analysis may be performed to look for potential infectious causes of the seizure, and a metabolic and toxic screen should be done because many seizures are due to metabolic or toxic insults. Common causes of seizures in adults include cerebral infarction, trauma, infection, and alcohol and drug withdrawal.

When using antiepileptic drugs (AEDs), monotherapy is preferred. It is now possible to obtain drug levels at the trough (i.e., just before the next dose of medication), which often helps to keep the medications to a minimum. The choice of AEDs can vary greatly from one institution to another. According to recent guidelines from the American Academy of Neurology, patients with newly diagnosed epilepsy who require treatment can be started on stan-

dard AEDs, such as carbamazepine, phenytoin, valproic acid, phenobarbital, or one of the newer AEDs, including lamotrigine, gabapentin, oxcarbazepine, or topiramate. AED choice depends heavily on individual patient characteristics. Historically, for generalized seizures, valproic acid is a good first choice, with phenytoin as an alternate option (Fig. 12.3). For partial seizures, carbamazepine is the drug of choice, with valproic acid as an alternative. For certain seizure types, specific drugs have been known to be particularly effective. Examples include ethosuximide for typical absence seizures, valproic acid for juvenile myoclonic epilepsy, and magnesium sulfate for toxemia of pregnancy. The newer AEDs, such as gabapentin, lamotrigine, topiramate, felbamate, and tiagabine, are more widely used now than in previous years. Refer to Table 12.10 for an overview of the different antiepileptic drugs.

Surgical treatment of epilepsy is an option for some patients at specialized centers where it is possible to document that the epilepsy is refractory to medical treatment while going through a detailed neuropsychological evaluation and extensive EEG monitoring that helps with anatomical mapping before the surgery. Vagal nerve stimulation may also help certain patients who have intractable seizures, although the mechanism of action is unknown, and the efficacy is not well established.

Epilepsy in pregnancy can be challenging. Because all AEDs are potentially teratogenic, a general rule is to keep AEDs at an absolute minimum, especially during first-trimester organogenesis. All female seizure patients of childbearing years should be maintained on folate to minimize the risk of neural tube defects. Severe seizures are probably worse for the fetus than any AED because of the potential for anoxic injury to the fetus. The risks versus the benefits must be weighed for each patient when individualizing treatment plans. The rules for stopping AEDs have been learned from experience. A long seizurefree period (about 4 years) is recommended. A normal EEG at the time AEDs are discontinued and a normal brain MRI predict a better long-term seizurefree outcome. Nonetheless,

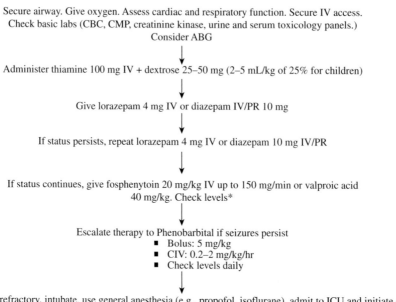

Secure airway. Give oxygen. Assess cardiac and respiratory function. Secure IV access.
Check basic labs (CBC, CMP, creatinine kinase, urine and serum toxicology panels.)
Consider ABG

↓

Administer thiamine 100 mg IV + dextrose 25–50 mg (2–5 mL/kg of 25% for children)

↓

Give lorazepam 4 mg IV or diazepam IV/PR 10 mg

↓

If status persists, repeat lorazepam 4 mg IV or diazepam 10 mg IV/PR

↓

If status continues, give fosphenytoin 20 mg/kg IV up to 150 mg/min or valproic acid
40 mg/kg. Check levels*

↓

Escalate therapy to Phenobarbital if seizures persist
- Bolus: 5 mg/kg
- CIV: 0.2–2 mg/kg/hr
- Check levels daily

↓

If status becomes refractory, intubate, use general anesthesia (e.g., propofol, isoflurane), admit to ICU and initiate continuous
EEG monitoring

Figure 12.4   Treatment of Status Epilepticus.
*Check antiepileptic levels 1-2 hours after the completion of the loading dose. Goal serum phenytoin levels are 10-20 μg/ml for the total levels and 1-2 μg/ml for the free levels. Goal serum valproic levels are 50-100 μg/ml for the total levels.

the risk of seizure recurrence in the "best" group of patients is still about 30%.

Seizures can be associated with a sudden alteration of consciousness that may interfere with the activities of daily living or put the patient in a dangerous situation. In general, patients should not drive unless the seizures are under control. Each state within the United States, as well as other countries, has specific rules about what is meant by the phrase "seizure free for a long enough period." Generally, this period ranges between 6 and 12 months without a seizure while on an appropriate AED regimen. Some states require that the physician report such cases to the Registry of Motor Vehicles; in other states, this is not necessary. Familiarity with local laws on this subject is recommended. Other activities such as swimming, bathing, operating heavy machinery, and climbing great heights are usually not regulated specifically, but should be avoided when unsupervised.

Patients with epilepsy have an increased risk of sudden death. Many causes are possible; however, most deaths are due to an autonomic storm with consequent cardiac arrhythmias.

STROKE

A stroke is the sudden or rapid onset of a neurologic deficit in a vascular territory caused by an underlying cerebrovascular disease lasting longer than 24 hours. A transient ischemic attack (TIA) is the same, but it lasts less than 24 hours. Of note, a proposed new definition of a TIA is a "brief episode of neurologic dysfunction caused by a focal disturbance of brain or retinal ischemia, with clinical symptoms typically lasting less than 1 hour, without evidence of infarction." Common diseases and conditions associated with stroke include atherosclerosis, lipohyalinosis (arteriolar sclerosis), cerebral embolism, arterial dissection, fibromuscular dysplasia, berry aneurysm, vascular malformations, and vasculitis. Hypercoagulable states may be associated with thrombosis-prone conditions.

All strokes are divided into two subtypes: ischemic and hemorrhagic strokes. Ischemic strokes themselves are subdivided into two groups: thrombotic and embolic. Thrombotic stroke is subdivided into those caused by large-vessel disease and those caused by small-vessel disease. The large vessels that may be a cause of thrombotic strokes are the carotid arteries (anterior circulation), or the vertebral and basilar arteries (posterior circulation). Small vessels can also thrombose, causing small infarcts deep in the brain, known as lacunes. Embolic stroke is divided into cardiac- and arterial-source emboli. Cardiac-source emboli are generally larger and more likely to produce serious stroke deficits. Emboli tend to affect midsized cerebral vessels, resulting in middle cerebral artery syndrome, anterior cerebral artery syndrome, and posterior cerebral artery syndrome.

Hypercoagulable states are subdivided into two types: primary and secondary. The primary hypercoagulable states are disorders that involve endogenous anticoagulant mechanisms, such as protein S and protein C deficiency, antithrombin III deficiency, and various fibrinolytic disorders. Secondary hypercoagulable states include

TABLE 12.10

INDICATIONS AND ADVERSE EFFECTS OF COMMON ANTIEPILEPTIC MEDICATIONS

Medication	Partial and Secondary Generalized Seizures	Primary Generalized Seizures (Tonic-Clonic)	Absence Seizures	Myoclonic Seizures	Adverse Effects
Phenytoin (Dilantin)	✓	✓			Ataxia, dizziness, encephalopathy, thyroid dysfunction, hirsutism, gingival hyperplasia, rash, osteomalacia, coagulation disorders
Carbamazepine (Tegretol)	✓	✓			Drowsiness, dizziness, ataxia, diplopia, rash, tremor, weight gain, hyponatremia, leukopenia
Oxcarbazepine (Trileptal)	✓	✓			Somnolence, headache, hyponatremia, weight gain
Phenobarbital	✓	✓	✓	✓	Sedation, ataxia, mood changes, risk of dependency
Valproic acid (Depakote)	✓	✓	✓	✓	Nausea, vomiting, cognitive disturbance, weight gain, polycystic ovarian syndrome, thrombocytopenia, increased bleeding times, tremor
Ethosuximide		✓	✓		Gastrointestinal symptoms, drowsiness, ataxia, extrapyramidal symptoms
Clonazepam (Klonopin)	✓	✓	✓	✓	Sedation, withdrawal symptoms, seizure exacerbations
Gabapentin (Neurontin)	✓				Drowsiness, dizziness, ataxia, tremor, vomiting
Lamotrigine (Lamictal)	✓	✓			Rash, headache, ataxia, depression, psychosis
Levetiracetam (Keppra)	✓				Somnolence, dizziness, psychosis, mood changes
Vigabatrin	✓	✓	✓	✓	Visual field constriction, mood change, weight gain, tremor
Topiramate (Topamax)	✓	✓			Dizziness, ataxia, tremor, weight loss, diplopia, cognitive dysfunction
Tiagabine (Gabitril)	✓				Dizziness, fatigue, flulike symptoms, ataxia, depression
Zonisamide (Zonegran)	✓				Sedation, mental slowing, weight loss, oligohidrosis, risk of heat stroke

antiphospholipid antibody syndrome, paraneoplastic (Trousseau's) syndrome, and various rheologic problems, such as those caused by immobility, obesity, and pressure from artificial surfaces.

Hemorrhagic strokes are divided into two types: bleeding that occurs into the brain parenchyma, also known as an intracerebral hemorrhage (ICH), or bleeding that takes place in the subarachnoid space, also known as subarachnoid hemorrhage (SAH). ICHs caused by hypertension typically occur deep in the brain, particularly in the putamen, thalamus, pons, and cerebellum. ICHs caused by a rupture of fragile arteries affected by amyloid (congophilic angiopathy) tend to be lobar and closer to the surface of the brain, where the affected pial vessels are plentiful. SAH commonly is due to the rupture of a congenital (berry) aneurysm or of an abnormal vascular malformation, such as an arteriovenous malformation (AVM), capillary malformation, or venous malformation.

The diagnosis of stroke or TIA can be determined by a clinical evaluation and confirmed by imaging. The clinical history for deficits in each of the major cerebral territories is fairly characteristic. When the ophthalmic artery is involved, patients complain of transient or permanent episodes of monocular blindness known as amaurosis fugax. Anterior cerebral artery ischemia produces contralateral leg weakness with relative sparing of the arm and face. The middle cerebral syndrome consists of hemiparesis that is worse in the face and hand than in the leg. Vertebral artery occlusions tend to cause infarction in the cerebellum and lateral medulla, producing ipsilateral ataxia, facial numbness, Horner's syndrome, hoarseness, and vertigo with contralateral body numbness. This syndrome, when it affects the lateral medulla, is known as Wallenberg's syndrome. Basilar artery disease is divided into mainstem basilar disease and basilar branch disease. Mainstem basilar disease tends to produce episodes of progressive tetraparesis, dysarthria, dysphagia, ataxia, and eye movement abnormalities, as well as changes in the level of consciousness. Basilar branch disease tends to produce episodic or progressive contralateral hemiparesis with ipsilateral cranial nerve findings. The top of the basilar syndrome is a characteristic cerebral embolism syndrome in which a sudden loss of consciousness occurs. When patients awaken, there could be a major abnormality in vision, such as blindness, with denial of deficit (Anton's syndrome) or a visual agnosia (Balint's syndrome), often with a major visual field cut, such as a hemianopsia. The differential diagnosis of strokes should always include complicated migraine, postictal paresis (Todd's paresis), hypoglycemia, conversion disorder, subdural hematoma, and brain tumors.

Refer to Table 12.11 to review the various stroke syndromes.

In the setting of a suspected acute stroke, the deficits should be assessed by a careful neurologic examination. Several scales have been developed to quantify the severity of the neurologic deficit; the National Institutes of Health Stroke Scale is most often used. The history is crucial—the exact time of symptom onset helps determine whether the patient is a candidate for intravenous (IV) or intra-aortic (IA) thrombolytic therapy. If the time of symptom onset is unclear, the time the patient was last seen normal is used as "time zero." Blood pressures should be closely monitored, and the patient should be placed on telemetry to monitor for arrhythmias. Laboratory testing during the acute period should include an Accu-Chek (because hypoglycemia can cause strokelike symptoms), a CBC, a complete metabolic panel (CMP), a coagulation panel, and cardiac enzymes. Patients with acute or chronic renal failure or patients with IV dye contrast allergies are not candidates for the studies requiring dye injection. In these cases, a noncontrast CT or an emergent noncontrast MRI of the brain and magnetic resonance angiography (MRA) of the carotids and circle of Willis should be arranged. Based on the results of the diagnostic studies and the time window, the stroke patient may be a candidate for IV or IA thrombolytic therapy.

Various noninvasive studies are available for evaluating cerebral vasculature, including ultrasound evaluation of the carotids, transcranial Doppler for the vertebral and middle cerebral intracranial arteries, MRA, CT angiography, nuclear flow studies, functional imaging such as positron emission tomography (PET), single-photon emission CT, and functional MR. Stroke centers are frequently using magnetic resonance (MR) diffusion and perfusion imaging in the assessment of acute stroke. MR diffusion sequences indicate areas of infarcted tissue, whereas MR perfusion sequences indicate areas of the brain that are not adequately perfused or territories "at risk." MR diffusion and perfusion sequences can assess the extent of the penumbra, which is brain tissue that is not adequately perfused but remains viable if blood flow can be quickly re-established. CT perfusion and angiography may be used to

TABLE 12.11

ACUTE STROKE SYNDROMES

Artery Involved	Syndrome
Anterior cerebral artery (ACA)	Motor and/or sensory deficit (foot ≫ face, arm) Grasp, sucking reflexes Abulia, paratonic rigidity Gait apraxia
Middle cerebral artery (MCA)	Dominant hemisphere: aphasia, motor and sensory deficit (face, arm ≫ leg > foot), may be complete hemiplegia if the internal capsule is involved, homonymous hemianopia Nondominant hemisphere: neglect, anosognosia (ignorance of deficits), motor and sensory deficit (face, arm > leg > foot), homonymous hemianopia
Posterior cerebral artery	Homonymous hemianopia; alexia without agraphia (if dominant hemisphere, unable to understand written words but can still write); visual hallucinations, sensory loss, choreoathetosis, pain (with thalamic involvement); paresis of vertical eye movements; CN III palsy, motor deficits
Internal carotid artery	Progressive or stuttering onset of MCA syndrome, occasionally ACA syndrome as well as insufficient collateral flow
Vertebrobasilar system	Cranial nerve palsies Crossed sensory deficits Diplopia, dizziness, vertigo, nausea, vomiting, dysarthria, dysphagia Limb and gait ataxia Motor deficits Coma and bilateral signs indicate basilar artery stenosis
Penetrating vessels (lacunar syndromes)	Pure motor hemiparesis Pure sensory deficit Pure sensory-motor deficit Hemiparesis ataxia Dysarthria/clumsy hand syndrome

delineate those areas of brain tissue having poor flow and that are at risk for infarction—this imaging modality is being used more in the setting of an acute stroke because it is faster to obtain and is more widely available. Conventional angiography remains the gold standard to assess emboli localization, to exclude an aneurysm or AVM, and to exclude vasculitis. When cerebral emboli are suspected, a cardiac ultrasound evaluation is part of the workup. Transesophageal echocardiography has been demonstrated to be superior to transthoracic studies for demonstrating a potential cardiac source for cerebral emboli.

The treatment of acute stroke involves the maintenance of euvolemia and a minimization of fluids that contain free water to avoid cerebral edema, nothing by mouth for a day or two to avoid aspiration, and moderate blood pressure control. Sudden drops in blood pressure due to hypovolemia or antihypertensive agents may make the symptoms worse if cerebral blood flow is impaired as a result of extracranial or intracranial stenosis. Steroids are not only ineffective, but also probably dangerous in the context of acute strokes.

IV thrombolytic therapy is being used in many stroke centers to treat acute strokes. Intravenous tissue plasminogen activator (IV-tPA) is an FDA-approved treatment for acute stroke that has been shown to be beneficial when given in the first 3 hours after stroke onset (0.9 mg/kg of body weight, with 10% of the dose administered as a bolus and the rest infused over 1 hour for a maximum total dose of 90 mg). There are strict inclusion and exclusion criteria (Table 12.12) to be eligible for IV-tPA. Symptomatic hemorrhages after IV-tPA usually occur within the first 24 hours after treatment and are often associated with protocol violations. At certain stroke centers, there are intra-arterial therapies that have been shown to be beneficial if used within a 6-hour period from symptom onset. Multiple

devices for the mechanical removal of clots are currently being investigated for use in the 0- to 6-hour time window. Newer MRI and CT imaging techniques are being investigated to expand the available time window for thrombolysis and mechanical clot removal.

Carotid endarterectomy is considered for patients with symptomatic and asymptomatic stenosis of 60% to 99%. Patients who are symptomatic and have higher degrees of stenosis benefit more than those who are asymptomatic with less stenosis. Carotid angioplasty and stenting with distal emboli protection for high-risk patients was approved by the FDA in 2005. Catheter-guided techniques allow interventionalists to treat lesions that are not amenable to surgery.

Antiplatelet therapy is a mainstay of treatment for stroke unless a high-risk condition such as atrial fibrillation is present. Atrial fibrillation warrants consideration of systemic anticoagulation (heparin, warfarin) to prevent further strokes. Anticoagulation is relatively contraindicated in unreliable or alcoholic patients, in persons who have active infective endocarditis (due to risk of mycotic aneurysms) or a known blood dyscrasia, and in patients who are at risk for falls. Warfarin, aiming for an international normalized ratio (INR) of 2 to 3, is used in patients with known significant risk factors for cerebral embolism, such as atrial fibrillation, patent foramen ovale, myocardial infarction with a dyskinetic left ventricular wall, and cardiomyopathy. Higher-dose warfarin with an INR >3 is indicated in patients having antiphospholipid antibody syndrome and mechanical heart valves.

Antiplatelet therapy appears to be effective in reducing the risk of stroke and death in patients with past strokes. The most effective dose of aspirin is still not known. The lowest proven effective dose is 30 mg/day, but most neurologists prescribe either 81 or 325 mg/day. For patients who

---

TABLE 12.12

INCLUSION AND EXCLUSION CRITERIA FOR THE ADMINISTRATION OF IV-tPA

Inclusion Criteria	Exclusion Criteria
Onset of symptoms <3 hours	Systolic BP >185 mm Hg, diastolic BP <110 mm Hg
Screening NIH stroke scale	Rapidly resolving symptoms
CT scan of brain without hemorrhage	Seizure at onset
and early infarction less than one-third	Stroke within 3 months
MCA territory	Head trauma within 3 months
	GI of urinary tract hemorrhage within 3 months
	Noncompressible arterial puncture within 7 days
	Anticoagulants or heparin within 48 hours
	Elevated PTT or PT >15
	Platelet count <100,000
	Glucose <50 or >400

BP, blood pressure; MCA, middle cerebral artery; NIH, National Institutes of Health; PT, PTT, partial thromboplastin time.
Adapted from The National Institute of Neurological Disorders and Stroke rt-PA Stroke Study Group. Tissue plasminogen activator for acute ischemic stroke. *N Engl J Med* 1995;333:1581–1587.

are "aspirin failures," a combination of dipyridamole and aspirin (Aggrenox) or clopidogrel (Plavix) may be used for stroke prevention. Warfarin has not been shown to reduce the risk of recurrent stroke if the mechanism of stroke is unknown. The combination of dipyridamole and aspirin has been shown to significantly reduce the risk of stroke when compared to both placebo and aspirin therapy.

The treatment of subarachnoid (SA) hemorrhage includes surgical clipping or intra-arterial coiling of the offending aneurysm at the earliest possible time to prevent further SA bleeding. Antispasm therapy consists of hydration, calcium channel blocker therapy (primarily Nimodipine), blood pressure augmentation, and hemodilution. Hydrocephalus and seizures are other complications of SAH that may be life threatening and need to be urgently treated.

PERIPHERAL NEUROPATHY

The peripheral nerve is a mixed nerve that contains at least two major types of afferent fibers and two major types of efferent fibers. The afferent fibers include small-diameter unmyelinated fibers carrying nociceptive sensations, such as pain and temperature information, and large-diameter myelinated fibers carrying nonnociceptive information, such as proprioception, vibration sense, position sense, and touch to the spinal cord or brainstem. The efferent fibers consist of small-diameter unmyelinated fibers carrying autonomic information and large-diameter myelinated fibers carrying motor information to muscles. Neuropathy is a disorder of the nerve and can include all or some of the four major fiber types, including effects on the myelin sheaths of the large-diameter fibers, both efferent and afferent. In general, diseases of the roots, known as radiculopathies, are "lumped together" with neuropathies in the same category of illness.

There are three types of pathology that affect peripheral nerves: infarction or compression of the nerve, which produces mononeuropathy; axonal degeneration, which produces polyneuropathy; and segmental demyelination, which produces polyneuropathy or mononeuropathy.

When a patient presents with tingling, numbness, weakness, or autonomic changes, the possibility of a peripheral neuropathy should be considered. The rate of onset and progression of the illness is extremely important because some neuropathies progress rapidly and are life threatening, whereas others are slow or nonprogressive. Because the peripheral nerve is predictably susceptible to toxic metabolic insults, a careful history of any known toxins, such as metals, solvents, and glue, is also important. Drugs are often toxic to peripheral nerves; therefore, in taking a history, inquiry should be made about the use of quinine derivatives, phenytoin, glutethimide, gold, hydralazine, isoniazid, nitrofurantoin, and vincristine. This list is not complete, however, and any drug is potentially

neurotoxic. A history of recent immunizations, such as those against influenza, rabies, typhoid, or smallpox, may also be responsible for some of the immune-mediated demyelinating neuropathies. Recent infections, particularly gastrointestinal infections that might be due to *Campylobacter*, are particularly important because immune reactions against this organism are known to cause certain kinds of neuropathy. The history of underlying malignancy is also important because a number of paraneoplastic and nutritional neuropathies exist, and a family history is particularly important because about a third of patients with chronic neuropathy of unknown cause are eventually found to have a familial form of the syndrome.

The clinical picture is generally divided into the major categories of the syndrome of mononeuropathy and the syndrome of polyneuropathy. Mononeuropathy involves the loss of motor or sensory function in the distribution of one nerve or asymmetrically in multiple nerves (in which case it is known as mononeuropathy multiplex) associated with pain and loss of appropriate reflexes. The pain and loss of reflexes may or may not be present, depending on the nerve that is affected. In polyneuropathy, a loss of motor or sensory function occurs symmetrically, in a distribution that usually affects the longest nerves first. This so-called "dying-back phenomenon" is extremely accurate and helpful in distinguishing axonal polyneuropathy from mononeuropathy or demyelinating diseases. In axonal polyneuropathy, the loss of reflexes affects the longest nerves first, and pain is variable, depending on the cause and nature of the neuropathic disease.

Among the neuropathies, one of the most common forms is compression or entrapment neuropathy. Sometimes these neuropathies are related to amyloid, acromegaly, or hypothyroidism, but usually they are associated with recurrent trauma or are completely cryptogenic. Any nerve that is susceptible to such an injury could suffer this kind of problem, but the most common are carpal tunnel syndrome of the median nerve at the wrist, the peroneal nerve at the knee, the radial nerve in the arm, the ulnar nerve at the elbow, and the lateral femoral cutaneous nerve (meralgia paresthetica) in the inguinal ligament. Mononeuritis and mononeuritis multiplex are commonly seen in systemic vasculitic diseases; in various vasculopathy syndromes, such as diabetes mellitus; in some hyperviscosity circumstances, such as Waldenström's syndrome, multiple myeloma, and polycythemia; in certain toxic circumstances, particularly those caused by lead; in some infectious diseases, particularly those caused by herpes zoster or leprosy; and sometimes cryptogenically or postinfectious, such as Bell's palsy. Among the polyneuropathies, segmental demyelination is seen in the postinfectious or postimmunization syndrome of Guillain-Barré, now known as acute inflammatory demyelinating polyneuropathy (AIDP). A chronic form also exists, known as chronic inflammatory demyelinating polyneuropathy (CIDP). Metachromatic leukodystrophy and Krabbe's disease are inherited forms of segmental demyelinating polyneuropathy having CNS myelin involvement as well. Genetically, the most common form is known as Charcot-Marie-Tooth (CMT) disease. Axonal degeneration-type polyneuropathy is the most common of all. It can be associated with vitamin deficiencies sometimes associated with alcohol abuse, such as thiamine, B_6, and folate. It is also seen with diabetes mellitus, hepatic failure, renal failure, paraneoplastic syndromes, diphtheria, amyloidosis, porphyria, and with exposures to a large number of toxins. It can be genetically determined or immune mediated, as when it is associated with monoclonal gammopathy of unknown significance and in the so-called POEMS (polyneuropathy, organomegaly, endocrinopathy, monoclonal gammopathy, and skin changes) syndrome seen in osteosclerotic myeloma. Last, axonal degeneration may be completely cryptogenic, as is the case with many motor neuron diseases. Refer to Table 12.13 for causes of peripheral neuropathy.

Laboratory studies in patients with a peripheral neuropathy are directed at revealing the underlying cause. They should include a CBC, CMP, urine and serum toxicology screens, heavy metal screening, ANA and ENA panels, ESR, fasting lipid panel, an oral glucose tolerance test, monoclonal proteins (serum and urine), thyroid-stimulating hormone, rapid plasma reagent test, rheumatoid factor, vitamin B_{12}, and folate levels. An electromyogram (EMG) may reveal evidence of denervation in the affected muscles and can be used to determine whether any motor units remain under voluntary control. Nerve conduction studies permit conduction velocities to be measured in motor and sensory fibers. In demyelinating forms of neuropathy, the EMG reveals little or no evidence of denervation, but there is evidence of a conduction block or marked slowing of maximal conduction velocities in the affected nerves. In the axonal neuropathies, denervation is revealed, especially in the distal extremities, but maximal nerve conduction velocity is normal or slowed only slightly.

The treatment of neuropathy depends a great deal on the underlying cause. The best protocol is to treat the underlying condition, such as reversing vitamin deficiencies, treating diabetes mellitus, discontinuing medications that are toxic to nerves, or treating an underlying malignancy. For uncomplicated forms of neuropathy, tricyclic antidepressants (i.e., amitriptyline), selective serotonin reuptake inhibitors (i.e., Cymbalta), gabapentin (Neurontin), topiramate (Topamax), and pregabalin (Lyrica) can be started to relieve neuropathic pain and titrated up as necessary. Steroids can be beneficial in certain categories of neuropathy, such as Bell's palsy and CIDP. Plasmapheresis has been demonstrated to be useful in AIDP, CIDP, and possibly in certain paraneoplastic neuropathies. IV immunoglobulin may also be effective for AIDP, CIDP, and paraneoplastic neuropathies. Hospitalization for respiratory support is often necessary for patients with severe AIDP; therefore, plasmapheresis can be used frequently during that period.

TABLE 12.13

CAUSES OF PERIPHERAL NEUROPATHY

- Idiopathic inflammatory neuropathies
- Acute idiopathic polyneuropathy (Guillain-Barré syndrome)
- Chronic inflammatory demyelinating polyneuropathy
- Metabolic and nutritional neuropathies
- Diabetes
- Hypothyroidism
- Acromegaly
- Uremia
- Liver disease
- Vitamin B_{12} deficiency
- Infective and granulomatous neuropathies
- AIDS
- Leprosy
- Diphtheria
- Sarcoidosis
- Sepsis and multiorgan failure
- Vasculitic neuropathies
- Polyarteritis nodosa
- Rheumatoid arthritis
- Systemic lupus erythematosus
- Neoplastic and paraproteinemic neuropathies
- Compression and infiltration by tumor
- Paraneoplastic syndromes
- Paraproteinemias
- Amyloidosis
- Drug-induced and toxic neuropathies
- Alcohol
- Sensory neuropathies: chloramphenicol, cisplatin, pyridoxine, Taxol, Taxotere, ethambutol, hydralazine, metronidazole
- Motor neuropathies: dapsone, imipramine, certain sulfonamides
- Mixed sensory and motor: amiodarone, chloroquine, disulfiram, gold, indomethacin, isoniazid, phenytoin, vincristine
- Hereditary neuropathies
- Idiopathic: hereditary motor and sensory neuropathies, hereditary sensory neuropathies, Friedreich's ataxia, familial amyloidosis
- Metabolic: porphyria, metachromatic leukodystrophy, Krabbe's disease, abetalipoproteinemia, Tangier disease, Refsum's disease, Fabry's disease
- Entrapment neuropathies

Last, genetic counseling is often useful for patients with a known genetically determined neuropathy.

MOVEMENT DISORDERS

Disorders of movement are divided into two major categories: those characterized by too little movement (hypokinetic disorders) and those characterized by too much movement (hyperkinetic disorders). Hypokinetic disorders fall into three major syndromes: paralysis, rigidity, and akinesia. Refer to Table 12.14 for details.

Many movement disorders are characterized by too much movement. Tremor is the most common hyperkinetic movement disorder; it refers to an oscillating

TABLE 12.14

HYPOKINETIC DISORDERS

Abnormal Movement	Description	Subtypes and Comments
Paralysis (paresis when incomplete)	Inability to use limb voluntarily	Upper motor neuron (supranuclear)—weakness of voluntary effort in a limb Lower motor neuron (infranuclear)—inability of limb to move under any circumstance, with associated muscle atrophy and wasting Upper and lower motor neuron—motor neuron disease (i.e., amyotrophic lateral sclerosis)
Rigidity	Abnormal stiffness in a muscle	Spasticity—velocity-dependent stiffness in patients who have upper motor neuron disease Lead-pipe stiffness—not velocity dependent and seen in extrapyramidal disorders such as Parkinson's disease Paratonic stiffness—can be seen in frontal lobe diseases such as hydrocephalus or Alzheimer's disease
Akinesia/bradykinesia	Delay between beginning of effort to make movement and start of movement Slowness of movement	Tendency not to move produces a rigid appearance of face and body, decreased blink count, decreased arm swing

involuntary movement around some fulcrum. Tremors may be proximal or distal, fast or slow, and are generated by synchronous or asynchronous activity at a joint. It is useful from a clinical perspective to divide all tremors into two categories: those that are obvious when resting, known as a repose or resting tremor, and those that are present with action, known as an intention tremor. Among the tremors at rest, one group improves with action, and one group worsens and changes in character with action. A resting tremor that is relieved by action is most likely due to Parkinson's disease. The tremor is slow and alternating at about three or four cycles per second at rest. With action, the tremor reduces in amplitude and frequency. Patients are often aware of the fact that their tremor is better when moving. A resting tremor that is exaggerated with action is known as a rubral or cerebellar outflow tremor and is often due to a disease in the white matter superior cerebellar peduncle as it crosses the midbrain on its way to the lateral thalamus. Patients with MS or head trauma are particularly susceptible to having a rubral tremor. Among the action tremors, some are present only with goal-directed action, such as pointing at a particular goal. This intention tremor is due to cerebellar disease either in the cerebellum itself or in fibers going to or coming from the cerebellum. Action tremors that are activated simply by a particular position (i.e., the antigravity posture) are known as postural action tremors. The physiological (normal) tremor is an example of a postural action tremor. This type of tremor can be exaggerated by the use of medication that activates β-receptors in muscle or that leads to increased amounts of circulating catecholamines in the blood. Thus, caffeine, theophylline, asthma medications, and catecholamine reuptake inhibitors all exaggerate physiological tremor and make it a symptom. A somewhat slower tremor that occurs with postural action is known as essential tremor. It tends to run in families,

beginning asymmetrically and progressing slowly over many years. Refer to Tables 12.14 and 12.15 for an overview of the hyperkinetic disorders.

Parkinson's may be induced by drugs that block dopamine receptors in the CNS, particularly those neuroleptic drugs used in psychiatric circumstances. Parkinson's is often associated with other degenerative diseases of the nervous system, such as progressive supranuclear palsy and multisystem atrophy, strionigral degeneration, and olivopontocerebellar atrophy. These disease states are grouped into a category termed "Parkinson's-plus syndromes," which are often less responsive to medications and carry a poorer prognosis than typical Parkinson's disease. Refer to Table 12.16 for an overview of these Parkinson's-plus syndromes.

Parkinson's is sometimes familial, but it is usually a sporadic illness. It can be seen in association with the deposition of certain minerals in the basal ganglia, as in the case of Wilson's disease (copper), Fahr's disease (calcium and magnesium), Hallervorden-Spatz disease (iron), and miner's Parkinsonism (manganese). Parkinson's may be toxic, as occurs with intoxication with N-methl-phenyl-1, 2, 3, 6-tetrahydropydropyridine and even may be metabolic, as in subacute necrotizing encephalomyelopathy of Leigh and other mitochondrial diseases.

Parkinson's disease is caused by a cryptogenic loss of pigmented cells in the substantia nigra, resulting in a subsequent loss of dopamine in the striatum. Motor symptoms begin when there is a loss of approximately 60% of pigmented cells. Parkinson's disease is a clinical diagnosis, and the onset of symptoms is typically asymmetric. The classic features include (a) resting tremor, usually a pill-rolling tremor; (b) bradykinesia—slow movements, difficulty initiating movements; (c) cogwheel rigidity; and (d) shuffling gait with a stooped posture.

TABLE 12.15

HYPERKINETIC DISORDERS

Abnormal Movement	Causes	Description
Tremor	Essential tremor Parkinson's disease, disorders and drugs that cause parkinsonism	Movements are regular and alternating or oscillatory Classified as resting, intention, postural, or physiological
Fibrillation	Neuropathic disease	Smallest possible movement disorder—only seen on electromyelogram testing Consists of firing of one muscle fiber within a muscle belly occurring without command
Fasciculation	Anxiety (hyperventilation) Metabolic disorders (hypomagnesia) Amyotrophic lateral sclerosis (if upper and lower motor neuron signs)	Firing of all muscle fibers connected to one motor neuron (a motor unit)
Myoclonus/asterixis	Metabolic encephalopathies (renal and hepatic failure), pulmonary disease, or the use of opiates Prion disease	Nonrhythmic, rapid, nonsuppressible, shocklike twitches occur, sometimes in multiple muscles simultaneously
Athetosis	Huntington's disease, encephalitis, hepatic encephalopathy Drugs (e.g., cocaine, amphetamines, antipsychotics)	Movements are nonrhythmic, slow, writhing, sinuous, primarily in distal muscles; alternating postures of the proximal limbs often blend continuously to produce a flowing stream of movement Athetosis often occurs with chorea as choreoathetosis
Chorea	Huntington's disease, thyrotoxicosis, systemic lupus erythematous affecting the central nerve system (CNS), rheumatic fever, tumors, or infarcts of the caudate nucleus Pregnancy, often in women who had rheumatic fever Age older than 60 years (as senile chorea) Drugs (e.g., antipsychotics—tardive chorea)	Movements are nonrhythmic, jerky, rapid, and nonsuppressible, primarily in distal muscles or the face Sometimes abnormal movements merge imperceptibly into purposeful or semipurposeful acts that mask the involuntary movements Chorea often occurs with athetosis
Dystonias	Primary (idiopathic) Degenerative or metabolic CNS disorders (e.g., Wilson's disease, Hallervorden-Spatz disease, various lipidoses, multiple sclerosis, cerebral palsy, stroke) Drugs, most often antipsychotics (e.g., phenothiazines, thioxanthenes, butyrophenones) or antiemetics Repetitive motions (writer's cramp)	Nonrhythmic sustained muscle contractions occur, often distorting body posture Can be focal, segmental, or generalized Focal: writer's cramp Segmental: torticollis, blepharospasm Generalized: hereditary forms (dopamine responsive dystonias)
Hemiballismus	Usually, damage to the subthalamic nucleus or nuclei due to hemorrhagic or ischemic strokes, metastatic tumors, cysts, infectious disorders, or inadvertent tissue damage during neurosurgery	Movements are nonrhythmic, rapid, nonsuppressible, violent, and flinging; they occur unilaterally, primarily in the proximal arm
Tics	Tourette's syndrome, Huntington's disease, primary dystonia, neuroacanthocytosis, Hallervorden-Spatz disease, infections, stroke, obsessive-compulsive disorder Drugs (e.g., methylphenidate, cocaine, amphetamines) Toxins	Movements are idiosyncratic, nonrhythmic, rapid, suppressible, and repetitive; they occur almost unconsciously Tics can be suppressed only for brief periods and with conscious effort Tics may be simple or complex Simple tics (e.g., eye blinking) often begin as nervous mannerisms in childhood or later, and then disappear spontaneously Tics tend to be more complex than myoclonus and less flowing than chorea

Patients with early or mild parkinsonian symptoms or those who are younger than 65 years are often treated with central dopamine agonists such as pramipexole (Mirapex) or ropinirole (Requip), rather than dopamine replacement with carbidopa/levodopa (Sinemet). The early initiation of these agents can delay the need for carbidopa/levodopa for years and decreases the number of patients who develop dyskinesias. Levodopa is used in the later stages of the disease or if patients fail dopamine agonists. Catechol-O-methyltransferase inhibitors decrease

TABLE 12.16

PARKINSON'S-PLUS SYNDROMES ("MULTISYSTEM ATROPHIES")

Disorder	Major Manifestations	Ocular Findings	Parkinsonian Symptoms	Dementia
Shy-Drager syndrome	Orthostatic hypotension without reflex tachycardia, resulting in syncope; autonomic features (impotence, sweating, incontinence); fasciculations and muscular atrophy	Extra ocular palsy, iris atrophy	Rigidity, tremor, akinesia	No
Striatonigral degeneration	Initial Parkinson's followed by autonomic dysfunction; hypotonia, syncope, incontinence		Often initial; poorly responsive to levodopa	
Olivopontocerebellar atrophy	Sporadic or familial; initial cerebellar symptoms (ataxia, tremor); lateral parkinsonism (often mild) and autonomic failure		Late, often mild	Yes
Progressive supranuclear palsy	Usually in males, often starts with akinesia; predominant truncal rigidity; falls; dysarthria	Vertical gaze palsy, slowing of downward vertical saccades	Akinesia is the most prominent feature; truncal rigidity	Yes (subcortical dementia)
Corticobasal degeneration	Rapidly progressive akinetic-rigid syndrome; asymmetric; alien limb syndrome; severe gait ataxia		Asymmetric, akinetic-rigid	
Lewy body dementia	Prominent dementia; progressive cognitive impairment; abnormal response to neuroleptics		Gait impairment with falls	Prominent

the peripheral metabolism of levodopa by the gut and liver, thereby increasing the amount available for the CNS; these are used as adjunctive therapy to levodopa. Stalevo, a combination of levodopa, carbidopa, and entacapone (Comtan), has been shown to be effective in patients with advanced Parkinson's disease. In patients having predominately tremor, anticholinergics such as trihexyphenidyl (Artane) or benztropine (Cogentin) may be used. Amantadine (Symmetrel) improves central dopamine release and may be used alone or in combination with the anticholinergics or levodopa. Given the high incidence of side effects to these medications, all drugs should be initiated slowly and titrated to the lowest possible effective dose. In patients with psychiatric manifestations of Parkinson's disease (in particular, hallucinations), clozapine (Clozaril) may be helpful because it will not worsen motor symptoms.

Deep brain stimulation of areas involved in the pathophysiology of Parkinson's disease is usually reserved for patients who become refractory to conventional medical therapy. Recent advancements in stereotactic techniques have made the placement of electrodes into deep regions of the brain less risky for patients. Electrodes are typically placed in the subthalamic nucleus or the globus pallidus. The advantages of electrical stimulation in these areas include improvement of all parkinsonian symptoms, a reduction in medications, and the potential of neuroprotection.

Treatment of chorea is difficult unless levels of the offending drug, such as hormonal birth control, can be reduced. Antidopamine therapy using a central dopamine receptor antagonist, such as haloperidol (Haldol), is sometimes useful, but haloperidol often produces Parkinson's and other side effects. Cholinergic therapy using a centrally acting acetylcholine precursor such as choline or lecithin or a cholinergic agonist such as deanol (Deaner), or anticholinesterase therapy using physostigmine or donepezil, is occasionally beneficial. Myoclonus can be treated with serotonergic agonists, such as 5-hydroxytryptophan and carbidopa, or with centrally acting serotonin reuptake inhibitors, such as fluoxetine (Prozac). Dystonia is difficult to treat unless it happens to be a dopamine-responsive dystonia. Otherwise, injection of the affected muscles with small doses of botulinum toxin is often helpful. Tardive dyskinesia, whether it be dystonia, athetosis, chorea, or akathisia, is often best treated by discontinuing the offending drug, even though to do so may transiently increase the movement disorder. Sometimes a small benefit can be obtained by using a centrally acting catecholamine-depleting drug, such as reserpine or tetrabenazine.

Tics are best ignored and not treated at all unless they are particularly bothersome. Developmental tics will disappear spontaneously. Severe tic disorder can be treated in a manner similar to the treatment of obsessive-compulsive disorders or sometimes with haloperidol or clonidine.

DISEASES OF MYELIN

Myelin is a lipoprotein that allows underlying axons to conduct impulses at a much more rapid rate due to saltatory (jumping) conduction. Peripheral myelin is made by Schwann cells, and central myelin is made by oligodendrocytes. In both cases, myelin is a lipoprotein composed of 70% lipid and 30% protein. The myelin sheath is actually a modified plasma membrane. Demyelination refers to an acquired illness that causes a loss of myelin, while other elements of the nervous system are relatively intact. The most common CNS demyelinating disease is multiple sclerosis (MS). Other CNS demyelinating diseases are optic neuropathy, transverse myelitis, acute disseminated encephalomyelitis, neuromyelitis optica (Devic's disease), and progressive multifocal leukoencephalopathy. MS is a disease of CNS myelin that is manifested by attacks separated in both time and space: lesions must occur in more than one location, and they must have occurred at more than one time. The disease has an interesting epidemiology in that it most tends to affect populations that are farthest from the equator. Initially, this was believed to be due to a possible infectious etiology of the disease, but it appears more probably because of a genetic predisposition for what is probably an autoimmune demyelinating process. The pathology consists of perivenular inflammation, with demyelination limited completely to the CNS. The current view is that MS is probably an immune-mediated illness for which a genetic predisposition exists to some triggers in the environment, such as otherwise benign viral illnesses.

The diagnosis is based on the clinical history of multiple lesions in space and time. There are a set of criteria to help with making the diagnosis using both clinical and imaging information. Refer to Table 12.17 for details.

No single diagnostic test for MS exists at this time. The spinal fluid is abnormal in 90% of patients, an elevated γ-globulin level is found in about 75% of cases, and more than 5 lymphocytes/mm^3 are found in about 50% of cases. MRI is the most useful and diagnostic study, but even it is not perfectly sensitive and specific for the diagnosis of MS. Patients with MS may have one attack and never have any trouble again, they may have multiple attacks from which they relatively recover, or the disease may progress unremittingly. The treatment of relapsing-remitting MS has been studied in the greatest detail because this is the most common form of the disease. It is generally believed that IV methylprednisolone should be given for acute attacks at a dose of about 1 g/day for 5 days. Strong evidence now suggests that β-interferon reduces the attack rate in the relapsing-remitting form of the disease by about 20%. Three forms of β-interferon are presently available: β-interferon 1A (Avonex) is given intramuscularly once a week, β-interferon 1A (Rebif) is given subcutaneously three times per week, and β-interferon 1B (Betaseron) is given subcutaneously every other day. Another medication, glatiramer acetate (Copaxone), is a synthetic polypeptide that is administered daily subcutaneously; it is roughly as effective as the interferons.

TABLE 12.17

2005 REVISED MCDONALD MULTIPLE SCLEROSIS DIAGNOSTIC CRITERIA

Clinical (Attacks)	Objective Lesions	Additional Requirements to Make Diagnosis
2 or more	2 or more	None. Clinical evidence alone will suffice; additional evidence desirable but must be consistent with multiple sclerosis (MS)
2 or more	1	Dissemination in space by MRI or two or more MRI lesions consistent with MS plus positive cerebrospinal fluid (CSF) or await further clinical attack implicating other site
1	2 or more	Dissemination in time by MRI or second clinical attack
1	1	Dissemination in space by MRI or two or more MRI lesions consistent with MS plus positive CSF *and* dissemination in time by MRI or second clinical attack
0 (progression from onset)	1 or more	Disease progression for 1 year (retrospective or prospective) *and* two out of three of the following: ■ Positive brain MRI (nine T2 lesions or four or more T2 lesions with positive visual-evoked potentials) ■ Positive spinal cord MRI (two or more focal T2 lesions) ■ Positive CSF

Adapted from Polman et al. Diagnostic criteria for multiple sclerosis: 2005 revisions to the "McDonald" criteria. *Ann Neurol* 2005;58:840–846.

TABLE 12.18

OTHER DEMYELINATING DISEASES OF THE NERVOUS SYSTEM

Disease	Description
Central Demyelinating Diseases	
Optic neuritis	Condition due to inflammation of the optic nerve in one or both eyes, which can lead to sudden vision loss.
Devic disease (neuromyelitis optica)	Condition characterized by inflammation of the optic nerve and spinal cord, which may result in temporary blindness, muscle weakness or paralysis. Can be extremely aggressive.
Transverse myelitis	Acute demyelinating illness that affects the spinal cord, leading to pain, weakness or paralysis. Treated with a short course of intravenous methylprednisolone.
Acute disseminated encephalomyelitis (Weston-Hurst disease)	Disorder due to inflammation of the brain and spinal cord, which may result in headache, delirium, seizures and coma. Usually monophasic. Can be severe and even fatal following a viral illness or immunization.
Progressive multifocal leukoencephalopathy	Caused by an infection of the oligodendrocyte with the JC virus. Pathogenic in immunocompromised patients (e.g., patients with lymphoma, leukemia, or HIV, or on chronic immunosuppressive therapy. No known effective treatment and is usually lethal in a matter of months.
Peripheral Demyelinating Diseases	
Acute inflammatory demyelinating polyneuropathy (AIDP)	Usually postinfectious disease. Can be life threatening. Course shortened with use of plasmapheresis or intravenous (IV) immunoglobulin therapy. Many patients require some period of respiratory support, but 95% of patients will recover more than 95% of their original neurologic state.
Chronic inflammatory demyelinating polyneuropathy	Formerly believed to be a chronic form of the AIDP; now considered a different immune-mediated disease. Slowly progressive or episodic and never affects respiratory musculature. Treated with immunosuppression using steroids or the episodic use of IV immunoglobulin. Sometimes secondary to an underlying malignancy or plasma cell dyscrasia. When it is not, it is a chronic illness that often requires treatment for many years.

Symptomatic therapy to control spasticity includes baclofen, both orally and intrathecally. Limb weights, thalamic surgery, and thalamic stimulation may be used to help control ataxia. Carbamazepine, amitriptyline, gabapentin, and narcotics are used to treat pain associated with MS. Oxybutynin is used for bladder spasticity, and cholinomimetics are used for hypotonicity of the bladder. The serotonin reuptake inhibitors and tricyclic drugs are used to treat the depression associated with the disease, and amantadine is used to treat fatigue. Treating underlying infections, such as urinary tract infections, is also extremely useful in reducing the severity and number of attacks. Several experimental treatments, including use of oral myelin, oral interferons, oral glatiramer, and other immune system modulators, are under investigation, but they are not clinically available for general use at this time. In severely resistant patients with progressive disease, more radical immune modulation includes the use of cyclophosphamide, azathioprine, and methotrexate.

Optic neuropathy is a demyelinating disease of the optic nerve and may or may not be part of the general syndrome of MS. Patients present with pain in the eye, loss of visual acuity with particularly severe loss of the ability to see red (red desaturation), and a reduction in the reaction of pupils to direct light, which is best compared with a reaction to consensual light (the Marcus-Gunn deafferented pupil).

In managing a patient who shows signs of this syndrome, the possibility of temporal arteritis, tumor in the optic nerve, toxic amblyopia from cyanide exposure or vitamin deficiency, and Leber hereditary optic neuropathy (a mitochondrial disease) should be excluded. A relationship exists between optic neuropathy and MS, but it is not a 1:1 relationship. About 20% of patients with optic neuropathy eventually develop MS, and this percentage is probably greater in women. About 40% of MS patients have had clinical optic neuritis, and more than 80% have had subclinical optic neuritis, as judged by visual-evoked responses. The treatment is IV methylprednisolone; about one-third of the patients recover completely, about one-third recover partially, and one-third do not recover at all. Refer to Table 12.18 for more details about other demyelinating diseases.

SLEEP DISORDERS

Sleep is an active physiological state that is regulated by the brain, homeostatic drive, and circadian rhythms. The adult sleep cycle typically lasts for 90 to 110 minutes, and consists of non–rapid eye movement and rapid eye movement (REM) sleep. The function of sleep is still not fully known, but deep sleep (delta sleep) is believed to be physically restorative, and REM sleep is believed to help consolidate memories, especially procedural memories.

Excessive daytime sleepiness (EDS) is a common complaint for many patients. The most common cause of

EDS is insufficient sleep. Common sleep disorders to consider when evaluating EDS include obstructive sleep apnea syndrome (OSAS), restless legs syndrome (RLS), circadian rhythm disorders, and narcolepsy.

OSAS is characterized by recurrent episodes of upper airway collapse (complete or partial). Many patients with OSAS snore loudly and have been told that they stop breathing during sleep. Risk factors for OSAS include the male gender, large neck circumference (>17 inches), obesity, a crowded posterior oropharynx, and retrognathia. Patients with untreated moderate to severe sleep apnea (apnea-hypopnea index >15) have an increased risk of developing hypertension. They also have an increased risk of having a heart attack or stroke. Many patients will state that daytime sleepiness or tiredness is a problem, whereas others may complain of having a decreased quality of life due to interrupted sleep.

The evaluation of patients with suspected OSAS consists of a complete history and physical examination followed by an overnight polysomnogram (PSG). During a routine PSG, multiple physiological parameters are monitored: EEG, EMG, limited ECG, eye movements, oxygen saturation, airflow, respiratory effort, and leg movements. The treatment for some patients with mild OSAS consists of weight loss if obesity is a problem or positional therapy if most of the respiratory events occur when the patient is in the supine position. A dental referral for an adjustable oral appliance may be helpful if retrognathia is present. Continuous positive airway pressure (CPAP) is indicated for patients with moderate to severe OSAS. If CPAP cannot be tolerated, the patient may be a candidate for upper airway surgery.

Narcolepsy is characterized by EDS and sleep attacks, which are brief episodes of sleep that can occur anytime during the day. Some patients with narcolepsy have cataplexy, which is a bilateral loss of muscle tone that is usually triggered by a strong emotion (laughter or anger). Episodes of cataplexy are typically short, and consciousness is preserved throughout the episode. An overnight PSG (to rule out other sleep disorders that may be contributing to EDS) followed by a multiple sleep latency test (MSLT) the day after (to objectively assess sleep and REM latencies) should be performed. A positive MSLT would show that the mean sleep latency over five nap trials was ≤8 minutes and that there were two or more sleep-onset REM periods. A normal MSLT would show that the mean sleep latency is ≥10 minutes with zero to one sleep-onset REM period. Treatments of choice for narcolepsy are CNS stimulants such as modafinil (Provigil) or methylphenidate (Ritalin). In addition, short scheduled naps are often helpful in managing EDS.

RLS is a clinical diagnosis that can affect 10% of the general population. Not all patients with RLS need to be treated. Over time, patients may have a hard time falling asleep or may have periodic limb movements during sleep that interfere with sleep quality, with a difficulty falling

TABLE 12.19

SECONDARY CAUSES OF RESTLESS LEG SYNDROME

- End-stage renal disease with or without hemodialysis
- Iron deficiency with or without anemia
- Pregnancy
- Peripheral neuropathy
- Diabetes
- Vitamin B_{12} deficiency
- Folate deficiency
- Drug effects (tricyclic antidepressants, selective serotonin reuptake inhibitors, H_1-antihistamines, typical and atypical neuroleptics, lithium, antinausea medications)

asleep. There are four essential criteria that are needed to make a diagnosis of RLS: (a) an urge to move the legs that may be due to an uncomfortable sensation in the legs, (b) the urge to move the legs begins or worsens during periods of rest or inactivity, (c) the urge to move the legs is partially or completely relieved by moving them, and (d) the urge to move the legs is worse in the evening or nighttime. A PSG is only needed if there is a suspicion for sleep disordered breathing. Iron deficiency has been linked with RLS and a ferritin level <50 mcg/L is significant for patients with RLS. Many studies have shown that treatment with oral iron supplements can improve RLS symptoms. Dopamine agonists (pramipexole and ropinirole) are the treatment of choice for RLS. Nonpharmacologic treatments include counterstimulation (rubbing legs, hot or cold baths, ice packs); regular exercise (not after 7 pm); stretching; mental activities; and avoidance of caffeine, alcohol, and nicotine near bedtime. Primary RLS is more likely to be familial and is more common than secondary RLS. There are many secondary causes of RLS that should be considered (Table 12.19).

REVIEW EXERCISES

QUESTIONS

1. A 50-year-old woman complains of headaches. She has never had headaches before and has no history of neurologic or psychiatric disease. The headaches began about 6 weeks before and are not severe, but they seem to be getting worse and are beginning to worry her. They wax and wane throughout the day without any particular pattern. They respond well to aspirin but seem to return when the aspirin wears off. They do not wake her from sleep, nor do they cause nausea or vomiting. No neurologic prodrome is present, and she cannot think of anything that exacerbates the pain. It is difficult to localize the headache, and it is not pulsating in character. The pain sometimes improves when her husband massages her neck. No significant past medical, family, or social history is taken. She takes no drugs and does not drink alcohol or smoke. General physical examination is normal, as is the mental status and cranial nerve examination. Motor examination shows a slight but definite pronation of the left arm on extension of upper limbs. Careful sensory examination shows some extinction to double simultaneous stimulation on the left. Coordination is normal. Reflexes are symmetric and of average amplitude. Both plantars are flexor. Which of the following is the most appropriate next step?

a) Reassurance
b) Prescribe paroxetine
c) Lumbar puncture
d) CT of the head without contrast
e) MRI of the head with gadolinium

Answer and Discussion

The answer is d. This case raises many important issues encountered in the management of a patient complaining of headache. In this particular case, the history itself is worrisome and is enough to warrant further testing. Although the headaches are mild, they are different for this patient than her usual pattern. This is probably the most important part of the history in a headache patient. Headaches that have changed in quality are more worrisome than severe headaches that are the same as always. The fact that the headaches respond to mild analgesic medication or to massage should not be reassuring to the physician. All sorts of pains respond to analgesic medication, and this in and of itself does not mean that the cause of the headache is benign. Of the greatest importance is the abnormality in the neurologic examination. A slight but definite pronation of the left arm on extension of the upper limbs indicates a mild left hemiparesis. A positive neurologic examination in the presence of headache should always lead to further evaluation. In some centers, it may be possible to do an MRI, but CT scanning is a more widespread and available technology. For this patient, there is really no reason to obtain skull radiographs or any other noninvasive evaluation other than a CT scan. The CT scan may be done without contrast, at which time a lesion may be found. If nothing is found, a decision about injecting contrast can be made later.

2. A 68-year-old man is complaining that his handwriting is deteriorating and that his hands shake when he tries to drink from a glass or coffee cup. He has no significant past medical history and no family history of neurologic or psychiatric disease. He does not drink alcohol or smoke. His only medication is Sinemet 10/100 four times a day given to him by a physician whom he saw once while on vacation in Florida 2 years before. A physician friend of the patient has been rewriting the prescription since then. His general examination is normal. On motor examination, he is noted to have a rather expressionless face and sits rigidly in his chair with arms flexed, bent slightly forward. Tone is diffusely increased with "cogwheeling." Power is normal. There is a 2- to 3-second alternating tremor noted in both hands while he is seated. When asked to extend his hands, this tremor becomes finer but more rapid. On finger-nose-finger testing, the tremor intensifies, but no dysmetria is noted. When he attempts to write, the tremor becomes severe, leading to illegible script. Sensory examination is intact. Reflexes are average and symmetric. Both plantars are extensor. His gait is shuffling but with a narrow base. He has difficulty getting started, but, once he is going, he walks quite well although slightly bent forward. Which of the following is the most appropriate treatment plan for this patient's tremors?

a) Begin metoprolol.
b) Begin primidone.
c) Increase the Sinemet dose.
d) Decrease the Sinemet dose.
e) Recommend moderate alcohol consumption.

Answer and Discussion

The answer is d. This 68-year-old man has two separate problems. The first is a tendency not to move, known as akinesia or bradykinesia. This gives him the expressionless face and accounts for his sitting rigidly in a chair with his arms flexed and bent slightly forward. This akinesia is sometimes referred to as Parkinsonism. In addition to the akinesia, he shows the classic tremor of Parkinsonism, which is characterized as a slow alternating tremor with a frequency of about three cycles per second. This tremor is most prominent in the position of repose and improves when the limb moves into action. When a tremor is superimposed on rigidity, the phenomenon of cogwheeling develops. The tremor of his Parkinson's disease is probably not bothering him because it is present only in repose and improves on action. His major complaint concerned deterioration of handwriting. In fact, he is complaining about a second tremor, some form of postural tremor, which could be either an essential tremor or an exaggerated physiological tremor. Tremor is defined as an alternating movement around some fulcrum. Tremors may be proximal or distal, rapid or slow, synchronous or alternating. They may be greatest in the position of repose or on action. Action tremors are subdivided into goal-directed action tremor, which is present only when the patient attempts to make a projected precise movement, and postural action tremors, which occurs when the affected limb attains an antigravity posture, such as raising the hand. Physiological tremor is a rapid postural action tremor, and is most prominent in the extremities distally and interferes with carrying out fine motor activity, such as writing. It is caused by the peripheral action of catecholamines or their agonists on receptors in muscle. It is usually not symptomatic, but it may become symptomatic, in which case it is called exaggerated physiological tremor. Physiological tremor is exaggerated by situations that increase the sensitivity of peripheral catecholamine receptors or increase the amount of circulating catecholamines. Such circumstances include anxiety, hyperthyroidism, or the use of drugs that functionally raise the circulating catecholamine levels, such as antiasthma medications, lithium carbonate, theophylline, and caffeine. This tremor is treated best by reducing the exacerbating factors or, if necessary, with a small dose of beta-blocker. Alcohol is also effective against this tremor, but it is not recommended as a therapy. The second form of postural tremor is known as essential tremor. It is slightly slower than the physiological tremor, is also present in the extremities most commonly, may occur in families, and may develop only in older people (senile essential tremor). Treatment consists of either beta-blockade or use of the antiepileptic drug primidone (Mysoline). Evidence suggests that the incidence of essential tremor is higher in patients with Parkinsonism than in age-matched controls; that is, it may be true that action tremor is part of Parkinson's disease. It is also possible that this man has an exaggerated physiological tremor, possibly caused by the peripheral metabolism of Sinemet to norepinephrine, which then acts on receptors in the muscle. A tremor study done in an experienced neurophysiology laboratory might be helpful in distinguishing these two types of tremor, but a therapeutic trial of reduction in Sinemet may work just as well. In this case, the first choice would be to decrease or discontinue his Sinemet. If there was no effect on the tremor, then treatment with primidone or beta-blocker would be appropriate.

3. A 43-year-old mother of four presents to the office with complaints of headache, neck pain, some dizziness, and nausea. She has a history of chronic tension headaches and low-back pain. She works as a pharmaceutical representative and reports spending a lot of time in her car. She has been seeing a chiropractor on and off for 20 years to treat her chronic symptoms, but despite a visit to the chiropractor yesterday, her headache remained. She reported nausea right after the visit. While cooking dinner that night she reported dizziness. "I turned my head to the left, and the room started spinning and I felt nauseous. It lasted only a second." Today she reports similar episodes of spinning that have lasted longer periods associated with nausea. Physical examination reveals a normal vascular exam without bruits. There is no hearing deficit. Neurologic exam is

significant for horizontal nystagmus and mild left eyelid ptosis. Which of the following is the most likely cause of her vertigo?
a) Benign positional vertigo
b) Vestibular neuritis
c) Cerebrobasilar stroke
d) Migraine
e) Cholesteatoma

Answer and Discussion

The answer is c. Vertigo is defined as an illusion of movement and always reflects a disorder of the vestibular system. Vertigo originating from the central nervous system tends to spare hearing, produce less torsional vertigo, and be associated with other brainstem symptoms and signs, such as double vision, dysarthria, and ataxia. The horizontal nystagmus is concerning for cerebrobasilar stroke and consistent with her recent neck manipulation by her chiropractor. Although uncommon, extreme or abrupt twisting of the neck can damage the inner layer of vertebral arteries.

4. A 23-year-old man presents to your office after recently being discharged from the hospital for new-onset seizures and a diagnosis of epilepsy. He is currently taking valproic acid as prescribed and denies any seizures for the past 2 weeks. He works as an electrician and drives a company van to and from his jobs. He is often climbing ladders and working with "live" wires. Which of the following is the most accurate statement in regard to returning to normal daily activities?
a) He should not be driving until he has been seizure free for 6 to 12 months.
b) As long as his valproic acid level is therapeutic, he may return to normal activities, including driving.
c) Epileptics, regardless of seizure control, should not climb ladders or work with heavy machinery.
d) He will need approval from the Bureau of Motor Vehicles and a special driver's license to return to his job.

Answer and Discussion

The answer is a. Seizures can be associated with a sudden alteration of consciousness that may interfere with the activities of daily living or put the patient in a dangerous situation. In general, patients should not drive unless the seizures are under control. Each state within the United States, as well as other countries, has specific rules about what is meant by the phrase "seizure free for a long enough period." Generally, this period ranges between 6 and 12 months without a seizure while on an appropriate antiepileptic drug regimen. Some states require that the physician report such cases to the Registry of Motor Vehicles; in other states, this is not necessary. Familiarity with local laws on this subject is recommended. Other activities such as swimming, bathing, operating heavy machinery, and climbing great heights are usually not regulated specifically, but should be avoided when unsupervised.

5. A 65-year-old man presented to the emergency department after awakening with right-sided weakness. His family says that for about a year he has complained of brief episodes of blurred vision in his left eye. On the evening before admission, he had a short period of word-finding difficulty, which cleared after about 5 minutes, and he seemed to be normal when he retired for the night. On examination, his blood pressure is 160/100 mm Hg. The neurologic examination shows a mild degree of naming difficulty and mild pronation of the right arm on extension of the limb. Circumduction of the right leg occurs when walking, and mild deficits to all sensory modalities can be discerned on the right side. Reflexes are 2+ on the left and 1+ on the right, and a right-sided Babinski's sign is present. Carotid pulses are faint but palpable bilaterally without bruits. Flow in the external carotid branches on the face cannot be estimated clinically. During the examination, he has a 5-minute episode of dense right hemiplegia and mutism, from which he recovers and returns to his baseline state as described. Which of the following is the most accurate statement?

a) This patient has a right middle cerebral artery disorder.

b) Given the resolution between attacks, any impending stroke is likely to be mild.

c) The physical examination yields little information about the severity of carotid disease.

d) Dynamic palpations of facial pulses can distinguish a tight stenosis from occlusion of the internal carotid artery.

e) Neurodiagnostic studies must be performed in all patients with transient ischemic attacks.

Answer and Discussion

The answer is c. This patient is complaining of episodes of transient ischemic attacks (TIAs). A TIA is defined as the sudden onset of a neurologic deficit that fits a vascular territory and lasts less than 24 hours. This patient's spell fits a disorder in the distribution of a left middle cerebral artery. Although the spells seem mild and completely disappear between attacks, one should not feel comfortable that this does not foreshadow a serious subsequent stroke. There is no way to predict, based on the severity of the attack or its quality, whether a patient will go on to develop a stroke and whether this stroke will be severe or mild. The physical examination yields little information about the severity of carotid disease. The presence or absence of a cervical bruit is nearly useless, although bruits often represent vascular disease; however, the bruit may be on the wrong side (as in this patient) or not present at all if flow through a tight stenosis is slowed sufficiently. Dynamic palpations of facial pulses are a way of evaluating the direction of flow in the external carotid branches in the face. With a tight stenosis or occlusion of the internal carotid distal to the takeoff of the external carotid, it is often possible to demonstrate reversed flow in the branches of the external carotid artery of the face. This test, however, does not distinguish between a tight stenosis and an occlusion, an important distinction because surgical intervention is possible only in a case of tight stenosis, not in a case of total occlusion. Once it is recognized that this patient is undergoing TIAs in the distribution of the left carotid, the most difficult decision will involve which maneuver should be carried out next. Some experienced physicians would not investigate such a patient any further but would simply give the patient aspirin. Most experienced neurologists and neurosurgeons probably would carry out some form of neurodiagnostic study to evaluate the carotid. The simplest test, which gives the most information, is a magnetic resonance angiogram. This obtains a reasonably good angiogram at the lowest risk. If a tight carotid stenosis is found, most experienced neurologists would recommend a carotid endarterectomy done by an experienced neurosurgeon or vascular surgeon. If the carotid is occluded, most physicians would recommend the use of aspirin in an attempt to prevent further TIAs, which may be due to platelet emboli from the distal stump of the occlusion. If no carotid disease is found, a careful evaluation of the heart would follow, including transesophageal echocardiography, a set of blood cultures, and a careful cardiac examination, probably including a Holter monitor study.

SUGGESTED READINGS

Brott T, Bogousslavsky J. Treatment of acute ischemic stroke. *N Engl J Med* 2000;343(10):710–722.

French JA, Kanner AM, Bautista J, et al. Efficacy and tolerability of the new antiepileptic drugs I: treatment of new onset epilepsy: report of the Therapeutics and Technology Assessment Subcommittee and Quality Standards Subcommittee of the American Academy of Neurology and the American Epilepsy Society. *Neurology* 2004;62:1252–1260.

Gamaldo CE, Earley CJ. Restless legs syndrome: a clinical update. *Chest* 2006;130(5):1596–1604.

Hughes RAC, Wijdicks EFM, Barohn R, et al. Practice parameter: immunotherapy for Guillain-Barré syndrome: report of the Quality Standards Subcommittee of the American Academy of Neurology. *Neurology* 2003;61:736–740.

Krumholz A, Wiebe S, Gronseth G, et al. Practice parameter: evaluating an apparent unprovoked first seizure in adults (an evidence-based review): report of the Quality Standards Subcommittee of the American Academy of Neurology and the American Epilepsy Society. *Neurology* 2007;69:1996–2007.

McDonald WI, Compston A, Edan G, et al. Recommended diagnostic criteria for multiple sclerosis: guidelines from the International Panel on the Diagnosis of multiple sclerosis. *Ann Neurol* 2001;50(1):121–127.

Silberstein SD. Practice parameter: evidence-based guidelines for migraine headache (an evidence-based review): report of the Quality Standards Subcommittee of the American Academy of Neurology. *Neurology* 2000;55:754–762.

Silberstein SD, Lipton RB, Goadsby PJ. *Headache in Clinical Practice*, 2nd ed. London: Taylor & Francis, 2002.

Suchowersky O, Reich S, Perlmutter J, et al. Practice parameter: diagnosis and prognosis of new onset Parkinson disease (an evidence-based review): report of the Quality Standards Subcommittee of the American Academy of Neurology. *Neurology* 2006;66: 968–975.

Van der Worp H, van Gijn J. Acute ischemic stroke. *N Engl J Med* 2007;357(6):572–579.

Weinstein JN, Tosteson TD, Lurie JD, et al. Surgical vs nonoperative treatment for lumbar disk herniation: the Spine Patient Outcomes Research Trial (SPORT) observational cohort. *JAMA* 2006;296:2451–2459.

Chapter 13

Sexually Transmitted Diseases

Kristin A. Englund   Carlos M. Isada

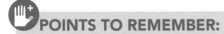

POINTS TO REMEMBER:

- Complications arising from nongonococcal urethritis include epididymitis and reactive arthritis. Partner notification is important because female sexual partners are at high risk for chlamydial infection and its complications.

- In women, gonococcal infections are often asymptomatic.

- An increasing spread of quinolone-resistant *Neisseria gonorrhoeae* has occurred to the extent that quinolone use is not recommended.

- Twenty to 25% of the U.S. adult population is infected with genital herpes.

- In all 50 states and the District of Columbia, adolescents can receive medical care for sexually transmitted diseases without parental consent.

Sexually transmitted diseases (STDs) remain among the most common problems encountered in the practice of general internal medicine. Despite their ubiquity, STDs remain a diagnostic and therapeutic challenge. This chapter focuses on the clinical manifestations, diagnosis, and treatment of the classic STDs, with emphasis on common clinical syndromes and their differential diagnoses. The topics of vaginitis and genital warts are also discussed. Treatment recommendations are based on the 2006 guidelines from the Centers for Disease Control and Prevention (CDC).

URETHRITIS AND CERVICITIS

Urethritis

In sexually active men, urethritis is characterized by dysuria and discharge of purulent material from the urethra. It is traditionally divided into two types: gonococcal and nongonococcal. Diagnostic testing to identify the offending pathogen is presently recommended because (a) both infections are reportable to state health departments, (b) treatment compliance may be better with a specific diagnosis, and (c) partner notification and treatment may be improved. The CDC recommends that if the diagnostic means are not available, patients should be treated for both gonococcal and chlamydial infections, although establishing a specific microbiological diagnosis is preferred.

Nongonococcal Urethritis

Etiology and Clinical Manifestations

Chlamydia trachomatis is the most common cause of nongonococcal urethritis (NGU), accounting for approximately 50% of cases, although the frequency is variable, depending on the case series. In males who have NGU but test negative for *C. trachomatis*, establishing an etiology is often difficult. *Ureaplasma urealyticum, Trichomonas vaginalis*, and herpes simplex virus (HSV) account for approximately 15% of cases. No etiologic diagnosis is found in up to 35% of cases.

NGU tends to have a more indolent presentation compared with gonococcal urethritis. The incubation period of NGU is 1 to 3 weeks. A mucoid or watery discharge from the urethra is the typical clinical presentation, although up to 25% of infected men may be asymptomatic. Fevers and chills are unusual, and symptoms of urinary tract infection are usually absent; patients may have some dysuria or itching, but hematuria, urinary frequency, or pelvic pain are unusual.

Complications arising from NGU include epididymitis and reactive arthritis. Partner notification is important because female sexual partners are at high risk for chlamydial infection and its complications.

Laboratory Diagnosis

It is important to objectively confirm the presence of urethritis in all suspected cases, particularly because some patients may present with vague or nonspecific genital symptoms. Urethritis can be diagnosed on clinical grounds alone when a purulent urethral discharge is found on physical examination, either on initial inspection or by milking the penis from the base to the glans. In less clear cases, however, urethritis can also be diagnosed by either of the following: (a) presence of five or more polymorphonuclear leukocytes per oil immersion field on a smear of a urethral swab specimen, or (b) a positive leukocyte esterase test from a first-void urine specimen or first-void urine with ≥ 10 white blood cells (WBCs) per high-power field. Although the leukocyte esterase test is convenient, a positive test result should be confirmed with a Gram-stained smear of a urethral swab specimen.

NGU is confirmed when a male meets one or more of the previous criteria and shows no evidence of gram-negative intracellular diplococci on Gram stain. Urethra specimens should be submitted routinely for detection of *N. gonorrhoeae* and *C. trachomatis*. A number of different nucleic acid amplification systems are available that are more sensitive than traditional culture techniques, particularly for *C. trachomatis*. Persons who present with nonspecific genitourethral symptoms and who fail to meet objective criteria for urethritis should still be tested for *C. trachomatis* and *N. gonorrhoeae* because if infection is minimally symptomatic, antibiotic treatment is generally deferred. In some instances, the empiric treatment of urethral symptoms in the absence of documented urethritis may be considered if the patient is unlikely to return for follow-up if contacted.

Therapy

Regimens presently recommended by the CDC for the treatment of NGU include:

- Doxycycline, 100 mg orally twice daily for 7 days, or
- Azithromycin, 1 g orally (single dose)

  Alternative regimens include:

- Erythromycin base, 500 mg orally four times daily for 7 days, or
- Erythromycin ethylsuccinate, 800 mg orally four times daily for 7 days, or
- Ofloxacin (Floxin), 300 mg orally twice daily for 7 days, or
- Levofloxacin, 500 mg orally once daily for 7 days

Mucopurulent Cervicitis

Etiology and Clinical Manifestations

The major infectious causes of mucopurulent cervicitis (MPC) include *C. trachomatis, N. gonorrhoeae*, and HSV. In many women, however, no organism is isolated. The CDC recommends that patients with MPC have cervical specimens tested for *C. trachomatis* and *N. gonorrhoeae*.

In sexually active women, MPC is the counterpart to urethritis in men. It is characterized by a yellow endocervical exudate that can be seen in the endocervical canal or on a swab of cervical secretions. In many women, the infection is minimally symptomatic or completely asymptomatic; others may have abnormal vaginal bleeding after intercourse. Serious complications of MPC include pelvic inflammatory disease (PID), tubal infertility, ectopic pregnancy, and chronic pelvic pain.

Laboratory Diagnosis

The diagnosis of MPC is supported by the visualization of yellow or green endocervical mucopus on a white swab (positive swab test result). The utility of the Gram stain of an endocervical swab specimen for confirming MPC is somewhat controversial. The presence of ten or more polymorphonuclear leukocytes per high-powered field of a Gram-stained specimen of endocervical mucopus correlates with the presence of recognized infectious causes of MPC. This test has a number of limitations, however, including a poor positive predictive value; it is not as clinically useful as the Gram stain of urethral exudates in males with urethritis. It is important to emphasize that most women with *C. trachomatis* or *N. gonorrhoeae* infection *do not* have active MPC.

Therapy

The therapy of MPC should be guided by the results of specific testing for *C. trachomatis* or *N. gonorrhoeae*. In patients unlikely to return for follow-up, treatment for both pathogens should be initiated. Treatment should cover both organisms if the likelihood of infection with either organism is high in a particular population. Current population-specific treatment recommendations from the CDC include the following:

- If there is a high prevalence of both *C. trachomatis* and *N. gonorrhoeae* (as in many STD clinics), treat for both agents.
- If the incidence of *N. gonorrhoeae* is low in the population and the likelihood of *C. trachomatis* is high, treat for chlamydial infection only.
- If both infections are uncommon, and if the likelihood of compliance for a return visit is good, await test results to guide specific therapy.

Chlamydia trachomatis Infection

Epidemiology and Clinical Manifestations

C. trachomatis is the most common bacterial STD in the United States. Approximately 2.8 million Americans are infected with this organism each year. The majority of these infections are asymptomatic, with asymptomatic infection in three-fourths of women with documented infection and about one-half of males. Teenage girls and young women are particularly predisposed to infection because the cervix has not fully matured. In women, the organism first infects the cervix and/or urethra. *C. trachomatis* may produce a variety of clinical syndromes, including urethritis, cervicitis, and proctocolitis in men who have sex with men (MSM). Approximately 40% of untreated infections in women progress from the cervix to involve the fallopian tubes or the uterus. *C. trachomatis* is a major contributing pathogen in women with PID, particularly in those with multiple reinfections. A number of women with PID suffer long-term complications, such as chronic pelvic pain, ectopic pregnancy, and infertility (about one-fifth). In addition, women with chlamydial infection are five times more likely to develop HIV if they become exposed. For these reasons, the CDC has expanded its recommendations for chlamydia screening among women. The CDC recommends routine annual screening for *C. trachomatis* in all sexually active adolescents and sexually active women 25 years of age or younger, including those who are asymptomatic. Annual screening is also recommended for older women with risk factors for infection, such as a new sexual partner or multiple partners. Because many of these infections are asymptomatic, the CDC recommends aggressive treatment for patients with *C. trachomatis* infection, as well as for their partners, even if asymptomatic, particularly those who have new or multiple sexual partners or who do not consistently use barrier contraceptives. Some women

with apparently uncomplicated cervical *C. trachomatis* infections are likely to have subclinical upper reproductive tract involvement and are thus at high risk for PID, ectopic pregnancy, and infertility. The treatment of such cervical infections likely reduces these sequelae.

Therapy

Current recommendations from the CDC for the treatment of uncomplicated chlamydial infection include the following regimens:

- Doxycycline, 100 mg orally twice daily for 7 days, or
- Azithromycin, 1 g orally (one dose)

The efficacy of doxycycline and azithromycin is comparable, provided the patient is adherent to the 7-day regimen of doxycycline. Azithromycin has the advantage of single-dose administration, which is particularly attractive in noncompliant patients. However, doxycycline has a longer history of safety, efficacy, and use, and is much less expensive.

Alternative regimens for the treatment of chlamydial infection include:

- Ofloxacin, 300 mg orally twice daily for 7 days, or
- Erythromycin base, 500 mg orally four times daily for 7 days, or
- Erythromycin ethylsuccinate, 800 mg orally four times daily for 7 days, or
- Levofloxacin, 500 mg orally for 7 days.

Ofloxacin and levofloxacin have been proven effective against *C. trachomatis*, but clinical trials have shown no advantage in efficacy compared with doxycycline. Both fluoroquinolones are expensive and have no dosing advantages over doxycycline. Other fluoroquinolones are not as yet recommended.

A routine test of cure for chlamydia soon after treatment with doxycycline or azithromycin (less than 3 weeks) is not recommended; the value of early retesting has not been proven and some of the nucleic acid–based tests for *C. trachomatis* may remain positive at 3 weeks despite microbiological eradication by traditional culture methods.

In contrast, it is now recommended by the CDC that women with documented chlamydial infections undergo routine rescreening 3 to 12 months after the completion of treatment. This guideline was issued due to the high prevalence of chlamydia found in women who had been diagnosed and treated in the preceding months, presumably from reinfection rather than failure of the initial antibiotic course.

The sexual partners of patients with chlamydial infection should be referred for evaluation and treatment. All partners of symptomatic patients with chlamydial infection should be treated if the last sexual contact with the index patient occurred within 30 days from the onset of the index patient's symptoms. If the index patient is asymptomatic, all sexual partners whose last sexual contact with the index patient occurred within 60 days of diagnosis should be evaluated and treated. In partners of index patients who fulfill neither of these criteria, the most recent sexual partner of the index patient should be treated even if the last sexual contact occurred beyond these time intervals.

For pregnant women with chlamydial infection, the CDC recommends the following regimen:

- Azithromycin, 1 g orally as a single dose, or
- Amoxicillin, 500 mg orally three times daily for 7 days

An alternative regimen includes:

- Erythromycin base, 500 mg orally four times daily for 7 days, or
- Erythromycin base, 250 mg orally four times a day for 14 days, or
- Erythromycin ethylsuccinate, 800 mg orally four times a day for 7 days, or
- Erythromycin ethylsuccinate, 400 mg orally four times a day for 14 days

Retesting at 3 weeks after completion of the treatment regimen is recommended in pregnancy. Doxycycline, ofloxacin, and erythromycin estolate are contraindicated during pregnancy.

GONOCOCCAL INFECTION

Gonorrhea

Gonorrhea remains endemic in the United States, despite public health measures to track and eradicate the infection. It is estimated that more than 600,000 new cases occur annually in this country. In men, gonococcal infection is usually sufficiently symptomatic for patients to seek medical care. In women, gonococcal infections are often asymptomatic, and a significant proportion of symptoms is nonspecific and may be confused with common vaginal or bladder infections. Women are at risk for complications such as PID, infertility, and ectopic pregnancy. Because of this, the CDC recommends screening high-risk women for gonorrhea, even if asymptomatic.

Therapy

Several factors influence the therapy of patients with suspected or confirmed gonococcal infection. Over the past 20 years, resistant strains of *N. gonorrhoeae* have become increasingly common. These include penicillinase-producing and tetracycline-resistant organisms, as well as strains with chromosomally mediated resistance to multiple antimicrobial agents. In recent years, an increasing spread of quinolone-resistant *N. gonorrhoeae* has occurred to the extent that quinolone use is not recommended. In addition, patients with gonococcal infection are frequently coinfected with *C. trachomatis*, thus making empiric therapy for this infection mandatory for most individuals. This strategy of dual therapy is usually accompanied by specific labora-

tory testing for *C. trachomatis*; however, in some situations, testing for chlamydia in persons with gonococcal infection may be deferred because of financial constraints. In most circumstances, it is recommended that persons with gonococcal infection be treated and tested for chlamydia.

The current CDC treatment recommendations for uncomplicated urethral, endocervical, and rectal gonorrhea are as follows:

- Ceftriaxone, 125 mg intramuscularly (IM) (single dose, 99.1% cure), or
- Cefixime (Suprax), 400 mg orally (single dose, 97.1% cure) (available in the United States only as a suspension)

Alternative regimens for uncomplicated gonococcal infection include:

- Spectinomycin (Trobicin), 2 g IM (single dose) (not available in the United States), or
- Injectable cephalosporin: ceftizoxime (Cefizox), cefotaxime (Claforan), cefotetan (Cefotan), or cefoxitin (Mefoxin), or
- Cefuroxime (Ceftin), 1 g orally (single dose)

For severe PCN or cephalosporin-resistant patients, a single 2-g dose of azithromycin can be used for uncomplicated gonococcal infections, but the CDC does not recommend widespread use of this because there is concern for the rapid development of azithromycin resistance.

In recent years, the CDC has reported a significant increase in quinolone-resistant *N. gonorrhoeae* (QRNG). In 2002, the CDC recommended that fluoroquinolones should be avoided in patients whose gonorrhea was acquired in Asia, Hawaii, other Pacific islands, California, and some other areas of the world such as England and Wales. In 2004, the CDC noted that local and national data showed a 5% prevalence of QRNG in MSM. This led to the 2004 recommendation that fluoroquinolones not be used to treat known or suspected gonorrhea in MSM, unless susceptibility testing or tests of cure were available. In April 2007, the CDC again updated their recommendations to completely eliminate fluoroquinolone use for gonococcal treatment because QRNG levels had reached 13.3% nationally, 8.6% excluding California and Hawaii.

Management of Sexual Partners

All sexual partners of symptomatic individuals with gonococcal infection should be evaluated and treated for both gonorrhea and chlamydial infection if their last sexual contact with the index patient was within 30 days of the onset of the patient's symptoms. If the index patient has no symptoms, sexual partners whose last sexual contact with the index patient was less than 60 days from the diagnosis should be evaluated and treated. In circumstances in which no partners fulfill these criteria, the most recent sexual partner should be treated, even if the last sexual contact took place beyond these time periods.

TABLE 13.1

CLINICAL MANIFESTATIONS OF DISSEMINATED GONOCOCCAL INFECTION

Common	Unusual	Rare
Fever	Endocarditis	Pneumonia
Leukocytosis	Meningitis	Adult respiratory distress syndrome
Skin lesions	Perihepatitis	
Tenosynovitis		Osteomyelitis
Polyarthralgia		
Oligoarthritis		
Hepatitis		
Myopericarditis		

Disseminated Gonococcal Infection

Etiology and Clinical Manifestations

In the past, disseminated gonococcal infection (DGI) was invariably produced by penicillin-susceptible strains of *N. gonorrhoeae*. In more recent years, however, documented cases of DGI due to penicillinase-producing strains and QRNG have been described. In this unique clinical syndrome, patients may exhibit a number of clinical manifestations, as summarized in Table 13.1.

The differential diagnosis of patients with suspected DGI includes infections such as meningococcemia, endocarditis, septic arthritis, infectious tenosynovitis, and other bacteremias; seronegative arthritides such as Reiter's syndrome, ankylosing spondylitis, psoriatic arthritis, and dermal vasculitis; and collagen vascular diseases such as systemic lupus erythematosus.

Diagnosis

The diagnosis of DGI should be suspected in individuals with the classic hemorrhagic pustules and symptoms of tenosynovitis or oligoarthritis. Skin lesions may be relatively asymptomatic and should be carefully sought. Usually, less than ten lesions are evident. In those with suspected DGI, cultures for *N. gonorrhoeae* should be obtained from skin lesions, joint fluid, blood, and mucosal surfaces such as the urethra, cervix, rectum, and pharynx. The diagnostic sensitivity of culture, Gram stain, and immunofluorescent testing are summarized in Table 13.2.

Therapy

The treatment for DGI should be initiated in the hospital with the administration of ceftriaxone, 1 g IM or intravenously (IV) every 24 hours, based on CDC recommendations in 2006. Alternative regimens include cefotaxime, 1 g IV every 8 hours, or ceftizoxime, 1 g IV every 8 hours. For patients allergic to β-lactam agents, the acceptable alternative is spectinomycin. Twenty-four to 48 hours after improvement, the patient can be switched to an oral regimen such as cefixime, 400 mg twice a day (400-mg tablet or by suspension 200 mg/5 mL), or cefpodoxime, 400 mg orally twice daily. This oral regimen should be continued to complete at least 1 week of therapy. Fluoroquinolones should only be used if culture and susceptibility data can be obtained.

Genital Ulceration With Regional Lymphadenopathy

The syndrome of genital ulceration with regional lymphadenopathy is characteristic of five of the six classic STDs: primary syphilis, primary genital HSV infection, chancroid, lymphogranuloma venereum (LGV), and granuloma inguinale (donovanosis) (Table 13.3). Of note, gonorrhea is not a cause of this syndrome. Genital ulcers are frequently misdiagnosed as to cause when the history and physical examination are used alone; thus, laboratory tests are important to confirm the clinical suspicion. An increased risk of HIV infection is associated with each of these infections. HIV testing should be performed in the management of patients who have genital ulcers caused by *Treponema pallidum* or *Haemophilus ducreyi*, and it should be considered in those who have ulcers caused by HSV.

Genital HSV infection is the most common cause of the syndrome of genital ulceration with regional lymphadenopathy in the United States. Based on serologic studies, it is estimated that approximately 50 million individuals in the United States are infected with HSV type 2 (HSV-2). The second most common cause of this syndrome in the United States is primary syphilis. Other infectious causes (the so-called minor venereal diseases), although common in other parts of the world, are relatively uncommon in the United States, although outbreaks have been reported. The diagnostic evaluation of patients with genital

TABLE 13.2

DISSEMINATED GONOCOCCAL INFECTION: DIAGNOSIS

Site	Patients With Positive Test Results (%)		
	Culture	Gram Stain	Immunofluorescence
Skin lesions	10	10	60
Joint fluid	20–30	10–30	25
Blood	10–30	—	—
Mucosal (pharynx, urethra, cervix, rectum)	80–90	—	—

TABLE 13.3

GENITAL ULCERATION WITH REGIONAL LYMPHADENOPATHY: SUMMARY OF CLINICAL MANIFESTATIONS

Genital Lesions	Incubation (days)	Type	Pain	Number	Duration
Primary syphilis	3–90	Clean ulcer, raised	No	Usually single	3–6 weeks
Primary herpes simplex virus	1–26	Grouped papules, vesicles, pustules, ulcers	Yes	Often multiple	1–3 weeks
Chancroid	1–21	Purulent ulcer, shaggy border	Yes	Single in men, multiple in women	Progressive
Lymphogranuloma venereum	3–21	Papule, vesicle, ulcer	No	Usually single	Few days
Granuloma inguinale	8–80	Nodules, coalescing granulomatous ulcers	No	Single or multiple	Progressive

Inguinal Adenopathy	Onset	Pain	Type	Frequency	Constitutional Symptoms
Primary syphilis	Same time	No	Firm	80%, 70% bilateral	Absent
Primary herpes simplex virus	Same time	Yes	Firm	80%, usually bilateral	Common
Chancroid	Same time	Yes	Fluctuant, may fistulize	50%–65%, usually unilateral	Uncommon
Lymphogranuloma venereum	26 weeks later	Yes	Indurated, fluctuant, may fistulize	Unilateral, one-third bilateral	Common
Granuloma inguinale	Variable		Suppurating pseudobubo	10%	15%

ulceration and regional lymphadenopathy is summarized in Table 13.4.

Primary Herpes Simplex Virus Infection

Etiology and Clinical Manifestations

Genital herpes may be produced by either HSV type 1 (HSV-1) or HSV-2. In the United States, HSV-2 accounts for the majority of cases of genital HSV, although in some groups (particularly teenage populations), almost 30% of cases may be from HSV-1. In other parts of the world, such as Japan, HSV-1 produces the majority of cases. The presence of HSV-2 antibody indicates prior anogenital infection (symptomatic or not) because HSV-2 is a very rare cause of

TABLE 13.4

GENITAL ULCERS: RECOMMENDED DIAGNOSTIC EVALUATION

Serologic test for syphilis
Dark-field examination or direct immunofluorescence test for *Treponema pallidum*
Culture or antigen test for herpes simplex virus

In Selected Cases
- Culture for *Haemophilus ducreyi*
- Lymphogranuloma venereum titers
- Biopsy for Donovan bodies

oral herpes infections. In contrast, the presence of HSV-1 antibodies is very common in the general population due to prior oral herpes infections; thus, it is not useful in distinguishing orolabial from anogenital herpes.

The incubation period after exposure for primary genital HSV infection is 1 to 26 days, with an average of 1 week. Before lesions appear, patients may complain of burning or pruritus. The initial lesions are grouped papules, which are often painful. They progress to vesicles and pustules, and then form small, clean-based ulcerations. Inguinal lymphadenopathy, usually bilateral, is apparent at the same time as the genital lesions in approximately 80% of patients. The nodes are firm and painful.

Primary genital HSV infection may be a systemic illness, and constitutional symptoms are common. Patients frequently complain of low-grade fever, malaise, headache, and fatigue. In severe cases, patients with primary HSV infection may present with aseptic meningitis, pelvic radiculomyelitis, flank pain simulating pyelonephritis, or abdominal pain resembling a surgical abdomen.

Based on recent studies using newer techniques for serologic testing, it is estimated that 20% to 25% of the adult U.S. population is infected with genital herpes. Many infections go unrecognized by both physicians and patients. The majority of genital herpes cases do not present in a "classic" manner. About 10% to 20% of persons with genital herpes will have genital ulcers, 10% to 20% will be asymptomatic, and 60% will have atypical symptoms such as genital itching, back pain, leg pain, vaginal discharge, and other nonspecific symptoms.

Diagnosis

Although the presence of grouped vesicles in the genital region is nearly pathognomonic for HSV infection, many patients present later in the course of the infection, when vesicles have already ulcerated. Thus, laboratory confirmation is important in many instances. Several methods are available for confirming the presence of HSV in genital ulcerations. The *Tzanck smear* evaluates cytologic detection of cellular changes and is insensitive and non–type specific. It is rarely used today. Definitive diagnosis is still established by the isolation of HSV in tissue culture, a technique available in most laboratories. In most cases, the turnaround time to isolation of the virus is short (relative to other viruses, such as varicella zoster virus or cytomegalovirus) because HSV grows rapidly and well in tissue culture systems. Alternative methods for HSV detection include several enzyme immunoassays that identify HSV-1 and HSV-2 antigen directly in clinical specimens. HSV can also be detected using the polymerase chain reaction (PCR) technique. It should be noted that a number of patients with primary HSV-2 or HSV-1 genital infection will be culture negative, particularly if the lesions have already crusted. False-negative cultures are even more common with recurrent genital HSV.

Serologic studies may be useful in certain patients with culture-negative primary infections. The detection of specific HSV immunoglobulin M (IgM) strongly suggests recent infection. However, IgM antibody may also be detectable in some individuals during recurrent episodes of genital HSV infection. A fourfold rise in HSV immunoglobulin G (IgG) between the acute and convalescent periods is also diagnostic of a primary HSV episode.

Recently, newer serologic tests with high specificity for the detection of HSV-2 and HSV-1 antibodies have been made commercially available. Older serologic tests for HSV-2 and HSV-1 lacked specificity and had limited clinical utility. Newer tests are based on the detection of the HSV-specific glycoprotein G2 for HSV-2 infection and glycoprotein G1 for HSV-1 infection; the sensitivity is in the range of 80% to 98%, and specificity is about 96%. These glycoprotein-based tests are useful in diagnosing culture-negative HSV-2 infections. Type-specific serologic tests can also be used to identify persons with atypical symptoms and to evaluate the sex partners of persons with genital herpes infections. Screening of the general population is not recommended.

Therapy

First Episode of Herpes Simplex Virus Infection

The first episode of HSV infection should be treated for 7 to 10 days with one of the following regimens:

- Acyclovir (Zovirax), 400 mg three times daily, or
- Acyclovir (Zovirax), 200 mg five times daily, or

- Famciclovir (Famvir), 250 mg orally three times daily, or
- Valacyclovir (Valtrex), 1 g orally twice daily

Longer treatment courses may be necessary in some cases. Patients with severe disease or with complications of primary HSV infection such as pneumonitis, encephalitis, or hepatitis may be treated with acyclovir, 5 mg/kg IV every 8 hours for 5 to 7 days. Acyclovir shortens the course of primary HSV infection and accelerates viral clearance and healing of ulcers. It has no effect, however, on the rate of subsequent recurrences. The drug is active only against replicating virus and does not target latent HSV. Topical acyclovir is less effective than acyclovir given orally.

The safety of acyclovir in pregnancy has not been definitively established, although limited available data do not show an increased risk of major birth defects in those exposed to acyclovir during the first trimester. Thus, acyclovir may be used in pregnant women with first-episode genital herpes and severe recurrent HSV disease. Data for valacyclovir or famciclovir are too limited to be able to make recommendations during pregnancy

Recurrent Episodes

Recurrences of genital HSV infection are common and problematic. Recurrent attacks are less frequently associated with regional lymphadenopathy and constitutional symptoms than primary HSV infection. In addition, genital lesions associated with recurrent episodes heal more quickly than do those of primary HSV infection. False-negative cultures for HSV are more common than with primary infection, and it is estimated that, on average, only 20% of cultures are positive during a recurrence.

In addition to recurrent ulcers, persons with genital herpes frequently demonstrate asymptomatic shedding of the virus, which is potentially transmissible to a susceptible partner. More than 90% of persons with genital HSV-2 shed live virus at some point after the primary infection. In the first few years after primary infection, it is estimated that virus is shed on 10% to 20% of days in the absence of visible lesions.

The number of recurrences is highly variable. Recurrences are much more common with genital infection from HSV-2 than HSV-1. On average, persons with genital HSV-2 experience four outbreaks in the first year following primary infection, which subsequently decreases by 0.5 outbreaks per year for subsequent years; however, this is only an average rate, and the actual number in an individual person is difficult to predict.

The optimal therapy for recurrent attacks remains controversial. Data from large studies suggest that acyclovir is of limited benefit when recurrent episodes are treated individually, shortening the duration of viral shedding and the time to crusting of lesions by less than 1 day. No beneficial effect is seen on the rate of recurrences. In severe recurrent disease, some individuals start acyclovir at the start of the prodrome and continue therapy for 5 days. Possible regimens include

- Oral acyclovir, 400 mg three times daily for 5 days, or
- Acyclovir, 800 mg twice daily for 5 days, or
- Acyclovir, 800 mg three times daily for 2 days

Alternative regimens include:

- Famciclovir, 125 mg orally twice daily for 5 days, or
- Famciclovir, 1,000 mg twice daily for 1 day, or
- Valacyclovir, 500 mg orally twice daily for 3 days, or
- Valacyclovir, 1.0 g once daily for 5 days

Daily Suppressive Therapy

Another approach for patients with frequent severe recurrences is daily suppressive acyclovir therapy. Studies have shown that individuals with frequent recurrences of HSV infection, defined as six or more outbreaks per year, may have a 75% reduction in the number of recurrences using daily suppressive therapy. Chronic suppression using acyclovir appears to be safe for up to 6 years, and for 1 year with famciclovir and valacyclovir; however, the U.S. Public Health Service recommends a 1-year course followed by reassessment of the need for daily therapy. Acyclovir-resistant HSV has been isolated from patients on suppressive therapy, but this has not been clearly associated with treatment failure. One limitation of daily suppressive therapy is its lack of long-term benefit; the frequency of outbreaks often returns to baseline once acyclovir is discontinued. Recommended regimens for daily suppressive therapy include:

- Acyclovir, 400 mg orally twice daily, or
- Famciclovir, 250 mg orally twice daily, or
- Valacyclovir, 500 mg orally daily, or 1 g orally daily

Genital Herpes Treatment in AIDS

Severe progressive HSV infections were commonly seen in individuals with AIDS in the era before highly active antiretroviral therapy (HAART). Fortunately, these infections are less common with the advent of HAART. Progressive genital and perianal ulcers with proctocolitis may be due to either HSV-1 or HSV-2 in persons with HIV. When HSV proctitis occurs, it may be quite debilitating, with anorectal pain, bloody stools, and fever. In patients with advanced immunodeficiency and HSV proctitis, recurrences are common. Such patients with AIDS are often placed on chronic suppressive acyclovir therapy. This has led to reports of the emergence of acyclovir-resistant HSV mutants. Recurrent episodes are often suppressed using daily acyclovir, especially if severe or associated with HSV proctitis. The dosage of acyclovir in this setting is controversial. In 2006, the CDC recommended acyclovir, 400 to 800 mg orally two to three times daily; famciclovir, 500 mg orally twice a day; or valacyclovir, 500 mg orally twice a day. For episodic treatment of genital herpes in HIV, several regimens may be used for 5 to 10 days, including:

- Acyclovir, 400 mg orally three times daily, or
- Famciclovir, 500 mg orally twice daily, or
- Valacyclovir, 1 gram orally twice daily

If lesions fail to heal while on appropriate therapy, the possibility of a drug-resistant HSV isolate should be considered, and culture should be obtained for susceptibility testing. Acyclovir-resistant HSV isolates are also usually cross-resistant to famciclovir and valacyclovir, and generally require alternative treatments such as foscarnet and cidofovir. This problem seems to have decreased with the advent of antiretroviral therapy.

CHANCROID

Etiology and Clinical Manifestations

Chancroid is caused by *H. ducreyi*, a gram-negative coccobacillus. Although uncommon in the United States, its worldwide incidence may exceed that of syphilis. In the 1980s, there was a marked increase in reported chancroid cases, mostly clustered in Florida, New York City, California, and Boston. The reported incidence of chancroid has declined over the past two decades, but that is likely due to underreporting. Chancroid and other genital ulcerative diseases are known cofactors for HIV transmission, and an estimated 10% of patients who have chancroid could be coinfected with *T. pallidum* or HSV.

After exposure, the incubation period for chancroid is 1 to 21 days, with an average of 7 days. Chancroid ulcers are painful, deep, shaggy, and friable, and their borders are undermined. Ulcers are commonly single in men but multiple in women.

Regional adenopathy occurs simultaneously with the ulcer and is seen in 50% to 65% of patients. The nodes are quite tender and tend to be unilateral. In addition, they tend to become fluctuant and can easily fistulize. The combination of a painful ulcer with suppurative inguinal lymphadenopathy is almost diagnostic of chancroid. Constitutional symptoms are uncommon.

Diagnosis

The isolation of *H. ducreyi* from an active genital ulcer is the only definitive means of confirming the diagnosis of chancroid. Special media and culture techniques are required to isolate this fastidious organism, and this special media is not widely available in the United States. Gram stain of an ulcer specimen may be misleading because of the presence of polymicrobial flora colonizing genital ulcers, and culture confirmation remains the gold standard. The sensitivity of culture isolation of *H. ducreyi* from active genital ulcers is variable, ranging from 50% to 80%, depending on the culture medium employed. It is important to note that *H. ducreyi* is almost never isolated from aspiration of inguinal buboes. Alternatives to culture confirmation have been described, but are investigational.

A probable diagnosis of chancroid can be made if the following criteria are met:

- One or more painful genital lesions
- No evidence of syphilis (a negative dark-field examination or negative rapid plasma reagin test result more than 7 days after onset of the ulcer)
- No evidence of HSV (clinically or by testing)

Therapy

Regimens recommended by the CDC for the treatment of chancroid include:

- Azithromycin (Zithromax), 1 g orally (single dose), or
- Ceftriaxone (Rocephin), 250 mg IM (single dose), or
- Ciprofloxacin (Cipro), 500 mg orally twice daily for 3 days
- Erythromycin, 500 mg orally three times daily for 7 days

For individuals with chancroid who are coinfected with HIV, some experts recommend the erythromycin regimen. Because a definitive diagnosis is difficult to make, patients should be re-evaluated 3 to 7 days after treatment is started to assure response. Patients should also be tested for HIV and syphilis when diagnosed with probable or definitive chancroid.

LYMPHOGRANULOMA VENEREUM

Etiology and Clinical Manifestations

LGV is caused by *C. trachomatis*, serovars L1, L2, or L3. The incubation period for LGV is variable, ranging from 3 to 21 days. The genital lesion is not striking and may be missed by both patients and physicians. It is usually single and painless and may be a papule, vesicle, or ulcer. It resolves within several days.

The key to the diagnosis of LGV is the nature of the regional adenopathy, not the genital lesion. Inguinal lymphadenopathy in LGV develops 2 to 6 weeks after the primary lesion, but in rare cases, the genital lesion may still be present. The nodes are matted, fluctuant, and large. Typically, they are painful. Adenopathy is unilateral in two-thirds of patients and bilateral in the remainder. Fistulas have been described, especially after diagnostic needle aspiration. Constitutional symptoms such as fever, headache, myalgia, and malaise are often prominent.

In 2004, the CDC reported 92 confirmed cases of LGV proctitis in the Netherlands identified over 17 months. The symptoms mimicked Crohn's disease, with these men who practiced anal intercourse having bloody diarrhea, mucous or purulent anal discharge, and tenesmus.

Diagnosis

Serologic titers for LGV may be useful in selected cases. The complement fixation test result is positive in most patients with active LGV at titers of 1:64 or higher. Titers become positive between 1 and 3 weeks after infection. Occasionally, high complement fixation titers have been found in individuals with other chlamydial infections and in asymptomatic individuals. Titers less than 1:64 are suggestive but not diagnostic of LGV. It is difficult to demonstrate a classic fourfold rise in specific antibody titer in LGV because of the late presentation in many patients.

Therapy

Doxycycline, 100 mg orally twice daily for 21 days, is the treatment of choice for LGV. An alternative regimen is erythromycin, 500 mg orally four times daily for 21 days. Treatment is the same in HIV-infected patients.

GRANULOMA INGUINALE (DONOVANOSIS)

Etiology and Clinical Manifestations

Granuloma inguinale, also termed *donovanosis*, is caused by the gram-negative bacillus *Calymmatobacterium granulomatis*. It is quite rare in the United States, but in many tropical and developing countries, such as India, the Caribbean islands, and southern Africa, it is endemic. The epidemiology and pathogenesis of donovanosis in the United States (and endemic countries as well) are poorly characterized. The precise role of sexual transmission is unclear, but repeated anal intercourse appears to be a risk factor for rectal and penile lesions in homosexual couples. Available data suggest that the infection is only mildly contagious.

The incubation period varies from 8 to 80 days. The lesion or lesions initially appear as subcutaneous nodules that later erode. Ulcerations forming above the nodules are painless, clean, and granulomatous. Granulation tissue often appears "beefy red" and with occasional contact bleeding. The lesions are most common on the glans or prepuce in men and on the labial area in women. The ulcers progressively enlarge in a chronic destructive fashion. They may be misidentified as carcinoma of the penis, chancroid, condyloma latum of secondary syphilis (when perianal lesions are present), and other causes of genital ulceration. Constitutional symptoms are usually absent.

Infection with *C. granulomatis* does not produce true regional lymphadenopathy. Instead, the granulomatous process in the genitals may extend into the inguinal region, causing further fibrosis and granulation tissue (pseudobuboes). These pseudobuboes are present in only 10% of patients with donovanosis and are variably painful.

Diagnosis

The diagnosis of granuloma inguinale is difficult, but can be confirmed by finding the characteristic *Donovan's bodies* in a crush preparation of fresh granulation tissue from a genital ulcer, which is spread over a clean microscope slide, air-dried, and stained with Wright or Giemsa stain. Donovan's bodies are multiple, darkly staining intracytoplasmic bacteria (*C. granulomatis*) found within the vacuoles of large mononuclear cells. They can also be identified in formal biopsy specimens with the use of standard light microscopy. There are no serologic or PCR tests available.

Therapy

There are limited studies on treatment, but granuloma inguinale typically responds well to doxycycline, 100 mg orally twice daily. Alternative regimens include azithromycin 1 g orally per week, trimethoprim-sulfamethoxazole, double-strength (160 mg trimethoprim/800 mg sulfamethoxazole) tablet orally twice daily, ciprofloxacin 750 mg orally twice daily, or erythromycin base 500 mg orally four times daily. All antibiotics are continued until the lesions are completely healed, usually 21 days or more. In pregnancy, erythromycin is recommended. HIV-infected individuals with granuloma inguinale are treated in the same manner as otherwise healthy individuals.

SYPHILIS

Primary Syphilis

Etiology and Clinical Manifestations

Syphilis is caused by the spirochete *T. pallidum*. The incubation period ranges from 3 to 90 days (mean, 21 days). The syphilitic chancre is typically a single, painless ulcer with raised and indurated borders. The base of the ulcer is clean and usually without purulence. However, up to one-third of syphilitic ulcers may be mildly painful. Development of the ulcer is usually slow. In the absence of treatment, chancres persist for up to 6 weeks. Constitutional symptoms are usually absent.

Inguinal lymphadenopathy is present in approximately 80% of patients with primary syphilis. The onset of lymphadenopathy usually occurs at the same time as the genital lesion. Characteristically, the adenopathy is painless (like the chancre), and the nodes are firm. In 70% of patients, the adenopathy is bilateral.

Diagnosis

The definitive methods of diagnosing early syphilis are dark-field examination and direct fluorescent antibody tests on active lesions or tissue biopsies. Serologic tests for syphilis, commonly used, are not diagnostic. A presumptive diagnosis of active syphilis can be made with one of various serologic tests, which are classified as nontreponemal and treponemal. Nontreponemal tests include the Venereal Disease Research Laboratory (VDRL) and rapid plasma reagin (RPR) tests. Treponemal tests include the fluorescent treponemal antibody absorption test, the microhemagglutination assay for antibody to *T. pallidum*, and the *T. pallidum* immobilization test.

Both positive treponemal and nontreponemal test results are necessary to presumptively diagnose syphilis in the absence of direct tests on primary lesions. As a rule, treponemal test results stay positive for life after the initial infection, whether appropriate therapy has been administered. Because treponemal test results do not correlate with disease activity, they are usually reported as either positive or negative. In contrast, nontreponemal test results do correlate with disease activity, reaching high titers with primary infection or recent reinfection and decreasing over time after appropriate therapy. Nontreponemal test results are reported as quantitative titers. The adequacy of therapy can be determined using serial RPR (or VDRL) tests; ideally, the same test in the same laboratory should be followed sequentially.

In primary syphilis, the VDRL test result is positive in approximately 70% of patients, and the RPR test result is positive in approximately 80%. Thus, it is important to realize that a substantial number of patients with a typical syphilitic chancre may have a negative nontreponemal test result. Treponemal test results may also be negative early on in primary syphilis. The percentage of positive test results for the fluorescent treponemal antibody absorption test is 85%; for the microhemagglutination assay for antibody to *T. pallidum*, 65%; and for the *T. pallidum* immobilization test, 50%. Thus, the diagnosis of primary syphilis should be considered in patients with lesions compatible with a chancre, even if nontreponemal and treponemal tests are negative.

All patients with syphilis, regardless of stage, should be tested for HIV according to the CDC recommendations.

Secondary and Tertiary Syphilis

Clinical Manifestations and Laboratory Diagnosis

In the absence of specific therapy, clinical manifestations may develop, in addition to genital ulceration with regional adenopathy. Secondary syphilis may present up to 2 years after the initial infection. Common clinical manifestations of secondary syphilis are summarized in Table 13.5. The most common manifestation is rash, and clinicians must consider secondary syphilis in all patients with unexplained rash, especially if accompanied by a risk history to suggest the diagnosis. The rash may be protean in its appearance, but involvement of the palms of the hands and soles of the feet should suggest the diagnosis.

Patients with syphilis and clinical signs suggesting either meningitis or uveitis should be fully evaluated for

TABLE 13.5

CLINICAL MANIFESTATIONS OF SECONDARY SYPHILIS

Manifestation	Cases (%)
Skin	90
Mouth and throat	35
Genital lesions	20
Constitutional symptoms	70
Central nervous system	
Asymptomatic	8–40
Symptomatic	1–2

Modified and used with permission from Mandell GL, Bennett JE, Dolin R, eds. *Mandell, Douglas and Bennett's Principles and Practice of Infectious Diseases*, 5th ed. Philadelphia: Churchill Livingstone, 1999.

neurosyphilis or luetic uveitis, with testing including lumbar puncture and slit-lamp examination. During primary or secondary syphilis, invasion of the cerebrospinal fluid (CSF) by *T. pallidum* is common, and abnormalities in the CSF can often be demonstrated. However, if primary or secondary syphilis is treated appropriately, neurosyphilis develops in only a small percentage of patients. The CDC does not recommend routine lumbar puncture in patients with primary or secondary syphilis, unless signs or symptoms of neurologic or ophthalmic involvement are present.

The natural history of untreated secondary syphilis is spontaneous resolution after 3 to 12 weeks, although viable organisms persist. VDRL, RPR, and treponemal test results are positive in nearly 100% of patients with secondary syphilis. In the absence of specific treatment, patients enter a stage of asymptomatic infection termed *latency*. They are classified as having *early-latent* disease if they are asymp-

tomatic and have acquired infection within the past year. Those without symptoms and with infection of more than 1 year's duration are said to have *late-latent* syphilis. In asymptomatic patients with a positive serology, it may be difficult to distinguish early- from late-latent disease.

Tertiary syphilis may produce cardiac or neurologic disease, as well as a variety of less common manifestations. The most common cardiac manifestation is aortitis. Neurologic manifestations of tertiary syphilis may include meningovascular syphilis, tabes dorsalis, and generalized paresis. *Gummatous syphilis* is a rare manifestation of late syphilis in which granulomatous lesions present as space-occupying lesions in a variety of organs such as liver, bone, central nervous system, respiratory tract, and bowel.

Therapy

Primary, secondary, and early-latent syphilis is treated with a single dose of benzathine penicillin G, 2.4 million U IM. For penicillin-allergic patients, the alternative is doxycycline, 100 mg orally twice daily for 2 weeks, or tetracycline, 500 mg orally four times daily for 2 weeks. Later stages of syphilis require more prolonged therapy. Current treatment recommendations for the respective stages of syphilis are summarized in Table 13.6.

Syphilis and HIV Infection

In HIV-infected individuals, syphilis can be highly aggressive. Patients may progress from primary to tertiary disease over the course of several years rather than several decades, as occurs in non–HIV-infected individuals. Several important caveats regarding syphilis in HIV-infected patients are summarized in Table 13.7. All individuals who present with syphilis should be offered HIV testing. In younger individuals who present with unexplained stroke,

TABLE 13.6

TREATMENT RECOMMENDATIONS FOR THE DIFFERENT STAGES OF SYPHILIS

Stage	Recommended	Alternative
Primary	Benzathine PCN G, 2.4 million U IM × 1 dose	Doxycycline, 100 mg PO BID, or tetracycline,[a] 500 mg PO QID for 2 weeks
Secondary	Benzathine PCN G, 2.4 million U IM × 1 dose	Doxycycline, 100 mg PO BID, or tetracycline,[a] 500 mg PO QID for 2 weeks
Early latent (<1 year)	Benzathine PCN G, 2.4 million U IM × 1 dose	Doxycycline, 100 mg PO BID, or tetracycline,[a] 500 mg PO QID for 2 weeks
Late latent (>1 year)	Benzathine PCN G, 2.4 million U IM weekly for 3 weeks	Doxycycline, 100 mg PO BID, or tetracycline,[a] 500 mg PO QID for 4 weeks
Gummas	Benzathine PCN G, 2.4 million U IM weekly for 3 weeks	Doxycycline, 100 mg PO BID, or tetracycline,[a] 500 mg PO QID for 4 weeks
Cardiovascular	Benzathine PCN G, 2.4 million U IM weekly for 3 weeks	Doxycycline, 100 mg PO BID, or tetracycline,[a] 500 mg PO QID for 4 weeks
Neurosyphilis	Aqueous PCN G, 18–24 million U IV daily for 10–14 days	Procaine PCN G, 2.4 million U IM daily; probenecid, 500 mg QID for 10–14 days

BID, twice a day; IM, intramuscularly; IV, intravenously; PCN, penicillin; PO, orally; QID, four times a day.
[a] Avoid tetracycline during pregnancy.

Progression to tertiary syphilis may occur rapidly (several years).
Neurosyphilis should always be considered in HIV-infected patients with neurologic disease.
When findings suggest syphilis at any stage but serologic test results are negative, diagnosis with biopsy, dark-field examination, or direct fluorescent antibody staining should be pursued.

Treatment
- Use penicillin.
- No changes in therapy for early syphilis.
- Consider cerebrospinal fluid examination in all patients with clues and HIV infection.
- Follow-up with Venereal Disease Research Laboratory or rapid plasma reagin test at 3, 6, 9, 12, and 24 months; if titers fail to decrease fourfold after 6 months, treat again and perform lumbar puncture.

meningovascular syphilis in the setting of unrecognized HIV infection should be considered in the differential diagnosis, along with infective endocarditis and more common causes of stroke.

VAGINAL INFECTIONS

Etiology and Clinical Manifestations

Vaginal discharge is a common complaint in primary care practice, accounting for approximately 10 million office visits annually in the United States. Vaginal signs and symptoms are nonspecific, however, and more serious conditions such as cervical neoplasia, MPC, and PID may mimic vaginitis. The most common causes of vaginitis include bacterial vaginosis (BV; i.e., nonspecific vaginitis), *Trichomonas vaginalis* vaginitis, and yeast vulvovaginitis due to *Candida albicans* and other yeasts.

The symptoms of vaginitis are rarely specific enough to suggest a precise etiologic diagnosis. Nevertheless, the common clinical manifestations of the respective causes of vaginitis are summarized in Table 13.8.

Diagnosis

The diagnostic evaluation of patients with suspected vaginitis should include the microscopic examination of vaginal secretions, testing of secretions for pH, and application of 10% potassium hydroxide to secretions to elicit a fishy odor (whiff test). The results of these tests may distinguish the respective causes, as summarized in Table 13.9.

BV may be caused by *Gardnerella vaginalis*, mycoplasmas, and, occasionally, anaerobic bacteria. Criteria for the clinical diagnosis of BV include the following:

- Gray homogeneous discharge adherent to the vaginal epithelium and cervix
- Fishy odor
- pH 4.5
- Clue cells
- Positive whiff test

Therapy

The sexual partners of individuals with BV do not require treatment. Recommended regimens for the therapy of BV include the following antibiotics:

- Metronidazole, 500 mg orally twice daily for 7 days, or
- Clindamycin 2% cream (Cleocin), 5 g intravaginally at bedtime for 7 days, or
- Metronidazole, 0.75% gel, 5 g intravaginally once a day for 5 days

Alternative regimens include:

- Clindamycin, 300 mg orally twice daily for 7 days, or
- Clindamycin ovules, 100 g intravaginally once at bedtime for 3 days

TABLE 13.8

VAGINAL INFECTIONS: CLINICAL MANIFESTATIONS

	Normal Vagina	Yeast Vaginitis	Trichomoniasis	Bacterial Vaginosis
Etiology	—	*Candida albicans*, other yeasts	*Trichomonas vaginalis*	*Gardnerella vaginalis*, mycoplasmas, anaerobes
Symptoms	—	Itching, irritation, discharge	Malodorous discharge, often profuse	Malodorous discharge
Discharge				
Color	Clear or white	White	Yellow	White or gray
Consistency	Nonhomogeneous, floccular	Clumped, adherent plaques	Thin, homogeneous, frothy	Homogenous, coats vaginal mucosa
Inflammation of vulva/introitus	—	Vaginal erythema, vulvar dermatitis	Vaginal erythema, strawberry cervix	None

Modified and reproduced with permission from Paavonen J, Stamm WE. Sexually transmitted diseases: lower genital tract infections in women. *Infect Dis Clin North Am* 1987;1:179–198.

TABLE 13.9

VAGINAL INFECTIONS: DIAGNOSIS

	Normal Vagina	Yeast Vaginitis	Trichomoniasis	Bacterial Vaginosis
pH	<4.5	<4.5	≥4.5	≥4.5
Ammonia odor with 10% potassium hydroxide	None	None	Usually present	Present
Microscopy	Epithelial cells, lactobacilli	Leukocytes, epithelial cells; yeast, mycelia, pseudo-mycelia in up to 80%	Leukocytes, motile trichomonads in 80%–90%	Clue cells, few leukocytes, profuse mixed flora

Modified and reproduced with permission from Paavonen J, Stamm WE. Sexually transmitted diseases: lower genital tract infections in women. *Infect Dis Clin North Am* 1987;1:179–198.

Bacterial vaginosis has been linked with a number of pregnancy complications, including chorioamnionitis, preterm birth, premature rupture of membranes, and others. Treatment is recommended for all pregnant women who are symptomatic. Women at high risk for preterm delivery should be screened and treated, even if asymptomatic. Treatment of asymptomatic BV in pregnant women not at high risk for preterm delivery is more controversial. The CDC has recommended against the use of topical agents during pregnancy for BV. The recommendations for the treatment for BV during pregnancy are as follows:

- Metronidazole, 500 mg orally two times daily for 7 days, or
- Metronidazole, 250 mg orally three times daily for 7 days, or
- Clindamycin, 300 mg orally twice daily for 7 days

Trichomoniasis

The protozoan *T. vaginalis* can cause vaginitis in females and NGU in males, and can be asymptomatic. Wet preparations are often used to identify the motile trichomonas protozoan in vaginal samples, but have a sensitivity of approximately 50% to 70%. They are even less sensitive for male infections. Culture is the most sensitive and is available for vaginal secretions, urine, and male urethral swabs. An immunochromatographic dipstick (OSOM) is available for point-of-care testing, as is AFFIRM, a nucleic acid probe test that detects *T. vaginalis, G. vaginalis,* and *C. albicans.*

For the treatment of trichomonas infection, metronidazole, 2 g orally (single dose), is recommended. Tinidazole at a dose of 2 g orally in a single dose is also recommended and is available in the United States, but is substantially more expensive than metronidazole and no more efficacious. An alternative regimen is metronidazole, 500 mg orally twice daily for 7 days. Metronidazole gel is not recommended for trichomonas due to poor efficacy, although it is approved for BV. Sexual partners should also be treated.

Trichomonas infection in pregnancy has been associated with a variety of adverse outcomes. It is not clear, however, whether treatment of asymptomatic trichomoniasis in pregnancy decreases adverse outcomes. The recommended regimen in pregnancy is 2 g of metronidazole given as a single dose; the CDC feels that no clear teratogenic effect of metronidazole has been shown.

The recommended regimens for the treatment of vulvovaginal candidiasis include the following agents:

- Butoconazole 2% cream (Femstat), 5 g intravaginally for 3 days, or
- Butoconazole 2% cream, 5 g sustained-release, single intravaginal application, or
- Clotrimazole 1% cream, 5 g intravaginally for 7 to 14 days, or
- Clotrimazole, 100-mg vaginal tablet for 7 days, or
- Clotrimazole, 100-mg vaginal tablet, two tablets for 3 days, or
- Miconazole (Monistat) 2% cream, 5 g intravaginally for 7 days, or
- Miconazole, 200-mg vaginal suppository for 3 days, or
- Miconazole, 100-mg vaginal suppository for 7 days, or
- Miconazole, 1,200-mg vaginal suppository, single dose, or
- Nystatin, 100,000-U vaginal tablet, one tablet daily for 14 days, or
- Terconazole (Terazol) 0.4% cream, 5 g intravaginally for 7 days, or
- Terconazole 0.8% cream, 5 g intravaginally for 3 days, or
- Terconazole, 80-mg suppository once daily for 3 days, or
- Tioconazole 6.5% ointment (Vagistat-1), 5 g intravaginally in a single application, or
- Fluconazole (Diflucan), 150 mg orally as a single dose

Sexual partners do not require treatment (unless balanitis is present). Pregnant women are treated in the same manner as nonpregnant women.

GENITAL WARTS

Etiology and Clinical Manifestations

More than 100 strains or types of human papillomavirus (HPV) exist, and more than 30 types can infect the genital tract. They have been broadly classified into low-risk (e.g., HPV-6 and -11) and high-risk (e.g., HPV-16, -18, -31, -33, -35) types on the basis of their association with cancer. HPV-6 and -11 are the most common types found in external genital warts. Most visible genital warts are associated with low-risk HPV types. Occasionally, visible warts are associated with the high-risk types, but this is much less common.

Genital warts are one of the most commonly diagnosed STDs in the United States, with an estimated prevalence of 20 million cases and an incidence of 6 million new infections annually. About 50% of sexually active persons in the United States will acquire genital HPV infection at some point. Genital warts accounted for more than one-third of the total cost for STDs in the United States in 1995. The sexual and behavioral risk factors associated with genital HPV infections include multiple sexual partners, sex with a person with warts, or anoreceptive intercourse (for intra-anal but not perianal warts). Condoms do not completely protect against HPV transmission, especially in women.

Most HPV infections are subclinical and asymptomatic, but lesions that do occur usually appear between 3 weeks and 8 months after infection of genital tract cells. Genital warts affect a variety of sites, including the penis, scrotum, vulva, perineal and perianal areas, pubic area, and crural folds. HPV types that cause external genital warts can also cause warts in the vagina or cervix and inside the urethra or anus. Persons who practice anal receptive intercourse are at risk for developing intra-anal warts; this is in contrast to perianal warts, which can develop as an extension of genital warts, unrelated to anal intercourse. Intraurethral warts may cause terminal hematuria or intermittent spotting. Genital warts may occur as discrete lesions or may coalesce into confluent plaques. Four morphologic types exist:

- Condyloma acuminatum: cauliflower shaped, usually on moist surfaces
- Smooth papular: dome shaped, usually on dry surfaces
- Keratotic: thick horny layer, possibly resembling a common wart or seborrheic keratosis, usually on dry surfaces
- Flat to slightly raised, flat-topped papular: on any mucosal or cutaneous surface

A strong association exists between infection with certain types of HPV and anogenital cancer. Bowenoid papulosis, almost always associated with HPV-16 or HPV-18, is characterized by dome-shaped or flat papules 1 to 5 mm in size that may be hyperpigmented or bluish hued. Histologic examination of these papules shows high-grade squamous intraepithelial lesions. Buschke-Löwenstein tumor, a form of verrucous squamous cell carcinoma, is perhaps the only neoplastic lesion associated with low-risk HPV types. Cervical, vulvar, and perianal intraepithelial neoplasia and carcinomas of the vulva, cervix, anus, and penis have all been associated with HPV, mostly types 16 and 18.

Diagnosis

Clinical trials have demonstrated that diagnosis based on clinical examination is reliable and consistent with histologic diagnosis. Bright light and magnification may assist in the diagnosis of flat or small warts. The application of a 3% to 5% acetic acid solution to genital tissues for 5 to 10 minutes (acetowhite test) before examination may be useful in populations with a high prevalence of warts and for the identification of flat-topped warts that may be particularly difficult to visualize. However, this test is not recommended for routine screening. Biopsy is not routinely required but should be considered when:

- One or more lesions are indurated, ulcerated, or fixed to underlying structures.
- An individual lesion is >10 mm.
- The diagnosis is in doubt.
- Lesions are unresponsive to standard therapy.
- Lesions are pigmented.
- The condition worsens during therapy.
- The patient is immunocompromised.

The American Cancer Society and American College of Obstetricians and Gynecologists guidelines recommend annual cervical Papanicolaou (Pap) smear screening for women ages 21 to 30 years, and then every 2 to 3 years for women ages 30 years and older if three consecutive annual Pap tests are negative. Only one FDA-cleared test exists for the detection of HPV DNA, the Digene Hybrid Capture II. The HPV DNA test may be performed by (a) cocollecting a specimen; (b) using a supplied swab at the time of the Pap test, if conventional cytology is used; (c) reflex testing, if liquid-based cytology is used and enough residual material is available in the cytology test vial; or (d) scheduling a separate follow-up appointment when the Pap test report results are known. If the high-risk HPV DNA test is positive, women are referred immediately for colposcopy and, if indicated, directed cervical biopsy.

Patients with genital warts and their partners should be screened for other STDs. Because women with external genital warts have a greater probability of exposure to high-risk oncogenic HPV types, these women and the female partners of men with warts should be screened annually for cervical cancer using a Pap smear until receiving three negative test results. Subsequent screening should be considered. There are no guidelines for anal cancer screening, but patients with perianal warts, HIV-infected patients, and patients with a history of anoreceptive intercourse should be asked about symptoms of perianal pruritus, rectal pain, or hematochezia, and anal cytology should also be considered.

Therapy

External genital warts are usually asymptomatic, but depending on their size, number, and location, they may be painful, friable, or pruritic and may interfere with normal function. In addition, they may be socially stigmatizing and emotionally distressing. Although unpredictable, some warts may resolve spontaneously, but regression is often followed by disease recurrence. In most patients, however, warts either remain unchanged or increase in size and number, especially during pregnancy and immune deficiency. Currently available therapies may eliminate the warts, but not the infection, and may not decrease infectivity. No simple, routinely effective therapies are available, and this often makes the treatment of genital warts a frustrating experience for both patients and clinicians. Most treatment modalities have similar efficacy. The size, location, number, and character of the warts affect treatment decisions, as do coexisting medical conditions (e.g., pregnancy or immune deficiency).

Patient-controlled therapies are best suited for patients who desire more control over their care; they are usually less invasive and require patient education. Their safety and efficacy have not been established in pediatric patients and pregnant women. One commonly used agent is 0.5% podofilox solution or gel (Condylox), which should be applied twice daily for 3 consecutive days. This cycle is repeated weekly until the warts are gone, but no longer than 4 weeks. Another agent is 5% imiquimod (Aldara) cream applied at bedtime on 3 alternating days per week until the lesions clear, or for 16 weeks. The cream is washed off 6 to 10 hours after application.

Physician-applied therapies include:

- Trichloroacetic acid or bichloracetic acid applied every 1 to 2 weeks, or
- Podophyllin resin (10%–25%) in tincture of benzoin applied one to two times weekly for six treatments, or
- Cryotherapy with liquid nitrogen applied by cryoprobe, spray, or loosely wound cotton on a wooden applicator (this requires training for proper administration), or
- Office surgery, including curettage, electrosurgery, and fine-scissor or tangential shave excision (these require equipment and significant training)

Complex destructive modalities include laser or intralesional interferon. These require in-depth training and are not recommended for first-line treatment. Systemic interferon is not efficacious. Treatment should be changed or the patient should be referred when:

- Three treatment sessions have resulted in no improvement.
- Complete clearance has not occurred after six treatment sessions.

- Continued treatment would extend beyond the manufacturer's recommendations for patient-applied therapies.

Immune compromise decreases the likelihood of spontaneous regression and responsiveness to conventional therapies, and increases the likelihood of relapse. In HIV-infected patients, the ulcerations caused by therapy increase the risk of transmission of HIV and other STDs to sexual partners.

An integral component of therapy for patients with genital warts is counseling. Many patients respond to the appearance of warts with a strong mix of emotions, ranging from embarrassment to anger to fear. Genital warts can damage a patient's feelings of self-esteem and interactions with sexual partners. Worry about the possibility of cancer or transmission of the disease to sexual partners or to a newborn during delivery can also cause anguish. Clinicians can be sensitive to these concerns by addressing them with both verbal reassurance and written information. A nonjudgmental attitude is critical to the success of counseling, which is aimed at preventing or alleviating the significant emotional, psychological, and social sequelae that may result from the disease.

HPV PREVENTION

There is one quadrivalent vaccine (Gardasil) available that offers protection against HPV-16 and -18 (the two types of HPV that cause 80% of cervical cancer in the United States) and HPV-6 and -8 (the types of HPV most commonly causing genital warts). This vaccine has demonstrated efficacy of more than 90% against persistent infection with either HPV-16 or HPV-18 in women who have received all three doses of the vaccine. It is approved for use in females ages 9 to 26 years and is a series of three vaccines given at 0, 2, and 6 months. Because the vaccine does not protect against all high-risk types of HPV that could lead to cervical cancer, Pap smears must still be performed routinely even in those sexually active girls and women who have been vaccinated. It is optimal to get the vaccine series completed before girls or women begin sexual activity and are potentially exposed to HPV. However, because it is unlikely that a woman would have been exposed to all four types of HPV protected by the vaccine, even those with prior sexual exposure or evidence of abnormal Pap smears or genital warts may benefit from the vaccine. Screening for HPV is not necessary before vaccination.

ADOLESCENTS

In all 50 states and the District of Columbia, adolescents can receive medical care for STDs without parental consent. Laws regarding vaccinations of adolescents and parental consent vary by state.

REVIEW EXERCISES

QUESTIONS

1. A 19-year-old man has a low-grade fever, tender inguinal adenopathy, and grouped vesicles on his penis. He has never had a sexually transmitted disease before, and he has a new female partner. How should this patient be managed?

a) Acyclovir cream applied to the lesions three times daily until resolution

b) No therapy because trials have failed to demonstrate efficacy in this setting

c) Acyclovir, 400 mg orally three times daily; famciclovir, 250 mg orally three times daily; or valacyclovir, 1 g orally twice daily for 7 days

d) Acyclovir, 5 mg/kg intravenously every 8 hours

e) None of the above

Answer and Discussion

The answer is c. The patient has primary herpes simplex virus infection. Topical agents have no role in therapy, and intravenous therapy is reserved for patients who experience complications of primary HIV infection, such as pneumonitis, encephalitis, or hepatitis. The patient should receive some form of treatment because therapy partially relieves symptoms and accelerates healing. Newer antivirals are now available as alternatives to acyclovir.

2. A 26-year-old man has a several-weeks-old penile lesion with new inguinal adenopathy. On examination, a single nontender ulcer is present. Bilateral palpable inguinal nodes are present, which are also nontender. Rapid plasma reagin test results are negative. The most likely diagnosis is

a) Lymphogranuloma venereum

b) Chancroid

c) Primary syphilis

d) Variant herpes simplex virus infection

e) Granuloma inguinale

Answer and Discussion

The answer is c. Rapid plasma reagin (RPR) test results are positive in primary syphilis in only 70% of patients. Thus, a negative RPR result does not rule out the diagnosis. The five options listed constitute the differential possibilities for the syndrome of genital ulcers with regional adenopathy. The three most common etiologies in the United States are HIV, syphilis, and chancroid.

3. A 44-year-old man has had a painful penile ulcer for several weeks. He is HIV negative but has frequent prostitute exposure. He has tender inguinal lymph nodes on the right, which appeared at the same time as the genital ulcer. He has seen several physicians, apparently without a diagnosis. On examination, the node is

fluctuant and has a fistula with pus. Which of the following would be effective treatment?

a) Azithromycin, 1 g orally twice daily for 7 days

b) Ceftriaxone, 250 mg intramuscularly once

c) Ciprofloxacin, 500 mg orally once

d) All of the above

e) None of the above

Answer and Discussion

The answer is b. The correct diagnosis is chancroid. One intramuscular dose of ceftriaxone is a recommended regimen. Azithromycin is another option, but a single dose is sufficient, rather than a 7-day course of therapy. Ciprofloxacin is effective but needs to be given twice daily for 3 days. Finally, erythromycin can be used at a dose of 500 mg orally four times daily for 7 days.

4. A 27-year-old woman comes to the office because her boyfriend was recently diagnosed with genital herpes. She is sexually active without condoms but is asymptomatic. Pelvic examination is normal. She is requesting some type of evaluation for herpes. What is the most appropriate next step?

a) Oral acyclovir for 7 to 10 days

b) Tzanck smear of the cervix

c) Glycoprotein G–based herpes simplex virus (HSV) serologies

d) HSV nucleic acid testing from blood and cervix

Answer and Discussion

The answer is c. The Centers for Disease Control and Prevention has recently advocated the use of type-specific glycoprotein G–based serologic tests for the diagnosis of genital herpes in certain circumstances, particularly in suspected cases that are culture negative. A positive herpes simplex virus type 2 antibody test is indicative of infection with anogenital herpes at some time in the past. The antibody test may be useful in partner evaluation, although pretest counseling is important. The test is not recommended for routine screening in the population but should be available to anyone requesting testing.

5. A 60-year-old woman is seen on referral for a positive Venereal Disease Research Laboratory (VDRL) test result. She is asymptomatic, except for mild memory loss. She recalls having had syphilis as a teenager but was never treated. Cerebrospinal fluid (CSF) examination shows no white blood cells, normal protein, and normal glucose; the CSF VDRL is nonreactive. How should she be managed next?

a) Erythromycin, 250 mg orally four times daily for 2 weeks

b) Hospitalization and treatment with aqueous crystalline penicillin G at 12 million U intravenously daily for 14 days

c) Benzathine penicillin G, 2.4 million U intramuscularly (IM) once
d) Benzathine penicillin G, 2.4 million U IM each week for 3 weeks

Answer and Discussion

The answer is d. The patient has late-latent syphilis. The recommended therapy is 3 weekly IM doses of benzathine penicillin G. In penicillin-allergic patients, doxycycline or tetracycline should be given for 4 weeks.

6. Which of the following statements about secondary syphilis is false?
a) Rash is the most common clinical manifestation.
b) Erythromycin is the treatment of choice in penicillin-allergic patients.
c) Up to 20% of patients have a genital lesion evident.
d) Nontreponemal test results are almost always positive.

Answer and Discussion

The answer is b. Doxycycline, not erythromycin, is the treatment of choice for secondary syphilis in penicillin-allergic patients. All the other statements are correct. Of note, the presence of the primary chancre should not divert from the diagnosis. The rash can manifest in many different ways, but by the time it is present, nontreponemal test results are positive almost 100% of the time, making the diagnosis relatively easy, if considered.

7. A 19-year-old sexually active man (HIV negative) has dysuria and a urethral discharge. He has a new partner. Gram stain of the discharge shows >10 white blood cells per oil immersion field. Which of the following statements is false?
a) He should be specifically tested for *Chlamydia trachomatis*.
b) He should be specifically tested for *Neisseria gonorrhoeae*.
c) If the patient is unreliable for follow-up, he should be treated with antibiotics empirically.
d) This condition could be caused by herpes simplex virus.
e) Asymptomatic infection is rare.

Answer and Discussion

The answer is e. Many men and women with urethritis/mucopurulent cervicitis are minimally symptomatic or asymptomatic. Causative agents include *N. gonorrhoeae, C. trachomatis*, herpes simplex virus, *Trichomonas vaginalis*, and *Ureaplasma urealyticum*. If a patient is unreliable, he should be treated empirically to help prevent further spread of the infection to other sexual partners.

8. A 19-year-old man presents with a painful urethral discharge. He denies any history of prior sexually transmitted disease. Gram stain of the discharge shows white blood cells with intracellular gram-negative diplococci. The next step is
a) No treatment until cultures of the discharge are finalized
b) Ciprofloxacin, 500 mg orally once
c) Ceftriaxone, 125 mg intramuscularly (IM) once and azithromycin 1 g orally once
d) Ceftriaxone, 250 mg IM once
e) None of the above

Answer and Discussion

The answer is c. The patient has gonorrhea. Gram stain is diagnostic, so there is no need to await culture results. Due to the prevalence of quinolone-resistant *Neisseria gonorrhoeae*, empiric ciprofloxacin use is not appropriate. The lower dose of ceftriaxone is sufficient and empiric therapy for chlamydial infection should always be used concurrently with antigonococcal therapy.

9. Which of the following statements is false regarding human papillomavirus infection?
a) Human papillomavirus type 6 is the most common type associated with external genital warts.
b) External genital warts are one of the most commonly diagnosed sexually transmitted diseases in the United States.
c) Condoms completely protect against herpes simplex virus transmission.
d) Screening for cervical cancer is recommended in patients with genital warts.

Answer and Discussion

The answer is c. Condoms do not completely protect against human papillomavirus (HPV) transmission. Genital warts are one of the most common sexually transmitted diseases in the United States. HPV-6 and -11 are considered low-risk and HPV-16 and -18 high-risk for cervical cancer. Thus, all female patients with genital warts should be screened.

10. A 35-year-old woman complains of a several-day history of malodorous vaginal discharge. On pelvic examination, a gray homogeneous discharge is present. Examination of the discharge reveals a pH of 6. Gram stain shows clue cells. The most likely diagnosis is
a) Trichomoniasis
b) *Chlamydia trachomatis* infection
c) Bacterial vaginosis
d) Yeast vulvovaginitis
e) None of the above

Answer and Discussion

The answer is c. Gram stain shows clue cells, which are characteristic of bacterial vaginosis. Trichomoniasis can also cause an increased vaginal pH, but does not demonstrate clue cells on the wet-mount preparation. Neither of these findings is present in vaginal yeast infections or chlamydial cervicitis.

SUGGESTED READINGS

General

Brown TJ, Yen-Moore A, Tyring SK. An overview of sexually transmitted diseases: part I. *J Am Acad Dermatol* 1999;41:511–532.

Brown TJ, Yen-Moore A, Tyring SK. An overview of sexually transmitted diseases: part II. *J Am Acad Dermatol* 1999;41:661–677.

Cates W Jr. Estimates of the incidence and prevalence of sexually transmitted diseases in the United States. American Social Health Association Panel. *Sex Transm Dis* 1999;26(Suppl 4): S2–S7.

Centers for Disease Control and Prevention. Update to CDC's *Sexually Transmitted Diseases Treatment Guidelines, 2006*: fluoroquinolones no longer recommended for treatment of gonococcal infections. *MMWR Morb Mortal Wkly Rep* 2007;56(14):332–336.

Centers for Disease Control and Prevention. Sexually transmitted diseases treatment guidelines. *MMWR Morb Mortal Wkly Rep* 2006;55(RR-11):1–93.

Czelusta A, Yen-Moore A, Van der Straten M, et al. An overview of sexually transmitted diseases: part III. Sexually transmitted diseases in HIV-infected patients. *J Am Acad Dermatol* 2000;43:409–432.

Genital Ulcer Disease

DiCarlo RP, Martin DH. The clinical diagnosis of genital ulcer disease in men. *Clin Infect Dis* 1997;25:292–298.

Dillon SM, Cummings M, Rajagopalan S, et al. Prospective analysis of genital ulcer disease in Brooklyn, New York. *Clin Infect Dis* 1997;24:945–950.

Herpes Simplex Virus Infection

Diaz-Mitoma F, Sibbald RG, Shafran SD, et al. Oral famciclovir for the suppression of recurrent genital herpes: a randomized, controlled trial. *JAMA* 1998;280:887–892.

Leung DT, Sacks SL. Current recommendations for the treatment of genital herpes. *Drugs* 2000;60:1329–1352.

Marques AR, Straus SE. Herpes simplex type 2 infections—an update. *Adv Intern Med* 2000;45:175–208.

Mertz GJ, Loveless MO, Levin MJ, et al. Oral famciclovir for suppression of recurrent genital herpes simplex virus infection in women: a multicenter, double-blind, placebo-controlled trial. *Arch Intern Med* 1997;157:343–349.

Reitano M, Tyring S, Lang W, et al. Valacyclovir for the suppression of recurrent genital herpes simplex virus infection: a large-scale dose range-finding study. *J Infect Dis* 1998;178:603–610.

Sacks SL, Aoki FY, Diaz-Mitoma F, et al. Patient-initiated, twice daily oral famciclovir for early recurrent genital herpes: a randomized, double-blind multicenter trial. *JAMA* 1996;276: 44–49.

Tetrault I, Boivin G. Recent advances in management of genital herpes. *Can Fam Physician* 2000;46:1622–1629.

Wald A. New therapies and prevention strategies for genital herpes. *Clin Infect Dis* 1999;28(Suppl 1):S4–S13.

Whitley RJ, Kimberlin DW, Roizman B. Herpes simplex viruses. *Clin Infect Dis* 1998;26:541–545.

Chancroid

Lewis DA. Diagnostic tests for chancroid. *Sex Transm Infect* 2000; 76:137–141.

Mertz KJ, Weiss JB, Webb RM, et al. An investigation of genital ulcers in Jackson, Mississippi, with use of a multiplex polymerase chain reaction assay: high prevalence of chancroid and human immunodeficiency virus infection. *J Infect Dis* 1998;178:1060–1066.

Schmid GP. Treatment of chancroid, 1997. *Clin Infect Dis* 1999; 28(Suppl 1):S14–S20.

Lymphogranuloma Venereum

Centers for Disease Control and Prevention. Lymphogranuloma venereum among men who have sex with men—Netherlands, 2003–2004. *MMWR Morb Mortal Wkly Rep* 2004;53(42):985–988.

Heaton ND, Yates-Bell A. Thirty-year follow-up of lymphogranuloma venereum. *Br J Urol* 1992;70:693–694.

Donovanosis

Hart G. Donovanosis. *Clin Infect Dis* 1997;25:24–32.

Syphilis

Augenbraun MH, Rolfs R. Treatment of syphilis, 1998: nonpregnant adults. *Clin Infect Dis* 1999;28(Suppl 1):S21–S28.

Blocker ME, Levine WC, St. Louis ME. HIV prevalence in patients with syphilis, United States. *Sex Transm Dis* 2000;27:53–59.

Clyne B, Jerrard DA. Syphilis testing. *J Emerg Med* 2000;18:361–367.

Genc M, Ledger WJ. Syphilis in pregnancy. *Sex Transm Infect* 2000; 76:73–79.

Larsen SA, Steiner BM, Rudolph AH. Laboratory diagnosis and interpretation of tests for syphilis. *Clin Microbiol Rev* 1995;8:1–21.

Singh AE, Romanowski B. Syphilis: review with emphasis on clinical, epidemiologic, and some biologic features. *Clin Microbiol Rev* 1999;12:187–209.

Urethritis and Cervicitis

Burstein GR, Zenilman JM. Nongonococcal urethritis: a new paradigm. *Clin Infect Dis* 1999;28(Suppl 1):S66–S73.

Molodysky E. Urethritis and cervicitis. *Aust Fam Physician* 1999; 28:333–338.

Chlamydia Infection

Burstein GR, Gaydos CA, Diener-West M, et al. Incident *Chlamydia trachomatis* infections among inner-city adolescent females. *JAMA* 1998;280:521–526.

Fenton KA. Screening men for *Chlamydia trachomatis* infection: have we fully explored the possibilities? *Commun Dis Public Health* 2000;3:86–89.

Howell MR, Quinn TC, Gaydos CA. Screening for *Chlamydia trachomatis* in asymptomatic women attending family planning clinics: a cost-effectiveness analysis of three strategies. *Ann Intern Med* 1998;128:277–284.

Magid D, Douglas JM Jr, Schwartz JS. Doxycycline compared with azithromycin for treating women with genital *Chlamydia trachomatis* infections: an incremental cost-effectiveness analysis. *Ann Intern Med* 1996;12:389–399.

Weber JT, Johnson RE. New treatments for *Chlamydia trachomatis* genital infection. *Clin Infect Dis* 1995;20(Suppl 1):S66–S71.

Gonorrhea

Centers for Disease Control and Prevention. Update to CDC's *Sexually Transmitted Diseases Treatment Guidelines, 2006*: fluoroquinolones no longer recommended for treatment of gonococcal infections. *MMWR Morb Mortal Wkly Rep* 2007;56(14):332–336.

Human Papillomavirus Infection

Cutts FT, Franceschi S, Goldie S, et al. Human papillomavirus and HPV vaccines: a review. *Bull World Health Organ* 2007;85(9):719-726.

Alexander KA, Phelps WC. Recent advances in diagnosis and therapy of human papillomaviruses. *Expert Opinion Invest Drugs* 2000;9:1753–1765.

Beutner KR, Reitano MV, Richwald GA, et al. External genital warts: report of the American Medical Association consensus conference. *Clin Infect Dis* 1998;27:796–806.

Beutner KR, Wiley DJ, Douglas JM, et al. Genital warts and their treatment. *Clin Infect Dis* 1999;28(Suppl 1):S37–S56.

Palefsky JM. Human papillomavirus-related tumors. *AIDS* 2000;14(Suppl 3):S189–S195.

Severson J, Evans TY, Lee P, et al. Human papillomavirus infections: epidemiology, pathogenesis, and therapy. *J Cutan Med Surg* 2001;5:43–60.

Vaginal Infections

Egan ME, Lipsky MS. Diagnosis of vaginitis. *Am Fam Physician* 2000;62:1095–1104.

Haefner HK. Current evaluation and management of vulvovaginitis. *Clin Obstet Gynecol* 1999;42:184–195.

Joesoef MR, Schmid GP, Hillier SL. Bacterial vaginosis: review of treatment options and potential clinical indications for therapy. *Clin Infect Dis* 1999;28(Suppl 1):S57–S65.

Petrin D, Delgaty K, Bhatt R, et al. Clinical and microbiological aspects of *Trichomonas vaginalis. Clin Microbiol Rev* 1998;11:300–317.

Reef SE, Levine WC, McNeil MM, et al. Treatment options for vulvovaginal candidiasis, 1993. *Clin Infect Dis* 1995;20(Suppl 1):S80–S90.

Sobel JD. Bacterial vaginosis. *Annu Rev Med* 2000;51:349–346.

Sobel JD. Vaginitis. *N Engl J Med* 1997;337:1896–1903.

Chapter 14

Human Immunodeficiency Virus Infections and Acquired Immunodeficiency Syndrome

Wendy S. Armstrong   Alan J. Taege

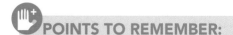

POINTS TO REMEMBER:

- A percutaneous exposure through a needlestick injury or intravenous drug use results in transmission 0.4% or 0.67% of the time, respectively.

- The symptoms of acute HIV infection are self-limited and most likely correlate with viremia.

- The evaluation of fever of unknown origin or unexplained weight loss should always include an HIV test, even in elderly patients without identified risk factors.

- Routine health maintenance care appropriate for the individual's age must not be overlooked, including breast, colon, and prostate cancer screening as per current guidelines.

AIDS is caused by the retrovirus known as HIV. The virus primarily targets CD4+ T-helper lymphocytes, depleting the immune system and leading to a state of immunodeficiency. As the immune system deteriorates and the CD4+ count approaches 200 cells/mm^3, opportunistic infections often occur.

The clinical syndrome of AIDS was first described in 1981, when a cluster of cases of *Pneumocystis carinii* (now *P. jirovecii*) pneumonia (PCP) was noted in a group of homosexual men.[1] The causative agent, HIV, was identified in 1984. By 1987, the first medication to treat HIV, azidothymidine (AZT; Retrovir) became available. Currently, more than 20 medications in five drug classes are available to be used in combination cocktails of three or more drugs often referred to as highly active antiretroviral therapy (HAART).

Two genetic types of HIV have been identified, HIV type 1 (HIV-1) and HIV type 2 (HIV-2). HIV-1 is the predominant type throughout the world. HIV-2 appears to be concentrated in West Africa, with small numbers of cases noted in France, Portugal, Angola, and Mozambique. HIV-2 appears to be less easily transmitted, results in disease that progresses more slowly, and is believed to be less virulent.[2,3]

HIV-1 is divided into three groups, designated group M (composed of subtypes or clades A–K), N, and O. In the United States, 98% of HIV-1 is group M, subtype B.[2,3]

EPIDEMIOLOGY

It is estimated that nearly 34 million people worldwide were living with HIV through the end of 2006.[4] Of this number, the adult population accounted for more than 31 million cases, whereas 2.3 million were children younger than 15 years. The epidemic has claimed nearly 25 million lives since its onset in 1981, of which 4.5 million were children. An estimated 14 million children are orphans because of the epidemic.

Sub-Saharan Africa has borne a disproportionate number of cases of HIV/AIDS, in part attributable to poverty, gender inequalities, political upheaval, and an inconsistent or absent public health infrastructure. These factors and others result in unavailable or severely fragmented medical care. This region has an estimated 22.5 million people living with HIV/AIDS, 61% of whom are female. In East Asia, Eastern Europe, and Central Asia, the number of individuals diagnosed with HIV had increased by 21% since 2004.[4] Globally, the most common means of acquiring HIV is through heterosexual contact. All age groups are affected, with the largest number of cases occurring between the ages of 20 and 50 years, the most productive years of life. Males and females are represented equally in case numbers.

An estimated 1.2 million people are living with HIV/AIDS in the United States. More than 500,000 people have died from AIDS. The vast majority of cases are in adults, whereas less than 5,000 children are currently living with HIV/AIDS. Males comprise 74% of cases; females account for 26%. The most common mode of transmission in the United States is male-to-male sexual contact (49%), followed by high-risk heterosexual contact (32%), and then injection drug use (14%). Mother-to-child transmission (which occurs prenatally, during birth, or postnatally via breast feeding) makes up a small group of cases in the United States. Rare cases occur through transfusion of blood products.[4,5,5a]

Although African Americans constitute slightly more than 12% of the U.S. population, nearly 40% of all cases of HIV/AIDS have occurred in this group.[6] In the most recently available statistics, African Americans accounted for 49% of new cases in 2005. From 1999 to 2002, African American females represented 72% of the new cases among women with HIV.[6] Hispanics represent 18% of HIV/AIDS cases, and Caucasians account for 31% of the total. See Tables 14.1 to 14.3 for various summaries of the statistics.

Individuals between the ages of 25 and 45 years account for nearly two-thirds of all cases in the United States. A re-

cent alarming trend demonstrates increasing numbers of infections in the 15- to 25-year age group. The majority of cases are clustered along the coastal areas, with major metropolitan areas having the largest numbers of cases.[5,5a] The epidemic has steadily infiltrated all areas of the country, both urban and rural.

PATHOPHYSIOLOGY

The HIV viruses belong to the lentivirus subfamily of the RNA retroviruses. The genetic material is contained in two copies of single-stranded RNA. Like most retroviruses, the HIV genome consists of three structural genes: *gag*, *pol*, and *env*. The *gag* gene codes for viral capsid proteins, *env* for the viral envelope proteins, and *pol* for the proteins responsible for viral replication, including the RNA-dependent DNA polymerase known as reverse transcriptase (RT). In addition, other regulatory genes are present, including *nef, rev, tat, vpr, vpu,* and *vif*.

Most commonly, transmission of the virus occurs after a breach in the integument or mucous membranes. HIV infection occurs when the envelope subunit gp120 binds both the human CD4 T-cell receptor, found primarily on lymphocytes and monocyte-derived macrophages, and one of two chemokine receptors, CCR5 or CXCR4. The viral envelope then fuses with the host cell, allowing the release of the viral core into the host cell. Viral RNA is transcribed by RT into DNA, which is then incorporated into the host

TABLE 14.2

HIV INFECTION: ETHNICITY

White	31%
African American	49%
Hispanic	18%

From Centers for Disease Control and Prevention, Divisions of HIV/AIDS Prevention. Available at: www.cdc.gov/hiv/resources/factsheets/At-A-Glance.htm.

TABLE 14.3

HIV INFECTION: MODE OF TRANSMISSION

MSM	49%
Heterosexual	32%
IDU	14%
MSM/IDU	4%
Other	1%

IDU, intravenous drug use; MSM, men who have sex with men.
From Centers for Disease Control and Prevention. Cases of HIV Infection and AIDS in the United States and Dependent Areas, 2005. HIV/AIDS Surveillance Report, Vol. 17, Revised June 2007. Available at: www.cdc.gov/hiv/topics/surveillance/resources/reports/2005report/pdf/2005SurveillanceReport.pdf.

TABLE 14.1

HIV INFECTION: GENDER

Male	74%
Female	26%

From Centers for Disease Control and Prevention, Divisions of HIV/AIDS Prevention. Available at: www.cdc.gov/hiv/resources/factsheets/us.htm.

genome by the viral protein integrase. Once viral gene expression occurs, the resultant polyproteins are cleaved by the viral protease, and production of mature virions can occur. These then bud from the infected cell and propagate the infection.[7]

Initial infection is characterized by a dramatic loss in memory CD4+ T cells residing in the gut-associated lymphoid tissue (GALT). Over time, infected persons have a slow, progressive loss of additional CD4+ lymphocytes, which leads to increasing degrees of immune suppression. The rate of CD4+ cell loss is variable and depends on viral and host factors. After the initial infection, on average, persons lose 40 to 80 cells/mm^3/year.[8] A subset of individuals will progress rapidly. Five percent of infected persons, known as long-term nonprogressors, will have little or no progression of clinical disease or decline in CD4 counts over 10 years, even without antiretroviral therapy.[9]

Transmission of the virus occurs via exposure to infected body fluids. These include, but are not limited to, blood, semen, vaginal fluid, and breast milk. The most common modes of transmission are sexual contact (male-male or heterosexual sex), parenteral exposure to blood and blood products, and vertical transmission during pregnancy. The magnitude of risk depends on the exposure. For example, the risk of HIV transmission from a known HIV-positive source from receptive anal intercourse is 0.1% to 0.3%, whereas receptive vaginal intercourse carries a risk per episode of 0.08% to 0.2%. A percutaneous exposure through a needlestick injury or intravenous drug use results in transmission 0.4% or 0.67% of the time, respectively.[10] The risk of vertical transmission from mother to fetus without any preventive therapy is approximately 25%.[11] The efficiency of transmission increases with greater degrees of viremia in the source patient and the presence of concurrent sexually transmitted diseases.

SIGNS AND SYMPTOMS

Acute HIV Infection

It is estimated that 40% to 90% of individuals infected with HIV experience the clinical syndrome of HIV seroconversion known as acute/primary HIV infection or acute retroviral syndrome. In one prospective study, among those with symptoms at the time of seroconversion, 95% sought medical care. Nevertheless, acute HIV infection is rarely diagnosed, partly because the symptoms are protean. The onset of illness is between 2 and 6 weeks after viral transmission and is believed to correlate with peak viremia, often in excess of 1 million viral copies/mL. Fever (mean, 38.9°C), rash, lymphadenopathy, and nonexudative pharyngitis are each present in more than 70% of individuals (Table 14.4). Most often, the rash is reminiscent of a viral exanthem, with erythematous maculopapular lesions on the face and trunk, although many types of lesions have been described.

TABLE 14.4	
ACUTE HIV INFECTION: FREQUENCY OF ASSOCIATED SIGNS AND SYMPTOMS	
Fever—96%	Headache—32%
Lymphadenopathy—74%	Nausea and vomiting—27%
Pharyngitis—70%	Hepatosplenomegaly—14%
Rash—70%	Weight loss—13%
Myalgia or arthralgia—54%	Thrush—12%
Diarrhea—32%	Neurologic symptoms—12%

Adapted with permission from the DHHS Panel on Antiretroviral Guidelines for Adults and Adolescents—A Working Group of the Office of AIDS Research Advisory Council (OARAC). Guidelines for the Use of Antiretroviral Agents in HIV-1-Infected Adults and Adolescents. January 29, 2008. Available at: www.aidsinfo.nih.gov/ContentFiles/AdultandAdolescentGL.pdf.

Headache with or without cerebrospinal fluid (CSF) pleocytosis, myalgias, and gastrointestinal symptoms are also common. Although present in only 5% to 20% of patients, oral or genital ulcers can be an important diagnostic clue. Laboratory abnormalities, specifically leukopenia, thrombocytopenia, and elevated transaminases are not uncommon. Opportunistic infections, such as mucocutaneous candidiasis and PCP, may present during acute HIV infection as a result of transient but dramatic CD4 cell count depletion due to the high level of viremia.[12]

The symptoms of acute HIV infection are self-limited and most likely correlate with viremia. After reaching high levels, the viral load declines to a steady state or set point, and the peripheral CD4 count rebounds. HIV-1–specific cytotoxic T lymphocytes are present in high titer and appear to play an important role in controlling viral replication. The magnitude of the viral set point and the severity of initial symptoms predict disease progression. Whether early antiretroviral treatment is beneficial remains controversial. Regardless, recognition of this syndrome has obvious implications for public health. One study using mathematical modeling suggests that the 25% of HIV-infected individuals in the United States who are unaware of their HIV status account for 54% of new HIV infections.[12a] Furthermore, acute HIV infection is postulated to be a time of markedly increased transmission risk.[12b]

Chronic HIV Infection

A variety of historical details, findings on physical examination, and laboratory abnormalities should prompt testing to identify individuals with established HIV infection. As expected, these findings are more prominent in patients with more advanced disease. Frequently, the initial diagnosis of HIV infection is made when the patient develops an AIDS indicator condition (Table 14.5).[13] The astute clinician, however, can often detect signs and symptoms of HIV infection earlier in the course of disease, thus allowing access to appropriate therapy and prophylaxis prior to the development of significant illness.

TABLE 14.5

AIDS INDICATOR DISEASES

Candidiasis, invasive
Cervical cancer, invasive
Coccidioidomycosis, extrapulmonary
Cryptococcosis, extrapulmonary
Cryptosporidiosis of longer than 1 month duration
Cytomegalovirus disease outside lymphoreticular system
Dementia, HIV
Encephalopathy, HIV related
Herpes simplex infection of longer than 1 month duration or visceral
Salmonella bacteremia, recurrent
Histoplasmosis, extrapulmonary
Isosporiasis of longer than 1 month duration
Kaposi's sarcoma
Lymphoma: primary central nervous system
Non-Hodgkin's lymphoma
Mycobacterial disease, disseminated or extrapulmonary
Mycobacterium tuberculosis infection
Nocardiosis
Pneumocystis carinii pneumonia
Pneumonia, recurrent (>1 episode/year)
Progressive multifocal leukoencephalopathy
Strongyloidiasis, extraintestinal
Toxoplasmosis, cerebral
Wasting syndrome due to HIV

Physicians must conduct a thorough, nonjudgmental assessment of risk factors for HIV infection. Testing should be offered to individuals with a history of intravenous drug use, sexually transmitted diseases including human papillomavirus (HPV), hemophilia, and receipt of blood products between 1977 and 1985. Men who have had sex with men, sex workers, and heterosexual persons with multiple partners are also at high risk, as are the sexual partners of high-risk or HIV-infected individuals. Mental illness and incarceration may serve as markers for high-risk behavior, as does a history of hepatitis B or C infection. At present, the Centers for Disease Control and Prevention advocates HIV testing for all individuals between the ages of 13 and 64 years at least once, with additional annual tests for those with risk behaviors, including unprotected sex with a partner who is unaware of their HIV status.[13a]

A history of certain illnesses can also be suggestive of HIV infection. Infections such as active tuberculosis, recurrent community-acquired pneumonia, esophageal candidiasis, and either multidermatomal herpes zoster or zoster in younger adults should lead to HIV testing. Neoplastic diseases such as B-cell lymphoma, severe anal or cervical dysplasia, or invasive carcinoma and Kaposi's sarcoma (KS) are indications for HIV testing, as is idiopathic dilated cardiomyopathy. The evaluation of fever of unknown origin or unexplained weight loss should always include an HIV test, even in elderly patients without identified risk factors.

Various findings on physical examination may suggest coexisting HIV infection. An examination of the skin can be particularly revealing. Seborrheic dermatitis or molluscum contagiosum are common in early disease, as is psoriasis. Oral candidiasis and oral hairy leukoplakia can be seen, typically with CD4 counts <500 cells/mm^3. Generalized lymphadenopathy is common. Recurrent or severe lesions of herpes simplex virus may be indicative of underlying HIV infection. Neurologic findings such as unexplained peripheral neuropathy or dementia are suggestive.

On laboratory evaluation, idiopathic thrombocytopenia (ITP), unexplained anemia, neutropenia, and/or leukopenia are frequent early clues to underlying HIV infection.

DIAGNOSIS

Multiple tests have been developed to aid in the serologic diagnosis of HIV-1 and -2. Samples of blood, urine, and oral secretions have been used for testing. The standard approach employs a two-step process using the enzyme-linked immunosorbent assay (ELISA or EIA) and the Western blot (WB).[14] Both are designed to detect antibodies to HIV. The EIA is a highly sensitive screening test, which when positive is repeated for verification. A positive EIA is only presumptive evidence of infection by HIV and should never be accepted as definitive by itself. It must be followed and confirmed by a WB. Most individuals develop a positive EIA approximately 2 weeks after infection, with the vast majority seroconverting in 4 weeks. Rapid screening tests that can give results in 20 minutes or less are also EIAs and require WB confirmation. Currently, four tests are available: OraQuick Advance Rapid HIV-1/2 Antibody Test (OraSure Technologies, Inc., Bethlehem, PA), Uni-Gold Recombigen (Trinity Biotech, Wicklow, Ireland), Reveal G$_2$ (MedMira, Inc., Halifax, Nova Scotia), and Multispot HIV-1/HIV-2 (BioRad Labs, Hercules, CA). False-positive EIAs occur as a result of cross-reacting antibodies (common HLA antigens), chronic renal failure, malignancies, severe liver disease, vaccination, or autoreactive antibodies (i.e., ANA).

The WB is an immunoblot electrophoretic assay that measures antibodies to the HIV gene products of *env*, *pol*, and *gag* (including the p24 antigen). A positive study is defined as one in which bands to two of the following three proteins are present: the envelope proteins gp41 and gp120/160, and the viral capsid protein p24. A negative WB has no positive bands, but a study with any positive bands that do not meet the previous criteria is considered indeterminate. Indeterminate assays are usually caused by nonspecific cross-reacting proteins, HIV-2 infection, pregnancy, transfusions, malignancy, autoimmune diseases, or connective tissue diseases. Indeterminate assays can also occur in early seroconversion. A repeat assay should be performed within 2 to 4 weeks to evaluate the progression or regression of the test result. Additional bands on follow-up testing are suggestive of evolving seroconversion. In a low-risk population, stable persistent indeterminate tests are usually of no clinical consequence. When in doubt, an expert in the field of HIV disease should be consulted.[15]

INITIAL EVALUATION

The advances in therapy and prevention during the past 10 years have transformed HIV into a chronic, but often treatable, disease. As such, the initial encounter should not only be an important data gathering session, but also an opportunity to establish a long-term relationship with the patient. The initial evaluation should include a very detailed comprehensive history and physical examination, coupled with appropriate lab and x-ray tests.

A thorough medical history is critical. Particular attention should be directed to common HIV-related symptoms such as unexplained fevers, night sweats, weight loss, rashes and other skin lesions, diarrhea, weight loss, oral or vaginal candidiasis, oral ulcers, herpes zoster, visual changes, paresthesias or weakness, changes in mental status, or symptoms of depression.

A complete and nonjudgmental sexual history is necessary, including sexual practices, number and type of partners, use of condoms, and previous or current sexually transmitted diseases. A thorough history of substance abuse should be obtained, including the drug abused, route administered, and method of acquiring illicit substances. Patients should also be specifically asked about alcohol abuse and crystal methamphetamine, which can be overlooked on history. Caregivers must also inquire about domestic violence, both physical and emotional. The patient's sexual partners or needle-sharing partners must be notified of their potential HIV exposure, although this can be done anonymously.

Travel and residential history may be pertinent. Those living in endemic geographic locales may be at risk for various infections (e.g., histoplasmosis in the Ohio and Mississippi River valleys or coccidioidomycosis in the southwestern United States).

A routine vaccination history should be recorded including adult vaccinations such as hepatitis A and B vaccine and tetanus vaccinations. Previous purified protein derivative (PPD) testing and tuberculosis exposure or treatment should be included in the record. Because of the increased risk of acquisition and reactivation, annual PPD skin tests are recommended. Induration ≥ 5 mm is considered a positive test in an HIV-infected individual.

Throughout the interview, the knowledge base of the patient should be noted and educational needs assessed, with subsequent planning to address these needs. The educational needs of the patient's partners and/or family members should also be considered and addressed.

The physical examination must also be thorough. The skin examination may reveal seborrheic dermatitis, KS, psoriasis, or extensive folliculitis. Evidence of cytomegalovirus retinitis on funduscopic examination suggests advanced disease. If the examiner does not feel adept at funduscopy, referral to an ophthalmologist is appropriate. Oral findings may include thrush, KS, aphthous ulcers, or oral hairy leukoplakia (OHL). Dental hygiene and dental health should be noted, with appropriate care or referral planned. The size and location of enlarged lymph nodes are important. Varying degrees of generalized lymphadenopathy are common in HIV, but focal lymphadenopathy that persists or enlarges may require further evaluation. Pelvic and rectal examination should be directed toward evidence of candidiasis, sexually transmitted diseases, or malignancy. Because HIV-infected patients have higher rates of cervical dysplasia, carcinoma in situ, and frank cervical carcinoma than in the general population, two normal Papanicolaou (Pap) tests should be obtained 6 months apart, after which annual testing is routine. All abnormalities should be pursued aggressively. Men should be specifically evaluated for genital HPV, regardless of sexual orientation. Most clinicians recommend annual anal Pap smears to aid in early detection of anorectal carcinoma.

Laboratory testing is an important aspect of the evaluation of an HIV-positive patient. Table 14.6 lists those baseline tests that are recommended. If the patient presents with an anonymous HIV test result, the HIV serology should be repeated and confirmed.

Lymphocytopenia is often noted on the complete blood count but HIV-related leukopenia, thrombocytopenia, or anemia may also be present. Abnormal liver tests may suggest further pathology including viral hepatitis or opportunistic infections. Underlying renal insufficiency may be present and would suggest further evaluation.

Testing for syphilis with a nontreponemal test (rapid plasma reagin or Venereal Disease Research Laboratory) and for hepatitis (hepatitis A, B, and C serologies) is essential because these infections are seen with greater frequency in patients with HIV infection. Toxoplasma immunoglobin G (IgG) serologies should be sent to determine whether the patient is at risk for reactivation of this protozoan.

HIV-infected patients have higher rates of cardiovascular disease. In addition, some of the medications are associated with hyperlipidemia. For these reasons, baseline lipid profiles should be obtained.

The CD4+ count and HIV viral load are important prognostic indicators. Patients with high viral loads (typically >100,000 copies/cc) experience a more rapid progression

---

TABLE 14.6

THE INITIAL EVALUATION: LABORATORY TESTING

Complete blood count with diff	CD4+ count
Chemistry	HIV viral load
Rapid plasma reagin/Venereal Disease Research Laboratory	HIV genotype
Urinalysis	
Hepatitis A, B, and C serologies	Cytomegalovirus IgG
Glucose-6-phosphate dehydrogenase[a]	Toxoplasma IgG
	Lipid profile

IgG, immunoglobin G.
[a]When indicated.

TABLE 14.7

CENTERS FOR DISEASE CONTROL AND PREVENTION HIV CLINICAL STAGING

CD4+ Count (mm³)	Asymptomatic	Symptomatic	AIDS Indicator
≥500	A1	B1	C1
200–499	A2	B2	C2
<200	A3	B3	C3

of their disease and more frequent complications. The CD4+ count is also used for staging purposes (Table 14.7). The numerical aspect of staging is determined by the CD4+ cell count (1: CD4 ≥500 cells/mm³, 2: CD4 = 200–499 cells/mm³, and 3: CD4 <200 cells/mm³), whereas the letter designations of A, B, or C refer to symptoms associated with HIV disease or indicator illnesses. Category A patients are asymptomatic, whereas category C patients have experienced an AIDS indicator condition (Table 14.5). Most, but not all, AIDS indicator conditions occur when the CD4+ count drops to <200 cells/mm³. By definition, a CD4+ count of 200/mm³ is an AIDS indicator event. Category B patients are symptomatic but have not experienced an AIDS indicator condition. Category B patients may have herpes zoster, persistent or recurrent thrush, persistent or recurrent vaginal candidiasis, constitutional symptoms, prolonged unexplained diarrhea (>1 month), ITP, OHL, cervical dysplasia, or neuropathy. Some degree of variation may be noted in CD4+ counts and viral loads between testing sessions, as well as between laboratories. It is important to establish a trend with respect to counts and to attempt to use the same laboratory for testing.

Newly infected patients are increasingly acquiring drug-resistant virus. Currently, baseline HIV resistance testing (HIV genotype) is recommended in all newly diagnosed patients. This information may be used to guide current or future drug therapy.

THERAPY

The appropriate treatment of the HIV-infected individual requires much more than a consideration of antiretroviral therapy. Preventive care is essential to treating the HIV-infected patient. Some infections can be minimized by avoiding uncooked and undercooked foods such as seafood, eggs, and meats; abstaining from drinking lake and river water; avoiding contact with animals with diarrhea and litter boxes; and the institution of careful handwashing. Patients with CD4 counts >200 cells/mm³ should receive the pneumococcal vaccine, updated every 5 years, with consideration for vaccination in all patients regardless of CD4 counts. The influenza vaccine is recommended, as is hepatitis B vaccination if the patient is seronegative. Although hepatitis A vaccination is indicated if the patient has existing hepatitis B or C, most practitioners favor

vaccinating all seronegative individuals. Tetanus boosters are indicated every 10 years. At present, live vaccines are not recommended in patients with advanced disease. The safety of these vaccines, which include varicella, measles-mumps-rubella, and yellow fever, in patients with preserved CD4+ T-cell counts is unknown and can be considered individually. The inactivated vaccines for typhoid (Typhim Vi capsular polysaccharide) and polio (inactivated polio vaccine) should be administered when required, rather than the live vaccines.[16]

Routine health maintenance care appropriate for the individual's age must not be overlooked, including breast, colon, and prostate cancer screening as per current guidelines. Smoking cessation should be addressed. Aggressive control of cardiovascular risk factors is necessary. Annual ophthalmologic and dental visits are recommended.

The identification of a durable power of attorney and a discussion of advanced directives are valuable early in disease. Mental health or substance abuse treatment programs should be offered if needed. Consultation with a nutritionist experienced in HIV care and a social worker is beneficial.

Patients with advanced HIV disease require prophylaxis to prevent opportunistic infections (Table 14.8). At CD4 counts <200 cells/mm³ or CD4+ ≤14, PCP prophylaxis should be initiated promptly because the incidence of disease approaches 20% per year. The first-line agent is trimethoprim-sulfamethoxazole (TMP-SMX), one double-strength tablet daily. Dapsone (100 mg/day) is recommended for patients who are TMP-SMX intolerant and not glucose-6-phosphate dehydrogenase deficient. When the CD4 count falls to <100 cells/mm³, patients with positive *Toxoplasma gondii* IgG serologies require prophylaxis to prevent reactivation. Daily TMP-SMX is again the drug of choice. Patients on dapsone require the addition of pyrimethamine. Although *Mycobacterium avium* complex (MAC) prophylaxis is recommended at CD4 counts <50 cells/mm³, initiation is never emergent, and active MAC disease should be ruled out prior to starting prophylaxis if the patient has any suggestive symptoms. The most common regimen is azithromycin 1,200 mg/week. More detailed information can be obtained from the U.S. Public Health Service and Infectious Diseases Society of America Guidelines for the Prevention of Opportunistic Infections Among HIV-Infected Persons—2002.[16]

TABLE 14.8

PRIMARY PROPHYLAXIS AGAINST OPPORTUNISTIC INFECTIONS

Pathogen	Indication	Drug of Choice	Alternatives
Pneumocystis carinii	CD4 count <200/μL or oropharyngeal candidiasis	TMP-SMZ, 1 SS or DS tablet daily	Dapsone, pyrimethamine, leucovorin, aerosol pentamidine, atovaquone, TMP-SMZ 3× week
Mycobacterium tuberculosis[a,b]	TST positive (5 mm) or prior positive TST without treatment or contact with active case	INH, 300 mg daily, plus pyridoxine, 50 mg daily, for 9 months; INH, 900 mg, plus pyridoxine, 100 mg 2× week for 9 months; or rifampin, 600 mg, plus pyrazinamide, 15–20 mg/kg, daily for 2 months [c]	Rifabutin, 300 mg, plus pyrazinamide, 15–20 mg/kg, daily for 2 months; or rifampin, 600 mg daily, for 4 months
INH-resistant M. tuberculosis	Same as previous; high probability of exposure to INH-resistant tuberculosis	Rifampin, 600 mg, plus pyrazinamide, 20 mg/kg, daily for 2 months[c]	Rifabutin plus pyrazinamide daily for 2 months, or rifampin or rifabutin daily for 4 months
Toxoplasma gondii	CD4 count <100/μL and IgG antibodies to Toxoplasma	TMP-SMZ, 1 DS tablet, daily	Low-dose TMP-SMZ; dapsone plus pyrimethamine plus leucovorin; atovaquone pyrimethamine plus leucovorin daily
Mycobacterium avium complex[b]	CD4 count <50/μL	Clarithromycin, 500 mg BID, or azithromycin, 1,200 mg, weekly	Rifabutin daily or azithromycin weekly plus rifabutin daily
Varicella zoster virus	Significant exposure in seronegative patient or patient with no history of chickenpox or shingles	VZIG, 5 vials IM, 96 hours after exposure	None

BID, twice daily; DS, double strength; IgG, immunoglobin G; IM, intramuscularly; INH, isoniazid; SS, single strength; TMP-SMZ, trimethoprim-sulfamethoxazole; TST, tuberculin skin test; VZIG, varicella zoster immunoglobulin.
[a]Consult USPHS/IDSA document for recommendations on prophylaxis of INH-resistant or multidrug-resistant M. tuberculosis. Guidelines for Prevention and Treatment of Opportunistic Infections in HIV-Infected Adults and Adolescents. Modified with permission from Centers for Disease Control and Prevention.
[b]Pharmacokinetic interactions may occur when rifampin, rifabutin, or clarithromycin are administered concurrently with protease inhibitors or nonnucleoside reverse transcriptase inhibitors.
[c]Because of potential liver injury, the 9-month daily INH regimen is preferred unless the patient has been exposed to an INH-resistant strain or is unlikely to complete the course of therapy. Use the 2-month regimen with caution, especially in patients taking other medications associated with liver injury and those with alcoholism.
Modified with permission from Draft 2001 USPHS/IDSA guidelines for the prevention of opportunistic infections in persons infected with human immunodeficiency virus. Available at: www.aidsinfo.nih.gov/contentfiles/Adult_OI.pdf. Dosing modifications may be indicated for individuals with renal or hepatic dysfunction.

ANTIRETROVIRAL THERAPY

Over the past decade, the selection of highly active antiretroviral therapy (HAART) has become increasingly complex. The ideal time to start HAART therapy remains controversial. Many studies confirm that poorer outcomes are seen when antiretroviral therapy is initiated after the CD4+ T-cell count falls to <200 cells/mm^3. Therefore, all patients with symptomatic HIV disease or a CD4 count ≤200 should be offered HAART. Current U.S. Department of Health and Human Services (DHHS) recommendations (2007) suggest that treatment should be recommended to asymptomatic individuals with CD4+ T cells between 200 cells/mm^3 and 350 cells/mm^3, regardless of viral load. Some experienced clinicians advocate therapy in those with CD4+ T-cell counts >350 cells/mm^3 when the HIV RNA levels exceed 100,000 copies/cc, but most will defer HAART in this setting. In general, recent guidelines suggest initiat-

ing HAART later than previously recommended, due to the emerging problems of drug resistance and medication side effects, coupled with uncertain benefit. Most important, the decision to start HAART must be individualized in every case. Factors such as the rate of CD4 T-cell decline or rise in viral load and the readiness of the patient to initiate therapy are critical. Often, the decision to start therapy should be delayed in those with untreated depression or substance abuse. Because the guidelines and expert opinion change regularly based on ongoing studies, interested individuals should review the most current set of guidelines.[17]

Currently, five different antiretroviral drug classes are licensed: nucleoside/nucleotide reverse transcriptase inhibitors (NRTIs), nonnucleoside reverse transcriptase inhibitors (NNRTIs), protease inhibitors (PIs), entry and fusion inhibitors, and integrase inhibitors (Table 14.9). The NRTIs are nucleoside/nucleotide analogs and act as chain terminators that impair the process of reverse transcription

TABLE 14.9

CURRENTLY AVAILABLE ANTIRETROVIRAL AGENTS (2007)

Nucleoside Reverse Transcriptase Inhibitors
Zidovudine (AZT, Retrovir)
Didanosine (ddI, Videx)
Zalcitabine (ddC, Hivid)
Lamivudine (3TC, Epivir)
Stavudine (d4T, Zerit)
Abacavir (ABC, Ziagen)
Emtricitabine (FTC, Emtriva)

Nucleotide Reverse Transcriptase Inhibitors
Tenofovir (TDF, Viread)

Nonnucleoside Reverse Transcriptase Inhibitors
Nevirapine (Viramune)
Delavirdine (Rescriptor)
Efavirenz (Sustiva)

Protease Inhibitors
Ritonavir (Norvir)
Indinavir (Crixivan)
Saquinavir (Invirase, Fortovase)
Nelfinavir (Viracept)
Amprenavir (Agenerase)
Fosamprenavir (Lexiva)
Atazanavir (Reyataz)
Lopinavir/ritonavir (Kaletra)
Darunavir (Prezista)
Tipranavir (Aptivus)

Entry Inhibitors
Enfuvirtide (T20, Fuzeon)—fusion inhibitor
Maraviroc (Selzentry)—CCR5 antagonist

Integrase Inhibitors
Raltegravir (Isentress)

Combination Pills
Combivir (zidovudine/lamivudine)
Trizivir (zidovudine/lamivudine/abacavir)
Epzicom (abacavir/lamivudine)
Truvada (tenofovir/emtricitabine)
Atripla (tenofovir/emtricitabine/efavirenz)

of viral RNA into DNA. The NNRTIs inhibit reverse transcriptase by binding the RT enzyme and preventing its function. The PIs impair the packaging of viral particles into a mature virion capable of budding from the cell and productively infecting additional T lymphocytes. Finally, entry inhibitors prevent the virus from entering the cell. There are several types of entry inhibitors. Currently, two medications are approved: a fusion inhibitor, which impairs membrane fusion of the HIV virion to the T cell, thus preventing initial infection of the lymphocyte, and a CCR5 chemokine receptor antagonist, which blocks binding of the virus to the CD4 cell. Integrase inhibitors block DNA strand transfer preventing the integration of viral genetic material into the human genome. Additional agents are in development, including other entry inhibitors, integrase inhibitors, and maturation inhibitors. Initial therapy should always include a minimum of three

agents. No single regimen is appropriate for all patients. Recommended first-line regimens include two NRTIs and either an NNRTI or a PI. Regimens containing triple NRTIs have been shown to have higher rates of virologic failure and are therefore not recommended as first-line therapy, except in the rare instances when an NNRTI- or PI-containing regimen cannot or should not be used. The DHHS guidelines currently recommend one NNRTI-containing regimen (efavirenz + zidovudine/lamivudine or tenofovir/emtricitabine) and three PI-containing regimens (lopinavir/ritonavir twice daily or fosamprenavir + ritonavir twice daily or atazanavir + ritonavir) + (zidovudine/lamivudine or tenofovir/emtricitabine) for first-line therapy. Currently available protease inhibitors, with the exception of nelfinavir, are frequently prescribed in combination with low-dose ritonavir, a technique known as *boosting*. Ritonavir is a potent inhibitor of the CYP3A4 isoenzyme that is part of the cytochrome P450 system of hepatic metabolism. All PIs are substrates of this enzyme. As a result, low-dose ritonavir increases the trough and prolongs the half-life of the coadministered PI, thus enhancing the drug exposure and allowing for less frequent dosing. Many experts now believe that all first-line PI-containing regimens should use ritonavir-boosted PIs.[17,18]

The response to therapy should be carefully monitored. Patients on initial regimens should reach undetectable viral loads 16 to 24 weeks after initiating therapy. However, viral loads should be followed every 4 to 8 weeks immediately after starting the regimen. Failure to achieve an undetectable viral load or a rebound in plasma viremia after reaching this goal should lead to a careful assessment of the reasons for virologic failure. These considerations should include nonadherence, decreased drug absorption, drug-drug interactions altering drug metabolism, and the development of resistance. Resistance testing should be performed if alternative reasons for virologic failure are not apparent. The most critical and modifiable factor affecting success is patient adherence. Only 45% of patients taking 90% to 95% of their prescribed doses of antiretroviral medications will achieve viral suppression (<400 copies/cc) compared to 78% in those taking more than 95% of their doses.[19] Incomplete viral suppression leads to the development of drug resistance. Adherence to the antiviral regimen should be addressed at every visit with every physician in a detailed fashion, and the importance of careful adherence should be stressed.

The clinician must also be aware of side effects and toxicities that may occur due to the prescribed antiretroviral medications (Table 14.10). The most common and potentially serious include:

- Cytopenias, with the use of zidovudine
- Pancreatitis, with the use of didanosine
- Peripheral neuropathy, with the use of didanosine and stavudine

TABLE 14.10

SELECTED COMMON ADVERSE EVENTS (AEs) DUE TO ANTIRETROVIRAL AGENTS

Antiretroviral Class	Antiretroviral Drug	AE Unique to the Antiretroviral	AE Common Across the Class
Nucleoside/nucleotide reverse transcriptase inhibitors	Zidovudine (AZT, ZDV)	Anemia, neutropenia	Lactic acidosis with hepatic steatosis, lipoatrophy[a]
	Didanosine (ddI)	Peripheral neuropathy, pancreatitis	
	Zalcitabine (ddC)	Peripheral neuropathy	
	Stavudine (d4T)	Peripheral neuropathy	
	Lamivudine (3TC)		
	Abacavir (ABC)	Hypersensitivity syndrome	
	Tenofovir (TDF)	Fanconi's syndrome	
	Emtricitabine (FTC)		
Nonnucleoside reverse transcriptase inhibitors	Nevirapine (NVP)	Hepatitis	Rash
	Delavirdine (DLV)		
	Efavirenz (EFV)	Central nervous system symptoms	
Protease inhibitors	Indinavir (IDV)	Nephrolithiasis, unconjugated hyperbilirubinemia	Lipodystrophy,[a] gastrointestinal intolerance, hyperglycemia, lipid abnormalities
	Ritonavir (RTV)		
	Nelfinavir (NLV)		
	Saquinavir (SQV)		
	Amprenavir (APV)		
	Fosamprenavir (fAPV)		
	Atazanavir (ATV)[b]	Nephrolithiasis, unconjugated hyperbilirubinemia	
	Lopinavir/ritonavir (LPV)		
	Tipranivir (TPV)	Intracerebral hemorrhage	
	Darunavir (DRV)		
Entry inhibitors	Enfuvirtide (ENF)	Injection site reactions	
	Maraviroc		

[a]The role of various antiretroviral agents in the development of lipodystrophy is not fully understood.
[b]Lipid abnormalities appear to be less prominent with this agent.
Adapted with permission from the DHHS Panel on Antiretroviral Guidelines for Adults and Adolescents—A Working Group of the Office of AIDS Research Advisory Council (OARAC). Guidelines for the Use of Antiretroviral Agents in HIV-1-Infected Adults and Adolescents. January 29, 2008. Available at: www.aidsinfo.nih.gov/ContentFiles/AdultandAdolescentGL.pdf.

- Hypersensitivity, including rash, fever, and risk of death, with re-exposure to abacavir
- Rash, with the use of all NNRTIs
- Hepatitis, with the use of nevirapine
- Unconjugated hyperbilirubinemia or nephrolithiasis with the use of indinavir or atazanavir
- Gastrointestinal toxicity, including diarrhea and nausea, with the use of all protease inhibitors

More recently appreciated are the metabolic abnormalities that can occur in patients taking HAART. Hyperglycemia, hypercholesterolemia, and hypertriglyceridemia should be carefully monitored and treated (with attention to interactions between the protease inhibitors and many HMG CoA reductase inhibitors). Fat distribution abnormalities (lipodystrophy) are frequently noted, including wasting of the limbs and face (lipoatrophy) and enlargement of the dorsocervical fat pad and central obesity (fat accumulation). An increased risk of osteopenia and aseptic joint necrosis has been noted. Nucleo-side analogs, again notably stavudine, didanosine, and zidovudine, can lead to mitochondrial dysfunction due to the inhibition of mitochondrial γ-DNA polymerase. Like the etiology of lipoatrophy and other effects, mitochondrial dysfunction can also lead to potentially fatal lactic acidosis with hepatic steatosis. Early symptoms of this syndrome are protean, and include fatigue, abdominal pain and bloating, nausea and vomiting, tachypnea, and paresthesias. Elevated lactate levels establish the diagnosis; however, transaminase elevations may be suggestive. Treatment requires the discontinuation of the inciting drugs. In addition, significant drug interactions can occur between antiretroviral agents and commonly prescribed drugs; these interactions can lead either to drug toxicities or a reduction in levels of the drug or the antiretroviral agent, thus rendering them ineffective. For a complete listing of adverse effects, toxicities, and medication interactions, refer to the Guidelines for the Use of Antiretroviral Agents in HIV-1-Infected Adults and Adolescents.[17]

SPECIAL CIRCUMSTANCES: PREGNANCY

Pregnant women who are HIV-infected pose special treatment challenges. The risks of antiretroviral medications to the fetus are not fully known for all available agents. Most experts believe that, with a few exceptions as noted here, the benefits of therapy to the mother and the reduction in the risk of vertical transmission to the infant outweigh the risks of antiretroviral therapy. Currently, antiretroviral medications that are avoided in pregnancy include efavirenz (due to the occurrence of birth defects in monkeys) and the combination of stavudine and didanosine (increased risks of mitochondrial toxicity in pregnancy). The greatest amount of data in pregnancy exists for zidovudine, and it should be included as part of the treatment regimen when feasible.

Delivery by cesarean section at 38 weeks is recommended for women if the plasma viral load late in pregnancy exceeds 1,000 copies/cc. Current data suggest that women with viral loads below this level appear to have equivalent risks of mother-to-child transmission regardless of mode of delivery; that rate is <2%. All HIV-infected women should receive intravenous zidovudine during labor (or as a continuous infusion, beginning with a loading dose prior to planned cesarean section), and the infant should receive zidovudine for 6 weeks after birth. Women declining HAART in the second and third trimester should be encouraged to take zidovudine at a minimum, although single-drug therapy does increase the risk of developing resistant virus in the mother and potentially transmitting resistant virus to the infant. When used alone, this three-part zidovudine regimen has been shown to reduce the risk of mother-to-child transmission from 23% to 8%.[20] Pregnant women presenting in labor without documented HIV testing or prenatal care should be offered rapid HIV testing. Administration of antiretroviral medications to the mother and the child can reduce rates of maternal-to-child transmission even when initiated shortly before birth.

SPECIAL CIRCUMSTANCES: POSTEXPOSURE PROPHYLAXIS

Limited data suggest that treatment with antiretroviral medications immediately after exposure to potentially infectious material from an HIV-infected source may reduce the risk of seroconversion in the exposed individual. The data are largely derived from a single retrospective cohort study of zidovudine prophylaxis after occupational exposures. In this study, the risk of transmission was reduced by 81%. Animal data, scientific theory, and mother-to-child transmission studies all support the concept that postexposure prophylaxis may be beneficial. Guidelines have been established for occupational exposures, and extrapolation of these concepts to nonoccupational exposures is left to the treating physicians.

Exposures are evaluated based on risk of the exposure. Percutaneous exposures carry a greater risk of transmission than mucus membrane exposures. Exposures resulting from a deep injury, from a device on which blood was visible, or from a device that had been in the source patient's artery or vein also carry a greater risk of seroconversion. Fluids from source patients with advanced disease, as measured by disease activity or viremia, carry a higher risk of transmission than those from patients with earlier disease and lower-level viremia.

Based on these criteria, the exposure is rated as either a more or less severe percutaneous or mucus membrane exposure from a higher- or lower-risk source patient. Individuals sustaining percutaneous exposures or high-volume mucus membrane exposures from high-risk patients or severe percutaneous exposures from lower-risk patients are offered an expanded (three or more drug) prophylaxis regimen. Those with less severe percutaneous exposures or high-volume mucus membrane exposures from lower-risk patients or small-volume mucus membrane exposures from high-risk patients are offered basic (two-drug) prophylactic regimens. Individuals with small-volume mucus membrane exposures from low-risk patients can consider a basic regimen. Basic regimens contain two NRTIs. The most common are zidovudine/lamivudine or tenofovir/emtricitabine. Addition of a protease inhibitor is recommended when an expanded regimen is selected. The regimen should be initiated as soon as possible, ideally within 1 hour of the exposure, and continued for 28 days. Baseline HIV serologic tests should be obtained. Follow-up testing at 6 weeks, 3 months, and 6 months is recommended. Expert consultation should be sought if the source patient is known to have drug-resistant virus and postexposure prophylaxis regimens should be tailored accordingly.[21]

VACCINES

Vaccines have been one of the most effective means of combating and controlling infectious diseases. An extensive effort is under way to find such a treatment for HIV. Despite several vaccine trials evaluating both therapeutic and preventative vaccines, none has been found effective to date. Critical to this effort are ongoing attempts to seek an understanding of the basic immune correlates of protection from HIV. In addition, methods must be developed to deal with the marked genetic variability between different strains of HIV. Vaccines appear to hold the most promise for the world as a whole in conquering the HIV epidemic. Unfortunately, none appears to be on the horizon at this time.

OPPORTUNISTIC INFECTIONS

Many uncommon infections may occur in HIV patients as the disease progresses and cell-mediated immunity

TABLE 14.11

COMMON OPPORTUNISTIC INFECTIONS

Pneumocystis carinii (now *P. jiroveci*) pneumonia	Cytomegalovirus
Candida	*Myobacterium avium* complex
Herpes simplex virus	*Cryptococcus neoformans*
Human herpes virus type 8	*Histoplasma capsulatum*
Toxoplasma gondii	JC virus

deteriorates. Table 14.11 lists the more common opportunistic infections (OIs). As noted, toxoplasmosis, MAC, and PCP are targeted for primary prophylaxis (no evidence of active disease, but the patient is at risk). Secondary prophylaxis (ongoing treatment after acute infection has been diagnosed and treated) is indicated for PCP, toxoplasmosis, MAC, cryptococcosis, cytomegalovirus, histoplasmosis, and coccidioidomycosis. Although various OIs have occurred at higher CD4+ counts, in general, prophylaxis is not necessary in those with CD4 counts >200 cells/mm^3 or 14%. Table 14.12 lists OIs and the CD4+ count at which they are known to occur with increased frequency. With the arrival of HAART and subsequent improvement of the immune system through control of the virus (immune reconstitution), it has become possible to discontinue the use of primary and secondary prophylactic medications. Table 14.13 reviews the U.S. Public Health Service and Infectious Diseases Society of America Prevention of Opportunistic Infections Working Group guidelines for starting and stopping primary and secondary prophylaxis.[16]

A detailed discussion of all OIs is beyond the intent of this chapter. A brief overview of the salient aspects of the presentation and diagnosis of PCP, toxoplasmosis, MAC, and cryptococcosis follows.

PNEUMOCYSTIS JIROVECII PNEUMONIA

PCP is the most common pulmonary infection in HIV patients, typically occurring when the CD4+ T-cell count

TABLE 14.12

CD4+ CELL COUNT AND OPPORTUNISTIC INFECTIONS

CD4+/mm^3	Infection/Complication
<500	Varicella zoster virus, oral candida, tuberculosis, HSV, Kaposi's sarcoma (human herpes virus type 8)
<200	*Pneumocystis carinii* (now *P. jiroveci*) pneumonia, severe mucocutaneous HSV
<100	Toxoplasmosis, cryptococcosis, microsporidiosis
<50	Progressive multifocal leukoencephalopathy, cryptosporidiosis, *Myobacterium avian* complex, cytomegalovirus

HSV, herpes simplex virus.

is ≤200 cells/mm^3. Although the organism exists in cyst, tachyzoite, and sporozoite forms, it is taxonomically most closely associated with the fungi. Symptoms are nonspecific; insidious in onset; and include shortness of breath, dyspnea, nonproductive cough, fever, chest tightness, fatigue, and weight loss. The chest radiograph most commonly demonstrates interstitial infiltrates, although it may be normal in 20% of cases.[22] Spontaneous pneumothoraces may occur. Laboratory tests are of little assistance in the diagnosis. The serum lactate dehydrogenase (LDH) may be elevated but is nonspecific. An exercise desaturation test may reveal exercise-induced hypoxia, which may aid in the diagnosis of PCP. The diagnosis is based on clinical suspicion and the demonstration of the organisms on silver stain or by other means in the laboratory. Open-lung biopsy has been the gold standard, but more commonly bronchoscopy and bronchoalveolar lavage (BAL) are used, with yields of nearly 100%.[23] Expectorated or induced sputum samples generally have variable yields that are inferior to BAL. Treatment is TMP-SMX for 3 weeks. If the PO$_2$ is <70 mm Hg, a tapering dose of prednisone is recommended, starting at 40 mg twice daily. Alternate therapies include pentamidine and dapsone or trimethoprim. When acute therapy has been completed, secondary prophylaxis should be initiated.

TOXOPLASMA ENCEPHALITIS

T. gondii is an obligate intracellular parasite. The cat is the definitive host, whereas humans and other animals are secondary hosts. It is the most common cause of intracerebral lesions in HIV patients[24] and usually presents as encephalitis.

The clinical presentation is subacute and may include subtle progressive changes in mental status or neuropsychiatric function, focal motor weakness, coma, and seizures. Neuroimaging is very important in the diagnosis and characteristically reveals multiple intracranial ringenhancing lesions with surrounding edema. The lesions have a predilection for the basal ganglia. The differential diagnosis of toxoplasmosis includes central nervous system lymphoma, histoplasmoma, cryptococcoma, tuberculoma, bacterial abscesses, or metastatic carcinoma. A lumbar puncture often yields a nonspecific elevation of protein, minimal change in glucose, and mild mononuclear pleocytosis. Nearly all patients have a positive toxoplasma IgG serology, indicating prior exposure and subsequent risk for reactivation. Where available, polymerase chain reaction of the CSF for toxoplasma may be helpful. The demonstration of organisms on brain biopsy makes a definitive diagnosis, but biopsy is reserved for those cases that do not appear to respond to treatment or that have a negative baseline toxoplasma serology. First-line therapy of toxoplasmic encephalitis is pyrimethamine, sulfadiazine, and folinic acid. Alternative therapies include TMP-SMX, clindamycin, or

TABLE 14.13

INITIATION AND DISCONTINUATION OF PRIMARY PROPHYLAXIS

Pathogen	Criteria for Initiation	Criteria for Discontinuation	Criteria for Restarting
Pneumocystis carinii pneumonia	CD4+ <200 cells/μL or oropharyngeal candidiasis	CD4+ >200 cells/μL for $\geq$3 months	CD4+ <200 cells/μL
Toxoplasmosis	CD4 count <100/μL or IgG antibody to toxoplasma	CD4+ >200 cells/μL for $\geq$3 months	CD4 <100–200 cells/μL
Disseminated *Mycobacterium avium* complex	CD4 count <50/μL	CD4+ >100 cells/μL for $\geq$3 months	CD4 <100–200 cells/μL

Modified with permission from Draft 2001USPHS/IDSA guidelines for the prevention of opportunistic infections in persons infected with human immunodeficiency virus. Available at: www.aidsinfo.nih.gov/contentfiles/ Adult_186.pdf.

other macrolides combined with pyrimethamine. Initial treatment for 3 to 6 weeks is followed by secondary prophylaxis.

CRYPTOCOCCOSIS

Cryptococcus neoformans is an encapsulated dimorphic fungus that is ubiquitous in nature, found in the soil, and in high concentrations in pigeon feces. It is the most common cause of meningitis in HIV patients. Cryptococcal infections occur as CD4+ counts approach 100 cells/mm^3.

The clinical presentation is often subtle, with fever and headache. Meningoencephalitis may occur with altered mental status, headache, and fever. Despite a high burden of organisms, the inflammatory response is muted or absent. The CSF will usually have elevated protein, decreased glucose, and a pleocytosis that seems minor for the degree of disease present. The serum and CSF cryptococcal antigen and fungal culture are the best diagnostic tools. The CSF antigen will be present in more than 90% of meningitis cases, and the serum antigen will be present in 94% to 100% of cases.[25]

Treatment for 10 weeks starting with amphotericin B 0.7 mg/kg/day for 2 weeks, followed by fluconazole 400 mg daily is recommended.[26] Flucytosine may be added to the first 2 weeks of therapy. Initial therapy is followed by fluconazole prophylaxis. Alternatively, fluconazole may be used for the entire course of therapy.

MYCOBACTERIUM AVIUM COMPLEX

MAC is a rapid-growing mycobacterium that presents as a disseminated disease in advanced HIV, typically at CD4+ counts of <50/mm^3. The clinical syndrome is nonspecific, with a combination of several symptoms and findings that may include wasting, fever, night sweats, anorexia, diarrhea, enlarged liver and spleen, central and peripheral lymph node enlargement, or anemia. The organism may be cultured from blood, bone marrow, lymph nodes, or liver biopsy. The presence of the organism in stool or spu-

tum may indicate colonization or pathological disease. Although an elevated serum alkaline phosphatase is a nonspecific laboratory finding, it is frequently noted with MAC infection. The burden of organisms in the various tissues is usually massive. Prolonged therapy is necessary and includes at a minimum clarithromycin or azithromycin with ethambutol.

NATIONAL GUIDELINES

- DHHS Guidelines for the Use of Antiretroviral Agents in HIV-Infected Adults and Adolescents, December 4, 2007
- Public Health Service Task Force Recommendations for the Use of Antiretroviral Drugs in Pregnant HIV-1 Infected Women for Maternal Health and Interventions to Reduce Perinatal HIV-1 Transmission in the United States, October 12, 2006
- NPHRC/HRSA/NIH Guidelines for the Use of Antiretroviral Agents in Pediatric HIV Infection, October 26, 2006
- U.S. Public Health Service and Infectious Diseases Society of America Guidelines for the Prevention of Opportunistic Infections Among HIV-Infected Persons—2002, June 14, 2002
- Updated U.S. Public Health Guidelines for Management of Occupational Exposure to HIV and Recommendations for Postexposure Prophylaxis, September 30, 2005

REFERENCES

1. Pneumocystis pneumonia—Los Angeles. *MMWR Morb Mortal Wkly Rep* 1981;30:250–252.
2. Markovitz DM. Infections with human immunodeficiency virus type 2. *Ann Intern Med* 1993;118:211–218.
3. Weidle PJ, Ganea CE, Irwin KL, et al. Presence of human immunodeficiency (HIV) type 1, group M, non-B subtypes, Bronx, New York: a sentinel site for monitoring HIV genetic diversity in the United States. *J Infect Dis* 2000;181:470–475.
4. UNAIDS, World Health Organization. AIDS Epidemic Update, December 2006. Available at: http://www.unaids.org/en/knowledgecenter/HIVData/default.asp.
5. Centers for Disease Control and Prevention, Divisions of HIV/AIDS Prevention. Available at: www.cdc.gov/hiv/resources/factsheets/index.htm.

5a. Centers for Disease Control and Prevention. Cases of HIV Infection and AIDS in the United States and Dependent Areas, 2005. HIV/AIDS Surveillance Report, Vol. 17, Revised June 2007. Available at: http://www.cdc.gov/hiv/topics/surveillance/index.htm.

6. HIV/AIDS among African Americans. CDC Divisions of HIV/AIDS Prevention. Available at: www.cdc.gov/hiv/topics/aa/resources/factsheets/aa.htm.

7. Liang C, Wainberg MA. Virology of HIV. In: Cohen J, Powderly WG, eds. *Infectious Diseases*, 2nd ed. Edinburgh: Mosby, 2004:1251–1255.

8. Mellors JW, Mu-oz A, Giorgi JV, et al. Plasma viral load and CD4+ lymphocytes as prognostic markers of HIV-1 infection. *Ann Intern Med* 1997;126:946–954.

9. Cao Y, Qin L, Zhang L, et al. Virologic and immunologic characterization of long-term survivors of human immunodeficiency virus type 1 infection. *N Engl J Med* 1995;332:201–208.

10. Centers for Disease Control and Prevention. Management of possible sexual, injecting-drug-use, or other nonoccupational exposure to HIV, including considerations related to antiretroviral therapy. Public Health Service Statement. *MMWR Recomm Rep* 1998;47(RR17):1–14.

11. Sperling RS, Shapiro DE, Coombs RW, et al. Maternal viral load, zidovudine treatment, and the risk of transmission of human immunodeficiency virus type 1 from mother to infant. *N Engl J Med* 1996;335:1621–1629.

12. Kahn JO, Walker BD. Current concepts: acute human immunodeficiency virus type 1 infection. *N Engl J Med* 1998;339:33.

12a. Marks G, Crepaz N, Janssen RS. Estimating sexual transmission of HIV from persons aware and unaware that they are infected with virus in the USA. *AIDS* 2006;20:1447–1450.

12b. Zetola NM, Pilcher CD. Diagnosis and management of acute HIV infection. *Infect Dis Clin North Am* 2007;21:19–48.

13. 1993 Revised classification system for HIV infection and expanded surveillance case definition for AIDS among adolescents and adults. *MMWR Recomm Rep* 1992;41(RR17).

13a. Revised recommendations for HIV testing of adults, adolescents, and pregnant women in health-care settings. *MMWR Recomm Rep* 2006;55(RR-14):1–17.

14. Mylonakis E, Paliou M, Lally M, et al. Laboratory testing for infection with the human immunodeficiency virus: established and novel approaches. *Am J Med* 2000;109:568–576.

15. Centers for Disease Control and Prevention. Interpretation and use of the Western blot assay for serodiagnosis of human immunodeficiency virus type 1 infections. *MMWR Morb Mortal Wkly Rep* 1989;38(S7):1–7.

16. U.S. Public Health Service and Infectious Diseases Society of America Prevention of Opportunistic Infections Working Group. Guidelines for the Prevention of Opportunistic Infections Among HIV-Infected Persons—2002: Recommendations of the U.S. Public Health Service and the Infectious Diseases Society of America. June 14, 2008. Available at: http://aidsinfo.nih.gov/contentfiles/Adult_OI.pdf.

17. DHHS Panel on Antiretroviral Guidelines for Adults and Adolescents—A Working Group of the Office of AIDS Research Advisory Council (OARAC). Guidelines for the Use of Antiretroviral Agents in HIV-1-Infected Adults and Adolescents. January 29, 2008. Available at: www.aidsinfo.nih.gov/ContentFiles/AdultandAdolescentGL.pdf.

18. Yeni PG, Hammer SM, Hirsch MS, et al. Treatment for adult HIV infection: 2004 recommendations of the International AIDS Society–USA Panel. *JAMA* 2004;292:251–265.

19. Paterson DL, Swindells S, Mohr J, et al. Adherence to protease inhibitor therapy and outcomes in patients with HIV infection. *Ann Intern Med* 2000;133:21–30.

20. Perinatal HIV Guidelines Working Group. Public Health Service Task Force Recommendations for Use of Antiretroviral Drugs in Pregnant HIV-Infected Women for Maternal Health and Interventions to Reduce Perinatal HIV Transmission in the United States. July 8, 2008. Available at: http://aidsinfo.nih.gov/ContentFiles/PerinatalGL.pdf.

21. Centers for Disease Control and Prevention. Updated U.S. public health guidelines for management of occupational exposure to HIV and recommendations for postexposure prophylaxis. *MMWR Recomm Rep* 2005;54(RR09):1–17.

22. Brenner M, Ognibene FP, Lack EE, et al. Prognostic factors and life expectancy of patients with acquired immunodeficiency syndrome and *Pneumocystis carinii* pneumonia. *Am Rev Respir Dis* 1987;136:1199.

23. Broaddus V, Dake M, Stulbarg M, et al. Bronchoalveolar lavage and transbronchial biopsy for the diagnosis for pulmonary infections in patients with the acquired immunodeficiency syndrome. *Ann Intern Med* 1985;102:747.

24. Luft B, Remington J. Toxoplasmic encephalitis in AIDS. *Clin Infect Dis* 1992;15:211.

25. Chuck S, Sande M. Infections with *Cryptococcus neoformans* in the acquired immunodeficiency syndrome. *N Engl J Med* 1989;321:794.

26. Saag MS, Graybill RJ, Larsen RA, et al. Practice guidelines for the management of cryptococcal disease. *Clin Infect Dis* 2000;30:710–718.

Chapter 15

Infective Endocarditis

Thomas F. Keys   Alice I. Kim

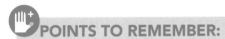

POINTS TO REMEMBER:

- A recent study demonstrated a high frequency of *Staphylococcus aureus* endocarditis secondary to preventable sources.

- Approximately 10% of patients with clinically suspected endocarditis will have negative blood cultures.

- Brain abscess and mycotic aneurysms are relatively infrequent. As a general rule, anticoagulation should be avoided because of the increased risk of intracranial bleeding. One may elect to continue anticoagulation in patients with mechanical heart valves, but dosing should be in the low therapeutic range to minimize the risk of bleeding.

Infective endocarditis (IE) remains a challenge to American medicine. The incidence has remained stable during the antibiotic era: an estimated 1 case per 1,000 hospital admissions, or approximately 8,000 cases per year. The most appropriate medical and surgical management for IE is a challenge in this era of great technology, but increasing restraints from third-party payers. Its prevention is a challenge because of the threat of nosocomial bacteremia from intravascular catheters or surgical wounds, which is often caused by antibiotic-resistant micro-organisms. Its medical treatment remains a challenge because of the relative lack of new or innovative antimicrobial agents that are needed to confront those enterococci and staphylococci that have become absolutely or relatively insensitive to vancomycin. This chapter discusses the epidemiology of IE, current diagnostic methods, pharmacologic and surgical treatments, persistent fever during therapy, neurologic complications, and preventive strategies.

EPIDEMIOLOGY

In the preantibiotic era, survival was rare after an attack of IE. With the introduction of effective chemotherapy beginning in the early 1940s and surgical intervention beginning in the late 1960s, the outcome of IE was no longer bleak (Table 15.1). Despite these striking advances, however, mortality remains around 20%. In part, this is because more patients are living longer with prosthetic heart valves, and intravenous drug abuse (IVDA) continues to be a problem. Furthermore, our technically complex health care system often exposes patients to nosocomial bloodstream infections that may result in endocarditis. In the modern era, death is usually not due to uncontrolled infection but more commonly to congestive heart failure (CHF) and mechanical failure of heart valves.

Although rheumatic valvulitis was historically considered a frequent predisposing disease to IE, times have changed (Table 15.2). Mitral valve prolapse, aortic sclerosis, and even bicuspid aortic valvular heart disease are more frequent factors. Prosthetic valvular heart disease accounts for approximately one-third of all cases of IE and is seen in 1% to 3% of patients undergoing valvular heart surgery. Thirty years ago, early-onset (within 1 year of surgery) prosthetic valve endocarditis (PVE) was often fatal; surgeons were reluctant to operate on patients who had active endocarditis involving freshly implanted heart valves. Mortality was reported at 90% in one series. Infection most often resulted from intraoperative contamination by nosocomial bacteria, especially *Staphylococcus epidermidis*, as well as by inexperience with surgical techniques. Despite advancing surgical expertise and standard antibiotic prophylaxis against staphylococci, early-onset PVE continues to be a problem, although mortality is now around 25% because of more aggressive surgical intervention combined with antibiotic therapy. In addition to valve replacement, preferably with homograft tissue, surgeons are successfully debriding and repairing native valves without replacement.

Late-onset PVE (at least 1 year after surgery) is much more frequent because more patients with prosthetic heart valves survive longer. Fortunately, these cases are usually caused by the same organisms as native valve endocarditis (NVE). Cure rates are nearly as good, and reoperation may not be necessary.

Pacemaker endocarditis, another complication of advancing technology, is usually caused by skin bacteria from a battery pack that migrate from a pocket infection or

TABLE 15.1

DECLINING INCIDENCE OF DEATH FROM INFECTIVE ENDOCARDITIS

Series	Years	Patients	Deaths (%)
Cates and Christie	1945–1949	442	44
Lerner and Weinstein	1939–1959	100	37
Pelletier and Petersdorf	1963–1972	125	37
Keys et al.	1981–1982	90	21
Sandre and Shafran	1985–1993	135	19

Data adapted from Cates JE, Christie RV. Subacute bacterial endocarditis: a review of 442 patients treated in 14 centers appointed by the Penicillin Trials Committee of the Medical Research Council. *QJM* 1951;20:93; Keys TF, Schaber D, Lever H, et al. Treatment of infective endocarditis. *Proceedings of the 14th International Congress on Chemotherapy, Kyoto, Japan.* Tokyo: University of Tokyo Press, June 25, 1985:1981–1982; Lerner PI, Weinstein L. Infective endocarditis in the antibiotic era. *N Engl J Med* 1966;274:199; Pelletier LL Jr, Petersdorf RG. Infective endocarditis: a review of 125 cases from the University of Washington Hospitals, 1963–1972. *Me Med* 1977;56:287–313; Sandre RM, Shafran SD. Infective endocarditis: review of 135 cases over 9 years. *Clin Infect Dis* 1996;22:276–286.

erosion through the skin. Early cases are usually caused by *Staphylococcus aureus* and late cases by *S. epidermidis*. Pacemaker leads may encapsulate into the ventricle, making explantation tedious and difficult.

A recent study demonstrated a high frequency of *S. aureus* endocarditis secondary to preventable sources. Of 59 cases reported from Duke University, 23 were caused by infected intravascular catheters and 14 from surgical wounds (Table 15.3). It has been estimated that 25% of vascular catheter–associated bacteremias caused by *S. aureus* result in endocarditis.

A significant risk factor for endocarditis is IVDA. Patients who use injection drugs tend to be younger and may be coinfected with HIV. IVDA-associated endocarditis is usually quite responsive to antibiotic therapy. The quoted overall mortality is around 10%.

PATHOGENESIS

IE usually follows endothelial trauma, as might occur from regurgitant blood flow or a high pressure gradient.

TABLE 15.2

UNDERLYING HEART DISEASE IN 60 PATIENTS WITH NATIVE VALVE ENDOCARDITIS

Lesion	Patients (n)	Prevalence (%)
Mitral valve prolapse	14	23
Aortic sclerosis	12	20
Bicuspid aortic valve	6	10
Miscellaneous	6	10
Rheumatic	5	8
Unknown	17	28

TABLE 15.3

FREQUENCY OF SOURCES RESPONSIBLE FOR ENDOCARDITIS DUE TO *STAPHYLOCOCCUS AUREUS*

Presumed Source	Cases (n)	
	Hospital	Community
Intravenous catheter	12	11
Hemodialysis fistula	2	5
Surgical wound	12	2
Other	1	1
None	0	13

Micro-organisms with adherence factors are preferentially attracted to these lesions and proliferate within a fibrin meshwork, resulting in vegetation. Adherence is promoted by dextran-producing streptococci. For example, *Streptococcus mutans* produces large concentrations of dextran and is commonly associated with endocarditis, whereas this is rarely caused by non–dextran-secreting organisms such as group A β-hemolytic streptococci.

MICROBIOLOGY

Viridans and other streptococci, including *Streptococcus bovis* and *Enterococcus faecalis*, are responsible for the largest percentage of endocarditis cases (Table 15.4). *Streptococcus mitis* is nutritionally deficient and requires vitamin B$_6$ and thio compounds for growth. It accounts for 10% of all cases of viridans endocarditis and tends to be less responsive to penicillin therapy. Occasionally, cases of group B streptococcal endocarditis occur, and they often present with major embolic events from vegetations. Rarely, *Streptococcus pneumoniae* may cause endocarditis. This has been reported in alcoholic men, who may present with the Osler triad of pneumonia, meningitis, and endocarditis; mortality is high.

In several recent studies, endocarditis due to *S. aureus* has surpassed viridans group streptococci as the leading cause

TABLE 15.4

NATIVE VALVE ENDOCARDITIS MICROBIOLOGY

Organism	Cases (%)
Streptococcus viridans	30–40
Enterococcus species	5–10
Other streptococci	10–25
Staphylococcus aureus	10–27
Coagulase-negative staphylococci	1–3
Gram-negative bacilli	2–13
Fungi	2–4
Other	5
"Culture negative"	5–24

TABLE 15.5

EARLY-ONSET PROSTHETIC VALVE ENDOCARDITIS MICROBIOLOGY

Organism	Cases (%)
Staphylococcus epidermidis	35
Staphylococcus aureus	17
Streptococcal species	8
Diphtheroids	10
Gram-negative bacilli	16
Fungi	11
Other	3

of IE. *S. aureus* endocarditis may result in a sepsis syndrome with a fulminating coagulopathy.

Metastatic foci of infection occur in the brain, lungs, liver, and kidneys. Overall, this infection has the highest mortality when cases related to IVDA are excluded. *S. aureus* is also a common cause of early-onset PVE, although not as frequently as *S. epidermidis* (Table 15.5). Although historically related to intraoperative contamination from skin bacteria, infections of vascular catheters and surgical wounds are now more important sources of infection. Endocarditis due to *Staphylococcus lugdunensis* has recently been emphasized in the literature. This organism, first described in 1988, is coagulase negative, but may be confused with *S. aureus* in the laboratory. Although usually very susceptible to penicillin, isolates appear highly virulent. Cases present acutely, and infection is associated with a very high mortality rate. In one series, death was certain unless patients underwent emergency valve replacement. *S. epidermidis*, the most frequent cause of early-onset PVE, is almost always resistant to methicillin (Staphcillin) or oxacillin, but has a more favorable prognosis.

The HACEK group of fastidious gram-negative microorganisms occasionally causes endocarditis. HACEK is an all-inclusive term for endocarditis due to *Haemophilus, Actinobacillus, Cardiobacterium, Eikenella,* and *Kingella* species of bacteria. Clinically, these cases are characterized by a subacute or chronic course and often present with embolic lesions from large vegetations.

Most cases of fungal endocarditis occur in patients who are receiving prolonged antibiotics or parenteral nutrition through central vascular catheters. Such patients may also be immunocompromised. The most common species is *Candida albicans,* followed by *Candida parapsilosis.* Endocarditis due to *Histoplasma capsulatum* or *Aspergillus* species is rare.

Finally, unusual cases of endocarditis should be considered when standard microbiological techniques fail to provide a diagnosis. Q fever endocarditis, due to *Coxiella burnetii,* usually has an atypical presentation. Patients may not have fever but frequently have underlying valvular heart disease and are on immunosuppressive therapy. Vegetations are rarely detected on echocardiogram. Routine blood cultures are negative. Serologic studies are reasonably specific, and an alerted microbiology laboratory may recover the organism from buffy-coat cultures. *Bartonella henselae* may also cause endocarditis. This infection, often of the homeless and alcoholic population, is difficult to diagnose. Blood cultures are negative, but serology may be helpful. Studies using the polymerase chain reaction technique on resected valve tissue may provide the diagnosis if the technology is available.

DIAGNOSIS

The diagnostic clues noted by Sir William Osler in 1908 remain true today: remittent fever with a valvular heart lesion, embolic findings, skin lesions, and progressive cardiac changes. In 1981, Von Reyn et al. reported the benefit of strict definitions for managing cases and comparing outcomes. The use of echocardiography improved the specificity of diagnosis, and, in 1984, Durack et al. from Duke University, proposed updated criteria that have now been accepted for diagnosis:

- Positive valve culture or histology
- Two major criteria: typical organism, persistent bacteremia, positive blood culture or anti-phase IgG antibody titer for *C. burnetii,* positive echocardiogram for vegetations, abscess, or valve dehiscence
- Five of six minor criteria: predisposing lesions or IVDA, temperature >38°C, vascular events (emboli, infarcts, mycotic aneurysm, hemorrhages), immunologic phenomena (glomerulonephritis, Osler's nodes, Roth spots, rheumatoid factor), suggestive echocardiogram, positive blood culture or serology
- One major and three minor criteria

Transesophageal echocardiography is more sensitive and specific than transthoracic echocardiography for detecting vegetations and other lesions, such as ring abscesses and valve dehiscence (Table 15.6).

The clinical features of patients with PVE are not much different from those with NVE (Table 15.7). Fever, skin lesions, a newly appreciated heart murmur, and splenomegaly occur with equal frequency. Weight loss may be more common in NVE, however, presumably because patients are sicker longer before they seek medical attention.

The most important laboratory study to confirm a clinical diagnosis of endocarditis is the blood culture. In a landmark study reported by Werner et al. (1967), a clear majority of patients with suspected bacterial endocarditis had positive blood cultures within a period of 2 days, provided that they had not been on antibiotics recently. Therefore, one need not collect more than three blood cultures during a 24-hour period unless antibiotics are already on board. More sophisticated blood culture techniques have also improved the recovery of organisms: BACTEC system (Johnston Laboratories, Inc., Towson, MD) for staphylococcal

TABLE 15.6

ECHOCARDIOGRAM DETECTION OF VEGETATIONS IN PATIENTS WITH INFECTIVE ENDOCARDITIS

Study	Year	Patients	TTE	Sensitivity (%) TEE
Daniel et al.	1987	69	78	94
Mugge et al.	1989	91	58	90
Shively et al.	1991	16	44	94
Birmingham et al.	1992	31	30	88

TEE, transesophageal echocardiography; TTE, transthoracic echocardiography.
Data adapted from Birmingham GD, Rahko PS, Ballantyne F III. Improved detection of infective endocarditis with transesophageal echocardiography. *Am Heart J* 1992;123:774–781; Daniel WG, Mugge A, Grote J, et al. Comparison of transthoracic and transesophageal echocardiography for detection of abnormalities of prosthetic and bioprosthetic valves in the mitral and aortic positions. *Am J Cardiol* 1993;71:210–215; Mugge A, Danile WG, Frank G, et al. Echocardiography in infective endocarditis: reassessment of the prognostic implications of vegetation size determined by the transthoracic and transesophageal approach. *J Am Coll Cardiol* 1989;14:631–638; Shively BK, Gurule FT, Roldan CA, et al. Diagnostic value of transesophageal compared with transthoracic echocardiography in infective endocarditis. *J Am Coll Cardiol* 1991;18:391–397.

species and the ISOLATER system (E.I. duPont de Nemours and Company, Wilmington, DE) for gram-negative bacilli and yeasts. Other laboratory features, although nonspecific, may suggest the diagnosis. These include an elevated erythrocyte sedimentation rate, a positive rheumatoid factor, proteinuria, and circulating immune complexes.

TREATMENT

Pharmacologic Treatment

In the preantibiotic era, IE was a fatal disease. Now, penicillin, often in combination with gentamicin, remains a cornerstone of therapy for endocarditis caused by susceptible streptococci (Table 15.8). For penicillin-allergic pa-

TABLE 15.7

CLINICAL FINDINGS IN 90 PATIENTS WITH INFECTIVE ENDOCARDITIS

Symptom	NVE (%) ($n = 60$)	PVE (%) ($n = 30$)
Fever	75	87
Weight loss	52	20
Skin lesions	51	47
New murmur	33	33
Splenomegaly	20	20

NVE, native valve endocarditis; PVE, prosthetic valve endocarditis.

TABLE 15.8

THERAPY OF NATIVE VALVE ENDOCARDITIS: PENICILLIN-SENSITIVE STREPTOCOCCI

Antibiotic	Regimen	Duration (weeks)
Penicillin G	12–18 MU IV daily	4
Ceftriaxone	2 g IV daily	4
Ceftriaxone + gentamicin	2 g IV daily 3 mg/kg IV daily	2
Vancomycin	1 g IV every 12 hours	4

MU, million units.
Doses assume normal renal function. Minimum inhibitory concentration ≤ 0.1 μg/mL.

tients, vancomycin is substituted. Intravenous ceftriaxone (Rocephin), given once a day for 4 weeks, has been reported to cure penicillin-sensitive streptococcal endocarditis. More recently, ceftriaxone in combination with gentamicin has proved successful with only 2 weeks of therapy. This is not recommended, however, for patients who have PVE, major embolic complications, or symptoms lasting longer than 2 months. In one series reported from the Mayo Clinic, 24% of all patients required valvular heart surgery within 5 to 36 days after beginning treatment. Therefore, careful follow-up is essential, especially if patients are discharged from the hospital to complete antibiotic therapy at home.

For streptococci that are relatively insensitive to penicillin (minimum inhibitory concentration 0.12–0.5 μg/mL), penicillin or ceftriaxone is used. The penicillin dosage is increased, and antibiotics are continued for 4 weeks (Table 15.9). Gentamicin is given for the first 2 weeks. The treatment of enterococcal endocarditis is longer, using ampicillin or penicillin with gentamicin for 6 weeks. Vancomycin may be substituted for penicillin, provided that the isolate is susceptible. For vancomycin-resistant

TABLE 15.9

THERAPY OF NATIVE VALVE ENDOCARDITIS FOR PENICILLIN-INSENSITIVE STREPTOCOCCI[a] OR ENTEROCOCCI[b]

Antibiotic	Regimen	Duration (weeks)
Penicillin G	24 MU IV daily	4–6[c]
+Gentamicin	1 mg/kg IV/IM every 8 hours	2–6[c]
Ceftriaxone	2 g IV/IM every 24 hours	
+Gentamicin	1 mg/kg IV/IM every 8 hours	
Vancomycin	1 g IV every 12 hours	4–6
+ Gentamicin[d]	1 mg/kg IV/IM every 8 hours	4–6

MU, million units.
Doses assume normal renal function.
[a]Minimum inhibitory concentration = 0.1–0.5 μg/mL.
[b]Minimum inhibitory concentration >0.5 μg/mL.
[c]Prolonged therapy for enterococci.
[d]Gentamicin with vancomycin only for enterococci.

TABLE 15.10

THERAPY OF PROSTHETIC VALVE STAPHYLOCOCCAL ENDOCARDITIS

Isolate	Antibiotic	Regimen	Duration (weeks)
MSSA or MSSE	Oxacillin	2 g IV every 4 hours	≥ 6
	+ Gentamicin	1 mg/kg IV/IM every 8 hours	First 2
	+ Rifampin	300 mg PO every 8 hours	≥ 6
MRSA or MRSE	Vancomycin	1 g IV every 12 hours	≥ 6
	+ Gentamicin	1 mg/kg IV/IM every 8 hours	First 2
	+ Rifampin	300 mg PO every 8 hours	≥ 6

MRSA, methicillin-resistant *Staphylococcus aureus*; MRSE, methicillin-resistant *Staphylococcus epidermidis*; MSSA, methicillin-sensitive *Staphylococcus aureus*; MSSE, methicillin-sensitive *Staphylococcus epidermidis*.
Doses assume normal renal function.

enterococci, anecdotal success has been reported using quinupristin-dalfopristin or linezolid.

The therapy for NVE caused by methicillin-susceptible staphylococci is oxacillin or cefazolin for 4 to 6 weeks. If the organism is methicillin resistant, vancomycin is substituted. Gentamicin can be added for the first 3 to 5 days. Although this may shorten the duration of bacteremia, it does not improve the cure rate and, if continued longer, may cause renal toxicity.

Antibiotic therapy for staphylococcal PVE must be more aggressive because of the greater likelihood of treatment failure or relapse (Table 15.10). Oxacillin is prescribed for at least 6 weeks, with gentamicin for the first 2 weeks. If the isolate is methicillin resistant, vancomycin is substituted for oxacillin. Rifampin is added, providing the organism is susceptible.

Endocarditis caused by *S. aureus* associated with IVDA is generally more responsive to short-course antibiotic therapy. In one study, a cure rate of 89% was reported using a 2-week course of intravenous cloxacillin alone.

The current recommended treatment for the HACEK group of gram-negative bacteria is ceftriaxone or ampicillin-sulbactam or ciprofloxacin for 4 weeks (Table 15.11). Patients with late-onset PVE may often be cured medically without valve surgery.

TABLE 15.11

THERAPY OF ENDOCARDITIS DUE TO HACEK[a] MICRO-ORGANISMS

Antibiotic	Regimen	Duration (week)
Ceftriaxone	2 g IV every 24 hours	4
Ampicillin-sulbactam	3 g IV every 6 hours	4
Ciprofloxacin	1 g PO every 2 hours or 400 mg IV every 12 hours	4

[a]HACEK, *Haemophilus, Actinobacillus, Cardiobacterium, Eikenella,* and *Kingella* species of bacteria.
Doses assume normal renal function.

Patients with fungal endocarditis generally have a poor prognosis. In one study, only 30% of patients survived despite aggressive antifungal therapy, often in combination with surgery. My colleagues and I recently reported a 67% survival rate in treating cases of fungal PVE. The mainstay of therapy was aggressive surgery accompanied by intravenous amphotericin B (Fungizone) and followed by lifelong suppression with oral azole compounds such as fluconazole (Diflucan) or itraconazole (Sporanox).

Approximately 10% of patients with clinically suspected endocarditis will have negative blood cultures. A trial of empiric therapy can be considered using ampicillin-sulbactam plus gentamicin for NVE or vancomycin plus gentamicin and cefepime and rifampin for early and late PVE. Approximately 50% of these patients respond, as the typical organisms may not be recovered from the blood but may still be within vegetations. A common reason is that prior antibiotic treatment has suppressed growth in blood cultures. If a patient remains ill despite empiric therapy, however, one must look for an unusual organism or a noninfectious cause of endocarditis.

Surgical Treatment

Death from IE is usually due to CHF, often accompanied by valve dysfunction. In the past quarter century, aggressive surgery has been the most important advance in therapy. Surgery during acute infection does not increase mortality; in fact, restoration of a failing pump improves function and outcome. Valve dysfunction causing moderate to severe CHF (New York Heart Association class III or IV) is a strong indication for urgent surgery, as are endocardial abscesses. These frequently involve the aortic root, a valve ring, or the ventricular septum. Other conditions favoring surgery include vegetations >1 cm in diameter and failure or relapse of medical therapy due to organisms such as *S. aureus, Pseudomonas aeruginosa,* or *Candida* species.

Even if surgery is not required during the period of antimicrobial therapy, it may be required later, when heart failure develops because of valve damage from

TABLE 15.12

PERSISTENT FEVERS DURING TREATMENT OF INFECTIVE ENDOCARDITIS

Reason	Patients	%
Annular abscesses	11	26
Pulmonary or systemic emboli	7	17
Drug hypersensitivity	7	17
Myocarditis	3	7
Intravenous site infection	2	5
Other	6	14
Unknown	6	14

endocarditis. In one study, 47% of patients required surgery, usually within 2 years after completing medical therapy.

Complications of Treatment

A significant number of patients will have persistent fever during treatment (Table 15.12). Annular or ring abscesses may cause fever and are a strong indication for surgery. Other causes of prolonged fever during therapy include myocarditis, pulmonary and systemic emboli, drug hypersensitivity, and intravenous site infections.

Major neurologic complications from endocarditis are fortunately rare (Table 15.13). However, they can present difficult and sometimes vexing management dilemmas. Leading causes are stroke, encephalopathy, and retinal emboli. Brain abscess and mycotic aneurysms are relatively infrequent. As a general rule, anticoagulation should be avoided because of the increased risk of intracranial bleeding. One may elect to continue anticoagulation in patients with mechanical heart valves, but dosing should be in the low therapeutic range to minimize the risk of bleeding. Fortunately, most cases of mycotic aneurysm do not require surgery and resolve after appropriate medical therapy.

TABLE 15.13

NEUROLOGIC COMPLICATIONS IN NATIVE VALVE ENDOCARDITIS (NVE) AND PROSTHETIC VALVE ENDOCARDITIS (PVE)

Complication	NVE (%) (n = 13)	PVE (%) (n = 62)
Stroke	15	21
Encephalopathy	9	8
Retinal emboli	3	3
Headache	4	3
Mycotic aneurysm	3	—
Abscess	1	2
Meningitis	1	2
Seizures	1	—
Total	37	39

PREVENTION

The need for and adequacy of antibiotic prophylaxis to prevent IE continues to be debated. In 1986, Bayliss et al. observed that a presumed dental portal of entry was recognized less than 20% of the time. In two-thirds of cases, no portal of entry could be determined. Further controversy was stimulated by a recently published case-control study from the greater Philadelphia area (Table 15.14). Controls were matched for age, sex, and neighborhood. Information was collected through structured telephone interviews and outside medical and dental records. Patients with cases of endocarditis were no more likely than controls to have had recent dental procedures, with a procedure rate of around 20% (similar to the finding in the Bayliss study). One interesting caveat was present: Six cases of endocarditis were preceded by dental extraction, although none was noted in the control group. More important, however, cardiac risk factors dominated endocarditis cases. Mitral valve prolapse, congenital heart disease, rheumatic valvular heart disease, previous cardiac surgery, a history of IE, and a known heart murmur were nearly six times more frequent in endocarditis patients than in the control group.

The American Heart Association's (AHA) most recent guidelines for prophylaxis were published in 2007 to address the controversies that continue to exist regarding the efficacy of antibiotic prophylaxis in preventing IE. The new guidelines are simplified and focused on the prevention of endocarditis in those patients with the highest risk of morbidity and mortality from the infection. Considerations that led to revisions of the guidelines included the lack of data to support the causal relationship of bacteremias resulting from dental, gastrointestinal (GI) tract, or genitourinary (GU) tract procedures in the development of IE, as well as risks associated with antibiotic therapy, including potential adverse effects and increasing rates of drug-resistant micro-organisms.

In the previous 1997 AHA recommendations, patients were stratified into risk categories for the development of IE with antibiotic prophylaxis recommended for those in the high- and moderate-risk groups. In the most recent guidelines, however, prophylaxis is directed and limited to those individuals who are at highest risk of adverse outcomes from endocarditis (Table 15.15). The following

TABLE 15.14

DENTAL AND CARDIAC RISK FACTORS FOR INFECTIVE ENDOCARDITIS

Risk Factor	Cases (n = 273)	Controls (n = 273)
Dental prophylaxis	24	23
Extractions	6	0
Gingival surgery	1	0
History of endocarditis	17	1
Cardiac valvular surgery	37	2
Mitral valve prolapse	52	6

TABLE 15.15

CARDIAC CONDITIONS THAT PROPHYLAXIS WITH DENTAL PROCEDURES IS RECOMMENDED

- Prosthetic cardiac valve or prosthetic material used for cardiac valve repair
- Previous infective endocarditis
- Cardiac transplantation recipients who develop cardiac valvulopathy
- Congenital heart disease (CHD)
  - Unrepaired cyanotic CHD, including palliative shunts and conduits
  - Completely repaired congenital heart defect with prosthetic material or device, whether placed by surgery or by catheter intervention, during the first 6 months after the procedure
  - Repaired CHD with residual defects at the site or adjacent to the site of prosthetic patch or prosthetic device

Adapted from Wilson W, Taubert KA, Gewitz M, et al. Prevention of infective endocarditis: guidelines from the American Heart Association. *Circulation* 2007;116:1753–1754.

TABLE 15.16

PROCEDURES FOR WHICH ENDOCARDITIS PROPHYLAXIS IS REASONABLE FOR PATIENTS IN TABLE 15.15

- All dental procedures that involve manipulation of gingival tissue or the periapical region of teeth or perforation of the oral mucosa[a]
- Invasive procedure of the respiratory tract that involves incision or biopsy of the respiratory mucosa or procedure to treat an established infection such as drainage of abscess or empyema
- Surgical procedure that involves infected skin, skin structure, or musculoskeletal tissue

[a]The following procedures and events do not need prophylaxis: routine anesthetic injections through noninfected tissue, taking dental radiographs, placement of removable prosthodontic or orthodontic appliances, adjustment of orthodontic appliances, and placement of orthodontic brackets. Shedding of deciduous teeth, and bleeding from trauma to the lips or oral mucosa.
Adapted from Wilson W, Taubert KA, Gewitz M, et al. Prevention of infective endocarditis: guidelines from the American Heart Association. *Circulation* 2007;116:1736–1754.

cardiac conditions are targeted for prophylaxis: (a) patients with prosthetic cardiac valves; (b) previous history of IE; (c) patients with unrepaired cyanotic congenital heart disease (CHD), as well as those recently repaired CHD (within the first 6 months) with prosthetic material or device and those with residual defects after repair; and (d) cardiac transplant recipients who develop cardiac valvulopathy. Of note is the exclusion of patients with mitral valve prolapse (MVP) in the most updated recommendations. The rationale behind this change is that although MVP is a common predisposing position to IE, the incidence of IE in this population is actually low and is not usually associated with the adverse outcomes compared to the other cardiac conditions listed previously.

Another change from previous recommendations has been the indications for which prophylaxis are recommended. Currently, only those with the previously mentioned cardiac conditions should receive prophylaxis in the following procedures: (a) all dental procedures that involve manipulation of gingival tissue or the periapical region of teeth or perforation of the oral mucosa; (b) invasive procedures of the respiratory tract that involve incision or biopsy of the respiratory mucosa or drainage of infective focus, such as abscess or empyema; and (c) any surgical procedure that involves infected skin, skin structure, or musculoskeletal tissue. Prophylaxis for GI or GU procedures is no longer recommended (Table 15.16).

Amoxicillin remains the oral prophylactic antibiotic of choice. If the patient is unable to take oral medication, either ampicillin or cefazolin or ceftriaxone may be used. For patients allergic to penicillin or ampicillin, oral alternatives include cephalexin, clindamycin, or the macrolides (azithromycin or clarithromycin). For penicillin- or ampicillin-allergic patients unable to take oral medication, cefazolin or ceftriaxone, or clindamycin can be substituted. Of note, procedures involving known

TABLE 15.17

PROPHYLACTIC REGIMENS

Situation	Agent	Regimen: Single Dose 30 to 60 Minutes Before Procedure
Oral	Amoxicillin	2 g
Unable to take orally	Ampicillin	2 g IM/IV
	Cefazolin or ceftriaxone	1 g IM/IV
Penicillin allergy—oral	Clindamycin	600 mg
	Cephalexin	2 g
	Azithromycin or clarithromycin	500 mg
Penicillin allergy—unable to take oral	Cefazolin or ceftriaxone	1 g IM/IV
	Clindamycin	600 mg IM/IV

IM, intramuscularly; IV, intravenously.
Adapted from Wilson W, Taubert KA, Gewitz M, et al. Prevention of infective endocarditis: guidelines from the American Heart Association. *Circulation* 2007;116:1736–1754.

or suspected infection with staphylococci should include an agent active against this species such as an anti-staphylococcal penicillin or cephalosporin. However, in hospitals with a high prevalence of methicillin-resistant staphylococci (*S. aureus* and *S. epidermidis*) or those with β-lactam allergy, vancomycin or clindamycin should be used (Table 15.17).

For patients undergoing cardiac valve surgery, perioperative prophylaxis with a first- or second-generation cephalosporin is recommended.

Antibiotic prophylaxis should be administered in a single dose 30 to 60 minutes before the procedure. If the dose is inadvertently not given before the procedure, the dose may be given up to 2 hours after the procedure. For those undergoing cardiac valve surgery, the antibiotic infusion should be completed within 30 minutes of the skin incision with a second dose given if the surgical procedure exceeds 4 hours in duration and discontinued within 48 hours postoperatively.

REVIEW EXERCISES

QUESTIONS

1. Probable infective endocarditis by the Duke Criteria Diagnosis
a) Typical organism
b) Persistent bacteremia
c) Classic skin/mucosal lesions

(1) a, b
(2) a, c
(3) b, c
(4) a, b, c

Answer
The answer is (1).

2. Predictable organisms causing early-onset prosthetic valve endocarditis
a) *Staphylococcus epidermidis*
b) *Staphylococcus aureus*
c) Vancomycin-resistant *Enterococcus* species

(1) a
(2) a, b
(3) a, c
(4) a, b, c

Answer
The answer is (2).

3. Unusual causes of endocarditis: diagnosis by polymerase chain reaction
a) *Coxiella burnetii*
b) *Tropheryma whippelii*
c) *Bartonella* species

(1) a, b

(2) a, c
(3) b, c
(4) a, b, c
Answer
The answer is (4).

4. Presumptive therapy of late-onset prosthetic valve endocarditis
a) Penicillin + gentamicin
b) Penicillin + vancomycin
c) Penicillin + vancomycin + gentamicin
d) Vancomycin + gentamicin

(1) a
(2) b
(3) c
(4) d
Answer
The answer is (3).

5. Infective endocarditis: indication(s) for surgery
a) Congestive heart failure
b) Vegetations on echocardiogram
c) Ring abscesses

(1) a
(2) a, b
(3) c
(4) a, b, c
Answer
The answer is (3).

6. Infective endocarditis: indications for prophylaxis
a) Probable mitral valve prolapse
b) Prosthetic valvular heart disease
c) History of infective endocarditis

(1) a
(2) a, b
(3) b, c
(4) a, b, c
Answer
The answer is (3).

7. History of penicillin allergy: alternatives for dental prophylaxis
a) Vancomycin
b) Cephalexin
c) Clindamycin
d) Azithromycin

(1) a, b
(2) c, d
(3) b, c, d
(4) a, b, c, d
Answer
The answer is (3).

SUGGESTED READINGS

Baddour LM, Wilson WR, Bayer AS, et al. Infective endocarditis: Diagnosis, antimicrobial therapy, and management of complications. *Circulation* 2005;111:e394–e433.

Bayliss R, Clarke C, Oakley CM, et al. Incidence, mortality and prevention of infective endocarditis. *J R Coll Physicians Lond* 1986;20:15–20.

Dajani AS, Taubert KA, Wilson W, et al. Prevention of bacterial endocarditis: recommendations by the American Heart Association. *JAMA* 1997;277:1794–1801.

Douglas A, Moore-Gillon J, Eykyn S. Fever during treatment of infective endocarditis. *Lancet* 1986;1:1341–1343.

Durack DT, Lukes AS, Bright KD, et al. New criteria for diagnosis of infective endocarditis: utilization of specific echocardiographic findings. *Am J Med* 1994;96:200–209.

Fowler VG, Sanders LL, Kong LK, et al. Infective endocarditis due to *Staphylococcus aureus. Clin Infect Dis* 1994;28:106–114.

Hoesley CJ, Cobbs CG. Endocarditis at the millennium. *J Infect Dis* 1999;179(Suppl 2):S360–S365.

Melgar GR, Nasser RM, Gordon SM, et al. Fungal prosthetic valve endocarditis in 16 patients. *Medicine* 1997;76:1–10.

Murray HW, Roberts RB. *Streptococcus bovis* bacteremia and underlying gastrointestinal disease. *Arch Intern Med* 1978;138:1097–1099.

Sexton DJ, Tenenbaum MJ, Wilson WR, et al. Ceftriaxone once daily for 4 weeks compared with ceftriaxone plus gentamicin once daily for 2 weeks for treatment of endocarditis due to penicillin-susceptible streptococci. *Clin Infect Dis* 1998;27:1470–1474.

Strom BL, Abrutyn E, Berlin JA, et al. Dental and cardiac risk factors for infective endocarditis. *Ann Intern Med* 1998;129:761–769.

Von Reyn CF, Levy BS, Arbeit RD, et al. Infective endocarditis: an analysis based on strict case definitions. *Ann Intern Med* 1981;94:505–518.

Werner AS, Cobbs CG, Kaye D, et al. Studies on the bacteremia of bacterial endocarditis. *JAMA* 1967;202:127–131.

Wilson W, Taubert KA, Gewitz M, et al. Prevention of infective endocarditis: guidelines from the American Heart Association. *Circulation* 2007;116:1736–1754.

Chapter 16

Pneumonias

Steven K. Schmitt

 POINTS TO REMEMBER:

- *Staphylococcus aureus* should be sought in the setting of aspiration or as a result of influenza in the nursing home. There are increasing reports of pneumonia due to methicillin-resistant *S. aureus* in patients with little or no hospital contact.

- Pathogens such as *Mycoplasma, Chlamydophila,* and viruses can present in a subacute fashion with low-grade fever, nonproductive cough, constitutional symptoms, and absent or diffuse findings on lung examination.

- Although aspiration more commonly affects the right lung because of tracheobronchial anatomy, both lungs can be affected simultaneously. The affected site may depend on position at the time of aspiration.

- The sputum culture remains a controversial tool but is still recommended to help tailor therapy. It may prove particularly helpful in identifying resistant nosocomial bacterial pathogens.

- When a patient is hospitalized with pneumonia, blood cultures drawn within 4 hours may improve clinical outcome.

- Clindamycin is preferred over penicillin for the treatment of community-acquired aspiration pneumonia because of its superiority in the treatment of oral anaerobes such as *Bacteroides melaninogenicus.* Amoxicillin/clavulanic acid also provides excellent coverage in this setting.

- Five to 15% of pneumococcal isolates in many areas of the United States exhibit high-level penicillin resistance, with several areas reporting 35% of isolates with at least intermediate resistance.

Sir William Osler described pneumonia as the "captain of the men of death".[1] Although the advent of the antimicrobial age has somewhat reduced this rank, pneumonia remains the eighth leading cause of death in the United States. In 2004, the age-adjusted death rate due to pneumonia was 20.3 per 100,000 persons. Estimates of the incidence of pneumonia range from 4 to 5 million cases per year, with about 25% requiring hospitalization. Because pneumonia crosses the boundaries of all internal medicine subspecialties, a discussion of difficult issues regarding diagnosis, antimicrobial selection, treatment setting, and prevention is appropriate.

ETIOLOGY OF PNEUMONIA

Pathogenesis

Six mechanisms have been identified in the pathogenesis of pneumonia in immunocompetent adults:

- Inhalation of infectious particles
- Aspiration of oropharyngeal or gastric contents
- Hematogenous deposition
- Invasion from infection in contiguous structures
- Direct inoculation
- Reactivation

The inhalation of infectious particles is probably the most important pathogenic mechanism in the community. It is believed to be particularly contributory in pneumonia due to *Legionella* species and *Mycobacterium tuberculosis*.

The aspiration of oropharyngeal or gastric contents is by far the most prevalent pathogenetic mechanism in cases of nosocomial pneumonia, with a variety of factors contributing to this risk. Swallowing and epiglottic closure may be impaired by neuromuscular diseases or stroke. States of altered consciousness, such as in chemical sedation, delirium, coma, or seizures, can also depress swallowing, the gag reflex, and closure of the epiglottis. In addition, endotracheal and nasogastric tubes may interfere with these anatomical defenses. Finally, impaired lower esophageal sphincter function and nasogastric and gastrostomy tubes increase the risk of the regurgitation of gastric contents. Fortunately, aspiration rarely leads to overt bacterial pneumonitis. It is probable that the nature of the resident flora, the size of the inoculum, and underlying diseases may determine which aspirations result in lung infection.

Direct inoculation rarely occurs as a result of surgery or bronchoscopy but may play a role in the development of pneumonia in patients supported with mechanical ventilation. The hematogenous deposition of bacteria in the lung is also uncommon but is responsible for some cases of pneumonia due to *Staphylococcus aureus*, *Pseudomonas aeruginosa*, and *Escherichia coli*. The reactivation of latent infection likely plays an important role in the development of pneumonia due to cytomegalovirus and *M. tuberculosis*. The direct extension of infection to the lung from contiguous areas such as the pleural or subdiaphragmatic spaces is rare.

Once bacteria reach the tracheobronchial tree, infectivity may be enhanced by defects in local pulmonary defenses. The cough reflex can be impaired by stroke, neuromuscular disease, sedatives, or poor nutrition. Mucociliary transport is depressed with the aging process, dehydration, morphine, atropine, prior infection with influenza virus, tobacco smoking, and chronic bronchitis. Anatomical derangements, including emphysema, bronchiectasis, and obstructive mass lesions, can also hinder clearance of organisms. Proteolytic enzymes, such as neutrophil elastase, are released by inflammatory cells recruited to infected areas of the pulmonary tree, thus altering the bronchial epithelium and ciliary clearance mechanisms as well as stimulating excess mucus production.

Bacteria in the tracheobronchial tree may encounter a blunted cellular and humoral immune response, thus increasing the risk of pneumonia. For example, granulocyte chemotaxis is reduced with aging, diabetes mellitus, malnutrition, hypothermia, hypophosphatemia, and corticosteroid administration. Absolute granulocytopenia may be caused by cytotoxic chemotherapy. Alveolar macrophages may be rendered dysfunctional by corticosteroids, cytokines, viral illnesses, and malnutrition. Diminished antibody production or function can be the sequelae of hematologic malignancies, such as multiple myeloma or chronic lymphocytic leukemia.

Pathological Agents

Despite the emergence of several newer pathogens as causes of community-acquired pneumonia, *Streptococcus pneumoniae* remains the most commonly identified pathogen. A variety of other pathogens have been reported to cause pneumonia in the community, with their order of importance depending on the location and population studied. These include long-recognized pathogens such as *Haemophilus influenzae*, *Mycoplasma pneumoniae*, and influenza A, along with newer pathogens such as *Legionella* species and *Chlamydophila pneumoniae*. Other common causes in the immunocompetent patient include *Moraxella catarrhalis*, *M. tuberculosis*, and aspiration pneumonia.

The following organisms are the causative agents in the 50% to 70% of cases for which a cause is identified:[2]

- *S. pneumoniae*, 20% to 60%
- *H. influenzae*, 3% to 10%
- *S. aureus*, 3% to 5%
- Gram-negative bacilli, 3% to 10%
- *Legionella* species, 2% to 8%
- *M. pneumoniae*, 1% to 6%
- *C. pneumoniae*, 4% to 6%
- Viruses, 2% to 15%
- Aspiration, 6% to 10%
- Others, 3% to 5%

Whereas pneumonias arising in the nursing home can be caused by community-acquired pathogens, higher percentages are caused by pathogens seen with relatively low frequency in the community. *S. aureus* should be sought in the setting of aspiration or as a result of influenza in the nursing home. There are increasing reports of pneumonia due to methicillin-resistant *S. aureus* (MRSA) in patients with little or no hospital contact. Gram-negative organisms are also more prominent.

Because of the different pathogenetic mechanisms leading to its development, nosocomial pneumonia is caused by a group of micro-organisms quite different from those causing community-acquired pneumonia. Organisms known to colonize the respiratory tree of hospitalized patients, such as *S. aureus* and enteric gram-negative organisms of the genuses *Pseudomonas, Enterobacter, Citrobacter, Serratia, Acinetobacter,* and *Stenotrophomonas,* are commonly isolated. Outbreaks of *Legionella* pneumonia and tuberculosis have also occurred in nursing homes and hospitals.

DIAGNOSIS OF PNEUMONIA

Because the clinical syndromes characterizing pneumonic infections caused by various agents frequently overlap with each other and with many noninfectious processes, the diagnosis of pneumonia can be challenging. The diligent clinician can narrow the differential diagnosis, however, by considering the place of acquisition and patient characteristics along with diagnostic tests.

Place of Acquisition

The differential diagnosis of pneumonia acquired in the community is quite different from that acquired in the nursing home or hospital.

A residence and travel history can help focus the differential diagnosis of pneumonia. Coccidioidomycosis should be considered in patients developing pneumonia on return from the southwestern United States. A patient developing pneumonia after a trip to Southeast Asia may have melioidosis or tuberculosis. A patient infected with HIV living in New York City with cough, fever, and night sweats may have multidrug-resistant tuberculosis. Residents of the desert southwestern United States with pneumonia and exposure to rodent excreta should be evaluated for the Hantavirus pulmonary syndrome. A person returning from an area with an active outbreak of severe acute respiratory syndrome (SARS) should be tested for SARS coronavirus.

Clinical Presentation

Typical bacterial pathogens such as *S. pneumoniae, H. influenzae,* and the enteric gram-negative organisms usually present acutely with high fever, chills, tachypnea, tachycardia, productive cough, and examination findings localized to a specific lung zone. In contrast, atypical pathogens such as *Mycoplasma, Chlamydophila,* and viruses can present in a subacute fashion with low-grade fever, nonproductive cough, constitutional symptoms, and absent or diffuse findings on lung examination. Rapid progression of disease can be seen in severe pneumococcal, staphylococcal, or *Legionella* pneumonia. The overlap between the presentations of typical and atypical pathogens, however, weakens the specificity of these categorizations considerably.

Certain extrapulmonary physical findings can provide clues to the diagnosis. Poor dentition and foul-smelling sputum may indicate the presence of a polymicrobial lung abscess. Bullous myringitis can accompany infection with *M. pneumoniae.* An absent gag reflex or altered sensorium raises the question of aspiration. Encephalitis can complicate pneumonia with *M. pneumoniae* or *Legionella pneumophila.* Cutaneous manifestations of infection can include erythema multiforme (*M. pneumoniae*), erythema nodosum (*C. pneumoniae* and *M. tuberculosis*), or ecthyma gangrenosum (*P. aeruginosa*).

Patient Characteristics

The age of the patient can play an important role in disease etiology and presentation. Older patients often have humoral and cellular immunodeficiency as a result of underlying diseases, immunosuppressive medications, and aging. They are more frequently institutionalized with anatomical problems that inhibit the pulmonary clearance of pathogens. The presentation is often more subtle than in younger adults, with more advanced disease and sepsis despite minimal fever and sputum production. More prolonged antimicrobial therapy is often required.

The occupation and hobbies of the patient can provide important clinical clues. For example, exposure to construction sites or old buildings with accumulations of bat or bird droppings can predispose to pneumonias due to *Histoplasma capsulatum* or *Cryptococcus neoformans.* Hunters who skin their own rabbits may be exposed to *Francisella tularensis.* Farmers working with stored hay may be exposed to *Aspergillus* species, as may patients who smoke marijuana. Laboratory workers handling the SARS coronavirus can develop disease with this pathogen.

Underlying diseases are a critical part of the history of the patient with pneumonia. Risk factors for HIV infection should be sought in the clinical history. HIV increases the risk for pneumonias due to common bacterial pathogens, as well as opportunistic pathogens such as *Pneumocystis carinii,* cytomegalovirus, and *Mycobacterium avium-intracellulare.* Fungal pneumonias caused by *H. capsulatum, Coccidioides immitis,* and *C. neoformans* have been seen in HIV-infected patients in appropriate epidemiologic settings and can have especially severe courses. Neutropenic patients are especially prone to fungal pneumonias, such as those caused by *Aspergillus* species. Patients treated with prolonged courses of immunosuppressive medications, such as corticosteroids, are at risk for pulmonary infections with various viral, fungal, and mycobacterial agents. Alcoholism predisposes individuals to aspiration pneumonia, with mixed gram-positive and gram-negative aerobic and anaerobic flora, as well as to tuberculosis. *M. catarrhalis*, *H. influenzae*, and *S. pneumoniae* are more likely in those with chronic obstructive pulmonary disease (COPD). Diabetic patients are more prone to staphylococcal infections. Patients with functional or surgical asplenia are prone to infection with encapsulated organisms such as *S. pneumoniae* and *H. influenzae*. Patients treated with tumor necrosis factor inhibitors are at risk for reactivation of tuberculosis and endemic mycoses such as histoplasmosis.

Radiography

A cornerstone of diagnosis is the chest radiograph, which usually reveals an infiltrate at presentation. This finding, however, may be absent in the dehydrated patient during the first 24 to 48 hours of rehydration. Also, the radiographic manifestations of chronic diseases such as congestive heart failure, COPD, and malignancy may obscure the infiltrate of pneumonia.

Although radiographic patterns are usually nonspecific, they can suggest a microbiological differential diagnosis. Lobar consolidation or a large pleural effusion suggests a bacterial pathogen. Cavitation may be found in bacterial abscesses, as well as mycobacterial, fungal, or nocardial infections. Pneumonias caused by *S. pneumoniae* may present as a lobar or bronchopneumonia. Gram-negative and staphylococcal pneumonias can cause consolidation and cavitation. The infiltrate that progresses rapidly from a single lobe to multiple lobes should raise suspicion of *L. pneumophila*.

Although aspiration more commonly affects the right lung because of tracheobronchial anatomy, both lungs can be affected simultaneously. The affected site may depend on position at the time of aspiration. Aspiration, while recumbent, will commonly lead to clinical and radiographic pneumonia in the posterior segments of the upper lobes and superior segments of the lower lobes. Upright aspiration usually affects the lung bases.

When diffuse interstitial infiltrates predominate in the absence of clinical evidence of fluid overload, pneumonias caused by viruses or *P. carinii* should be considered in the differential diagnosis.

Cultures

A Gram-stained sputum specimen can also provide critical information in choosing empiric therapy. Unfortunately, sputum is frequently difficult to obtain from elderly patients because of a weak cough, obtundation, and dehydration. Inhaled nebulized saline may help mobilize secretions. Nasotracheal suctioning can sample the lower respiratory tract directly, but this technique risks oropharyngeal contamination and is therefore of lesser value. A sputum specimen is believed to reflect lower respiratory secretions when more than 25 white blood cells (WBCs) and less than 10 epithelial cells are seen in a low-powered microscopic field. When such a specimen also shows a predominant organism, it lends a high positive predictive value for the choice of appropriate antimicrobial therapy. Other stains, such as the acid-fast stain for mycobacteria, modified acid-fast stain for *Nocardia*, or the toluidine blue and Gomori methenamine silver stains for *P. carinii*, may prove useful when historically indicated. The direct fluorescent antibody staining of sputum, bronchoalveolar lavage fluid, or pleural fluid may help identify *Legionella* species.

The sputum culture remains a controversial tool but is still recommended to help tailor therapy. It may prove particularly helpful in identifying resistant nosocomial bacterial pathogens. Expectorated morning sputum specimens can also be sent for mycobacterial culture when a compatible clinical syndrome is noted.

When a patient is hospitalized with pneumonia, blood cultures drawn within 4 hours may improve clinical outcome.

When these procedures fail to yield a microbiological diagnosis, and when the patient fails to respond to empiric antibiotic therapy, more invasive diagnostic techniques may be indicated. Fiber-optic bronchoscopy allows the use of several techniques in the diagnosis of pneumonia. Bronchoalveolar lavage with saline can obtain deep respiratory specimens for the gamut of stains and cultures mentioned previously. A transbronchial biopsy of infiltrated lung parenchyma can reveal alveolar or interstitial pneumonitis, viral inclusion bodies, and invading fungal or mycobacterial organisms. The protected brush catheter is used to quantitatively distinguish between tracheobronchial colonizers and pneumonic pathogens. When recovered secretions contain 10^3 colony-forming units (cfu)/mL of a bacterial pathogen, lower respiratory infection should be suspected.

In some centers, minibronchoalveolar lavage is another method used in the diagnosis of nosocomial pneumonia. This procedure is performed through the nonbronchoscopic passage of a telescoping catheter through the endotracheal tube. Several recent articles have suggested a high culture concordance between this method and the bronchoscopic protected-brush catheter technique.

A more substantial amount of lung tissue may be obtained for culture and histologic examination using thoracoscopic or open-lung biopsy. Because these procedures can carry considerable morbidity, their timing in the diagnostic algorithm is controversial. They are usually reserved for the deteriorating patient with a pneumonia that defies diagnosis by less invasive techniques.

Serologic Testing

Serologic testing for such pathogens as *Legionella* species, *Mycoplasma* species, and *C. pneumoniae* should include sera drawn in both acute and convalescent phases for comparison. A fourfold increase in the immunoglobulin G (IgG) titer is suggestive of recent infection with these organisms. Immunoglobin M (IgM) assays are prone to false positives, but can provide evidence of acute infection. A single IgM titer of $\geq 1{:}16$ is judged to be diagnostic of acute infection with *C. pneumoniae*.

A sensitive enzyme immunoassay has been developed for the detection of *L. pneumophila* antigen in urine. Because the antigen persists for prolonged periods after infection, it is difficult to differentiate between past and current infections when using this assay. A similar urine antigen test has been developed for the detection of *S. pneumoniae*, and it may be used to augment standard techniques of culture and Gram staining.

A urinary assay for the detection of *H. capsulatum* antigen is also available and can be a useful diagnostic adjunct to traditional fungal complement fixation and immunodiffusion test batteries.

Molecular Techniques

Powerful molecular techniques are being applied to the early diagnosis of pneumonia. DNA probes have been used for the detection of *Legionella* species, *M. pneumoniae*, and *M. tuberculosis* in sputum. These probes have excellent sensitivity and specificity, but can produce some false-positive results. The polymerase chain reaction (PCR) has been shown to be a sensitive tool for the early detection of *M. tuberculosis* in sputum specimens. Given the large percentage of pneumonia cases for which no microbial etiology is identified, it is likely that molecular tools will eventually be applied to the identification and antimicrobial susceptibility testing of nearly all agents of pneumonia.

TREATMENT OF PNEUMONIA

Hospitalization

Health care budgetary constraints have given rise to a number of studies addressing the issue of hospitalization in community-acquired pneumonia. A recent study[3] validated a risk scale, the Pneumonia Severity Index, for mortality in community-acquired pneumonia. Patients younger than 50 years of age without significant coexisting diseases or vital sign abnormalities were assigned to risk group I. All others were grouped in classes II (≤ 70 points), III (71–90 points), IV (91–130 points), and V (>130 points) using a system assigning points for age, residence, coexisting diseases, physical examination findings, and laboratory abnormalities:

- Age: males, 1 point per year; females, 1 point per year minus 10
- Nursing home resident, 10 points
- Coexisting illnesses: neoplastic disease, 30 points; chronic renal disease, 10 points; congestive heart failure, 10 points; chronic liver disease, 20 points; cerebrovascular disease, 10 points
- Physical findings: respiratory rate 30 breaths/minute, 20 points; systolic blood pressure <90 mm Hg, 20 points; pulse 125 beats/minute, 10 points; temperature $40°C$ or $<35°C$, 15 points; altered mental status, 20 points
- Diagnostic tests: PaO_2 <60 mm Hg, 10 points; hematocrit $<30\%$, 10 points; blood urea nitrogen >30 mg/dL, 20 points; pleural effusion on chest radiograph, 10 points; sodium <130 mM, 20 points; glucose >250 mg/dL, 10 points; arterial pH <7.35, 30 points

Patients in the first three risk classes had less than 1% mortality, with steep increases to 9.3% in class IV and 27.0% in class V. Less than 6% of patients in the first three groups treated as inpatients required intensive care unit admission, and less than 10% of patients in the first two groups treated as outpatients were subsequently hospitalized. Although these data can help in patient assessment, the decision to admit must ultimately be individualized to each patient encounter.

Pharmacologic Treatment

With concerns about antimicrobial overuse, health care costs, and bacterial resistance increasing, pharmacologic therapy should always follow the confirmation of the diagnosis of pneumonia and should always be accompanied by a diligent effort to identify an etiologic agent. When the history, chest radiograph, and Gram-stained sputum fail to suggest a specific cause for pneumonia, a trial of empiric antibiotics is warranted. Antibiotic therapy is best initiated after obtaining appropriate specimens for culture, when appropriate. The choice of antimicrobial is dictated by severity of illness, treatment setting, and comorbid diseases. Table 16.1 provides a framework for the initial therapy of community-acquired pneumonia, based on the consensus recommendations of the Infectious Disease Society of America (IDSA) and American Thoracic Society (ATS).[4]

In the outpatient treatment of pneumonia, the IDSA/ATS guidelines recommend the use of an oral macrolide or tetracycline for previously healthy individuals. The guidelines recommend the use of a newer fluoroquinolone (i.e., levofloxacin, gatifloxacin, or moxifloxacin), or a beta-lactam plus a macrolide, for outpatients with comorbid diseases or risks for resistant pathogens. The use of the newer fluoroquinolones as first-line agents for pneumonia should be considered in the context of emerging resistance to these agents. If HIV infection is a suspected comorbidity, then strong consideration should be given

TABLE 16.1

ANTIBIOTIC THERAPY FOR COMMUNITY-ACQUIRED PNEUMONIA IN IMMUNOCOMPETENT ADULTS

Setting	Patient	Common Pathogens	Empiric Therapy
Outpatient	No comorbid diseases; no recent prior antibiotic therapy	*Streptococcus pneumoniae* *Mycoplasma pneumoniae* *Chlamydophila pneumoniae* viruses *Haemophilus influenzae*	A macrolide or doxycycline
	Having comorbid disease; recent prior antibiotic therapy	*S. pneumoniae* viruses *H. influenzae* Gram-negative bacilli[b] *Staphylococcus aureus*[b]	Fluoroquinolone alone or a newer macrolide plus a β-lactam[a]
Inpatient	Not severely ill	*S. pneumoniae* *H. influenzae* Polymicrobial Anaerobes *S. aureus* *C. pneumoniae* viruses	A macrolide and cefotaxime or ceftriaxone or a β-lactam/β-lactamase inhibitor[c]; a fluoroquinolone[d] alone
	Severely ill	*S. pneumoniae*[e] *Legionella* Gram-negative bacilli *M. pneumoniae* viruses *S. aureus*[f]	Azithromycin or a fluoroquinolone[c] and cefotaxime, ceftriaxone, or a β-lactam/β-lactamase inhibitor

[a]High-dose amoxicillin, high-dose amoxicillin-clavulanate, cefpodoxime, cefprozil, or cefuroxime.
[b]In most cases, patients with pneumonias due to these organisms should be hospitalized.
[c]Piperacillin-tazobactam or ampicillin-sulbactam.
[d]Levofloxacin, gatifloxacin, moxifloxacin.
[e]Critically ill patients in areas with significant rates of high-level pneumococcal resistance and a suggestive sputum Gram stain should receive vancomycin or a newer quinolone pending microbiological diagnosis.
[f]Critically ill patients suspected of having community-acquired methicillin-resistant *Staphylococcus aureus* respiratory infections should receive vancomycin or linezolid pending microbiological diagnosis.
Modified from Mandell LA, Wunerink RG, Anzueto A, et al. Infectious Diseases Society of America/American Thoracic Society consensus guidelines on the management of community-acquired pneumonia in adults. *Clin Infect Dis* 2007;44:S27–S72.

to the inclusion of trimethoprim-sulfamethoxazole in the treatment regimen.

When patients with community-acquired pneumonia require hospitalization but are not critically ill, intravenous therapy with cefotaxime, ceftriaxone, or a β-lactam/β-lactamase inhibitor combination plus a macrolide is warranted. Newer fluoroquinolones provide a monotherapeutic option. When the pneumonia is severe, empiric intravenous therapy should include cefotaxime, ceftriaxone, or a β-lactam/β-lactamase inhibitor combination (the latter is preferred if resistant gram-negative pathogens are suspected) plus either azithromycin or a newer fluoroquinolone. When community-acquired MRSA is a consideration on the basis of history and diagnostic studies, vancomycin or linezolid may be added. Daptomycin, which also has good activity against MRSA, is not used in pneumonia because of poor lung tissue penetration. Intravenous antibiotics may be switched to oral antibiotics when the patient is stable and afebrile, provided that the patient can adhere to the selected regimen and has adequate swallowing and gastrointestinal function.

Because gram-negative organisms predominate in pneumonia acquired in hospital settings, an agent possessing antipseudomonal activity (e.g., an antipseudomonal cephalosporin or penicillin, β-lactam/β-lactamase inhibitor, imipenem, or a fluoroquinolone) and an aminoglycoside are usually used. When nosocomial pneumonia is severe, and the institution has a significant percentage of methicillin-resistant staphylococci, consideration should be given to the empiric addition of vancomycin or linezolid until culture data excluding the presence of these pathogens can be obtained. If the hospitalized patient is also neutropenic, and the response to antibacterials is suboptimal, some consideration should be given to the early addition of antifungal therapy.

Clindamycin is preferred over penicillin for the treatment of community-acquired aspiration pneumonia because of its superiority in the treatment of oral anaerobes such as *Bacteroides melaninogenicus*. Amoxicillin/clavulanic acid also provides excellent coverage in this setting. When large-volume aspiration is documented in the hospital, a β-lactam/β-lactamase inhibitor combination or the combination of clindamycin and an antipseudomonal agent should be used.

When the diagnostic techniques described previously yield a specific causative agent for the pneumonia, special effort should be made to narrow the spectrum of activity used as early as possible. Overuse of broad-spectrum agents encourages the development of resistance and should be avoided whenever possible.

Despite a lack of controlled data specifically addressing length of therapy, many cases of community-acquired pneumonia are adequately treated with 10 to 14 days of therapy. Given concern for resistance and cost, there is considerable interest in shorter course, in the range of 5 to 7 days. Certain organisms (e.g., *Legionella*, *S. aureus*, *Pseudomonas*, or *C. pneumoniae*) may require longer courses. Similarly, patients with comorbidities that compromise local (COPD) or systemic (hematologic malignancy) immunity may take longer to clear their illness.

With concern for health care costs on the rise, much attention has been given to the oral treatment of pneumonia. Fully oral and intravenous-to-oral "switch" therapies offer potential reductions in length of stay, antibiotic administration costs, complications of venous access, and disruption of families and careers. Many antibiotics are well absorbed from the gastrointestinal tract, lending further credence to the notion of effective oral treatment. Because well-controlled, risk-stratified data comparing oral and intravenous therapies are few, appropriate patient populations and treatment settings for oral therapy are yet to be fully defined. Better data exist for the use of switch therapies for the stabilized patient who has good gastrointestinal and swallowing function and adequate social support, and such regimens have gained wide acceptance.

SPECIFIC PATHOGENS

Certain emerging pathogens have been the subject of considerable research in recent years. Given their importance, they are worthy of special attention.

Streptococcus pneumoniae

Although the pneumococcus is a familiar enemy, it has become even more formidable in recent years. The exact incidence of pneumococcal pneumonia is unknown, but it has been estimated at 1 to 2 per 1,000 persons per year in the United States. It is more common in the elderly, with incidence estimates ranging from 14 to 46 per 1,000 persons per year. Untreated mortality has been estimated at about 30%.

Although pneumococci have traditionally been exquisitely sensitive to penicillin, strains of the organism possessing low- or high-level resistance to penicillin have established a foothold in many communities. The Centers for Disease Control and Prevention (CDC) states that 5% to 15% of pneumococcal isolates in many areas of the United States exhibit high-level penicillin resistance, with several areas reporting 35% of isolates with at least intermediate resistance. Some of these strains are multiply resistant, with resistance to multiple cephalosporins, erythromycin, tetracyclines, and trimethoprim-sulfamethoxazole. No strains resistant to vancomycin have been isolated. This has led to the recommendation by several authorities that empiric therapy for life-threatening disease suspected or proven to be due to pneumococci include vancomycin or a newer fluoroquinolone (in nonmeningeal disease) until susceptibility patterns are known. Because peak penicillin levels in high-dose intravenous therapy reach 50 to 60 μg/mL, many authorities believe that pneumonia due to pneumococci that are inhibited by a minimum concentration (MIC) of 0.12 to 2 μg/mL of penicillin can be treated with high-dose penicillin (150,000–200,000 U/kg/day in divided doses). Ceftriaxone or cefotaxime may be used for strains with reduced susceptibility to penicillin (MIC >1 μg/mL), providing the MIC for these agents is <2 μg/mL. If the penicillin MIC is >4 μg/mL (penicillin-resistant *S. pneumoniae*) and the cephalosporin MIC is also elevated, then vancomycin and the newer fluoroquinolones are the treatments of choice. Whenever possible, vancomycin should be changed to β-lactam therapy because of both improved efficacy and the continuing emergence of vancomycin resistance among gram-positive pathogens such as enterococci and staphylococci.

Legionella Species

Although difficult to visualize on sputum Gram stain and slow to grow even on specialized culture media, members of the *Legionella* genus frequently leave several epidemiologic clues helpful to the diagnosis of Legionnaire's disease. Most frequently occurring in the spring or summer months, Legionnaire's disease can occur sporadically or in epidemics in settings with recirculated air, such as hotels, airplanes, and hospitals. It can occur in adults of all ages but is more common in middle-age and elderly persons. A prodrome of malaise, myalgia, and headache is frequently present, sometimes accompanied by gastrointestinal symptoms such as watery diarrhea, nausea, or abdominal pain. The pneumonia is often explosive, with nonproductive cough, high fever, shaking chills, tachycardia, and tachypnea. Focal findings on lung examination and chest radiograph (initially patchy areas of bronchopneumonia) can progress within hours to a multilobe process. Confusion and disorientation can be present.

Laboratory evaluation can also yield information useful in the diagnosis. Left-shifted leukocytosis may be present on the complete blood count. Elevated liver function tests, azotemia, hypophosphatemia, hyponatremia, and hypoxemia may be seen, but none of these findings are pathognomonic for legionellosis. Urinalysis may reveal hematuria.

The sputum Gram stain in *Legionella* pneumonia usually reveals many WBCs but no predominant organism. Culture is best attempted with charcoal-yeast extract agar, but sensitivities of 50% to 70% are common. Therefore, a variety of alternative tests has been developed to support the diagnosis. Serology is 70% to 96% sensitive and more than 95% specific, but results may not be available for several days. Sputum-direct fluorescent antibody testing is likewise highly specific, but quite technique dependent, with sensitivities of 25% to 80% reported. DNA probing of sputum specimens is expensive, available only in a few laboratories, and relatively insensitive (50%–65%). Urinary antigen testing is sensitive (75%–90%), uniformly specific, and may turn positive as early as 72 hours into the illness. It only detects *L. pneumophila* type 1, however, which accounts for 80% of cases of legionellosis. The test fails to distinguish acute from remote infection because antigenuria may be present for up to 1 year after infection. The IDSA recommends culture and urinary antigen testing as the primary diagnostic modalities for *Legionella* pneumonia. However, empiric therapy for legionellosis may still be warranted when the clinical setting is appropriate, despite extensive negative testing.

Recent guidelines have moved toward the use of azithromycin or quinolones (including respiratory quinolones or ciprofloxacin) in the treatment of legionellosis. Many authorities advocate the addition of rifampin, which also offers good intracellular penetration. A lengthy course (at least 3 weeks) may be required for cure.

Chlamydophila pneumoniae

Predicted more than 40 years ago by epidemiologic studies of psittacosislike infections with no exposure to birds, *C. pneumoniae* has been recognized since 1986 as a pathogen distinct from *C. psittaci* and having person-to-person respiratory transmission. Current seroepidemiology suggests that *C. pneumoniae* accounts for about 10% of all cases of community-acquired pneumonia, with a seroprevalence in the United States of about 50%. Data indicate that most adults are exposed during the teenage years, outside the home. Outbreaks have been reported to spread somewhat more slowly than influenza through closed populations such as military recruits and college students.

The clinical presentation of respiratory infections due to *C. pneumoniae* is frequently nonspecific. Cough (productive or nonproductive) and sore throat are common, occurring in more than 80% of patients. A clinical clue present in only 30% of cases is hoarseness, which is present in less than 5% of patients with mycoplasmal or viral infections. Mild fever and leukocytosis are common. The presentation on lung examination and chest radiography is usually that of a localized infiltrate. The illness is usually indolent, although severe pneumonias can occur in elderly and immunocompromised adults.

Culture diagnosis is uncommon because the organism is difficult to cultivate. The diagnosis is made more commonly by serology, with IgM titers ≥1:16 or a fourfold titer increase considered diagnostic.

Both tetracyclines and macrolides have been shown to have excellent in vitro activity against *C. pneumoniae* and are considered the treatment agents of choice despite a relative paucity of clinical data. Alternatives to these agents may include quinolones such as levofloxacin, gatifloxacin, and moxifloxacin.

Mycoplasma pneumoniae

Like *C. pneumoniae*, *M. pneumoniae* accounts for 5% to 20% of community-acquired pneumonia, with slow spread through closed populations. It produces a syndrome of low-grade fever, nonproductive cough, and pharyngitis. Headache and otalgia are also frequently reported. The most common respiratory syndrome is bronchitis, with up to one-fourth of these patients proceeding to pneumonia. Radiographic presentations range from single to multilobe, with patchy infiltrates. Uncommon but sometimes severe extrapulmonary manifestations can include hemolytic anemia, myocarditis, pericarditis, meningoencephalitis, monoarthritis or polyarthritis, and erythema multiforme.

The culture of *M. pneumoniae* requires broth medium and a 7- to 10-day span of time, so it is usually not performed. Diagnosis is serologic, with specific IgM positivity, IgG titers ≥1:256, or a fourfold increase in IgG titer considered diagnostic. The cold agglutinin test is nonspecific but supports the diagnosis of mycoplasmal infection when a high titer (≥1:128) is present.

Therapy consists of the administration of a macrolide, tetracycline, or fluoroquinolone for at least 14 days.

Community-Acquired MRSA

In the past several years, a new strain of MRSA has been observed to cause tissue-invasive disease, including pneumonia, in patients with little or no hospital contact. This strain, designated USA 300, causes a severe, rapidly progressive, necrotizing pneumonitis.[5] Its pathogenicity appears to be mediated by cytotoxins, including the Panton-Valentine leukocidin. When community-acquired MRSA is suspected as a cause of pneumonia, antibiotic therapy should include vancomycin or linezolid. Some authorities add clindamycin to deter toxin production.

Influenza and Other Viruses

In some series of community-acquired pneumonia, no etiologic agent was established in 40% to 50% of cases. It is likely that a portion of these is due to viral agents, which are an underdiagnosed cause of pneumonia. Among immunocompetent adults, influenza viruses (especially influenza

A) are the most common causes of viral pneumonia. Mainly occurring between October and March, influenza pneumonia is characterized by nonproductive cough, wheezing, myalgia, sore throat, and fever. Chest radiographs may show localized or diffuse patchy infiltrates. The diagnosis is established by serology or by swab collection of nasopharyngeal cells for culture or rapid antigen detection, such as direct immunofluorescent staining. Rapid methods, which can provide an answer in minutes to hours, are perhaps most useful when treatment is contemplated. The standard treatment of influenza A pneumonia has been amantadine or the less toxic rimantadine. Two newer agents, zanamivir and oseltamivir, have activity against both influenza A and influenza B. If given soon after the onset of symptoms, these drugs can shorten the duration of symptoms and viral shedding by 1 to 2 days. Much international concern has been directed toward the possibility of a pandemic of influenza arising from avian strains.

When the patient with suspected or documented influenza develops a secondary, more acute phase of illness with high fever and productive cough, bacterial superinfection must be considered. *S. aureus*, *S. pneumoniae*, and *H. influenzae* are the most common causes of pneumonia in this setting.

Adenoviruses have been demonstrated to cause pneumonia in military recruits. Along with adenoviruses, respiratory syncytial virus, influenza virus, and parainfluenza virus can cause viral pneumonia in immunocompromised patients. Direct immunofluorescent staining of the nasopharyngeal cells provides the most rapid diagnostic method.

Hantavirus Pulmonary Syndrome

In 1993, a cluster of 24 patients living in the Four Corners area of New Mexico, Arizona, Colorado, and Utah developed acute respiratory failure following an influenzalike illness. Twelve of these patients died, leading to the isolation of a new pathogen in the Hantavirus family, the Sin Nombre virus. Subsequent epidemiologic investigation of the illness caused by this agent suggests that it is transmitted to humans by exposure to the excreta of the deer mouse (*Peromyscus maniculatus*). The geographic range of this disease has grown steadily since its characterization, and cases have been noted in several regions of the United States.

Fever, myalgia, nausea, vomiting, and abdominal pain mark the prodromal phase of the disease, lasting 3 to 6 days. Upper respiratory symptoms are uncommon. The cardiopulmonary phase is heralded by progressive cough and dyspnea, with tachypnea, tachycardia, fever, and severe hypotension. Laboratory evaluation reveals thrombocytopenia, abnormal coagulation parameters, and leukocytosis, sometimes with atypical lymphocytosis. Renal failure is rare, but ventilatory failure is common, with 88% of patients requiring mechanical ventilation. The chest radiograph progresses rapidly to diffuse interstitial edema. Lung pathology reveals evidence of vascular permeability without parenchymal necrosis.

The diagnosis is serologic, with demonstration of IgM or a fourfold increase in IgG antibodies. Treatment is largely supportive. Ribavirin, either in the intravenous or aerosolized form, has been proposed by some as a potential therapy, but controlled data to support the use of this toxic drug are lacking.

Severe Acute Respiratory Syndrome

An outbreak of severe respiratory disease spread from southern China worldwide within several weeks of first reports in early 2003. A novel virus, SARS coronavirus, was quickly identified, and diagnostic tests were developed. The outbreak was aggressively controlled by quarantine methods.

The CDC case definition of SARS requires an epidemiologic exposure to the virus, either by travel, close contact, or occupation, within 10 days of developing the prodromal symptoms of headache, chills, myalgias, and malaise. The more severe syndrome of high fever, cough, dyspnea, and radiographic abnormalities follows in some cases. The diagnosis involves the exclusion of and empiric therapy for severe CAP while awaiting the results of diagnostic testing by serology and PCR of blood, respiratory, or stool specimens. Specific treatment has not yet been defined and is currently supportive in nature.

PERFORMANCE MEASURES

As part of the quality movement in health care, certain parts of the IDSA/ATS practice guidelines have been adopted as pay-for-performance measures by insurance payers. Among the measures adopted are assessment of oxygenation, screening for pneumococcal vaccination, blood cultures before first antibiotic dose, assessment for smoking cessation, antibiotics within 4 hours of arrival at the hospital, and correct choice of antibiotics.

PREVENTION OF PNEUMONIA

Simple, low-technology solutions such as handwashing and cough etiquette are critical to prevention of spread of respiratory pathogens. Given the increased resistance among pneumococci and the undiminished importance of influenza as a respiratory pathogen, emphasis on immunization against these agents should be intensified. Immunization can play a critical role in the prevention of pneumonia, particularly in immunocompromised and older adults. The influenza vaccine is formulated and administered annually. Given the risk of postinfluenza bacterial superinfection in elderly and immunocompromised individuals, this vaccine should be given to all patients in these groups, except those allergic to eggs.

The pneumococcal vaccine, containing polysaccharide antigens of the 23 strains responsible for 88% of cases of bacteremic pneumococcal disease, has been shown to be 60% to 70% effective in immunocompetent patients. Side effects are rarely serious and consist of local pain and erythema, which occur in up to 50% of recipients. Patients who are immunosuppressed and those with severely debilitating cardiovascular, pulmonary, renal, hepatic, or diabetic disease may not have sustained titers of protective antibody and should be considered for revaccination after 6 years.

Selective digestive decontamination uses a combination of antibacterial and antifungal agents in an attempt to reduce gastrointestinal and oropharyngeal colonization with micro-organisms. The simultaneous administration of these agents as an oral paste and a nasogastric suspension has been shown to reduce the incidence of nosocomial pneumonia in some studies but without a convincing improvement in morbidity, mortality, or length of intensive care unit stay.

Nosocomial pneumonia is frequently preventable, and recent guidelines from the CDC address strategies to reduce the incidence of this entity. Handwashing and barrier precautions are stressed as strategies to reduce patient-to-patient transmission of respiratory pathogens by health care workers in the intensive care unit. Many hospitals now employ teams to evaluate swallowing function and aspiration risk. The modified barium swallow can help establish the types of liquid and solid foodstuffs likely to be aspirated. Elevation of the upper airway to above the level of the stomach and the use of jejunostomy (rather than gastrostomy) tubes for enteral feeding can help diminish aspiration risk in patients with incompetent lower esophageal sphincters. Finally, careful attention to pulmonary toilet can assist debilitated persons in clearing tracheobronchial secretions.

REVIEW EXERCISES

QUESTIONS

1. A 58-year-old woman presents with a 3-week history of nonproductive cough and hoarseness. She reports a temperature of 100.4°F. She is not short of breath and has no chills or sweats. She has a smoking history of 20 packs per year but quit 20 years ago. She lives at home with her husband, who is asymptomatic. She has had several antibiotics in the past week, of which she comments, "I felt a little better after the clarithromycin, but not much, so my doctor changed me to cefuroxime, and I felt worse." On examination, she appears healthy. She has a low-grade fever at 38°C, but her vital signs are otherwise normal. The physical examination is

unremarkable. Laboratory evaluation is notable only for a normal white blood cell count with a mild left shift. Chest radiograph reveals a subtle right-sided infiltrate. The most appropriate next step in the care of this patient would be

a) Admission for high-dose intravenous erythromycin
b) Outpatient therapy with oral doxycycline
c) Admission for intravenous ceftriaxone
d) Outpatient therapy with oral ciprofloxacin
e) Home intravenous antibiotic therapy with piperacillin/tazobactam

Answer and Discussion

The answer is b. The patient presents with a subacute, indolent illness and radiographic evidence of community-acquired pneumonia. No risk factors for mortality are present, and admission is probably not warranted. Piperacillin/tazobactam has no activity against common atypical bacterial organisms. Ciprofloxacin has poor activity against gram-positive organisms and should not be used in this setting. Correct therapeutic options include oral tetracyclines, macrolides, levofloxacin, gatifloxacin, or moxifloxacin. In this case, the symptom of hoarseness and partial response to clarithromycin raise suspicion for *C. pneumoniae* as a pathogen. Doxycycline is preferred in this setting.

2. A 23-year-old college student presents in late December with a 5-day history of nonproductive cough and shortness of breath. He notes that a number of fellow students have had respiratory illnesses over the past 2 months. He has recently tested HIV negative. Physical examination shows that he is in good physical condition. His temperature is 38.3°C, his heart rate is 120 beats/minute, his respiratory rate is 22 breaths/minute, and his blood pressure is 90/60 mm Hg. The examination is otherwise remarkable only for a few scattered rales at the lung bases. On laboratory evaluation, he is hypoxemic with a PO_2 of 76. The white blood cell count is 14,000/mm^3, with a marked left shift. His hemoglobin is 8.3 g/dL, and his peripheral smear shows red cell fragments. Chest radiograph reveals bilateral patchy lower lobe infiltrates.

The patient deteriorates soon after admission, requiring mechanical ventilation and pressors. Chest radiography reveals a progression of the infiltrates to involve all five lung lobes. A Swan-Ganz catheter is placed, revealing a high systemic vascular resistance but a low cardiac output.

The most appropriate empiric antimicrobial therapy for this patient is

a) Trimethoprim-sulfamethoxazole 5 mg/kg intravenously (IV) every 6 hours
b) Doxycycline 100 mg IV every 12 hours

c) Piperacillin/tazobactam 3.375 g IV every 6 hours

d) Azithromycin 500 mg intravenously every day plus ceftriaxone 1 g IV every day

e) Clindamycin 900 mg IV every 8 hours plus ceftazidime 1 g IV every 8 hours

Answer and Discussion

The answer is d. The patient is acutely and severely ill with a community-acquired process. By IDSA guidelines, appropriate therapy consists of a macrolide or fluoroquinolone and ceftriaxone, cefotaxime, or β-lactam/β-lactamase inhibitor combination. Because he is HIV negative and acutely ill, trimethoprim-sulfamethoxazole would not provide adequate coverage for either atypical or serious gram-negative pathogens. Likewise, neither piperacillin-tazobactam nor the combination of clindamycin and ceftriaxone would cover atypical pathogens. Intravenous doxycycline alone would not cover all likely typical bacterial pathogens. Of the provided answers, only the combination of azithromycin and ceftriaxone would treat severe pneumonia due to both *Legionella* and typical bacterial pathogens.

This patient presents with several clinical clues to the correct diagnosis. He presents with a nonproductive cough and low-grade fever, suggesting an atypical pathogen. His sputum Gram stain shows no predominant organism, despite a fulminant process. He has evidence of hemolytic anemia and cardiac dysfunction. His *Mycoplasma* IgM titer was strongly positive, illustrating the potentially severe complications of this ordinarily indolent pathogen.

3. A 66-year-old man with a history of non-Hodgkin's lymphoma presents with a 2-week history of dry cough and low-grade fever in January. He has a pet parakeet, and a grandchild has a respiratory illness. His lung exam is remarkable for a few rales at the lung bases. His chest x-ray (CXR) initially reveals a faint infiltrate in both lung bases.

The patient is admitted to the hospital, and levofloxacin is administered intravenously. Despite this therapy, the patient's respiratory status worsens over the first 48 hours of hospitalization. He is admitted to the intensive care unit and requires mechanical ventilation. A repeat CXR shows reticulonodular infiltrates throughout both lung fields.

Which of the following are causes of failure to respond to therapy in community-acquired pneumonia?

a) Wrong diagnosis

b) Empyema

c) Poor adherence to medical regimen

d) a and c

e) a, b, and c

Answer and Discussion

The answer is e. Several factors can contribute to failure to respond to initial antibiotic therapy in community-acquired pneumonia. First, one should consider the correctness of the diagnosis. A number of diagnoses may lead to pulmonary infiltrates, including noninfectious diseases such as heart failure. Host factors such as empyema, immunodeficiency, and bronchial tree obstruction may slow the response to antibiotics. It is also important to consider difficulties with the regimen itself: Is this the wrong drug or dose? Is the patient adhering to the regimen? The clinician must also place less common microbial pathogens in the differential diagnosis, as some pathogens do not respond to standard antibiotic regimens. Finally, certain pathogens, such as *Legionella* species and *Streptococcus pneumoniae*, may cause overwhelming infection that may not immediately respond to antibiotics.

In this circumstance, the patient is immunocompromised by virtue of his lymphoma. He has a pet parakeet and might have pneumonia caused by an unusual pathogen, such as *C. psittaci*. He has a granddaughter with a respiratory illness, but it is January, raising the question of viral pathogens such as influenza, respiratory syncytial virus, adenovirus, parainfluenza virus, and others. Given his rapid decline, bronchoscopy is likely indicated to obtain a specimen for staining and culture for a broad range of pathogens. Serology may be useful to help diagnose infection with *Chlamydia* species or other atypical pathogens, such as *Legionella* and *Mycoplasma* species.

4. A 67-year-old woman with a history of steroid-dependent asthma is admitted to the hospital with fever (temperature 37.9°C), cough, and myalgia. Chest radiography reveals an increase in interstitial markings bilaterally, and a nasopharyngeal swab is polymerase chain reaction positive for influenza A. Because of immune suppression, the patient is treated with oseltamivir. The patient experiences resolution of fever and myalgia and improved cough over the first 2 hospital days, but fever recurs and is accompanied by productive cough and chills on the third hospital day. On examination, the patient looks acutely ill. Her temperature is 38.5°C, pulse is 126 beats/minute, respiratory rate is 3 breaths/minute, and blood pressure is 90/58 mm Hg. There are coarse crackles heard at the left lung base. Chest radiography now reveals a dense lobar infiltrate at the left base. Which of the following is not an appropriate measure in the care of this patient?

a) Blood cultures

b) Sputum Gram stain and culture

c) Intravenous vancomycin
d) Replace oseltamivir with amantadine
e) Intravenous linezolid

Answer and Discussion

The answer is d. This patient, who is seemingly recovering from acute influenza A, suffers a relapse of symptoms with a more acute presentation. The primary concern is for a bacterial superinfection in the lungs. *Staphylococcus aureus* and *Streptococcus pneumoniae* are important pathogens in this setting; community-acquired methicillin-resistant *S. aureus* (CA-MRSA) is a concern in this toxic-appearing patient. Blood and sputum studies are clearly indicated to identify a pathogen and direct therapy. Intravenous vancomycin and linezolid are therapeutic options for CA-MRSA. Given the clinical course and radiographic change, it is unlikely that a change in antiviral therapy will have an effect on the patient's course.

5. A 45-year-old man with Crohn's disease treated with infliximab presents in December with an increasing nonproductive cough and fever over the past 2 weeks. He denies myalgia but has considerable fatigue. He is prescribed a 5-day course of oral levofloxacin without any improvement. He seeks care again for worsening symptoms. On examination, he looks chronically ill and is actively coughing without sputum production. The patient's temperature is 37.7°C, and vital signs are otherwise normal. The lung examination is clear. A chest radiograph suggests scattered small nodules diffusely.

Which measure is not appropriate in the care of this patient?

a) Protein purified derivative skin testing
b) Bronchoscopy with bronchoalveolar lavage and transbronchial biopsy
c) Fungal complement fixation and immunodiffusion serology battery
d) *Histoplasma* urinary antigen
e) *Streptococcus pneumoniae* urinary antigen

Answer and Discussion

The answer is e. Therapy with tumor necrosis factor inhibitors such as infliximab has been associated with reactivation of tuberculosis and endemic mycoses such as histoplasmosis. In this setting, protein purified derivative skin testing, *Histoplasma* urinary antigen testing, and fungal serology battery are clearly indicated. Because skin and serologic testing can yield delayed or no diagnosis, bronchoscopy can be critical to obtain diagnostic specimens and direct antimicrobial therapy. The patient's subacute illness and the radiographic pattern are less consistent with "typical" bacterial pathogens such as *Streptococcus pneumoniae*, and pneumococcal urinary antigen testing is not indicated for this patient.

REFERENCES

1. Osler W. *Principles and Practice of Medicine.* New York: Appleton, 1892.
2. Bartlett JG, Mundy LM. Community-acquired pneumonia. *N Engl J Med* 1995;333:1618–1624.
3. Fine MJ, Auble TE, Yealy DM, et al. A prediction rule to identify low-risk patients with community-acquired pneumonia. *N Engl J Med* 1997;336:243–250.
4. Mandell LA, Wunerink RG, Anzueto A, et al. Infectious Diseases Society of America/American Thoracic Society consensus guidelines on the management of community-acquired pneumonia in adults. *Clin Infect Dis* 2007;44:S27–S72.
5. Pogue M, Burton S, Kreyling P, et al. Severe methicillin-resistant *Staphylococcus aureus* community-acquired pneumonia associated with influenza—Louisiana and Georgia, December 2006–January 2007. *MMWR Morb Mortal Wkly Rep* 2007;56:325–329.

SUGGESTED READINGS

Ailani RK, Agastya G, Mukunda BN, et al. Doxycycline is a cost-effective therapy for hospitalized patients with community-acquired pneumonia. *Arch Intern Med* 1999;159:266–270.
American Thoracic Society/Infectious Disease Society of America. Guidelines for the management of adults with hospital-acquired, ventilator-associated, and healthcare-associated pneumonia. *Am J Respir Crit Care Med* 2005;171:388–416.
Butler JC, Peters CJ. Hantaviruses and Hantavirus pulmonary syndrome. *Clin Infect Dis* 1994;19:387–395.
Cassiere HA, Fein AM. Duration and route of antibiotic therapy in community-acquired pneumonia: switch and step-down therapy. *Semin Respir Infect* 1998;13:36–42.
Centers for Disease Control and Prevention. Guidelines for prevention of nosocomial pneumonia. *MMWR Morb Mortal Wkly Rep* 1997;46:1–85.
Friedland IR, McCracken GH. Management of infections caused by antibiotic-resistant *Streptococcus pneumoniae*. *N Engl J Med* 1994;331:377–382.
Grayston JT, Campbell LA, Kuo CC, et al. A new respiratory tract pathogen: *Chlamydia pneumoniae* strain TWAR. *J Infect Dis* 1990;161:618–625.
Marrie TJ. Community-acquired pneumonia. *Clin Infect Dis* 1994; 18:501–513.
Marrie TJ. *Mycoplasma pneumoniae* pneumonia requiring hospitalization, with emphasis on infection in the elderly. *Arch Intern Med* 1993;153:488–494.
McEachern R, Campbell GD. Hospital-acquired pneumonia: epidemiology, etiology, and treatment. *Infect Dis Clin North Am* 1998;12:761–769.
Murray HW, Masur H, Senterfit LB, et al. The protean manifestations of *Mycoplasma pneumoniae* infection in adults. *Am J Med* 1975;58:229–242.
Rello J, Quintana E, Ausina V, et al. Incidence, etiology, and outcome of nosocomial pneumonia in mechanically ventilated patients. *Chest* 1991;100:439–444.
Scheld WM, Mandell GL. Nosocomial pneumonia: pathogenesis and recent advances in diagnosis and therapy. *Rev Infect Dis* 1991;13(Suppl):743–751.
Stout JE, Yu VL. Legionellosis. *N Engl J Med* 1997;337:682–687.

Chapter 17

Infections in the Ambulatory Setting

Sherif B. Mossad

Antimicrobial agents are more widely prescribed in the ambulatory setting in the United States than in Europe; only 3 of 27 European countries use more antibiotics, and this use is mainly characterized by a shift toward newer antibiotics, including fluoroquinolones and macrolides. Guidelines for judicious use of antibiotics for infections encountered in the ambulatory setting have been published. The efficacy data for low-cost antimicrobials, defined as $15 or less, have been shown to be similar to higher-cost antimicrobials. Estimates of the prevalence of allergic reactions to antibiotics vary widely. Antibiotics account for about half of all cutaneous drug eruptions.

ACUTE INFECTIOUS DIARRHEA

Acute diarrhea is defined as having more than three liquid stools (more than 200 g) per day for a period of less than 14 days. Acute infectious diarrhea (AID) is second only to the common cold in frequency of health care–related visits. AID is more common during the winter months, with an average incidence of 1.4 episodes per person a year. AID results in about 900,000 hospitalizations and 6,000 deaths annually in the United States. The mortality rate is much higher in the developing world, particularly among infants.

Viruses, such as noroviruses, rotaviruses, and Norwalk-like viruses, cause most cases of AID. In the United States, bacterial causes of AID in adults, in order of frequency, are *Campylobacter, Salmonella, Shigella,* and *Escherichia coli* O157:H7 (Shiga toxin–producing *E. coli* [STEC]).

The most important step in evaluating a patient with AID is to differentiate between inflammatory and noninflammatory causes. Symptoms suggestive of inflammatory AID include fever, presence of blood in stools, and tenesmus. Because most cases of AID are self-limited, laboratory investigation is not indicated for patients presenting within 24 hours of illness, unless they have one of the previously described symptoms. Testing for fecal leukocytes using microscopy or an immunoassay for lactoferrin may be used if the history is equivocal. Stool cultures are grossly overused, making the cost per positive result greater than $1,000. The incubation period between exposure to the presumed culprit food and the onset of illness may offer some clues for specific etiologic diagnoses (Table 17.1), but significant overlap occurs, thus making this an inaccurate measure. Epidemiologic clues, such as the type of food consumed, recent hospitalization, recent travel, regional outbreaks, and day care exposure, can be very helpful in narrowing down the differential diagnosis. Similarly, clinical clues, such as fever, bloody stools, and dysentery, as well as host-related defenses and immune defects should offer further clues to the etiologic diagnosis.

Rehydration is the most important measure in the management of AID. Ample evidence refutes the misconception that the bowels need to rest in AID. Oral rehydration suffices in most cases, using home remedies such as soups and Gatorade. Glucose-containing electrolyte solutions are preferred over hyperosmolar fluids. A standard oral rehydration formulation is recommended by the World Health Organization, particularly in resource-poor areas. Bismuth subsalicylate and kaolin-pectin are effective antidiarrheal agents. The antimotility agent's loperamide and diphenoxylate should be avoided in cases of bloody diarrhea, particularly those proven to be due to STEC. Antimicrobial agents are effective in the treatment of travelers' diarrhea, shigellosis, *Clostridium difficile*–associated diarrhea, and, when given early, in cases of campylobacteriosis. A concern exists for prolonged fecal shedding in cases of salmonellosis

Conflict of interest: Dr. Mossad is the cite primary investigator for a multicenter study sponsored by Hoffman-LaRoche, the manufacturer of oseltamivir (Tamiflu)

TABLE 17.1

INCUBATION PERIOD FOR VARIOUS CAUSES OF AID

Less Than 6 Hours	6 to 24 Hours	16 to 72 Hours
Staphylococcus aureus	*Clostridium perfringens*	Noroviruses, enterotoxigenic
Bacillus cereus	*B. cereus*	*Escherichia coli, Vibrio, Salmonella, Shigella, Campylobacter, Yersinia,* STEC, *Giardia, Cyclospora, Cryptosporidium*

TABLE 17.2

CLASSIFICATION AND MICROBIOLOGY OF UTI

Acute Cystitis and Acute Pyelonephritis	Catheter-Related UTI	Prostatitis
Escherichia coli (80%) (may be clonal)	*E. coli*	*E. coli*
Staphylococcus saprophyticus (10%)	*Proteus*	*Proteus*
Klebsiella	*Candida*	*Providencia*
Enterobacter	*Enterococcus*	*Klebsiella*
Proteus	*Pseudomonas*	*Enterobacter*
Enterococcus	*Klebsiella*	*Pseudomonas*
	Enterobacter	*Citrobacter*
	Staphylococcus aureus	*Enterococcus*
		S. aureus and *Staphylococcus epidermidis*

treated with antibiotics. Antimicrobial therapy is contraindicated in cases of STEC infection because some studies have shown that this increases the risk of serious complications. Trimethoprim-sulfamethoxazole (TMP-SMX), or fluoroquinolones, such as ciprofloxacin are appropriate empiric options, when indicated. Macrolides should be used when quinolone-resistant campylobacteriosis is suspected, such as in travelers returning from Southeast Asia. Oral metronidazole and stopping of systemic antibiotics are the treatment for *C. difficile* colitis. Healthy adults should be treated for 3 days (10 days for the latter infection) in most cases, but immunocompromised patients usually require a longer duration of therapy. Advising travelers about appropriate eating and drinking habits is crucial in preventing travelers' diarrhea. Prophylactic bismuth subsalicylate decreases the incidence of travelers' diarrhea, but causes blackening of the tongue and stools. Self-treatment with empiric antibiotics is recommended for travelers with AID, but prophylactic antibiotics are not recommended for most travelers. Rifaximin is a nonabsorbable antibiotic that has been shown to be effective in preventing diarrhea in travelers to Mexico, but is currently not approved for this indication by the U.S. Food and Drug Administration.

POINTS TO REMEMBERS:

- Most cases of acute diarrhea in the United States are viral in origin and treated with rehydration.

- Diagnosis depends on incubation period, epidemiologic, and clinical clues.

- Empiric antibiotics used for inflammatory and travelers' diarrhea include fluoroquinolones or TMP-SMX.

URINARY TRACT INFECTIONS

Urinary tract infection (UTI) results in 7 million visits to outpatient clinics and 100,000 hospitalizations annually, with an estimated cost to the health care system of $1.6 billion. UTI may be classified into four categories: acute cystitis, acute pyelonephritis, catheter related, and prostatitis. *E. coli* is the most common causative organism in these categories, but the distribution of other causative agents varies (Table 17.2).

Acute Cystitis

The first step in the management of acute cystitis is to differentiate this from cervicitis, vaginitis, and urethritis. If symptoms of cystitis (frequency, dysuria, urgency) are most prominent, one should ask about other symptoms suggestive of upper UTI, such as fever, chills, and flank pain. Next, risk factors for having complicated cystitis should be evaluated. These include having symptoms for 14 days, most UTI in men, diabetics, renal transplant recipients, other immunosuppressed individuals, and during pregnancy. In addition, patients with history of urinary stone, and those with anatomical genitourinary abnormalities should also be considered to have a potentially complicated UTI.

The detection of pyuria by leukocyte esterase test or urine microscopy, as well as the detection of bacteriuria by nitrite test or urine Gram staining, have low sensitivity and positive predictive value and high specificity and negative predictive value for the diagnosis of UTI. Both tests have their limitations and perform better when used together. Vaginal contamination may cause false-positive leukocyte esterase test, and high urine protein or glucose may cause false-negative test. UTI caused by gram-positive cocci or yeast, low dietary nitrate, rapid transit, and low bacterial count may all cause false-negative nitrite test. Using a decision aid that includes the presence of dysuria, leukocytes, and nitrates would reduce unnecessary antimicrobial prescriptions by 40% and urine cultures by 59%. Routine urine culture is not indicated for the management of simple cystitis, and empiric therapy is appropriate.

The first line of therapy remains TMP-SMX or trimethoprim alone, with fluoroquinolones, nitrofurantoin, and fosfomycin considered as second-line agents. Despite these recommendations published by the Infectious Diseases Society of America in 1999, the use of quinolones for the treatment of uncomplicated UTI increased significantly from 1996 to 2001, with quinolones being prescribed in 48% and sulfas in 33% of UTI visits. In addition, approximately one-third of the quinolones used were broader spectrum agents. Due to the high rate of antimicrobial resistance in the pathogens causing UTI to penicillins and cephalosporins, these agents are not recommended for empiric therapy. Even in women infected by susceptible organisms, beta-lactam agents may not be as effective as the recommended first-line agents, due to their inferior ability to eradicate vaginal *E. coli*, thus allowing reinfection.

The following factors increase the risk of antimicrobial resistance to TMP-SMX:

- Local resistance pattern to TMP-SMX of >20%
- Recent use of TMP-SMX
- Current use of any antimicrobial agents
- Recent hospitalization
- Recurrent UTI
- Estrogen exposure for contraception or hormone replacement
- Diabetes mellitus

Single-dose therapy has been advocated for women, but a high failure rate may be seen with associated occult upper urinary tract infection or with certain organisms such as *Staphylococcus saprophyticus*. Treatment for 3 days is appropriate for most women. Treatment for 7 to 10 days is recommended for most men, diabetics, and renal transplant recipients; during pregnancy; in patients older than 65 years; in women who concomitantly use cervical diaphragms; in patients with symptoms lasting more than 7 days and who have known antimicrobial resistance. Options for recurrent cystitis in women are continuous prophylaxis, postcoital prophylaxis, or self-initiated therapy. The latter option has been well studied and proven reliable.

Acute Pyelonephritis

Risk factors associated with acute pyelonephritis in healthy women include frequency of sexual intercourse in the preceding 30 days, having a new sexual partner in the previous year, recent spermicide use, UTI, or incontinence, diabetes mellitus, and UTI history in the mother. The differential diagnosis for acute pyelonephritis includes renal calculi and renal infarction. The majority of patients with acute pyelonephritis have more than 10^5 colony-forming units (CFU)/mL of organisms on urine culture; in fact, 20% may have 10^2 to 10^5 CFU/mL. Blood cultures are positive in 15% to 20% of patients ill enough to require hospitalization. Discordance between blood and urine cultures occurs in less than 3% of cases, however. Empiric outpatient an-

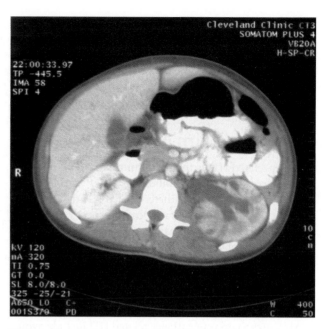

Figure 17.1 Left pyelonephritis and intrarenal abscess.

tibiotic therapy includes either oral fluoroquinolones or TMP-SMX for 7 to 14 days. Hospitalization and initial parenteral antimicrobial therapy is advised in patients presenting with nausea and vomiting and in diabetic and immunosuppressed individuals.

Empiric parenteral antibiotic choices include ampicillin in conjunction with gentamicin, fluoroquinolones, and third-generation cephalosporins. A change to oral antimicrobial therapy can be made as soon as oral intake is restored. Extending antimicrobial therapy beyond 2 weeks will not benefit uncomplicated cases of pyelonephritis, even in bacteremic patients. The persistence of symptoms despite appropriate antimicrobial therapy for more than 48 to 72 hours warrants an imaging study, such as ultrasonography or CT (Fig. 17.1), to look for intrarenal abscess or evidence of obstruction. Antimicrobial resistance may be seen with any urinary pathogen, particularly *Pseudomonas aeruginosa* and enterococci. The latter organisms may need combination antimicrobial agents or longer-duration therapy. If no anatomical defect that could be corrected is detected, a "test of cure" urine culture is recommended 1 to 2 weeks after the completion of therapy.

Asymptomatic Bacteriuria

For men, this is defined as the isolation of a single bacterial strain from a clean-catch voided urine in a quantitative count $\geq 10^5$CFU/mL. For women, this has to occur on two consecutive specimens. For men or women who are catheterized, a quantitative count $\geq 10^2$CFU/mL of a single organism in one specimen fulfills the definition. Even if a person with asymptomatic bacteriuria also has pyuria, this in and of itself does not constitute an indication for antimicrobial therapy. Screening for and treatment of asymptomatic bacteriuria is indicated in pregnancy and before urologic procedures in which mucosal bleeding is anticipated, including transurethral resection of the prostate. Women with diabetes mellitus who have asymptomatic bacteriuria are not at increased risk for faster decline in renal function or the development of hypertension.

Catheter-Related UTI

Catheter-related UTI is the most common nosocomial infection, accounting for 1 million cases per year. Pyuria is strongly associated with catheter-related UTI due to gram-negative bacilli, but not gram-positive cocci or yeast. In addition, bacteriuria with as few as 100 CFU/mL may be indicative of infection in catheterized patients. Because most patients with catheter-related UTI do not have urinary symptoms, one should obtain urine culture and consider empiric therapy for UTI if a catheterized patient develops signs of sepsis that cannot be otherwise explained.

Measures to prevent catheter-related UTI include avoiding catheterization in the first place, following strict aseptic insertion techniques, using a closed drainage system, using nitrofurazone-coated or silver-coated catheters, discontinuing catheterization as soon as the indication resolves, or using alternatives such as condom or suprapubic catheters.

Acute Bacterial Prostatitis

About one-fourth of men are diagnosed with prostatitis during their lifetime. Patients with acute bacterial prostatitis present with symptoms suggestive of cystitis, associated with deep pelvic pain and constitutional symptoms. In such cases, the prostate gland is swollen and extremely tender on digital rectal exam. Prostate massage should be avoided in these patients because it may precipitate bacteremia; urine culture suffices. An infection is not present in most patients with chronic symptoms. The "four-cup" localization culture test should be used in these patients to differentiate between chronic bacterial prostatitis, chronic nonbacterial prostatitis, or chronic pelvic pain syndrome. Similar to acute cystitis, empiric therapy for bacterial prostatitis includes TMP-SMX or fluoroquinolones; however, the recommended duration of therapy is 4 weeks for acute cases and 6 to 12 weeks for chronic cases.

POINTS TO REMEMBERS:

- Before prescribing treatment for UTI, consider other causes of urinary frequency, differentiate between simple cystitis and pyelonephritis, and determine whether UTI is simple or complicated.

- TMP-SMX remains the first-line antibiotic for simple cystitis, and TMP-SMX or a quinolone for acute pyelonephritis.

- Screening for and treatment of asymptomatic bacteriuria is indicated in pregnancy and before urologic procedures in which mucosal bleeding is anticipated.

UPPER RESPIRATORY TRACT INFECTIONS

Antibiotic prescriptions for upper respiratory tract infection (URTI) account for 30% of all antibiotics prescribed for adults, with a total annual cost of $726 million. Fortunately, after years of extensive educational interventions to both physicians and the public, recent surveys have shown a downward trend in the proportion of patients diagnosed with the common cold or bronchitis who are prescribed antibiotics. However, the use of broad-spectrum antimicrobial agents in these patients has actually increased by threefold. Physicians in training have lower antimicrobial prescribing rates than practicing physicians. Several symptoms predictive of physicians prescribing antibiotics for URTI, such as production of yellow sputum, sore throat, fever, and colored nasal discharge, actually have poor predictive evidence in the literature for the efficacy of the prescribed antibiotics. One-third of patients with colds mistakenly think that antibiotics can make them get better faster or can prevent a more serious illness. Several studies have shown the importance of a personal explanation of the lack of efficacy and the potential adverse effects of antibiotics to patients presenting with nonspecific URTI. In addition, counseling patients about the cost of antibiotics, the false sense of security created by taking them, and the increasing problem of antimicrobial resistance resulting from selective pressure and elimination of normal flora is also very important. Clinical decision support systems have been shown to reduce overall antimicrobial use in primary care settings and improve appropriateness of antimicrobial selection for acute respiratory tract infections. A study done in Japan showed that minimal use of antibiotics for adults with URTI resulted in improvement in 97% of patients and in patient satisfaction in 95% at 15 days.

Infectious Mononucleosis Syndrome

Epstein-Barr virus (EBV) is the most common cause of a "monolike" illness, consisting of the triad of fever, sore throat, and lymphadenopathy. Several other infectious agents can produce a similar illness, including cytomegalovirus, HIV, human herpesvirus 6, parvovirus B-19, toxoplasmosis, and group A β-hemolytic streptococcus (GABHS). Patients with EBV infection may also present with fatigue, which can last for 3 weeks or more, headache, and myalgia. Physical examination findings include generalized lymphadenopathy in 95% of cases, pharyngitis with occasional palatal petechiae in 80%, splenomegaly in 50%, and hepatomegaly and jaundice in 10%; the latter two being more commonly seen in adults than adolescents. A maculopapular rash is noted on presentation in 5% to 10% of cases, and this rash is more likely to develop in patients who receive ampicillin or amoxicillin for presumed GABHS pharyngitis. Large, lobulated "atypical" lymphocytes are often seen on peripheral blood smear. Mild to moderate leukopenia, thrombocytopenia, and hemolytic anemia may also be seen during the acute illness. Liver function abnormalities occur in up to 80% of patients, particularly in older adults. Monospot test detects heterophile antibodies in 70% to 90% of cases within 1 to 5 weeks of the onset of illness. Specific EBV IgM is positive with acute infection and usually wanes within 3 months, whereas EBV IgG remains positive, often for life. This is a self-limited illness, so treatment is only supportive. Treatment with antiviral agents is not recommended. Corticosteroids are only useful in cases associated with severe pharyngeal edema. Patients should be advised to avoid contact sports for 4 weeks to avoid splenic rupture. Confirmed association exists between EBV and oral hairy leukoplakia and certain types of lymphoma, particularly following organ transplantation, and nasopharyngeal carcinoma. More recently, a relation between EBV and multiple sclerosis has been suggested by epidemiologic studies.

Influenza

In the United States, annual influenza epidemics infect 5% to 20% of the population, resulting in 25 million health care visits, 140,000 hospitalizations (approximately 16% of cases), and 40,000 to 60,000 deaths (approximately 0.6% of cases), with an average cost of $12 million. Epidemics in the Northern Hemisphere occur between the months of September and March. They usually start in school children and then spread to the rest of the community. Transmission occurs by small-particle aerosols from infected persons. Viral shedding peaks within 2 to 3 days of infection, but may last for 1 week or more. Yearly minor antigenic changes, or *antigenic drift,* in the viral glycoprotein hemagglutinin allow for the viral evasion of immunologic protection built up from influenza infections or immunizations in preceding seasons, thus resulting in annual epidemics. Major changes in viral antigenic composition, or *antigenic shift,* however, result in pandemics.

Patients typically present with sudden diffuse or throbbing headache, high fever, severe myalgia, and dry cough. Sore throat and rhinorrhea may occur, but the systemic symptoms are much more pronounced. The presence of sneezing among older patients actually argues against the diagnosis of influenza. Patients with underlying chronic medical conditions such as chronic obstructive lung disease and congestive heart failure are at risk for developing serious complications due to exacerbation of their underlying illness or bacterial superinfection. Bacterial pneumonia after influenza is commonly caused by *Streptococcus pneumoniae* or *Staphylococcus aureus*, including methicillin-resistant *S. aureus* (MRSA), and usually develops several days or weeks later. The gold standard to confirm the diagnosis for epidemiologic purposes is either viral culture or acute and convalescent serology. Because these measures are not practical for clinical use, several rapid diagnostic tests have been developed, including direct fluorescent antigen detection, enzyme immunoassay, and polymerase chain reaction. Rapid diagnostic tests also reduce unnecessary use of antibacterial agents.

The adamantanes amantadine and rimantadine are not currently recommended for use due to a high rate of resistance (96%) of influenza A H3N2 to these agents, and they have no intrinsic activity against influenza B. The neuraminidase inhibitors zanamivir and oseltamivir are active against both influenza A and B, are better tolerated than the adamantanes, and are associated with a much lower risk of developing viral resistance. For maximum benefit, zanamivir or oseltamivir should be started within 1 to 2 days of the onset of illness. When used early in the course of influenza, studies have shown them to shorten the duration of illness by 1 to 2 days and to significantly decrease the severity of symptoms. These benefits are more evident in patients infected with influenza A than B and in those presenting with severe illness.

Vaccination remains the primary preventive measure against influenza. The trivalent, inactivated, intramuscular vaccine is recommended for children ages 6 to 59 months, adults 50 and older, pregnant women, residents of chronic care facilities, patients with medical conditions that put them at risk of influenza-related complications regardless of age, and all health care providers, household contacts of the aforementioned groups, and contacts of children younger than 6 months. It is well tolerated, and, contrary to false belief by some patients, it cannot cause influenza. The live-attenuated, cold-adapted, intranasal influenza vaccine is as effective as the inactivated vaccine in adults and even more effective in children ages 12 to 59 months, but is only approved for use in healthy persons ages 2 to 49 years. Several large studies have shown that influenza vaccine is effective in preventing illness, hospitalization, and death, and that vaccination is cost effective. Vaccination rates in the United States have improved during the past decade but are still suboptimal, with only 20% to 69% of people for whom the vaccine is indicated being immunized. Vaccination rates can be boosted by educating health care providers, educating patients, and implementing evidence-based measures, such as automatic reminders and standing orders. Influenza vaccination of health care providers should be monitored as a patient safety quality measure, and feedback on specific vaccination rates of both health care providers and their patients should be provided. Although the neuraminidase inhibitors have been effective in preventing influenza, they should not be regarded as a substitute to vaccination.

The ongoing H5N1 avian influenza epizootic that started in the Far East has now involved multiple countries in Asia, Europe, and Africa, causing more than 300 human cases, half of which have died. In the event of an H5N1 pandemic, extrapolating data from the 1918–1919 influenza pandemic, about 1 billion people worldwide would become ill and 62 million would die (96% of them in the developing world), increasing global mortality by 114%. The U.S. Department of Health and Human Services is stockpiling human H5N1 influenza vaccine, oseltamivir and zanamivir, in anticipation of an avian influenza pandemic. Social distancing measures such as school closures and travel restrictions will be required to slow the course of a pandemic.

Acute Rhinosinusitis

Annual crude prevalence rate of acute sinusitis in adults is 14% to 16%, with approximately 20 million cases per year in the United States. The majority of cases are due to viruses, with only about 40% caused by bacteria, including *S. pneumoniae, Haemophilus influenzae, Moraxella catarrhalis,* and *S. aureus.* Paranasal sinus ostial blockade due to mucosal edema is usually preceded by a nonspecific upper respiratory viral infection, but only about 2% of colds are complicated by bacterial sinusitis. Other predisposing factors include nasal allergies, deviated nasal septum, ciliary dysfunction, and immune deficiency.

Characteristic clinical features include maxillary toothache, unilateral facial pain or tenderness, purulent nasal discharge, decreased transillumination, and, most important, lack of response to decongestants for 7 to 10 days. CT is more informative and priced comparably to plain radiography. However, viral and bacterial sinusitis have similar radiologic appearance. CT should only be done to rule out serious complication or to define the anatomy before an anticipated corrective surgery. Most cases of acute sinusitis presenting to the primary care physician do not require CT, sinus endoscopy, or sinus aspiration.

Most cases of mild sinusitis improve with topical intranasal steroids and topical or systemic nasal decongestants, without antimicrobial therapy. In fact, one-third of patients with acute sinusitis have some residual symptoms lasting 10 days or more, whether they received nasal steroids, antibiotics, or placebo. However, both antibiotics and nasal steroids are being prescribed more often than their published efficacies would encourage. First-line antimicrobial agents recommended for moderate and severe cases include amoxicillin, TMP-SMX, and doxycycline for 7 to 10 days. Alternatives include cefpodoxime, cefuroxime, cefdinir, and macrolides. Amoxicillin-clavulanate, levofloxacin, and moxifloxacin should be reserved as second-line agents in patients who do not improve with one of the first-line agents administered for 3 to 5 days, or if the symptoms return within 2 weeks. Patients who do not improve with a second-line antimicrobial

agent should be referred to an ear, nose, and throat specialist in consideration for sinus endoscopy or aspiration for culture-directed therapy, or surgical intervention.

Streptococcal (Tonsillo) Pharyngitis

The differential diagnosis for someone presenting with sore throat includes pharyngitis, epiglottitis, thyroiditis, and gastroesophageal reflux disease. The most important question to answer in a patient presenting with pharyngitis is whether it is caused by GABHS, a readily treatable infection, which may prevent suppurative and immunologic complications. Viruses, such as rhinovirus and coronavirus, cause the majority of cases of pharyngitis, and other bacteria, including group C β-hemolytic streptococci, *Corynebacterium diphtheriae, Neisseria gonorrhoeae, Arcanobacterium haemolyticum, Chlamydia pneumoniae,* and *Mycoplasma pneumoniae* each cause a small percentage of cases. The Centor criteria—fever, tonsillar exudate, tender anterior cervical lymphadenopathy, absence of cough, and exposure within 2 weeks to someone with GABHS pharyngitis—increase the diagnostic likelihood of GABHS infection. In adults, streptococcal rapid antigen detection test is 90% sensitive and 95% specific, whereas culture is 97% sensitive and 99% specific. Testing for GABHS remains underused, and empiric antimicrobial treatment, even in patients with three or four Centor criteria, results in antibiotic overuse. Unfortunately, clinicians adhere to guidelines for management of pharyngitis in less than 30% of cases. It is prudent not to test for GABHS and not to prescribe antibiotics in patients at low risk for streptococcal pharyngitis according to the Centor criteria. In the United Kingdom, a 50% decrease in the rate of prescribing antibiotics was not accompanied by an increase in hospital admissions for peritonsillar abscess or rheumatic fever.

Oral penicillin for 10 days is the treatment of choice. Alternatives include intramuscular penicillin, oral first-generation cephalosporins, and oral macrolides.

Acute Tracheobronchitis

This illness is characterized by cough, with or without sputum production, lasting 1 to 3 weeks. Other commonly associated symptoms include wheezing, coryza, and constitutional symptoms. Viruses such as influenza A and B, parainfluenza, respiratory syncytial virus, rhinovirus, coronavirus, and adenovirus cause the majority of cases. Fewer than 10% of cases are caused by *Bordetella pertussis, Bordetella parapertussis, M. pneumoniae,* and *C. pneumoniae* (TWAR). In otherwise healthy patients presenting with cough, pneumonia can be reasonably excluded if the vital signs are normal and if clinical signs of consolidation, such as rales and egophony, are absent. Purulence of sputum is a poor predictor of bacterial infection. Chest radiography should be reserved for patients with comorbid conditions, those with abnormal vital signs or clinical signs of consolidation, or those with persistent symptoms for more than 3 weeks. A normal C-reactive protein can reasonably exclude pneumonia, but may be elevated in the presence of several other infectious and noninfectious conditions. If cough lasts more than 6 weeks, postnasal drip, asthma, and gastroesophageal reflux disease account for the majority of causes. Antibiotics are only recommended for confirmed pertussis, mycoplasma, chlamydia, or acute exacerbation of chronic bronchitis. Most cases resolve spontaneously. Selective β-agonist bronchodilators and antitussive agents may offer symptomatic relief. Other measures used to treat nonspecific URTI, such as vaporizers, and acetaminophen may also be used.

Acute Otitis Externa and Acute Otitis Media

Acute otitis externa occurs in 10% of adults. Risk factors include aggressive cleaning of ear canal, swimming, ear devices such as the iPod, and diabetes mellitus. One-third of cases are polymicrobial, with causative organisms including *S. aureus*, *Pseudomonas*, *Candida*, and *Aspergillus*. Itching, earache, drainage, and swelling of the external canal and auricle are the main features. Treatment is by initiating topical eardrops of acetic acid, neomycin/polymyxin/clotrimazole, or steroids and removing impacted cerumen. Malignant "necrotizing" otitis externa due to *Pseudomonas aeruginosa* is seen in diabetics.

Acute otitis media occurs in 0.25% of adults. Risk factors include younger age, smoking, allergic rhinitis, and immune deficiency. Causative organisms include respiratory syncytial virus, influenza virus, rhinovirus, *Streptococcus pneumoniae*, *Haemophilus influenzae*, *Moraxella catarrhalis*, and *Mycoplasma pneumoniae*, which may be associated with bullous formation. Patients present with fever, earache, decreased hearing, and drainage. A fluid level behind the tympanic membrane may be visualized by otoscopy. Treatment includes decongestants, analgesics, and antibiotics such as amoxicillin or macrolides in cases of suppurative otitis media. A "wait-and-see prescription" for antibiotics approach substantially reduced unnecessary use of antibiotics without deleterious effects. Potential complications include mastoiditis, meningitis, and epidural abscess.

POINTS TO REMEMBER:

- American College of Physicians Guidelines recommend considering antibiotics for patients with URTI in
  - Patients with moderate or severe sinusitis accompanied by maxillary toothache, unilateral face pain, purulent discharge, decreased transillumination, and poor response to 7 to 10 days of decongestants
  - Patients with pharyngitis associated with positive streptococcal rapid antigen test, suspected GABHS based on three to four Centor criteria, unilateral tonsillitis, or peritonsillar abscess
  - Patients with acute bronchitis, only if pneumonia cannot be excluded clinically

- In patients with a "monolike" illness, large, lobulated "atypical" (reactive) lymphocytes are often seen on peripheral blood smear.

- Neuraminidase inhibitors are currently the only recommended class of antivirals for treatment and prevention of influenza. Vaccination remains the first line of defense.

SOFT TISSUE INFECTIONS

Cellulitis

Cellulitis is infection involving the skin and subcutaneous tissues. Incidence rises with age, and more cases occur during the warm summer months, possibly due to increased outdoor activities. Risk factors include diabetes mellitus, arterial or venous insufficiency, and tinea pedis. Patients whose saphenous veins have been harvested for coronary artery bypass surgery and those who undergo mastectomy and axillary lymph node dissection for breast cancer are at increased risk of recurrent cellulitis due to lymphatic disruption and lymphedema. Recurrence within 2 years may occur in up to 20% of cases, particularly when involving the pretibial area, and in patients with ipsilateral dermatitis and history of malignancy. Differentiating staphylococcal from streptococcal cellulitis is not possible on clinical grounds alone, so empiric antimicrobial coverage should include an agent active against both types of organisms, such as oral dicloxacillin, intravenous oxacillin, and oral or intravenous first-generation cephalosporins, depending on the severity of illness. The generally accepted course of therapy is 7 to 14 days, or 3 days beyond clinical resolution. Elevation and rest of the involved limb is necessary to reduce edema. Patients with chronic limb edema and lymphedema are advised to use elastic support stockings after cellulitis resolves to avoid recurrence. Interdigital epidermophytosis should be treated with topical antifungal agents. Cellulitis surrounding a decubitus ulcer or a diabetic foot ulcer is likely to be polymicrobial, so a broad-spectrum antimicrobial agent such as ampicillin-sulbactam is appropriate. Pain or tenderness extending outside the area of erythema, crepitus, and loss of sensations in the inflamed area should raise suspicion for necrotizing fasciitis, which warrants immediate surgical consultation. *H. influenzae* causes buccal cellulitis, so treatment with a third-generation cephalosporin is appropriate. Confirmed Group A streptococcal cellulitis is best treated using penicillin combined with clindamycin to overcome the inoculum effect, which is a stationary micro-organism growth phase that makes penicillin less effective. Beta-lactam agents are bactericidal, which may result in lysis of bacteria and toxins release. Clindamycin is a bacteriostatic agent, which acts synergistically by inhibiting protein and bacterial toxin synthesis.

Cellulitis and recurrent furunculosis due to community-acquired MRSA USA 300 clone have been expanding problems lately. Risk factors include participation in contact sports, and both conditions are seen more frequently in prisoners, soldiers, injection drug users, men who have sex with men, native Americans, and patients with recent antibiotic exposure or hospitalization within the preceding 12 months. Oral antimicrobial options include tetracycline, TMP-SMX, clindamycin, linezolid, and rifampin when used in conjunction with another agent. Incision and drainage of soft tissue abscesses that are smaller than 5 cm in length may be sufficient treatment, with no need for antibiotics.

Rapidly progressive cellulitis in immunocompromised patients, particularly cirrhotics, who are exposed to saltwater or who eat raw oysters should raise the suspicion for *Vibrio vulnificus* as the etiologic agent. Hemorrhagic bullae are characteristically seen in infections by this organism. Bacteremic cases are fatal in 30% to 50% of cases. Doxycycline is the treatment of choice, and thorough cooking of seafood remains the only effective preventive measure.

Cellulitis due to *Aeromonas hydrophila* is another serious form of cellulitis also seen more frequently in cirrhotics and cancer patients who are exposed to fresh water. Some reports linking this infection to medicinal leeches have been published. Other manifestations of infection by this organism include gastroenteritis and spontaneous bacterial peritonitis. Ciprofloxacin is the treatment of choice.

Erysipeloid, caused by *Erysipelothrix rhusiopathiae*, is usually an occupational infection that occurs in healthy people handling meat products or saltwater fish. A violaceous lesion that spreads peripherally and has a raised border and central clearing is characteristic. Ulceration usually does not develop, and this infection is almost always localized to the site of inoculation. It responds well to penicillin therapy.

Hot tub folliculitis due to inadequate chlorination is typically due to *P. aeruginosa*. Cryptococcal cellulitis is seen almost exclusively in immunocompromised patients.

Several mimics of cellulitis exist, including stasis dermatitis, insect bites, acute gout, deep venous thrombosis, fixed drug eruption, pyoderma gangrenosa, and Sweet's syndrome.

POINTS TO REMEMBER:

- If erysipelas cannot be clinically differentiated from cellulitis, antimicrobial coverage for both streptococci and staphylococci should be used.
- Contrary to paronychia or felon, incision and drainage is contraindicated for herpetic whitlow be-

cause this may result in viremia or secondary bacterial infection.

- Antifungal therapy for onychomycosis takes several weeks, so microbiological documentation is required.

Erysipelas

Erysipelas is infection involving the superficial skin and cutaneous lymphatics. Older literature indicated the face to be the most common site of occurrence, but more recent studies show the lower extremities to account for 80% of cases. Incidence has increased lately, possibly due to loss of collective immunity. Classic features of erysipelas that distinguish it from cellulitis are the sharp demarcating edge and palpable induration "peau d'orange." Sometimes, however, it is not possible to distinguish both clinically. Blood culture and surface culture are rarely positive in erysipelas, and aspirating the leading edge for culture is of low yield. A rising antistreptolysin O titer may be helpful in confirming the diagnosis. Almost all cases of erysipelas are caused by GABHS and are treatable with penicillin, or macrolides in allergic patients. Some cases of bullous erysipelas are caused by MRSA. Patients with lymphedema or venous insufficiency are at risk for recurrent erysipelas in up to 30% of cases.

Bites

Almost one-half of all Americans are bitten at some point during their lifetime by an animal or by another person. Humans are most frequently bitten by, in order, dogs, cats, wild animals, and other humans. When it comes to potential complications of bites, however, this order is reversed. The majority of human bites occur over the weekend or on a public holiday in males consuming alcohol, with the ear being the most common target followed by the upper limb (clenched fist). When bite wounds get infected, *Pasteurella multocida* is the organism seen most frequently in cat bites, α-hemolytic streptococci in dog bites, and *Eikenella corrodens* in human bites. In addition, *S. aureus* and mixed anaerobic organisms are seen in approximately 30% of infected bites. In fact, the bacteriologic analysis of infected dog and cat bites yields a median of five bacterial isolates per culture. Cat scratch disease due to *Bartonella henselae* may also follow a bite.

Radiographic studies should be considered when fracture or an impacted foreign body, such as a tooth fragment, is suspected, or if the bite is close to a joint. If the bite is less than 8 hours old and does not appear to be clinically infected, culture from the wound is not recommended. Most bite wounds should be left open with delayed closure. Irrigation, debridement, elevation, and immobilization are important steps in managing any bite wound. A tetanus booster is recommended if the patient has not received one within the preceding 10 years. Rabies vaccine is not recommended for dog or cat bites occurring in the United States, but should be considered for rodent or wild animal bites. The antimicrobial agent of choice in infected bites is amoxicillin-clavulanic acid. For penicillin-allergic individuals, tetracyclines or a combination of a quinolone and clindamycin are reasonable alternatives. First-generation cephalosporins are not an appropriate choice.

Prophylactic antibiotics in clinically uninfected wounds are recommended only in those involving severe crush injuries, involving joints or bones, near prosthetic joints, or on the hands. In addition, any bite in immunocompromised patients who are at risk for developing more serious infections should be treated with antibiotics. Prompt surgical intervention is imperative for any deep hand or facial bite that becomes infected.

Herpetic Whitlow

Autoinoculation by herpes simplex virus (HSV) type 1 as a complication of oral herpes or by HSV type 2 as a complication of genital herpes may result in herpetic whitlow, particularly with an antecedent trauma to the nail cuticle. Exposure may also occur during manual sexual contact or in health care workers exposed to oral lesions. The pain associated with this condition is severe and out of proportion to the physical findings. Systemic symptoms and regional lymphadenopathy are common. Lesions may mimic bacterial infections, such as paronychia, which is an infection of the epidermis bordering the nail, and felon, which is an infection of the distal phalanx pad. Treatment with antiviral agents, such as acyclovir, may shorten illness if started within 48 hours of the onset. Contrary to paronychia or felon, incision and drainage is contraindicated for herpetic whitlow because this may result in viremia or secondary

bacterial infection. To avoid occupational exposure, respiratory therapists and dental hygienists should wear gloves when exposed to oral secretions. Unfortunately, recurrence occurs in up to 30% of patients, so either suppressive therapy or treatment during the prodromal stage may be beneficial.

Onychomycosis

Fungal infection of fingernails and toenails is a very common condition, accounting for approximately half of all nail problems. The distal subungual form is more common than the proximal subungual, superficial, or total dystrophic forms. Most cases are caused by either *Trichophyton rubrum* or *Trichophyton mentagrophytes*. Risk factors include increasing age, familial predisposition, diabetes mellitus, peripheral arterial occlusive disease, HIV infection, other immunocompromising conditions, and possibly genetic factors. Exposure may occur at public spas or pools. Concomitant tinea pedis is present in almost half the patients with onychomycosis. Even though this infection is frequently perceived as a cosmetic problem, it may have psychological, social, and medical consequences, the direst of which is diabetic foot infection, which may lead to amputation. Other conditions, such as psoriasis, may resemble onychomycosis. This, together with the fact that treatment is both lengthy and costly, has led most health insurance companies to require mycologic confirmation of the diagnosis before reimbursing the cost of treatment. This confirmation may be accomplished by using either a potassium hydroxide preparation of the nail bed scrapings or fungal culture. Systemic antifungal treatment is generally much more effective than topical therapies, such as ciclopirox nail varnish. Older antifungal agents, such as griseofulvin and ketoconazole, have been largely replaced by safer and more effective options, such as itraconazole and terbinafine. The

TABLE 17.3

INFECTIONS IN THE AMBULATORY SETTING: SUMMARY

Condition	Etiology	Treatment
AID	Viral	Rehydration
	Bacterial	Quinolone or TMP-SMX
Acute cystitis	*Escherichia coli*	TMP-SMX
Acute pyelonephritis	*E. coli*	Quinolone or TMP-SMX
Catheter-related UTI	*E. coli*	Quinolone or TMP-SMX
Acute prostatitis	*E. coli*	Quinolone or TMP-SMX
Infectious mononucleosis	EBV	Symptomatic
Influenza	Influenza A and B	Zanamivir or oseltamivir
Acute rhinosinusitis	*Streptococcus pneumoniae*	Amoxicillin
Acute (tonsillo) pharyngitis	GABHS	Penicillin
Acute bronchitis	Viral	Beta-agonists
Cellulitis	*Staphylococcus aureus* and streptococci	Penicillinase-resistant penicillin or first-generation cephalosporin
Erysipelas	GABHS	Penicillin
Herpetic whitlow	HSV types 1 and 2	Acyclovir
Onychomycosis	*Trichophyton rubrum*	Terbinafine or itraconazole

duration of therapy is 12 weeks for toenails and 6 weeks for fingernails. Intermittent "pulse" therapy with itraconazole for 1 week per month has been shown to be both efficacious and cost effective. Patients should be reminded that continued improvement is expected for several weeks after completing the course of therapy. Unfortunately, relapse may occur in approximately 15% of cases, and may be prevented by avoiding hyperhidrosis and early treatment of athlete's foot.

Several other important topics on infections in the ambulatory setting, such as community-acquired pneumonia, sexually transmitted diseases, hepatitis, and tuberculosis, are discussed in other chapters of this book.

SUMMARY

Table 17.3 summarizes the signs and symptoms and treatment of the infectious diseases presented in this chapter.

REVIEW EXERCISES

QUESTIONS

1. A 30-year-old healthy woman presents with nonbloody diarrhea that has persisted for less than 24 hours. She has nausea and abdominal cramping, but no fever or tenesmus. No recent travel is noted, and her exam is normal. You should
a) Ask her if other family members are affected.
b) Check fecal leukocytes by microscopy or lactoferrin.
c) Collect stools for bacterial culture and rotavirus polymerase chain reaction.
d) Tell her to avoid antidiarrheal agents such as loperamide.
e) Start empiric ciprofloxacin.

Answer and Discussion
The answer is a. If AID can be linked to the ingestion of a certain meal, such as in a family outbreak setting, the incubation period can be helpful for diagnosis (**Table 17.1**). Certain foods are also linked to particular infections: undercooked poultry and campylobacteriosis, undercooked hamburger and STEC, seafood and *Vibrio* species, improperly refrigerated fried rice and *Bacillus cereus*, fresh soft cheeses and *Listeria monocytogenes*, contaminated eggs and *Salmonella* species, unrefrigerated potato salad and *S. aureus* (preformed enterotoxin), and undercooked pork and *Yersinia enterocolitica*. The most likely cause in this case is a viral infection.

Because this illness is less than 24 hours in duration and is not associated with inflammatory features, the detection of fecal leukocytes and stool cultures are not indicated at this time. Rotavirus polymerase chain reaction should not be used in routine clinical care. Oral rehydration is the appropriate management here. Anti-

motility agents such as loperamide and diphenoxylate may be used here if needed because the diarrhea is not bloody. Empiric antimicrobials are indicated for moderate to severe travelers' diarrhea, and febrile, community-acquired, inflammatory diarrhea, particularly in immunocompromised patients, unless STEC is suspected on epidemiologic grounds. Severe nosocomial diarrhea in patients receiving systemic antibiotics or chemotherapeutic agents should also be treated empirically with metronidazole, pending the results of a *C. difficile* toxin assay. Persistent diarrhea for more than 10 days should raise the concern of protozoal pathogens, such as *Giardia* and *Cryptosporidium*; empiric therapy with metronidazole, pending stool microscopy or immunoassay, is reasonable in this setting.

2. A 22-year-old woman presents with dysuria and foul-smelling urine for 24 hours. No fever or suprapubic or flank pain is present. She had a similar episode in the past year. She uses spermicide-coated condoms and diaphragms for contraception. Her exam is normal. You should
a) Collect urine for culture.
b) Order ultrasound of the urinary bladder and kidneys.
c) Prescribe trimethoprim-sulfamethoxazole for 7 days.
d) Advise her to avoid vaginal spermicides.
e) Advise against future self-treatment or prophylaxis.

Answer and Discussion
The answer is d. The microbiology of acute uncomplicated cystitis in women is predictable, so empiric antimicrobial therapy would be appropriate. Collecting urine for culture should be considered if empiric therapy fails. Ultrasound of the urinary bladder may be useful in cases with persistent symptoms to rule out the presence of stone or diverticulum. Renal ultrasound should be considered if a clinical suspicion for upper UTI is present. Treatment with TMP-SMX for 3 days is appropriate in most women; extending therapy for 7 days may be considered in patients with persistent symptoms. The use of vaginal spermicides is a known risk factor for UTI; women with recurrent UTI should be advised to use another form of contraception. Once the diagnosis is established, antimicrobial self-treatment at the onset of dysuria and postcoital prophylaxis are reasonable options for this young woman with recurrent cystitis.

3. A 20-year-old college student presents with fever, sore throat, myalgia, splenomegaly, and generalized lymphadenopathy. Which of the following is true?
a) HIV testing should be considered. Treatment is symptomatic.
b) A vaccine could have prevented this illness. Specific therapy is indicated if presenting within 48 hours.

c) *S. pneumoniae* and *H. influenzae* are likely causes. Amoxicillin remains the first-line agent.

d) Fever, tonsillar exudate, tender anterior cervical lymphadenopathy, and absence of cough increase the likelihood of group A β-hemolytic streptococcus (GABHS) infection.

e) Rhinovirus is the most common cause. No diagnostic tests are needed.

Answer and Discussion

The answer is a. In the appropriate setting, patients presenting with mononucleosis-type illness should be questioned about their sexual practices because the acute retroviral syndrome has a similar presentation. HIV antibody test is usually negative during the acute illness and may require several weeks or months to become positive. An accurate diagnosis requires a plasma HIV RNA test or HIV p24 antigen detection. This has clear clinical and public health implications because a large proportion of HIV-infected people are not aware of their HIV status; thus, they may present at a later stage of disease, while continuing to transmit infection to others. The Centers for Disease Control and Prevention currently recommends the "opt-out" HIV screening approach, where assent is inferred unless the patient declines testing. The statement in b) refers to a patient with influenza, an illness that, unlike infectious mononucleosis, may be preventable with a vaccine and is treatable with specific antiviral agents. The statement in c) refers to a patient with acute sinusitis, which is not associated with splenomegaly or generalized lymphadenopathy. The statement in d) refers to a patient with "strep throat," a form of pharyngitis more common in children than adults and associated with certain clinical features that do not include splenomegaly or generalized lymphadenopathy. The statement in e) could apply to a patient with nonspecific upper respiratory tract infection (common cold) or bronchitis; these illnesses are gradual in onset and, again, not associated with splenomegaly or generalized lymphadenopathy.

4. A 60-year-old diabetic woman with history of varicose veins has mild fever and painful, ill-defined redness at an erosion over her tibia. Which of the following is true?

a) Blood cultures are rarely positive. Penicillin is the drug of choice.

b) Herpes simplex is in the differential diagnosis. Ask about sexual practices.

c) Hospital admission for intravenous antibiotics, MRI, and surgical consultation are warranted.

d) Initiate antimicrobial coverage for streptococci and penicillinase-producing staphylococci.

Answer and Discussion

The answer is d. Risk factors for soft tissue infection in this woman include diabetes and varicose veins. The portal of entry for the causative organism is likely the erosion overlying her tibia. The ill-defined redness is more consistent with cellulitis than erysipelas. It is true that blood cultures are usually not positive in most cases of cellulitis, but treatment with penicillin would only be appropriate for erysipelas. Herpes simplex virus infection is not a consideration here, and sexual activity is not a risk factor for cellulitis. Even though one might consider admission to the hospital to initiate intravenous antimicrobial therapy and observe clinical improvement, surgical consultation would only be warranted for this case if necrotizing fasciitis is clinically or radiologically suspected. Topical antifungal therapy may be considered here only if tinea pedis is present.

SUGGESTED READINGS

Goossens H, Ferech M, Coenen S, et al. Comparison of outpatient systemic antibacterial use in 2004 in the United States and 27 European countries. *Clin Infect Dis* 2007;44:1091–1095.

Gruchalla RS, Pirmohamed M. Antibiotic allergy. *N Engl J Med* 2006;354:601–609.

Hansen LA, Vermeulen LC, Bland S, et al. Guideline for low-cost antimicrobial use in the outpatient setting. *Am J Med* 2007;120:295–302.

Acute Infectious Diarrhea

Centers for Disease Control and Prevention. Diagnosis and management of food borne illness: a primer for physicians and other health care professionals. *MMWR Morb Mortal Wkly Rep* 2004;53(RR-4).

Dupont HL, Jiang Z-D, Okhuysen PC, et al. A randomized, double-blind, placebo-controlled trial of rifaximin to prevent travelers' diarrhea. *Ann Intern Med* 2005;142:805–812.

Guerrant RL, Van Gilder T, Steiner TS, et al. Practice guidelines for the management of infectious diarrhea. *Clin Infect Dis* 2001;32:331–350.

Hill DR, Ericsson CD, Pearson RD, et al. The practice of travel medicine: guidelines by the Infectious Diseases Society of America. *Clin Infect Dis* 2006;43:1499–1539.

Musher DM, Musher BL. Contagious acute gastrointestinal infections. *N Engl J Med* 2004;351:2417–2427.

Thielman NM, Guerrant RL. Acute infectious diarrhea. *N Engl J Med* 2004;350:38–47.

Urinary Tract Infections

David RD, DeBlieux PMC, Press R. Rational antibiotic treatment of outpatient genitourinary infections in a changing environment. *Am J Med* 2005;118:7–13.

Hooton TM, Besser R, Foxman B, et al. Acute uncomplicated cystitis in an era of increasing antibiotic resistance: a proposed approach to empirical therapy. *Clin Infect Dis* 2004;39:75–80.

Johnson JR, Kuskowski MA, Wilt TJ. Systematic review: antimicrobial urinary catheters to prevent catheter-associated urinary tract infection in hospitalized patients. *Ann Intern Med* 2006;144:116–126.

Kallen AJ, Welch HG, Sirovich BE. Current antibiotic therapy for isolated urinary tract infections in women. *Arch Intern Med* 2006;166:635–639.

Katchman EA, Milo G, Paul M, et al. Three-day vs longer duration of antibiotic treatment for cystitis in women: systematic review and meta-analysis. *Am J Med* 2005;118:1196–1207.

Koya S, Many WJ Jr, Halanych JH. Managing urinary tract infections in adults in primary care. *Resid Staff Physician* 2006;52:15–21.

Liu H, Mulholland SG. Appropriate antibiotic treatment of genitourinary infections in hospitalized patients. *Am J Med* 2005;118:14–20.

McIsaac WJ, Moineddin R, Ross S. Validation of a decision aid to assist physicians in reducing unnecessary antibiotic drug use for acute cystitis. *Arch Intern Med* 2007;167:2201–2206.

Nicolle LE, Bradley S, Colgan R, et al. Infectious Diseases Society of America guidelines for the diagnosis and treatment of asymptomatic bacteriuria in adults. *Clin Infect Dis* 2005;40:643–654.

Schaeffer AJ. Clinical practice: chronic prostatitis and the chronic pelvic pain syndrome. *N Engl J Med* 2006;355:1690–1698.

Scholes D, Hooton TM, Roberts PL, et al. Risk factors associated with acute pyelonephritis in healthy women. *Ann Intern Med* 2005;142:20–27.

Taur Y, Smith MA. Adherence to the Infectious Diseases Society of America guidelines in the treatment of uncomplicated urinary tract infection. *Clin Infect Dis* 2007;44:769–774.

Warren JW, Abrutyn E, Hebel R, et al. Guidelines for antimicrobial treatment of uncomplicated acute bacterial cystitis and acute pyelonephritis in women. *Clin Infect Dis* 1999;29:745–758.

Wilson ML, Gaido L. Laboratory diagnosis of urinary tract infections in adult patients. *Clin Infect Dis* 2004;38:1150–1158.

Upper Respiratory Tract Infections

Aagaard E, Gonzales R. Management of acute bronchitis in healthy adults. *Infect Dis Clin North Am* 2004;18:919–937.

Beigel JH, Farrar J, Han AM, et al. Avian influenza A (H5N1) infection in humans. *N Engl J Med* 2005;353:1374–1385.

Bisno AL, Gerber MA, Gwaltney JM Jr, et al. Practice guidelines for the diagnosis and management of group A streptococcal pharyngitis. *Clin Infect Dis* 2002;35:113–125.

Bisno AL, Peter GS, Kaplan EL. Diagnosis of strep throat in adult: are clinical criteria really good enough? *Clin Infect Dis* 2003;35:126–129.

Call S, Vollenweider MA, Hornung CA, et al. Does this patient have influenza? *JAMA* 2005;293:987–997.

Ebell MH. Epstein-Barr virus infectious mononucleosis. *Am Fam Physician* 2004;70:1279–1287.

Falsey AR, Murata Y, Walsh EE. Impact of rapid diagnosis on management of adults hospitalized with influenza. *Arch Intern Med* 2007;167:354–360.

Fiore AE, Shay DK, Haber P, et al. Advisory Committee on Immunization Practices (ACIP), Centers for Disease Control and Prevention (CDC). Prevention and control of influenza. Recommendations of the Advisory Committee on Immunization Practices (ACIP). *MMWR Morb Mortal Wkly Rep* 2007;56(RR-6):1–54.

Humair JP, Revaz SA, Bovier P, et al. Management of acute pharyngitis in adults: reliability of rapid streptococcal tests and clinical findings. *Arch Intern Med* 2006;166:640–644.

Hurt C, Tammaro D. Diagnostic evaluation of mononucleosis-like illnesses. *Am J Med* 2007;120:911.e1–911.e8.

Leskinen K, Jero J. Acute complications of otitis media in adults. *Clin Otolaryngol* 2005;30:511–516.

Lindbaek M. Acute sinusitis: to treat or not to treat? *JAMA* 2007;298:2543–2544.

Linder JA, Chan JC, Bates DW. Evaluation and treatment of pharyngitis in primary care practice: the difference between guidelines is largely academic. *Arch Intern Med* 2006;166:1374–1379.

Mossad SB. Influenza update 2007–2008: vaccine advances, pandemic preparation. *Cleve Clin J Med* 2007;74:889–894.

Nichol KL. Improving influenza vaccination rates among adults. *Cleve Clin J Med* 2006;73;1009–1015.

Piccirillo JF. Acute bacterial sinusitis. *N Engl J Med* 2004;351:902–910.

Samore MH, Bateman K, Alder SC, et al. Clinical decision support and appropriateness of antimicrobial prescribing: a randomized trial. *JAMA* 2005;294:2305–2314.

Sande MA, Gwaltney JM. Acute community-acquired bacterial sinusi-

tis: continuing challenges and current management. *Clin Infect Dis* 2004;39:S151–S158.

Sharp HJ, Denman D, Puumala S, et al. Treatment of acute and chronic rhinosinusitis in the United States, 1999–2002. *Arch Otolaryngol Head Neck Surg* 2007;133:260–265.

Small CB, Bachert C, Lund VJ, et al. Judicious antibiotic use and intranasal corticosteroids in acute rhinosinusitis. *Am J Med* 2007;120:289–294.

Snow V, Mottur-Pilson C, Cooper RJ, et al., for the American College of Physicians-American Society of Internal Medicine. Principles of appropriate antibiotic use for acute pharyngitis in adults. *Ann Intern Med* 2001;134:506–508.

Snow V, Mottur-Pilson C, Gonzales R, for the American College of Physicians-American Society of Internal Medicine. Principles of appropriate antibiotic use for treatment of nonspecific upper respiratory tract infections in adults. *Ann Intern Med* 2001;134:487–489.

Snow V, Mottur-Pilson C, Gonzales R. Principles of appropriate antibiotic use for treatment of acute bronchitis in adults. *Ann Intern Med* 2001;134:518–520.

Snow V, Mottur-Pilson C, Hickner JM, for the American College of Physicians-American Society of Internal Medicine. Principles of appropriate antibiotic use for acute sinusitis in adults. *Ann Intern Med* 2001;134:495–497.

Spiro DM, Tay KY, Arnold DH, et al. Wait-and-see prescription for the treatment of acute otitis media: a randomized controlled trial. *JAMA* 2006;296:1235–1241.

Tomii K, Matsumura Y, Maeda K, et al. Minimal use of antibiotics for acute respiratory tract infections: validity and patient satisfaction. *Intern Med* 2007;46:267–272.

van Balen FAM, Smit WM, Zuithoff NPA, et al. Clinical efficacy of three common treatments in acute otitis externa in primary care: randomised controlled trial. *Br Med J* 2003;327:1201–1205.

Weintrob AC, Giner J, Menezes P, et al. Infrequent diagnosis of primary human immunodeficiency virus infection: missed opportunities in acute care settings. *Arch Intern Med* 2003;163:2097–2100.

Wenzel RP, Fowler AA III. Acute bronchitis. *N Engl J Med* 2006;355:2125–2130.

Soft Tissue Infections

Botek G. Fungal nail infection: assessing the new treatment options. *Cleve Clin J Med* 2003;70:110–114.

Clark DC. Common acute hand infections. *Am Fam Physician* 2003;68:2167–2176.

Daum RS. Skin and soft-tissue infections caused by methicillin-resistant *Staphylococcus aureus*. *N Engl J Med* 2007;357:380–390.

Elewski BE. Onychomycosis: treatment, quality of life, and economic issues. *Am J Clin Dermatol* 2000;1:19–26.

Faergemann J, Baran R. Epidemiology, clinical presentation and diagnosis of onychomycosis. *Br J Dermatol* 2003;149(Suppl 65):1–4.

Falagas ME, Vergidis PI. Narrative review: diseases that masquerade as infectious cellulitis. *Ann Intern Med* 2005;142:47–55.

Henry FP, Purcell EM, Eadie PA. The human bite injury: a clinical audit and discussion regarding the management of this alcohol fuelled phenomenon. *Emerg Med J* 2007;24:455–458.

King MD, Humphrey BJ, Wang YF, et al. Emergence of community-acquired methicillin-resistant *Staphylococcus aureus* USA 300 clone as the predominant cause of skin and soft-tissue infections. *Ann Intern Med* 2006;144:309–317.

Krasagakis K, Samonis G, Maniatakis P, et al. Bullous erysipelas: clinical presentation, staphylococcal involvement and methicillin resistance. *Dermatology* 2006;212:31–35.

McNamara DR, Tleyjeh IM, Berbari EF, et al. Incidence of lower-extremity cellulitis: a population-based study in Olmsted County, Minnesota. *Mayo Clin Proc* 2007;82:817–821.

McNamara DR, Tleyjeh IM, Berbari EF, et al. A predictive model of recurrent lower extremity cellulitis in a population-based cohort. *Arch Intern Med* 2007;167:709–715.

Swartz MN. Cellulitis. *N Engl J Med* 2004;350:904–912.

Taplitz RA. Managing bite wounds: currently recommended antibiotics for treatment and prophylaxis. *Postgrad Med* 2004;116:49–52, 55–56, 59.

Chapter 18

Oncologic Emergencies

Tarek Mekhail   David J. Adelstein

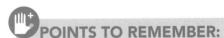

POINTS TO REMEMBER:

- Patients with superior cava obstruction usually present with complaints of neck and facial swelling, dyspnea, and cough.

- The prognosis of patients with superior vena cava syndrome depends entirely on the prognosis of their underlying disease.

- The diagnosis of spinal cord compression must be anticipated: Once neurologic dysfunction develops, it is rarely reversible.

- Bone metastases may develop in up to 50% of patients with malignancy, and 5% to 10% of patients with bone metastases develop pathological long-bone fractures.

- Malignant pleural effusions may develop in one of two ways: (a) direct deposition of tumor metastases on the pleural surface, with a resultant exudation of pleural fluid; or (b) tumor involvement of mediastinal lymph nodes, producing lymphatic obstruction and pleural fluid accumulation.

- Rapid cell death results in a number of metabolic disturbances that define the syndrome of tumor lysis syndrome, including hyperkalemia, hyperuricemia, hyperphosphatemia, and hypocalcemia (due to precipitation of calcium phosphate).

Malignancies can produce medical emergencies from both local and metastatic disease. This discussion focuses on some of the common structural problems associated with cancer, such as superior vena cava syndrome, spinal cord compression, malignant ascites, and tumor lysis syndrome.

A number of malignancy-related metabolic and endocrinologic conditions are also emergencies, including hyponatremia, hypoglycemia, acute renal failure, and ectopic hormone production. Hematologic emergencies include leukopenia and hyperleukocytosis; thrombocytopenia and thrombocytosis; and polycythemia, hyperviscosity, and disseminated intravascular coagulation. These syndromes are not addressed in this chapter.

SUPERIOR VENA CAVA SYNDROME

The superior vena cava is a thin-walled, low-pressured, vascular structure rigidly confined to the mediastinum and surrounded by lymph nodes. It is readily occluded or thrombosed by any distortion of the normal architecture. Fortunately, an extensive collateral network exists, allowing for decompression and venous return. Patients with superior cava obstruction usually present with complaints of neck and facial swelling, dyspnea, and cough. Physical examination is notable for distended jugular veins; prominent superficial venous collaterals; and edema of the face, shoulders, and arms.

The diagnosis is usually made at the bedside. Chest radiography may reveal mediastinal widening or a right hilar mass. Further delineation of the anatomical abnormality can be obtained via CT, contrast venography, or ultrasonography. The differential diagnosis should include congestive heart failure, pericardial tamponade/constriction, and pulmonary hypertension.

Although the clinical presentation of superior vena cava syndrome is often dramatic, death from superior vena cava obstruction alone is not well described. Overall, the prognosis of patients with this syndrome depends entirely on the prognosis of their underlying disease.

Symptomatic measures, such as diuretics and elevation of the head of the bed, are usually sufficient and allow time for an accurate etiologic diagnosis. The etiology of superior vena cava syndrome includes the following:

- Malignancy
- Small cell and non–small-cell lung cancer
- Lymphoma

- Thrombosis
- Fibrosis
- Substernal goiter
- Syphilitic aneurysm

Most patients with superior vena cava obstruction have malignancy. Lung cancer, particularly small cell carcinoma, is the cause in most cases. Malignant lymphoma is also commonly responsible. Many patients now develop superior vena cava syndrome as a result of the more frequent use of central venous catheters.

An accurate etiologic diagnosis is crucial, and tissue confirmation is required to verify the presence of malignancy. Despite fears to the contrary, invasive diagnostic procedures carry little additional risk in these patients. Although it was recommended in the past, radiation therapy before the histologic confirmation of malignancy is inappropriate and may confound accurate histologic diagnosis. Several cancers commonly implicated are potentially curable with appropriate treatment, thus justifying an aggressive diagnostic and therapeutic approach.

Clinical improvement occurs in most patients, although this improvement may largely result from the development of adequate collateral circulation. Anticoagulation has not been used extensively, except when thrombosis has resulted from a central venous catheter. The treatment plan should generally be based on the tumor histology and disease extent, not just on the presence of superior vena cava obstruction. Radiation therapy is most appropriate in those patients with non–small cell lung cancer or other neoplasms unresponsive to chemotherapy. Patients with small cell lung cancer or lymphoma, however, can be treated primarily with chemotherapy, with the expectation of a rapid response.

Although clinical improvement can be expected in 70% to 95% of patients, radiologic evidence of recanalization and patency of the superior vena cava at postmortem examination is much less frequent. It is the development of adequate collateral circulation that allows for this symptomatic resolution, despite continued superior vena caval obstruction.

SPINAL CORD COMPRESSION

Neoplastic epidural spinal cord compression (ESCC) is a common complication of cancer that causes pain and sometimes irreversible loss of neurologic function. In adults, the tip of the spinal cord usually lies at the L1 vertebral level; below this level, the lumbosacral nerve roots form the cauda equina, which floats in cerebrospinal fluid. Because the pathophysiology of compression of the thecal sac at the level of the cauda equina does not differ significantly from that of more rostral compression, compression of the cauda equina is still generally referred to by the slightly inaccurate name of ESCC.

Spinal cord compression resulting from malignancy usually occurs in patients with incurable disease and is responsible for serious morbidity. Indeed, treatment success is usually measured by whether a patient remains ambulatory and continent. The diagnosis of spinal cord compression must be anticipated: Once neurologic dysfunction develops, it is rarely reversible.

Most often, spinal cord compression arises from a metastasis that involves the vertebral body and extends to produce an anterior epidural cord compression. However, hematologic neoplasms such as lymphoma and myeloma may produce ESCC by direct extension from a paravertebral mass without bone involvement. The thoracic spine represents the most common site of cord compression, and the lesions are often multiple.

Etiology

The most common tumors responsible include:

- Lung cancer
- Breast cancer
- Prostate cancer
- Myeloma
- Lymphoma

The gastrointestinal tumors metastasize to bone less frequently and are therefore relatively less likely to cause this syndrome.

Pathophysiology

The pathophysiology of spinal cord compression is shown in Figure 18.1.

Clinical Picture

The symptomatic hallmark of spinal cord compression is back pain. Although a common symptom, its presence in association with known spinal metastases mandates further evaluation. The presence of a symptomatic radiculopathy or myelopathy in a patient with malignancy is also a clear indication for further evaluation. Although epidural cord compression is the most common cause of

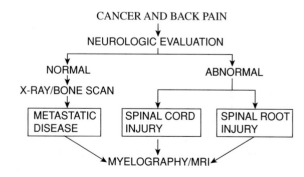

Figure 18.1 Cancer and back pain neurologic evaluation.

myelopathic symptomatology in a patient with malignancy, the following etiologies must also be considered:

- Intradural or intramedullary tumor
- Carcinomatous meningitis
- Radiation myopathy
- Paraneoplastic syndrome

Diagnostic options include

- Neurologic examination
- Plain films
- Bone scan
- Complete myelogram
- CT
- MRI with contrast required if intramedullary tumor suspected

The results of neurologic examination are often normal in these patients. If abnormal, however, the findings may be useful in localizing the level of cord disease. Either an MRI scan or complete myelography is required for diagnosis. Although most patients with spinal metastases and a radiculopathy or myelopathy will have evidence of epidural lesions, cord compression will also be found in a significant number of patients with spinal metastases and back pain alone.

Prevention

A retrospective analysis of 150 patients with metastatic prostate cancer conducted to determine whether early detection with MRI of the spine and treatment of clinically occult spinal cord compromise (SCC) facilitate preservation of neurologic function was conducted. The results suggest that prophylactic radiotherapy for patients with back pain or radiologic SCC without neurologic deficit may facilitate preservation of neurologic function. Thus, MRI surveillance for SCC may be important for some cancer patients with bone metastases.

Treatment

Once myelopathic signs have developed, the treatment of spinal cord compression is imperfect. Nonambulatory patients rarely recover the ability to ambulate. When diagnosed early, however, the preservation of neurologic function is the rule.

1. *Steroids* should be initiated, and radiation and surgical consultation should be obtained as soon as possible. Corticosteroids appear to have a short-term benefit. Guidelines for their use include:
   - Prevent secondary pathological changes
   - Dexamethasone 10 mg followed by 4 mg q6hr
   - High-dose steroids may help for quick pain control
2. *Radiation* is indicated in most patients. Radiation can shrink the tumor within days. Stereotactic radiosurgery, which has long been used in the treatment of intracranial lesions, has recently been applied to the spine and

enables the effective treatment of metastatic lesions. Although a relatively new technique, the use of stereotactic radiosurgery in the spine has advanced rapidly in the past decade. Spinal stereotactic radiosurgery is an effective and safe modality for the treatment of spinal metastatic disease. Future challenges involve the refinement of noninvasive fiducial tracking systems and the discernment of optimal doses needed to treat various lesions. In addition, dose-tolerance limits of normal structures need to be further developed. Increased experience will likely make stereotactic radiosurgery of the spine an important treatment modality for a variety of metastatic lesions.

3. *Surgery:* A randomized study that compared surgery followed by radiotherapy to radiotherapy alone in patients presenting with spinal cord compression secondary to metastatic disease indicated that direct decompressive surgery plus postoperative radiotherapy is superior to radiotherapy alone, resulting in a greater likelihood of being ambulatory at the end of treatment. Surgical decompression is especially indicated in the following situations:
   - No histologic diagnosis is available.
   - Rapid development of neurologic dysfunction occurs.
   - Progression occurs during radiation therapy.
   - Recurrence develops after completion of radiation therapy.
   - Spinal instability is present.
   - Retropulsion of a bony fragment is present.

Chemotherapy may be indicated in chemosensitive disease, particularly in children. Chemotherapy can be used in combination with radiotherapy for the treatment of spinal cord compression, or alone in adults who are not surgical or radiation candidates, but who have chemosensitive tumors, such as lymphoma, small cell carcinoma, myeloma, and germ cell tumors.

In general, the key to a successful outcome in this neurologic emergency is early diagnosis, although a patient's overall prognosis is more dependent on the natural history of the malignancy. The preservation of neurologic function is of obvious importance in this group of patients.

BONE METASTASES

Bone metastases may develop in up to 50% of patients with malignancy, and 5% to 10% of patients with bone metastases develop pathological long-bone fractures. The most frequent primary tumors metastasizing to bone are:

- Breast cancer
- Prostate cancer
- Lung cancer
- Multiple myeloma (almost invariably involves bone)
- Kidney cancer
- Malignancies of gastrointestinal origin

Marrow-containing bone, such as the vertebral bodies, pelvis, ribs, and femurs, are the most common sites of bone involvement.

Pain is the most common manifestation of bone metastases and is found in up to 75% of patients. Asymptomatic bone disease may be found during staging procedures or at another unsuspected site during an evaluation for bone pain.

Radionuclide bone scans are sensitive in the detection of bone metastases but are relatively nonspecific. However, patients with purely lytic bone disease, as in multiple myeloma, may have normal bone scans. Plain radiographs, although considerably less sensitive, are quite specific. Radiographic abnormalities have been described as purely lytic (myeloma, kidney, or thyroid), predominantly blastic (prostate), or mixed lytic and blastic (breast and lung). CT and MRI scans may be useful for specific indications, particularly in better defining disease of the spine and pelvis.

Biopsy confirmation of a bone metastasis may be required if the abnormality represents the first sign of tumor recurrence or in the presence of a single or otherwise unusual bone abnormality. Multiple bone lesions, in the setting of widely disseminated disease, do not require histologic verification.

The treatment of bone metastases is considered palliative. Treatment goals include relief of pain and preservation of function.

Surgery is usually required for the adequate repair of a pathological fracture and is often recommended for those patients with radiographic evidence of an impending fracture. The indications for prophylactic surgical intervention, particularly involving a weight-bearing bone (e.g., the femur), include a lytic bone lesion with a diameter of >2 to 3 cm or with more than 50% cortical destruction.

Radiation therapy will relieve pain in up to 90% of patients and may prevent progression of bone destruction or even allow for healing. Its value is limited, however, in patients with widespread bone involvement.

Hormonal therapy in patients with breast and prostate cancer, chemotherapy in patients with breast and prostate cancer, and chemotherapy in patients with hematologic neoplasms and other chemotherapy-sensitive diseases are often effective in achieving temporary control. Recent studies have demonstrated the efficacy of intravenous bisphosphonates in reducing skeletal complications in patients with both multiple myeloma and metastatic breast cancer to bone.

In widespread disease with multiple sites of painful bone involvement, hemibody radiation or the systemic administration of radioisotopes has been used.

MALIGNANT EFFUSIONS

Pleural Effusions

Malignant pleural effusions may develop in one of two ways: (a) direct deposition of tumor metastases on the pleural surface, with a resultant exudation of pleural fluid; or (b) tumor involvement of mediastinal lymph nodes, producing lymphatic obstruction and pleural fluid accumulation. The second mechanism has been described in some patients with lymphoma and lung cancer.

The most common diagnoses in patients with malignant pleural effusions include:

- Breast cancer
- Lung cancer
- Lymphoma
- Ovarian cancer
- Adenocarcinoma of unknown primary site

Although the effusion may be asymptomatic in up to 25% of patients, the clinical presentation includes dyspnea, cough, and chest pain.

Patients may have a pre-existing malignancy or may present with a malignant effusion as the first manifestation of disease. An accurate diagnostic confirmation and differentiation from a benign pleural effusion are of obvious prognostic and therapeutic importance.

A thoracentesis with pleural fluid cytology is often the easiest diagnostic maneuver. Biochemical analysis of the pleural fluid may be suggestive but is nonspecific. A closed pleural biopsy may add to the diagnostic yield. Thoracoscopy has recently emerged as an excellent diagnostic tool for pleural effusions. If neoplastic, appropriate treatment is often possible at the time of thoracoscopy as well. It is important to recognize the diagnostic difficulty posed by patients with mesothelioma. Cytology and needle biopsy are often nondiagnostic or confusing in such patients, and thoracoscopy, or even thoracotomy, are usually needed.

Treatment strategies include:

- Thoracentesis
- Pleural sclerosis
- Pleurectomy
- Pleuroperitoneal shunts
- Radiation therapy
- Systemic chemotherapy/hormones

Patients with malignant pleural effusions are usually incurable, and their management strategy should be palliative. Thoracentesis alone is of only temporary benefit unless effective systemic treatment is available, such as in lymphoma or breast cancer. Patients with non–small cell lung cancer will usually require chest tube drainage and pleural sclerosis if permanent control of the effusion is to be expected. The intrapleural instillation of agents such as doxycycline, talc, quinacrine, bleomycin, and various other chemotherapeutic agents has been associated with a successful outcome in 70% to 85% of patients. Those patients with continued fluid reaccumulation despite pleural sclerosis may require pleurectomy or the use of a pleuroperitoneal shunt. Radiation therapy is unfortunately of limited value, except when administered to the mediastinum in patients with extensive mediastinal lymphoma.

Malignant Pericardial Effusions

Cardiac involvement by malignancy is often an asymptomatic autopsy finding and has been reported in 10% to 15% of patients with malignancy. It is clinically important only if it results in cardiac dysfunction, the most common manifestation being pericardial tamponade. This complication is not usually the first manifestation of malignancy and has been reported most frequently in patients with the following diseases:

- Lung cancer
- Breast cancer
- Leukemia/lymphoma
- Melanoma
- Sarcoma

The etiology may reflect either direct extension from mediastinal tumor (as in lymphoma and lung cancer) or hematogenous dissemination. Despite the dramatic presentation of patients with pericardial tamponade, several of the responsible malignancies are potentially curable, even when involving the heart. As such, an aggressive approach to diagnosis and management is imperative. It is also important that malignant pericarditis be distinguished from both the acute and chronic pericarditis occurring after radiation therapy and from the cardiomyopathy that can result from anthracycline use.

The presence of clinical signs or symptoms suggestive of pericarditis or pericardial tamponade mandates urgent evaluation. Diagnostic options include echocardiography, pericardiocentesis, and pericardial biopsy. Echocardiography is usually diagnostic and can be followed rapidly by a diagnostic/therapeutic pericardiocentesis. Cytologic examination may be positive in 80% of patients with neoplastic involvement. In those patients with lymphoma, however, especially after radiation therapy, pericardial biopsy may be needed for diagnosis.

Treatment strategies include:

- Closed drainage/intrapericardial sclerosis
- Pleuropericardial window/subxiphoid pericardiotomy
- Pericardiectomy
- Radiation therapy
- Systemic chemotherapy

Multiple treatment options have been described. Closed pericardial drainage alone or drainage with intrapericardial sclerosis using doxycycline, talc, or any of several chemotherapeutic agents has proved remarkably effective and often represents the procedure of first choice. If unsuccessful, or if the diagnosis is uncertain, a surgical approach using either a pleuropericardial window or a subxiphoid pericardiotomy has been recommended. Patients with radiosensitive tumors can often be effectively treated using mediastinal radiation therapy. Systemic chemotherapy is appropriate in those patients with sensitive diseases.

MALIGNANT ASCITES

The development of ascites in any patient requires a vigorous evaluation for etiology. Ascites is considered malignant if it arises from the metastatic deposition of tumor on peritoneal surfaces with the resultant exudation of fluid. Ascites may develop in a patient with malignancy from a number of other causes, however, including:

- Hepatic failure due to tumor replacement
- Chemotherapy toxicity
- Myocardial or pericardial disease
- Vena, caval, or hepatic venous obstruction
- Infection

Obviously, the therapeutic approach depends on the etiology of the ascites.

In patients with ovarian or gastrointestinal cancer, malignant ascites may be either the presenting manifestation of the disease or an end-stage complication. In other tumors, such as breast cancer or lymphoma, malignant ascites usually reflects the progression of an established malignancy.

The diagnostic evaluation includes paracentesis with cultures and cytologic analysis. Abdominal CT scan or ultrasonography is often needed to define the presence of any hepatic abnormality. Rarely, an open peritoneal biopsy may be required.

Therapeutic options in patients with cytologically positive malignant ascites have been limited and relatively unsuccessful:

- Medical management
- Paracentesis
- Intracavitary radiocolloids
- Intraperitoneal chemotherapy
- Systemic chemotherapy
- Peritoneovenous shunts

Unlike patients with malignant pleural or pericardial effusions, palliation is difficult. Medical management, including diuresis and salt restriction, has provided only marginal benefit. Repeated paracentesis is an unsatisfactory solution; it is inconvenient for patients and results in significant protein loss and the risk of infection. The intracavitary administration of radioactive colloids has been attempted in the past with mixed results. Intracavitary sclerosing agents, such as those used for pleural effusions, make little theoretical sense and are generally not beneficial.

Some interest has arisen in the use of intraperitoneal chemotherapy, particularly in neoplasms such as ovarian cancer. However, drug penetration is limited, and in the presence of bulky, intraperitoneal tumor, this intervention has not been very successful. In patients with breast cancer, ovarian cancer, or lymphoma, systemic chemotherapy may be effective and is indicated.

For those patients with refractory ascites unresponsive to other measures, peritoneovenous shunting has been moderately effective. Generally, such patients have limited life expectancy and achieve significant palliative benefit from this procedure. Although shunt occlusion is frequent, the development of carcinomatosis or of a coagulopathy has not been common.

TUMOR LYSIS SYNDROME

Tumor lysis syndrome (TLS) is a serious complication of malignancy that can be life threatening. TLS is associated with rapid cell death that is usually triggered by chemotherapy, although it can occur spontaneously. Rapid cell death results in a number of metabolic disturbances that define the syndrome of TLS, which include:

- Hyperkalemia
- Hyperuricemia
- Hyperphosphatemia
- Hypocalcemia (due to precipitation of calcium phosphate)

These metabolic derangements can ultimately lead to acute renal failure.

Lactate dehydrogenase level is used as a marker for the degree of tumor lysis.

Etiology

The tumors most frequently associated with the TLS are the poorly differentiated lymphomas, such as Burkitt's lymphoma, and the leukemias, particularly acute lymphoblastic leukemia and, less often, acute myeloid leukemia.

Posttreatment TLS has also been described in patients with multiple myeloma, breast cancer, medulloblastoma, sarcomas, ovarian cancer, squamous cell carcinoma of the vulva, and small cell lung cancer.

Most affected patients receive combination chemotherapy, but steroids alone may be sufficient in patients with lymphoma and lymphoblastic leukemia.

Pathogenesis

Spontaneous Tumor Lysis Syndrome

Spontaneous TLS occurs prior to initiation of therapy. These patients have increased uric acid production and hyperuricosuria due to the high rate of tumor cell turnover, resulting in uric acid crystallization in renal tubules. Uric acid crystallizes in acidic urine, and urine alkalinization may be useful in decreasing the risk of uric acid nephropathy.

After Initiation of Therapy

The use of allopurinol before the onset of antitumor therapy has reduced, but not eliminated, the incidence of acute uric acid nephropathy. Acute renal failure following therapy is now more frequently associated with severe *hyperphosphatemia*. Calcium phosphate deposition in the renal parenchyma and vessels may contribute to the decline in renal function in this setting. Calcium phosphate deposition is enhanced in alkaline medium; therefore, if urine alkalinization was started prior to initiation of chemotherapy, it should be stopped with the start of chemotherapy, and hydration maintained by normal saline infusion alone.

An important distinction between spontaneous tumor lysis and that occurring after therapy is the lack of hyperphosphatemia in the spontaneous form. It has been postulated that rapidly growing neoplasms with high cell turnover rates can lead to high uric acid levels through rapid nucleoprotein turnover but that the tumor is able to reuse released phosphorus for resynthesis of new tumor cells. In contrast, the acute increase in uric acid levels associated with chemotherapy is due to cell destruction; in this setting, no new cancer cells are available to reuse the large amounts of released phosphorus.

In rare cases of TLS, acute renal failure is induced by xanthinuria because high-dose allopurinol prevents the metabolism of xanthine to uric acid.

Management

Effective management of TLS is a combination of prophylaxis, prevention, and appropriate dialytic treatment.

Prophylaxis

Prophylaxis should start at least 2 days before receiving chemotherapy or radiation for a malignancy with rapid cell turnover. Drugs of choice include:

- Allopurinol: Give orally 600 to 900 mg/day. For those unable to receive oral medications, intravenous allopurinol could be used.
- Rasburicase: Rasburicase is indicated for the initial management of plasma uric acid levels in pediatric patients with leukemia, lymphoma, and solid malignancies who are receiving chemotherapy expected to result in tumor lysis. In contrast to allopurinol, which decreases formation of new uric acid by inhibition of xanthine oxidase, rasburicase, a recombinant urate oxidase, converts existing uric acid into allantoin. Therefore, it has a more rapid effect in lowering uric acid. In a head-to-head, randomized comparison in patients receiving cytoreductive chemotherapy who were at risk of developing TLS, uric acid fell more rapidly and to a significantly lower level with rasburicase compared with allopurinol. All patients who had hyperuricemia at study entry achieved uric acid levels <8 mg/dL by 4 hours with rasburicase. Median time for the allopurinol arm to achieve uric acid level <8 mg/dL was 23.9 hours.
- Fluids: Intravenous hydration should be given to maintain a high urine output (>2.5 L/day).
- Alkalinization of urine: The role of urinary alkalinization with acetazolamide and sodium bicarbonate is less

clear. Alkalinization converts uric acid to the more soluble urate salt, thereby diminishing the tendency to uric acid precipitation. However, experimental studies suggest that hydration with saline alone is as effective as alkalinization in minimizing uric acid precipitation. Furthermore, alkalinization has the potential disadvantage of promoting calcium phosphate deposition in patients with marked hyperphosphatemia and is therefore not recommended.

Treatment

Acute Uric Acid Nephropathy Prior to Chemotherapy

Therapy after the onset of acute renal failure consists of:

- Allopurinol (if it has not already been given)
- Fluids and a loop diuretic in an attempt to wash out the obstructing uric acid crystals
- Sodium bicarbonate should not be given at this time because it is difficult to raise the urine pH in this setting
- Hemodialysis to remove the excess circulating uric acid should be used in those patients in whom a diuresis cannot be induced

The prognosis for complete recovery is excellent if treatment is initiated rapidly. Studies have shown that oliguria due to acute uric acid nephropathy responds rapidly to hemodialysis with the initiation of a diuresis as the plasma uric acid level falls to 10 mg/dL.

Acute Renal Failure Following Chemotherapy

Marked hyperphosphatemia is usually the precipitating factor in this setting. The rapid recovery of renal function in the oliguric patient requires normalization of phosphorus (and uric acid) levels. The phosphate burden in these patients can vary from 2 to 7 g/day; as a result, it is frequently necessary to perform hemodialysis at 12- to 24-hour intervals. Continuous arteriovenous hemodialysis (CAVHD) with a high dialysate flow rate and continuous venovenous hemofiltration may also be effective. Phosphorus clearance using CAVHD can reach 40 mL/minute at a dialysate flow rate of 4 L/hour. This can lead to the removal of up to 10 g/day of phosphorus without the rebound hyperphosphatemia often seen after intermittent hemodialysis.

HYPERCALCEMIA OF MALIGNANCY

Hypercalcemia is the most common life-threatening metabolic disorder in patients with cancer.

Pathophysiology

The pathophysiological characteristics of hypercalcemia in the setting of cancer are:

- Parathyroid hormone–related protein: most common
- Vitamin D_3

- Cytokines: transforming growth factor-α and -β, tumor necrosis factor, interleukin 6
- Osteolytic bone lesions

Treatment

The treatment of hypercalcemia of malignancy follows the same guidelines as hypercalcemia of other causes. Adequate intravenous hydration is mandatory to avert declining renal function and the reabsorption of calcium. Bisphosphonates play an important role in the treatment of hypercalcemia of malignancy.

REVIEW EXERCISES

QUESTIONS

1. A 55-year-old woman smoker is seen in the emergency room complaining of several days of increasing facial fullness, orthopnea, and swelling in her neck and hands. Physical examination is notable for obvious facial swelling, with conjunctival edema, jugular venous distention, and symmetric swelling of both upper extremities. Fullness is present in both supraclavicular fossae, but there is no clear lymph node enlargement, and the lungs are clear. The patient is tachycardic, but no gallop, murmur, or rub is present. No hepatomegaly, ascites, or pedal edema is present. Chest radiography reveals a right hilar mass. The patient is admitted to the hospital at midnight, and you order which of the following?

a) An emergency upper extremity venogram
b) An emergency CT scan of the chest
c) An emergency echocardiogram
d) Diuretics and elevation of the head of the bed until the morning

Answer and Discussion

The answer is d. The clinical diagnosis of superior vena cava syndrome is clear. Although the presentation is dramatic, it is not life threatening, and the initial management is symptomatic. Emergency diagnostic procedures are rarely indicated.

2. The next morning, the patient feels better, although she remains quite edematous and cannot lie flat. You order the following test to determine the etiology of the patient's superior vena cava syndrome:

a) CT scan of the chest
b) Thyroid scan
c) Serologic test for syphilis
d) Upper extremity venogram
e) All of the above

Answer and Discussion

The answer is a. Malignancy is the most common cause of superior vena cava syndrome and is suggested by this patient's chest radiograph. Further anatomical definition of the process with a CT scan is in order.

3. You are called by the radiologist that afternoon with the results of the chest CT scan. This study reveals a large right hilar and mediastinal mass, with evidence of compression of the superior vena cava. Your response is which of the following?
a) Expeditiously proceed to bronchoscope or mediastinoscopy to establish the tissue diagnosis.
b) Recognize the risk of invasive diagnostic procedures in patients with superior vena cava syndrome and order sputum cytology.
c) Identify this as an incurable malignancy and refer the patient for urgent radiation therapy.
d) Identify this as an incurable malignancy and refer the patient for hospice care.

Answer and Discussion
The answer is a. Invasive diagnostic procedures do not pose any increased risk in patients with superior vena cava syndrome. Although the etiology is likely to be malignant, several of the potential malignant diagnoses are curable with appropriate treatment, and this treatment may include chemotherapy. Aggressive and expeditious attempts to establish a histologic diagnosis are indicated so that the most effective treatment can be initiated in an organized fashion.

4. The patient proves to have squamous cell carcinoma of the lung and receives a course of mediastinal radiation therapy. The patient does quite well, noting rapid improvement in both the symptoms and signs of her superior vena cava obstruction. A staging workup subsequently demonstrates evidence of asymptomatic bone metastases in rib, femur, and multiple vertebral bodies. Because the patient is feeling well, she declines any discussion of chemotherapy and is followed in your office. Four months later, the patient calls you with the complaint of a 2-week history of increasing midback pain. The patient is fully ambulatory, but the pain is causing difficulty sleeping. The patient specifically denies any weakness in the lower extremities, radicular pain, or incontinence. You would do which of the following?
a) Suggest a course of acetaminophen with codeine.
b) Order an elective bone scan.
c) Refer the patient for radiation therapy to the spine.
d) Order an MRI of the entire spine.

Answer and Discussion
The answer is d. Spinal metastases have already been demonstrated in this patient. The new development of pain suggests the possibility of spinal cord compression and mandates the performance of a whole-spine MRI.

5. Your patient has heard about MRI scans and does not

want one. Angry that you suggested it, the patient cancels her appointment and begins to take her husband's analgesics. Three days later, you call the patient and are told by her husband that she has fallen several times and is now having difficulty walking. You insist that the patient come to the hospital and obtain an emergent MRI scan, which she then does. The MRI reveals extensive midthoracic vertebral body replacement by tumor, with evidence of spinal cord compression. By the time the patient gets to the hospital, she is unable to walk and has had a single episode of urinary incontinence. You begin high-dose corticosteroids, hospitalize the patient, and recommend which of the following?
a) Immediate neurosurgical intervention.
b) Intravenous morphine and hospice referral.
c) Immediate radiation therapy.

Answer and Discussion
The answer is a or c. Both surgery and radiation may be used in this situation. Surgery is particularly indicated in patients in whom the neurologic weakness develops more acutely (within hours), when histologic diagnosis is not established, when there is a failure of radiation, or when compression occurs secondary to retropulsion of a bone fragment.

6. The patient is treated with radiation therapy and, somewhat to your surprise, makes a significant recovery. The patient regains almost full leg strength and can ambulate with minimal assistance. Physical therapy has been started, but new discomfort is noted in the patient's right hip during treatment. You order plain films that reveal a large lytic lesion of the right hip with cortical involvement but no fracture. In consideration of the patient's deteriorating medical condition, limited ambulatory ability, and life expectancy, you recommend which of the following?
a) Pain medication with continued physical therapy and partial weight bearing
b) Pain medication, physical therapy with partial weight bearing, and radiation therapy to the affected hip
c) Surgical stabilization of the right hip with pain medication and subsequent physical therapy

Answer and Discussion
The answer is b or c. Specific treatment of painful bone disease is almost always indicated. Decisions about the best specific treatment (i.e., radiation therapy or surgery) must consider all facets of the patient's medical condition and disease extent.

7. Your patient elects to not have surgery but undergoes the radiation and physical therapy with some success. The patient has limited ambulation but is managing at home with a walker. Over the next 6 weeks, the patient gradually improves but then returns to see you in the office, concerned about increasing exertional dyspnea.

On examination, the patient is afebrile, has a resting tachycardia, but has no facial swelling and no jugular venous distention. No pleural or pericardial rub is present, although diminished breath sounds are noted at the right base. Neither hepatomegaly, ascites, nor pedal edema is identified. The hemoglobin is 11.2 g/dL, and chest radiography reveals a new, large, right pleural effusion. The most likely diagnosis is which of the following?

a) Malignant pleural effusion
b) Radiation-induced pleuritis
c) Congestive heart failure
d) Radiation-induced pericardial constriction
e) Pulmonary embolus with infarction

Answer and Discussion

The answer is a. Although all answers are in the differential diagnosis, the absence of a pleural or pericardial rub makes a malignant pleural effusion most likely.

8. In the office, you perform a 1-L thoracentesis for slightly bloody fluid, which on analysis proves exudative. Cultures are negative, and cytologies are not diagnostic. The patient feels immediately better after the thoracentesis but returns to the office 3 days later with increasing dyspnea and recurrence of this effusion. Your next step is which of the following?

a) Repeat the thoracentesis with cytology.
b) Repeat the thoracentesis with cytology and perform a closed pleural biopsy.
c) Refer the patient for thoracoscopy.
d) Refer the patient for chest tube drainage and pleural sclerosis.

Answer and Discussion

The answer is d. In a patient this sick, it may be most prudent to forego further aggressive attempts to confirm the likely diagnosis of a malignant pleural effusion and to proceed directly to appropriate management.

9. In patients with spinal cord compression, which of the following is the best predictor of posttreatment neurologic function?

a) Level of cord compression
b) Degree of cord compression on MRI scans
c) Duration of neurologic symptoms prior to treatment
d) Pretreatment neurologic function

Answer and Discussion

The answer is d. Pretreatment neurologic function is the best predictor of posttreatment function, hence the importance of early diagnosis and management.

10. Tumor lysis syndrome is associated with all the following, *except*

a) Hypercalcemia
b) Hyperkalemia
c) Hyperphosphatemia
d) Hyperuricemia

Answer and Discussion

The answer is a. Tumor lysis syndrome is associated with decreased serum calcium.

SUGGESTED READINGS

Adelstein DJ. Managing three common oncologic emergencies. *Cleve Clin J Med* 1991;58:457–458.

Adelstein DJ, Hines JD, Carter SG, et al. Thromboembolic events in patients with malignant superior vena cava syndrome and the role of anticoagulation. *Cancer* 1988;62:2258–2262.

Aelony Y, King R, Boutin C. Thoracoscopic talc poudrage pleurodesis for chronic recurrent pleural effusions. *Ann Intern Med* 1991;115:778–782.

Ahmann FR. A reassessment of the clinical implications of the superior vena cava syndrome. *J Clin Oncol* 1984;2:961–969.

Alcan KE, Zabetakis PM, Marino ND, et al. Management of acute cardiac tamponade by subxiphoid pericardiotomy. *JAMA* 1982;247:1143–1148.

Berenson JR, Lipton A. Use of bisphosphonates in patients with metastatic bone disease. *Oncology* 1988;12:1573–1579.

Byrne TN. Spinal cord compression from epidural metastases. *N Engl J Med* 1992;327:614–619.

Coleman RE. Skeletal complications of malignancy. *Cancer* 1997; 80(Suppl):1588–1594.

Daw HA, Markman M. Epidural spinal cord compression in cancer patients: diagnosis and management. *Cleve Clin J Med* 2000;67: 497–504.

Gilbert RW, Kim JH, Posner JB. Epidural spinal cord compression from metastatic tumor: diagnosis and treatment. *Ann Neurol* 1978;3: 40–51.

Glover DJ, Glick JH. Managing oncologic emergencies involving structural dysfunction. *CA Cancer J Clin* 1985;35:238–251.

Goldman SC, Holcenberg JS, Finklestein J, et al. A randomized comparison between rasburicase and allopurinol in children with lymphoma or leukemia at high risk for tumor lysis. *Blood* 2001;97:2998–3003.

Gough IR, Balderson GA. Malignant ascites: a comparison of peritoneovenous shunting and nonoperative management. *Cancer* 1993;71:2377–2382.

Hausheer FH, Yarbro JW. Diagnosis and treatment of malignant pleural effusion. *Semin Oncol* 1985;12:54–75.

Helms SR, Carlson MD. Cardiovascular emergencies. *Semin Oncol* 1989;16:463–470.

Hillner BE, Ingle JN, Berenson JR, et al. American Society of Clinical Oncology guideline on the role of bisphosphonates in breast cancer. *J Clin Oncol* 2000;18:1378–1391.

Lacy JH, Wieman TJ, Shively EH. Management of malignant ascites. *Surg Gynecol Obstet* 1984;159:397–412.

Loblaw DA, Laperriere NJ. Emergency treatment of malignant extradural spinal cord compression: an evidence-based guideline. *J Clin Oncol* 1998;16:1613–1624.

Maranzano, Latini P, Checcaglini F, et al. Radiation therapy in metastatic spinal cord compression. *Cancer* 1991;67:1311–1317.

Markman M. Common complications and emergencies associated with cancer and its therapy. *Cleve Clin J Med* 1994;61:105–114.

Nielson OS, Munro AJ, Tannock IF. Bone metastases: pathophysiology and management policy. *J Clin Oncol* 1991;9:509–524.

Okamoto H, Shinkai T, Tamakido M, et al. Cardiac tamponade caused by primary lung cancer and the management of pericardial effusion. *Cancer* 1993;71:93–98.

Patchell PA, Tibbs PA, Regine WF, et al. Direct decompressive surgical treatment of spinal cord compression caused by metastatic cancer: a randomized trial. *Lancet* 2005;366(9486):6438.

Posner MR, Cohen GI, Skarin AT. Pericardial disease in patients with cancer: the differentiation of malignant from idiopathic and radiation-induced pericarditis. *Am J Med* 1981;71:407–413.

Press OW, Livingston R. Management of malignant pericardial effusion and tamponade. *JAMA* 1987;257:1088–1092.

Rodichok LD, Harper GR, Ruckdeschel JC, et al. Early diagnosis of spinal epidural metastases. *Am J Med* 1981;70:1181–1188.

Ruckdeschel JC, Moores D, Lee JY, et al. Intrapleural therapy for malignant pleural effusions: a randomized comparison of bleomycin and tetracycline. *Chest* 1991;100:1528–1535.

Sahn MA. Malignant pleural effusions. *Clin Chest Med* 1985;6:113–125.

Schiff D, O'Neill BP, Wang CH, et al. Neuroimaging and treatment implications of patients with multiple epidural spinal metastases. *Cancer* 1998;83:1593–1601.

Schraufnagel DE, Hill R, Leech JA, et al. Superior vena caval obstruction—is it a medical emergency? *Am J Med* 1981;70:1169–1174.

Spiess JL, Adelstein DJ, Hines JD. Multiple myeloma presenting with spinal cord compression. *Oncology* 1988;45:88–92.

Tong D, Gillick L, Hendrickson FR. The palliation of symptomatic osseous metastasis: final results of the study by the Radiation Therapy Oncology Group. *Cancer* 1982;50:893–899.

Tsang TSM, Seward JB, Barnes ME, et al. Outcomes of primary and secondary treatment of pericardial effusion in patients with malignancy. *Mayo Clin Proc* 2000;75:248–253.

Venkitaraman R, Barbachano Y, Deanrnaley DP, et al. Outcome of early detection and radiotherapy for occult spinal cord compression. *Radiother Oncol* 2007;85(3):469–472.

Weissman DE. Glucocorticoid treatment for brain metastases and epidural spinal cord compression: a review. *J Clin Oncol* 1988;6:543–551.

Willson JKV, Masaryk TJ. Neurologic emergencies in the cancer patient. *Semin Oncol* 1989;16:490–503.

Chapter 19

Gynecologic, Prostate, and Testicular Cancers

Chad Michener   *Jorge Garcia*

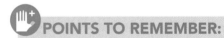 **POINTS TO REMEMBER:**

- Human papillomavirus testing in addition to the Papanicolaou smear is now recommended for screening of cervical cancer in women older than 30 years.

- Uterine cancer is the most common gynecologic cancer, causing approximately 6% of all malignancies and accounting for 3% of all cancer deaths in women.

- Most women with endometrial cancer are diagnosed at an early stage and are often cured by surgery with or without radiation therapy.

- Recently, intraperitoneal chemotherapy with cisplatin and paclitaxel was shown to improve overall survival by 16 months when compared to intravenous administration in women with optimally debulked ovarian cancer.

- To date, most patients with newly diagnosed prostate cancer present with organ-confined disease as a result of a positive screening test.

- To date, there is no randomized prospective evidence to suggest that one modality of local definitive treatment for localized prostate cancer is superior to the other one (i.e., surgery vs. radiation).

- Although chemotherapy confers a high cure rate for testicular cancer (more than 80% for good and intermediate-risk patients), patients live long enough to experience late toxicities.

GYNECOLOGIC CANCERS

Cervical Cancer

Cervical cancer is one of the few cancers in history where a successful screening test has been implemented to save countless lives. Since the introduction of the Papanicolaou (Pap) smear more than 50 years ago, the incidence of invasive cervical cancer in the United States has declined from more than 30 cases per 100,000 women per year to approximately 9 cases per 100,000 women per year.

One of the major reasons that screening is beneficial is that the change from normal cervical epithelium to invasive cancer generally follows a stepwise progression from mild to severe dysplasia and eventually to invasive cancer if left untreated. Pap screening allows clinicians to identify women with abnormal cytology that need additional evaluation with diagnostic colposcopy and biopsies. Histologic confirmation of dysplasia allows clinicians to intervene before the lesion progresses to invasive cancer. Therefore, the decrease in invasive cervical cancer has led to a concomitant increase in the number of cases of cervical dysplasia. Several etiologic factors are associated with carcinoma of the cervix, including early initial sexual activity, multiple sexual partners, and prior venereal infections. Experimental and epidemiologic data have provided strong evidence that infection with the human papillomavirus (HPV), particularly subtypes 16 and 18, is important in the pathogenesis of this malignancy. More recently, it has been shown that individuals with AIDS or other immunocompromised states have a high risk for the development of carcinoma of the cervix.

The strong association between HPV infection and cervical dysplasia and cervical cancer has led to a new paradigm in the way we perform cervical cancer screening. HPV testing in addition to the Pap smear is now recommended for screening of women older than 30 years. Several studies have demonstrated the excellent negative predictive value of HPV testing. In fact, a negative HPV test combined with a negative Pap smear has a negative predictive value of nearly 100% for severe dysplasia and cervical carcinoma. We now have a more complete understanding of the well-defined pathways leading to development of cervix cancer, from dysplasia to carcinoma in situ (cytologic features of neoplasia, but without an invasion through the basement membrane) to invasive carcinoma. This progression from mild to severe changes is the reason that Pap smear screening works well using an annual screening test. Although the traditional Pap smear has only 70% sensitivity for detecting early intraepithelial neoplastic changes, slow progression and repetitive smears have allowed us to catch most significant lesions. Liquid-based cytology has higher sensitivity with similar specificity. However, false-negative smear results can be observed in the presence of inflammation, necrosis, or hemorrhage, so all areas observed to be abnormal on visual inspection must be examined via biopsy, regardless of the Pap smear findings.

Standard treatment of carcinoma in situ of the cervix is surgery (usually total abdominal hysterectomy). Young women wanting to have children may be treated with cervical conization and extremely careful follow-up provided the margins of the cone specimen are negative. Invasive cervical carcinoma is typically treated with surgery, chemoradiation, or a combination of the two modalities. Historically, chemotherapy was used mainly in patients with far advanced and recurrent disease. Although responses are observed and may modestly influence survival, they are generally of short duration (<4–6 months). Of far greater impact are results reported from several randomized trials, which have demonstrated that the use of cisplatin-based chemotherapy in combination with external beam radiation therapy followed by intracavitary brachytherapy significantly improves overall survival in women with locally advanced cervix cancer.

Overall prognosis is based mainly on stage at diagnosis and is the only gynecologic cancer where staging remains clinical rather than surgical. The importance of finding cancerous changes as soon as possible in the natural history of this disease is highlighted by the fact that the long-term survival for individuals who are diagnosed as having carcinoma in situ is more than 98% to 99% compared to approximately 65% survival in patients with locally advanced disease. Although the addition of chemotherapy to radiation has improved survival, the best option for survival is prevention and early detection. The U.S. Food and Drug Administration recently approved an HPV vaccine for the prevention of HPV-6, -11, -16, and -18. HPV-16 and -18 are responsible for nearly 70% of all cervical cancers in the United States, and vaccination against these four subtypes may offer cross-protection against other related subtypes. Current recommendations are to vaccinate all females between the ages of 9 and 26 years.

Endometrial Cancer

Uterine cancer is the most common gynecologic cancer, causing approximately 6% of all malignancies and accounting for 3% of all cancer deaths in women. The incidence of the disease is approximately three times higher than that of cervix cancer. Suggested risk factors include:

- Age
- Late menopause and early menarche
- Obesity
- Diabetes
- Hypertension

Unopposed estrogen from any source has the potential to cause endometrial cancer. In fact, unopposed exogenous estrogen use has been shown to increase the incidence of endometrial cancer. In contrast, the risk of the disease appears to be decreased by the administration of progesterone. Thus, the use of combination estrogen and progesterone may decrease the risk of endometrial cancer in women receiving this regimen.

The Pap smear identifies approximately 15% to 20% of women with endometrial carcinoma but *is not* a screening test for endometrial cancer. In most patients, the diagnosis is made through a more extensive evaluation of evacuated tissue after a fractional dilatation and curettage, or direct biopsy. The most common presentations in women with endometrial cancer are:

- Bleeding abnormalities (90%)
- Abnormal discharge
- Pyometra (fever, pain, discharge)
- Pelvic mass

Concern has been raised regarding the risk of endometrial cancer in individuals receiving tamoxifen, either as a treatment for breast cancer or as a preventive strategy for this malignancy. Women taking tamoxifen who experience any abnormal vaginal bleeding should undergo a careful gynecologic evaluation. Currently, no evidence suggests that a more rigorous screening program is required in this clinical setting. In addition, prophylactic hysterectomy is not recommended for women receiving tamoxifen.

One additional risk factor for endometrial carcinoma is family history. Patients with strong family history of colon and uterine cancer should be considered potential carriers of gene mutations in the hereditary nonpolyposis colorectal cancer syndrome. Women from these families carry a 40% risk of endometrial and 10% risk of ovarian cancer during their lifetime. Patients believed to be at risk should be referred for genetic counseling and can be followed with surveillance or undergo prophylactic surgery.

Endometrial cancer is staged surgically and includes hysterectomy, bilateral salpingo-oophorectomy, and evaluation of the pelvic and para-aortic lymph nodes. Fortunately, most women with endometrial cancer are diagnosed at an early stage and are often cured by surgery with or without radiation therapy. Patients with high-risk histologic subtypes, such as papillary serous or clear cell carcinomas, and those with metastatic disease may be treated with adjuvant chemotherapy, radiation, or both. Recurrent endometrial carcinoma may be treated with chemotherapy or may be responsive to hormonal therapy using a progestational agent alone or alternating cycles of progestational agents and tamoxifen. Estrogen and progesterone receptor status is predictive of response to hormonal therapy.

Ovarian Cancer

Although ovarian cancer is less common than either cancer of the cervix or uterus, it causes more deaths each year in the United States than both of these other gynecologic malignancies combined. Unfortunately, no effective screening test for detecting early stage disease exists, so less than 10%

to 20% of patients are diagnosed with localized disease. Intensive research efforts have been undertaken at a number of centers to find a reliable screening test for ovarian cancer. These have focused on vaginal ultrasonography, circulating tumor markers (e.g., CA-125), and combination testing using imaging and circulating tumor markers. Unfortunately, this has not led to an increase in the percentage diagnosed at an early stage. Therefore, screening may be used in patients who have an increased risk for the development of ovarian cancer (i.e., strong family history), but it cannot be recommended for use in the general population.

Although many etiologic factors have been proposed for the development of ovarian cancer (including disordered endocrine function), none has been strongly associated with the disease. It has been noted that approximately 5% to 10% of all women with ovarian cancer have a family history of the malignancy, suggesting the importance of genetic factors. Two genetic abnormalities, *BRCA-1* and *BRCA-2*, have been demonstrated to be responsible for the large majority of cases of hereditary ovarian cancer. Mutations in *BRCA-1* carry up to a 50% risk of ovarian cancer by age 70 years, whereas a mutation in *BRCA-2* carries up to 25% risk. In addition, these women have a more than 70% risk of breast cancer in their lifetime. Several studies have shown a significant reduction (nearly 95%) in ovarian cancers in women who undergo prophylactic bilateral salpingo-oophorectomy (PBSO). These women also have up to 50% reduction in breast cancer risk if the PBSO is performed at a premenopausal age. To date, there is no association of the far less common ovarian germ cell, sex cord stromal, or borderline tumors with mutations in the *BRCA* genes. Fortunately, these tumors carry a more favorable prognosis than their invasive epithelial ovarian cancer counterparts because many are diagnosed at an early stage.

Typical symptoms for ovarian cancer are related to the gastrointestinal and urinary tracts because ovarian cancer tends to remain largely confined to the peritoneal cavity for most of its natural history. These symptoms may include bloating, abdominal swelling, early satiety, abdominal pain, and urinary urgency or frequency. Unfortunately, these are nonspecific complaints and are often signs of advanced stage disease; however, they should be considered in the differential in women with these complaints.

Initial therapy for ovarian cancer is surgical in most cases. Several large retrospective analyses have shown a survival advantage for women who have their tumor cytoreduced to <1 cm in greatest dimension (optimally debulked) prior to initiation of chemotherapy. Therefore, patients should have the opportunity for surgical consultation prior to initiation of any chemotherapy.

In the unusual situation in which ovarian cancer is found to be confined to one ovary (stage 1), complete surgical staging without adjuvant chemotherapy can be a reasonable treatment option. However, unstaged patients who undergo salpingo-oophorectomy have more than a 30% risk of being upstaged once they undergo thorough surgical staging. Long-term survival in stage 1 ovarian cancer is more than 80% to 90%.

Several well-designed, randomized, controlled trials have revealed that the combination of a platinum agent (carboplatin or cisplatin) plus a taxane (paclitaxel or docetaxel) results in superior objective response rates, progression free survival, and overall survival, compared with nonplatinum, nontaxane regimens previously employed in the management of advanced epithelial ovarian cancer. Approximately 70% to 80% of patients experience objective and subjective evidence of a response to chemotherapy, and more than 50% are found to have no clinical evidence of disease at the completion of therapy. Unfortunately, the disease ultimately recurs in most of these individuals.

Recently, intraperitoneal chemotherapy with cisplatin and paclitaxel was shown to improve overall survival by 16 months when compared to intravenous administration in women with optimally debulked ovarian cancer. This clinical benefit comes at the cost of higher toxicity and lower quality of life scores during therapy and in the first 6 months after completion of therapy. Despite the controversy surrounding this study, consideration should be given to this regimen until we have clinical data supporting equivalence of other regimens.

In women with persistent or recurrent ovarian cancer after initial chemotherapy, second-line chemotherapy regimens can be used. Various regimens are available to clinicians, but a trial of platinum should be considered as the initial second-line agent in women who are believed to be platinum sensitive (more than 12 months and possibly 6 months out from completion of first-line therapy). In view of the extended survival (often in excess of 5 years) for many patients, even with documented progression following primary therapy, it is appropriate to consider ovarian cancer a "chronic disease process," where *cure* is not the ultimate anticipated outcome, but where *prolonged survival of good or excellent quality* is a highly realistic goal of disease management.

MALE GENITOURINARY CANCERS

Prostate Cancer

Prostate cancer is the second leading cause of death in men in the United States. It is expected that more than 186,320 new cases will be diagnosed in 2008. With the widespread availability of serum prostate-specific antigen (PSA) testing, the incidence of prostate cancer detection has increased. Adjusting for age, the lifetime risk for developing prostate cancer in men ages 40 to 59 years is 1 in 6, whereas men ages 60 to 79 years will have a 1 in 7 chance of being diagnosed with this malignancy.

Subclinical prostate cancer is even more common than clinical disease, with 15% to 45% of autopsies in men without any known history of cancer during their life demon-

strating the malignancy. This observation raises the important question of the clinical relevance of finding asymptomatic prostate cancer on screening tests in men with a life expectancy of less than 10 years. Overall, prostate cancer is a slowly growing malignancy. Thus, simply finding microscopic cancer in an elderly individual should not necessarily be an indication to treat. The diagnosis of prostate cancer is most often suspected after finding an elevated serum PSA. Less commonly, a diagnostic evaluation is instituted due to abnormal findings on digital rectal examination (DRE). However, the gold standard for prostate cancer diagnosis is a transrectal ultrasound with prostate biopsies. Although the number of biopsies required for an accurate diagnosis remains a controversial topic, a standard 10- to 12-core biopsy scheme has been suggested by some as the best schema to optimize cancer detection.

To date, most patients with newly diagnosed prostate cancer present with organ-confined disease as a result of a positive screening test. When symptomatic, prostate cancer can cause urinary urgency, nocturia, frequency, and hesitancy; these symptoms are also present in men with benign prostatic hypertrophy (BPH) and are more likely to be caused by BPH than cancer. The routes of spread once cancer has gone beyond the prostate are first to the pelvic and retroperitoneal lymph nodes, and then to the bone and bone marrow. Other uncommon sites of involvement include visceral organs such as lung and liver.

The following are risk factors for prostate cancer:

- Age older than 50 years
- African American race
- Family history
- Twofold risk with one first-degree relative diagnosed with prostate cancer
- Ninefold risk with two first-degree relatives diagnosed with prostate cancer

Among the factors not proven to confer an increased risk are dietary fat and history of vasectomy.

Notwithstanding its near ubiquitous application in the United States, the utility of PSA screening remains highly controversial. Screening for prostate cancer involves the same goals as screening for any other disease: the detection of early disease in a patient who would suffer from or die of the disease and in whom treatment of early disease prevents mortality and morbidity. To date, there is no prospective randomized trial evidence demonstrating that screening improves prostate cancer–specific or overall survival. Proponents most frequently extrapolate benefit from observational studies that have used different statistical designs to evaluate a heterogeneous population of patients at risk for developing prostate cancer. Another important point to make is that the true sensitivity and specificity of PSA screening remains unknown given that the gold standard (i.e., careful pathological evaluation of the entire prostate) is not feasible. Attempts to improve the utility of PSA screening by use of PSA kinetics have become a focus of contemporary studies. Among the strategies tested, PSA velocity (change over time) is used by many practicing urologists because it appears to be more specific than a single PSA value cut-off of 4 ng/mL, and when measured years before prostate cancer diagnosis, it also appears to predict survival. Unfortunately, one of its limitations is that after adjusting for PSA level, PSA velocity cannot independently predict prostate cancer.

Despite these controversial issues, most medical organizations in the United States recommend starting PSA screening at age 40 years for high-risk patients, such as African Americans and patients with a family history (first-degree relatives) of prostate cancer. For other patients, screening is recommended to start at age 50 years. In contrast, however, elderly men and those with significant comorbid illnesses with limited life expectancy should rarely, if ever, undergo screening.

The recommended screening technique requires both serum PSA (it is important to draw the PSA *before* performing a DRE) and DRE.

It is also important to remember other reasons why PSA values can be elevated in men older than 40 years:

- BPH
- Infection, specifically prostatitis
- Any inflammation or irritation of the prostate cancer (e.g., immediately following a DRE or a needle biopsy of the prostate)

The following represent indications for performing a prostate biopsy:

- Abnormal DRE: Induration of the prostate, either unilaterally or bilaterally, or the finding of a nodule. An abnormal DRE regardless of the PSA requires a biopsy.
- Elevated PSA velocity: The PSA velocity is the rate of rise of the PSA. Any increase in PSA of >0.75 ng/mL/year has a more than 90% specificity for the detection of prostate cancer, and such patients should be biopsied.
- Elevated free-to-total PSA ratio: The free-to-total PSA can help distinguish BPH from cancer. Men with BPH have a higher fraction of free or unbound PSA. Those with prostate cancer have more PSA bound to α-1 antichymotrypsin. A free-to-total PSA <0.15 warrants a prostate biopsy.

To date, the role of CT scan, bone scan, positron emission tomography (PET) scan, or a prostate-specific membrane antigen radioimmunoscintigraphy scan in early diagnosis of prostate cancer remains unknown.

Summary on Screening

Existing data fail to support the widespread application of PSA-based prostate cancer screening. In those subsets of men at very high risk of developing aggressive tumors (significant family history and African American race), screening may be prudent. In contrast, however, elderly men and

those with significant comorbid illnesses with limited life expectancy should rarely if ever undergo screening. While we wait for the final results from the American PLCRO Trial and the European Randomized Study of Screening for Prostate Cancer, PSA screening should be considered a risk–benefit procedure that should be discussed with patients, not administered as an accepted, data-driven practice.

Clinical Findings and Treatment of Prostate Cancer

The most common presenting symptom of prostate cancer is the absence of any symptoms because most men are detected after screening. Patients with symptoms often present with obstructive voiding symptoms (nocturnal frequency, a slow urinary stream, hesitancy, dribbling, and frequent urinary tract infections). Additional symptoms include:

- Hematospermia or decreased ejaculatory volume due to seminal vesicle involvement
- Impotence due to neurovascular bundle invasion
- Pedal edema or lymphedema due to lymph node metastases
- Bone pain due to bone metastases
- Constitutional symptoms, including malaise, anorexia, and weight loss

The physical examination for patients with prostate cancer includes abnormalities on the DRE, such as induration, nodules, and extension of disease to the seminal vesicles superiorly or to the pelvic sidewall laterally. It is important to remember that the DRE is commonly normal. Bony tenderness may occur in the vertebral column or the pelvic bones.

Treatment modalities for localized prostate cancer include:

- Radical prostatectomy
- Radiation therapy
- Brachytherapy (interstitial implantation of radioactive seeds)
- Radiation plus hormone therapy for patients with locally advanced disease (i.e., those with prostate cancer beyond the prostate that has not spread to lymph nodes or bone)

To date, there is no randomized prospective evidence to suggest that one modality of local definitive treatment is superior to the other one (i.e., surgery vs. radiation). For patients with advanced (systemic) prostate cancer, the mainstay of therapy is the suppression of testosterone production. There is no difference between "medical" (using luteinizing hormone-releasing hormone [LHRH] agonist agents) and surgical castration (bilateral orchiectomy) with regard to efficacy, clinical outcome, or side effects. Other therapies commonly used in this cohort of patients are the antiandrogens, agents capable of inhibiting the binding of the active metabolite of testosterone (DHT) to the androgen receptor (ER) within the nucleus of the prostate cancer cell.

The most commonly used LHRH agonists are goserelin and leuprolide. Similarly, (bicalutamide, flutamide, and nilutamide) are the most common nonsteroidal antiandrogens used in the United States. Despite its benefits, androgen deprivation has a number of side effects that can significantly impact a patient's quality of life. These side effects include:

- Hot flashes
- Gynecomastia
- Impotence
- Anemia
- Osteoporosis

Osteoporosis, in particular, is a side effect of long-term hormone therapy for which screening is appropriate, especially for those men who have additional risk factors for osteoporosis.

Another important side effect of androgen deprivation relates to its ability to significantly increase the risk for developing diabetes, coronary artery disease, and even sudden cardiac death. Treatment for patients with castrate-resistant prostate cancer has also evolved significantly in the past several years. Treatment options for patients with advanced disease, once believed to be a futile endeavor, have changed significantly with the understanding that new interventions, including secondary hormonal manipulations, chemotherapy, and a variety of new investigational approaches have clear anticancer effects. Systemic palliative chemotherapy has become standard for patients with metastatic castrate-resistant prostate cancer. Patients for whom chemotherapy is appropriate are men with a good performance status who have progressive symptomatic disease despite the use of hormonal therapy. Large randomized trials have established docetaxel as the main chemotherapy agent for this patient population.

Testicular Cancer

Testicular cancer, or germ cell tumors (GCTs), account for 1% of all male malignancies, and it is estimated that 8,090 new cases will be diagnosed in the United States in the year 2008. Despite its overall curability, approximately 380 men in the United States are expected to die this year as a consequence of GCTs. Although GCT is an uncommon malignancy, it is the most common malignancy among men ages 15 to 35 years. The classification of testicular cancer includes seminoma and nonseminoma. The latter includes embryonal, choriocarcinoma, teratoma, and mixed tumors. Seminoma accounts for 40% of all GCTs, while non–seminoma germ cell tumors (NSGCTs) account for 60%.

Testicular cancer differs from almost all other cancers in several aspects. First, testicular cancer is a cancer for which serum tumor markers (α-fetoprotein, β-human chorionic gonadotropin [HCG], and lactate dehydrogenase [LDH]) are uniquely helpful. For example, an elevated α-fetoprotein defines a testicular cancer as a non-seminoma—that is, this marker predicts histologic subtype. In addition, the rate of decline of markers during treatment has prognostic predictive value. Second, testicular cancer is routinely curable even when metastatic. Third, patients with residual or growing masses after chemotherapy, usually teratomas, can be cured with surgical resection.

Although risk factors for the development of this disease are largely unknown, the risk of developing GCT is greater in the following settings:

- Cryptorchidism; confers a 20- to 40-fold risk.
- Disgenetic gonads; for example, Klinefelter's syndrome (47-XXY) is associated with mediastinal GCTs.
- Prior contralateral testis cancer; confers a 500-fold risk of second testis cancer 3 to 5 years following the primary case.
- The contribution of orchitis, testicular trauma, or irradiation to the genesis of GCT is unknown, but it has been postulated that the final pathway common to these associations is testicular atrophy with increased follicle-stimulating hormone drive. There is growing support for the concept of transplacental damage to the fetal gonad by maternal estrogen levels as a contributing causative agent of germ cell cancer.
- Extragonadal GCTs appear to arise as a consequence of the malignant transformation of residual midline germinal elements, usually in the mediastinum or retroperitoneum, but occasionally in other locations such as the sacrococcygeal region and the pineal gland. Whether these residual germinal elements are a consequence of abnormal germ cell migration is not known, and other factors that may contribute to the development of extragonadal GCT have not been identified.

For testicular cancer, no specific screening algorithm has been recommended by large public health groups. Conversely, men ages 15 years and older should perform a testicular self-examination on a yearly basis. This recommendation, however, has not been tested in formal clinical trials.

The most common presentation of testicular cancer is testicular swelling (>70%). A commonly held misconception is that testicular cancers are painless and that painful testicular masses need not be evaluated for malignancy. In fact, testicular pain is a presenting feature of 18% to 46% of patients with GCT. A patient who presents with this symptom should undergo a testicular ultrasound to help differentiate a solid mass from a hydrocele or possibly a hernia. Acute pain may be associated with torsion of the neoplasm and infarction or bleeding in the tumor. Signs and symptoms indistinguishable from acute epididymitis have been observed in up to one-fourth of patients with testicular neoplasms. Approximately 25% of patients with advanced disease can have symptoms referable to their metastases. The most common sites of spread include the retroperitoneal lymph nodes, lungs, and mediastinum.

Such lesions can present with an abdominal mass, shortness of breath, or even hemoptysis. Less common sites of spread include bone, liver, and brain. For a patient with an undifferentiated cancer, the finding of an isochromosome 12P in the tumor tissue is diagnostic of a GCT.

Any patient with a testicular mass or abnormal ultrasonography, or both, should have testicular carcinoma ruled out by a unilateral radical transinguinal orchiectomy. Orchiectomy is the definitive procedure for both pathological diagnosis and local control of the primary tumor, and, in some cases, may be a curative procedure. Transscrotal biopsies are contraindicated due to violation of tissue planes that may allow additional lymphatic routes of metastatic spread.

The physical examination of the testicles is performed by fully palpating all areas of the testicle between thumb and fingers. Testicular masses are firm to hard, and generally, the scrotal sac is normal in appearance unless there is a large mass causing distension. Patients with testicular masses must have a careful and complete physical examination, including examination for lymphadenopathy, intra-abdominal masses, hepatomegaly, bone tenderness, and pulmonary abnormalities.

The first step after the histologic confirmation of a GCT is to determine the extent of the disease (staging) so that appropriate therapy may be undertaken. An assessment of risk of metastases (in the case of local disease) or response to systemic therapy (in the case of advanced disease) using the results of histopathological, biochemical, and radiographic evaluations should be an integral element of the staging process.

Prognosis in testicular cancer depends on the following factors:

- Histology; seminoma tends to have a slightly better prognosis
- Primary site; mediastinal primary tumors carry a worse prognosis
- Nonpulmonary visceral metastases
- Degree of elevation of tumor markers

The management of early disease "clinical stage I GCT" is in part dependent on an assessment of the risk of occult nodal metastases. The treatment of choice for seminoma includes a radical orchiectomy followed by either close surveillance or low-dose radiation therapy (25–35 Gy) to the pelvic and retroperitoneal lymph nodes. Consideration should be given to tumor size (>4 cm) and rete testis invasion when discussing treatment options with patients. One or two cycles of single-agent carboplatin have also been explored as adjuvant therapy; however, it is not standard of care in the United States.

For nonseminoma, the treatment of choice includes radical orchiectomy followed by close surveillance of retroperitoneal lymph node dissection, assuming that the tumor markers normalize after the radical orchiectomy. Controversy over the optimal management of clinical stage I non-

seminomatous GCT has prompted a search for prognostic factors that can be used to predict the risk of occult nodal involvement. Histologic subtype, local tumor extension, and vascular or lymphatic invasion have all been shown to correlate with occult nodal metastases. If these patients still have elevated tumor markers, they should receive chemotherapy.

Patients who undergo retroperitoneal lymph node dissection and are found to have microscopic cancer cells in those lymph nodes appear to have a lower likelihood of recurrence when two cycles of adjuvant chemotherapy are administered. For advanced-stage testicular cancer (overt disease in the pelvic or retroperitoneal lymph nodes or distant metastases), chemotherapy is the initial treatment of choice. Patient risk stratification (primary site, other metastatic sites, and level of tumor markers) should be taken into account when selecting chemotherapy treatment for these patients.

Although chemotherapy confers a high cure rate for testicular cancer (more than 80% for good and intermediate-risk patients), patients live long enough to experience late toxicities. Fatal toxicities only occur in 1% to 5% of testis cancer patients. The most commonly observed toxicities while on chemotherapy are dose and drug related and include:

- Pulmonary fibrosis; most often related to bleomycin
- Acute leukemia; most often related to etoposide
- Oligospermia or azoospermia
- Raynaud's phenomenon
- Infertility, azoospermia and oligospermia
- Peripheral neuropathy, ototoxicity; most often related to cisplatin
- Metabolic syndrome; related to cisplatin

REVIEW EXERCISES

QUESTIONS

1. A 24-year-old woman presents for an annual gynecologic exam. She has never had a Papanicolaou (Pap) smear and has been sexually active since age 19 years with five lifetime partners to date. She has not had any pregnancies or sexually transmitted diseases. What do you recommend regarding her gynecologic screening and care?
a) No screening currently necessary
b) Pap smear alone
c) Pap smear and human papilloma virus (HPV) testing
d) Pap smear and HPV vaccine
e) None of the above

Answer and Discussion

The answer is d. Pap smear screening should begin by age 21 years, or 3 years after the onset of sexual activity.

The recommendation for screening young women for cervical cancer is annual Pap testing alone. Pap and HPV testing should be used in women older than 30 years, when most transient HPV infections have cleared. However, current recommendations are to vaccinate all women ages 11 to 12 years, catch up vaccination for women ages 13 to 26 years, and consideration for vaccination of girls ages 9 to 10 years.

2. A 56-year-old female had a recent diagnosis of breast cancer. She underwent breast lumpectomy with negative lymph nodes and negative margins, breast irradiation, and is now on Tamoxifen. Due to the increased risk of endometrial cancer with Tamoxifen use, you recommend
a) Hysterectomy ± bilateral salpingo-oophorectomy
b) An endometrial biopsy at least every 6 months while on Tamoxifen therapy
c) Annual ultrasound screening while on Tamoxifen
d) Evaluation only if symptoms arise
e) Oral progesterone therapy

Answer and Discussion
The answer is d. Studies have not shown any benefit to screening women taking Tamoxifen with either ultrasound or biopsy. Common symptoms include vaginal bleeding or discharge and should be evaluated, preferably with biopsy, or ultrasound measurement of the endometrial thickness.

3. A 74-year-old obese white female presents with vaginal bleeding. You do an endometrial biopsy and find a grade 1 endometrial carcinoma. She asks about her primary mode for therapy, and you tell her
a) Whole pelvic radiation is the primary treatment modality in women older than 70 years.
b) Hysterectomy, oophorectomy, and staging are the best initial approaches.
c) A trial of progesterone and repeat biopsy in 3 months would have high cure rates.
d) Concomitant chemoradiation has been shown to improve survival in locally advanced endometrial cancer.
e) None of the above.

Answer and Discussion
The answer is b. Current standard of care for women with endometrial cancer is surgical staging with hysterectomy, salpingo-oophorectomy, and staging lymph node sampling. Radiation can be used as primary therapy in medically inoperable patients, and hormonal therapy can be used cautiously in young women who want to preserve their fertility. There is currently no data to support chemoradiation in endometrial cancer.

4. A healthy 42-year-old patient asks about screening for ovarian cancer. She has no symptoms suggestive of the

disease, and the results of her physical examination are normal. You should
a) Ask about her family history of ovarian and breast cancers.
b) Strongly recommend yearly screening until at least age 70 years.
c) Recommend a CA-125 blood test and transvaginal ultrasonography.
d) Recommend consultation for prophylactic oophorectomy.
e) None of the above.

Answer and Discussion
The answer is a. Currently, no evidence suggests that screening for ovarian cancer reduces mortality from this malignancy. If there are multiple women with breast or ovarian cancer, particularly at young ages, these women should be referred for genetic counseling and testing. High-risk patients can then be offered screening. However, it can certainly be argued that screening at least has the potential for detecting the disease at an earlier point in time when therapy may be more effective. A woman undergoing such screening must be informed of the limited data supporting this therapeutic strategy.

5. A 53-year-old patient with abdominal bloating and a large pelvic mass, carcinomatosis, and CA-125 of 1,340 U/mL presents to discuss paracentesis results showing adenocarcinoma. She asks for your recommendation regarding treatment. Which one of the following would be the best recommendation in this setting?
a) Refer for colonoscopy and esophagogastroduodenoscopy.
b) Begin neoadjuvant chemotherapy while awaiting surgical consultation.
c) Give six cycles of cisplatin or carboplatin plus paclitaxel, and then repeat abdominal imaging to assess response.
d) Referral for surgical tumor resection followed by cisplatin or carboplatin plus Ataxane.
e) None of the above.

Answer and Discussion
The answer is d. The standard treatment for advanced ovarian cancer is surgical debulking, followed by cisplatin or carboplatin, plus paclitaxel chemotherapy regimen. No evidence suggests that neoadjuvant chemotherapy or chemotherapy alone is more beneficial than the surgery plus chemotherapy. Colonoscopy and esophagogastroduodenoscopy would not be appropriate given the amount of information available in this scenario.

6. A 19-year-old patient has an advanced germ cell tumor of the ovary, which has spread to the omentum. All gross disease is removed at the time of surgery. Which one of the following statements concerning this tumor is correct?

a) Using cisplatin-based chemotherapy, this individual's chances of survival are between 10% and 20%.
b) The administration of chemotherapy will almost certainly result in sterility.
c) Compared with epithelial ovarian cancers, germ cell tumors of the ovary have a superior survival.
d) Dysgerminomas have the worst prognosis among the germ cell tumors of the ovary.
e) None of the above.

Answer and Discussion
The answer is c. The overall prognosis of germ cell tumors of the ovary is excellent, certainly compared with epithelial ovarian cancer.

7. Which of the following is true regarding prostate cancer screening?

a) High-risk men should begin annual screening at age 35 years.
b) Proper screening includes a digital rectal exam followed by prostate-specific antigen measurement.
c) Spiral CT scan or prostate-specific membrane antigen radioimmunoscintigraphy scanning are alternative options for screening.
d) Men with a life expectancy of less than 10 years should not be screened.
e) There are not data supporting screening for prostate cancer.

Answer and Discussion
The answer is d. High-risk men (African Americans or men with a positive family history of prostate cancer) should begin annual screening at age 40 years; average-risk men should begin screening at age 50 years. Proper screening includes prostate-specific antigen measurement *before* performance of a digital rectal exam (DRE) because the DRE can cause a false-positive elevation of the prostate-specific antigen. Spiral CT scanning, positron emission tomography scanning, or prostate-specific membrane antigen scanning have no established role in screening for prostate cancer. Men with an estimated life expectancy of less than 10 years do not benefit from screening because many such patients have clinically unimportant disease (i.e., prostate cancer that will cause neither morbidity nor mortality in their remaining life span).

8. All of the following men should be referred for prostate biopsy *except*

a) A 47-year-old man with a prostate-specific antigen (PSA) of 2.1 who feels well and has a firm area on the right lobe of the prostate
b) An 84-year-old man with a PSA 6.8, free-to-total PSA of 0.25, nocturia for 15 years, and a diffusely enlarged prostate but no new symptoms

c) A 65-year-old man with a PSA of 5.5, malaise, low-grade fever, dysuria with an enlarged and tender prostate
d) A 61-year-old man with yearly PSAs of 2.2, 2.6, 2.9, and 3.9 who feels well and has a normal prostate examination
e) b
f) c
g) b and c

Answer and Discussion
The answer is g. The patient with a PSA of 2.1 (a) has an abnormal digital rectal examination (DRE). Any man in screening who has an abnormal DRE should be referred for a prostate biopsy. The 84-year-old man (b) most likely has benign prostatic hypertrophy, given the free-to-total PSA ratio of 0.25. Those men with a free-to-total PSA of <0.15 have a significantly higher risk of prostate cancer. This patient probably should not have been screened. The 65-year-old man with malaise, fever and dysuria, and a tender prostate gland (c) likely has prostatitis and should return to the office in 2 months for a repeat PSA once the infection has resolved. Therefore, this patient should also not be referred for a prostate biopsy. The 61-year-old man with the rising PSA and a normal prostate exam (d) has a PSA velocity that exceeds 0.75 ng/mL/year during the last year of screening (PSA rising by 1.0 ng/mL), which puts this patient at high risk for prostate cancer despite the fact that his PSA remains in a normal range.

9. A 63-year-old man presents with a screening prostate-specific antigen of 6.7, no symptoms, and a nodule on the right lobe of the prostate. Transrectal ultrasound and biopsy confirms adenocarcinoma in both lobes of the gland. Treatment options include all of the following, *except*

a) Radical prostatectomy
b) Orchiectomy
c) Radiation therapy, plus 2 years of hormone therapy
d) Radiation therapy (external beam or interstitial implantation of radioactive seeds)
e) Hormones followed by radical prostatectomy
f) b and e

Answer and Discussion
The answer is f. Radical prostatectomy (a) and radiation therapy (d) are standard treatments for patients with localized disease. Radiation therapy with a defined duration (e.g., 2 years) or hormone therapy (c) is standard therapy for a patient with locally advanced disease (i.e., cancer that has spread outside the capsule of the prostate into the seminal vesicles). Orchiectomy (b) is an excellent option for systemic prostate cancer (i.e., cancer that has spread to lymph nodes or to bone). The alternative option for androgen ablation is luteinizing

hormone-releasing hormone agonists (e.g., leuprolide or goserelin). The patient in question likely still has organ-confined or locally advanced disease for which orchiectomy is not an appropriate initial therapy. Similarly, there are no data supporting the use of neoadjuvant hormones prior to surgery.

10. A 67-year-old man, 4 years status postprostatectomy presents with low back pain and tenderness. His prostate-specific antigen is 185, and a bone scan is positive in multiple areas. The most appropriate treatment is
a) Orchiectomy
b) Radiation therapy to the prostate bed followed by orchiectomy
c) Chemotherapy with docetaxel
d) Bicalutamide (Casodex) followed by goserelin (Zoladex) subcutaneously every 3 months
e) a or d

Answer and Discussion
The answer is e. Orchiectomy (a) or bicalutamide followed by goserelin (d) represent appropriate initial hormone therapy for patients with systemic disease from metastatic prostate cancer. Bicalutamide is given before goserelin for approximately 10 days to prevent the stimulation of prostate cancer growth that accompanies the transient surge in testosterone production that occurs shortly after the initiation of luteinizing hormone-releasing hormone agonists (goserelin or leuprolide). The great majority of men have rapid systematic relief, with a radiographic response as well. Radiation to the prostate bed (b) has no role for a patient with metastatic cancer, and therefore, would be performed prior to orchiectomy. Chemotherapy (c) is appropriate for the patient whose disease progresses on hormone therapy.

11. Which of the following are side effects of hormone therapy for advanced prostate cancer?
a) Anemia
b) Osteoporosis
c) Impotence
d) Diabetes mellitus type 2
e) All of the above
f) a and c

Answer and Discussion
The answer is e. Anemia, osteoporosis, and impotence are important side effects of hormone therapy for prostate cancer. Three months of androgen deprivation have shown to increase the risk to develop diabetes mellitus, coronary artery disease, and myocardial infarction. The anemia is usually mild and does not require therapy. Osteoporosis is a significant side effect, however, which can lead to compression fractures or fractures of long bones. Men on hormone therapy

must be monitored for this complication, and appropriate therapy should be instituted early because these men frequently have multiple risk factors for osteoporosis. Impotence occurs essentially uniformly in men treated with either orchiectomy or luteinizing hormone-releasing hormone agonists. Few of these men respond to therapy with phosphodiesterase-type 5 inhibitors (e.g., sildenafil).

12. A 28-year-old baseball star presents with a painless left testicular mass. Physical exam is otherwise normal. α-Fetoprotein is >400. The most appropriate next step is
a) Testicular ultrasound
b) Ultrasound-guided transscrotal testicular biopsy
c) Inguinal orchiectomy
d) Trial of antibiotics
e) Whole body positron emission tomography scan

Answer and Discussion
The answer is a. Testicular ultrasound (a) is the initial diagnostic test of choice for any patient who presents with a testicular mass. Although one might argue that an α-fetoprotein level of 400 in a young man with a testicular mass is essentially diagnostic of testicular cancer, an ultrasound is still an important first step followed by radical inguinal orchiectomy (c). A transscrotal testicular biopsy (b) is contraindicated due to the violation of tissue planes, which allows alternate lymphatic avenues of metastasis. A trial of antibiotics (d) is not warranted in a patient who has a painless left testicular mass and no testicular tenderness to suggest epididymitis or some other infectious etiology. A whole body positron emission tomography scan (e) is not a staging procedure at the initial diagnosis of testicular cancer. CT scanning of the chest, abdomen, and pelvis is the standard staging workup, but would not be pursued before a diagnosis has been confirmed.

13. A 21-year-old man with stage III nonseminomatous germ cell tumor requires chemotherapy. Which of the following might you *not* expect as a late toxicity?
a) Pulmonary fibrosis
b) Biliary sclerosis
c) Azoospermia
d) Acute leukemia
e) Raynaud's phenomenon
f) Myocardial infarction

Answer and Discussion
The answer is b. Curative chemotherapy for testicular cancer and other malignancies can cause important late toxicities. Biliary sclerosis, however, is not a known late toxicity. Pulmonary fibrosis (a) occurs in a small fraction and a small percentage of patients treated with bleomycin, most of whom are asymptomatic. However, approximately 1% of patients have

significant symptoms. Another subgroup of patients develops pulmonary nodules that can be mistaken for lung metastases. Oligospermia (c) commonly exists before the diagnosis of testicular cancer but certainly has a much higher prevalence after the administration of chemotherapy. Acute leukemia (d) is a well-known late sequela of several different types of chemotherapy. Patients with testicular carcinoma receive etoposide, which is one of the agents known to cause this complication. Raynaud's phenomenon (e) occurs in a small subset of patients as well.

14. A 22-year-old man with testicular cancer comes back to your office 5 months after a radical inguinal orchiectomy and chemotherapy for nonseminomatous germ cell tumor. The patient feels well and has no complaints. His markers (α-fetoprotein, β-HCG, and LDH) normalized with treatment and remain normal. A mass is palpated in the left midabdomen. This mass is most likely

a) A mature teratoma, best treated with surgical resection
b) Recurrent testicular cancer, best treated with high-dose chemotherapy and autologous stem cell rescue
c) Seminoma, best treated with radiation therapy
d) Chemotherapy-induced chloroma (solid tumor manifestation of acute leukemia), best treated with radiation and chemotherapy

Answer and Discussion

The answer is a. Mature teratoma (a) is a well-known phenomenon that can occur after the successful treatment of nonseminomas, particularly those that contain a component of teratoma. Such a mass is generally curable with surgical resection. Left untreated, these masses can degenerate into malignant teratomas that are not curable. Recurrent testicular cancer (b) can certainly occur but is an unusual phenomenon and, in the setting of tumor markers that remain normal, would be highly unlikely. Seminoma (c) would similarly be extremely unusual after chemotherapy for a nonseminoma. Chemotherapy-induced acute leukemia (d) is a well-described complication of chemotherapy but

occurs with a latency of 2 to 9 years. In addition, a patient with acute leukemia and tumor bulk consisting of a chloroma would not generally be asymptomatic.

ACKNOWLEDGMENTS

The authors want to thank David Peereboom, MD, and Maurie Markman, MD, for their work on previous editions and for their critical review of the original manuscript.

SUGGESTED READINGS

Gynecologic Cancers

Armstrong DK, Bundy B, Wenzel L, et al. Intraperitoneal cisplatin and paclitaxel in ovarian cancer. *N Engl J Med* 2006;354(1):34–43.
Cannistra SA, Niloff JM. Cancer of the uterine cervix. *N Engl J Med* 1996;334:1030–1038.
Kauff ND, Barakat RR. Risk-reducing salpingo-oophorectomy in patients with germline mutations in *BRCA1* or *BRCA2* (review). *J Clin Oncol* 2007;25(20):2921–2927.
Markman M. Optimizing primary chemotherapy in ovarian cancer. *Hematol Oncol Clin North Am* 2003;17:957–968.
Morris M, Eifel PJ, Lu J, et al. Pelvic radiation with concurrent chemotherapy compared with pelvic and para-aortic radiation for high-risk cervical cancer. *N Engl J Med* 1999;340:1137–1143.
Rubin SC, Sutton GP, eds. *Ovarian Cancer*, 2nd ed. Philadelphia: Lippincott Williams & Wilkins, 2001.
Wright TC, Massad LS, Dunton CJ, et al. 2006 consensus guidelines for the management of women with abnormal cervical cancer screening tests. *Am J Obstet Gynecol* 2007;197(4):346–355.

Male Genitourinary Cancers

Abeloff, Armitage, Niederhuber, et al. *Clinical Oncology*, 3rd ed. Elsevier 2004:2175–2214.
Bill-Axelson A, Holmberg L, Ruutu M, et al. Radical prostatectomy versus watchful waiting in early prostate cancer. *N Engl J Med* 2005;352(19):1977–1984.
Loblaw DA, Virgo KS, Nam R, et al. American Society of Clinical Oncology. Initial hormonal management of androgen-sensitive metastatic, recurrent, or progressive prostate cancer: 2006 update of an American Society of Clinical Oncology practice guideline. *J Clin Oncol* 2007;25(12):1596–1605. Epub 2007 Apr 2.
Nelson WG, De Marzo AM, Isaacs WB. Prostate cancer. *N Engl J Med* 2003;24;349(4):366–381.
Tannock IF, de Wit R, Berry WR, et al. Docetaxel plus prednisone or mitoxantrone plus prednisone for advanced prostate cancer. *N Engl J Med* 2004;351(15):1502–1512.

Chapter 20

Leukemia

Matt Kalaycio

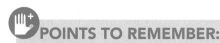

POINTS TO REMEMBER:

- The treatment of Hodgkin's disease often uses alkylating agents, and myelodysplastic syndrome/acute myelogenous leukemia is the most common secondary malignancy associated with the treatment of Hodgkin's disease.

- Chronic lymphocytic leukemia (CLL) may be complicated in several important ways:

  - Infection. Patients with CLL are predisposed to a variety of infections.

  - Autoimmune phenomena. These usually manifest as cytopenias (immune thrombocytopenic purpura).

  - Richter's transformation. Transformation into diffuse, large B-cell lymphoma.

- Patients who present with the clinical features of chronic myelogenous leukemia, but lack detectable *BCR/ABL*, often have another myeloproliferative disorder, such as myelofibrosis or chronic myelomonocytic leukemia.

- Imatinib mesylate was developed as a specific inhibitor of the *bcr/abl* tyrosine kinase. In patients refractory to, or intolerant of, interferon, imatinib results in a 100% hematologic remission and at least a 50% cytogenetic remission.

- Acute promyelocytic leukemia (APL) is also characterized by an unusual coagulopathy. The coagulopathy has traditionally been considered a form of disseminated intravascular coagulation. The APL coagulopathy, however, manifests with normal levels of antithrombin III, and bleeding is the major complication.

- When considered as a whole, studies clearly demonstrate the ability of hematopoietic growth factors to reduce the duration of neutropenia without increasing the risk of relapse.

The leukemias are hematopoietic malignancies that result in bone marrow failure or immune system dysfunction. Often thought of as either acute or chronic, and myeloid or lymphocytic, the leukemias are in fact a heterogeneous group of malignancies that differ in their molecular pathophysiology, if not always in their histology. These differences are being exploited in modern treatment protocols to improve survival and cure rates. This chapter strives to describe the various leukemias, explain their unique characteristics, and discuss their diagnosis and management.

ETIOLOGY

The etiology of the vast majority of leukemias is unknown. Clearly, environmental exposures to chemicals such as benzene and ionizing radiation increase the risk of acute leukemia. No environmental agent, however, has been demonstrated to increase the risk of chronic lymphocytic leukemia (CLL).

In some cases, the etiology of leukemia is known. Several hematologic disorders may transform into acute leukemia. The most common disorder to transform is myelodysplastic syndrome (MDS), but patients with myeloproliferative disorders and aplastic anemia are also at risk. MDS is discussed in greater detail later, but approximately one-third of MDS transforms into acute myelogenous leukemia (AML).

Cancer patients who survive after treatment with chemotherapy are at risk for the subsequent development of high-risk MDS. The risk is particularly high for patients treated with long courses, or high doses, of alkylating agents such as melphalan, busulfan, and cyclophosphamide. The treatment of Hodgkin's disease often includes such agents, and MDS/AML is the most common secondary malignancy associated with the treatment of Hodgkin's disease. Autologous stem cell transplantation for breast cancer or lymphoma may also be complicated by MDS/AML in as many as 10% to 15% of survivors. In contrast, the AML that results from exposure to epipodophyllotoxins, such as etoposide, generally develops in the absence of MDS and has different characteristics, as discussed in the Secondary Leukemia and Myelodysplastic Syndromes sections.

Congenital syndromes such as Down and Klinefelter's syndromes often increase the risk of subsequent acute leukemias. A genetic predisposition to some leukemias may also exist, particularly childhood acute lymphoblastic leukemia (ALL).

CHRONIC LYMPHOCYTIC LEUKEMIA

CLL is the most common adult leukemia in Western society. This leukemia increases in incidence with increasing age, and no other etiologic factor has been implicated. Patients are often asymptomatic at diagnosis and require no therapy. Patients often present with lymphadenopathy. An excisional biopsy of the involved lymph nodes demonstrates histologic changes identical to diffuse, small cell lymphocytic lymphoma. There is no meaningful difference in the pathophysiology, complications, and management of CLL and small cell lymphocytic lymphoma, and they are usually considered as a single entity.

Important prognostic information can be determined at diagnosis. Several staging systems have been devised that predict survival based on the extent of disease at diagnosis (Table 20.1). Those patients with low-risk disease often require no therapy and die of unrelated causes. Those patients with high-risk disease have shorter than expected survival, but treatment is not known to alter this fact. Other prognostic factors have been suggested, such as lymphocyte doubling time, ZAP-70 expression, and β_2-microglobulin levels but none significantly alters treatment recommendations.

CLL may be complicated in several important ways:

- Infection. Patients with CLL are predisposed to a variety of infections.

- Autoimmune phenomena. These usually manifest as cytopenias (immune thrombocytopenic purpura).
- Richter's transformation. Transformation into diffuse, large B-cell lymphoma.

Infections are managed as they occur, but prevention with vaccinations and possibly intravenous immunoglobulins is often appropriate. Autoimmune cytopenias, such as immune thrombocytopenic purpura and autoimmune hemolytic anemia, are treated with corticosteroids, as they would be in benign presentations. Richter's transformation carries a poor prognosis but is treated as any other large cell lymphoma.

The treatment for CLL is usually successful in inducing at least partial remissions. The elimination of all detectable disease, however, occurs less often, and relapse is inevitable. Traditionally, single-agent alkylating agents, such as chlorambucil, have been used with good effect and minimal side effects. More recently, purine analogs, such as fludarabine, have been shown to increase the remission rate, but at the expense of increased side effects. Survival rates do not seem improved, however, and fludarabine-based therapy is usually reserved for healthier patients.

The prognosis for patients who no longer respond to fludarabine is poor, with a median survival of less than 2 years. The treatment for relapsed disease may consist of alkylating agents, purine analogs, or monoclonal antibodies, such as alemtuzumab (Campath), alone or in combination. The role of allogeneic hematopoietic stem cell transplantation is undefined.

HAIRY CELL LEUKEMIA

Hairy cell leukemia is an uncommon, chronic, B-cell malignancy with unique features. In the United States, 400 to 600 cases are diagnosed each year; the median age of patients is 50 years, with a 4:1 male predominance.

TABLE 20.1

STAGING SYSTEMS FOR CHRONIC LYMPHOCYTIC LEUKEMIA

Clinical Features	Rai	Modified Rai	Binet	Survival (years)
Lymphocytosis only	0	Low risk		>10
Enlargement of less than three areas[a]			A	>10
Enlarged lymph nodes	I			8
Enlarged liver, spleen, or both	II			6
Enlarged lymph nodes + spleen + liver		Intermediate risk		7
Enlargement of three areas[a]			B	5
Hgb <11	III			2.5
Plts <100K	IV			2.5
Hgb <11 and plts <100K		High risk		1.5
Hgb <10, plts <100K, or both			C	2.5

Hgb, hemoglobin; Plts, platelets.
[a]The three areas include cervical, axillary, and inguinal lymph nodes; spleen; and liver.

Symptoms attributable to pancytopenia or splenomegaly are often present. The leukocyte differential and peripheral smear demonstrate a relative or absolute lymphocytosis with characteristic hairy cells. The bone marrow biopsy is usually hypercellular, with a diffuse infiltrate of hairy cells and increased reticulin, collagen, and fibrosis. Although immunoglobulin levels are normal, antibody-dependent cellular cytotoxicity and cellular immunity are impaired. These immune defects, in association with neutropenia and a characteristic monocytopenia, often lead to unusual infections (e.g., mycobacterial and fungal infections).

Splenectomy improves pancytopenia in two-thirds of patients. Although this procedure temporarily removes the site of platelet and white cell sequestration, it does not prevent continued malignant lymphocyte proliferation, marrow infiltration, or eventual relapse. Patients treated with interferon obtain a partial remission, but relapse within 1 to 2 years after the discontinuation of therapy. Nucleoside analogs have demonstrated promising results. A single cycle of 2-chlorodeoxyadenosine induces prolonged complete and partial remissions in 80% and 20% of patients, respectively.

CHRONIC MYELOGENOUS LEUKEMIA

Extensive knowledge of the molecular pathophysiological basis for chronic myelogenous leukemia (CML) has led to exciting treatment advances. CML is characterized by the Philadelphia chromosome, t(9;22). The translocation of the ABL oncogene from chromosome 9 to juxtapose the BCR gene on chromosome 22 results in a unique, chimeric fusion gene, BCR/ABL, which results in a chimeric protein with autonomous tyrosine kinase activity. This activity directly results in the activation of several intracellular processes that stimulate cellular proliferation and inhibit apoptosis. The malignant clone expands to the exclusion of normal clones and eventually leads to the clinical manifestations of the disease.

Patients may be asymptomatic at presentation, but often present with fever, sweats, weight loss, and bone pain. Physical examination often reveals splenomegaly. Masses composed of hematopoietic tissue—chloromas—may be detected anywhere and signify more advanced disease.

The peripheral blood smear reveals a left-shifted neutrophilic leukocytosis with basophilia and perhaps circulating blasts. Red cell and platelet counts may be either increased or decreased. The diagnosis is confirmed by the demonstration of BCR/ABL by cytogenetic analysis or molecular techniques. Patients who present with the clinical features of CML, but lack detectable BCR/ABL, often have another myeloproliferative disorder, such as myelofibrosis or chronic myelomonocytic leukemia. These patients have a poorer prognosis.

CML inevitably transforms to AML, or *blast crisis*, in the absence of therapy designed to eliminate the leukemic clone. The transformation is often heralded by an accelerated phase of disease, characterized by worsening symptoms, progressive splenomegaly, chloromas, and clonal evolution (additional cytogenetic abnormalities in addition to the Philadelphia chromosome). The median survival of patients with untreated CML is 5 to 6 years.

The treatment for CML was strictly palliative in the not-too-distant past. Hydroxyurea effectively controls symptoms and blood counts, but does not suppress the Philadelphia chromosome and, therefore, does not prolong survival or delay blast crisis. Interferon-α also controls symptoms and blood counts. Importantly, however, interferon can suppress the Philadelphia chromosome and thereby improve survival and delay blast crisis. Some patients with low-risk disease have complete suppression of their Philadelphia chromosome, which may translate into prolonged disease-free survival and potential cure. Interferon, however, does not effectively suppress the Philadelphia chromosome in the majority of patients and has significant side effects. Therefore, most patients are not cured by interferon.

Imatinib mesylate was developed as a specific inhibitor of the *bcr/abl* tyrosine kinase. In patients refractory to, or intolerant of, interferon, imatinib results in a 100% hematologic remission and at least a 50% cytogenetic remission. In accelerated phase disease and blast crisis, imatinib also results in high complete hematologic remission rates, although the cytogenetic remission rate is lower, and relapse is common with more advanced disease. These dramatic results generally occur in the absence of significant side effects. In addition to being better tolerated, imatinib proved superior to the combination of interferon and cytarabine in inducing remission and preventing progression in a large prospective, randomized clinical trial in newly diagnosed patients in the chronic phase. Thus, the treatment of choice in patients with CML is imatinib.

After 5 years of therapy, nearly 90% of patients treated with imatinib remain in chronic phase with no evidence of progressive disease. Some patients, in particular those with more advanced disease, do not respond to imatinib or relapse after an initial response. Most of these patients develop mutations in the BCR/ABL gene that confers resistance to the effects of imatinib. However, newer tyrosine kinase inhibitors, such as dasatinib and nilotinib, may inhibit the imatinib-resistant *bcr/abl* tyrosine kinase and allow for long remissions.

Although the discovery of the tyrosine kinase inhibitors represents a major advance in the treatment of CML, the only treatment known to cure CML is allogeneic stem cell transplantation. Patients with chronic phase CML transplanted within 1 year of diagnosis have a 50% to 70% chance of cure, whether their donor is a human leukocyte antigen (HLA)–matched sibling or matched unrelated donor. Results are worse for more advanced disease, but cure is still possible even for blast crisis. However, transplantation is associated with high treatment-related morbidity and mortality. Given the spectacular results achievable with imatinib, stem cell transplant is now deferred until patients become resistant to the tyrosine kinase inhibitors.

ACUTE LEUKEMIAS

Gone are the days when clinicians could think of the acute leukemias as either myeloid (AML) or lymphoid (ALL). The French-American-British (FAB) classification system, which subclassified AML and ALL into histologic subtypes, has lost usefulness in the face of newer prognostic categories. Furthermore, the histologic subtypes are subject to poor interobserver agreement and, with the exception of acute promyelocytic leukemia (APL), do not clearly influence treatment decisions. Newer information derived from the study of molecular pathogenesis, cytogenetic and immunophenotypic analyses, and the results of clinical trials have delineated many distinct acute leukemias, each with a specific phenotype and clinical manifestation.

Acute Promyelocytic Leukemia

The translocation of the promyelocytic leukemia (PML) oncogene on chromosome 15 to the retinoic acid receptor-α (RARα) gene on chromosome 17 results in a novel chimeric fusion protein that binds DNA and interferes with hematopoietic cell differentiation. Normally, RARα binds to DNA, where it regulates cellular proliferation with other regulatory proteins. The PML/RARα nuclear-binding protein irreversibly binds corepressor proteins that effectively inhibit the cellular processes necessary for differentiation. Under the inhibition of PML/RARα, the affected leukemic cell's maturation is arrested in the blast or promyelocyte stage. Thus, apoptosis is inhibited and the leukemic blasts accumulate, which ultimately leads to the clinical manifestations of APL. All-*trans* retinoic acid (ATRA) binds to PML/RARα, induces the unbinding of the corepressors, and allows for subsequent differentiation and apoptosis of the leukemic clone.

The recognition of the molecular pathogenesis of APL is important in that it represents a paradigm for the leukemic transformation of hematopoietic stem cells. Other leukemias caused by translocations have similar pathogeneses. Future treatments for these leukemias will probably involve the inhibition or reversal of these leukemogenic pathways.

APL is characterized by a distinct blast morphology, immunophenotype, and karyotype. The blasts often display numerous Auer rods and show at least some evidence of early differentiation, such as cytoplasmic granules. The blasts also express a distinct pattern of cell surface proteins: CD34$^-$, CD33$^+$, HLA-DR$^-$, and CD13$^+$. Most other myeloid leukemias express HLA-DR and may or may not express CD34. Finally, the pathognomonic feature of APL is the presence of t(15;17) by cytogenetic analysis.

APL is also characterized by an unusual coagulopathy. The coagulopathy has traditionally been considered a form of disseminated intravascular coagulation. The APL coagulopathy, however, manifests with normal levels of antithrombin III, and bleeding is the major complication. One study suggests that the coagulopathy stems from an overexpression of annexin II on the APL blast surface. Annexin II results in the overproduction of plasmin, which may explain the hemorrhagic diathesis. The coagulopathy is treated with intensive transfusion support, including platelets, cryoprecipitate, and fresh-frozen plasma. Before ATRA, as many as 30% of patients with APL died from hemorrhage. ATRA reduces the hemorrhagic complications by differentiating the blasts into neutrophils, rather than killing them as chemotherapy does.

The treatment of APL is also different from that applied to other leukemias. APL is uniquely sensitive to the differentiating effects of ATRA. ATRA alone induces an 80% to 90% complete remission rate. In combination with standard chemotherapy, particularly anthracyclines such as daunorubicin and idarubicin, 60% to 80% of patients in remission are cured. Patients who are older than 60 years or present with a white blood count (WBC) >10,000/μL have a worse prognosis, but cure is still possible. For patients who relapse, arsenic trioxide induces a second complete remission in approximately 85% of patients, who are then eligible for potentially curative treatment with an autologous or allogeneic hematopoietic stem cell transplant. The role of arsenic trioxide in less advanced APL is currently under study.

Core-Binding Factor Leukemia

These leukemias are characterized by translocations that disrupt the function of core-binding factor (CBF), a nuclear-binding protein that regulates hematopoiesis in a fashion similar to that of RARα. CBF is composed of two subunits, each of which can be affected by chromosomal translocations that result in leukemogenesis.

One leukemogenic translocation is t(8;21), which juxtaposes the AML1 oncogene to the ETO oncogene, creating a chimeric and leukemogenic CBFα subunit. The resulting leukemia is characterized morphologically by the relatively common observance of Auer rods. Unlike APL, however, this leukemia expresses CD34, CD33, and HLA-DR. Lymphoid antigens, particularly CD19, may also be expressed, with no impact on prognosis. The coexpression of CD56, when present, does connote a worse prognosis, as it does when expressed on other leukemias. Clinically, this leukemia is often associated with granulocytic sarcomas (chloromas).

Another well-characterized translocation is inv(16). This abnormality inverts the CBFβ subunit on the q arm of chromosome 16 to the *MYH11* gene on the p arm. The resulting chimeric CBFβ/MYH11 protein can also be formed by t(16;16) and is leukemogenic in a fashion similar to t(8;21). This leukemia, however, has a unique morphology: The blasts are myelomonocytic, displaying nuclear clefts and cytoplasmic vacuolization. Importantly, dysplastic eosinophils are also evident in marrow aspirates. Thus, this particular leukemia has been referred to as *acute myelomonocytic leukemia with eosinophilia*.

Both t(8;21) and inv(16) result in leukemias that are exquisitely sensitive to cytarabine. Both are almost always induced into remission using standard chemotherapy. However, additional cycles of high-dose cytarabine are needed to maintain remission. With appropriate treatment, the CBF leukemias are curable in 60% to 70% of cases.

Secondary Leukemia and the Myelodysplastic Syndromes

The MDSs are malignancies of hematopoietic stem cells that generally occur in the older patient population. They usually present as asymptomatic cytopenias and often as macrocytic anemias. They are characterized by inexorable progressively worsening bone marrow failure, but they do not necessarily result in transformation to acute leukemia or death. Treatment is supportive, with blood transfusions and antibiotics for neutropenic infections. Younger patients, however, should be offered potentially curative allogeneic hematopoietic stem cell transplant.

One study has characterized the prognosis of patients with MDS (Table 20.2). The International Prognostic Scoring System uses cytopenias, age, blast percentage, and cytogenetics to classify patients into prognostic groups. Lower-risk disease carries a more favorable prognosis and probably has a different pathophysiology. These patients are generally treated with supportive care, and bone marrow transplant is delayed until the time of progression to more advanced disease. However, some patients may reduce their transfusion requirement by treatment with lenalidomide, an immunomodulating agent. This is particularly true for patients with MDS characterized by a 5q– chromosomal deletion. Thus, the identification of patients with MDS has become more important now that treatments exist that can improve their quality of life.

Higher-risk MDS tends to transform into acute leukemia. The secondary leukemias are those that are preceded by hematologic disorders such as MDS or by exposure to stem cell toxins, such as benzene, ionizing radiation, and cytotoxic chemotherapy. Historically, the difference between MDS and AML was made by arbitrary cut-offs for blast percentage. However, high-risk MDS and secondary leukemia share enough characteristics to be considered the same disease regardless of blast percentage. Demethylating agents such as 5-azacytidine and decitabine can treat these patients. These drugs induce remission in a minority of patients, but tend to delay progression to acute leukemia and may prolong survival.

Secondary leukemia is characterized by cytogenetic abnormalities that often involve chromosomes 5 and 7. These

TABLE 20.2

INTERNATIONAL PROGNOSTIC SCORING SYSTEM FOR MYELODYSPLASTIC SYNDROMES

Marrow Blast Percentage	Score
<5	0
5–10	0.5
11–20	1.5
21–30	2.0
Cytogenetic features (karyotype)	
Good prognosis	0
Intermediate prognosis	0.5
Poor prognosis	1.0
Cytopenias (Hemoglobin <10, Absolute Neutrophil Count <1,500, Platelets <100K)	
0 or 1	0
2 or 3	0.5

Overall Score + Cytogenetic + Cytopenia Scores)	Median Survival (years)
Low = 0	5.7
Low intermediate = 0.5 or 1.0	3.5
High intermediate = 1.5 or 2.0	1.2
High = >2.5	0.4

Good prognosis: normal, –Y only, 5q– only, 20q– only; intermediate prognosis: +8, single miscellaneous abnormality, double abnormalities; poor prognosis: complex abnormalities, abnormal chromosome 7.

leukemias are difficult to induce into remission, and survival is short. In fact, secondary leukemias are uniformly fatal in the absence of allogeneic stem cell transplant. These leukemias are also difficult to cure with transplant and are associated with a high relapse rate.

An exception to the rule of poor prognosis in secondary leukemias is the 5q– syndrome. This syndrome tends to occur in female subjects. The syndrome usually presents as a mild anemia, but may also be associated with thrombocytosis. Unlike the other leukemias associated with abnormalities of chromosome 5, the 5q– syndrome carries with it a favorable long-term prognosis, with little likelihood of transformation into acute leukemia. As indicated previously, lenalidomide is especially effective in the treatment of patients with 5q– abnormalities.

Another unique secondary leukemia is characterized by abnormalities of chromosome 11q23. Prior exposure to epipodophyllotoxins, such as etoposide used in the treatment of childhood ALL, is associated with an increased risk of leukemias that harbor 11q23 abnormalities, such as t(9;11). Unlike the secondary leukemias induced by alkylating agents (i.e., melphalan), these leukemias are not preceded by a myelodysplastic phase. They are more easily induced into remission; however, similar to the other secondary leukemias, survival is short, and transplant is necessary for cure.

Acute Myelogenous Leukemia in the Older Adult

The incidence of AML increases dramatically with increasing age. Most patients with AML, in fact, are older than 60 years. In many respects, AML in the older adult is no different from secondary AML. Both are characterized by dysplastic morphology and harbor similar chromosomal derangements. Both are also characterized by a poor prognosis. The poor prognosis stems from both a more drug-resistant leukemic clone and the inability of older patients to withstand the rigors of induction chemotherapy. To this end, clinical trials have explored the role of adjuvant therapies designed to reduce the morbidity of chemotherapy in this patient population.

A series of clinical trials studied the potential role of hematopoietic growth factors in reducing the period of neutropenia after chemotherapy. When considered as a whole, these studies clearly demonstrate the ability of hematopoietic growth factors to reduce the duration of neutropenia without increasing the risk of relapse. However, no clear survival benefit was demonstrated. Although the hematopoietic growth factors are not considered standard therapy, they are often used to reduce the risk of infection in patients at high risk.

All older patients with AML either fail initial chemotherapy or have a relapse. No effective therapy has been found for these patients. An anti-CD33 monoclonal antibody was linked to calicheamicin, a chemotherapeutic agent too toxic to give as a single agent. The resulting molecule, ozogamicin gemtuzumab, effectively targets CD33$^+$ cells, such as leukemic blasts. For older patients with relapsed AML, approximately 30% achieve a second remission using ozogamicin gemtuzumab.

Precursor B-Cell Acute Lymphoblastic Leukemia

Precursor B-cell ALL is the most common subtype of ALL and is the subtype generally associated with childhood ALL. Whereas ALL in children is curable in as many as 80% of cases, the same is not true in adult populations. The major contributing factor to poor outcome in adult populations is that adult ALL is associated with adverse clonal cytogenetic abnormalities such as t(9;22) and t(4;11).

ALL typically presents as an acute illness with bone marrow failure, constitutional symptoms, and variable degrees of lymphadenopathy and splenomegaly. The diagnosis is suspected by a histologic review of blood and marrow specimens, but ALL cannot be distinguished reliably from AML on the basis of morphology alone. The best way to discriminate the lineage of acute leukemia is with flow cytometry of the leukemic blasts to determine their immunophenotype. Whereas AML blasts typically express CD33, CD13, and HLA-DR, pre–B-cell ALL blasts typically express CD10, CD19, and tDt.

The treatment of ALL is typically based on the combination of vincristine and prednisone. An anthracycline, such as daunorubicin, is usually included with or without other agents such as L-asparaginase and cyclophosphamide. Remissions are achieved in approximately 80% of patients with any one of a number of induction regimens. Despite intensive postremission treatment, most patients relapse. The risk of relapse increases with increasing WBC at diagnosis, increasing age, and the presence of adverse, clonal cytogenetics such as t(9;22) and t(4;11). At relapse, adult patients require allogeneic stem cell transplant for cure.

ALL tends to involve sanctuary sites, such as the central nervous system (CNS), more often than does AML. Although the risk of CNS involvement is less in adults compared with children, prophylactic CNS treatment with intrathecal doses of chemotherapy, and sometimes whole brain radiotherapy, is recommended in most modern treatment regimens.

Precursor T-Cell Acute Lymphoblastic Leukemia

T-cell ALL needs to be considered as a separate entity from pre–B-cell ALL due to its distinct clinical presentation, natural history, and response to treatment. Morphologically, T-cell ALL is indistinguishable from lymphoblastic lymphoma (LBL). There are subtle histologic differences between T-cell and pre–B-cell ALL. However, both T-cell ALL and LBL can be distinguished from pre–B-cell ALL by immunophenotype. As might be expected, pre–B-cell ALL expresses B-cell antigens such as CD19 and CD 20, but both T-cell ALL and LBL express T-cell antigens such as CD2, CD3, CD4, CD5, CD7, and CD8. T-cell ALL and LBL express similar antigens.

In fact, the only difference between T-cell ALL and LBL is the degree of marrow infiltration. They are both characterized by mediastinal masses and tend to occur in young men. Both are treated identically, with similar results. Most investigators consider them as the same illness.

T-cell ALL, and therefore LBL, has a better prognosis than does pre–B-cell ALL. Relapse only occurs in 30% to 40% of patients with T-cell ALL. Modern treatment regimens that maximize survival in T-cell ALL include cyclophosphamide and higher doses of cytarabine, in addition to intensive CNS prophylaxis.

Mature B-Cell Lymphoblastic Leukemia

Mature B-cell lymphoblastic leukemia is characterized by an extremely aggressive, rapidly proliferating population of blasts that are identified by translocations of the *c-myc* oncogene, as occurs in t(8;14) and t(8;22), among others. The blasts have a distinct morphology that, in the FAB classification system, was labeled L3, or Burkitt's leukemia. The immunophenotype is also distinctive in that surface immunoglobulin is detected, but the cytogenetic abnormality is diagnostic. This leukemia tends to invade the CNS early and requires prophylactic CNS treatment.

Untreated, or treated improperly, B-cell ALL is rapidly fatal, with a short survival time. However, with appropriate, intensive, short-course chemotherapy, cure is the rule rather than the exception.

MANAGEMENT OF ACUTE LEUKEMIA

Despite the distinctive nature of the individual acute leukemias, some management principles are shared by all of them. Bone marrow failure is universal in the acute leukemias, as a consequence of the leukemia and its treatment. The management of the resulting pancytopenia is critical to the success of any treatment program.

Neutropenic Fever

The incidence of infection increases with more profound and prolonged neutropenia, particularly as the absolute neutrophil count falls to $<500/\mu L$. At this degree of neutropenia, the risk of rapidly fatal septicemia is quite high. In contrast to other situations, a fever in the setting of severe neutropenia must be treated empirically to reduce the risk of infectious mortality.

The onset of fever in the neutropenic host should prompt a clinical evaluation looking for a source of infection and the collection of blood and other bodily fluids for culture. Once the cultures are obtained, antibiotics that cover gram-negative organisms are started empirically (including *Pseudomonas aeruginosa*). The gram-negative organisms are not the most common infections in this setting, but they are the most virulent. This fact has prompted the study of prophylactic antibiotics for neutropenic patients. The most commonly used agents are the fluoroquinolones, which have been shown to reduce the incidence of gram-negative infections, but have not been clearly demonstrated to reduce infectious mortality or improve survival.

Gram-positive infections are the most common organisms identified in modern series. These infections are typically less aggressive, however, and empiric therapy is not mandatory. A gram-positive infection becomes even more likely in the setting of prophylactic antibiotics or an indwelling central venous catheter. Vancomycin is often added to other empiric antibiotics in these situations.

The initial empiric antibiotic regimen of choice depends in large part on the susceptibility patterns of bacteria in the patient's hospital. Whatever regimen is chosen, however, should be broad-spectrum enough to cover a wide variety of organisms, including *P. aeruginosa*. Common regimens include broad-spectrum penicillin, such as piperacillin in combination with an aminoglycoside. In some situations, monotherapy using agents such as imipenem is appropriate. Cephalosporins should probably be avoided because their long-term use tends to increase the inci-

dence of infections with vancomycin-resistant strains of enterococcus.

If the fever resolves, the antibiotics should be continued until the neutropenia resolves. The aminoglycosides, however, may require replacement after approximately 2 weeks of therapy to avoid ototoxicity. If a specific organism is identified, antibiotics can be changed accordingly. Persistent or recurrent fever in the setting of appropriate broad-spectrum antibiotics suggests fungal infection.

Fungal infections, particularly with *Aspergillus* species, contribute greatly to the infectious morbidity and mortality of patients with prolonged neutropenia. These organisms are notoriously difficult to isolate in culture, but early treatment improves outcome. Therefore, presumed fungal infections must be treated empirically. Fever persisting for more than 4 days in the setting of neutropenia and appropriate antibacterials should be treated with empiric antifungal agents. Traditionally, amphotericin B has been the treatment of choice in this situation, but newer agents such as voriconazole and caspofungin may be safely substituted.

Another situation in which fungal infection should be considered is a fever that develops as the neutropenia is resolving. Hepatosplenic candidiasis often presents in this fashion, in association with elevations of alkaline phosphatase. CT of the liver and spleen is recommended to demonstrate the typical hypodense parenchymal lesions. Although biopsy of the lesions is recommended for confirmation, the constellation of symptoms and signs in the right setting calls for empiric antifungal therapy.

Other infections are also possible but are either less likely or less likely to be fatal. *Herpes simplex* infections often complicate the therapy of acute leukemia, and seropositive patients should be treated with prophylactic acyclovir. *Cytomegalovirus* infections are less common but should be suspected if no other source of infection is identified. *Pneumocystis carinii* complicates the treatment of ALL enough to warrant prophylactic treatment with trimethoprim-sulfamethoxazole.

Transfusion Support

Although a decision to transfuse should be individualized, certain guidelines pertaining to transfusion support should be followed to avoid complications.

The risks of serious spontaneous bleeding increase rapidly as the platelet count falls to $<10,000/\mu L$. Platelet transfusions for platelet counts of $<10,000$ to $20,000/\mu L$ are therefore warranted. These compromised patients are at risk for transfusion-associated graft-versus-host disease resulting from the transfer of lymphocytes in blood products; these patients, especially bone marrow transplantation candidates, should receive irradiated blood products. Patients may acquire cytomegalovirus through blood transfusions; therefore, previously unexposed patients, especially bone marrow transplantation candidates, should receive cytomegalovirus-seronegative or (preferably) leukocyte-reduced blood products.

Leukocyte reduction is generally performed by filtration. Filtered blood products are associated with less risk of febrile transfusion reactions and may reduce the incidence of alloimmunization. Some authorities suggest that all blood products should be filtered, but this is particularly important in immunocompromised individuals because leukocyte reduction decreases the rate of viral transfer.

Refractory thrombocytopenia caused by alloimmunization may occur in approximately 20% of patients with acute leukemia. No increased incidence exists with cumulative platelet transfusion exposure. Single-donor or HLA-matched platelets may have an increased survival time and may, therefore, be of benefit in this situation.

Red blood cell transfusions should also be filtered and irradiated for the same reasons pertaining to platelet transfusions.

The benefit of granulocyte transfusion is uncertain. The only potential indication for granulocyte transfusion is the patient with a documented infection that is susceptible, but not responding, to appropriate antibiotics.

REVIEW EXERCISES

QUESTIONS

1. A 35-year-old woman presents to the emergency room with 24 hours of fever and chills. In addition, she complains of increasing fatigue, dyspnea on exertion, and spontaneous bruising.

On physical examination, she appears ill; her vitals are temperature 39.5°C, blood pressure 80/40 mm Hg, pulse 140 beats/minute, respiration rate 22 breaths/minute, petechiae on soft palate, no lymphadenopathy, clear lungs, tachycardia, I/VI systolic ejection murmur, no abdominal mass or hepatosplenomegaly, and scattered petechiae, especially on lower extremities.

Her laboratory values are hemoglobin, 8.7; platelets, 14,000; white blood cells, 3,000, with 2% neutrophils, 45% lymphocytes, and 53% blasts; international normalized ratio, 1.1; partial thromboplastin time, 23; and fibrinogen, 345.

Her peripheral blood smear shows normochromic, normocytic anemia; thrombocytopenia; rare neutrophils; and many blasts.

The best course of action is to immediately
a) Withhold antibiotics until the source of infection is identified.
b) Fluid resuscitate and start piperacillin and gentamicin.
c) Fluid resuscitate and give granulocyte transfusion.
d) Perform bone marrow aspirate and biopsy.

Answer and Discussion
The answer is b. This patient has life-threatening sepsis and must be admitted for fluid resuscitation; a quick evaluation including blood cultures; and the administration of empiric, broad-spectrum intravenous antibiotics. She is anemic, thrombocytopenic, has spontaneous bruising, and is at risk for life-threatening hemorrhage; therefore, she needs transfusion with red blood cells and platelets. There is no clear role for granulocyte transfusions.

2. Which of the following is needed to make the diagnosis and predict prognosis?
a) Histologic examination of the blasts
b) Immunophenotype of the blasts
c) Cytogenetic analysis
d) All of the above

Answer and Discussion
The answer is d. All these tests are needed. The morphology of the blasts may be diagnostic in itself. Histochemical staining may also be indicated to improve diagnostic precision. Immunophenotyping is the most important test to determine cell lineage (acute myelogenous leukemia vs. acute lymphoblastic leukemia) and may help with prognosis. Cytogenetics is the most important predictor of outcome next to age.

3. A 25-year-old man presents to the emergency room complaining of dyspnea on exertion for several days. Recently, he has noted frequent nasal congestion and occasional epistaxis. He denies fevers, night sweats, and weight loss, and has noted a rash on his legs. He denies any hospitalizations or history of transfusions.

On physical examination, you find a well-developed man in no acute distress; temperature 36.8°C, blood pressure 126/74 mm Hg, respiration rate 20 breaths/minute; his oral mucosa has a few petechial hemorrhages, the skin of the pretibial area is covered with petechial hemorrhages, and no palpable lymphadenopathy or splenomegaly is present; he is otherwise normal.

His laboratory values are hemoglobin, 8.3; platelets, 32,000; white blood cells, 1,100, with 1% neutrophils, 73% lymphocytes, 13% monocytes, and 13% blasts; prothrombin time, 20; international normalized ratio, 2.1; partial thromboplastin time, 40; and fibrinogen, 90.

His peripheral smear shows pancytopenia, circulating blasts with Auer rods, and occasional schistocytes. A bone marrow aspirate and biopsy is hypercellular with 85% blasts and immature granulocytes.

The most important next step is to
a) Confirm the diagnosis with cytogenetic analysis.
b) Start piperacillin and gentamicin.
c) Transfuse platelets and fresh-frozen plasma.
d) Start chemotherapy.

Answer and Discussion
The answer is d. This patient probably has acute promyelocytic leukemia, given the obvious Auer rods and evidence of a significant coagulopathy. Both plasma and platelets are needed to reduce the incidence of fatal hemorrhage. In the absence of fever or other signs of infection, antibiotics are not recommended for neutropenia. Prophylactic antibiotics are controversial but have not consistently been shown to improve survival. Urgent therapy is needed, but chemotherapy may precipitate a worsening of the coagulopathy. All-*trans* retinoic acid is usually started before chemotherapy in order to reduce the incidence of severe bleeding.

4. A 29-year-old woman presents to your office for a Papanicolaou smear. She is asymptomatic and has a normal physical examination except for a moderately enlarged spleen.

Her laboratory values are hemoglobin, 11.9; platelets, 671,000; and white blood cells, 227,000, with 55% neutrophils, 7% metamyelocytes, 19% myelocytes, 2% promyelocytes, 2% blasts, 1% eosinophils, 7% basophils, and 3% lymphocytes. A bone marrow chromosome analysis shows 46,XX, t(9;22).

The most important next step is to
a) Immediately hospitalize.
b) Start chemotherapy.
c) Tissue-type the patient and her siblings to consider bone marrow transplantation.
d) Start imatinib.

Answer and Discussion
The answer is d. This patient's signs, symptoms, complete blood count, and bone marrow are characteristic of chronic myelogenous leukemia (CML). The t(9;22) is the Philadelphia chromosome, which secures the diagnosis. The high white blood cell count requires neither leukophoresis nor hospitalization. Unlike a high blast count, a high neutrophil count does not increase the risk of leukostasis and hyperviscosity syndrome. Hydroxyurea, and other chemotherapeutic agents, will not prevent the progression of CML to blast crisis. The only known curative therapy is bone marrow transplant, but this procedure carries a significant risk of early mortality. Because imatinib induces long-lasting remissions in the majority of patients, transplant is usually deferred until the time imatinib and other tyrosine kinase inhibitors fail.

5. A 35-year-old man with acute myelogenous leukemia has been severely neutropenic for 10 days and has been febrile with temperatures >38.5°C for the past 5 days. He has been on piperacillin, gentamicin, and vancomycin for 8 days. No localizing signs of infection are present on examination, and all cultures are negative to date. The most appropriate course of action would be to

a) Continue current antibiotics.
b) Change antibiotics to imipenem.
c) Add voriconazole.
d) Draw fungal cultures and continue current antibiotics.

Answer and Discussion
The answer is c. As the duration of neutropenia increases, the risk of fungal infection increases. This is particularly true in the setting of broad-spectrum antibacterials. This patient is at high-risk for fungal infection. The current antibiotics are failing, thus continuing them with no other changes is inappropriate. A change to imipenem might cover additional bacterial pathogens, but does not address the risk of fungal infection. Fungal infections are difficult to isolate. Clinical studies have clearly demonstrated the importance of *empiric* antifungal therapy. Thus, voriconazole is the correct choice.

6. A 75-year-old man with a 5-year history of untreated, chronic lymphocytic leukemia presents with fatigue and a peculiar craving for ice. Examination reveals generalized, but small peripheral lymphadenopathy and a barely palpable spleen tip. His laboratory values are white blood cells, 34,000; hemoglobin, 5.2; and platelets, 133,000; reticulocytes 2%; direct Coombs' test negative; and lactate dehydrogenase and bilirubin normal. The peripheral blood smear demonstrates normocytic red cells and no polychromasia. The most likely cause of anemia in this patient is
a) Pure red cell aplasia
b) Autoimmune hemolytic anemia
c) Bone marrow infiltration with leukemia
d) Gastrointestinal bleeding

Answer and Discussion
The answer is d. Chronic lymphocytic leukemia (CLL) is a fairly common lymphoproliferative disorder in the older patient population. Although CLL may be the direct cause of anemia in some patients, it is important to remember that these patients are also at risk for other problems as well. This particular patient has pica, a very specific symptom of iron-deficiency anemia. Even though the red cells are not microcytic, iron-deficiency anemia is still possible, especially if the onset is relatively rapid. Pure red cell aplasia is another possibility, but less likely given the indolent nature of the patient's leukemia and the presence of pica. Similarly, infiltration of the marrow with leukemia in an untreated patient would not likely be enough to induce this degree of anemia given the nonbulky lymph nodes, modest splenomegaly, and modest leukocytosis. The absence of microspherocytes, reticulocytosis, and a negative Coombs' test make autoimmune hemolytic anemia (AIHA) the least likely cause of anemia in this patient, but AIHA is a common cause of anemia in patients with CLL.

SUGGESTED READINGS

Cassileth PA, Harrington DP, Appelbaum FR, et al. Chemotherapy compared with autologous or allogeneic bone marrow transplantation in the management of acute myeloid leukemia in first remission. *N Engl J Med* 1998;339:1649–1656.

Cazzola M, Malcovati L. Myelodysplastic syndromes—coping with ineffective hematopoiesis. *N Engl J Med* 2005;352:536–538

Chiorazzi N, Rai KR, Ferrarini M. Chronic lymphocytic leukemia. *N Engl J Med* 2005;353:804–815.

Greenberg P, Cox C, LeBeau MM, et al. International prognostic scoring system for evaluating prognosis in myelodysplastic syndromes. *Blood* 1997;89:2079–2088.

Grimwade D, Walker H, Oliver F, et al. The importance of diagnostic cytogenetics on outcome in AML: analysis of 1,612 patients entered into the MRC 10 trial. *Blood* 1998;92:2322–2333.

Mayer RJ, Davis RB, Schiffer CA, et al. Intensive post-remission chemotherapy in adults with acute myeloid leukemia. *N Engl J Med* 1994;331:896–903.

O'Brien SG, Guilhot F, Larson RA, et al. Imatinib compared with interferon and low-dose cytarabine for newly diagnosed chronic-phase chronic myeloid leukemia. *N Engl J Med* 2003;348:994–1004.

Pui CH, Relling MV, Downing JR. Acute lymphoblastic leukemia. *N Engl J Med* 2004;350:1535–1548.

Rai KR, Petersen BL, Appelbaum FR, et al. Fludarabine compared with chlorambucil as primary therapy for chronic lymphocytic leukemia. *N Engl J Med* 2000;343:1750–1757.

Saven A, Piro L. Newer purine analogues for the treatment of hairy-cell leukemia. *N Engl J Med* 1994;330:691–697.

Schiffer CS. BCR-ABL tyrosine kinase inhibitors for chronic myelogenous leukemia. *N Engl J Med* 2007;357:258–265.

Warrell RP, deThe H, Wang Z, et al. Acute promyelocytic leukemia. *N Engl J Med* 1993;329:177–189.

Chapter 21

Disorders of Platelets and Coagulation

Christy J. Stotler   Steven R. Deitcher   Roy L. Silverstein

POINTS TO REMEMBER:

- The *activated partial thromboplastin time (aPTT)* is a clot-based test that measures the time for recalcified plasma to clot in the presence of anionic phospholipids and an activator of the contact system (usually diatomaceous earth, kaolin, or silica). It assesses the integrity of the so-called intrinsic and common pathways (factors XI, X, IX, VIII, V, and II, and fibrinogen).

- The *prothrombin time (PT)* measures the ability of recalcified plasma to clot in the presence of anionic phospholipids and tissue factor. It is primarily sensitive to deficiency of the vitamin K–dependent factor VII and is widely employed to monitor the oral anticoagulant warfarin.

- The first step in evaluating a prolonged PT and PTT is a mixing study in which patient plasma is mixed 1:1 with pooled normal plasma. Complete correction of the PT or PTT indicates a factor deficiency whereas persistent prolongation or only partial correction indicates a circulating factor inhibitor or lupus anticoagulant.

- An initial panel of testing is often helpful in raising several key questions, which will then help the assessing physician guide further laboratory testing. These should include a complete blood count with differential to evaluate the platelet count and for evidence of any other cytopenias or elevated counts, an examination of the peripheral blood smear to evaluate platelet size and detect the presence of microangiopathic changes in red blood cells, and a PT and aPTT to evaluate the coagulation cascade.

■ *Von Willebrand disease (vWD)* is the most common inherited bleeding disorder of primary hemostasis, affecting up to 1% of the general population by some estimates. It is caused by quantitative or qualitative abnormalities in von Willebrand factor (vWF), a very large multimeric glycoprotein encoded by a single gene on chromosome 12.

■ Platelet dysfunction is a common complication of *uremia* and is multifactorial in origin. Uremia can alter prostaglandin metabolism, induce a storage poollike platelet defect, and induce abnormalities in the interaction between vWF and platelet receptors.

■ The approach to the hypercoagulable patient should include a comprehensive clinical evaluation to guide management of the acute thrombosis, screen patients age appropriately for an underlying malignancy, and determine which patients will benefit from further special coagulation testing.

The role of hemostasis is to prevent exsanguination. A normally functioning human hemostatic system accomplishes this by promoting thrombus formation at the site of vascular injury and simultaneously maintaining blood in a fluid state, thus avoiding pathological thrombosis. The major components of normal hemostasis are the vascular endothelium, platelets, proteins of the coagulation cascade, and the plasminogen (fibrinolytic) system. Red blood cells (RBCs), white blood cells, and shear forces generated by blood flow also play a supporting role. Precise integration of the steps in this process sustains the careful balance between a prohemorrhagic and a prothrombotic state. In understanding the physiology of normal hemostasis, we can recognize aberrancies in either quantitative or qualitative components of the system that result in abnormalities of hemostasis.

NORMAL HEMOSTASIS

The initial phase of hemostasis is termed *"primary hemostasis"* and involves formation of a *platelet plug* at the site of a vascular injury. It requires *vascular endothelial cells, platelets,* and components of the subendothelial connective tissue matrix, most important, *von Willebrand factor* (vWF) and fibrillar *collagen.* The intact vascular endothelium normally provides an effective anticoagulant barrier between circulating platelets and the highly thrombogenic subendothelium. On its surface are receptors for antithrombotic and profibrinolytic proteins, heparin sulfate, and ADPase, an enzyme that degrades ADP, thereby limiting platelet activation. Endothelial cells are also a source of nitric oxide and prostacyclin, which inhibit platelets and promote smooth muscle relaxation and vasodilatation. With vascular injury, the normally antithrombotic endothelium is lost or rendered dysfunctional, and quiescent "resting" platelets become exposed to the subendothelial matrix (Fig. 21.1). There they encounter vWF, an extremely large glycoprotein that is synthesized by endothelial cells. Under conditions of high shear stress, platelets stick to vWF molecules via a platelet receptor known as the GPIb/IX complex and form a monolayer on the exposed subendothelial matrix in a process termed *platelet adhesion.* Other platelet receptors, including integrins and GP6, are also involved in platelet adhesion. Adhesion is enhanced by further interaction of platelets with exposed collagen. Signals generated by platelet adhesive interactions and signals mediated by soluble agonists, such as thrombin, epinephrine, ADP, and thromboxane A2, which are present locally at sites of vascular injury, convert resting platelets to an *activated* state. This results in a dramatic change in shape, synthesis and

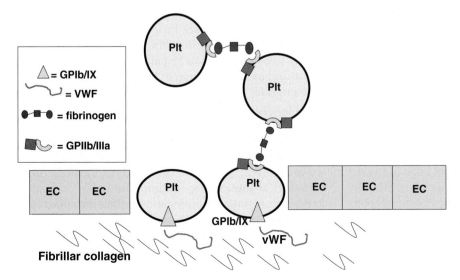

Figure 21.1 Primary hemostasis. Resting platelets stick to exposed von Willebrand factor via GPIb/IX and to fibrillar collagen in exposed subendothelial matrix after injury. Once platelets are activated, they are cross-linked by fibrinogen binding to GPIIb/IIIa. (See Color Fig. 21.1.)

secretion of thromboxane A2, release of granular contents including ADP, and activation of a platelet surface receptor for fibrinogen, called glycoprotein IIb/IIIa or integrin $\alpha_{IIb}\beta_3$. Fibrinogen is a large, multivalent circulating plasma protein that can bind $\alpha_{IIb}\beta_3$ receptors on adjacent platelets. The net result of these reactions is recruitment of additional platelets to the site of injury and formation of a cross-linked "plug" of *aggregated* platelets that "seals" the injury. Under pathological conditions, such as rupture of an atherosclerotic plaque, the plug can become occlusive, leading to tissue ischemia and infarction. Stability of the platelet plug is controlled by numerous factors, including blood flow and the secondary hemostasis system described as follows.

The second phase of the hemostatic response, termed *secondary hemostasis*, involves the formation of an insoluble *fibrin thrombus* (commonly referred to as a *clot*) at the site of injury. This is controlled by a series of enzymatic reactions (*coagulation cascade*) that generate the active serine protease, thrombin (factor IIa), from its circulating precursor, prothrombin (factor II). These steps occur simultaneously with those of primary hemostasis and require the presence of an anionic phospholipid surface (e.g., the activated platelet surface) and calcium. The critical enzymes of the coagulation cascade (factors XI, X, IX, VII, and II) are serine proteases synthesized as inactive zymogens by the liver. Factors II, VII, IX, and X share the unique feature of containing a cluster of the modified amino acid, gamma-carboxyglutamic acid (gla) at their amino termini. The gla domain is required for coagulation factor binding to anionic phospholipid surfaces; without it, their activity is essentially zero. Gla is formed by posttranslational enzymatic addition of a carboxyl group to glutamic acid (glu) in a reaction that requires the reduced form of vitamin K. The coumarin class of anticoagulant drugs (e.g., warfarin) inhibits the generation of reduced vitamin K and thus prevents synthesis of functional enzymes.

As shown in **Figure 21.2**, secondary hemostasis is initiated when blood comes into contact with a transmembrane protein called *tissue factor* (TF) that is expressed on cells in the subendothelial matrix and on cells of most parenchymal tissues. Its expression can also be induced on leukocytes and endothelial cells in response to injury and inflammation. TF is also frequently expressed by cancer cells. TF forms a complex with coagulation factor VIIa, and the complex functions as an efficient enzyme to convert factor X to its active form Xa. Xa then interacts with a cofactor, factor V, on anionic phospholipid surfaces forming the so-called prothrombinase complex, which rapidly converts prothrombin to *thrombin*. This initial burst of thrombin generation (formerly called the "extrinsic" pathway because TF is not a normal component of circulating blood) is further amplified by TF/VIIa-mediated conversion of factor IX to its active form IXa. IXa then interacts with a cofactor, factor VIII, on anionic phospholipid surfaces,

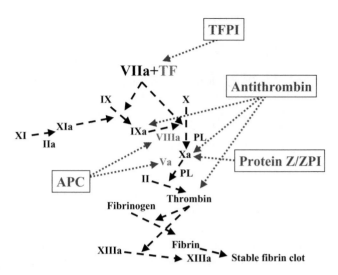

Figure 21.2 Secondary hemostasis. The procoagulant zymogens and enzymes are shown in black and their cofactors in blue. The major anticoagulant systems are in red. (See Color Fig. 21.2.)

forming the so-called tenase complex, which rapidly converts X to Xa. Thrombin further promotes its own production by enzymatically activating the two cofactors, V and VIII, and by converting factor XI to its active form, XIa, which can directly activate factor IX. Recent studies have demonstrated that TF-bearing microparticles (MPs) may contribute to the initiation of thrombin generation. MPs are small, membrane-bound vesicles that bud off cells (including monocytes, platelets, endothelial cells, and cancer cells) during cellular activation and/or apoptosis. MPs generated from monocytes are rich in TF and have been shown to accumulate in the developing thrombus after a vascular injury.

Once formed, thrombin proteolyses fibrinogen, releasing two small peptides and converting the molecule from a highly soluble dimer to an insoluble polymer termed *fibrin*. The polymer is relatively unstable. However, through the action of a transglutaminase enzyme, factor XIIIa, the fibrin strands are covalently cross-linked to one another to form a stable fibrin mesh. Factor XIIIa is converted from its inactive precursor by thrombin. Thrombin thus plays a pivotal role in hemostasis by participating in platelet activation and in multiple steps of fibrin generation. As such, it is a target for commonly used antithrombotics, including heparin, argatroban, lepirudin, and bivalirudin, as well as drugs in development (e.g., dabigatran).

The thrombin-generating coagulation cascade is tightly regulated by a system of natural *anticoagulants*, shown in red in **Figure 21.2**. This effectively prevents generation of pathological thrombi by confining thrombus formation to the sites of vascular injury and limiting thrombus size. The four major natural anticoagulants are *antithrombin* (formerly antithrombin III), *activated protein C (APC)*, tissue factor pathway inhibitor (TFPI), and protein Z–dependent

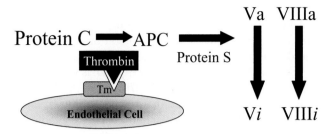

Figure 21.3 Protein C anticoagulant system. The vitamin K–dependent protease-activated protein C (APC) is activated by thrombin when thrombin is bound to a cofactor, thrombomodulin (Tm), expressed on the surface of endothelial cells. APC then halts thrombin generation by proteolytically cleaving and inactivating two critical cofactors of the coagulation cascade, factors Va and VIIIa. (See Color Fig. 21.3.)

inhibitor. As its name suggests, antithrombin inactivates thrombin, but also has activity against the serine protease coagulation factors Xa, IXa, and XIa. The activity of antithrombin is greatly enhanced by endogenous endothelial heparin sulfate and pharmacologic heparins, including low molecular weight heparins (LMWHs) and synthetic pentasaccharides.

The protein C system (Fig. 21.3) is activated when thrombin binds to an endothelial cell surface protein called *thrombomodulin*. This changes the specificity of thrombin so that it proteolyses and thereby activates the vitamin K–dependent circulating zymogen protein C. APC then inhibits further thrombin formation by cleaving and inactivating the two coagulation cofactor proteins, factors V and VIII. The activity of APC is enhanced by its cofactor, protein S. The protein Z system is a recently described regulator of thrombin generation that consists of a vitamin K–dependent cofactor, protein Z, and a protease inhibitor, Z-dependent protease inhibitor. TFPI is a lipoprotein-associated, factor Xa–dependent inhibitor of the TF/VIIa complex.

Fibrinolysis is the enzymatic process that dissolves the formed thrombus, allowing restitution of normal blood flow and facilitating completion of endothelial healing. Plasmin, the active fibrin dissolving enzyme, is formed from its precursor plasminogen by the action of one of two physiological plasminogen activator (PA) enzymes, urinary-type PA (uPA) or tissue-type PA (tPA). During thrombus formation, plasminogen is bound to fibrin and integrated into the new thrombus. uPA and tPA are released from adjacent uninjured endothelium, leukocytes, or epithelium and convert fibrin-bound plasminogen to plasmin. The kinetic efficiency of tPA on plasminogen not bound to fibrin is very low, making it fairly clot specific. Fibrin degradation results in release of fibrin fragments, including those containing the cross-linked "D domains" (so-called D-dimers) of the original fibrin molecule. Circulating D-dimers serve as a marker for the presence of thrombus and active fibrin degradation. The fibrinolytic system is

itself regulated and localized by two protease inhibitors, $\alpha 2$-antiplasmin and plasminogen activator inhibitor-1 (PAI-1). PAI-1 binds and inactivates circulating uPA and tPA, whereas $\alpha 2$-antiplasmin binds to freely circulating plasmin released during clot breakdown, preventing generalized fibrinolysis.

Alterations in the quantitative and qualitative status of any element within the hemostatic system can have significant biological effects. Platelet deficiency (thrombocytopenia) or functional defects in platelet adhesion, activation, or aggregation are associated with an inability to form an adequate primary platelet plug. These conditions can lead to significant mucocutaneous bleeding and posttraumatic hemorrhage. In contrast, a marked increase in platelet count (thrombocytosis) and accentuated or inappropriate platelet aggregation are associated with thromboembolic events. Deficiencies of components of the coagulation cascade are associated with variable degrees of bleeding tendency, usually involving bleeding into joints and muscles or posttraumatic hemorrhage. Insufficient or functionally abnormal vWF is associated with alterations of both primary and secondary hemostasis because it has a role in both processes—first in anchoring platelets to sites of vascular injury, and second as a carrier molecule for coagulation factor VIII. Elevated levels of procoagulant factors VIII, II, XI, and VII are recognized risk factors for vascular disease and thrombosis. A deficiency of natural anticoagulant proteins, such as protein C or S, or antithrombin is associated with venous thromboembolic disease. Inadequate tPA or plasminogen, or excess plasma levels of PAI-1, have been linked to thrombosis. A deficiency of factor XIII or of the fibrinolytic inhibitors $\alpha 2$-antiplasmin and PAI-1 cause clot instability and may precipitate delayed bleeding after trauma. The balance between these opposing groups of proteins, not the level of any individual factor, seems to be the most critical to hemostatic regulation.

COAGULATION TESTS

The *activated partial thromboplastin time (aPTT)* is a clot-based test that measures the time for recalcified plasma to clot in the presence of anionic phospholipids and an activator of the contact system (usually diatomaceous earth, kaolin, or silica). It assesses the integrity of the so-called intrinsic and common pathways (factors XI, X, IX, VIII, V, II, and fibrinogen). The aPTT can be prolonged by a deficiency or abnormality of any of these factors or by a circulating inhibitor such as heparin, autoantibodies to factor VIII, or the lupus anticoagulant. Although the aPTT is prolonged by a deficiency of factor XII, this protein does not play a major role in physiological coagulation, and patients with deficiency states do not have a bleeding disorder. The *activated clotting time (ACT)* measures the time to clot whole blood drawn into a tube containing an activator of the contact system such as kaolin. It is sensitive to heparin therapy in a linear fashion and is used as a bedside test to monitor regional heparinization, such as during cardiac bypass surgery. The *prothrombin time (PT)* measures the ability of recalcified plasma to clot in the presence of anionic phospholipids and tissue factor. It is primarily sensitive to deficiency of the vitamin K–dependent factor VII and is widely employed to monitor the oral anticoagulant warfarin. In such cases, the PT value is "normalized" to account for varying potencies of the tissue factor reagent and is expressed as the *international normalized ratio (INR)*. Generally, both PT and aPTT will be normal as long as a factor level in the patient's plasma is above 30% to 40% of normal. This allows a wide range of "normal" values detected by these assays before a deficiency is detected. For this reason, any abnormality in PT or aPTT merits attention, especially when surgery is anticipated. The first step in evaluating prolongation of either PT or aPTT is a *mixing study* in which patient plasma is mixed 1:1 with pooled normal plasma. Correction of the PT or aPTT to normal indicates a factor deficiency, whereas absence of complete correction indicates the presence of a circulating factor inhibitor or lupus anticoagulant. In the setting of low-avidity factor inhibitors, the mixing study may correct initially but not correct if the mixed sample is allowed to incubate at 37°C for 1 to 2 hours before testing. *Thrombin time (TT)* simply measures the time for plasma to clot after addition of thrombin. This assesses the final step in the common pathway, the conversion of fibrinogen to fibrin. It is prolonged in the setting of fibrinogen deficiency (hypofibrinogenemia), fibrinogen dysfunction (dysfibrinogenemia), and elevated levels of fibrin degradation products, and in the presence of heparin or direct thrombin inhibitors. *Fibrinogen levels* can vary significantly because fibrinogen is an acute phase reactant and can be very high in acute severe illnesses. The *platelet count* screens for both states of platelet deficiency (thrombocytopenia) and platelet excess (thrombocytosis). Artifactual thrombocytopenia is a falsely low platelet count that can occur as a result of an unusual ex vivo response to the anticoagulants used in blood collection tubes. This can be diagnosed by the presence of platelet clumping on a *peripheral blood smear* and by documenting normal platelet counts in blood drawn into an alternative anticoagulant. Peripheral smears also reveal evidence for microangiopathic hemolysis (schistocytes and helmet cells), which should prompt the clinician to assess for disseminated intravascular coagulation (DIC), vasculitis, and thrombotic thrombocytopenia purpura (TTP). The *bleeding time (BT)* assay measures the time for bleeding to cease after inflicting a defined skin wound. It reflects the elements involved in primary hemostasis (platelet plug formation) and is an excellent, but heavily operator-dependent, assessment of platelet function. It prolongs in a linear fashion as the platelet count falls from $100,000/\mu L$ to $20,000/\mu L$ and therefore is not useful to detect functional platelet defects in the setting of thrombocytopenia. The BT does not predict risk of surgery- or procedure-related bleeding and should not be used for those purposes. Recently, in vitro assays performed on whole blood have been introduced as noninvasive tests of platelet function. One example, the *platelet function analyzer (PFA)-100*, is widely available and may be preferred to the BT for vWF and platelet defect screening. Rapid quantitative and semiquantitative assays for circulating *D-dimer* are now widely available. Elevated levels reflect the concomitant activation of the coagulation and fibrinolytic pathways, and a normal assay essentially rules out the presence of DIC and acute venous thrombosis.

Diagnostic Approach to Patient With Suspected Bleeding Disorder

The clinical setting and associations between bleeding and certain disease states are critically important to appreciate in order to arrive at a correct diagnosis. For these reasons, a thorough clinical history should be the first step in evaluating a patient with a suspected hemostatic defect. This includes the patient's age, gender, racial background, and personal and family history of abnormal bleeding, with particular attention to dental, obstetric, and surgical histories. A thorough drug history is essential, including nonprescription and "alternative" therapies. The onset and course of bleeding (e.g., immediate and delayed) should be elucidated, as should the sites (e.g., mucosal, gastrointestinal, skin, muscle, joint) and characteristics of the bleeding (e.g., petechial, purpura, ecchymoses, hematomas).

An initial panel of testing is often helpful in raising several key questions that will then help the assessing physician guide further laboratory testing. These should include a CBC with differential to evaluate the platelet count and, for evidence of any other cytopenias or elevated counts, an examination of the peripheral blood smear to evaluate platelet size and detect the presence of microangiopathic changes in RBCs, and a PT and aPTT to evaluate the coagulation cascade. The results of these screening tests in the context of the history and physical examination should in most cases define whether further evaluation is needed and whether it should focus on platelet or coagulation system parameters.

Disorders of Primary Hemostasis

Disorders of primary hemostasis occur when there is either a qualitative of quantitative defect in any of the components of normal primary hemostasis, that is, *platelets*, the *blood vessel wall*, or *vWF*. Patients with disorders of primary hemostasis typically experience mucocutaneous or gingival bleeding, petechiae, epistaxis, ecchymoses, and excessive bleeding associated with dental procedures and/or childbirth.

Von Willebrand disease (vWD) is the most common inherited bleeding disorder of primary hemostasis, affecting up to 1% of the general population by some estimates.

It is caused by quantitative or qualitative abnormalities in vWF, a very large multimeric glycoprotein encoded by a single gene on chromosome 12. vWF is secreted constitutively into the circulation at low levels by endothelial cells and is also synthesized by megakaryocytes. It is stored in platelet granules and in the Weibel-Palade bodies of endothelial cells from which it is secreted locally in response to vascular injury. As previously mentioned, vWF functions as both a carrier molecule for coagulation factor VIII and to recruit and adhere platelets to an area of vascular injury. Because of this latter function, vWD can be thought of as a disorder of platelet function. vWD most commonly presents in a heterozygous state involving inheritance of a single copy of a null mutation (type 1 vWD) with blood levels of vWF circulating at ~50% of normal. Very rarely, it presents in the homozygous null state (type 3 vWD) in which case levels of both vWF and factor VIII are <5% of normal. Qualitative or functional defects of vWF are collectively termed type 2 vWD.

In type 1 vWD, which accounts for ~80% of cases, all sizes of vWF multimers are present in reduced amounts. Patients typically present with mucocutaneous, gingival, or posttraumatic bleeding, or menorrhagia. Those patients with only mild to moderate reductions in their vWF activity levels may be clinically asymptomatic. Conversely, patients with type 3 vWD present with severe and often life-threatening bleeding episodes and, due to the associated very low levels of factor VIII, can display hemarthroses or deep tissue bleeds, akin to a hemophilialike presentation, in addition to severe mucocutaneous bleeding.

Mutations causing type 2 vWD are categorized into subtypes based on the specific functional abnormality of the protein. Type 2A mutations result in absence of high molecular weight vWF multimers and in impaired interaction between vWF and platelets. Type 2B mutations create a variant of vWF, which has increased affinity for platelet glycoprotein Ib. The consequence of this is a variable degree of platelet agglutination and an increase in platelet clearance from the circulation, resulting in a mild thrombocytopenia. Type 2M mutations result in impaired interaction between vWF and platelets due to a specific defect in the GPIb binding domain of vWF. Type 2N mutations are located in the factor VIII binding domain of vWF and cause a marked decreased affinity for factor VIII. These patients have normal multimeric distributions, normal levels of vWF, and normal ristocetin cofactor activities, but have extremely low levels of factor VIII. Accordingly, some males who have been diagnosed as mild hemophiliacs actually have this form of vWD. This disorder is also called *autosomal hemophilia*.

Acquired vWD can occur as a result of development of autoantibodies (inhibitors) against vWF and has been described in association with B-cell malignancies, myeloproliferative disorders, hypothyroidism, and intestinal angiodysplasias. Patients with specific cardiac defects, such as tight aortic stenosis that are associated with extremely high intravascular shear forces, may develop an acquired vWD due to shear-induced binding of vWF to the platelet surface.

When vWD is suspected, an initial screening evaluation should include BT (or PFA-100), platelet count, PT, and aPTT. Some patients with very mild type 1 vWD, however, may have normal screening laboratory tests. More severe disease usually manifests with a prolonged bleeding time and aPTT. If clinical suspicion is high or if the screening tests are abnormal, further evaluation is based on measuring circulating levels of vWF protein antigen (vWF:Ag), assessing vWF multimer structure by electrophoresis, and measuring factor VIII coagulant activity (VIII:C) and vWF functional activity (vWF:risto). The latter is based on the ability of the antibiotic ristocetin to induce vWF binding to GPIb on fixed platelets, which results in their agglutination. Diagnosis of vWD is made difficult because vWF is an acute phase reactant and thus levels are often increased in the setting of acute and chronic inflammatory states. Also, the *vWF* gene is regulated by estrogen so that pregnancy, menses, oral contraceptives, and postmenopausal estrogen use can increase vWF levels, masking mild deficiencies of the protein. If initial testing is negative, but clinical suspicion remains high, then retesting should be performed at a future date when confounding factors may have resolved.

Treatment of vWD depends on the underlying defect. Patients with mild to moderate type I and IIA syndromes may respond well to treatment with desmopressin (DDAVP), an analog of vasopressin. DDAVP stimulates release of vWF from the Weibel-Palade bodies of endothelial cells, producing an immediate rise in plasma levels of vWF and factor VIII. The effects of DDAVP are short lived, lasting only 1 to 24 hours, and additional doses may result in a decreased response due to development of tachyphylaxis. Hyponatremia can rarely result from DDAVP infusions. In patients with a severe vWF deficiency or in patients undergoing major surgery, DDAVP alone may be inadequate, and vWF replacement therapy may be necessary. DDAVP should be avoided in patients with type IIB disease because its use has been associated with thrombotic complications. Cryoprecipitate is a blood product that contains concentrated fibrinogen, vWF, and factors VIII and XIII, and is a therapeutic option for some patients. Due to the potential risk of transfusion-related transmission of infectious agents, purified factor VIII/vWF concentrates such as Humate-P are usually recommended in situations where DDAVP is not appropriate. In acquired vWD, factor VIII/vWF concentrate infusions usually produce a short-lived response due to the presence of anti-vWF antibodies. In acute bleeding situations, immunosuppressive therapy with corticosteroids or high-dose intravenous immunoglobulin (IVIG) may decrease production of anti-vWF antibodies, allowing concentrates to work and hemostasis to be achieved.

Disorders of Platelet Function

Bernard-Soulier syndrome is an autosomal recessive disorder in which platelet glycoprotein Ib, the receptor for vWF, is absent or deficient. Accordingly, a severe defect in platelet adhesion occurs. Like vWD, it is characterized by abnormal ristocetin agglutination; however, unlike vWD, this abnormal response is not corrected by the addition of normal vWF. Bernard-Soulier syndrome is also characterized by moderate thrombocytopenia and the presence of large platelets in the circulation ("macrothrombocytopenia").

Glanzmann's thromboasthenia is an autosomal recessive disorder in which platelet glycoprotein IIb/IIIa, the receptor for fibrinogen is absent or deficient. Platelets from these patients fail to aggregate in response to all agonists (except ristocetin), resulting in a severe bleeding disorder.

Other inherited disorders of platelet function are the group of *storage pool disorders* in which patients have inherited defects in production and/or secretion of platelet dense or α-granules. **α-Granule deficiency**, also called **gray platelet syndrome**, presents clinically as a mild bleeding abnormality, whereas dense granule storage pool disorders cause a more severe bleeding tendency. They are often associated with congenital disorders of other organ systems, such as immune deficiencies (Wiskott-Aldrich syndrome), skeletal anomalies (TAR [thrombocytopenia with absent radia] syndrome), and oculocutaneous albinism (Hermansky-Pudlak syndrome).

Treatment of inherited platelet disorders is reserved for active hemorrhage or prophylactically for planned surgical procedures. In all cases, platelet transfusions from normal donors are effective for severe bleeding. For minor oral bleeding, mouthwash with ε-aminocaproic acid (Amicar) can be useful. DDAVP is effective for patients with storage pool disorders in improving hemostasis for most surgical procedures.

Acquired disorders of platelet function usually occur in three clinical scenarios—in association with *drugs that affect platelet function*, due to an *underlying systemic disease* (e.g., renal or liver failure), or as a result of a *disorder of hematopoiesis* (myeloproliferative and myelodysplastic disorders). Rarely, paraproteins produced in patients with multiple myeloma or Waldenström's macroglobulinemia can affect platelet function by binding to the platelet surface nonspecifically and interfering with adhesion and/or aggregation. Platelet function can also be disturbed as a result of contact with artificial membranes, such as those used for extracorporeal oxygenation during cardiopulmonary bypass.

Drugs are the most common cause of acquired platelet dysfunction and a careful drug history should be obtained from all patients with a bleeding disorder. Aspirin and nonsteroidal anti-inflammatory drugs (NSAIDs) are by far the most common culprits. Aspirin impairs platelet function by acetylating cyclo-oxygenase enzymes (COX-1 and COX-2), thereby blocking production of thrombox-

ane A2, a potent platelet agonist. Aspirin acts irreversibly, and its effect therefore lasts for the life of the platelet (7–10 days), whereas the NSAIDs reversibly impair COX function, and, therefore, their effects depend on the half-life of the drug. Other drugs, including furosemide, verapamil, hydralazine, methylprednisolone, and cyclosporin A, may also have weak anti-COX activity. Tricyclic antidepressants, cocaine, lidocaine, chlorpromazine, propranolol, cephalosporins, penicillins, and alcohol can interfere nonspecifically with platelet membrane function and produce a mild bleeding disorder. Inhibition of platelet phosphodiesterase activity occurs with caffeine, dipyridamole, aminophylline, and theophylline, and results in a mild platelet functional deficit. The platelet glycoprotein IIb/IIIa inhibitors abciximab, tirofiban, and eptifibatide have a dramatic effect on platelet aggregation, produce a severe functional platelet deficit, and are therefore used therapeutically only for short-term indications such as acute coronary interventions. Drugs that irreversibly block the platelet ADP receptor include ticlopidine and clopidogrel, and are now in widespread use for secondary prevention of atherothrombotic disorders. These agents, like aspirin, lead to prolongation of BT and are associated with increased risk of bleeding. Both ticlopidine and clopidogrel have also been associated with the development of TTP (see Thrombotic Thrombocytopenia Purpura section). The primary intervention for drug-induced platelet dysfunction associated with bleeding is to stop the offending agent. Usually, observation alone, with time allowed for platelet turnover, is adequate. It is rare that platelet transfusions are necessary. The possible exception is the platelet dysfunction experienced during cardiopulmonary bypass, which is often severe and multifactorial in nature. Drugs known to interfere with platelet function exacerbate the defects produced by cardiopulmonary bypass–induced platelet activation and storage granule content depletion. In this setting, aprotinin may improve platelet survival and function by inactivating plasmin, and Amicar may reduce bleeding by decreasing plasmin production.

Platelet dysfunction is a common complication of *uremia* and is multifactorial in origin. Uremia can alter prostaglandin metabolism, induce a storage poollike platelet defect, and induce abnormalities in the interaction between vWF and platelet receptors. The uncleared metabolic product, guanidinosuccinic acid, also inhibits platelet function by inducing endothelial cell nitric oxide release. The first approach to the uremic patient with bleeding problems is to ensure adequate dialysis. However, in severe situations, DDAVP, conjugated estrogens, and cryoprecipitate have been shown to improve hemostasis. Platelet transfusions are required only in instances of life-threatening hemorrhage. Patients with acute and chronic *liver disease* often have a multifactorial coagulopathy related to platelet dysfunction, reduced production of coagulation factors and fibrinolytic inhibitors, reduced clearance of fibrin degradation products (FDPs), thrombocytopenia related to hypersplenism, and abnormalities in the structure of fibrinogen (dysfibrinogenemia).

Thrombocytopenia

Normal hemostasis requires an adequate number of functional platelets, generally more than 80,000 to 100,000/μL of blood. Many processes and disorders can result in thrombocytopenia and evaluation can be guided by categorizing etiologies as either *decreased production* or *increased destruction* of platelets, or an abnormal *sequestration* of platelets within the spleen.

Sequestration

In a normal individual, approximately 20% of platelets are held within the spleen. Any condition that produces splenomegaly can significantly increase this percentage and therefore lower circulating platelet counts. If the platelet life span is normal, splenomegaly alone should not reduce the platelet count to <40,000 to 50,000/μL. If the platelet count is lower than this level, a concurrent problem in platelet production or destruction should be sought. In disease states where there is both splenomegaly and a reduced platelet survival due to development of an autoantibody to platelets (e.g., lymphoproliferative and autoimmune disorders), a splenectomy may be an effective treatment modality to increase the number of circulating platelets. Splenectomy is not as effective in patients with advanced liver disease. In this context, the bleeding tendency is usually a multifactorial problem. In patients with advanced myeloproliferative syndromes, especially myelofibrosis, a markedly enlarged spleen with extramedullary hematopoiesis develops in which the spleen is both sequestering and producing platelets. In the thrombocytopenic patient with myelofibrosis, the balance between production and sequestration is often difficult to assess, and splenectomy carries the potential risk of worsening an already severe thrombocytopenia by removing the site of extramedullary hematopoiesis.

Decreased Platelet Production

An insult to or abnormality of megakaryocytes within the marrow, the cells responsible for platelet production, can result in thrombocytopenia. Sometimes a source of the insult is easily identifiable, such as radiation therapy or chemotherapy in cancer patients; recent viral infections; or exposures to toxins such as benzenes, insecticides, and gold salts. Deficiencies in vitamin B$_{12}$ or folic acid cause ineffective megakaryocyte production and may be suspected in malnourished patients or those with a history of significant alcohol consumption. Alcohol itself is a toxin to the marrow. Hematopoietic malignancies, metastatic carcinoma, and certain infections such as tuberculosis are associated with platelet production defects due to bone marrow infiltration. Diagnosis of platelet production defects, if not obvious from the medical history, usually requires examination of the bone marrow aspirate and/or biopsy, which will reveal a relative paucity of megakaryocytes and may

detect the presence of an infiltrative process. Congenital disorders associated with defects of platelet production are usually diagnosed before adulthood and include Fanconi's anemia, TAR (thrombocytopenia with absent radius) syndrome, May-Hegglin anomaly, and Wiskott-Aldrich syndrome. Rubella infection or maternal use of thiazide diuretics during pregnancy can cause congenital megakaryocyte hypoplasia and thrombocytopenia in the newborn.

Increased Platelet Destruction

Thrombocytopenia due to shortened platelet survival can be extremely severe and is generally due to either immune-mediated clearance of circulating platelets or pathological platelet consumption related to excessive or inappropriate activation of prothrombotic mechanisms. Evaluation of platelet destruction disorders begins with a thorough history to identify underlying disorders, recent exposures to drugs or blood products, or recent viral infections. Examination of the bone marrow may be indicated and reveals increased numbers of megakaryocytes.

Immune Purpura

Immune-mediated platelet destruction can be either alloimmune or autoimmune in nature. The latter can be idiopathic or related to drugs, infections, lymphoproliferative disorders, or systemic autoimmune disorders. In general, platelet transfusions are not indicated for patients with immune purpura; however, in the setting of severe active bleeding, platelet transfusions should not be withheld.

Drug-Related Thrombocytopenia ("Drug Purpura")

Many drugs have been associated with immune-mediated thrombocytopenia. The prototypic examples are quinine and quinidine products that act as haptens, triggering production of drug-dependent antiplatelet antibodies that mediate rapid clearance of platelets from the circulation. Other drugs associated with autoantibody formation are sulfonamides, gold salts, penicillin, and α-methyldopa. Drug-related thrombocytopenia generally presents 7 to 14 days after initiating the drug but can occasionally occur much later. The resulting thrombocytopenia can be quite severe but usually responds to cessation of the offending agent. In some cases, a short course of high-dose corticosteroids may be indicated to hasten recovery. *Heparin-induced thrombocytopenia (HIT)* is a unique example of drug-induced purpura that deserves special attention because of the potentially devastating thrombotic complications that may arise. It is discussed in more detail in the Thrombotic Disorders section.

Immune Purpura Associated With Lymphoproliferative, Autoimmune, and Infectious Disorders

Hodgkin and non-Hodgkin's lymphoma and chronic lymphocytic leukemia have been associated with development of autoantibodies to platelets. In these cases, the thrombocytopenia usually responds to treatment of the underlying malignancy. Antiplatelet antibodies can also be triggered by infections such as infectious mononucleosis, viral hepatitis, histoplasmosis, HIV, and Lyme disease. For this reason, laboratory evaluation of any patient presenting with an autoimmune thrombocytopenia should include testing for HIV and viral hepatitis. Initiation of antiviral therapy in these situations often significantly ameliorates the thrombocytopenia. Autoimmune thrombocytopenia often accompanies systemic autoimmune syndromes, such as systemic lupus erythematosus (SLE) and rheumatoid arthritis. In fact, thrombocytopenia may be the only sign heralding the onset of lupus. When immune thrombocytopenia occurs simultaneously with autoimmune hemolytic anemia, the term Evan's syndrome is applied.

Idiopathic/Immune-Mediated Thrombocytopenic Purpura (ITP)

ITP, that is, autoimmune platelet destruction in the absence of an underlying immune, infectious, or malignant disorder, is a diagnosis of exclusion. ITP can occur at any age, but persons 20 to 40 years of age are most commonly affected, and it occurs in women more frequently than in men. Most adults with chronic ITP have antiplatelet immunoglobin G (IgG) antibodies in their serum and coating their platelets (so-called platelet-associated immunoglobulin), but these are not usually useful as diagnostic tests. Typically, patients present with a petechial rash on their lower extremities and are then found to have very low platelet counts; counts of $<10,000/\mu L$ are not uncommon. Patients may also experience epistaxis, gum bleeding, and hemorrhagic bullae in the oropharynx and occasionally life-threatening gastrointestinal or intracerebral bleeding may occur. High doses of corticosteroids (e.g., 1 mg/kg prednisone) is the initial treatment of choice for adults with chronic ITP when associated with active bleeding or low ($<30,000/\mu L$) platelet counts. A response to steroids occurs in approximately two-thirds of patients and is usually seen within 7 to 14 days. Patients who respond should be continued on full doses for 2 to 4 weeks before initiating a slow taper. Splenectomy (preferably via laparoscopic technique) should be considered for the ~50% of patients who are refractory to corticosteroids, or who relapse when the daily dose of prednisone is tapered to <10 mg. Approximately one-half to two-thirds will maintain platelet counts in a reasonable range (e.g., $>60,000/\mu L$) after splenectomy. If possible, pneumococcal and *Haemophilus influenzae* vaccines should be administered 2 to 3 weeks prior to splenectomy. In those patients who remain refractory despite steroids and splenectomy, several alternative treatments are available. High-dose IVIG may induce a rapid increase in platelet count of variable duration. The exact mechanism of action of IVIG is unclear but likely results from the blockade of immunoglobulin Fc receptors on reticuloendothelial cells. An alternative to IVIG for patients whose blood type is Rh+ is infusion of anti-D immunoglobulin. This is often complicated by mild to moderate hemolysis, but the infusion is a much lower volume than IVIG and is associated with fewer systemic side effects. Danazol, an attenuated androgen, has been associated with therapeutic responses in ITP and may be especially useful in elderly patients who are not candidates for splenectomy or in those who relapse following splenectomy, although it may take 1 to 2 months of therapy before seeing a therapeutic response. Antibody-targeted therapy against CD20-bearing B cells (Rituximab) is being used with increasing frequency, and success rates of 50% or more have been reported. Recent experimental studies with thrombopoietic agents have shown surprising activity in patients with ITP, and these may soon become available for refractory patients. The favorable effect of thrombopoietic agents in ITP supports experimental evidence of inappropriately low thrombopoietin levels and a platelet production deficiency that accompanies enhanced platelet clearance in this condition. It should be noted that although some patients with ITP have incomplete responses to all therapeutic modalities mentioned, many maintain a good quality of life with thrombocytopenia in the range of 30,000 to $60,000/\mu L$, without any specific therapy required. As a "last resort" for the severely refractory patients, immunosuppressive agents (e.g., vincristine, azathioprine, cyclophosphamide, cyclosporin A, and even combination chemotherapy) have been shown to be helpful in case reports. However, these have significantly greater toxicities, including myelosuppression and neurotoxicity.

Posttransfusion Purpura

Post-transfusion purpura is an uncommon alloimmune condition that results from exposure to blood products, most commonly, packed RBCs or platelets. It is typically seen in multiparous women or in heavily transfused men or women. In this situation, when transfusion recipients who lack the platelet antigen PL^{A-1} are exposed to PL^{A-1}-positive blood, a brisk anamnestic immune response to the antigen develops, and 5 to 7 days later, the patients become suddenly and profoundly thrombocytopenic. The mechanism of the acute platelet destruction is not well understood, but one hypothesis is that the transfused platelets expressing PL^{A-1} antigen adhere to the patient's PL^{A-1} negative platelets, which are then destroyed as innocent bystanders. The anti-PL^{A-1} antibody can be detected in the patient's plasma, and further transfusions are contraindicated unless they are specifically tested for PL^{A-1} negativity. The thrombocytopenia is usually severe, and bleeding is common. Treatment with corticosteroids and IVIG is usually effective in aborting the immune response.

Consumptive Thrombocytopenias

Thrombocytopenia can result from platelet consumption associated with severe traumatic hemorrhage and massive red cell transfusion, and platelet transfusions must be used in this scenario. Patients with massive bilateral venous thrombosis of the ileofemoral systems or with large aortic aneurysms may also develop a mild to moderate thrombocytopenia from localized platelet consumption. A group of syndromes associated with systemic microvascular thrombosis, including TTP, hemolytic uremic syndrome, HELLP syndrome, and DIC are also paradoxically associated with thrombocytopenia and are described in more detail later in this chapter.

Thrombotic Thrombocytopenia Purpura

TTP is an acute syndrome seen most commonly in younger patients, with women more commonly affected than men. The classic presentation consisting of the pentad of fever, thrombocytopenia, renal failure, neurologic symptoms, and microangiopathic hemolytic anemia is seen in only 40% of patients. The presence of severe thrombocytopenia with microangiopathic hemolytic anemia (i.e., schistocytes on peripheral blood smear and elevated serum lactate dehydrogenase [LDH]) are considered sufficient for diagnosis. Typically, on initial presentation, the PT and aPTT tests are normal, distinguishing TTP from severe DIC. The pathogenesis of TTP involves a deficiency of ADAMTS13, a vWF-cleaving protease that is required to process newly synthesized vWF molecules to their physiological form. Most commonly, the deficiency is due to circulating autoantibodies to the protease, but rare cases of hereditary deficiency states have been described. The decrease in protease activity results in ultra-large vWF multimers remaining in the circulation, and these in turn promote uncontrolled platelet adhesion and aggregation.

- The classic "pentad" of TTP is only present in 40% of patients at diagnosis.
- Thrombocytopenia, schistocytes on a peripheral smear, and an elevated LDH are considered sufficient for diagnosis, and plasmapheresis should be initiated.
- TTP occurs due to deficiencies of vWF-cleaving protease, ADAMTS13.
- Platelet transfusions in TTP are contraindicated, except in the case of life-threatening bleeding, because they are believed to "feed the fire" and usually result in a rapid clinical decline.

The schistocytes that form in this disease are a result of mechanical fragmentation of RBCs as they flow past intra-arteriolar platelet thrombi. The thrombocytopenia that develops in TTP can be severe, and patients often experience significant bleeding complications, even in the face of often severe microvascular thrombosis. Platelet transfusions in patients with TTP can be associated with a rapid clinical decline and are contraindicated unless bleeding is life threatening. Mortality approaches 100% in untreated TTP, but treatment with plasmapheresis to remove the ultra-large vWF multimers and plasma exchange with fresh-frozen plasma (FFP) to replenish vWF-cleaving proteases induces remission in nearly all patients with idiopathic TTP. Many patients with TTP relapse after successful treatment, but most can be treated successfully with repeated courses of plasmapheresis and exchange. Immunosuppressive therapies and splenectomy may be effective for patients with multiple relapses or who become refractory to plasmapheresis. TTP can also occur in association with drugs (ticlopidine and, less commonly, clopidogrel, quinine, and mitomycin C), severe lupus, HIV disease, pregnancy, and allogeneic organ transplantation. In drug-related cases, stopping the offending agent usually leads to remission. Transplant, HIV, and lupus-related TTP carry an extremely poor prognosis.

HELLP Syndrome

HELLP syndrome is a pregnancy-associated disorder in which **H**emolysis, **E**levated **L**iver enzymes, and **L**ow **P**latelets occur. It presents most frequently during the third trimester of pregnancy but will occasionally present earlier and, in about 30% of cases, can present postpartum. Patients complain of nausea, fatigue, and epigastric or right upper quadrant pain. A small portion of patients with pre-eclampsia can develop HELLP syndrome. The thrombocytopenia and hemolytic anemia seen in this disorder is generally more severe than is seen in pre-eclampsia. The cornerstone of treatment is delivery of the fetus, which typically halts the process rapidly. Occasionally, HELLP evolves into overt TTP following delivery; this scenario is life threatening and usually portends a poor outcome.

Hemolytic Uremic Syndrome

Hemolytic uremic syndrome is a TTP-like disorder in which renal signs and symptoms predominate, and neurologic signs are rare. It is most commonly seen in children who develop bloody diarrhea in response to *Escherichia coli* O157:H7 infection. In adults infected with *E. coli* O157:H7, renal involvement is less pronounced; however, although outcomes in children are very good and treatment is only supportive care, mortality in adults is much higher and, for this reason, should be treated with plasma exchange and hemodialysis.

Disseminated Intravascular Coagulation

Disseminated intravascular coagulation (DIC) is a complex, consumptive coagulopathy associated with a variety of medical and surgical disease states. DIC itself is not a disease, but like fever is a manifestation of an underlying disorder. It is an exaggerated, poorly controlled systemic response to illness in which procoagulant mechanisms are activated, intravascular fibrin is produced, small vessel thrombosis occurs, and ischemic organ damage results. A compensatory fibrinolysis develops, and combined with the exhaustion of coagulation factors and thrombocytopenia, a hemorrhagic diathesis may occur. Conditions associated with acute DIC include obstetric disorders such as abruption placenta and retained dead fetus, bacterial sepsis, massive tissue injury due to burns or trauma, and acute promyelocytic leukemia. Although acute DIC primarily presents as a hemorrhagic disorder, the bleeding results from coagulation factor deficiencies and thrombocytopenia caused by diffuse organ-based microvascular thromboses. A more indolent chronic DIC can be seen in patients with solid tumors, systemic vasculitic disorders, and large abdominal aortic aneurysms. In patients with DIC, the PT and aPTT are usually prolonged, fibrinogen levels are either low or found to be decreasing on serial measurements, and FDPs (e.g., D-dimer) are present in increased concentration in the circulation. Antithrombin, along with other natural anticoagulants, is also consumed, and thus these levels are also diminished. The TT is prolonged due to the presence of FDPs and low fibrinogen levels, and platelets are consumed, causing a thrombocytopenia that can be severe. Fibrin strands laid down in the microvasculature shear passing RBCs, causing microangiopathic hemolysis. The cornerstone of treatment for DIC is the identification and amelioration of the precipitating cause. Rapid reversal of the inciting event with supportive care may suffice. However, if bleeding occurs, transfusion of cryoprecipitate as a source of fibrinogen, FFP as a source of clotting factors, and platelets to correct the thrombocytopenia may be effective. The infusion of antithrombin concentrates in patients with severe DIC may be appropriate in some circumstances, but, unfortunately, these infusions are often begun too late to accomplish more than improvement in laboratory parameters without impacting patient outcome. Activated protein C concentrate has been used as an adjunctive treatment in patients with severe sepsis who exhibit DIC but who are not thrombocytopenic. In patients who have thrombotic events associated with chronic DIC, particularly in association with malignancy, warfarin therapy is often unsuccessful in preventing further events, and, in this situation, use of chronic heparin or LMWH should be considered.

Abnormalities of Vessel Walls and Subcutaneous Tissues

Ehlers-Danlos syndrome is a group of disorders caused by abnormal collagen synthesis. Patients with this syndrome exhibit fragile, velvety, stretchable skin and hyperextensible joints. They experience easy bruisability but rarely demonstrate severe bleeding complications. *Pseudoxanthoma elasticum* is a rare inherited defect in which the elastic fibers within the vessel wall become calcified. Calcified vessels rupture, causing severe gastrointestinal, genitourinary, and menstrual bleeding, and spontaneous retinal hemorrhages. Physical examination often reveals xanthomalike lesions over flexural regions such as neck and axilla, and angioid streaks in the retina. Close control of blood pressure and hypercholesterolemia is very important in these patients. Easy bruisability and the risk of postpartum hemorrhage are said to be increased in **Marfan's syndrome**, caused by a mutation in the fibrillin gene on chromosome 15. **Hereditary hemorrhagic telangiectasia** (HHT; formerly Osler-Weber-Rendu syndrome) is an autosomal dominantly inherited disorder resulting in a defect of endothelial cells in arterioles, venules, and capillaries. The disorder is characterized by multiple telangiectasias of the skin and mucous membranes that become evident as pa-

tients progress through puberty into young adulthood. It may result in significant bleeding complications. *Scurvy* is an acquired disorder of vitamin C deficiency, resulting in weakened and abnormal collagen. Patients exhibit perifollicular petechiae, easy bruisability, and poor wound healing. Patients at risk for scurvy are those at risk for other forms of malnutrition, for example, elderly patients with cognitive deficits, substance abusers, mentally ill patients, and people on unusual diets. Chronic steroid use can cause *steroid-induced purpura* due to thinning of the connective tissues. *Senile purpura* is the term used to describe easy bruisability in elderly patients in whom no specific defects in platelet function or coagulation factors are apparent. This condition is usually mild and due to skin fragility. It is more common in women than men and is associated with history of frequent sun exposure and tobacco use.

Patients with vascular purpura or structural abnormalities of the vessel wall or subcutaneous tissues often have normal laboratory values. Routine screening should include a platelet count, PT, and aPTT. If the diagnosis is not clear from the patient's history and physical examination, further studies of platelet function may be indicated. Management of patients with HHT is often difficult, for as the disease becomes more prominent through adulthood, blood loss from multiple sources occurs continuously and can be difficult to control. Appropriate iron replacement should be instituted to support an adequate production of red cells to keep up with continued losses. For patients who have a reversible disorder such as vitamin C deficiency, vitamin C supplementation of 200 to 500 mg daily should be recommended. Otherwise, patients should be cautioned against the use of aspirin and nonsteroidals, urged to try to avoid minor trauma, and offered reassurance.

DISORDERS OF SECONDARY HEMOSTASIS

Disorders of secondary hemostasis involve abnormalities of components of the coagulation cascades. Patients with disorders of secondary hemostasis generally have preserved platelet function and, therefore, although they experience muscle hematomas, hemarthroses, and excessive bleeding with severe trauma, significant blood loss from minor cuts or abrasions is unusual.

Inherited Disorders of Secondary Hemostasis

Hemophilia A (factor VIII deficiency) and **hemophilia B** (factor IX deficiency or Christmas disease) are both X-linked recessive disorders. As such, these hemophilias arise almost exclusively in males, with sons of male hemophiliacs having a normal phenotype and daughters being obligatory carriers of the trait. Women who are hemophilia carriers are usually asymptomatic but have a 50% chance of having an affected son and a 50% chance of having a carrier daughter. Women can only have true hemophilia A or B in the setting of Turner's syndrome (XO), unusual patterns of X chromosome inactivation (lyonization) in the liver, or if the father is a hemophiliac and the mother is a carrier. The incidence of hemophilia A and B is about 1:10,000 and 1:30,000 live male births, respectively. This disease has a relatively high spontaneous mutation rate, and as many as one-third of hemophiliacs may not have a family history of the disorder. The clinical severity of hemophilia A generally parallels the factor VIII activity level. Hemophiliacs with factor VIII activity levels of <1% are classified as severe, those with levels between 1% and 5% of normal as moderate, and those with levels >5% as mild. Patients with severe disease are often diagnosed in infancy due to frequent spontaneous bleeds into joints, muscles, and other organs. Patients with moderate to mild disease have less risk of unprovoked hemorrhage but still carry a significant risk of life-threatening hemorrhage with trauma or surgery. Due to repetitive episodes of hemarthroses, patients experience significant morbidity concomitant with the development of a chronic arthropathy ("target joint") from cartilage destruction. Intracranial hemorrhage accounts for 20% to 30% of deaths in hemophiliacs. Patients with suspected hemophilia are diagnosed based on an elevated aPTT and a normal PT and BT. The aPTT will correct completely when patient's plasma is mixed with normal plasma in a 1:1 ratio. Assays for specific coagulation factor activities can then be performed to make the definitive diagnosis. Treatment involves specific factor replacement. Although cryoprecipitate and FFP may still be used as a replacement source of factor VIII for patients with mild disease, virally inactivated, monoclonal antibody purified plasma-derived and recombinant factor VIII concentrates are the preferred therapeutic agents for most patients with hemophilia A. DDAVP can affect a rapid release of endogenously synthesized factor VIII from the Weibel-Palade bodies of endothelial cells, but due to development of tachyphylaxis, use of DDAVP is usually reserved for patients with mild hemophilia. Prophylactic factor VIII replacement therapy is used for patients undergoing surgical procedures and is now often provided to children to prevent devastating joint disease. In hemophilia B, both plasma-derived and recombinant factor IX concentrates are available in the United States. Advances in gene transfer technology hold promise as a means of converting some patients with severe hemophilia into less symptomatic moderate forms.

Factor XI deficiency (hemophilia C) is inherited in an autosomal recessive fashion and is more prevalent in persons of Ashkenazi Jewish descent. Patients with homozygous deficiency states have factor XI levels ranging from <1% in severe forms to ~20% in milder forms. Bleeding risk is extremely variable and, surprisingly, does not relate precisely to the levels of circulating factor XI. The best predictors of bleeding in patients with factor XI deficiency are a past history or family history of excessive bleeding with trauma, childbirth, or surgery (including dental

procedures). Patients who have undergone surgery successfully in the past without bleeding in the absence of factor replacement can probably be managed conservatively for future surgeries. When needed, FFP is used for factor XI replacement.

The major adverse effect of plasma-derived factor concentrates for all hemophilias has been the transmission of infectious viruses. A significant number of hemophilia patients who received factor replacement in the 1970s and 1980s were infected with HIV, hepatitis B virus, and hepatitis C virus (HCV). Current viral inactivation methods, combined with a generally safer blood supply, have practically eliminated the risk of HIV and HCV transmission. However, nonlipid-enveloped viruses, such as hepatitis A and parvovirus B19, have continued to be detected in these products, and for this reason, recombinant factor concentrates have gained popularity. Importantly, despite the fear of viral illness, bleeding remains the most significant source of morbidity and mortality in hemophilia patients not infected with HIV or HCV.

Hypofibrinogenemia/Dysfibrinogenemia

Fibrinogen is synthesized in the liver and is encoded for by three genes localized to chromosome 4. Null mutations in any of these genes can produce a hypofibrinogenemic state and a mild hemophilia. Homozygosity for null mutations can produce afibrinogenemia, which causes both platelet dysfunction (because fibrinogen is essential in platelet aggregation) and a coagulopathy. Most described mutations in fibrinogen genes result in the production of an abnormal fibrinogen molecule (dysfibrinogenemia). Some mutations produce molecules that are unable to polymerize to insoluble fibrin, in which case patients exhibit a bleeding diathesis. Treatment of hypofibrinogenemia or dysfibrinogenemia is reserved for episodes of uncontrolled bleeding or surgical prophylaxis and is generally accomplished by transfusion of cryoprecipitate. Rarely, mutations can render the fibrinogen molecule resistant to plasmin proteolysis and lead to a thrombotic phenotype.

Factor XIII deficiency is a rare autosomal recessive disorder in which factor XIII is produced in insufficient amounts, resulting in a fibrin clot that cannot be cross-linked and stabilized. Diagnosis of factor XIII deficiency is made by demonstrating increased solubility of a plasma clot when placed in 6M urea. Bleeding is typically delayed, occurring 24 hours after trauma or surgery, and patients often present shortly after birth with bleeding from the umbilical stump or circumcision site. Treatment of factor XIII deficiency is accomplished by infusions of cryoprecipitate, although purified factor may soon be available. Factor XIII has a very long circulating half-life, and infusions are generally effective for up to 1 month.

Fibrinolytic disorders are rare bleeding disorders in which increased plasmin activity leads to accelerated lysis of thrombi and unstable clots. Congenital deficiencies of the major inhibitor of the fibrinolytic cascade, α2-plasmin inhibitor, have been reported. Excess production of plasminogen activators can induce a profibrinolytic state and is seen occasionally in patients with urologic disorders and cancer.

Acquired Disorders of Secondary Hemostasis

Liver Disease

The bleeding disorder associated with liver disease is multifactorial in nature. The liver is the exclusive synthetic machinery for almost all coagulation factors, with the exception of vWF, factor VIII, and tPA. The liver also plays a role in clearing activated factors from the circulation and in producing the natural anticoagulants, antithrombin and protein C. A prolongation of the PT heralds the onset of hepatic failure. Factor VII has a very short half-life of about 6 hours, and a liver with deteriorating function cannot sustain adequate production of this rapidly disappearing factor. For this reason, in severe liver disease, the PT is the first to prolong. With worsening hepatic synthetic function, all factor levels decrease, and both PT and aPTT become prolonged. Treatment is complicated by the numerous defects of hemostasis. FFP contains all coagulation factors, but massive transfusions of FFP are generally required to correct a severe coagulopathy and often result in fluid overload.

Vitamin K Deficiency

Vitamin K–dependent gamma carboxylation of coagulation factors II, VII, IX, and X and proteins C, S, and Z is essential for their full activity. Vitamin K deficiency initially affects factor VII due to its short half-life and prolongs the PT, but as other factor levels decline, the aPTT will also lengthen. Vitamin K deficiency is seen in patients with malabsorption syndromes such as pancreatitis, short bowel syndrome, sprue, or small bowel states of bacterial overgrowth such as sometimes accompany use of broad-spectrum antibiotics. It can also be seen in patients with extremely poor dietary intake of green leafy vegetables. Certain drugs such as cholestyramine or mega doses of vitamins A and E can impede absorption or metabolism of vitamin K. Coagulopathy due to vitamin K deficiency can be distinguished from that due to liver failure or DIC by measuring the levels of three coagulation factors: a vitamin K–dependent factor (e.g., factor IX), a non–vitamin K–dependent factor (e.g., factor V), and a nonhepatic synthesized factor (factor VIII). If levels of all three are low, the diagnosis is most likely DIC. If factor VIII is normal, but the other two are low, liver failure is likely. If factor VIII and V are both normal and factor IX is low, the likely diagnosis is vitamin K deficiency. Dietary deficiencies of vitamin K can be easily replenished with daily oral supplementation of 5 to 10 mg (Fig. 21.4 and Table 21.1). However, in patients with malabsorption syndromes, the subcutaneous route should be considered. The most common cause of fully functional vitamin K deficiency is the therapeutic use of *oral anticoagulant drugs* of the coumarin family, such as

	Liver Disease	DIC	Vit K deficiency
Factor IX	↓	↓	↓
Factor VIII	normal	↓	normal
Factor V	↓	↓	normal

Figure 21.4 Diagnostic approach to patient with elevated prothrombin time/activated partial thromboplastin time. Measuring the activities of a hepatic synthesized vitamin K–dependent coagulation factor (factor IX); a non–vitamin K–dependent, hepatic synthesized factor (factor V); and a nonhepatic, non–vitamin K–dependent factor (factor VIII) allows one to distinguish liver failure, disseminated intravascular coagulation, and vitamin K deficiency.

warfarin. These agents inhibit vitamin K epoxide reductase, thus preventing regeneration of the active, reduced form of the vitamin. If a patient taking warfarin is bleeding, or if the effects of warfarin need to be rapidly reversed as in the case of need for emergent surgery, FFP can be given to immediately restore coagulation factor levels and normalize the PT. Dosing of FFP is based on the formula described in the next paragraph. A patient with a greater than target PT/INR from warfarin who is not bleeding can be approached in two ways. Either warfarin can be withheld, allowing the PT/INR to drift slowly into the target range, or a small dose of vitamin K (1–2 mg) can be given orally to bring the PT/INR to therapeutic range more rapidly. Vitamin K can also be given intravenously (IV), although there is a small risk of anaphylactoid reactions. Coagulation factor levels begin to improve within a few hours of an IV dose of vitamin K.

Dose calculations of FFP or coagulation factor concentrates to reverse coagulopathy are based on plasma volume (PV) determined by the patient's weight and hematocrit using the formula:

$$\text{(Desired factor level (U/mL)} - \text{Current level)} \times \text{PV}$$
$$= \text{Volume of FFP (mL) to be infused}$$

The PV is calculated as

$$(40 \text{ mL/kg} \times \text{Wt}) \times (1 - \text{Hct})/(1 - 0.44)$$

For a patient whose INR is within the target range of 2 to 3 or higher, the effective current level of factor VII can

TABLE 21.1

DIFFERENCE BETWEEN VITAMIN K DEFICIENCY, LIVER FAILURE, AND DISSEMINATED INTRAVASCULAR COAGULATION

A minimum of three coagulation factors should be measured:
- Vitamin K–dependent factor (e.g., factor IX)
- Non–vitamin K–dependent factor (e.g., factor V)
- Nonhepatic synthesized factor (e.g., factor VIII)

be considered 0 to 0.05. The target level depends on the clinical circumstances; for life-threatening hemorrhage or emergency surgery, correction to 100% is reasonable (i.e., 1 U/mL), whereas for lesser degrees of bleeding or postoperative states, correction to 50% is usually adequate. Thus, for an 80-kg man with an INR of 4.0 and a hematocrit of 30%, the amount of FFP needed to restore factor levels to 50% would be

$$(0.5\,\text{U/mL} - 0.05) \times [(40\,\text{mL/kg} \times 80\,\text{kg}) \times \\ (1 - 0.3/1 - 0.44)] = 1{,}800\,\text{mL}\ (\text{i.e.,} \sim 7\text{–}8\,\text{U of FFP})$$

Factor VII has the shortest half-life of the coagulation factors (about 6 hours), so dosing needs to be repeated at frequent intervals until the bleeding stops or, in the case of warfarin reversal, until vitamin K has been repleted or warfarin eliminated from the body. This same formula can be used to calculate FFP requirements for patients with liver failure and to calculate coagulation factor concentrate doses in patients with hemophilia.

Acquired Inhibitors of the Coagulation Cascade

One of the most devastating adverse effects of factor VIII replacement is the development *factor VIII inhibitors*, which are neutralizing alloantibodies which develop because the immune system recognizes the replacement factor as a foreign protein. Interestingly, patients with hemophilia B rarely develop inhibitors, whereas inhibitors develop in ~20% of hemophilia A patients after as few as 9 to 30 exposures to replacement therapy. These occur predominantly in the pediatric population and are treated with various strategies, including use of high doses of factor VIII, "bypass" agents such as recombinant factor VIIa (NovoSeven) or an activated prothrombin complex concentrate, and/or immunosuppression.

Occasionally, factor VIII inhibitors arise de novo as autoantibodies in patients with no prior history of hemophilia. This disorder is rare but potentially lethal and is seen most typically in elderly patients and in the postpartum period. Patients with factor VIII inhibitors demonstrate an aPTT, which either corrects transiently or does not correct during a mixing study. Generally, the first line of therapy is immunosuppression with corticosteroids. If patients are actively bleeding, quantifying the inhibitor by obtaining a titer using a modification of the aPTT called the Bethesda assay helps determine treatment options. Patients with titers of <5 to 10 Bethesda U/mL can be treated with factor VIII concentrates, although larger initial and maintenance doses than used in hemophilia A may be necessary. When the titer of the factor inhibitor exceeds 10 Bethesda U/mL, factor VIII concentrates alone may not correct the coagulopathy; in this situation, bypass agents should be considered.

An unusual but severe coagulopathy has been described in postoperative patients exposed to intraoperative "fibrin glue." Some of these preparations contain bovine factor V and/or thrombin, and following exposure to this product alloantibodies are formed that cross-react with human proteins.

Recombinant factor VIIa (NovoSeven) has been used "off-label" as a general hemostatic agent in situations of severe surgical or traumatic bleeding or other life-threatening hemorrhagic states not responsive to conventional therapy. Because VIIa is active only when complexed to TF, its action is limited to sites of vascular injury or developing thrombi, and therefore, the risk of systemic thrombosis associated with its use is limited. Nevertheless, it is important to note that use of recombinant factor VII for these indications has not been validated by controlled trials and is not approved by the U.S. Food and Drug Administration.

THROMBOTIC DISORDERS

Thrombophilia refers to any inherited or acquired abnormality of the hemostatic system that places a person at increased risk for developing venous or arterial thromboses. Among the most important of these risk factors is age; the risk of VTE increases exponentially beginning at about age 55 years, and by age 80 years, incidence rates are nearly 1/100 per year, about 1,000-fold higher than for those age 45 years or younger. Other important risk factors are tobacco use, obesity, cancer, diabetes, heart failure, pregnancy and the puerperium, trauma, surgery (especially orthopedic and neurologic), hospitalization for serious medical illness, immobility, indwelling venous catheters, and certain pharmacologic agents, including estrogens and cancer chemotherapy. Pathophysiological mechanisms underlying VTE were described in the 19th century by Virchow as a "triad" of vascular injury, venous stasis, and inherent problems of blood fluidity. We know now that vascular injury can include endothelial cell "activation" by cytokines or components of pathogens, and that blood fluidity is influenced by a delicate balance among a large array of pro- and anticoagulant molecules. Studies of patients with inherited thrombophilias have led to a model in which even subtle perturbations of this balance can increase thrombotic risk by severalfold.

Usually, it is the interaction of several risk factors and not one alone that tips the regulatory balance resulting in thromboses. Any approach to the hypercoagulable patient should include a comprehensive clinical evaluation, not only to guide acute thrombosis management and screen patients for an underlying malignancy, but also to help determine which patient will benefit most from special coagulation laboratory testing. This evaluation should include an assessment of risk factors described previously and prior history or family history of thrombosis or recurrent fetal loss. Knowledge of a patient's age at time of first thrombosis; the location of the thrombosis; and whether the thromboses involved the venous system, arterial vascular tree, or both are also important pieces of information.

Indications for a full evaluation for an inherited defect in a patient with VTE are controversial and may include:

- A single unprovoked thrombotic event
- Recurrent thrombotic events
- A strong family history of thromboembolic disease or a family member with a known history of a hypercoagulable disorder
- Thrombosis in an unusual site (e.g., cerebral venous sinus, retinal vein, or portal/mesenteric veins)
- History of recurrent, otherwise unexplainable miscarriages

Testing should be avoided during an acute episode of thrombosis because protein levels may be transiently low as a result of consumption, and anticoagulants may interfere with testing results.

SPECIFIC HYPERCOAGULABLE STATES

Factor V Leiden is a mutation in the factor V gene creating a substitution of glutamine for arginine at position 506. This produces a factor V molecule that cannot be fully cleaved by APC, hence the condition is also called the "syndrome of activated protein C resistance." The prevalence of the mutation in the general population is highly variable, being highest (5%) in persons of northern European descent, but rare in persons of Hispanic, African, or Asian heritage. Patients who are homozygous for the abnormality generally have a strong family history, a higher risk of VTE, and may present at a young age. Heterozygous individuals have a four- to sixfold increased risk of VTE. Women with factor V Leiden have an increased risk of fetal loss. Although thromboses in unusual sites such as the cerebral vein are described, unprovoked deep vein thrombosis (DVT) or DVT in the setting of pregnancy or estrogen use is still the most common presentation.

Prothrombin gene mutation is a point mutation (G20210A) in the 3' untranslated region of the prothrombin gene on chromosome 11 is associated with a three- to fivefold increased risk of VTE, probably as a result of modest elevation in plasma prothrombin levels. Prothrombin levels are not, however, a reliable means of diagnosing this disorder. This mutation is more common in Caucasian populations.

Antithrombin deficiency is inherited as an autosomal dominant disorder with heterozygous patients having antithrombin levels between 40% and 70% of normal. The abnormality is classified as type 1 if there is a decrease in the amount of the protein and as type 2 if the protein is dysfunctional (i.e., unable to bind to heparin). The trait increases the risk of thrombosis by 10- to 20-fold, and unusual sites of thromboses such as the cavernous sinus or brachial and mesenteric veins are not uncommon. Acquired antithrombin deficiency can occur in DIC or heparin administration, or with the use of the chemotherapeutic agent L-asparaginase. Treatment options include replacement therapy with antithrombin concentrates.

Protein C deficiency and protein S deficiency are autosomal dominant disorders. The homozygous states are associated with neonatal purpura fulminans, which is fatal within the first hours of life if not treated. Heterozygous individuals have variable presentation, with some developing recurrent venous thromboembolism beginning in the second to third decades of life. Diagnosis of protein S deficiency is difficult because 50% to 60% of protein S circulates in an inactive complex bound to C4b-binding protein, but it is free protein S levels that correlate best with thrombotic risk. C4b-binding protein is an acute phase reactant, and patients may develop functional deficiency of free protein S in the setting of chronic or acute inflammatory conditions. Protein C and S levels may also become low during pregnancy, nephrotic syndrome, DIC, and the use of warfarin and oral contraceptives.

Individuals with *persistently elevated levels of procoagulant proteins*, including coagulation *factors VIII, IX, XI,* and *prothrombin* are at two- to threefold increased risk for VTE. Many of these syndromes are likely to have a genetic component, but the details remain to be discovered. It is important to note that coagulation factor levels are influenced by acute thrombosis and by acute inflammatory states, so it is not helpful to measure them in the setting of an acute VTE.

Antiphospholipid antibody (APLA) syndrome is an autoimmune disorder characterized by the presence of circulating antibodies reactive with phospholipid-binding proteins and a constellation of clinical signs and symptoms that include arterial and/or venous thrombosis and/or recurrent fetal loss. APLAs are most commonly detected by enzyme-linked immunosorbent assay (ELISA) assays using cardiolipin as the antigen, but reactivity in fact is directed against specific proteins, such as prothrombin, protein C, or β_2-glycoprotein-I. Some APLAs prolong phospholipid-dependent coagulation tests, such as the aPTT or the more sensitive dilute Russel viper venom time (dRVVT), in which case they are known as "lupus anticoagulants" (LACs). Diagnosis of LACs is confirmed by showing that the prolonged clotting times do not correct when patient plasma is mixed 1:1 with normal plasma, but do correct when the patient plasma is adsorbed by incubation with purified phospholipids. In most cases, the anticoagulant activity of LAC is an in vitro artifact, although patients with LAC will occasionally demonstrate a bleeding diathesis. These cases are almost always associated with prolonged PT and with the presence of antiprothrombin antibodies. Not all APLAs have LAC activity, and not all LAC antibodies react positively in ELISA assays, so diagnostic testing requires both ELISA and LAC assays. Although APLAs are present in 5% to 15% of patients with SLE, they can also be seen in other clinical conditions, including malignancies, drug reactions (procainamide, quinidine, chlorpromazine), and HIV infection, and in otherwise healthy individuals. In the latter case, the syndrome is called primary APLA syndrome

(PAPS). In persons with an APLA who are asymptomatic, no specific therapy is required. The presence of APLA in a patient with idiopathic VTE is associated with high risk of recurrent thrombosis after discontinuing warfarin therapy, and for this reason, it is usually recommended that such patients receive long-term warfarin therapy. Women with APLA syndrome and recurrent spontaneous abortions are often managed with heparin-based anticoagulation during pregnancy to improve pregnancy outcome, even in the absence of a history of VTE. Thrombotic risk in APLA syndrome correlates with the titer and isotype of the antibody, with IgG antibodies carrying much more risk than immunoglobin M. The presence of LAC activity is also associated with increased risk.

Homocysteine is an intermediate product of methionine metabolism. It is converted to methionine by the B_{12}- and folate-dependent methylene-tetrahydrofolate reductase (MTHFR) enzyme or to cysteine by the B_6-dependent cystathionine-β-synthase. When one of these pathways is disrupted, an increase in homocysteine levels occurs. **Hyperhomocysteinemia** can be genetic due to common polymorphisms in MTHFR (C677T resulting in thermolabile MTHFR) or rare mutations in cystathionine-β-synthase, or acquired due to deficiencies of vitamin $B_{12,}$ folate, or $B_6.$ Hyperhomocysteinemia is associated with increased risk of both arterial and venous thrombosis, although the mechanisms underlying this risk are not known. Interestingly, even though supplementation of vitamins B_{12} and B_6, and particularly folate, has been shown to decrease levels of homocysteine, studies have not shown a corresponding decrease in thrombotic risk.

All malignancies confer an increased thrombotic tendency, but certain malignancies such as adenocarcinomas of the pancreas, colon, stomach, and ovaries, as well as primary brain tumors, are especially associated with thromboembolic events. Several prospective studies have shown that up to 10% to 15% of patients presenting with an otherwise unexplainable VTE have an underlying malignancy, but the utility of performing an extensive cancer search beyond standard age-appropriate screening in such patients has not been demonstrated. The pathogenesis of the thrombotic tendency is multifactorial in nature and, in some cases, may relate to release of procoagulant factors and microparticles from the tumor itself. Factors such as immobilization with blood stasis, tumor-related vascular compression, indwelling catheters, surgery, vascular toxic chemotherapy, and infection are also important contributors. Cancer-related thrombosis can be difficult to treat, and recent studies suggest that LMWHs may be more effective than warfarin for secondary prevention.

Bone marrow disorders such as paroxysmal nocturnal hemoglobinuria (PNH), polycythemia vera (PCV), and essential thrombocythemia (ET) predispose to arterial and venous thrombosis, including thrombi in unusual sites. The majority of individuals who develop an idiopathic portal vein or mesenteric vein thrombosis have one of these conditions. Aspirin is now standard of care for patients with PCV and ET, even in the absence of prior thrombotic events because of the high risk of arterial thrombosis. Chronic warfarin anticoagulation may be advocated in persons with PNH.

The pathogenesis of *HIT* involves formation of multi-molecular complexes between heparin and platelet factor 4 (PF4), a platelet α-granule protein that is released by platelets when they are activated. In some individuals exposed to heparin, IgG class antibodies are generated against this complex, which then binds to immunoglobulin Fc receptors expressed on platelets, leukocytes, and endothelial cells. This, in turn, leads to activation of these cells, followed by release of additional procoagulants and a marked increase in thrombin generation and platelet aggregation. Paradoxically, this leads to increased clearance of platelets with resultant thrombocytopenia, and a highly thrombogenic environment with increased risk for both arterial and venous thrombosis. Left untreated, as many as 50% of patients will develop clinically significant thrombi. A very modest fall in platelet count is common in the first few days of exposure to unfractionated heparin due to passive binding of heparin to platelets, causing a transient shortening of the platelet life span. This is clinically insignificant and should not be confused with the far more severe form of immune-mediated HIT (or HIT with thrombosis [HITT]). This syndrome typically develops between 5 and 14 days after starting heparin therapy. *A more than 50% drop in platelet count, even if the total platelet count is within normal limits, can signal the development of a heparin-induced antibody and mandates urgent action.* A drop in platelet count before day 5 of heparin exposure is unlikely to be HIT unless the patient has a recent prior exposure to heparin (within 3 months). Both functional and antigenic assays are available to detect HIT-IgG antibodies. These include platelet serotonin release assays and ELISA-based assays for heparin-dependent anti-PF4 antibodies. Both false-positive and false-negative results can occur, and for this reason, clinical diagnosis remains the "gold standard." Once diagnosed, all forms of heparin, including LMWHs, IV catheter flushes, and heparin-coated indwelling catheters, should be immediately discontinued, and because of the significant risk of a major thromboembolic event, therapy with a direct thrombin inhibitor such as lepirudin or argatroban should be started. DVT is the most frequently encountered thrombotic complication, followed by pulmonary embolism, cerebral sinus thrombosis, and adrenal vein thrombosis. Arterial thromboses, although less common than venous thromboses, do occur, and usually involve the extremities; however, stroke, myocardial infarction, and renal artery thrombosis have also been described. The direct thrombin inhibitors (DTIs) have a short half-life, effectively inactivate clot-bound thrombus, and can be monitored using the aPTT assay. Lepirudin, a recombinant protein, can induce clearance-inhibiting antibody production in up to 40% of patients and must be used with great care in the setting of even mild renal insufficiency. Argatroban is a synthetic lysine analog that does not cross-react with heparin, has a shorter half-life than lepirudin, can be monitored by the aPTT assay, and does not induce antibody formation. It is also safe in the setting of renal insufficiency but should be avoided in the setting of significant liver dysfunction. Warfarin anticoagulation should be discontinued during the acute phase of HIT because its use has been associated with severe skin and soft tissue necrosis. Considering the complexity of HIT diagnosis and treatment, early detection and HIT prevention must be emphasized. Patients receiving unfractionated heparin should have platelet count monitoring at baseline and then every third day between days 5 and 21 of heparin exposure. Surgical patients and patients with active atherosclerotic disease are at highest risk, probably because of chronic low levels of platelet activation and PF4 release. Patients with a history of HIT should not be re-exposed to heparin within 3 months of last exposure or if anti-PF4 antibody is still detectable.

TREATMENT OF VENOUS THROMBOEMBOLISM

Acute management involves immediate initiation of treatment with heparin or a heparin derivative, which should overlap by at least 5 days with a variable course of chronic treatment with oral anticoagulation, typically warfarin. For patients with severe iliofemoral DVT or massive pulmonary embolism, thrombolytic therapy can be effective at restoring blood flow and minimizing long-term sequelae. Combinations of pharmacologic agents (e.g., tPA) with catheter-based mechanical approaches are now readily available. The targets of the currently available antithrombotic agents are shown in **Figure 21.5**. Heparin acts as a potent activator of antithrombin, thus inhibiting factors IXa, Xa, and IIA, with a rapid onset of action but a short duration of activity. This makes it ideal for initial anticoagulation. Dosing

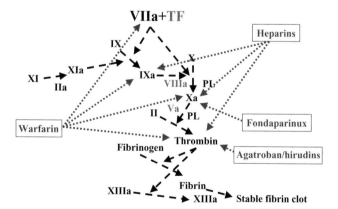

Figure 21.5 Anticoagulant drugs and their targets. Unfractionated heparin and low molecular weight heparins activate antithrombin (AT) and inhibit IX, Xa, and IIA. Warfarin, by inhibiting the vitamin K cycle, inhibits VII, IX, X, and II (but also inhibits anticoagulant proteins C, S, and Z). Fondaparinux is an AT-dependent inhibitor of Xa, and argatroban, lepirudin, and bivalirudin are direct thrombin inhibitors. (See Color Fig. 21.5.)

for hospitalized patients is typically initiated as a bolus of 80 U/kg in order to saturate all the binding sites, thereby allowing free heparin in the plasma to bind to and catalyze antithrombin activity. A continuous infusion of 16 to 18 U/kg/hour following the initial bolus maintains the balance between free and bound heparin. The aPTT is a simple and accurate measure of heparin activity, and most institutions have initiated a heparin dosing nomogram that guides titration of the dose until a therapeutic aPTT is achieved. It is important to monitor the platelet count for HIT in patients receiving more than 5 days of heparin. LMWH preparations and the pentasaccharide fondaparinux are at least as effective as unfractionated heparin for initial treatment of VTE, but have more predictable pharmacodynamics and pharmacokinetics. They can thus be safely administered subcutaneously once or twice daily without need for monitoring aPTT. For these reasons, treatment of most patients with uncomplicated VTE can now be accomplished in the outpatient setting. The antifactor Xa activity of LMWH exceeds their antithrombin activity by two- to threefold, and therefore, these agents generally do not cause a rise in aPTT. However, the risk of bleeding is similar to that of unfractionated heparin. It is important to be aware that LMWH remains active for 12 to 24 hours and that neither protamine nor FFP can fully reverse the effect. Also, LMWH is cleared renally, and therefore, patients with renal insufficiency require a dose adjustment in order to prevent excessive anticoagulation.

Patients with acute VTE require a period of long-term anticoagulation to prevent clot propagation and recurrent VTE. Oral warfarin, which inhibits synthesis of the vitamin K–dependent factors II, VII, IX, and X, is usually the drug of choice. Because it has no effect on proteins already carboxylated by vitamin K, full anticoagulation does not occur until the supply of functional factors has been exhausted, typically 5 to 7 days. Paradoxically, warfarin can promote clot formation due to its initial effect in decreasing the production of fully functional natural anticoagulant protein C. Patients with pre-existing deficiency of protein C are at particular risk and are prone to develop the syndrome of warfarin skin necrosis as a consequence. Patients with lower extremity DVT should be encouraged to resume physical activity as soon as feasible and to wear compression hose to minimize the degree of postphlebitic syndrome. This can be a debilitating condition with episodes of pain and swelling and is difficult to treat once established.

The data regarding ideal duration of therapy for DVT are variable, but recent studies suggest that a longer duration of anticoagulation after initial DVT may be associated with fewer recurrences. For a first episode of DVT, recommended duration of anticoagulation is usually 6 to 12 months. Risk factors for thrombosis should be assessed for and eliminated if feasible. However, if a second episode occurs, the general recommendation is that anticoagulation should be continued for at least 12 months and perhaps indefinitely.

REVIEW EXERCISES

QUESTIONS

1. At 2:00 am, a young woman presents to the emergency department of a small rural community hospital complaining of headache and fever. Except for some pallor, mild scleral icterus, and sleepiness, the physical exam is normal. The complete blood count report comes back with "low platelets" and a hematocrit of 28%. The prothrombin time/activated partial thromboplastin time and electrolytes are normal. The lab sends down the peripheral smear, which you examine under the microscope (Fig. 21.6).

The next best step is

a) Immediate broad-spectrum antibiotics for probable meningococcal sepsis

b) Platelet transfusions to control a probable intracerebral bleed

c) High-dose steroids for probable autoimmune thrombocytopenia with autoimmune hemolytic anemia (Evan's syndrome)

d) Immediate transfusions of fresh-frozen plasma

Answer and Discussion

The answer is d. The diagnosis of thrombocytopenia purpura (TTP) is easily made given the clear evidence of microangiopathic hemolysis (arrows show schistocytes on blood smear) associated with thrombocytopenia, fever, and neurologic signs/symptoms. With this degree of thrombocytopenia and hemolysis, a normal prothrombin time/activated partial thromboplastin time effectively rules out disseminated intravascular coagulation, thus making sepsis unlikely. Autoimmune hemolytic anemia does not produce schistocytes, but rather produces spherocytes. Platelet transfusions are relatively contraindicated in TTP because of their potential to aggravate thrombosis. Ideally, the patient

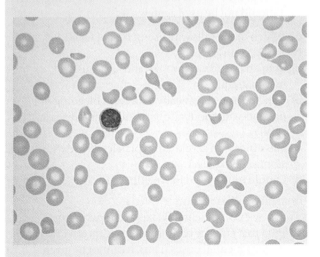

Figure 21.6   Platelets.

should receive plasmapheresis with fresh-frozen plasma (FFP) replacement; however, in the emergency setting in a rural emergency department, the first available treatment is transfusion with large volumes of FFP while making arrangements for transfer to an institution that can perform apheresis.

2. An asymptomatic 59-year-old woman was referred to you for preoperative clearance for a planned open colectomy. The routine laboratory examinations were all normal except for an elevated activated partial thromboplastin time (aPTT) of 57 seconds. She denied any history of excess bleeding or bruising. The lab calls you the next day to inform you that when they mixed her plasma 1:1 with pooled normal plasma, the aPTT was 43 seconds, normal being <31 seconds. Which of the following is most likely true?

a) The story is most consistent with mild von Willebrand disease, and the patient should be treated preoperatively with DDAVP (desmopressin).

b) The most likely diagnosis is "lupus anticoagulant," and the patient needs to receive perioperative thromboprophylactic therapy because of the increased risk of venous thromboembolism.

c) The woman likely has congenital factor XI deficiency and needs to have fresh-frozen plasma administered prior to surgery.

d) The woman most likely has an acquired, autoimmune factor VIII inhibitor and needs aggressive immune suppressive therapy prior to surgery.

Answer and Discussion

The answer is b. The aPTT would correct to normal if the patient had von Willebrand disease or congenital factor XI deficiency because the aPTT prolongs only if factor levels drop below ~40% of normal. Acquired factor VIII inhibitors are almost always associated with severe bleeding and bruising. Thus, the likely scenario here is lupus anticoagulant, a finding seen with the antiphospholipid syndrome. This is a significant risk factor for thrombosis, and the additional prothrombotic stress of general surgery mandates thromboprophylaxis.

3. Mr. Jones is a 77-year-old retired steel worker who is widowed and lives alone in a two-story house. He was brought to the emergency room (ER) by his daughter because of an extremely painful, swollen, red right leg. He believed that maybe he twisted his knee while walking down the stairs in his home, but when the pain and swelling did not improve after 24 hours and the swelling extended up into his thigh, he called his daughter who immediately brought him to the ER. A physical examination revealed normal vital signs; mild degenerative joint disease; and a swollen, erythematous right leg. A duplex Doppler was performed and revealed a large occlusive thrombus extending from the popliteal vein to the iliofemoral system. Chest x-ray and ECG were normal, and the physician in the infirmary gave him a prescription for enoxaparin and warfarin and referred him to your office. You saw him 3 days later, at which time his international normalized ratio was 2.8. You take a detailed history and discover that he has been feeling "poorly" for about 2 months. He notices a definite loss of energy, decreased appetite, and constipation. Physical examination reveals a rather frail elderly man with muscle wasting in the temporal region. Prostate is 3+ enlarged but without nodules. Stool is negative for occult blood. The remainder of the exam is negative except for the right leg, which is still swollen and tender, although no longer red. The most appropriate course of action at this point is to

a) Obtain colonoscopy.
b) Stop the enoxaparin because his international normalized ratio is now therapeutic.
c) Obtain thrombophilia panel, including factor V Leiden assay, to guide decision on duration of anticoagulation.
d) Obtain plasma anti-Xa assay to assess enoxaparin dosing because his leg is still swollen and tender.

Answer and Discussion

The answer is a. An underlying malignancy is the most likely etiology of his thrombophilia, and the presence of an inherited or other acquired thrombophilia is not likely to influence therapeutic decisions. Randomized trials showed that heparin therapy should always be extended for at least 5 days in patients with venous thromboembolism, even if the international normalized ratio (INR) is therapeutic. In fact, newer studies suggest that low molecular weight heparins are more effective than warfarin in long-term treatment of cancer-associated venous thrombosis. In this case, the rapid INR response is probably due to underlying vitamin K deficiency from malnutrition. Resolution of symptoms from severe deep vein thrombosis can take many days; persistent swelling at day 3 is not an indication of inadequate heparin effect.

4. Which of the following bleeding disorders can be present despite normal screening coagulation studies (PT, aPTT, and PFA-100)?

a) Mild von Willebrand disease
b) Mild hemophilia
c) Factor XIII deficiency
d) α-Antiplasmin deficiency
e) All of the above

Answer and Discussion

The answer is e. Mild coagulation factor deficiencies can be difficult to diagnosis because the screening assays are sensitive only to levels below 30% to 40% of

normal. Disorders of clot stability, including fibrinolysis defects (e.g., α2-antiplasmin deficiency) and abnormal fibrin clot cross-linking (factor XIII deficiency), will not affect prothrombin time or activated partial thromboplastin time. Von Willebrand factor levels fluctuate greatly and are sensitive to estrogen levels and acute inflammation so that platelet screening tests can be normal in patients with mild von Willebrand disease.

5. A 56-year-old man has an uneventful mitral valve replacement surgery. Heparin was given during the procedure and continued postoperatively. On the eighth postoperative day, he develops a painful, cold, pulseless leg. His activated partial thromboplastin time is subtherapeutic at 39 seconds. His platelet count is $55,000/\mu L$ (112,000 on postop day 1). The most important next step in his management is to

a) Obtain a vascular surgery consultation for revascularization.
b) Increase the dose of heparin to obtain a therapeutic activated partial thromboplastin time.
c) Perform platelet transfusion to increase count to $>100,000/\mu L$.
d) Discontinue all heparin immediately.
e) Begin warfarin and order anti-PF4 antibody test so that heparin can be safely stopped if the test is positive.

Answer and Discussion

The answer is d. If heparin-induced thrombocytopenia (HIT) is suspected, as it should be in this case of acute thrombosis in the setting of a 50% drop in platelet count, then it is critical to stop all heparin (including catheter flushes immediately) and initiate therapy with a direct thrombin inhibitor. Giving more heparin or infusing platelets are associated with worse outcomes. Vascular surgery may be helpful, but not before stopping the heparin. Warfarin has been associated with cutaneous thrombosis and necrosis in the setting of HIT and should not be used acutely.

6. Which of the following is not true of DDAVP (desmopressin)?

a) Is an analog of vasopressin and can cause hyponatremia
b) Can be given chronically to prevent bleeding in patients with moderate von Willebrand disease (vWD)
c) Has efficacy in several mild platelet disorders, such as storage pool defect
d) Should not be used in type IIb vWD

Answer and Discussion

The answer is b. Tachyphylaxis occurs with this drug so that efficacy typically disappears after two or three sequential doses. Thus, it cannot be given chronically. DDAVP can cause thrombosis and/or thrombocytopenia in patients with type IIB vWD and, thus, should not be used in that setting.

7. A 22-year-old sexually active college student is referred to you from the Student Health Service because of a low platelet count ($18,000/\mu L$) that was discovered when a complete blood count (CBC) was obtained to evaluate a rash on her lower extremities. She has been feeling otherwise well, but has noted some gum bleeding when she brushes her teeth over the past few days. She takes no medications other than a multivitamin. She had a normal CBC at the time of her college physical. The following would be an appropriate next step:

a) Immediately obtain bone marrow aspirate.
b) Begin therapy with intravenous immunoglobin G because her platelet count is so low.
c) Send out tests for hepatitis C and HIV.
d) Send out tests to rule out systemic lupus erythematosus.

Answer and Discussion

The answer is c. The most likely diagnosis is idiopathic/immune-mediated thrombocytopenic purpura (ITP), and in a young woman with no other likely cause of thrombocytopenia, a bone marrow aspirate is not necessary. Intravenous immunoglobin is not considered first-line therapy in the absence of major bleeding; rather, prednisone at 1 mg/kg/day would be the preferred medical therapy. Although lupus is associated with ITP, finding a positive ANA or anti-DNA would not change management. HIV and hepatitis C are not uncommon causes of ITP in young, sexually active patients and should always be ruled out.

8. You are called to the surgical intensive care unit to consult on a case of a 60-year-old chronic alcoholic who was admitted with a severe gastrointestinal bleed. After resuscitation with 4 units of packed red blood cells, he was noted to have a hemoglobin of 11 g/dL, an activated partial thromboplastin time (aPTT) of 90 seconds, a prothrombin time (PT) of 24 seconds, a platelet count of 90,000, and a bilirubin of 12. The lab reported that a 50:50 mix of his plasma with pooled normal plasma corrected both the aPTT and PT to normal. Appropriate therapeutic interventions include

a) Transfuse 2 units of fresh-frozen plasma now and repeat every 8 hours.
b) Administer low-dose heparin to stop the DIC process.
c) Administer high-dose steroids to raise the platelet count.
d) None of the above.

Answer and Discussion

The answer is d. This patient has a profound coagulopathy, likely due to hepatic failure, although a component of vitamin K deficiency could also be present.

There is no evidence to support disseminated intravascular coagulation. The modest thrombocytopenia is probably multifactorial in origin, including splenomegaly from portal hypertension and alcohol-related marrow toxicity; high-dose steroids are not likely to have a significant effect. The appropriate treatment is transfusion of fresh-frozen plasma, but he will need far more than 2 units to correct his severe factor deficiency, and dosing every 8 hours will not be adequate.

9. Ms. Smith is an 82-year-old widow who lives alone and has been brought to your emergency department by her niece who notes that her aunt has been "failing" for the past 2 to 3 months. Other than long-standing hypertension, the medical history is noncontributory. Physical examination reveals a sleepy, thin elderly woman with pedal edema, blood pressure of 190/110 mm Hg, and S3 gallop. Laboratory values are remarkable for hemoglobin of 7 g/dL, creatinine of 9.2, and blood urea nitrogen of 123. That evening, she develops a severe nose bleed that requires packing by the ear/nose/throat service and also notices bleeding external hemorrhoids. Which of the following can be used to improve her hemostasis?

a) Aggressive dialysis to resolve her uremic state
b) Packed red blood cell transfusion and erythropoietin to bring her hemoglobin to > 10 g/dL
c) Intravenous desmopressin
d) High doses of estrogen
e) All of the above

Answer and Discussion

The answer is e. Uremia is associated with a moderate to severe multifactorial bleeding diathesis that can be improved with dialysis and that responds partially to pharmacologic intervention with DDAVP (desmopressin) (can only be used acutely) or estrogen (can be used more chronically). One function of red blood cells is to "push" platelets to the outer edge of the column of flowing blood, maximizing their interaction with the vascular wall. Thus, the bleeding time is negatively influenced by severe anemia and can be improved by treating the anemia.

10. You are asked to see a 62-year-old man who is 4 days status post elective total hip replacement. He has been treated since the night before surgery with enoxaparin, 40 mg/day, but now has developed a symptomatic deep vein thrombosis on the same side as the surgery. Your plan is to increase the low molecular weight heparin dose and start warfarin until you recall that these drugs can adversely affect hypercoagulability testing. What tests do you order before beginning therapy?

a) Factor V Leiden, prothrombin gene mutation, and homocysteine level
b) Protein C, protein S, and antithrombin III levels

c) Lupus anticoagulant and anticardiolipin antibody levels

d) All of the above

e) None of the above

Answer and Discussion

The answer is e. The patient has a "provoked" or "situational" venous thrombosis associated with the hip surgery. Even in the setting of adequate thromboprophylaxis, venous thrombosis occurs at a frequency of 1% to 4%. The results of testing are unlikely to impact clinical decisions regarding the duration, intensity, or type of anticoagulation therapy in this setting.

SUGGESTED READINGS

Colman RN, Marder VJ, Clowes AW. *Hemostasis and Thrombosis: Basic Principles and Clinical Practice*, 5th ed. Philadelphia: Lippincott Williams & Wilkins, 2005.

Godeau B, Provan D, Bussel J. Immune thrombocytopenia purpura in adults. *Curr Opin Hematol* 2007;14:535–556.

Heit JA. Thrombophilia: common questions on laboratory assessment and management. *Hematology* 2007;(1):127–135.

Hillman RS, Ault KA, Rinder HM. *Hematology in Clinical Practice*, 4th ed. New York: McGraw-Hill Professional, 2005.

Kamal AH, Tefferi A, Pruthi RK. Concise review for clinicians: how to interpret and pursue an abnormal prothrombin time, activated partial thromboplastin time, and bleeding time in adults. *Mayo Clin Proc* 2007;82(7):864–873.

Loscalzo J, Schafer AI. *Thrombosis and Hemorrhage*, 3rd ed. Philadelphia: Lippincott Williams & Wilkins, 2003.

Warkentin TE. Think of HIT. *Hematology* 2006;(1):408–414.

Chapter 22

Anemia

Alan E. Lichtin

POINTS TO REMEMBER:

- The red blood cell (RBC) mass is maintained in humans as the result of a continuous production of differentiated erythrocytes, generated by erythroid progenitors and stimulated by the hormone erythropoietin. Iron and nutrients, such as vitamin B$_{12}$ and folate, are necessary for RBC production, and energy sources are required to maintain the RBC membrane for RBCs to survive an average of 120 days.

- If severe enough, all anemias result in symptoms of tissue hypoxia (i.e., the consequence of a low oxygen-carrying capacity of the blood). Therefore, several signs and symptoms are common to all anemias. Weakness, headache, feeling "cold," and exertional dyspnea are common nonspecific symptoms that may be mild if the anemia develops slowly.

- When anemia is detected, its analysis consists of obtaining old data, gathering an excellent history—especially a drug history—and using physical diagnostic and laboratory methods to classify the anemia and identify its underlying cause. The first step is always to exclude acute blood loss by history and physical examination, including stool guaiac for occult blood loss.

- The corrected reticulocyte count is a useful second test because it serves to divide anemias into two major categories: *hyperproliferative anemias* resulting from the loss or destruction of RBCs, with an associated increased bone marrow activity; and *hypoproliferative anemias*, resulting from decreased bone marrow production.

The red blood cell (RBC) mass is maintained in humans as the result of a continuous production of differentiated erythrocytes, generated by erythroid progenitors and stimulated by the hormone erythropoietin. Iron and nutrients, such as vitamin B_{12} and folate, are necessary for RBC production, and energy sources are required to maintain the RBC membrane for RBCs to survive an average of 120 days.

Anemia is defined as a reduction in the RBC mass as measured by either the hematocrit or the hemoglobin concentration. *Acquired anemia* is not a disease per se, but rather a sign or symptom of an underlying disease. Because the severity of the anemia does not correlate with the seriousness of the underlying disorder, each patient with anemia deserves a careful evaluation to determine the cause of the anemia.

CLINICAL FEATURES

Many of the clinical manifestations associated with an anemia are determined by the etiology of the underlying disease that is producing the anemia. If severe enough, all anemias result in symptoms of tissue hypoxia (i.e., the consequence of a low oxygen-carrying capacity of the blood). Therefore, several signs and symptoms are common to all anemias. Weakness, headache, feeling "cold," and exertional dyspnea are common nonspecific symptoms that may be mild if the anemia develops slowly. The presence of physical signs, such as pallor and tachycardia, can be severe but depends on the patient's previous cardiovascular status. Stress to the cardiovascular system may occur with mild anemia in patients with pre-existing cardiovascular disease; however, even a healthy person begins to have cardiovascular stress at hemoglobin levels of <10 g/dL, as a result of the increased cardiac output required to compensate for the reduced oxygen-carrying capacity of the blood.

EVALUATION

RBCs are made and destroyed constantly. Anemia results when this equilibrium cannot be maintained because of acute or chronic blood loss, failure to produce RBCs, or a shortening of the RBC life span. When anemia is detected, its analysis consists of obtaining old data, gathering an excellent history—especially a drug history—and using physical diagnostic and laboratory methods to classify the anemia and identify its underlying cause. The first step is always to exclude acute blood loss by history and physical examination, including stool guaiac for occult blood loss. Further analyses include a complete blood cell count (CBC) with red cell indices, including a calculation of the mean corpuscular volume (MCV), a review of the peripheral blood smear (PBS), and a corrected reticulocyte count. Results from these initial tests help determine whether more invasive or expensive testing is required, such as bone marrow aspiration and biopsy or immunoassays.

An important initial step in assessing anemia involves an examination of the PBS, the most cost effective of hematologic tests. It is useful to correlate the PBS with the RBC indices generated by an automated CBC. The RBC indices should never substitute for an examination of the PBS, however, because the statistical averaging that occurs with an automated CBC loses valuable information about small populations of RBCs. An examination of the PBS reveals more information about specific RBC morphology, dimorphic populations, inclusion bodies, and accompanying white blood cell (WBC) morphology, all of which are not available from an automated CBC.

The corrected reticulocyte count is a useful second test because it serves to divide anemias into two major categories: *hyperproliferative anemias* resulting from the loss or destruction of RBCs, with an associated increased bone marrow activity; and *hypoproliferative anemias*, resulting from decreased bone marrow production. When the underlying cause of an anemia is not readily apparent, the reticulocyte count can be invaluable in interpreting the blood smear and in making an initial assessment as to the etiology of the anemia.

Morphologically, hyperproliferative anemias are frequently macrocytic, with high MCVs resulting from the large size of reticulocytes; however, some anemias caused by chronic hemolysis may result in normocytic morphology or MCVs, which may be in the normal range as a result of averaging between macrocytic reticulocytes and smaller spherocytes. The PBS helps identify hemolytic anemias rapidly. The presence of spherocytes or schistocytes (fragmented RBCs) may indicate such acquired disorders as immune hemolysis, disseminated intravascular coagulation, or other forms of microangiopathic hemolysis. Inclusion bodies or sickle shapes may indicate hereditary disorders, such as enzymopathies or sickle cell disease. In hypoproliferative anemias, the smear and MCV can be even more informative when RBC size can serve to organize the differential diagnosis. Furthermore, WBC morphology is more likely to be altered in hypoproliferative anemias, in which multiple cell types within the bone marrow may be affected by the same disease process.

DIFFERENTIAL DIAGNOSES

Shortened Red Blood Cell Survival

The causes of shortened RBC survival include:

- Compensated acute blood loss occurring before depletion of iron stores
- Hemolytic anemias
- Immune and autoimmune disorders
- Drugs
- Membrane defects

- Hereditary spherocytosis
- Hereditary elliptocytosis
- Acquired paroxysmal nocturnal hemoglobinuria
- Congenital enzymopathies
- Pyruvate kinase deficiency
- Glucose-6-phosphate dehydrogenase (G6PD) deficiency
- Hemoglobinopathies (sickle cell disorders)
- Mechanical hemolysis
- Heart valves
- Disseminated intravascular coagulation
- Thrombotic thrombocytopenic purpura
- Infections (malaria)

Macrocytic Anemias (MCV >100 fl)

Contributing causes to macrocytic anemia include:

- Pernicious anemia (vitamin B_{12} deficiency)
- Folate deficiency
- Alcoholism
- Malabsorption
- Liver disease

Normochromic, Normocytic (MCV >80 fl, MCV <100 fl)

- Aplastic anemia
- Myelophthisic disorders
- Leukemias
- Lymphomas
- Myeloma
- Myelofibrosis
- Granulomatous diseases
- Lipid storage diseases
- Anemia of chronic disease (anemia of abnormal iron reutilization)
- Anemia of chronic renal failure
- Anemia of endocrine diseases
- Anemia of hepatic failure

Hypochromic Microcytic (MCV <80 fl)

- Iron deficiency
- Sideroblastic anemia
- Lead intoxication
- Thalassemias
- Anemia of chronic disease (advanced)

HYPERPROLIFERATIVE ANEMIAS

Hyperproliferative anemias are divided between processes that remove blood cells (i.e., bleeding) and those that destroy blood cells (i.e., hemolysis). The following sections discuss the three most common disorders resulting in RBC destruction: immune hemolysis, abnormal red cell content or architecture, and microangiopathic hemolysis (trauma to red cells).

Immune Hemolytic Disorders

Immune hemolytic processes can be crudely divided into *autoimmune* processes, in which the patient produces antibodies against RBC surface antigens, and *drug-induced* processes, in which the RBC is frequently an "innocent bystander" in an otherwise typical immune-mediated drug reaction.

All these disorders are characterized by an indirect hyperbilirubinemia, reticulocytosis, marrow erythroid hyperplasia, hemoglobinemia, and perhaps hemoglobinuria. The PBS may have spherocytes, and the haptoglobin protein level may be nearly undetectable because it is removed from the circulation after binding free heme. The Coombs' test will be "directly" positive if antibodies are detected on the patient's circulating RBCs, and it will be "indirectly" positive if antibodies capable of reacting to RBCs are detected only in the serum.

Immunoglobulin M–Induced Hemolysis

Immunoglobulin M (IgM) antibodies produce "cold agglutinin" disease because these antibodies usually only bind or lyse RBCs at lower temperatures. The IgMs are frequently directed against the I antigen or related RBC antigens and result in complement fixation and lysis at temperatures usually below body temperature. A common cause of cold agglutinins is cross-reactive IgMs resulting from infections (*Mycoplasma pneumoniae*, mononucleosis, cytomegalovirus). Lymphoproliferative diseases and connective tissue diseases can also produce cold agglutinins, some of which can generate difficult persistent hemolysis.

Immunoglobulin G–Induced Hemolysis

The immunoglobulin G (IgG) antibodies can also produce a hemolysis of RBCs; however, because they do so at body temperature, the hemolysis is usually clinically more serious. Also, because IgGs bind at warmer temperatures, they are referred to as *warm antibodies*. Although complement may be fixed by the IgGs, the antibody valency is generally inadequate to cause intravascular hemolysis. The RBCs are converted slowly into spherocytes and eventually removed extravascularly in the spleen.

IgG or warm antibody disease is much more likely to produce a clinically apparent anemia, which may be chronic and require treatment. Corticosteroids are the treatment of choice; frequently, these agents may already be in use to treat the connective tissue disease or lymphoma that may be the cause of the warm antibody. Splenectomy is effective treatment in about half of patients for whom corticosteroids fail.

When cold (IgM) hemolysis requires therapy, steroids may help, and plasmapheresis may be effective in reducing the intravascular titer of the antibody.

In either situation, a transfusion of RBCs is rarely indicated and always complicated by the difficulty of typing and crossing the patient with compatible blood.

DRUG-INDUCED IMMUNE HEMOLYSIS

Drugs can contribute to RBC hemolysis in four classic ways. All are diagnosed by taking a careful history.

- Hapten type. In patients receiving high doses of penicillins, hapten type occurs when the drug or its metabolites bind to the RBC and induce an immune response. The antibodies react to a RBC antigen-drug complex and therefore bind only to drug-coated RBCs.
- Quinidine type. The quinidine-type IgM antibody reaction is directed most frequently to the drug quinidine when the drug binds to plasma proteins. The antibody then cross-reacts with RBC antigens, resulting in acute hemolysis.
- α-Methyldopa type (Aldomet). The α-methyldopa–type reaction is similar to idiopathic warm antibody disease. By an unknown mechanism, one-fourth of patients receiving Aldomet (a drug rarely used now for hypertension) develop IgG autoantibodies directed against the Rh antigens, with 1% suffering some hemolysis. The drug itself is not involved in the antibody–RBC antigen reaction.
- Nonspecific reactions. In rare instances, drugs such as cephalosporins can coat the RBC membrane, resulting in the nonspecific binding of plasma proteins, which may make the Coombs' test positive. Hemolysis is rare.

The removal of the inciting drug is the appropriate treatment and frequently results in rapid improvement. Rarely, corticosteroids are necessary.

ABNORMAL RED BLOOD CELL CONTENT OR ARCHITECTURE (HEREDITARY DISORDERS CAUSING HEMOLYSIS, HEMOGLOBINOPATHY, ENZYMOPATHIES, AND CYTOSKELETAL DEFECTS)

The RBC is the most thoroughly studied entity in the human body because of its accessibility and quantity. The result has been a tremendous understanding, at the genetic and biochemical levels, of hereditary disorders af-

fecting hemoglobin (hemoglobinopathies), RBC enzymes (enzymopathies), and the RBC cytoskeleton and structural proteins (e.g., spectrin disorders resulting in hereditary spherocytosis).

Hemoglobinopathies and Sickle Cell Anemia

A point mutation of the β-globin chain at residue 6 substitutes a valine for glutamic acid, thereby altering the net charge and local conformation of the hemoglobin molecule (Hb S). The alteration in charge results in an instability of Hb S when in the deoxygenated state, resulting in insoluble aggregates. These aggregates precipitate into polymers of long rodlike fibers if the concentration of Hb S is sufficiently high. The propagation of these polymers distorts the normally pliant cell membrane into bizarre forms that resemble sickles. These sickle-shaped RBCs are the hallmark of a series of unstable hemoglobins that share a constellation of clinical problems, including hemolytic anemia, small vessel infarction, painful crises, and a predisposition to infections.

Hb S mutations follow recessive inheritance patterns, with the carrier state (sickle trait) being silent; however, patients heterozygous for Hb S, who also have an additional mutant hemoglobin, such as Hb C, D, or O, or thalassemia, manifest a clinically evident sickle syndrome. Diagnosis of Hb S or other hemoglobin mutants is made by electrophoresis of purified Hb. In addition, reducing agents that deprive cells of O_2 promote Hb polymerization and sickling, even in the cells of patients who are Hb AS heterozygotes, thus serving as a screening test (*sickle prep using sodium metabisulfite*).

The therapy of sickle cell anemia and crisis include hydration and analgesia, with early treatment of infections and judicious transfusions.

Enzymopathies

More than six enzymes involved in glycolysis and adenosine triphosphate production have been identified as hereditary defects capable of inducing hemolytic states. The most common is G6PD deficiency, which has more than 150 mutant forms. The mutations serve to decrease the half-life of the G6PD protein, which is essential for maintaining the reduced state of the hemoglobin in the RBC cytoplasm. With time, activity is lost, thus allowing the oxidation and precipitation of aging hemoglobin, with subsequent development of inclusion bodies (Heinz bodies) and hemolysis. Deficiency of G6PD is sex-linked and usually manifests in a male subject with episodic hemolysis following oxidative stresses associated with infections or drug ingestions. Because it is the "aged" RBCs that hemolyze, analysis for G6PD levels soon after the hemolytic episode may be misleading and should be delayed to allow the reaccumulation of older cells.

Cytoskeletal Defects

The cytoskeleton is a complex array of proteins that hold the RBC membrane at the edge of the cell. Its latticelike state allows the red cell to be pliant enough to navigate the tiny slits in the splenic sinusoids. If a problem is present within the lattice, such as an abnormal structure of spectrin, ankyrin, or band 4.1, a clinical phenotype results in abnormally shaped RBCs. These include hereditary spherocytosis, hereditary elliptocytosis, or hereditary pyropoikilocytosis. These individuals have anemia, elevated indirect hyperbilirubinemia, reticulocytosis, and erythroid hyperplasia of the bone marrow, and usually have mild spleen enlargement. After viral infections, anemia worsens and jaundice deepens, sometimes to the point of requiring transfusion. Bilirubin gallstones occur at a young age. Splenectomy ameliorates the anemia. Moderate to severely affected individuals often have both a cholecystectomy and a splenectomy by age 20 to 30 years.

Microangiopathy

Any disease state that leads to RBC trauma within the circulation can lead to microangiopathic hemolytic anemia. Irregularities of the surface of heart valves can produce fragmented RBCs (schistocytes) with elevations of lactate dehydrogenase, indirect hyperbilirubinemia, reticulocytosis, and anemia. This may occur after valve surgery and may be a reason that a second corrective surgery would be necessary. Thrombotic thrombocytopenic purpura (TTP) is a disorder in which platelet fibrin thrombi are found in small vessels, and when the RBCs traverse these areas, they become fragmented. Drugs such as cyclosporine, clopidogrel, and mitomycin can produce this. Microangiopathy can be found in persons with severe hypertension, collagen-vascular disease, and disseminated intravascular coagulation.

HYPOPROLIFERATIVE ANEMIAS

Hypoproliferative anemias include those diseases that interfere with RBC production or maturation and lead to an inappropriately low reticulocyte count. Historically, these anemias have been classified by RBC morphology and size. This classification frequently groups physiologically unrelated processes together, but this classification survives because it is an efficient means for clinically diagnosing these anemias.

Macrocytic Anemias

The two most important disorders in which the MCVs are elevated are vitamin B_{12} deficiency and folate deficiency. Macrocytosis may also be seen in myelodysplasia, alco-holism, liver disease, and persons receiving chemotherapy or phenytoin. The PBS is again valuable in identifying megaloblastic processes (B_{12} and folate deficiency) from processes that produce macrocytosis alone. Usually, not only are hypersegmented neutrophils present, but also the RBCs are pleomorphic, containing fragments and other signs of dyserythropoiesis.

Vitamin B_{12} and Folate Deficiency

Both vitamin B_{12} and folate are involved in DNA synthesis. A deficiency in either leads to dyssynchrony in nuclear and cytoplasmic maturation, producing the RBC macrocytosis and neutrophil hypersegmentation, which are the hallmarks of these disorders. In addition, vitamin B_{12} plays an important role in myelin production, and B_{12} deficiency leads to serious neurologic disorders. Because B_{12} and folate metabolism are closely connected, the administration of folate to B_{12}-deficient subjects bypasses and corrects the hematologic abnormalities of vitamin B_{12} deficiency without correcting the neurologic abnormalities. Indeed, the neurologic abnormalities can worsen irrevocably. It is therefore essential to diagnose B_{12} deficiency correctly and treat with vitamin B_{12} first, before administering any folate.

B_{12} Deficiency

Vitamin B_{12} is found in animal products, such as meat, chicken, and fish. On ingestion, B_{12} is bound by an intrinsic factor secreted by gastric parietal cells, and the B_{12} intrinsic factor complex passes into the distal ileum, where it is actively absorbed. B_{12} is then transported by transcobalamins into the liver for storage and then into the erythron. Absolute dietary deficiency can occur in strict ovo-lacto vegetarians. Parietal cell dysfunction occurs either through the autoimmune process of pernicious anemia or by surgical removal of the stomach. Ileal disease such as Crohn's disease or radiation enteritis, pancreatic insufficiency, blind loop syndromes, and ileal resections likewise result in failure to absorb the B_{12} intrinsic factor complex. Historically, the Schilling's test allowed for the discrimination between a gastric disorder and an ileal disorder, but it is not used now because the radioactive reagents are no longer made. Anti-intrinsic factor and antiparietal cell antibodies can be measured, but false negatives for pernicious anemia are frequent.

The clinical manifestations of B_{12} deficiency include symptoms attributable to anemia but also include disproportionate fatigue and subtle neurologic symptoms. Some B_{12}-deficient persons manifest only mild anemia or macrocytosis. Some of these patients may develop neuropsychiatric symptoms, neuropathies, or difficulties with unconscious proprioception. B_{12} deficiency can lead to "megaloblastic madness," in which patients even may become demented or disoriented.

The therapy for vitamin B_{12} deficiency is simply parenteral administration by monthly intramuscular injections of 100 to 1,000 μg of B_{12}, usually after initial repletion of body stores with an injection of 1 mg. This dose is sufficient to reverse the megaloblastosis within days. An improvement in erythropoiesis results in a lowering of serum iron because it is used rapidly and a lowering in serum lactate dehydrogenase, which is elevated as a result of ineffective erythropoiesis and intramedullary hemolysis.

Folate Deficiency

Many persons are at risk for relative or absolute folic acid deficiency. Those who have diets poor in fresh vegetables, have jejunal malabsorption, or take antagonistic drugs may develop low folic acid levels. Pregnant women are especially susceptible. Folic acid, like B_{12}, is also necessary for DNA synthesis and is important in one carbon transfer; however, unlike vitamin B_{12}, folate is poorly stored by the body and must be replenished continuously. Unlike liver stores of vitamin B_{12}, which may be sufficient for 2 to 5 years, folate stores are minimal, and florid deficiency can develop in 3 months or less.

The anemia of folate deficiency resembles the megaloblastosis of B_{12} deficiency. Diagnosis may be difficult because a small hospital meal, blood transfusion, or intravenous multivitamins may be sufficient to elevate serum levels, thus making any subsequent testing ambiguous. Because RBC folate levels are the last compartment to be replenished and normalized, measuring RBC folate can be diagnostic in situations in which treatment was initiated before diagnosis.

The most important aspect of folate deficiency is that folate is not involved in myelin production and cannot correct the neurologic deficit of B_{12} deficiency. Therefore, it is critical not to mistake vitamin B_{12} deficiency for folate deficiency.

NORMOCHROMIC NORMOCYTIC HYPOPROLIFERATIVE ANEMIAS AND ANEMIA OF CHRONIC DISEASE

The anemia of chronic disease can generate RBCs that are microcytic but more frequently may be normocytic. It is defined as an anemia associated with an underlying disorder when no other etiology for the anemia can be identified. Not surprisingly, it is the most common category for anemias within institutions or hospitals. This disorder is characterized by low serum iron, low total iron-binding capacity (transferrin), and a low percent of iron saturation. Often, however, a normal or high ferritin level is found, which, in the presence of a low total iron-binding capacity level, is diagnostic of anemia of chronic disease. It has been labeled by some as the *anemia of abnormal iron reutilization*.

Consistent with this, the bone marrow appears normocellular or slightly hypocellular, with poor hemoglobinization but significant iron within the marrow spaces. Patients with this anemia often have underlying neoplasms, inflammatory disorders, connective tissue diseases (lupus or rheumatoid arthritis), or infectious processes, such as osteomyelitis or tuberculosis. Increasing evidence suggests that cytokines and inhibitory growth factors released during such disease processes may directly inhibit erythropoiesis or make RBC progenitors relatively resistant to normal or mildly elevated erythropoietin levels. Efforts at treating these anemias with exogenous recombinant erythropoietin have met with modest success. The only effective therapy for this anemia remains the treatment of the underlying disorder.

Other forms of normochromic normocytic anemias tend to be uncommon and are usually associated with clinically obvious conditions, such as hypothyroidism and renal failure, or manifestations of pancytopenia. The anemia of renal failure deserves special mention because it represents an isolated deficiency of erythropoietin. Injections or infusions of recombinant erythropoietin correct this anemia as long as iron is given to support erythropoiesis. Recent studies have led to U.S. Food and Drug Administration labeling changes, warning not to allow hemoglobin to rise above 12 g/dL because there are increased rates of thromboembolic disease with higher hemoglobins.

HYPOCHROMIC MICROCYTIC HYPOPROLIFERATIVE ANEMIAS

The microcytic anemias can be characterized as anemias in which hemoglobin production is somehow deficient. This anemia may be the result of a hereditary inability to produce globin protein chains (thalassemia), to produce heme (sideroblastic anemias), or to supply the iron necessary for heme production (iron deficiency). Of these, iron deficiency is the most common form of impaired heme synthesis on a worldwide basis.

Iron Deficiency

Worldwide, dietary insufficiency and parasite infestations are leading causes for iron-deficiency anemia. In the United States, the diagnosis of iron deficiency in an adult requires a careful and diligent search for a pathological source of blood loss or iron malabsorption. Iron-deficiency anemia should be entertained in any anemic patient with microcytosis. Iron deficiency can also accompany other anemias, and if it presents with a macrocytic anemia, a dimorphic condition might exist on peripheral smear with normocytic indices. The red cell distribution width is an index that measures the variation in RBC size. As the red cell distribution width increases, the variation in RBC size increases, making it likely that anisocytosis (different sizes of red cells) or a dimorphic population of RBCs is present. In that situation, examination of the PBS is essential. In iron deficiency, the red cell distribution width is high, reflecting the hypochromia, microcytosis, poikilocytes, and fragments that are often present.

People at risk of iron deficiency include infants with low dietary intake, pregnant women, adolescents, and elderly persons. Individuals with celiac disease develop a combined iron and folate deficiency that can be treated with a glutenfree diet. Symptoms of iron deficiency include those common to other anemias, including weakness, lassitude, palpitations, and dyspnea on exertion; however, iron deficiency also produces some unique symptoms in rapidly proliferating tissue. Glossitis, stomatitis, gastric atrophy with abdominal pain, and fingernail changes are all associated. Pica, or a craving to eat abnormal substances such as ice, occurs for unexplained reasons.

Generally, the serum ferritin is the best test for screening for iron deficiency. If the ferritin is <30 ng/mL in a male patient or <10 ng/mL in a female patient, iron deficiency is present. Because ferritin is also an acute phase reactant, it may be falsely elevated. Even so, a value of <50 μg/mL in the face of inflammation is a strong indicator of iron deficiency. Iron deficiency can be quantified further by measuring the total iron-binding capacity and total iron level, with a calculated percent of transferrin saturation. Finally, the absence of iron within the bone marrow is another way to confirm iron deficiency.

Therapy is straightforward. Iron salts such as ferrous sulfate, gluconate, or fumarate can replete stores in 2 to 6 months. The initial step in treating iron-deficiency anemia, however, is to identify the underlying disease and/or source of blood loss, and then to correct it.

Thalassemias

The thalassemias are hereditary diseases in which an inadequate or unbalanced production of globin protein chains occurs. α-Thalassemia represents a deficiency in α-chain production, and β-thalassemia represents a reduction in β-chains. The pathological mechanisms responsible for the decreased protein production are generally the result of hereditary mutations, which either totally delete the genes or result in minimal or no globin RNA production. Afflicted persons have a lifelong microcytic hypochromic anemia that depends on the severity of the deficiency. Because there are four copies of the α-globin gene and two copies of the β-globin gene, variations in the production and the clinical spectrum of disease are vast. For instance, the total lack of α-globin is incompatible with life and results in death in utero during the second trimester. Lack of only one α-globin gene, however, can be clinically silent and difficult to diagnose. Between these two poles are patients with 50% or less β- or α-globin production who have mild anemias that may morphologically resemble iron

deficiency, but who obviously do not respond to iron therapy. Throughout the twenty-first century, clinicians have classified patients as having either thalassemia major, intermedia, or minor. These terms have no pathological basis and describe only the severity of the patient's anemia—major means a patient needs transfusions regularly to survive, and minor means the individual rarely, if ever, needs a transfusion.

In severe thalassemia, the clinical symptoms present in early childhood and are the result of ineffective erythropoiesis and bone marrow hypertrophy, along with anemia. Patients develop bony deformities from marrow hyperplasia and organomegaly from extramedullary hematopoiesis. Oddly, the clinical manifestations of thalassemia relate more to the degree of imbalance between α-globin and β-globin production, which leads to the precipitation of abnormal hemoglobins in the developing RBC and lysis within the marrow. Patients with severe disease rarely survive beyond the age of 30 years. Less severe thalassemias present with fewer manifestations of hyperplastic bones and bone marrow and with more of the classic symptoms and problems of chronic anemia.

The PBS in thalassemia is usually remarkable for hypochromic microcytic cells. Patients with severe disease have manifestations of precipitating hemoglobin in their RBCs, including inclusion bodies and cell fragments resulting from dyserythropoiesis, as well as bizarre forms. Patients with only anemia or thalassemia trait conditions have increased numbers of RBCs (>5 million/μL) and target cells but less often fragmented cells from severe intracellular hemoglobin precipitation.

The treatment of thalassemia involves the transfusion of RBCs in severely affected children to reduce their own endogenous bone marrow activity and thus avoid bony hypertrophy and extramedullary hematopoiesis. In adults with anemia, transfusion is again beneficial but can lead to severe iron overload, with consequent heart failure. Iron chelation is important, either with subcutaneous desferrioxamine or oral deferasirox. Finally, patients with thalassemia minor or trait rarely require transfusion but require diagnosis to avoid unnecessary investigations for incorrectly diagnosed iron deficiency.

REVIEW EXERCISES

QUESTIONS

1. A 31-year-old woman presents with complaints of fatigue, dyspnea on exertion, and tinnitus. The symptoms started 1 month ago. She had previously been in "perfect health." She has had three normal pregnancies. Her physical examination is remarkable for pallor. The hemoglobin concentration is 7.5 g/dL, the white blood cell count is 6,200, and her platelet count is 550,000/μL. After her last pregnancy 2 years ago, her hemoglobin was normal. Which of the following tests is the most appropriate first test in the initial evaluation of this patient's anemia?

a) Serum folate and vitamin B_{12} level
b) Review of the peripheral blood smear
c) Serum ferritin determination
d) Haptoglobin level
e) Coombs' direct and indirect tests

Answer and Discussion

The answer is b. A review of the peripheral blood smear (PBS) is the single most valuable first step in evaluating an acute anemia. The morphology of the red blood cells, the presence of polychromasia (reticulocytes), and platelet morphology can help focus the differential diagnosis and evaluation immediately. The differential diagnosis for this patient's acute or subacute anemia is broad and includes both gastrointestinal blood loss and diverse causes of hemolysis. The iron studies, folate and B_{12} levels, haptoglobin, and Coombs' test are premature and should be ordered according to results of the PBS review and reticulocyte count.

2. A 24-year-old Lebanese exchange student comes to the college infirmary with a 3-day history of upper respiratory infection symptoms, cough, purulent sputum, and a low-grade fever. His chest examination is clear, and he is given available trimethoprim-sulfamethoxazole (Bactrim) samples for clinical bronchitis. The following day, he returns with shortness of breath, severe abdominal pain, a high spiking fever, and dark urine. A complete blood count reveals a hemoglobin of 7 g/dL and a white blood cell count of 12,500. Peripheral blood smear has fragmented red blood cells, and distinct "bite cells" are present. The chest radiograph is normal. The patient is admitted to the hospital. Which of the following statements is true?

a) The Coombs' direct test will be positive.
b) The haptoglobin will be undetectable.
c) A sickle prep screen would be positive.
d) All of the above.

Answer and Discussion

The answer is b. This patient has clinical glucose-6-phosphate dehydrogenase (G6PD) deficiency with acute hemolysis, as manifested by the acute drop in hemoglobin, dark urine, and fragmentation on the peripheral blood smear. People of Mediterranean descent are more susceptible to rapid severe hemolysis, in contrast to people of African descent. The "bite cells" on the smear are pathognomonic for this condition, which was triggered by the oxidative stress of the sulfa drugs. The precipitating hemoglobin results in red blood cell (RBC) stromal damage and acute hemolysis. The haptoglobin level will be low if not undetectable because

of its binding to free hemoglobin and removal by the liver. The Coombs' tests, both direct and indirect, are negative because antibodies are not involved in this physical form of hemolysis. Although many antibiotics might produce immune hemolysis, the time course of acute onset within 24 hours goes against any immune process. The sickle preparation will be negative because the precipitation of hemoglobin results in inclusion bodies but not in polymerization with deformity of the RBC architecture. Sickle cells will not be seen unless this patient also has a hemoglobinopathy.

If the G6PD enzyme levels were measured, they would be near normal in the remaining young cells that survived and were not hemolyzed. As these cells age, the enzyme decays, and the enzyme levels drop, thus making these cells vulnerable to stress hemolysis. After acute hemolysis, however, the surviving cells usually have normal levels of enzyme.

3. A 48-year-old man presents with fatigue, weakness, diffuse nonlocalizing abdominal complaints, loss of libido, "funny sensations" in his arms and legs, and depression. He has attempted to medicate himself with "megadoses" of B-complex vitamins as well as vitamin E and α-carotene. He denies any recent alcohol consumption and has had no diarrhea or steatorrhea. He has never had surgery. Physical examination is remarkable for a chronically ill–appearing middle-age man. The only objective abnormalities include decreased sensation in the legs and decreased proprioception. Initial workup includes a complete blood count with a hemoglobin of 13 g/dL, mean corpuscular volume of 120, and white blood cell count of 4,500. Platelets were 220,000. The peripheral blood smear confirms macrocytosis and rare hypersegmented polys. Reticulocyte count is 0.5%. You measure serum B_{12} and folate levels because of the macrocytosis. Folate is >14 (normal >2.0) and B_{12} is 20 (normal >100). Which of the following statements is false?

a) Administration of folate can correct the anemia of B_{12} deficiency.
b) With severe vitamin B_{12} deficiency, pancytopenia can result.
c) Folate administration cannot correct the myelin production defects and neurologic deficits.
d) An oral vitamin B_{12} preparation (Geritol) would have been likely to prevent the patient's neurologic deficits.

Answer and Discussion

The answer is d. This patient most likely has pernicious anemia, an autoimmune disease directed against the intrinsic factor producing parietal cells of the gastric antrum. Almost all vitamin B_{12} deficiency is the result of malabsorption, either because of a lack of intrinsic factor (pernicious anemia) or because of a defective small bowel. Dietary deficiency is very rare and occurs almost exclusively in strict ovo-lacto vegetarians who consume no animal products (vegan). Oral vitamin B_{12} administration cannot overcome the deficit in malabsorption. Schilling's test, which measures the absorption of oral vitamin B_{12}, in the presence of exogenous intrinsic factor, can distinguish the etiology of the malabsorption.

Folate administration circumvents the B_{12} defect, in the production of thymidine and DNA synthesis. Therefore, anemia may be ameliorated, and only macrocytosis may exist. Folate does not correct the defect in myelin production, however, so neurologic deficits may exist without hematologic abnormalities.

4-6. Match the following patients with laboratory results (serum iron, total iron-binding capacity, transferrin serum saturation, and ferritin, respectively). (Normal values: serum iron, 60-160; total iron-binding capacity, 250-460; transferrin serum saturation, 24%−45%; ferritin, 20-300.)
a) 220, 260, 85%, 2,560
b) 200, 390, 51%, 840
c) 40, 210, 19%, 400
d) 20, 500, 4%, 12

4. A 65-year-old woman on nonsteroidal anti-inflammatory drugs for osteoarthritis with irregular, guaiac-positive stools

5. A 48-year-old man with polyarthritis, recent-onset diabetes, hyperpigmentation, and cirrhosis

6. A 59-year-old woman with long-standing rheumatoid arthritis and anemia

Answers and Discussion
4. d.
5. a.
6. c.
Serum ferritin and iron levels are frequently used to diagnose iron-deficiency states; however, ferritin is an acute phase reactant and may be elevated to a degree seen in iron overload states in response to inflammation and liver disease. A low serum iron in the presence of an elevated transferrin level and low ferritin are diagnostic of some element of iron deficiency. The ferritin may be falsely elevated in the case of acute inflammation, but rarely will it be >50 μg/L in the face of iron deficiency. In contrast, the iron level may be low, but if the transferrin level is not elevated and the ferritin is elevated or in the high normal range, then the condition of anemia of chronic disease is most likely present. Rheumatoid arthritis is the best described disease producing this situation. Finally, although in the iron overload condition of hereditary hemochromatosis, the ferritin may be extremely high, the transferrin saturation is a much more sensitive and accurate test.

7. For a patient with a chronic autoimmune hemolytic anemia (warm immunoglobin G antibody) associated with a connective tissue disease, all of the following are appropriate therapy, *except*
a) Daily oral prednisone
b) Plasmapheresis
c) Treatment of the underlying autoimmune disorder
d) Splenectomy

Answer and Discussion
The answer is b. Plasmapheresis has not been shown to reliably treat autoimmune hemolytic anemia.

8. Which of the following is the most important factor in inducing hemoglobin precipitation?
a) pH
b) O_2 partial pressure
c) Hb S concentration
d) Osmolality

Answer and Discussion
The answer is c. Although all may affect sickling, the Hb S concentration has the greatest effect on precipitation.

9. The least likely factor to produce vitamin B_{12} deficiency is
a) Pregnancy
b) Crohn's disease
c) Total gastrectomy for peptic ulcer disease
d) Strict vegetarian diet

Answer and Discussion
The answer is a. It takes a long time to deplete the body of B_{12} stores.

10. Which laboratory test is most likely to be elevated in iron-deficiency anemia?
a) Homocysteine
b) Total iron-binding capacity
c) Platelet count
d) Ferritin
e) All of the above

Answer and Discussion
The answer is b. Ferritin is low in iron deficiency. Homocysteine levels are unaffected. Platelet counts may be elevated, but total iron-binding capacity is almost always increased.

11. Chronic transfusion for the treatment of thalassemia major is associated with which of the following?
a) Cirrhosis
b) Cardiomyopathy
c) Hemosiderosis
d) All of the above

Answer and Discussion
The answer is d. This answer is self-explanatory.

SUGGESTED READINGS

Beutler E. The common anemias. *JAMA* 1988;259:2433–2437.

Buetler E. Discrepancies between genotype and phenotype in hematology: an important frontier. *Blood* 2001;98:2597–2602.

Campbell PJ, Green AR. The myeloproliferative disorders. *N Engl J Med* 2006;355:2452–2466.

Gladwin MT, Sachdev V, Jison ML, et al. Pulmonary hypertension as a risk factor for death in patients with sickle cell disease. *N Engl J Med* 2004;350:886–895.

Hebert PC, Fergusson DA. Red blood cell transfusions in critically ill patients. *JAMA* 2002;288:1525–1526.

Henry DH, Thatcher N. Patient selection and predicting response to recombinant human erythropoietin in anemic cancer patients. *Semin Hematol* 1996;33(Suppl 1):2–6.

Jongen-Lavrencic A, Peeters HRM, Vreugdenhil G, et al. Interaction of inflammatory cytokines and erythropoietin in iron metabolism and erythropoiesis in anaemia of chronic disease. *Clin Rheumatol* 1995;14:519–525.

May C, Rivella S, Chadburn A, et al. Successful treatment of murine β-thalassemia intermedia by transfer of the human β-globin gene. *Blood* 2002;99:1902–1908.

Means RT Jr, Krantz SB. Progress in understanding the pathogenesis of the anemia of chronic disease. *Blood* 1992;80:1639–1646.

Mills JL. Fortification of foods with folic acid—how much is enough? *N Engl J Med* 2000;342:1442–1445.

Pietrangelo A. Hereditary hemochromatosis—a new look at an old disease. *N Engl J Med* 2004;350:2383–2397.

Rosenfeld S, Follmann D, Nunez O, et al. Antithymocyte globulin and cyclosporine for severe aplastic anemia. *JAMA* 2003;289:1130–1135.

Roy CN, Enns CA. Iron homeostasis: new tales from the crypt. *Blood* 2000;96:4020–4026.

Smits LJM, Essed GGM. Short interpregnancy intervals and unfavourable pregnancy outcome: role of folate depletion. *Lancet* 2001;358:2074–2077.

Tefferi A. Myelofibrosis with myeloid metaplasia. *Med Prog* 2000;342:1255–1265.

Van Wijk R, van Solinge WW. The energy-less red blood cell is lost: erythrocyte enzyme abnormalities of glycolysis. *Blood* 2005;106:4034–4042.

Vincent JL, Baron J-F, Reinhart K, et al. Anemia and blood transfusion in critically ill patients. *JAMA* 2002;288:1499–1507.

Wald NJ, Law MR, Morris JK, et al. Quantifying the effect of folic acid. *Lancet* 2001;358:2069–2073.

Chapter 23

Breast Cancer

Halle C. F. Moore

POINTS TO REMEMBER:

- The estimated annual incidence of invasive breast cancer in the United States is in the range of 180,000 per year, and the death rate, although improving, remains higher than 40,000 per year in this country.

- For a woman, the estimated lifetime risk of being diagnosed with breast cancer is approximately 1 in 8.

- Familial breast cancer syndromes account for a minority of breast cancer cases. Pathological mutations in *BRCA-1* and *BRCA-2* are present in approximately 0.33% of the general population, but the frequency of mutations is higher in some groups such as the Ashkenazi Jewish population. Individuals with *BRCA-1* or *BRCA-2* mutations may have a >80% risk of developing breast cancer by age 70 years, particularly in families in which the penetrance of the gene is high.

- Other familial syndromes that account for a smaller proportion of inherited breast cancer include the Li-Fraumeni syndrome resulting from an inherited *p53* mutation, Cowden's disease, Muir-Torre syndrome, Peutz-Jeghers syndrome, and heterozygosity for the ataxia-telangiectasia gene.

- Mammography should never substitute for breast examination, and a normal mammogram does not rule out the possibility of cancer.

- The mainstay of breast cancer diagnosis, however, is biopsy, which may consist of fine-needle aspiration, core biopsy, or excisional biopsy.
- The most common histologic types of invasive breast cancer are infiltrating ductal carcinoma and infiltrating lobular carcinoma.
- Standard surgical treatment for invasive breast cancer includes either modified radical mastectomy (removal of the breast and an axillary lymph node dissection) or excision of the tumor (lumpectomy or partial mastectomy) with axillary dissection.

Currently, approximately 2.5 million American women are breast cancer survivors. Breast cancer is the most common serious cancer in American women. The estimated annual incidence of invasive breast cancer in the United States is in the range of 180,000 per year, and the death rate, although improving, remains higher than 40,000 per year in this country. A reduction in breast cancer mortality has been achieved over the past decades, presumably due to earlier detection and improved therapies. The median age at the time of breast cancer diagnosis is 63 years. Long-term survival following a diagnosis of breast cancer is common, and overall 5-year survival exceeds 85%.

RISK FACTORS AND SCREENING

The most common risk factor for breast cancer is female gender, with only approximately 1% of breast cancers occurring in men. For a woman, the estimated lifetime risk of being diagnosed with breast cancer is approximately 1 in 8. Hormonal factors appear to play an important role in the development of breast cancer. Factors associated with prolonged cyclic estrogen exposure, including early menarche, late menopause, nulliparity, and delayed parity, have been associated with an elevated risk of breast cancer. Postmenopausal hormone replacement therapy with a combination of estrogen and progesterone has been associated with an increase in breast cancer risk, particularly with prolonged use. Postmenopausal estrogen therapy alone (without progesterone) has not been clearly implicated in increasing breast cancer risk.

Other risk factors for breast cancer include exposure to therapeutic doses of ionizing radiation and certain findings identified on breast biopsy, including lobular carcinoma in situ (LCIS) and atypical hyperplasia. Breast cancer risk increases with increasing age, and approximately two-thirds of breast cancers are diagnosed in women older than the age of 55 years. For the most part, dietary links to breast cancer have not been clearly established, although increased alcohol intake has been associated with increased breast cancer risk. Increased mammographic breast density is a recently recognized risk factor for breast cancer, and an assessment of breast density is now routinely included in screening mammogram reports. Family history is also an important risk factor, particularly when the affected individual is young, has a first-degree or second-degree relative with breast cancer, or has bilateral breast cancer.

Familial breast cancer syndromes account for a minority of breast cancer cases. Pathological mutations in BRCA-1 and BRCA-2 are present in approximately 0.33% of the general population, but the frequency of mutations is higher in some groups such as the Ashkenazi Jewish population. Individuals with BRCA-1 or BRCA-2 mutations may have a >80% risk of developing breast cancer by age 70 years, particularly in families in which the penetrance of the gene is high. BRCA-1 is located on chromosome 17q21 and is also associated with a significantly increased risk of ovarian cancer, as well as other cancers, including prostate and colon cancers. BRCA-2 is located on chromosome 13 and has been associated with only a modestly increased risk of ovarian cancer, but with an increased risk of a greater variety of cancer types, including prostate, pancreatic, stomach cancers, and melanoma. Both mutations are inherited in an autosomal dominant pattern, although the penetrance of the mutations varies from family to family. No firm data demonstrate a survival benefit to aggressive screening for breast and ovarian cancer in women with known mutations in BRCA-1 or BRCA-2; however, screening often begins from age 25 years and may include clinical breast examination, screening mammography, pelvic examination, and ultrasonography every 6 to 12 months. MRI is also an accepted screening modality for individuals at particularly high risk for breast cancer but is costly. Prophylactic mastectomy and prophylactic oophorectomy procedures are frequently offered to BRCA carriers, but do not entirely eliminate the risk for developing cancer, and their impact on survival is unclear.

Other familial syndromes that account for a smaller proportion of inherited breast cancer include the Li-Fraumeni syndrome resulting from an inherited p53 mutation, Cowden's disease, Muir-Torre syndrome, Peutz-Jeghers syndrome, and heterozygosity for the ataxia-telangiectasia gene. These syndromes are characterized by a variety of clinical manifestations, including other cancer sites. Whereas the increased breast cancer risk in these patients should be recognized, other manifestations of these syndromes may dominate management of these individuals.

The goal of breast cancer screening is to reduce breast cancer mortality in the general population. Early detection before the development of symptomatic disease improves the potential for cure of breast cancer. The American Cancer Society recommends that women report to their health care provider any changes in how their breasts look or feel. Specifically, women should report the presence of a lump, swelling, skin irritation, dimpling, nipple pain, redness, or abnormal discharge. Clinical breast examination is recommended every 3 years from age 20 years until age 39 years. Women age 40 years and older should receive annual clinical breast examination along with annual mammography. Some controversy exists as to the precise benefit of screening in the 40-year to 49-year age group; however, annual mammography in conjunction with clinical breast examination appears to reduce breast cancer mortality by 25% to 30% in women between the ages of 50 and 69. An upper age cut-off for mammography has not been set, but the screening of elderly women should be individualized, with consideration of comorbid illnesses. Mammography should never substitute for breast examination, and a normal mammogram does not rule out the possibility of cancer. For women at particularly high risk for developing breast cancer, MRI screening may be considered in addition to mammography.

DIAGNOSIS AND LOCAL THERAPY

Once a suspicious lesion has been detected either through breast imaging or on breast examination, further evaluation is warranted. Diagnostic imaging, such as ultrasound, may be useful in differentiating solid from cystic lesions. MRI is also being used increasingly in the preoperative evaluation of breast cancer. The mainstay of breast cancer diagnosis, however, is biopsy, which may consist of fine-needle aspiration (FNA), core biopsy, or excisional biopsy. FNA is a relatively simple technique, which can be performed in the office and may confirm a suspicion of cancer. FNA may fail to differentiate between invasive and noninvasive cancer, and a negative FNA result does not rule out the possibility of cancer. An advantage of core needle biopsy over FNA is the ability to obtain enough tissue to evaluate histologic architecture and thus obtain important information about the pathology of the lesion. Excisional biopsy involves removal of the entire lesion of concern and may, at times, serve as the definitive procedure.

The most common histologic types of invasive breast cancer are infiltrating ductal carcinoma and infiltrating lobular carcinoma. The prognosis of both types of breast cancer is similar. Other less common histologies include medullary, tubular, metaplastic, squamous, adenoid cystic, and apocrine carcinomas. Rarely, other types of cancer such as lymphoma and sarcoma can present in the breast and are approached in accordance with their histology.

Noninvasive breast cancer, or ductal carcinoma in situ (DCIS), is an early form of breast cancer that, theoretically, should not have the ability to metastasize. It is characterized by a malignant epithelial proliferation that is contained within the ductal-lobular system of the breast. Simple mastectomy or local excision, followed in most cases by radiation therapy, is largely curative. LCIS is not a true cancer, but rather a histologic finding that is associated with an increased risk of breast cancer in either the affected or the contralateral breast. Excision of the LCIS does not appear to significantly alter subsequent cancer risk.

Standard surgical treatment for invasive breast cancer includes either modified radical mastectomy (removal of the breast and an axillary lymph node dissection) or excision of the tumor (lumpectomy or partial mastectomy) with axillary dissection. Ideally, surgical margins on the excised specimen should be free of both invasive cancer and DCIS. Radiation therapy is recommended for patients at high risk for local recurrence, and indications include breast-conserving surgery, large primary tumors (>5 cm), and extensive lymph node involvement (four or more). The role of the axillary dissection is in evolution and, although once regarded as crucial for local control, is now viewed primarily as a staging procedure. In an effort to limit the morbidity of a full axillary dissection, the sentinel lymph node procedure has been developed. This involves the injection of a radioactive tracer, a blue dye, or both into the affected area of the breast or subdermally to elicit the drainage pattern of the mammary lymphatics. Presumably, the first lymph nodes to pick up the dye or radioactive tracer would also have the highest likelihood of involvement with cancer and, if found to be normal, predict a high likelihood that no further cancer would be identified in the remaining axilla. The finding of tumor in a sentinel lymph node frequently prompts a full axillary lymph node dissection.

STAGING AND PROGNOSIS

Breast cancer staging uses the TNM (*Tumor*, *Node*, *Metastasis*) system outlined in Table 23.1. In general, stage I, II, and many stage III cancers are operable and considered to be *early breast cancer*. The term *locally advanced breast cancer* most often refers to stage IIIB or IIIC disease (which may or may not be operable), and metastatic breast cancer is stage IV. The staging evaluation to assess for the presence of distant disease typically includes chest radiography, a complete blood count, liver enzymes, and an optional bone scan. Additional studies such as abdominal and chest CT scans can be performed in patients perceived to be at relatively high risk for metastatic disease, including those with localizing symptoms, blood test abnormalities, or significant lymph node involvement. A positron emission tomography scan is also approved for use in breast cancer staging, but false-positive findings can be misleading.

Breast cancer mortality increases with the higher stage of disease. Adverse prognostic factors for early stage breast cancer include a greater number of axillary lymph nodes involved, larger tumor size, higher histologic grade of the tumor, negative hormone receptor (estrogen receptor [ER] and progesterone receptor [PR]) studies, and the presence

TABLE 23.1

AMERICAN JOINT COMMITTEE ON CANCER STAGING FOR BREAST CANCER: TNM SYSTEM

T (Primary Tumor Size)
Tis = Carcinoma in situ
T1 = Up to 2 cm in greatest diameter
T2 = Greater than 2 cm, but no greater than 5 cm
T3 = Greater than 5 cm
T4 = Tumor extends into skin or chest wall or inflammatory changes

N (Regional Lymph Nodes)
N0 = No regional lymph node involvement (includes lymph nodes with IHC-positive staining as long as no cluster is >0.2 mm)
N1 = Ipsilateral axillary metastasis involving one to three lymph nodes and/or internal mammary lymph node involvement detected by sentinel lymph node evaluation, but not clinically apparent
N2 = Involvement of four to nine ipsilateral axillary lymph nodes or no axillary involvement but clinically apparent internal mammary lymph nodes
N3 = Involvement of ten or more ipsilateral axillary lymph nodes, or involvement of any ipsilateral axillary lymph nodes plus clinically apparent internal mammary lymph node involvement, or any ipsilateral supraclavicular or infraclavicular lymph node involvement

M (Distant Metastases)
M0 = No detectable distant metastases
M1 = Any distant metastasis

Breast Cancer Stage Grouping

	T (Tumor)	N (Nodes)	M (Metastasis)
Stage 0	Tis	N0	M0
Stage 1	T1	N0	M0
Stage IIA	T0–1	N1	M0
	T2	N0	M0
Stage IIB	T2	N1	M0
	T3	N0	M0
Stage IIIA	T0–2	N2	M0
	T3	N1–2	M0
Stage IIIB	T4	N0-2	M0
Stage IIIC	Any T	N3	M0
Stage IV	Any T	Any N	M1

Adapted with permission from Singletary SE, Allred C, Ashley P, et al. Revision of the American Joint Committee on Cancer staging system for breast cancer. *J Clin Oncol* 2002;20:3628–3636.

of HER2/*neu* amplification. Younger patient age also appears to adversely affect prognosis.

ADJUVANT SYSTEMIC THERAPY

The goal of adjuvant systemic therapy for operable breast cancer is to increase the possibility of cure through the eradication of micrometastases. In general, adjuvant chemotherapy is considered for cancers measuring at least 0.5 to 1 cm or when axillary lymph node involvement is identified. Factors that influence the decision to proceed with chemotherapy include patient age and comorbid conditions, the histologic grade of the tumor, the presence or absence of estrogen receptors and progesterone receptors, as well as the anticipated absolute benefit from chemotherapy, which depends on the recurrence risk. In relative terms, traditional chemotherapy regimens can reduce the annual risk of recurrence by approximately 20% in women older than age 50 years and by approximately 35% in women

younger than age 50 years. The inclusion of newer agents in modern regimens should be associated with greater benefit to adjuvant chemotherapy. Individuals whose cancers are ER and PR negative may experience a greater benefit from chemotherapy than those that are hormone receptor positive.

Combination chemotherapy regimens commonly used in the adjuvant treatment of breast cancer are outlined in Table 23.2. The duration of adjuvant chemotherapy is typically 3 to 6 months. Common acute toxicities of adjuvant chemotherapy for breast cancer include varying degrees of nausea, vomiting, fatigue, myelosuppression, and alopecia. Long-term toxicities include the induction of premature menopause after cyclophosphamide-containing regimens, cardiac toxicity after anthracycline-containing chemotherapy, and neuropathy following use of the taxanes (paclitaxel or docetaxel). In addition, some chemotherapy drugs have been associated with an increase in the risk of acute leukemia, particularly when used in higher than standard doses.

TABLE 23.2

ADJUVANT CHEMOTHERAPY REGIMENS

CMF (cyclophosphamide, methotrexate, and 5-fluorouracil)
CAF (cyclophosphamide, doxorubicin, and 5-fluorouracil)
CEF (cyclophosphamide, epirubicin, and 5-fluorouracil)
AC (doxorubicin and cyclophosphamide)
AC>T (doxorubicin and cyclophosphamide followed by paclitaxel)
TAC (docetaxel, doxorubicin, and cyclophosphamide)
TC (docetaxel and cyclophosphamide)
AC>TH (doxorubicin and cyclophosphamide followed by paclitaxel and trastuzumab)
TCH (docetaxel, carboplatin, and trastuzumab)

The monoclonal antibody trastuzumab improves both disease-free survival and overall survival when added to chemotherapy in the treatment of patients whose tumors overexpress *Her2neu*. The most important toxicity of trastuzumab is cardiomyopathy, and this risk is increased in patients who are also receiving anthracycline chemotherapy.

Like adjuvant chemotherapy, adjuvant hormonal therapy is also used to improve the chance of cure following local therapy for breast cancer and is indicated for individuals whose cancers express estrogen, progesterone, or both receptors. Historically, tamoxifen, a selective estrogen receptor modulator (SERM), has been the most widely used hormonal treatment; a 5-year course of tamoxifen can reduce the annual risk of recurrence by nearly 50% in patients with ER-positive tumors and is effective regardless of menopausal status. Premenopausal women also benefit from ovarian ablation as adjuvant therapy; however, the value of ovarian ablation added to tamoxifen remains a matter of investigation. For postmenopausal women, the selective aromatase inhibitors, which prevent the peripheral conversion of adrenally produced androgens into estrogens, are also very effective in the adjuvant setting. Several large randomized clinical trials have demonstrated a benefit to using aromatase inhibitors either as an alternative to or in sequence with tamoxifen in postmenopausal hormone receptor–positive breast cancer. Ongoing studies are evaluating the safety and efficacy of aromatase inhibitors in combination with ovarian ablation in premenopausal hormone receptor–positive breast cancer.

Tamoxifen should also be considered for use in women with DCIS who have undergone breast conservation because this treatment reduces the risk of local recurrence as well as contralateral new primary breast cancers. The aromatase inhibitors are under investigation for the treatment of postmenopausal DCIS.

The common adverse effects of tamoxifen include vasomotor symptomatology and vaginal discharge. Long-term side effects of tamoxifen include increased risks of endometrial cancer, thromboembolic events, and cataracts. Tamoxifen has favorable effects on lipid profiles and on bone mineral density in postmenopausal women. Aromatase inhibitors are also associated with vasomotor symptoms but do not appear to have the same risk of uterine cancer or thromboembolism. Aromatase inhibitors can result in bone density loss and are associated with an increased incidence of musculoskeletal symptoms. For women with invasive breast cancer, the risks of hormonal therapy are generally more than offset by the survival advantage gained by preventing breast cancer recurrence. Their use in noninvasive breast cancer and in the setting of prevention needs to be considered more cautiously, given the lack of survival advantage in the latter situations.

FOLLOW-UP AND SURVEILLANCE FOR INDIVIDUALS WITH BREAST CANCER

Whereas screening for early stage (potentially curable) disease may have an important impact on survival, intensive surveillance to detect metastatic disease has not been shown to significantly affect outcome. The American Society of Clinical Oncology guidelines recommend that careful history and physical examination be performed every 3 to 6 months for 3 years after diagnosis, then every 6 to 12 months for the next 2 years, and annually thereafter. Patients should also continue annual mammography, and monthly breast self-examination. The routine use of tumor marker studies, other blood work, chest radiography, bone scans, or CT scans is not encouraged.

Because long-term survival after a diagnosis of breast cancer is common, it is important that patients continue to receive preventive medicine recommendations and undergo screening for treatable conditions. Examples include screening for colon cancer, cervical cancer, and osteoporosis, as well as preventive strategies for heart disease. Issues relating to menopause may be of particular concern for breast cancer survivors in whom hormone replacement therapy is generally contraindicated. Individuals who are at risk for inherited breast cancer syndromes should be offered genetic counseling.

METASTATIC BREAST CANCER

Once breast cancer metastasizes to organs outside the breast and local lymph nodes, cure is unlikely; however, average survival with metastatic breast cancer has improved significantly over the past several decades. Breast cancer tends to be responsive to a variety of therapies, including chemotherapy, hormonal therapy, and biological therapies. Treatment is directed at palliating symptoms and prolonging life. Because prolonged treatment is often required, selection of agents with favorable toxicity profiles is desirable.

TABLE 23.3

HORMONAL TREATMENT FOR METASTATIC BREAST CANCER

Antiestrogens
Tamoxifen
Toremifene
Fulvestrant (estrogen receptor downregulator)[a]

Ovarian Ablation[b]
Surgical oophorectomy
Gonadotropin-releasing hormone analogs

Selective Aromatase Inhibitors[a]
Anastrozole
Letrozole
Exemestane

Progestational Agents
Megestrol acetate

Androgens
Halotestin

[a]Active in postmenopausal women.
[b]Active in premenopausal women.

TABLE 23.4

CHEMOTHERAPY AGENTS ACTIVE IN METASTATIC BREAST CANCER

Capecitabine
Cyclophosphamide
Docetaxel
Doxorubicin
Epirubicin
5-Fluorouracil
Gemcitabine
Methotrexate
Vinorelbine
Paclitaxel
Ixabepilone
Carboplatin

For patients who have ER- and/or PR-positive metastatic disease, hormonal therapy is generally preferred over chemotherapy. Factors that predict a higher likelihood of response to hormonal therapy include a long disease-free interval before the development of metastatic disease and disease that is limited to bone, soft tissues, and pleura. In postmenopausal women, the selective aromatase inhibitors appear to be superior to tamoxifen as first-line therapy. Premenopausal women may benefit from removal of the ovaries or suppression of ovarian function with gonadotropin-releasing hormone agonists. Aromatase inhibitors can be considered in combination with ovarian ablation in premenopausal women. Tamoxifen may be given alone or in combination with ovarian ablation. In the metastatic setting, hormonal therapy should be continued as long as no evidence of disease progression is present. Patients whose disease has previously responded to a hormonal manipulation have a reasonable chance of responding to subsequent hormonal maneuvers. Commonly used hormonal therapies for metastatic breast cancer are listed in Table 23.3.

Individuals whose cancers are hormone receptor–negative, who have rapidly progressive or organ-threatening disease, and whose disease is no longer responding to hormonal therapy are candidates for chemotherapy. Chemotherapy drugs for metastatic disease may be given as single agents or in combination. Although the response rates are often higher with combinations of drugs, this does not always translate into a survival advantage and may expose patients to unnecessary toxicity. Patients with rapidly progressive visceral disease are most likely to benefit from combination therapy, whereas those with slower-paced disease may be successfully treated with single agents given sequentially. A variety of chemotherapy drugs have activity in metastatic breast cancer, and many of these are outlined in Table 23.4.

The current trend toward attempting to specifically target therapies to the cancer is exemplified by the development of trastuzumab for the treatment of *HER2/neu* overexpressing metastatic breast cancer. This monoclonal antibody therapy has a generally favorable toxicity profile and has activity in patients with *HER2/neu* overexpressing breast cancer. As in the adjuvant setting, a survival advantage is observed when trastuzumab is added to chemotherapy in appropriately selected patients. The tyrosine kinase inhibitor, lapatinib, is also active in combination with chemotherapy against *Her2neu* overexpressing breast cancer and is approved following progression on trastuzumab-containing therapy. Other biological therapies such as angiogenesis inhibitors and inhibitors of the epidermal growth factor receptor, have also demonstrated activity in the treatment of metastatic breast cancer.

Symptom control is another important aspect of managing metastatic breast cancer. Radiation therapy can be useful in palliating painful bony lesions or brain metastases and may be used to prevent an impending fracture or to treat spinal cord compression. Bisphosphonates, such as pamidronate and zoledronate, are useful in preventing skeletal complications from lytic bone metastases.

BREAST CANCER PREVENTION

Although no large randomized controlled trials have evaluated the effectiveness of prophylactic bilateral mastectomies for the prevention of breast cancer, a retrospective series from the Mayo Clinic suggested at least a 90% reduction in the risk of breast cancer using bilateral prophylactic mastectomy. For most women, however, breast cancer risk does not warrant this permanent and disfiguring option.

The effectiveness of tamoxifen for the prevention of breast cancer was demonstrated in a randomized controlled trial conducted by the National Surgical Adjuvant Breast

TABLE 23.5

BREAST CANCER RISK CRITERIA FOR NATIONAL SURGICAL ADJUVANT BREAST AND BOWEL PROJECT P-1

Female age 60 years or older
OR
Female ages 35–59 years with lobular carcinoma in situ on prior biopsy
OR
5-Year calculated breast cancer risk of at least 1.66%[a]

[a]Breast cancer risk is calculated using the Gail model, which takes into account the following variables: age, race, number of first-degree relatives with breast cancer, nulliparity or age at first live birth, number of prior breast biopsies, history of atypical hyperplasia on biopsy, and age at menarche.

and Bowel Project (NSABP). It had been previously observed that women receiving adjuvant tamoxifen for early stage breast cancer had fewer contralateral new primary breast cancers than those who did not receive tamoxifen, suggesting the drug's potential role as a preventive agent for women at high risk for breast cancer. The selection criteria used in the study, NSABP P-1, are outlined in Table 23.5. In this study, women randomized to receive 5 years of tamoxifen experienced a 49% reduction in the risk of developing invasive breast cancer at a median follow-up time of 54.6 months. Tamoxifen preferentially prevented hormone receptor–positive breast cancer, with no reduction in the development of hormone receptor–negative breast cancer. In addition, no difference in survival has been observed between patients who received and did not receive tamoxifen in the setting of prevention. A follow-up prevention study, NSABP P2, demonstrated that raloxifene, also a SERM, is similarly effective in reducing the risk of developing invasive breast cancer in postmenopausal women at increased risk with a lower risk of uterine cancer compared with tamoxifen. Aromatase inhibitors are also under investigation for the prevention of breast cancer in postmenopausal women at risk.

REVIEW EXERCISES

QUESTIONS

1–4. Choose the appropriate breast cancer screening/prevention strategy (in addition to regular breast self-examination) for each asymptomatic woman:

1. A 55-year-old perimenopausal woman with no family history of breast cancer or personal history of breast disease

2. A 52-year-old postmenopausal woman with lobular carcinoma in situ

3. A 30-year-old smoker whose great aunt had breast cancer at age 65 years

4. A 28-year-old woman whose sister had bilateral breast cancer in her 30s and mother had ovarian cancer in her 50s
a) Clinical breast examination every 3 years
b) Annual mammography and clinical breast examination
c) Clinical breast examination and mammography every 6 to 12 months and consideration of annual breast MRI examination
d) Annual mammography, clinical breast examination, and consideration of raloxifene for 5 years

Answers and Discussion
1. The answer is b. In women ages 50 to 69 years, annual mammography, in combination with clinical breast examination, appears to reduce breast cancer mortality.
2. The answer is d. Postmenopausal women at high risk for breast cancer, including those with lobular carcinoma in situ, can reduce the risk of developing breast cancer with the use of a selective estrogen receptor modulator, either tamoxifen or raloxifene, for 5 years. Individuals electing chemoprevention should continue regular screening with mammography and clinical breast examination.
3. The answer is a. This individual's breast cancer risk is not high enough to warrant intensive screening, and age-appropriate recommendations include breast self-examination and clinical breast examination every 3 years. A baseline mammogram could be considered at age 35 years; annual mammograms should begin at age 40 years.
4. The answer is c. This individual's family history is suggestive of a hereditary breast cancer syndrome, and intensive surveillance is appropriate. The value of tamoxifen for chemoprevention in this population is unclear. If this patient were to test positive for BRCA-1 or BRCA-2, counseling on the options of prophylactic mastectomies and/or oophorectomy (after completion of childbearing) is appropriate.

5–8. Choose the most appropriate management for each patient with metastatic breast cancer:

5. A 40-year-old premenopausal woman treated with chemotherapy alone for early stage hormone receptor–positive breast cancer 3 years ago develops diffuse bone pain and is found to have multiple lytic bone metastases.

6. A 45-year-old woman with hormone receptor–negative breast cancer involving lungs, who has been responding to chemotherapy, develops headache and slurred speech. She is found to have multiple brain metastases.

7. A 60-year-old woman with HER2/neu overexpressing hormone receptor–negative breast cancer is found to have liver metastases 9 months after the completion of adjuvant doxorubicin-containing chemotherapy.

8. A 65-year-old woman has just undergone pleurodesis for a malignant pleural effusion occurring 2 years after completing adjuvant tamoxifen for early stage breast cancer.
a) Refer to radiation therapy.
b) Begin a selective aromatase inhibitor.
c) Initiate trastuzumab in combination with taxane chemotherapy.
d) Recommend bilateral oophorectomy, tamoxifen, and monthly zoledronate.
e) Proceed with high-dose chemotherapy and stem cell transplant.

Answers and Discussion

5. The answer is d. Appropriate first-line hormonal therapy for a premenopausal woman with osseous metastatic breast cancer includes ovarian ablation, tamoxifen, or both. An aromatase inhibitor in combination with ovarian ablation would also be reasonable, but is not listed as an option. The addition of a bisphosphonate decreases the risk of fracture and other complications of lytic bone metastases.

6. The answer is a. Systemic treatment is unlikely to be effective for the treatment of symptomatic central nervous system metastases. Whole brain radiation is appropriate in this situation.

7. The answer is c. In *HER2/neu* overexpressing metastatic breast cancer, a survival advantage is observed when trastuzumab is combined with paclitaxel or docetaxel chemotherapy.

8. The answer is b. Hormonal therapy is appropriate for this patient having presumably hormone receptor–positive metastatic breast cancer limited to the pleura, and a selective aromatase inhibitor is the best option for this postmenopausal woman.

9. Which of the following factors in metastatic breast cancer predicts for response to hormonal therapy?
a) Prior response to tamoxifen
b) Young age
c) Hepatic involvement of breast cancer
d) Persistence of menses following adjuvant breast cancer therapy

Answer and Discussion

The answer is a. Response to hormonal therapy for metastatic disease is more likely with estrogen receptor/progesterone receptor–positive disease; long disease-free intervals; older age; disease that is limited to bone, soft tissues, and pleura; and disease that has previously responded to hormonal therapy.

10. Which of the following most clearly improves the cure rate for a 75-year-old woman who has undergone excision of a 2-cm estrogen receptor–positive left breast cancer?
a) Left axillary dissection or sentinel lymph node procedure
b) Bilateral mastectomy
c) Anastrozole 1 mg daily for 5 years
d) CMF (cyclophosphamide, methotrexate, and 5-fluorouracil) chemotherapy for 6 months

Answer and Discussion

The answer is c. Whereas an axillary node dissection or sentinel lymph node procedure is appropriate for the staging of breast cancer, a survival advantage to such procedures has not been established. Similarly, neither mastectomy nor bilateral mastectomy has demonstrated a survival benefit over breast-conserving surgery. The benefit of chemotherapy in women older than the age of 70 years with low-risk disease is unclear; however, a clear benefit in both survival and recurrence-free survival persists with endocrine therapy such as anastrozole.

11. Adjuvant chemotherapy for early stage breast cancer results in which of the following?
a) Prevention of or delay in progression to metastatic disease
b) Rapid reduction in cancer-related symptoms
c) Decrease in the risk of new primary breast cancers
d) All of the above

Answer and Discussion

The answer is a. The purpose of adjuvant chemotherapy is to reduce the risk of recurrence after surgical removal of the cancer. By definition, patients receiving adjuvant chemotherapy do not have symptomatic or detectable disease. Whereas adjuvant tamoxifen has been demonstrated to reduce the risk of contralateral new primary breast cancers, the same effect has not been established with chemotherapy.

12–17. For each of the following treatments used in patients with early breast cancer, match the associated potential long-term toxicity:
12. Tamoxifen

13. Anastrozole

14. Doxorubicin

15. Cyclophosphamide

16. Paclitaxel

17. Chest wall and axillary radiation therapy
a) Congestive heart failure
b) Premature menopause
c) Uterine cancer
d) Neuropathy
e) Lymphedema
f) Osteoporosis

Answers and Discussion

12. The answer is c. Tamoxifen has estrogen-like effects on the endometrium and, like estrogen, increases the risk of uterine cancer.

13. The answer is f. Because of profound lowering of estrogen levels, the aromatase inhibitors can result in bone density loss, increasing the risk of osteoporosis and fracture.

14. The answer is a. Doxorubicin is associated with cardiotoxicity. The effect is related to total (lifetime) dose of doxorubicin.

15. The answer is b. Alkylating agents, including cyclophosphamide, can cause ovarian failure. The risk is increased with higher patient age and higher cumulative drug dose.

16. The answer is d. Paclitaxel is associated with a peripheral neuropathy that preferentially affects the long nerves. This effect is usually reversible but may persist in some patients.

17. The answer is e. Local-regional radiation therapy is associated with an increased risk of lymphedema in the affected arm. The risk is increased with axillary radiation and with prior axillary dissection.

SUGGESTED READINGS

American Cancer Society. *Breast Cancer Facts & Figures 2007–2008.* Atlanta: American Cancer Society.

Baum M, Budzar AU, Cuzick J, et al. Anastrozole alone or in combination with tamoxifen versus tamoxifen alone for the treatment of postmenopausal women with early breast cancer. *Lancet* 2002;359:2131–2139.

Chlebowski RT, Hendrix SL, Langer RD, et al. Influence of estrogen plus progestin on breast cancer and mammography in healthy postmenopausal women: the Women's Health Initiative randomized trial. *JAMA* 2003;289:3243–3253.

Claus EB, Risch N, Thompson WD. Autosomal dominant inheritance of early-onset breast cancer: implications for risk prediction. *Cancer* 1994;73:643–651.

Collaborative Group on Hormonal Factors in Breast Cancer. Breast cancer and hormone replacement therapy: collaborative reanalysis of data from 51 epidemiological studies of 52,705 women with breast cancer and 108,411 women without breast cancer. *Lancet* 1997;350:1047–1059.

Coombes RC, Hall E, Gibson LJ, et al. A randomized trial of exemestane after two to three years of tamoxifen therapy in postmenopausal women with primary breast cancer. *N Engl J Med* 2004;350:1081–1092.

Cox CE, Haddad F, Bass S, et al. Lymphatic mapping in the treatment of breast cancer. *Oncology* 1998;17:1283–1292.

Early Breast Cancer Trialists' Collaborative Group. Polychemotherapy for early breast cancer: an overview of the randomized trials. *Lancet* 1998;352:930–942.

Early Breast Cancer Trialists' Collaborative Group. Tamoxifen for early breast cancer: an overview of the randomized trials. *Lancet* 1998;351:1451–1467.

Fisher B, Costantino JP, Wickerham DL, et al. Tamoxifen for the prevention of breast cancer: report of the National Surgical Adjuvant Breast and Bowel Project P-1 study. *J Natl Cancer Inst* 1998;90:1371–1388.

Fisher B, Dignam J, Wolmark N, et al. Tamoxifen in treatment of intraductal breast cancer: National Surgical Adjuvant Breast and Bowel Project B-24 randomized controlled trial. *Lancet* 1999;353:1993–2000.

Geyer CE, Forster J, Lindquist D, et al. Lapatinib plus capecitabine for Her2-positive advanced breast cancer. *N Engl J Med* 2006;355(26):2733–2743.

Goss PE, Ingle JN, Martino S, et al. A randomized trial of letrozole in postmenopausal women after five years of tamoxifen therapy for early-stage breast cancer. *N Engl J Med* 2003;349:1793–1802.

Grodstein F, Stampfer MJ, Colditz FA, et al. Postmenopausal hormone therapy and mortality. *N Engl J Med* 1997;336:1769–1775.

Hartmann LC, Schaid DJ, Woods JE, et al. Efficacy of bilateral prophylactic mastectomy in women with a family history of breast cancer. *N Engl J Med* 1999;340:77–84.

Hortobagyi GN, Theriault RL, Lipton A, et al. Long-term prevention of skeletal complications of metastatic breast cancer with pamidronate. *J Clin Oncol* 1998;16:2038–2044.

Hoskins KF, Stopfer JE, Calzone KA. Assessment and counseling for women with a family history of breast cancer: a guide for clinicians. *JAMA* 1995;273:577–585.

Jones SE, Savin MA, Holmes FA, et al. Phase III trial comparing doxorubicin plus cyclophosphamide with docetaxel plu cyclophosphamide as adjuvant therapy for operable breast cancer. *J Clin Oncol* 2006;24(34):5381–5387.

Khatcheressian JL, Wolff AC, Smith TJ, et al. American Society of Clinical Oncology 2006 update of the breast cancer follow-up management guidelines in the adjuvant setting. *J Clin Oncol* 2006;24:5091–5097.

Liede A, Karlan BY, Narod SA. Cancer risks for male carriers of germline mutations in *BRCA1* or *BRCA2*: a review of the literature. *J Clin Oncol* 2004;22:735–742.

MacMahon B, Cole P, Brown J. Etiology of human breast cancer. *J Natl Cancer Inst* 1973;50:21–42.

Morrow M, Schnitt SJ, Harris JR. In situ carcinomas. In: Harris JR, Lippman ME, Morrow M, et al., eds. *Diseases of the Breast.* Philadelphia: Lippincott-Raven, 1996:355–368.

Norton L, Slamon D, Leyland-Jones B, et al. Overall survival (OS) advantage to simultaneous chemotherapy (CRx) plus the humanized anti-HER2 monoclonal antibody Herceptin (H) in HER2-overexpression (HER2+) metastatic breast cancer (MBC) (abstract). *Proc Am Soc Clin Oncol* 1999;18:127a.

Piccart-Gebhart MJ, Procter M, Leyland-Jones B, et al. Trastuzumab after adjuvant chemotherapy in HER2-positive breast cancer. *N Engl J Med* 2005;353:1659–1672.

Romond EH, Perez EA, Bryant J, et al. Trastuzumab plus adjuvant chemotherapy for operable HER2-positive breast cancer. *N Engl J Med* 2005;353:1673–1684.

Rosen PP. Invasive mammary carcinoma. In: Harris JR, Lippman ME, Morrow M, et al., eds. *Diseases of the Breast.* Philadelphia: Lippincott-Raven, 1996:393–444.

Singletary SE, Allred C, Ashley P, et al. Revision of the American Joint Committee on Cancer staging system for breast cancer. *J Clin Oncol* 2002;20:3628–3636.

Smith I, Procter M, Gelber RD, et al. 2-Year follow-up of trastuzumab after adjuvant chemotherapy in HER2-positive breast cancer: a randomized controlled trial. *Lancet* 2007;369(9555):3–5.

Smith-Warner SA, Spiegelman D, Yaun S, et al. Alcohol and breast cancer in women: a pooled analysis of cohort studies. *JAMA* 1998;279:535–540.

Women's Health Initiative Investigators. Risks and benefits of estrogen plus progestin in healthy postmenopausal women: principal results from the Women's Health Initiative randomized controlled trial. *JAMA* 2002;288:321–333.

Chapter 24

Lymphoma

Brad L. Pohlman

HODGKIN LYMPHOMA

Hodgkin lymphoma (or Hodgkin's disease) is a malignant neoplasm involving primarily lymphoid tissue that has a characteristic histologic appearance including Reed-Sternberg (R-S) cells or their variants. Recent studies prove that the R-S cells arise from germinal center or post–germinal center B cells. The etiology of Hodgkin lymphoma is not known. Epidemiologic, serologic, and genetic studies have implicated Epstein-Barr virus in some cases. The American Cancer Society estimates that 8,220 new cases and 1,350 deaths will occur in the United States during 2008.

Clinical Presentation

The most common initial complaint is painless enlargement of cervical, supraclavicular, axillary, or, less often, inguinal lymph nodes. Most patients are asymptomatic, but up to one-third of patients have systemic B symptoms (i.e., fevers, night sweats, or weight loss). Some patients complain of cough, chest pain, dyspnea, or diminished exercise tolerance attributable to mediastinal or, less commonly, pericardial or pulmonary involvement. Infrequently, patients experience generalized or, less commonly, localized pruritus, which may be associated with a skin rash. Patients with a history of mononucleosis, autoimmune disease, or immunodeficiency, including HIV infection, have an in-creased incidence of Hodgkin lymphoma. The siblings of young adults with Hodgkin lymphoma also have an increased incidence.

Enlargement of supradiaphragmatic lymph nodes is present in most patients. Lymphadenopathy exclusively below the diaphragm occurs in only 5% to 10% of patients. Lymph nodes are usually firm, rubbery, mobile, and nontender. The spleen may be palpable. Laboratory abnormalities are not specific. A moderate to marked leukemoid reaction, monocytosis, eosinophilia, and thrombocytosis are common. Anemia resulting from impaired iron use, lymphopenia, and thrombocytopenia usually occur in patients with more advanced disease. Elevation of the erythrocyte sedimentation rate is present in approximately one-half of patients. Chest radiography commonly demonstrates mediastinal or hilar adenopathy.

Diagnosis and Staging

The diagnosis of Hodgkin lymphoma requires a biopsy of an involved lymph node or an extralymphatic site. If a superficial lymph node is not accessible, a percutaneous True-cut needle biopsy may occasionally be adequate. A fine-needle aspiration may be adequate to identify other malignancies, such as metastatic carcinoma, but this technique usually cannot distinguish Hodgkin lymphoma from non-Hodgkin lymphoma (NHL) or most benign etiologies. The histologic criteria for diagnosis include a disrupted nodal architecture, R-S cells or variants, and a nonmalignant reactive background. Two major types of Hodgkin lymphoma are recognized: classical (which includes the nodular sclerosis, mixed cellularity, lymphocyte-rich, and lymphocyte-depleted subtypes) and nodular lymphocyte predominant.

All sites of disease must be identified to stage, plan, and monitor therapy. The staging process should include a detailed history with particular attention to B symptoms, pruritus, HIV risk factors, and performance status; a complete physical examination, including the size of lymph nodes, liver, and spleen; laboratory evaluation, including a complete blood cell count and differential, erythrocyte

TABLE 24.1

ANN ARBOR STAGING SYSTEM

Stage	Definition
I	One lymph node region
II	Two or more lymph node regions on same side of diaphragm
III	Lymph node regions on both sides of diaphragm
IV	Extranodal sites
A	No B symptom
B	Any B symptom (i.e., fever, night sweats, or weight loss)

TABLE 24.3

PROGNOSTIC FEATURES IN HODGKIN LYMPHOMA

Poor Prognostic Features	Freedom From Progression (%)	Overall Survival (%)
0	84	89
1	77	90
2	67	81
3	60	78
4	51	61
Š5	42	56

Adapted from Hasenclever D, Diehl V. A prognostic score for advanced Hodgkin's disease. International Prognostic Factors Project on Advanced Hodgkin's Disease. *N Engl J Med* 1998;339:1506–1514.

sedimentation rate, liver tests, albumin, creatinine, calcium, and HIV screening (if risk factors are present); and imaging studies, including chest radiography, CT of the neck, chest, abdomen, and pelvis, and positron emission tomography (PET) scan. Patients with suspected advanced stage disease should have a bone marrow biopsy. The Ann Arbor staging system is shown in Table 24.1.

Treatment

The initial treatment of Hodgkin lymphoma depends primarily on the stage, but may also be influenced by the histologic subtype, prognostic features, and physician or patient preference. Historically, patients with stage I or II were treated with extensive radiation therapy. Currently, most of these patients are treated with chemotherapy followed by limited radiation therapy. Patients with stage III or IV are treated with chemotherapy followed occasionally by radiation therapy (primarily to sites of initially bulky disease). Patients who relapse after initial therapy may occasionally be cured with another chemotherapy regimen; however, high-dose therapy with autologous stem cell transplantation offers the best chance for long-term, diseasefree survival.

Prognosis

The prognosis for patients with newly diagnosed Hodgkin lymphoma is predicted by the stage and risk factors (Table 24.2). In early stage disease, these *are* bulky (especially mediastinal) adenopathy, older age, elevated sedimentation rate, and high number of involved nodal sites. Among patients with advanced stage disease, a prognostic score identified seven independent poor prognostic features: albumin level <4 g/dL, hemoglobin level <10.5 g/dL, male sex, stage IV disease, age 45 years or older, white blood cell count 15,000/mm^3 or higher, and lymphocyte count <600/mm^3 or <8%. The number of poor prognostic features predicts both freedom from progression and overall survival (Table 24.3).

Complications

In addition to relapse, patients who have been treated for Hodgkin lymphoma are susceptible to a variety of disease- and treatment-related complications. Because of disease-associated cell-mediated immunodeficiency, prior splenectomy, chemotherapy-induced neutropenia, or steroid administration, these patients are at risk for developing serious bacterial and fungal infections, varicella zoster, *Pneumocystis jiroveci* pneumonia, and other opportunistic infections. Up to 50% of patients who receive mantle irradiation develop clinical or subclinical hypothyroidism, which may not be apparent for several years. In addition, up to one-half of these patients develop benign, or rarely malignant, thyroid neoplasms 20 years or longer after treatment. Cardiopulmonary complications from chemotherapy, especially doxorubicin and bleomycin, and mantle irradiation may occur during or months to years after treatment. These complications are more likely to occur in patients who have received both chemotherapy and radiation therapy. Some chemotherapy regimens may cause temporary or permanent azoospermia in males and amenorrhea, sterility, or premature menopause in females. The risk of second malignancies after treatment of Hodgkin lymphoma is significantly higher than expected for age-matched controls. Ten percent to 20% of patients who receive extensive radiation therapy may subsequently develop solid tumors. The risk continues to increase with time. These tumors, which usually occur within the radiation field, include soft tissue sarcoma; melanoma; and cancer of the head, neck, lung, breast, gastrointestinal

TABLE 24.2

PROGNOSIS IN HODGKIN LYMPHOMA

Clinical Situation	Overall Survival (%)
Stage I–II without risk factors	90–95+
Stage I–II with risk factors	85–95+
Stage III–IV	50–90

tract, and urogenital tract. NHL develops in approximately 5% of patients. Myelodysplastic syndrome and acute non-lymphocytic leukemia occur mainly as complications of chemotherapy, particularly alkylating agents, in 3% to 10% of patients 2 to 10 years after treatment. The short- and long-term psychosocial sequelae of the diagnosis and treatment of Hodgkin lymphoma are often not discussed. These patients face problems with body image, self-esteem, marriage, interpersonal relationships, sexuality, insurability, employment, and socioeconomic advancement.

NON-HODGKIN LYMPHOMA

NHL is a heterogeneous group of malignant neoplasms arising from the immune system. Although these disorders are discussed together, they actually constitute an array of clinicopathological entities with widely variable features, behavior, treatment, and prognosis. The American Cancer Society estimates that 66,120 new cases and 19,160 deaths will occur in the United States in 2008. The incidence increases with age, and the median age is approximately 65 years.

Patients with inherited and acquired immunodeficiencies have a significantly increased risk of developing NHL. With few exceptions, the etiology of NHL is unknown. Epidemiologic studies have implicated irradiation, chemotherapy, and some environmental exposures. Table 24.4 presents infectious agents that have been strongly implicated in the pathogenesis of certain subtypes of NHL.

Clinical Presentation

Because NHL may involve any lymphatic or extralymphatic tissue, virtually any presenting symptom is possible. Most patients complain of painless enlargement of one or more superficial lymph nodes. This abnormality may have been present for weeks or months and may have been stable or progressing. Mediastinal lymphadenopathy may cause chest pain, cough, dyspnea, or superior vena cava syndrome. Splenomegaly, retroperitoneal, mesenteric, or pelvic lymphadenopathy may cause abdominal discomfort, early satiety, back pain, or lower extremity edema. Although extranodal involvement is often a manifestation of more extensive nodal disease, some extranodal sites may be the only site involved: *gastrointestinal tract lymphoma* may lead to abdominal pain or fullness, early satiety, symptoms of complete or partial bowel obstruction, hemorrhage, or perforation; *central nervous system lymphoma* may cause headaches, change in mental status, seizures, and focal neurologic deficits; and *cutaneous lymphoma* may result in localized or extensive lesions. Symptoms may be due to involvement of less common sites, such as bone, testis, spinal cord, orbit, and sinus. Patients may complain of symptoms of anemia or thrombocytopenia. Approximately 20% of patients have B symptoms (i.e., fever, night sweats, or weight loss).

The most common physical finding is single or multiple, firm, enlarged, nontender cervical, supraclavicular, axillary, inguinal, or epitrochlear lymph nodes. Splenomegaly is common. Occasionally, a mass may be palpable in the abdomen or pelvis. Waldeyer's ring may be involved. Extranodal involvement (e.g., skin, central nervous system, testis, bone, or orbit) may lead to abnormal findings.

The complete blood count is often normal; however, patients may have mild to moderate anemia (due to gastrointestinal involvement and hemorrhage, impaired iron utilization, bone marrow involvement, or autoimmune hemolysis), thrombocytopenia (resulting from bone marrow involvement, hypersplenism, or immune thrombocytopenic purpura), or, less commonly, leukopenia. Serum lactate dehydrogenase (LDH) may be mildly or markedly elevated. A monoclonal gammopathy may be present. Imaging studies may show lymphadenopathy, splenomegaly, or parenchymal lesions in any organ.

Diagnosis and Evaluation

The diagnosis of NHL requires a tissue biopsy. The World Health Organization classification recognizes more than 24 different types of NHL. The specific types are defined by histology, immunophenotype, and, occasionally, genotype. Recent studies have identified gene expression profiles (GEPs) that further divide some types of lymphoma (e.g., diffuse large B-cell lymphoma) into unique subsets with different prognoses. In the future, these GEPs may be used to guide therapy. For non-oncologists, the types of NHL can be divided into two broad categories: *indolent* and *aggressive*. Examples of each are listed as follows:

Indolent lymphomas

Follicular lymphoma
Small lymphocytic lymphoma
Extranodal marginal zone B-cell lymphoma of mucosa-associated lymphoid tissue (MALT)

TABLE 24.4

INFECTIOUS AGENTS STRONGLY IMPLICATED IN THE PATHOGENESIS OF CERTAIN SUBTYPES OF NON-HODGKIN LYMPHOMA

Infectious Agent	Non-Hodgkin Lymphoma Subtype
Epstein-Barr virus	Posttransplant lymphoproliferative disorder
	Burkitt lymphoma
Human T-cell lymphotrophic virus 1	T-cell leukemia/lymphoma
Human herpes virus 8	Primary effusion lymphoma
Helicobacter pylori	Gastric mucosa-associated lymphoid tissue lymphoma

Aggressive lymphomas

> Diffuse large B-cell lymphoma
> Peripheral T-cell lymphoma
> Lymphoblastic lymphoma
> Burkitt lymphoma

The indolent lymphomas account for approximately 50% of newly diagnosed cases. Eighty percent have stage III or IV. With few exceptions, these patients are incurable with conventional therapy. Paradoxically, they have a relatively long median survival of more than 10 years. The aggressive lymphomas account for the rest of cases. Approximately 50% of patients have stage III or IV. Patients with these subtypes are potentially curable with appropriate therapy.

The complete evaluation of these patients provides prognostic information and dictates management. The evaluation should include a detailed history, including age, performance status, and HIV risk factors; a complete physical examination, including lymph node regions, liver, and spleen; laboratory evaluation, including a complete blood cell count, differential, liver tests, creatinine, calcium, LDH, and HIV screening (if risk factors are present); imaging studies, including CT of the neck, chest, abdomen, and pelvis, PET scan, and occasionally other imaging studies (e.g., MRI) that may define other sites of disease; and bone marrow aspirate and iliac crest biopsy(ies). The stage is defined by the Ann Arbor system for Hodgkin lymphoma.

Treatment

The management of patients with NHL depends on the specific pathological type. Historically, patients with lymphoma have been treated with chemotherapy and/or radiation therapy. In 1997, rituximab was approved by the U.S. Food and Drug Administration (FDA) for the treatment of patients with B-cell NHL. This immunotherapeutic agent binds specifically to CD20 on benign and malignant B lymphocytes and leads to cell death by apoptosis, complement-dependent cytotoxicity, antibody-dependent cellular cytotoxicity, and possibly the generation of lymphoma antigen-specific T-cell response. Two radiolabeled monoclonal antibodies (yttrium 90 ibritumomab tiuxetan and iodine 131 tositumomab) were also recently approved for patients with B-cell NHL. Indeed, many novel targeted therapies (e.g., monoclonal antibodies, histone deacetylase inhibitors, proteosome inhibitors, immunomodulatory drugs, and other small molecules) have either been recently FDA approved or are under investigation for the treatment of NHL.

Gastric MALT lymphoma is a unique and uncommon variant of extranodal marginal zone B-cell lymphoma of MALT, which involves the stomach. Approximately 90% of cases are caused by *Helicobacter pylori*. Infection with this bacterium leads to chronic inflammation in the gastric mucosa, persistent lymphocyte stimulation, and development of an *H. pylori*–dependent (and subsequently independent) monoclonal B-cell proliferation. Remarkably, 50% to 70% of patients with localized gastric MALT lymphoma respond to anti–*H. pylori* therapy.

Most indolent lymphomas are considered incurable, and treatment is by definition palliative. A minority of patients may not require any treatment initially, and expectant monitoring of symptoms, physical findings, and radiographic abnormalities may be all that is required. When the patient develops deleterious signs or symptoms (e.g., bulky lymphadenopathy, pain, fever, night sweats, weight loss, anemia, or thrombocytopenia) or progressive disease with impending problems, treatment should be initiated. Patients with localized disease are treated with radiation therapy, chemotherapy, and/or immunotherapy, whereas patients with advanced stage disease are usually treated with chemotherapy and/or immunotherapy. Several, prospective, randomized studies in patients with indolent B-cell lymphoma have shown that the addition of rituximab to standard chemotherapy prolongs survival.

In contrast, many types of aggressive lymphoma are potentially curable. Therefore, treatment is initiated at the time of diagnosis. In general, patients with localized disease are treated with chemotherapy sometimes followed by involved field radiation therapy, whereas patients with advanced stage disease are treated with chemotherapy. Several prospective, randomized studies in patients with diffuse large B-cell lymphoma have shown that the addition of rituximab to standard chemotherapy improves survival. For patients who relapse after initial therapy, many salvage chemotherapeutic regimens are available. Patients who respond to salvage chemotherapy are often treated with high-dose therapy and autologous stem cell transplantation.

Prognosis

The prognosis of patients with newly diagnosed, aggressive NHL is predicted by the International Prognostic Index. This model recognizes five clinical features that independently predict a worse prognosis: age older than 60 years, LDH above normal level, performance status 2 to 4, stage III or IV, and more than one extranodal site of disease (Table 24.5).

TABLE 24.5

INTERNATIONAL PROGNOSTIC INDEX FOR AGGRESSIVE NON-HODGKIN LYMPHOMA

Poor Prognostic Features	Complete Response (%)	5-Year Survival (%)
0 or 1	87	73
2	67	51
3	55	43
4 or 5	44	26

Adapted from Anonymous. A predictive model for aggressive non-Hodgkin's lymphoma. The International Non-Hodgkin's Lymphoma Prognostic Factors Project. *N Engl J Med* 1993;329:987–994.

REVIEW EXERCISES

CASE 1

A 20-year-old woman presents with night sweats, 15-lb weight loss, and painless left neck lumps. Physical examination is remarkable only for multiple, nontender, rubbery, mobile, 1- to 2-cm left cervical lymph nodes. Laboratory studies reveal normocytic, normochromic anemia. CT of the neck confirms the presence of left cervical and supraclavicular lymphadenopathy.

1. Which procedure has the highest diagnostic yield?
a) Fine-needle aspiration of an enlarged lymph node
b) Core needle biopsy of an enlarged lymph node
c) Excisional biopsy of an enlarged lymph node

Answer and Discussion

The answer is c. The diagnosis of lymphoma requires histologic examination of a lymph node or involved tissue. The cytologic specimen provided by a fine-needle aspiration is usually inadequate to make a diagnosis of lymphoma, let alone determine the specific subtype. An excisional lymph node biopsy provides the most tissue for the pathologist to evaluate the lymph node and perform any indicated ancillary diagnostic studies.

2. Biopsy reveals classical Hodgkin lymphoma. CT of the chest, abdomen, and pelvis demonstrates thoracic lymphadenopathy and splenic lesions. What is the correct stage?
a) Stage IIA
b) Stage IIB
c) Stage IIIA
d) Stage IIIB

Answer and Discussion

The answer is d. Involvement of lymphoid tissue above and below the diaphragm indicates at least stage III. Both lymph nodes and spleen are considered lymphoid tissue. The presence of night sweats and weight loss (i.e., B symptoms) adds the letter B.

3. Which feature predicts a good prognosis?
a) Age 20 years
b) Female sex
c) Both age 20 years and female sex

Answer and Discussion

The answer is c. The International Prognostic Factors Project identified seven independent poor prognostic features among patients with newly diagnosed, advanced stage Hodgkin lymphoma: hypoalbuminemia, anemia, male sex, stage IV, age 45 years or older, leukocytosis, and lymphopenia.

CASE 2

A 78-year-old man complains of dyspepsia and 10-lb weight loss during the past several months. Eight years earlier, he had a gastrointestinal bleed that was attributed to ibuprofen-induced gastritis. His only medication is a baby aspirin. Physical examination is unremarkable. Laboratory studies are normal. Esophagogastroduodenoscopy shows erythema and ulcerations "consistent with medication-induced gastropathy." Biopsies unexpectedly reveal extranodal marginal zone B-cell lymphoma of mucosa-associated lymphoid tissue. Complete staging evaluation demonstrates no other evidence of lymphoma.

4. Which of the following statements is correct?
a) *Helicobacter pylori* is probably involved in the development of this patient's lymphoma.
b) *H. pylori* eradication may help his gastritis, but not his lymphoma.
c) *H. pylori* is the only infectious agent implicated in lymphomagenesis.

Answer and Discussion

The answer is a. *H. pylori* is demonstrable in 90% or more of patients with gastric mucosa-associated lymphoid tissue (MALT) lymphoma. The majority of patients with localized gastric MALT lymphoma respond to eradication of these bacteria. Other infectious agents (e.g., Epstein-Barr virus) have been implicated in the pathogenesis of several other types of lymphoma.

CASE 3

A 70-year-old woman complains of fatigue and progressive abdominal discomfort during the past 2 months and a "bulk" in her left abdomen during the past week. Her performance status is 1. Physical examination reveals a few 1-cm right axillary lymph nodes and a huge left lower quadrant mass. Laboratory studies include a white blood cell count of 15.4 with a normal differential, hemoglobin of 10.0, platelets of 370, and lactate dehydrogenase of 897 (normal, 100–220). CT of the chest, abdomen, and pelvis show a few slightly enlarged right axillary lymph nodes and massive retroperitoneal and mesenteric lymphadenopathy. CT-guided core needle biopsy demonstrates diffuse large B-cell lymphoma. Bone marrow biopsy shows no evidence of lymphoma.

5. Which of this patient's presenting features predict a good prognosis?
a) Age 70 years
b) Stage III
c) Elevated lactate dehydrogenase
d) Good performance status

Answer and Discussion

The answer is d. The International Non-Hodgkin Lymphoma Prognostic Factors Project identified five independent poor-risk features among patients with newly diagnosed, advanced stage, aggressive non-Hodgkin lymphoma: age older than 60 years, performance status 2 to 4, stage III or IV, elevated lactate dehydrogenase, and two or more extranodal sites of involvement.

SUGGESTED READINGS

Canellos GP, Anderson JR, Proper KJ, et al. Chemotherapy of advanced Hodgkin's disease with MOPP, ABVD, or MOPP alternating with ABVD. *N Engl J Med* 1992;327:1478–1484.

Coiffier B, Lepage E, Briere J, et al. CHOP chemotherapy plus rituximab compared with CHOP alone in elderly patients with diffuse large-B-cell lymphoma. *N Engl J Med* 2002;347:235–242.

Diehl V, Franklin J, Pfreundschuh M, et al. Standard and increased-dose BEACOPP chemotherapy compared with COPP-ABVD for advanced Hodgkin's disease. *N Engl J Med* 2003;348:2386–2395.

Fisher RI, Gaynor ER, Dahlberg S, et al. Comparison of a standard regimen (CHOP) with three intensive chemotherapy regimens for advanced non-Hodgkin's lymphoma. *N Engl J Med* 1993;328:1002–1006.

Fisher RI, LeBlanc M, Press OW, et al. New treatment options have changed the survival of patients with follicular lymphoma. *J Clin Oncol* 2005;23:8447–8452.

Hasenclever D, Diehl V. A prognostic score for advanced Hodgkin's disease. International Prognostic Factors Project on Advanced Hodgkin's Disease. *N Engl J Med* 1998;339:1506–1514.

Jaffe ES, Harris NL, Stein H, et al., eds. *World Health Organization Classification of Tumors: Pathology and Genetics of Tumors of Haematopoietic and Lymphoid Tissues.* Lyon, France: IARC Press, 2001.

McLaughlin P, Grillo-Lopez AJ, Link BK, et al. Rituximab chimeric anti-CD20 monoclonal antibody therapy for relapsed indolent lymphoma: half of patients respond to a four-dose treatment program. *J Clin Oncol* 1998;16:2825–2833.

Miller TP, Dahlberg S, Cassady JR, et al. Chemotherapy alone compared with chemotherapy plus radiotherapy for localized intermediate- and high-grade non-Hodgkin's lymphoma. *N Engl J Med* 1998;339:21–26.

Philip T, Guglielmi C, Hagenbeek A, et al. Autologous bone marrow transplantation as compared with salvage chemotherapy in relapses of chemotherapy-sensitive non-Hodgkin's lymphoma. *N Engl J Med* 1995;333:1540–1545.

Sekeres MA, Kalycio ME, Bolwell BE, ed. *Clinical Malignant Hematology.* New York: McGraw-Hill, 2007:503–831.

Shipp JA, for The International Non-Hodgkin's Lymphoma Prognostic Factors Project. A predictive model for aggressive non-Hodgkin's lymphoma. *N Engl J Med* 1993;329:987–994.

Chapter 25

Plasma Cell Disorders

Anuj Mahindra   Rachid Baz   Brian Bolwell

POINTS TO REMEMBER:

- Plasma cells are responsible for the production of immunoglobulins. Hence, plasma cell dyscrasias are characterized by the secretion of monoclonal immunoglobulins (also referred to as M protein, paraprotein, and monoclonal gammopathy).

- The presence of an M protein is usually associated with one of the following:
  - Multiple myeloma
  - Monoclonal gammopathy of undetermined significance (MGUS)
  - Waldenström's macroglobulinemia

- The clinical manifestations of plasma cell disorders may result from bone marrow infiltration by the malignant clone, impairment of humoral and cell-mediated immunity, damage from high levels of immunoglobulins or free light chains, and secretion of osteoclast activating factors with resultant bone damage.

- The clinical manifestations of multiple myeloma can be divided into three broad categories: plasma cell growth in bone marrow and skeletal disease, immunologic abnormalities, and effect of the abnormal paraprotein.

- MGUS occurs in about 3% of people older than 50 years of age and 5% of people older than 70 years.
- Myeloma differs from MGUS by the presence of end-organ damage.
- End-organ damage includes hypercalcemia, renal insufficiency, anemia, and lytic bone lesions.
- Unexplained bone pain, spontaneous fractures, elevated serum total protein, renal insufficiency and proteinuria, neuropathy, or recurrent infections should prompt for an evaluation for a plasma cell dyscrasia.
- Serum protein electrophoresis (SPEP) with immunofixation and urine protein electrophoresis (UPEP) with immunofixation should both be done as part of an initial workup.
- There is a low threshold for MRI of the spine in cases of suspected cord compression.
- Because 20% to 25% of patients will eventually progress to myeloma, evaluation for signs and symptoms and monitoring the SPEP and UPEP every 6 months is recommended. No treatment is indicated for patients with MGUS.
- Several agents have activity in multiple myeloma, including thalidomide, lenalidomide (immunomodulatory drugs), bortezomib (proteasome inhibitor), dexamethasone, melphalan, vincristine, doxorubicin, and hematopoietic stem cell transplantation.

Plasma cell dyscrasias are a group of neoplastic or potentially neoplastic disorders of hematopoietic cells known as plasma cells. Plasma cells are responsible for the production of immunoglobulins. Hence, plasma cell dyscrasias are characterized by the secretion of monoclonal immunoglobulins (also referred to as M protein, paraprotein, and monoclonal gammopathy).

The presence of an M protein is usually associated with one of the following:

- Multiple myeloma
- Monoclonal gammopathy of undetermined significance (MGUS)
- Waldenström's macroglobulinemia
- Primary amyloidosis

Rarely, the presence of a monoclonal protein is not associated with a plasma cell disorder but is noted in association with lymphoproliferative disorders (chronic lymphocytic leukemia, non-Hodgkin lymphoma), metastatic carcinoma, osteosclerotic myeloma or POEMS (Polyneuropathy, Organomegaly, Endocrinopathy, Monoclonal gammopathy, and Skin changes) syndrome, and the rare heavy-chain diseases.

The clinical manifestations of plasma cell disorders may result from bone marrow infiltration by the malignant clone, impairment of humoral and cell-mediated immunity, damage from high levels of immunoglobulins or free light chains, and secretion of osteoclast activating factors with resultant bone damage.

Unexplained bone pain, spontaneous fractures, severe osteoporosis, elevated serum total protein, unexplained renal insufficiency and proteinuria, neuropathy, or recurrent infections should prompt an evaluation for a plasma cell dyscrasia. Key summary features of the major plasma cell dyscrasias follow.

Multiple Myeloma

- Second most common hematologic malignancy—about 19,000 newly diagnosed cases in the United States annually
- Higher incidence for African Americans—about twice that of Caucasians
- Median age at diagnosis approximately 68 years, but 2% to 4% of patients are younger than 40 years of age

Monoclonal Gammopathy of Undetermined Significance

- Incidence increases with age. Affects about 3% of persons 50 years or older and 5% of persons 70 years or older
- Risk of progression to multiple myeloma (MM) or related disorder is about 1% per year
- Diagnostic criteria summarized in Table 25.1

Plasmacytoma

A solitary plasmacytoma—essentially, a solid tumor mass of plasma cells without systemic signs of MM—is found in 2% of patients. Solitary plasmacytomas of bone usually involve a vertebral body, whereas extramedullary plasmacytomas usually occur in the head and neck area.

Plasma Cell Leukemia

Primary plasma cell leukemia refers to the finding of >2,000/μL plasma cells in the peripheral blood at the time of diagnosis with MM. Secondary plasma cell leukemia occurs in end-stage MM. Plasma cell leukemia is associated with a poor prognosis.

Diagnostic and Staging Workup

Key aspects of the diagnosis and management of the plasma cell dyscrasias follow.

Routine laboratory tests include:

- Complete blood count and differential, peripheral blood smear
- Complete metabolic panel (includes calcium, albumin, and creatinine)
- Routine coagulation testing

TABLE 25.1

DIFFERENTIAL DIAGNOSIS AND DIAGNOSTIC CRITERIA FOR MONOCLONAL GAMMOPATHY OF UNDETERMINED SIGNIFICANCE (MGUS), SMOLDERING MULTIPLE MYELOMA (SMM), AND SYMPTOMATIC MULTIPLE MYELOMA

MGUS	SMM	Symptomatic Multiple Myeloma
Serum M protein <3g/dL and	Serum M protein ≥3g/dL or	Monoclonal gammopathy in serum and/or urine and
Bone marrow plasmacytosis <10% and	Bone marrow plasmacytosis ≥10% and	Monoclonal bone marrow plasma cells and/or a documented clonal plasmacytoma and
No related organ and tissue impairment	No related organ and tissue impairment	Related organ and tissue impairment*

*Related organ and tissue impairment (acronym—CRAB): hyperCalcemia: serum calcium >11.5 mg/dL (2.65 mmol/L), Renal dysfunction: serum creatinine >2 mg/dL (177 μmol/L or more), Anemia: hemoglobin <10 g/dL or 2 g/dL below the lower limit of normal, Bone disease (lytic lesions or osteopenia).

- Serum vitamin B_{12}, folate

  Myeloma-specific testing includes:

- SPEP, monoclonal protein analysis, and immunofixation
- 24-Hour urine collection for protein, urine protein electrophoresis, and immunofixation

(SPEP by itself is inadequate because some myeloma clones secrete only light chains, which are rapidly cleared from the plasma to the urine.)

- Serum β2 microglobulin, C-reactive peptide, and lactate dehydrogenase
- Bone marrow aspirate and biopsy with cytogenetics

  Imaging studies include:

- Skeletal bone survey (includes plain films of spine, pelvis, skull, humeri, and femurs); notably, MM is characterized by lytic bone lesions, which are not typically visualized on bone scan
- Bone mineral densitometry by DEXA scan at baseline
- Low threshold for MRI spine in case of suspicion of cord compression or significant back pain
- Echocardiography if anthracycline-based chemotherapy is planned or cardiac amyloidosis is suspected

Signs and Symptoms

The clinical manifestations of MM can be divided into three broad categories: plasma cell growth in bone marrow and skeletal disease, immunologic abnormalities, and effect of the abnormal paraprotein.

Plasma Cell Growth in Bone Marrow and Skeletal Disease

The most common presenting symptom of multiple myeloma is *bone pain*, usually involving the spine or chest. Diffuse osteoporosis is often seen radiographically. Characteristic myeloma changes are *lytic lesions* (rounded, punched-out areas of bone) found most commonly in vertebral bodies, the skull, ribs, and weight-bearing bones.

Importantly, lytic lesions are rarely found distal to the elbow or knees. Back pain can be secondary to bone marrow replacement, lytic lesions, vertebral compression fractures secondary to osteoporosis, and, occasionally, nonmalignant degenerative conditions.

Most *neurologic abnormalities* associated with MM result from direct extension of a skeletal tumor. *Spinal cord compression* occurs in 10% of patients. Although at diagnosis only a small subset of patients will have evidence of peripheral neuropathy on electrophysiological testing, peripheral neuropathy is more common in the setting of amyloidosis or Waldenström's macroglobulinemia.

Anemia is present in most patients and is generally due to decreased red blood cell production—either from marrow infiltration with plasma cells, from renal failure and resultant low erythropoietin levels, from chronic inflammation, or from vitamin B_{12} or iron deficiency. Rouleaux are often present on the peripheral smear. Leukopenia and thrombocytopenia are less common at presentation.

Immunologic Abnormalities

Patients with myeloma often suffer from repeated *infections*, similar to that seen in patients with reduced levels of immunoglobulins. An increased incidence of both gram-positive and gram-negative infections has been reported. Pneumonia is particularly common.

Effect of Abnormal Paraprotein

The *hyperviscosity* syndrome results from the presence of serum proteins with high intrinsic viscosity. This is most commonly associated with immunoglobulin M (IgM) paraprotein and less commonly with IgA paraprotein. High viscosity interferes with efficient blood circulation of the brain, kidneys, and extremities. Headache is common, and dizziness, vertigo, and symptoms of severe ischemia may result.

Peripheral neuropathy may occur due to occlusive changes in small vessels. In addition, high levels of M protein may interfere with coagulation factor function and levels as well as abnormal platelet function, and may result in bruising and purpura.

Renal dysfunction is noted in about 25% of patients at diagnosis and relates to the following etiologies: hypercalcemia, concomitant nephrotoxic agents (nonsteroidal anti-inflammatory drugs, intravenous contrast agents, aminoglycoside antibiotics), intravascular volume depletion, cast nephropathy (myeloma kidney), light-chain deposition disease, and amyloidosis. Therapy includes supportive care as well as therapy directed at the malignant plasma cell clone. Proteinuria is present in about 90% of patients with MM, and abnormal light chains (Bence-Jones protein) are found in 80% of patients.

Prognosis

Key prognostic features of the plasma cell dyscrasias are as follows:

- Despite recent advances, MM remains uniformly fatal.
- The presence of beta$_2$-microglobulin level at the time of diagnosis is the single best prognostic factor. Higher levels predict poor prognosis. This marker should not be used for diagnostic purposes because elevated levels are noted in patients with renal dysfunction, which may not be related to MM.
- C-reactive peptide and lactate dehydrogenase are also prognostic markers.
- Certain cytogenetic changes in the malignant plasma cell clone are powerful predictors of prognosis (e.g., deletion of chromosome 13 and the t (4; 14) predict poor outcomes.)

Staging

Traditionally, the Durie-Salmon staging system was used. This has been largely replaced by the International Staging System (ISS).

The simpler ISS uses beta$_2$-microglobulin (mg/dL) and albumin (g/dL) levels to define three stages:

1. Beta$_2$-microglobulin <3.5, albumin >3.5
2. Beta$_2$-microglobulin <3.5, albumin <3.5 or beta$_2$-microglobulin 3.5–5.5
3. Beta$_2$-microglobulin >5.5

Treatment

Key treatment points are summarized as follows:

- Monoclonal gammopathy of undetermined significance (MGUS)—Because 20% to 25% patients will eventually progress to myeloma, evaluation for signs and symptoms and monitoring the SPEP and UPEP every 6 months is recommended. No treatment is indicated for patients with MGUS. The bone marrow plasma cell percentage, the concentration of the monoclonal protein, and serumfree light-chain assays can be used to risk-stratify patients and identify a group of patients with a higher risk of developing MM.

- Smoldering multiple myeloma—About half the patients will progress to active MM. Patients are usually initially observed without therapy at more frequent intervals than patients with MGUS (usually every 3 months). Treatment is recommended only on progression to symptomatic/active myeloma.
- Solitary plasmacytoma—Radiation therapy to a solitary area can result in cure. Because there is an increased risk for systemic MM, monitoring is recommended using SPEP and UPEP.
- MM—MM is not curable with current treatments. The goal of treatment is palliation of symptoms, prevention of end-organ damage, and prolongation of survival.

Several agents have activity, including thalidomide, lenalidomide (immunomodulatory drugs), bortezomib (proteasome inhibitor), dexamethasone, melphalan, vincristine, doxorubicin, and hematopoietic stem cell transplantation.

Different combinations can be used depending on patient age, symptoms, stage, and comorbidities. For older patients, the combination of oral agents—melphalan, prednisone, and thalidomide—is often used first line, whereas a combination of thalidomide and dexamethasone is a frequently prescribed first-line therapy in younger patients (usually younger than 65 years of age).

Side effects of thalidomide include sedation, constipation, neuropathy, rash, thromboembolic events, and bradycardia. (Embryopathy is a well-recognized complication, making the drug contraindicated in women of childbearing age.) Side effects of lenalidomide include myelosuppression, diarrhea, rash, and thromboembolic events. Side effects of bortezomib therapy include myelosuppression (thrombocytopenia), peripheral neuropathy, and reactivation of herpes zoster.

Intravenous monthly bisphosphonate therapy (pamidronate, zoledronic acid) has been shown to decrease the skeletal-related complications of MM and may have effects on the plasma cell clone as well. Side effects of these agents include flulike symptoms (usually with the first dose), renal dysfunction, and the newly recognized osteonecrosis of the jaw.

AMYLOIDOSIS

Amyloidosis is characterized by extracellular deposition of pathological insoluble fibrillar proteins in organs and tissues. Categories include the following:

- Primary (AL)—with or without plasma cell and lymphoid neoplasms
- Secondary (AA)—associated with chronic infections or autoimmune disease
- Familial (ATTR)—associated with familial Mediterranean fever and others

- Aging-associated amyloidosis
- Amyloidosis of endocrine glands—with medullary thyroid carcinoma and multiple endocrine neoplasia type 2

Amyloid fibrils in primary amyloidosis are fragments of monoclonal immunoglobulin light chains. Why some immunoglobulin light chains form amyloid and others do not is not known.

There are approximately 1,500 to 3,000 new patients with amyloidosis diagnosed annually in the United States, with the median age of 65 years at onset.

Symptoms

Symptoms of amyloidosis are as follows:

- Initial symptoms are generally vague and nonspecific, including fatigue, malaise, and weight loss, usually resulting in diagnostic delays.
- The kidney and the heart are the most commonly affected organs.
- Renal involvement results in proteinuria, leading to nephrotic syndrome and renal failure.
- Cardiac involvement results in congestive heart failure (usually from diastolic dysfunction). Clinical clues include low voltage on the ECG, increased left ventricular wall thickness, and abnormal myocardial reflectivity (starry sky pattern) on echocardiography. Endomyocardial biopsy is required when histological diagnosis cannot be demonstrated in another organ.
- Autonomic and sensory neuropathy is common.
- Gastrointestinal symptoms include malabsorption or pseudo-obstruction, and hepatomegaly is common.
- Macroglossia occurs in about 20% of the patients.

Diagnosis

Key diagnostic features are summarized as follows:

- Biopsy of an involved organ will confirm the diagnosis.
- A subcutaneous abdominal fat aspirate stained with Congo red will be positive in about 85% of patients with primary amyloidosis.
- SPEP with immunofixation, UPEP with immunofixation, and bone marrow aspiration and biopsy are recommended.

Prognosis and Treatment

The prognosis of amyloidosis is variable and largely depends on the involved organ (worse for patients with cardiac involvement and best for patients with solitary renal involvement).

Dexamethasone-based therapy aimed at the plasma cell clone is the cornerstone of therapy. The addition of chemotherapy (melphalan), immunomodulary agents, and autologous stem cell transplantation are being investigated.

WALDENSTRÖM'S MACROGLOBULINEMIA

Key features include the following:

- Waldenström's macroglobulinemia (WM) is the result of the clonal proliferation of lymphoplasmacytic cells that produce monoclonal immunoglobulin M (IgM).
- The demonstration of IgM monoclonal protein is not synonymous with the diagnosis of WM as this can be seen in several lymphoproliferative disorders.
- WM is an uncommon disease with approximately 1,500 cases/year in the United States.
- The median age of individuals with WM is approximately 65 years. There is a slight male preponderance.

Diagnostic Criteria

Diagnostic criteria for WM include the following:

- IgM monoclonal protein of any concentration
- Bone marrow (BM) infiltration by small lymphocytes showing plasmacytoid/plasma cell differentiation
- An intertrabecular pattern of BM involvement

Clinical Features

Key clinical features of WM include the following:

- Results of tumor infiltration—lymphadenopathy, organomegaly, constitutional symptoms (fevers, weight loss)
- Consequences of monoclonal IgM—hyperviscosity, cryoglobulinemia, neuropathy, amyloidosis

Treatment and Prognosis

Multiple agents have activity in the treatment of WM, including purine analogs (fludarabine, pentostatin), alkylating agents (chlorambucil, cyclophosphamide), monoclonal antibodies (rituximab), and thalidomide. Therapy is palliative in nature and only recommended in the presence of symptoms or cytopenias.

REVIEW EXERCISES

QUESTIONS

1. A 68-year-old man is noted to have an elevated total protein level on a routine laboratory test done by his primary care physician. He is asymptomatic, has a normal complete blood count, serum creatinine AST/ALT, and calcium levels. A serum protein electrophoresis is ordered and reveals a monoclonal protein immunoglobin G Kappa measuring 0.5 g/dL. A skeletal survey is without evidence of lytic lesions. What should you recommend to this patient?

a) Bone scan
b) Observation
c) Treatment with thalidomide and dexamethasone
d) MRI of the spine
e) None of the above

Answer and Discussion
The answer is b. The abnormal serum protein electrophoresis (SPEP) with monoclonal protein in an asymptomatic patient with normal creatinine, calcium, and hemoglobin is suggestive of monoclonal gammopathy of unknown significance (MGUS). A bone marrow biopsy is not necessary in this patient because it is unlikely to diagnose multiple myeloma (MM).

Patients with MGUS are at risk of developing myeloma or a lymphoid neoplasm, with the risk of progression being about 1% a year and, hence, close observation with complete blood count, serum creatinine, calcium and SPEP and urine protein electrophoresis is recommended every 6 months, or if there is a change in symptoms.

Treatment with agents used in myeloma is not recommended in MGUS. An MRI of the spine is not recommended in this patient in the absence of bone/back pain. A bone scan is not usually helpful in MM because bone lesions are frequently purely lytic.

2. The previous patient is managed conservatively. Six years later, he is noted to have an elevation in his M protein, a mild increase in his serum creatinine and calcium, and back pain. A bone marrow biopsy reveals 14% monoclonal plasma cells, and a skeletal survey reveals multiple punched-out lesions (lytic lesions) in the skull and thoracic spine. An MRI of the spine does not reveal any cord compression. What should you do next?

a) Continue monitoring of his monoclonal gammopathy.
b) Start monthly intravenous bisphosphonate therapy.
c) Start therapy with melphalan and prednisone.
d) Prescribe ibuprofen for his bone pain.
e) Start therapy with melphalan, prednisone, and thalidomide, along with monthly intravenous pamidronate.

Answer and Discussion
The answer is e. The patient now fulfills the criteria for myeloma with >10% plasma cells in bone marrow, lytic bone lesions, and monoclonal protein in serum. He is symptomatic by virtue of skeletal lytic lesions, and therapy to his malignant plasma cell clone is recommended at this time. The use of melphalan, prednisone, and thalidomide is considered the first-line therapy of choice in this 74-year-old man. The addition of thalidomide to the combination of melphalan and prednisone increases the survival of patients and is thus superior to melphalan and prednisone alone.

In addition, bisphosphonate therapy is an important part of the management strategy because the bisphosphonates have been shown to decrease skeletal-related events.

Observation alone and bisphosphonate therapy alone would be inappropriate. Nonsteroidal anti-inflammatory drugs and intravenous contrast should be avoided in patients with monoclonal gammopathy of unknown significance and myeloma due to the potential of impairing renal function.

3. A 65-year-old man is diagnosed with multiple myeloma (MM). He had been planning dental extractions, but because of his new diagnosis decides to postpone the visit to the dentist. He receives intravenous pamidronate for MM. Nine months later, his tooth pain gets worse, and he has a tooth extraction done. He presents 1 month later again to his dentist with complaints of pain, swelling, and feelings of numbness of the jaw. Infection is suspected, and the patient is treated with antibiotics. The problem persists, and 3 weeks later, he has exposed bone at the site. What are the recommendations relevant to this condition?

a) Dental extractions should have been done prior to starting pamidronate.
b) Endodontic (root canal) therapy is preferable to extractions once a patient is on bisphosphonates.
c) Referral to oral maxillofacial surgeon or dental oncologist is recommended once the condition develops.
d) All of the above.

Answer and Discussion
The answer is d. The condition described is osteonecrosis of the jaw. The majority of reported cases of bisphosphonate-associated osteonecrosis of the jaw (BON) with the use of zoledronic acid and pamidronate have been associated with dental procedures such as tooth extraction; however, less commonly, BON appears to occur spontaneously in patients taking these drugs.

The risk for developing BON is much higher for cancer patients on intravenous bisphosphonate therapy than the risk for patients on oral bisphosphonate therapy. It is recommended that cancer patients

- Receive a dental examination prior to initiating therapy with intravenous bisphosphonates.
- Avoid invasive dental procedures while receiving bisphosphonate treatment. For patients who develop osteonecrosis of the jaw while on bisphosphonate therapy, dental surgery may exacerbate the condition.
- Dental infections should be managed aggressively and nonsurgically (when possible).

■ Endodontic therapy is preferable to extractions, and, when necessary, coronal amputation with root canal therapy on retained roots to avoid the need for extraction.

4. A 69-year-old man presents to his primary care physician with nonspecific complaints of fatigue and malaise. The symptoms are believed to be due to depression. He presents 3 months later with worsening fatigue, diarrhea, shortness of breath, and lower extremity edema. The chest x-ray is consistent with congestive heart failure. Laboratory evaluation includes a hemoglobin of 10 g/dL, creatinine of 2.2 g/dL, serum albumin of 2.9 g/dL, and 4 g of albuminuria per 24 hours. An echocardiogram reveals concentrically thickened ventricles with a starry sky appearance. Which of the following is true about his potential diagnosis?

a) Macroglossia can be seen in about 20% of the patients.

b) A subcutaneous fat pad aspirate stained with Congo red will be positive in about 85% of patients.

c) A cardiac biopsy is likely to be diagnostic.

d) All of the above.

Answer and Discussion

The answer is d. The patient's signs and symptoms are suggestive of amyloidosis. The diagnosis of amyloidosis is frequently missed initially. Initial symptoms tend to be nonspecific with fatigue, malaise, and weight loss. The kidney and heart are most commonly involved. The elevated serum globulin, abnormal hemoglobin and creatinine, and the echocardiogram findings are suggestive. Biopsy of involved organ will confirm the diagnosis. A less invasive option is subcutaneous fat aspirate or rectal biopsy stained with Congo red.

5. A 62-year-old man with history of multiple myeloma, hypertension, and benign prostatic hypertrophy undergoing treatment with thalidomide presents to his internist with complaints of low back pain and tingling and numbness in his feet after lifting his 30-lb dog. He also complains of difficulty urinating and believes that his dose of doxazosin needs to be readjusted. The next step should be

a) Give him a prescription for ibuprofen and a muscle relaxant.

b) Perform a urinalysis and increase the dose of doxazosin.

c) Reassure him that it is probably a strain and that a few days rest will take care of the problem.

d) Perform an immediate MRI of the spine.

e) Discontinue thalidomide.

Answer and Discussion

The answer is d. Cord compression is a real and devastating consequence of multiple myeloma. The threshold of suspicion should be low and, in the presence of signs and symptoms of potential cord involvement and a change in character of back pain, should warrant an MRI of the spine. Studies indicate that the eventual neurologic outcome depends on the speed of intervention. Once neurologic impairment sets in, the chances of full recovery diminish. Cord compression is an oncologic emergency, and a prompt radiologic evaluation and neurosurgical consultation are needed.

Although thalidomide can cause peripheral neuropathy, it should not result in exacerbation of back pain or urinary symptoms. Thus, discontinuing thalidomide should not result in improvement in his symptoms.

SUGGESTED READINGS

Attal M, Harousseau JL, Facon T, et al. Single versus double autologous stem-cell transplantation for multiple myeloma. *N Engl J Med* 2003;349:2495–2502.

Attal M, Harousseau JL, Stoppa AM, et al. A prospective, randomized trial of autologous bone marrow transplantation and chemotherapy in multiple myeloma. Intergroupe Francais du Myelome. *N Engl J Med* 1996;335:91–97.

Berenson JR, Crowley JJ, Grogan TM, et al. Maintenance therapy with alternate-day prednisone improves survival in multiple myeloma patients. *Blood* 2002;99:3163–3168.

Child JA, Morgan GJ, Davies FE, et al. High-dose chemotherapy with hematopoietic stem-cell rescue for multiple myeloma. *N Engl J Med* 2003;348:1875–1888.

Durie BG, Harousseau JL, Miguel JS, et al. International uniform response criteria for multiple myeloma. *Leukemia* 2006;20:1467–1473.

Jacobson JL, Hussein MA, Barlogie B, et al. A new staging system for multiple myeloma patients based on the Southwest Oncology Group (SWOG) experience. *Br J Haematol* 2003;122:441–450.

Jagannath S, Barlogie B, Berenson J, et al. A phase 2 study of two doses of bortezomib in relapsed or refractory myeloma. *Br J Haematol* 2004;127:165–172.

Kyle RA, Rajkumar SV. Multiple myeloma. *N Engl J Med* 2004;351:1860–1873.

Kyle RA, Therneau TM, Rajkumar SV, et al. A long-term study of prognosis in monoclonal gammopathy of undetermined significance. *N Engl J Med* 2002;346:564–569.

Rajkumar SV, Blood E, Vesole D, et al. Phase III clinical trial of thalidomide plus dexamethasone compared with dexamethasone alone in newly diagnosed multiple myeloma: a clinical trial coordinated by the Eastern Cooperative Oncology Group. *J Clin Oncol* 2006;24:431–436.

Rajkumar SV, Hayman SR, Lacy MQ, et al. Combination therapy with lenalidomide plus dexamethasone (Rev/Dex) for newly diagnosed myeloma. *Blood* 2005;106:4050–4053.

Richardson PG, Sonneveld P, Schuster MW, et al. Bortezomib or high-dose dexamethasone for relapsed multiple myeloma. *N Engl J Med* 2005;352:2487–2498.

Rifkin RM, Gregory SA, Mohrbacher A, et al. Pegylated liposomal doxorubicin, vincristine, and dexamethasone provide significant reduction in toxicity compared with doxorubicin, vincristine, and dexamethasone in patients with newly diagnosed multiple myeloma: a phase III multicenter randomized trial. *Cancer* 2006;106:848–858.

Rosen LS, Gordon D, Kaminski M, et al. Zoledronic acid versus pamidronate in the treatment of skeletal metastases in patients with breast cancer or osteolytic lesions of multiple myeloma: a phase III, double-blind, comparative trial. *Cancer J* 2001;7:377–387.

The National Comprehensive Cancer Network has delineated guidelines for the treatment of multiple myeloma at www.nccn.org.

Chapter 26

Review of Cellular Morphology

Karl S. Theil

CASE STUDIES

This chapter reviews some common and uncommon abnormalities of red blood cells (RBCs), white blood cells (WBCs), and platelets and selected infectious diseases that can be recognized by an experienced observer during review of the peripheral blood smear. Case histories are provided to frame each question to test your knowledge of cellular morphology. The answers to the questions posed in each case are listed at the end of the chapter. A discussion of the correct and incorrect answers for each question is provided in the text. Other details concerning individual disease entities and their treatment are discussed in their respective chapters.

Case 1

1. A 32-year-old male presented for evaluation of a microcytic anemia. His hemoglobin level was 11.5 g/dL,

and his mean corpuscular volume was 78 fL. Hemoglobin electrophoresis was abnormal and showed no hemoglobin A. The peripheral blood smear is shown (Fig. 26.1). The most likely diagnosis is
   a) Hemoglobin S-hereditary persistence of fetal hemoglobin
   b) Hemoglobin SC disease
   c) Hemoglobin CC disease
   d) Hemoglobin SS disease
   e) Hemoglobin S trait

Case 2

1. A 25-year-old male presented to the emergency room with fever and confusion. Laboratory data included white blood cell count 4.8×10^9/L, hemoglobin 7.5 g/dL, and platelet count 20×10^9/L. Prothrombin time and activated partial thromboplastin time were both normal. Based on review of the peripheral blood smear (Fig. 26.4), the most likely diagnosis is
   a) Idiopathic thrombocytopenic purpura
   b) Thrombotic thrombocytopenic purpura
   c) Autoimmune hemolytic anemia
   d) Disseminated intravascular coagulation
   e) Acute promyelocytic leukemia

Case 3

1. A 58-year-old woman presented with fatigue and malaise. Her hemoglobin level was 8.5 g/dL. Physical examination showed mild jaundice, splenomegaly, and generalized lymphadenopathy. The changes noted in the peripheral blood smear (Fig. 26.7) are most consistent with
   a) Cold agglutinin
   b) Clotted specimen
   c) Cryoglobulin
   d) Rouleaux
   e) Artifact

Case 4

1. A 23-year-old male graduate student presents to the emergency room with fever and chills. The peripheral blood smear (Fig. 26.10) is most consistent with
   a) Trypanosomiasis
   b) Babesiosis
   c) Borreliosis
   d) Malaria
   e) Artifact

Case 5

1. A 52-year-old male complaining of fatigue was found to have a white blood cell count 35.5×10^9/L and mild splenomegaly. In conjunction with the peripheral smear (Fig. 26.14), the most likely diagnosis is
   a) Infectious mononucleosis
   b) Leukemoid reaction
   c) Chronic lymphocytic leukemia
   d) Chronic myelogenous leukemia
   e) Acute myeloid leukemia

Case 6

1. A 58-year-old male who was evaluated for a routine physical examination was found to have moderate splenomegaly and no lymphadenopathy. His white blood cell count was 2.8×10^9/L, with 25% neutrophils and 75% "lymphoid" cells (Fig. 26.17). His hemoglobin level was 10.5 g/dL, and platelet count was 57×10^9/L. The most likely diagnosis is
   a) Waldenström's macroglobulinemia
   b) Chronic lymphocytic leukemia
   c) Hairy cell leukemia
   d) Prolymphocytic leukemia
   e) Myelodysplastic syndrome

Case 7

1. A 65-year-old male presented for his preretirement physical examination. Other than having a "cold" and feeling a little more tired than usual, he had no complaints. A complete blood cell count showed white blood cell count 50×10^9/L, hemoglobin 12 g/dL, and platelets 55×10^9/L. Considering the results of peripheral blood smear morphology (Fig. 26.18), the most likely diagnosis is
   a) Viral infection
   b) *Bordetella pertussis* infection
   c) Sézary syndrome
   d) Acute lymphoblastic leukemia
   e) Chronic lymphocytic leukemia

Case 8

1. A 19-year-old female presented to the university's health center with fatigue, sore throat, and cervical lymphadenopathy. A complete blood cell count showed white blood cell count 10.5×10^9/L and platelets 75×10^9/L. In conjunction with the peripheral blood smear (Fig. 26.20), the most likely diagnosis is
   a) Infectious mononucleosis
   b) Idiopathic thrombocytopenic purpura
   c) Non-Hodgkin lymphoma
   d) Acute myeloid leukemia
   e) Acute lymphoblastic leukemia

Case 9

1. A 20-year-old male undergraduate student presented with fever, petechial rash, and platelet count 25×10^9/L. Given the peripheral blood smear morphology (Fig. 26.24), the most likely diagnosis is
   a) Ehrlichiosis/anaplasmosis
   b) Disseminated histoplasmosis
   c) Candidal sepsis
   d) Meningococcemia
   e) Chediak-Higashi syndrome

Case 10

1. A 32-year-old asymptomatic woman was found to have a platelet count of 50×10^9/L. In conjunction with the peripheral blood smear (Fig. 26.27), the most likely diagnosis for the thrombocytopenia is
   a) Systemic lupus erythematosus
   b) Spurious thrombocytopenia
   c) Heparin-induced thrombocytopenia
   d) Idiopathic thrombocytopenic purpura
   e) Drug effect

RED BLOOD CELL MORPHOLOGY

Figure 26.1 demonstrates frequent *target cells* and distorted erythrocytes containing dense rhomboidal hemoglobin (Hb) C crystals. Target cells have a central dense staining

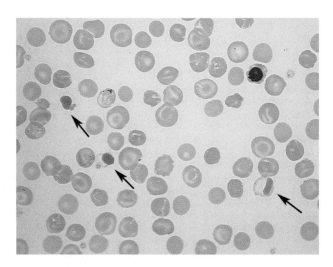

Figure 26.1 Peripheral blood smear: frequent target cells and hemoglobin C crystals (*arrows*). (See Color Fig. 26.1.)

TABLE 26.1
CONDITIONS ASSOCIATED WITH TARGET CELLS

Hemoglobinopathies
Thalassemias
Liver disease
Iron-deficiency anemia
Postsplenectomy
Artifact

area surrounded by a zone of otherwise normal RBC pallor. This appearance is attributed to an increased surface membrane to volume ratio, resulting from either excess membrane lipid or decreased cytoplasmic contents. Target cells can be seen in a variety of disorders (Table 26.1), but are notable in certain hemoglobinopathies, including Hb SC disease, Hb C disease, Hb S disease, Hb C trait, and Hb E trait.

Hb C crystals (Fig. 26.1, *arrows*) are observed in Hb C disease and Hb SC disease, but are not commonly found in Hb C trait. The crystals distort the RBC, concentrating the hemoglobin and leaving the rest of the cell with colorless cytoplasm surrounded by a thin membrane. Both Hb S and Hb C are due to a point mutation in the beta-globin gene at position 6 that normally codes for glutamic acid: substitution of lysine at this position results in Hb C, and substitution of valine results in Hb S. The peripheral blood smear in Hb S disease (Fig. 26.2) is characterized by classic "sickled" cells, target cells, polychromasia, and nucleated RBC. *Howell-Jolly bodies*, small round intracytoplasmic inclusions that are remnants of nuclear DNA, are found in children and adults reflecting hyposplenism or splenic atrophy. In patients with Hb SC disease, the peripheral smear shows target cells and irregular "boat-shaped" cells with misshapen hemoglobin crystals (Fig. 26.3); classic sickled cells or octahedral Hb C crystals are rare.

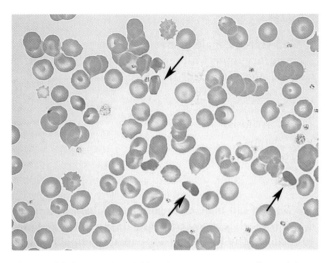

Figure 26.3 Peripheral blood smear: target cells and boat-shaped poikilocytes (*arrows*) in hemoglobin SC disease. (See Color Fig. 26.3.)

Sickle cell disease and Hb SC disease can be readily distinguished from Hb C disease by hemoglobin electrophoresis. Unlike patients with Hb S trait or Hb C trait who are heterozygous for an abnormal beta-globin gene, patients with Hb S disease, Hb C disease, or Hb SC disease have mutations affecting both beta-globin genes and cannot produce Hb A. Although patients who are doubly heterozygous for Hb S and hereditary persistence of fetal hemoglobin (HPFH) also lack hemoglobin A, they are not anemic, and their RBCs appear normocytic and normochromic. Patients with Hb S-HPFH are not symptomatic from a sickling condition due to the protective effect of fetal hemoglobin within each RBC that inhibits polymerization of Hb S.

The presence of numerous *RBC fragments* as shown in Figure 26.4 should prompt concern for a microangiopathic hemolytic anemia. RBC fragments, or schistocytes, can be observed in many conditions (Table 26.2); all are related

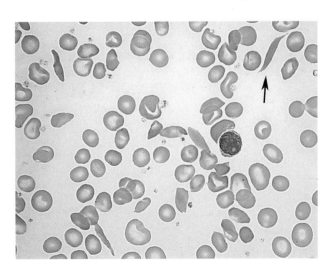

Figure 26.2 Peripheral blood smear in sickle cell disease showing polychromatophilic red blood cells and classic sickled cells (*arrow*). (See Color Fig. 26.2.)

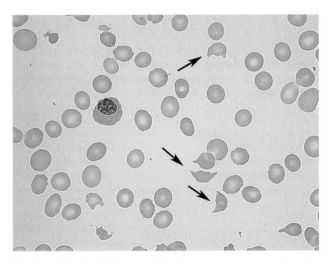

Figure 26.4 Peripheral blood smear: microangiopathic hemolytic anemias are characterized by the presence of red blood cell fragments (*arrows*). (See Color Fig. 26.4.)

TABLE 26.2

CONDITIONS ASSOCIATED WITH RED BLOOD CELL FRAGMENTS

Disseminated intravascular coagulation
Thrombotic thrombocytopenic purpura
Hemolytic-uremic syndrome
Damaged cardiac valve
Vasculitis
Malignant hypertension
Vascular malformation
Aortic aneurysm
Megaloblastic anemia
Severe burns
Malignancy
Improper sample collection (clotted catheter)

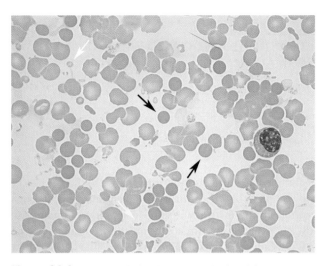

Figure 26.6 Peripheral blood smear: marked poikilocytosis with microspherocytes (*black arrows*) and red cell fragments (*white arrows*) following a severe burn. (See Color Fig. 26.6.)

to intravascular trauma to the RBC membrane. When there is concurrent thrombocytopenia, a diagnosis of disseminated intravascular coagulation, thrombotic thrombocytopenic purpura, or hemolytic uremic syndrome should be considered. The presence of circulating nucleated RBC precursors and polychromatophilia can be helpful in assessing the bone marrow response to peripheral RBC destruction. Other causes for RBC fragmentation, such as heart valve disease or metastatic carcinoma with intravascular spread, may not be associated with thrombocytopenia. Primary hematologic diseases, including megaloblastic anemia and acute promyelocytic leukemia (Fig. 26.5), can show schistocytes related to abnormal RBC production or consumptive coagulopathy. Patients with severe burns show marked poikilocytosis with *microspherocytes* and RBC fragments related to thermal trauma (Fig. 26.6). Samples collected through partially clotted intravascular catheters may have artifactual RBC fragmentation. Of note, idiopathic thrombocytopenic purpura is often associated with

severe thrombocytopenia, but RBC fragments are characteristically absent.

Variably sized clumps of RBC as shown in **Figure 26.7** are the hallmark of a *cold agglutinin*. Agglutination of RBC occurs in the presence of an IgM antibody that reacts optimally at cold temperatures (typically 4°C). When the antibody titer is high and the thermal amplitude of the antibody approaches body temperature, patients may suffer from cold agglutinin disease. Although most cold agglutinins are idiopathic, the IgM produced is occasionally related to a low-grade, B-cell lymphoproliferative disorder such as chronic lymphocytic leukemia, lymphoplasmacytic lymphoma, or marginal zone lymphoma, so it is important to review smears with cold agglutinins to rule out this possibility. Infectious mononucleosis (anti-i) and mycoplasma pneumonia (anti-I) may also be associated with cold

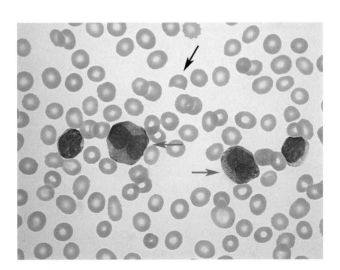

Figure 26.5 Peripheral blood smear in acute promyelocytic leukemia shows circulating blasts (*red arrows*). Severe thrombocytopenia and red cell fragments (*black arrow*) reflect a consumptive coagulopathy. (See Color Fig. 26.5.)

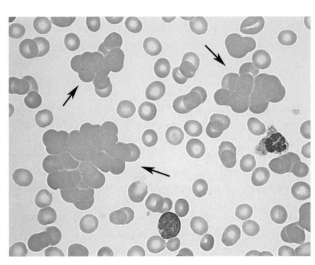

Figure 26.7 Peripheral blood smear: variably sized three-dimensional clumps of red blood cells (*arrows*) are the hallmark of a cold agglutinin. (See Color Fig. 26.7.)

TABLE 26.3

CONDITIONS ASSOCIATED WITH ROULEAUX FORMATION

Hypergammaglobulinemia due to chronic inflammation or liver disease
Lymphoproliferative disorders
Plasma cell myeloma
Monoclonal gammopathy

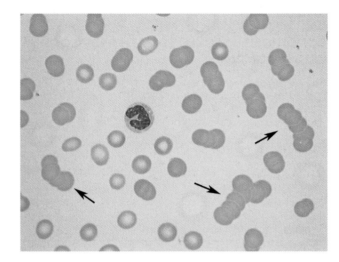

Figure 26.9 Peripheral blood smear shows red blood cells arranged as "stacks of coins" forming rouleaux (*arrows*). (See Color Fig. 26.9.)

agglutinins. Cold agglutinins interfere with RBC indices in the complete blood count: for a given hemoglobin concentration, the instrument spuriously underestimates the RBC count and overestimates the mean corpuscular volume (MCV), causing an elevated mean corpuscular hemoglobin and mean corpuscular hemoglobin concentration. Both the cellular agglutination and its effect on the RBC indices are abolished by warming the sample to 37°C.

Cold agglutinins are distinguished from *cryoglobulins* and *rouleaux* formation (Table 26.3). Cryoglobulinemia (Fig. 26.8) appears in peripheral blood smears as amorphous extracellular bluish deposits that may adhere to adjacent RBC; in some cases, the cryoprotein may take on a crystalline appearance. Cryoglobulins precipitate in cold temperatures, following specimen collection and processing, and redissolve on warming. Cryoglobulins can be quantitated and further classified according to protein composition. Most cryoglobulins are composed of immunoglobulin that is monoclonal (type I), polyclonal (type III), or mixed (type II). Neutrophils and monocytes may contain phagocytized cryoglobulin after specimens are cooled to room temperature. Rouleaux formation (Fig. 26.9) occurs in association with increased amounts of positively charged proteins, usually fibrinogen or gamma globulins. The positively charged proteins neutralize the negatively charged surface of RBC, allowing them to as-

sociate in the form of stacks of four or more cells. True rouleaux formation occurs even in the thin portion of the smear, whereas RBC in thicker portions of the smear normally appear artifactually arranged in a linear fashion. Rouleaux formation may be associated with spuriously low RBC counts and elevated MCV in automated hematology analyzers. Smears prepared from clotted specimens often have RBC and platelet clumps associated with fibrin strands.

A variety of micro-organisms can be identified based on careful review of the peripheral blood smear. Figure 26.10 shows several erythrocytes (*arrows*) infected with ring trophozoites of malaria, in this case *Plasmodium falciparum*. The ring forms have a red chromatin dot and blue cytoplasm. The various types of malaria cannot be speciated based on the presence of ring forms alone; other features, including presence or absence of other stages of

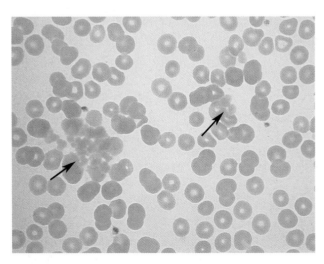

Figure 26.8 Peripheral blood smear shows amorphous extracellular light blue globules (*arrows*) in a patient with cryoglobulinemia. (See Color Fig. 26.8.)

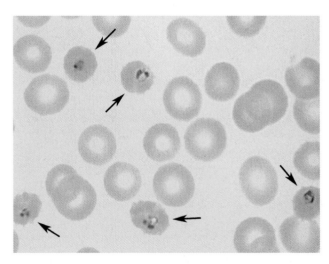

Figure 26.10 Peripheral blood smear shows several erythrocytes parasitized by ring trophozoites of malaria (*arrows*). (See Color Fig. 26.10.)

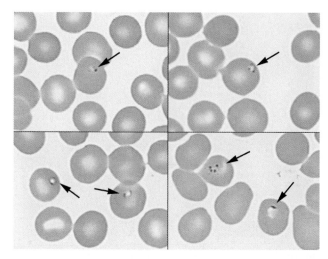

Figure 26.11 Peripheral blood smear in babesiosis shows small ring forms and characteristic tetrad form (*lower right*) within erythrocytes. (See Color Fig. 26.11.)

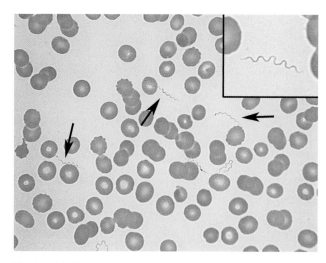

Figure 26.13 Peripheral blood smear in borreliosis shows extraerythrocytic spirochetes (*arrows*). (See Color Fig. 26.13.)

WHITE BLOOD CELL MORPHOLOGY

Blasts are not normally found in peripheral blood smears and can be recognized by a high nuclear:cytoplasmic ratio, immature, delicate chromatin, variably prominent nucleoli, and agranular cytoplasm (Fig. 26.14). Although morphology alone is not often reliable for distinguishing myeloid from lymphoid blasts, the presence of *Auer rods* (Fig. 26.14) is a useful marker of myeloid differentiation. Auer rods are formed from primary granules, are myeloperoxidase positive, and can be seen in high-grade myelodysplasia (refractory anemia with excess blasts type 2) and in acute myeloid, acute myelomonocytic, and acute erythroleukemia. Multiple Auer rods within blasts are a hallmark of acute promyelocytic leukemia (Fig. 26.15).

The peripheral blood smear in *chronic myelogenous leukemia* (CML) is characterized by a leukocytosis with

maturation, multiply parasitized cells, number of schizonts per infected cell, and size of parasitized RBC must be taken into account. The presence of ring forms (or gametocytes) alone, small rings, multiply parasitized RBC, and rings with two chromatin dots are features associated with *P. falciparum*. Potential look-alikes include babesiosis (Fig. 26.11) or platelets overlying RBC. *Babesia* spp. have one or more small ring forms within RBC, and can be distinguished from malaria by the presence of tetrad forms (Fig. 26.11) or extraerythrocytic ring forms. Trypanosomiasis, the cause of African sleeping sickness and Chagas' disease, is characterized by extracellular organisms with an undulating membrane, anterior flagellum, and a central kinetoplast (Fig. 26.12). *Borrelia recurrentis*, the spirochetal organism associated with epidemic relapsing fever, may be observed in peripheral blood (Fig. 26.13) during febrile episodes.

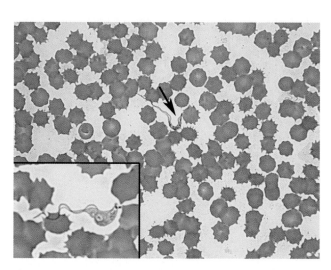

Figure 26.12 Trypanosomes (*arrow*) are extraerythrocytic parasites with an undulating membrane, central kinetoplast, and anterior flagellum. (See Color Fig. 26.12.)

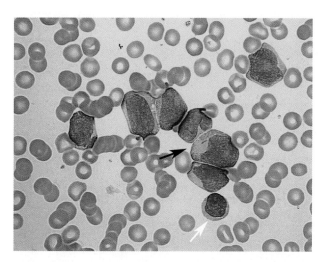

Figure 26.14 Peripheral blood smear with blasts and a lymphocyte (*white arrow*) from a case of acute myeloid leukemia. Auer rod (*black arrow*) within a blast is a distinctive feature associated with myeloid differentiation. (See Color Fig. 26.14.)

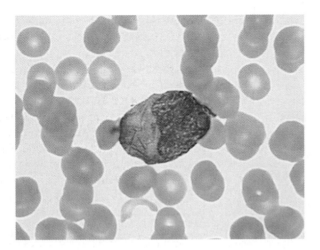

Figure 26.15 Multiple Auer rods within a blast in acute promyelocytic leukemia. (See Color Fig. 26.15.)

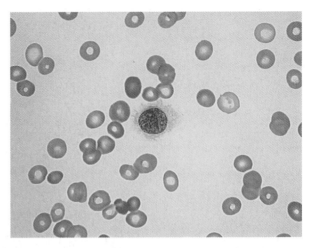

Figure 26.17 Peripheral blood smear in hairy cell leukemia shows a classic hairy cell with delicate cytoplasmic surface projections. (See Color Fig. 26.17.)

granulocyte predominance and left-shift in maturation with occasional circulating blasts (1%–2%) (**Fig. 26.16**). Eosinophilia, basophilia, and myelocyte and neutrophil predominance without dysplastic features are other distinguishing findings. There may be a significant thrombocytosis. The term neutrophilic *leukemoid reaction* refers to a granulocytosis (often >30 × 10⁹/L) with a left-shift in maturation; toxic granulation, vacuolization, and Döhle bodies are often present, but, in contrast to CML, circulating blasts are distinctly unusual. Leukemoid reactions are associated with inflammatory and infectious processes or growth factor therapy.

The lymphocytes in *hairy cell leukemia* have a classic morphology in peripheral blood smears. Hairy cells (**Fig. 26.17**) have delicate surface cytoplasmic projections and a cytoplasmic membrane that merges with the background. Nuclear chromatin is less condensed than a normal lymphocyte, and a single small nucleolus is often visible. Histochemical stains for detecting tartrate-resistant acid phosphatase characteristically present in

hairy cell leukemia have been replaced by flow cytometry for diagnosis. By flow cytometry, hairy cells are typically CD19+, CD20+, CD11c+, CD25+, CD103+, and CD123+, with monotypic kappa or lambda surface light-chain immunoglobulin. Bone marrow aspirates are often "dry taps" due to increased reticulin fibrosis, so identification of hairy cells in peripheral blood smears or marrow touch preps is critical for establishing a diagnosis. Hairy cell leukemia must be distinguished from other lymphoproliferative disorders, including chronic lymphocytic leukemia, prolymphocytic leukemia, lymphoplasmacytic lymphoma (Waldenström's macroglobulinemia), marginal zone lymphoma, and plasma cell leukemia.

The lymphocytes in *chronic lymphocytic leukemia* closely resemble normal mature lymphocytes, but have condensed, clumped, smudgy chromatin (**Fig. 26.18**). The cells are fragile, and are often smeared or smudged, forming so-called "basket cells" that are not suitable for differential counting. Because a lymphocytosis is present to a variable degree, morphology alone may not be diagnostic, and

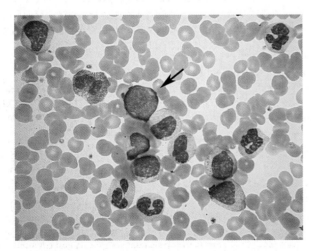

Figure 26.16 Peripheral blood smear in chronic myelogenous leukemia shows leukocytosis with left shift in granulocyte maturation, 1% to 2% circulating blasts (*arrow*), eosinophilia, and basophilia. (See Color Fig. 26.16.)

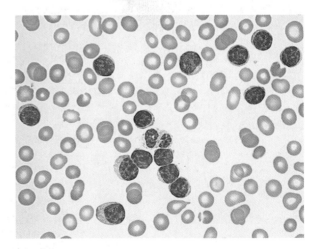

Figure 26.18 Peripheral blood smear in chronic lymphocytic leukemia shows a mature lymphocytosis with clumped smudgy chromatin. (See Color Fig. 26.18.)

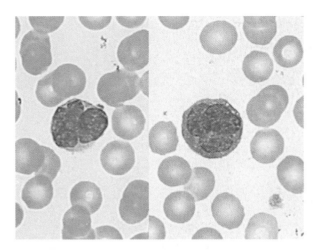

Figure 26.19 Sézary cells have characteristic convoluted nuclei. (See Color Fig. 26.19.)

distinction from a reactive lymphocytosis or other low-grade, B-cell lymphoproliferative disorder can be problematic. Flow cytometry in chronic lymphocytic leukemia reveals a clonal population of B lymphocytes that characteristically expresses CD19, CD20, CD5, CD23, and kappa or lambda (or neither) surface light-chain immunoglobulin (dim); expression of CD38 and/or ZAP-70 have been associated with a less favorable prognosis. There may be associated immune thrombocytopenia or hemolytic anemia. *Bordetella pertussis* infection in children is associated with a lymphocytosis of small lymphocytes that can resemble chronic lymphocytic leukemia, but the lymphocytosis is due to increased T cells, as shown by flow cytometry studies.

Sézary cells represent circulating abnormal T cells associated with the leukemic phase of mycosis fungoides. They are small to intermediate-size lymphocytes with characteristic convoluted, cerebriform nuclei (Fig. 26.19). Flow cytometry demonstrates an abnormal T-cell phenotype with expression of CD2, CD3, CD4, and CD5, but absence of CD7 (an early pan-T-cell marker) and CD26.

Reactive lymphocytes (Fig. 26.20) are a typical feature in viral infections such as infectious mononucleosis, cy-

TABLE 26.4

CONDITIONS ASSOCIATED WITH REACTIVE LYMPHOCYTES

Infectious mononucleosis
Cytomegalovirus
Viral hepatitis
Other viral infections
Drug reactions
Chronic inflammation

tomegalovirus, and hepatitis (Table 26.4). For the beginner, distinguishing reactive lymphocytes from monocytes or even blasts can be problematic. In a reactive process, there is a spectrum of lymphocyte morphologies ranging from small round cells to larger cells with basophilic cytoplasm and angular nuclei with clumped chromatin and small nucleoli, to plasmacytoid lymphocytes and large granular lymphocytes. Reactive lymphocytes have fragile cytoplasmic membranes that can be indented by adjacent RBCs or cause the cells to form smudges when the smear is prepared (Fig. 26.21). Serologic confirmation of viral infections is helpful in establishing a specific diagnosis. An eosinophilia may accompany the reactive lymphocytosis in drug reactions.

Blasts in *acute lymphoblastic leukemia* are small to intermediate in size with high nuclear:cytoplasmic ratios and variably prominent nucleoli (Fig. 26.22). In contrast to a reactive lymphocytosis, lymphoblast proliferations are more uniform in appearance. Anemia and thrombocytopenia are often present due to marrow infiltration. *Lymphoma cells* (Fig. 26.23) are slightly larger than normal lymphocytes, have clumped mature chromatin, high nuclear:cytoplasmic ratios, and often have irregular nuclear contours with indentations and clefts. Distinct nucleoli may or may not be visible.

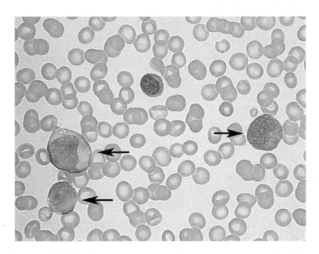

Figure 26.20 Reactive lymphocytes (*arrows*) as seen in infectious mononucleosis. (See Color Fig. 26.20.)

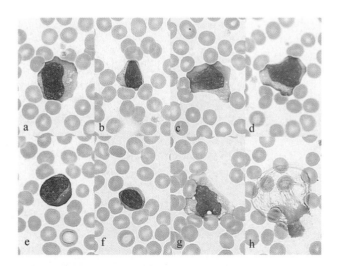

Figure 26.21 Reactive lymphocytes in infectious mononucleosis (**a–e**) contrasted with normal lymphocyte (**f**), monocyte (**g**), and smudge cell (**h**). (See Color Fig. 26.21.)

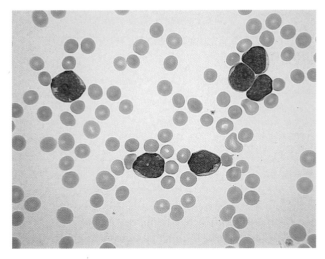

Figure 26.22   Peripheral blood in acute lymphoblastic leukemia shows a uniform population of small blasts. (See Color Fig. 26.22.)

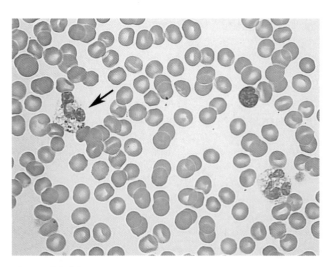

Figure 26.24   Peripheral blood smear with phagocytized bacteria (*arrow*) in a case of meningococcemia. (See Color Fig. 26.24.)

Although infrequent, the identification of neutrophils containing phagocytized bacteria (Fig. 26.24) or fungi (Fig. 26.25, *left panel*) in a peripheral blood smear can point to an overwhelming infection. Stained smears can be decolorized for Gram stain or other stains, and rapid diagnosis can be lifesaving. The presence of Howell-Jolly bodies in the smear may be a clue to an immunocompromised host who is at risk for infection with encapsulated organisms. Specimen collection from infected intravascular catheters or from infected heel sticks can introduce bacteria into the sample and need to be distinguished from true sepsis; a predominance of extracellular organisms may be noted in these situations. Ehrlichiosis and anaplasmosis are tickborne diseases due to small gram-negative coccobacilli that form microcolonies within monocytes and

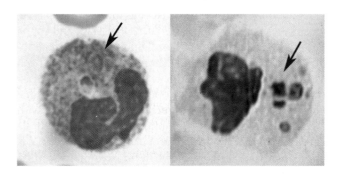

Figure 26.25   Peripheral blood smear with intracellular yeast in a case of disseminated histoplasmosis (*left*). Peripheral blood smear in anaplasmosis shows neutrophil with cytoplasmic morulae (*right*). (See Color Fig. 26.25.)

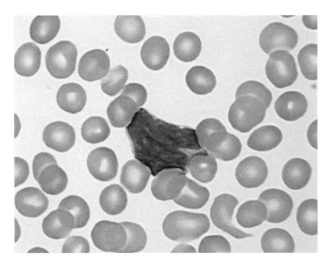

Figure 26.23   Follicular lymphoma cell in peripheral blood has clumped chromatin and indented nuclear outline with no visible nucleoli. (See Color Fig. 26.23.)

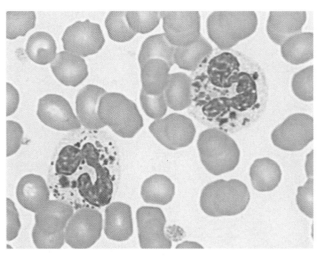

Figure 26.26   Peripheral blood smear in Chediak-Higashi syndrome shows abnormal cytoplasmic granulation. (See Color Fig. 26.26.)

neutrophils, respectively. The microcolonies are visualized as cytoplasmic inclusions in conventionally stained peripheral blood smears (Fig. 26.25, *right panel*).

Chediak-Higashi syndrome is a rare autosomal recessive condition characterized by abnormal cytoplasmic granulation in neutrophils (Fig. 26.26), lymphocytes, monocytes, and eosinophils, and a predisposition for recurrent pyogenic infections. The condition is usually recognized in childhood, and the abnormal cytoplasmic granulation should not be confused with intracellular organisms.

PLATELET MORPHOLOGY

Normal platelets are round to elliptical, have visible cytoplasmic azurophil granules, and range from 1 to 3 μm in diameter. Giant platelets are larger than normal RBCs. *Platelet satellitosis*, recognized when four or more platelets rosette around the periphery of individual neutrophils or monocytes, may be a cause for spurious thrombocytopenia (Fig. 26.27). The phenomenon is related to the presence of an IgG antibody directed against glycoprotein IIb/IIIa that binds to platelets in the presence of EDTA (the anticoagulant in the collection tube). The antibody-coated platelets bind to Fc receptors on neutrophils to produce the rosettes. In some cases, platelet phagocytosis may also be visible. *Platelet clumping* is another EDTA-related phenomenon in which platelets form aggregates in vitro (Fig. 26.28). The platelet clumps will not be enumerated as platelets in automated hematology analyzers, causing spuriously abnormal platelet counts. Performing a platelet count on blood collected in an alternate anticoagulant (sodium citrate, ammonium oxalate) can provide an accurate result in most circumstances. If clumping persists, a platelet cold agglutinin should be considered.

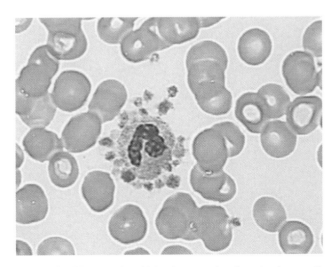

Figure 26.27 Peripheral blood smear showing platelet satellitosis. (See Color Fig. 26.27.)

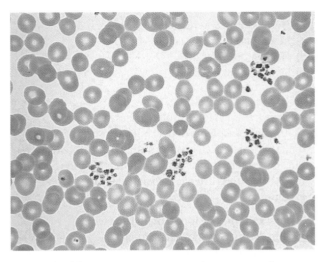

Figure 26.28 Platelet clumping can be a cause of spurious thrombocytopenia. (See Color Fig. 26.28.)

ANSWERS

1. c
2. b
3. a
4. d
5. e
6. c
7. e
8. a
9. d
10. b

REVIEW EXERCISES

QUESTIONS

1. Which of the following conditions is associated with rouleaux formation?
a) Thrombotic thrombocytopenic purpura
b) Plasma cell myeloma
c) Acute myeloid leukemia
d) Hereditary spherocytosis
e) Sézary syndrome

Answer and Discussion

The answer is b. Rouleaux formation is due to neutralization of the normal negative surface charge on red blood cells by positively charged plasma proteins such as a monoclonal immunoglobin G paraprotein associated with plasma cell myeloma. None of the other conditions listed is associated with chronic inflammation, hyperfibrinogenemia, or elevated gamma globulins.

2. Howell-Jolly bodies are expected in adult patients with
a) Sickle cell anemia
b) Sickle cell trait

c) Hemoglobin S-hereditary persistence of fetal hemoglobin

d) Hemoglobin C trait

e) Hemoglobin C disease

Answer and Discussion

The answer is a. Howell-Jolly bodies are evidence of functional asplenia or postsplenectomy state. Patients with sickle cell anemia undergo autosplenectomy due to vascular occlusion by sickled cells. None of the other conditions listed is associated with functional asplenia.

3. Auer rods may be found in patients with

a) Chronic myelogenous leukemia

b) Chronic lymphocytic leukemia

c) Infectious mononucleosis

d) Acute promyelocytic leukemia

e) Acute lymphoblastic leukemia

Answer and Discussion

The answer is d. Auer rods are typically observed in myeloid blasts and are characteristically present in bundles in acute promyelocytic leukemia. None of the other conditions listed is an acute myeloid leukemia or high-grade myelodysplastic syndrome.

4. Target cells are a feature associated with

a) Cold agglutinin

b) Cryoglobulin

c) Severe burn

d) Infectious mononucleosis

e) Thalassemia minor

Answer and Discussion

The answer is e. Target cells may be observed in patients with thalassemia, hemoglobinopathies, and liver disease. They may also be seen also postsplenectomy and as an artifact of slide preparation.

5. Which of the following conditions results in direct infection of red blood cells?

a) Histoplasmosis

b) Borreliosis

c) Babesiosis

d) Trypanosomiasis

e) Ehrlichiosis

Answer and Discussion

The answer is c. Babesiosis directly infects red blood cells (RBCs), where it undergoes asexual reproduction forming the characteristic tetrad. Ehrlichiosis infects granulocytes and monocytes. Histoplasmosis may be phagocytized by monocytes and granulocytes. Borrelia and trypanosomes may be observed in peripheral blood smears as extracellular organisms, but do not infect RBCs.

SUGGESTED READINGS

Bain BJ. *Blood Cells: A Practical Guide*, 4th ed. Oxford: Blackwell, 2006.

Glassy EF, ed. *Color Atlas of Hematology*. Northfield, IL: College of American Pathologists, 1998.

Chapter 27

Palliative Medicine: What Every Internist Ought To Know

Susan B. LeGrand

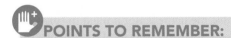

POINTS TO REMEMBER:

■ The Institute of Medicine defines palliative care as follows:

> Palliative Care seeks to prevent, relieve, reduce or soothe the symptoms of disease or disorder without affecting a cure.... Palliative care in this broad sense is not restricted to those who are dying or those enrolled in hospice programs.... It attends closely to the emotional, spiritual, and practical needs and goals of patients and those close to them.

■ Excellent palliative medicine requires skills in seven different areas:
  ■ Communication
  ■ Decision making
  ■ Symptom management
  ■ Prevention/management of complications
  ■ Psychosocial issues
  ■ Care of the imminently dying
  ■ Bereavement

■ Palliative care grew from the hospice movement and, as such, shares many key features. There are three fundamental differences.
  ■ *Life expectancy*: Hospice requires a limited life expectancy typically defined by Medicare or other insurances as less than 6 months. Palliative medicine has no such limitations.
  ■ *Goals of care*: Hospice care neither hastens death nor prolongs life. Palliative medicine is not limited in this way and may actively attempt to prolong life if consistent with the goals and values of the patient and family.
  ■ *Funding mechanisms*: Hospice care is a specific capitated benefit, whereas there is no specialized funding mechanism for palliative care.

In 2006, hospice and palliative medicine (HPM) was recognized as a subspecialty by the American Board of Medical Specialties. It set a unique precedent by being sponsored by ten specialties that obviously recognize the importance of this skill set to their diplomates. Palliative medicine focuses on ensuring the best quality of life for individuals living with advanced, ultimately terminal illness. The number of hospitals with palliative medicine services has increased steadily with guidance from the Center to Advance Palliative Care. The aging demographic guarantees ongoing need for this care. Despite this, education in the skill set for palliative medicine remains limited at best. Teaching in medical schools and residency programs is minimal, and supervision by faculty without the appropriate skills fails to reinforce what may have been learned in lectures or rotations. Nonetheless, primary palliative medicine skills are fundamental to good internal medicine and subspecialty care. This chapter defines palliative medicine, differentiates it from hospice care, and discusses the Medicare hospice benefit. It then focuses on the ethical issues at end of life and several key skills/controversies for primary palliative medical care. This is not a comprehensive review of these topics, and appropriate references for further review are included.

WHAT IS PALLIATIVE CARE?

The Institute of Medicine defines palliative care as follows:

> Palliative care seeks to prevent, relieve, reduce or soothe the symptoms of disease or disorder without affecting a cure.... Palliative care in this broad sense is not restricted to those who are dying or those enrolled in hospice programs.... It attends closely to the emotional, spiritual, and practical needs and goals of patients and those close to them.

HPM is the physician specialty that involves participation with other team members including nursing, social workers, pastoral care, and others to provide palliative care.

PALLIATIVE MEDICINE SKILL SET

Excellent palliative medicine requires skills in seven different areas:

- *Communication.* The ability to sensitively communicate prognosis, discuss goals of care when cure is not possible and explore an individual's hopes and values as end-of-life approaches is fundamental. It is necessary for good medical care in general and yet evidence that it is not well done abounds. All other skills depend on this being done properly.
- *Decision making.* To do everything requires no thought. Knowing what can be done and then deciding based on an individual's goals, values, disease status, etc. what should be done is much more complex.
- *Symptom management.* Knowledge of the different treatments (nonpharmacologic, pharmacologic, and interventional techniques) available to improve symptoms is fundamental. A 1,000 patient database found that on average, palliative medicine patients have 11 symptoms with a range of 1 to 27. Symptoms include both physical and psychological problems.
- *Prevention/management of complications.* This can be as simple as an air mattress in a cachetic patient to relieve pain and prevent decubitus ulcers to asking an orthopedic surgeon to prophylactically pin a high-risk lytic lesion in the arm of a cancer patient.
- *Psychosocial issues.* Management of social and practical concerns that affect patients and families is critical. A comprehensive assessment of family structure, dynamics, coping styles, cultural and religious influences, financial status, social support systems, etc. is invaluable in determining not only appropriate discharge plans but also facilitating better communication, decision making, and symptom control.
- *Care of the imminently dying.* Despite the common misconception that this is all palliative medicine does, it is a specific skill set that is clearly appropriate for every physician caring for acutely or chronically ill people.
- *Bereavement.* After the death of an individual in palliative care, the bereaved include not only the family members but the program staff, volunteers and if in a facility, their staff. The needs of these individuals are managed by bereavement support services in a team fashion.

Both hospice and palliative medicine identify their unit of care as patient and family (as defined by the patient). An advanced disease does not occur to just an individual but affects all those involved with that person. The emotional coping of the caregivers likewise impacts the health and symptoms of the patient. Effective exploration of goals of care, symptoms, coping strategies, decision making, etc., cannot occur without active understanding of the social and emotional circumstances of all involved. This fundamental need also leads to another key feature of both programs, an interdisciplinary team approach. The necessity of nursing, social work, and pastoral care involvement in identifying these issues cannot be overstated.

PALLIATIVE CARE VERSUS HOSPICE CARE

Palliative care grew from the hospice movement and as such shares many key features. There are three fundamental differences:

- *Life expectancy:* Hospice requires a limited life expectancy typically defined by Medicare or other insurances as less than 6 months. Palliative medicine has no such limitations.
- *Goals of care:* Hospice care neither hastens death nor prolongs life. Palliative medicine is not limited in this way and may actively attempt to prolong life if consistent with the goals and values of the patient and family.
- *Funding mechanisms:* Hospice care is a specific capitated benefit, whereas there is no specialized funding mechanism for palliative care.

Therefore, palliative medicine can be involved from the diagnosis of an advanced illness, assist in management of symptoms secondary to the illness and/or its treatment, and may then become the primary focus of care with ultimately a referral to hospice when appropriate.

HOSPICE CARE

One of the most misunderstood issues surrounding hospice is the question of life expectancy. Good hospice care requires time for relationships to develop between the patient/family and the team members, with a minimum of 90 days preferred. Currently, more than 30% of hospice patients die less than 2 weeks after referral. This is crisis intervention, not hospice care, although families may still express satisfaction with the care received. In the late 1990s, concern arose about abuse of hospice services with patients surviving for years on the Medicare benefit. Since then, the Office of the Inspector General (OIG) has tried to reassure physicians that they are not at risk of investigation with good faith estimates. The OIG acknowledges the difficulty of prognostication particularly with noncancer diagnoses. The hospice benefit was designed on a cancer model in which the disease trajectory follows a consistent downhill course once active treatment of the malignancy is no longer effective. Noncancer diagnoses such as congestive heart failure and chronic lung disease are more often characterized by periodic exacerbations with improvement, even though the overall course is progressive decline, and are therefore much more difficult to predict. Guidelines recommended by the National Hospice and Palliative Care Organization do not accurately predict a 6-month life expectancy but are commonly used by hospice agencies for documentation.

The question a referring physician should ask is not when the patient will die, but would they be surprised if death occurred within 6 months. If that would not be a surprise, and a primary focus on comfort would be an appropriate goal of care, then that person could be referred to hospice care. The physician is certifying to a probability that death will occur, not a guarantee. There is no penalty for patients who survive longer or a limit on the number of days an individual can be on the Medicare benefit. Prolonged time in hospice is an opportunity to reassess the original referral. Recertification every 2 to 3 months is required. If patients improve (or goals change) and they are truly no longer appropriate, they may revoke hospice and then readmit when/if decline occurs.

Most private insurers have benefits similar to Medicare. Some policies have a more limited approach with either a set number of visits or a specific dollar amount available. These require more discussion by social workers or discharge planners to create a useful service, often using home care benefits that may be less restricted. There are currently no "palliative medicine benefits" that are outside standard insurance payments (although under consideration by some companies). Physicians bill as they would any other patient, using the time spent rather than evaluation and management documentation for the prolonged counseling that may be required. Hospitalizations are coded using the primary diagnosis and any complications that occur, as one would any other admission.

Hospice, like an HMO, is a capitated benefit. Hospice is paid a set amount/day/patient to provide for all care related to the admitting diagnosis. For example, a patient with congestive heart failure admitted to hospice with a diagnosis of lung cancer will not have his heart medications paid for, but any medications/testing, etc., needed for the lung cancer will be covered. A patient admitted for heart failure would be provided their cardiac medications. Any care ordered for the admitting diagnosis is paid for by the hospice—laboratory tests, x-ray, durable medical equipment, hospitalization—from a current daily benefit of approximately $120 (exact amount varies by region). Longer stays in hospice help agencies recoup the initial costs involved in establishing care. The most cost-intense weeks are the first and last. Most hospices also have formularies of preferred medications to limit costs.

Another confusing issue is what the patient "gives up" when they go on hospice care. There is significant variability on what services hospices will provide. Each physician must learn the policies of the agencies they use. Some consider transfusion appropriate symptom management if it improves dyspnea/fatigue, whereas others consider it life-prolonging therapy and not part of hospice care. Ul-

timately, the decision to use a particular medication, hospitalization, or intervention is between the patient/family and their physician. They may always revoke hospice and return to their standard insurance if, after discussion, they want to receive something the hospice does not provide. Therefore, they do not "give up" anything.

Hospice Benefit versus Home Care

Hospice patients can actually be healthier in the short term than home care patients. To qualify for home care aide services, the first two criteria must be met:

- The patient must be home bound. Visits to the physician are allowed, but the ability to travel independently beyond the home setting will render the patient ineligible.
- The patient must have a skilled nursing need, such as a complicated dressing, physical therapy, short-term teaching for diabetic education, and/or new tube feedings.
- Any equipment requested must have a documented medical need, such as minimum oxygen saturation values for home oxygen support.

Because hospice is a capitated system, none of the previous criteria is required. Hospice patients may have a bed, a standard wheelchair, or oxygen if they think it is helpful. They may continue to travel or work if they want. Home care aides can be available to assist basic care needs, regardless of what other services are required. The involvement of the team may provide enough care to allow a person to remain in his or her home alone or for a family to continue to care for their loved one even when no skilled needs exist. The availability of 24/7 help on call with the potential for a home visit after hours also provides a sense of security that can prevent emergency room visits and hospitalizations.

ETHICAL CONCERNS AT END OF LIFE

The controversy surrounding Terry Schiavo in 2005 renewed debate on the ethics of withholding and withdrawing artificial nutrition and hydration (ANH). Numerous articles were written prior to and after her death. The legal issues were quite clear. A competent adult may refuse any and all medical interventions. A family member may make these decisions for an incompetent adult or child as outlined in state law. In the state of Florida, the spouse makes these decisions in the absence of a legal proxy. ANH has been defined both legally and medically as an intervention with no special status and may be discontinued or withheld like any other medical intervention. There is complete agreement on this within the various medical specialty groups (AMA, American College of Physicians, etc.) and the legal community, although certain religious communities may disagree.

In 2005, Pope John Paul commented that ANH must be provided and should never be discontinued in the persistent vegetative state (PVS). This seemed at odds with the 2001 U.S. Conference of Catholic Bishops Ethical and Religious Directives for Catholic Health Care Services, which stated

A person may forgo extraordinary or disproportionate means of preserving life. Disproportionate means are those that in the patient's judgment do not offer a reasonable hope of benefit or entail an excessive burden, or impose excessive expense on the family or the community.

There should be a presumption in favor of providing nutrition and hydration to all patients, including patients who require medically assisted nutrition and hydration, as long as this is of sufficient benefit to outweigh the burdens involved to the patient.

In a September 2007 clarification approved by Pope Benedict XVI, the Catholic Church stated that ANH should always be given and not withdrawn in the setting of PVS. PVS remains an uncommon reason for ANH, and this statement need not alter the decision making in other circumstances, but non-Catholic practitioners should be aware of this pronouncement.

ETHICAL CARE OF THE DYING AND PALLIATIVE SEDATION

Sensitive ethically appropriate care of the dying does not equate with a morphine drip. There are specific symptoms commonly associated with dying that need to be assessed and managed individually. The physician also has a responsibility to the family whose subsequent bereavement will be affected by how the dying process occurs and the education they receive in preparation for the death. The National Consensus Project for Quality Palliative Care has published clinical practice guidelines recommending the following seven steps in care of the imminently dying:

1. Recognize the transition to the actively dying phase when possible; communicate and document this appropriately to patient, family, and staff.
2. Address end-of-life concerns, hopes, fears, and expectations openly and honestly in a socially, culturally, and age-appropriate manner.
3. Assess and document with appropriate frequency the symptoms at end of life. Treatment is based on patient-family preferences.
4. Revise care plan to reflect the unique needs of the patient and family at this phase. Needs for higher intensity and acuity of care are met and documented.
5. Wishes for care setting at death are documented and met if possible. Any inability to meet this preference is reviewed and documented.

6. Family is educated regarding the signs and symptoms of approaching death in a developmentally and culturally appropriate manner.
7. Hospice care is offered if not already in place.

Signs and symptoms of death are similar, regardless of the specific underlying cause. In the last 48 hours of life, three problems predominate:

- *Pain*—If present, there may be crescendo pain, but it may not exist in all disease states.
- *Respiratory symptoms*—These include dyspnea and secretions.
- *Restlessness*—Otherwise termed terminal delirium.

Once it is clear that the dying process has actively begun, there are certain general recommendations:

- All medications except those needed for symptom management should be stopped. The only exception would be anticonvulsant medications if seizure is a significant risk. An alternative anticonvulsant, such as lorazepam, may be needed once swallowing problems occur.
- Medications for all potential symptoms (even if not yet present) should be ordered on an as needed (PRN) basis. If they are required frequently, then scheduled administration and/or continuous infusion may be needed. Even if rarely used, the efficacy of the dose should be assessed.
- As swallowing becomes impaired, alternative routes of administration will be required. In hospital settings, conversion to subcutaneous routes is preferable. In the home setting, rectal or sublingual administrations are acceptable alternatives. Hospice agencies can often advise on which products can be effectively used by these routes.
- Any lab or x-ray orders should be discontinued.
- Routine vital sign checks may be stopped. Because there is to be no action taken for changes, there is little role for these.

General Recommendations

Pain

Individuals with pre-existing pain concerns may develop pain crises as death approaches, necessitating a rapid increase in medication to re-establish adequate control. Those who have never had pain are unlikely to suddenly develop it in the last hours of life if basic needs such as bowels and bladder are addressed. Therefore, the common practice of starting a morphine infusion in those without pain (or dyspnea) for management of dying is incorrect. Morphine in the absence of a specific symptom may produce toxicity without benefit. Providing a PRN order for low-dose morphine (1 mg IV/SQ for the naïve) would give nurses an option if pain and/or dyspnea were to occur.

Respiratory Symptoms

Dyspnea in the last hours of life can be a difficult symptom to manage without sedation, which is to be discussed separately. Opioids are the medication of choice and will improve the sensation to a degree without sedation. Combination therapy with chlorpromazine in uncontrolled trials has also been helpful. Oxygen support is controversial but clearly contributes little other than normalization of oxygen saturation, when possible. Maintenance of a normal O_2 saturation frequently does not resolve dyspnea because mechanical issues such as muscle weakness rather than hypoxemia are the more important etiologic factors. Monitoring of oxygen saturation should be discontinued because the goal is comfort, not a particular level. Hypoxemia may allow endogenous opioids to occur and provide comfort, while maintenance of oxygen levels may prolong the dying process, which may not always be desired or kind. Opioids should not be used for sedation as noted.

Secretions, commonly called the death rattle, are a symptom of more concern to families than patients. In a study of family preference, 50% wanted management, whereas 50% were satisfied with education that it was a normal process and not distressing to the patient. Usually, treatment is reasonable. Positioning on either side can eliminate some sounds, but anticholinergic medications such as hyoscyamine, glycopyrrolate, or scopolamine have also been shown to help. These medications can be given via sublingual (hyoscyamine, glycopyrrolate), subcutaneous (glycopyrrolate), or transdermal (scopolamine) routes.

Terminal Delirium

This is the most common intractable symptom requiring sedation at end of life. Although maintaining consciousness is reasonable, when an individual is confused without reversible cause or if searching for a cause is not within the goals of care, then control of the symptom becomes primary. Easily treated causes such as fecal impaction and urinary retention should be excluded. Unfortunately, in the last days of life, adequate control may require sedation. It is quite distressing for families to see a loved one thrashing, moaning, or crying out, so treating the symptom is critical.

Differentiating pain and delirium can be difficult when patient report is not available. Moaning is not always pain. Physicians must use their best guess based on the physical appearance, pre-existing pain complaints, and family and nursing impressions. Medications used for sedation include the benzodiazepines, phenothiazines (particularly chlorpromazine), and barbiturates. Doses are titrated until comfort is achieved and then maintained either scheduled or PRN, depending on need. Because opioid medications can cause delirium, particularly if renal function is declining, increasing these medications for delirium may exacerbate the problem.

PALLIATIVE SEDATION THERAPY

Palliative sedation has been called many things to try to clarify the intent. These include terminal sedation and se-

dation of the imminently dying, but palliative sedation therapy (PST) has been recommended by an international panel convened to develop guidelines and standards. PST is defined as "the use of sedative medications to relieve intolerable suffering from refractory symptoms by a reduction in patient consciousness." Refractory symptoms are then defined as "symptoms for which all possible treatment has failed, or it is estimated that no methods are available for palliation within the time frame and the risk–benefit ratio that the patient can tolerate." The evidence base is and will likely remain limited given the practical and ethical difficulties of conducting studies in actively dying patients.

Although various attempts at guidelines exist, the following points are fundamental:

- The symptom must be intractable after appropriate attempts at palliative management. Whenever possible, this should include consultation with a palliative medicine specialist. Whether existential/psychosocial symptoms may be managed with sedation is extremely controversial.
- Interventional approaches to symptom management are either not available or not appropriate given the patient's status.
- Consent is obtained. For some individuals, maintenance of consciousness is paramount, despite what others might view as intractable suffering. Therefore, the institution of sedation requires patient consent when possible or family consent if the patient cannot.
- Medication is carefully titrated until a level of consciousness is obtained that provides symptom relief. The level of sedation need not be coma. The intent is symptom relief, not a specific level of consciousness and not hastening death.

PST may be maintained until death or may be a temporary respite from symptoms with a planned lessening to see if still required. Fluids should certainly be maintained in respite PST but should be discussed in continuous settings. Continuous deep PST is appropriate only in far advanced illness when death is expected in hours to days.

Medication Choices

There have been no controlled trials of medications for PST. The most commonly reported medications are benzodiazepines, particularly midazolam. There has also been a case series evaluating the sedating phenothiazine, chlorpromazine. Other agents such as phenobarbital or propofol have been used. Hospitals and hospices may have specific protocols for particular agents.

HYDRATION AT END OF LIFE

Hydration in the last days of life is a controversial subject, even within the field of palliative medicine. The debate centers on the burden–benefit ratio. A systematic review in 1997 found inadequate data from which to draw firm conclusions on the balance of burden and benefit. There is consensus that discontinuation of parenteral fluids in the dying is a legal and ethical choice. Parenteral fluid support is a medical intervention like any other that may be stopped if not appropriate to the patient and/or family goals of care. In looking at fluids in the last days of life, what is the goal? Do fluids help achieve that goal? Goals might include (a) comfort, (b) prevention/treatment of symptoms, and (c) prolongation of life.

Comfort

Do fluids contribute to comfort at end of life? An alternative question is does dehydration cause discomfort? Prospective evaluation of the intake in advanced cancer patients found that 60% drank <500 cc/day in the days prior to death. The only symptom experienced was dry mouth, and this was effectively managed with local measures. There was no difference in comfort level related to fluid consumption. Another study found that although 70% of dying cancer patients experienced thirst, it was satisfied with mouth care and small amounts of oral fluid. Therefore, fluids do not necessarily contribute to comfort, and dehydration may stimulate endogenous opioids, increasing comfort.

Fluids can cause discomfort in several ways: (a) the need for IV access, which may require repetitive sticks; (b) the development of edema because hypoalbuminemia is common; (c) increased frequency of urination, which may require painful movement or catheterization; and (d) accumulation of pulmonary secretions. If one looks at a goal of comfort only, then fluids probably cause more distress.

Prevention/Management of Symptoms

Those who advocate the use of fluids do so to achieve this goal. If renal insufficiency develops, some medications (particularly certain opioid metabolites) may accumulate and lead to neurotoxicity. Hydration can prevent or reverse this and potentially avoid an agitated delirium. In the setting of an unexplained deterioration in mental status, a time-limited trial of 1 to 1.5 L of fluid over 24 hours is reasonable. If mental status improves, then maintenance can continue. If there is no change, then fluids can be stopped.

Prolongation of Life

A question to ask is whether one is prolonging life or the dying process. There is little question that allowing dehydration to occur may shorten life if the expectancy is several weeks or more. In someone with hours or a few days to live, it is unlikely to change the time course. Fluids may however, prolong the dying process and the suffering.

- Arguments against hydration
  - The only symptom, dehydration, can be managed effectively with local measures
  - Increased discomfort from the IV access
  - Prolongation of the dying process
  - Increase in secretions/edema
- Arguments for hydration
  - Can administer via hypodermoclysis (subcutaneous) or proctoclysis (retention enema), avoiding the discomfort of IV
  - May improve delirium

The decision to use fluids in the dying must be individualized. Ultimately, the family must be able to live with whatever they choose. Physicians can counsel on the medical reality (i.e., dehydration not painful, etc.) that families often do not understand. The pros and cons should be sensitively discussed without bias based on the physician's personal belief system. If fluid support is continued, it should be at relatively low rates (1 L/day) to avoid excessive edema. The need can be readdressed at a later time, particularly if fluid accumulation in the lung should occur.

EFFECTIVE USE OF OPIOIDS

The decision of whether to use opioids for a particular person is beyond the scope of this chapter. The goal for this section is the correct use of opioids once initiated; therefore, fundamental principles are outlined. Physicians are encouraged to review the WHO guidelines for pain management that have been repeatedly validated. Successful pain control in 80% to 90% of cancer patients has been documented when these guidelines are used.

Definitions

Three troublesome definitions continue to interfere with appropriate management of pain, particularly in advanced disease:

- *Addiction.* Also called psychological dependence, addiction is a relatively rare occurrence in those without prior tendency to addictive behaviors. Certainly, in advanced malignancy and at end of life, this concern is irrelevant. Prior or current drug dependency does not prohibit use of opioids in these settings but does require careful follow-up, preferably by a specialist in the field.
- *Dependence.* Physical dependence necessitates a taper to prevent a withdrawal syndrome if/when a medication is no longer indicated. This is an aspect of the pharmacology of a particular medication and is not unique to opioids (selective serotonin reuptake inhibitors, benzodiazepines, barbiturates, etc.).
- *Tolerance.* The need for increasing dosage of medication for the same level of effect. Tolerance to the pain-relieving effects of opioids has been shown to be clinically irrelevant in malignancy, although may be more problematic in chronic nonmalignant pain. In malignancy, a need for increased medication is generally secondary to increased pain. Tolerance rapidly develops to

most side effects of opioids, with the notable exception of constipation.

Principles for Use of Opioid Medications

1. Perform careful pain assessment.
   - Assess for location, radiation, and description (i.e., sharp, burning, etc.).
   - Assess severity using any one of a variety of pain scales.
   - Elicit the time course (constant vs. intermittent) and any precipitating factors.
   - Assess and document each site/type of pain separately.
   - Document any past or present medication use, including degree and duration of response and side effects.
2. Choose a medication appropriate to the severity of the pain. See Figure 27.1.
   - Moderate or severe cancer-related pain (>4 on a scale of 0–10) should be managed with step 2 or 3 medications. Step 2 medications have a dose ceiling secondary to the combination product (acetaminophen or ASA) or toxicity (tramadol). Step 3 medications do not have a dose ceiling and may be increased as needed until adequate pain control is obtained.
   - It is not necessary to start at step 1 and progress to step 3, although this may be appropriate in nonmalignant pain. In cancer-related pain, the choice of medication is determined by the severity of the pain. For exam-

ple, a cancer patient whose baseline pain is 8 should receive morphine even if opioid naïve.
- Certain medications are *not* recommended for chronic pain management. These include the following:
  - *Meperidine.* Meperidine has a toxic metabolite that causes seizures and delirium. Some hospitals have removed it from their formulary completely to prevent usage. It has no advantage over other less toxic opioids.
  - *Agonist/antagonist agents.* Agonist/antagonist agents have ceiling effects and an increased incidence of psychotomimetic effects. Although they may be used in opioid-naïve individuals, their use in someone on chronic opioids can provoke withdrawal.
  - *Codeine.* Codeine is more constipating and has an increased incidence of psychotomimetic effects. It is a prodrug that requires metabolism to the active agent. Ten percent of the population lacks the enzyme needed for conversion.
  - *Propoxyphene.* Propoxyphene has been demonstrated to have no advantage over placebo in controlled trials. It is considered one of the most misused medications in the elderly.
3. Constant pain requires constant medication. This can be accomplished by sustained-release products or scheduled dosing of immediate-release products. A recent study of opioid errors (unpublished data) found this to be one of the more common problems with opioid prescribing. Despite constant pain, a person is given PRN pain medications. If treating an opioid-naïve person as an outpatient, initiation of PRN dosing for 24 to 48 hours to determine the need is reasonable if then promptly converted to sustained-release once dose has been determined.
4. The initial opioid chosen (± an adjuvant) should be titrated until a therapeutic effect is obtained or an intolerable side effect develops. Note the following:
   - There is no indication for more than one sustained-release opioid.
   - Immediate-release medications should be the same opioid when possible (exception: fentanyl).
5. Dosing should be based on the pharmacology of the medication, as well as the patient report of efficacy and duration of effect. Note the following:
   - Immediate-release opioid medications (excluding methadone) alone or in combination have an effective half-life of 3 to 4 hours. Therefore, every 4-hour dosing is preferred. Tramadol is dosed every 6 hours. Half-lives may be prolonged in the elderly, but PRN dosing should still be at the shorter interval. If the medication lasts longer, it will not be requested. If it does not, it will be available.
   - The oral sustained-release products are *never* dosed PRN. The most commonly prescribed medications (generic SR morphine, MS Contin, Oramorph, and

WHO's Pain Relief Ladder

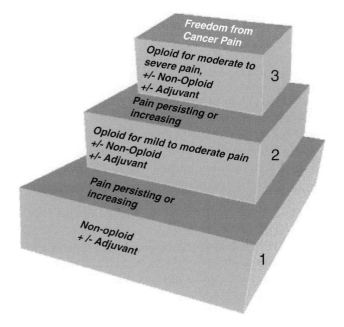

Figure 27.1 WHO's pain relief ladder. *Source:* Reproduced with permission from the World Health Organization. WHO's Pain Ladder. 2008. Available at: www.who.int/cancer/palliative/painladder/en/.

OxyContin) can usually be dosed every 12 hours. An occasional individual will experience end-of-dose failure with a consistent report of increased pain prior to each scheduled dose. This may be managed by an increase in dose or a change to an 8-hour schedule. Compliance is much better on twice-daily dosing. Similar problems can occur with transdermal fentanyl, with reports of worsening pain control on the third day. Patches may need to be changed at 48 to 60 hours. Changing patches more often than 48 hours is not recommended.

6. Patients on sustained-release medications or continuous parenteral infusions must also have immediate-release medications/bolus doses available for breakthrough pain.

7. Use of adjuvant analgesic agents—nonsteroidal anti-inflammatory drugs (NSAIDs), anticonvulsants, and tricyclic antidepressants—should be tailored to the specific characteristics of the pain. For example, adding an NSAID for musculoskeletal pain, an anticonvulsant or tricyclic for neuropathic pain, or a muscle relaxant/antispasmodic agent for cramps.

8. Frequent reassessment of the efficacy of the medication chosen, side effects, and need for breakthrough dosing is important because adjustments in management are frequently required. Patients should keep diaries of medication usage. Physicians must assess the baseline pain control, which includes the number of breakthrough doses required. The efficacy of the breakthrough dose should be assessed separately. If frequent breakthrough dosing is required, then an increase in scheduled medication may be appropriate. If breakthrough dosing is never needed, then a decrease in dose might be tolerated. When adjusting medications, phone call follow-up in several days with a clinic visit in 1 to 2 weeks is needed.

9. Anticipate and manage common side effects, particularly nausea, sedation, and constipation. Tolerance to these will develop with the exception of constipation. Patient education on the possibility of these side effects and the fact that they will resolve if given time can prevent premature discontinuation. Any patient started on opioid medications *must* also be placed on an aggressive bowel regimen, usually including a stool softener and a stimulant. Failure to start bowel regimens was another common error in a recent trial.

Choice of Opioid Medication

Despite small studies (often with pharmaceutical funding) that suggest superiority of one opioid or another for pain control or side effects, there are, in reality, minimal differences between opioids (exception methadone). There are, however, significant differences in cost. In the absence of clinically relevant efficacy or toxicity differences, cost should be a major factor in choosing medications. Most

individuals can be successfully managed with a less expensive opioid (i.e., generic morphine). If unacceptable side effects develop, then conversion to more expensive products such as sustained-release oxycodone or transdermal fentanyl would be appropriate. Patient report of "allergy" to morphine is more often a side effect, such as nausea or pruritus. Rechallenge is usually appropriate because tolerance will develop. If the prior reaction was delirium or confusion, then alternate medications should be used. Physicians prescribing opioids should know the relative costs of the products because an inability to afford the medication is a known cause of poor pain control.

SUMMARY

Care of those with advanced disease requires the same attention to detail needed throughout the life span. Sensitive communication that includes patient and families, honest discussion of the goals of care, and management of the symptoms of the disease are critical. The growth of palliative medicine as a field will increase the number of physicians skilled in this care, but the primary care specialist must learn to manage the majority of patients in this phase of life with consultation for the difficult. Dying is a normal part of life, not a physician failure, whereas dying unprepared with uncontrolled symptoms in a hospital when you wanted to be home *is* a physician failure.

REVIEW EXERCISES

QUESTIONS

1. Which of the following patients would not be appropriate for hospice care?
a) 45-year-old woman with metastatic breast cancer who is not going to receive any further chemotherapy
b) 85-year-old gentleman with widespread metastatic prostate cancer who wants to be Do Not Resuscitate (DNR) and has received his first dose of hormonal therapy
c) 74-year-old bed-confined and nonverbal dementia patient with a feeding tube whose family does not want to make him a DNR
d) 38-year-old man with type 1 diabetes complicated by kidney disease requiring dialysis and advanced, progressive HIV
e) 58-year-old man with ischemic cardiomyopathy and an implantable cardiac defibrillator (ICD) who wants to continue his cardiac medications

Answer and Discussion

The answer is b. Metastatic malignancy with no plans for therapy is almost always an appropriate hospice diagnosis. The only exception could be diseases with very slow progression such as carcinoid tumors and, occasionally, head and neck primaries. Medicare guidelines specifically state that hospices may not require a DNR order for admission. Dementia patients who have reached a functional state with one or less understandable words in 24 hours and an inability to independently get out of a chair have an average life expectancy of less than 6 months; therefore, that patient could be admitted to hospice. The dialysis patient will be admitted for a diagnosis other than his renal disease, so the hospice would not be responsible for it, and it may continue. Cardiac medications in heart failure are used to improve symptoms so they would be appropriate. The ICD can be turned off at a later date or not at all. The 85-year-old with prostate cancer has just started therapy with a high probability of response with life prolongation and so would be inappropriate for hospice.

2. Dr. X has personal religious beliefs that one should always provide and never discontinue artificial nutrition and hydration, regardless of the specific circumstances. He has been caring for an advanced dementia patient who did not complete a living will but did specify a legal medical proxy—his daughter. The nursing home has approached the daughter about placing a PEG tube because the patient has begun to lose weight. She has been reading on the Internet and questions whether there is any evidence that feeding tubes will make her father more comfortable. Of the following actions, which would be the least appropriate for Dr. X?
a) Transfer the care to a physician with different religious beliefs.
b) Explain that although he has particular religious beliefs, the evidence is that feeding tubes do not provide comfort and may actually cause distress.
c) Discuss his concern that her father will starve to death and be very uncomfortable without nutritional support.
d) Discuss her goals of care for her father and, if focused predominantly on comfort, suggest a hospice referral and further discussion of the role of nutritional support by the hospice team.
e) Support her reading of the literature and the lack of evidence of benefit without mentioning his religious beliefs.

Answer and Discussion
The answer is c.
Physicians with personal beliefs may not force their particular beliefs on other individuals, but they are also not required to provide care that they feel is ethically inappropriate. Therefore, because the evidence for feeding tubes in dementia does not support an improvement in quality of life, Dr. X should not use emotionally charged words such as "starve" to persuade a family member to his point of view. He may transfer the care

to another physician, allow the hospice team to have a conversation he personally feels uncomfortable with but maintain care of the patient, or present the evidence in an unbiased way. One can argue whether he should acknowledge his personal beliefs because the power imbalance between physician and family could be considered coercive, but this is preferred to allowing the bias to remain unspoken.

3. Mr. M is a 79-year-old man who has suffered a major intracerebral bleed. He was maintained on ventilator support for a week but has been successfully weaned. The team approaches the wife to discuss placing a feeding tube. She believes that her husband would not want to be sustained in this condition and requests that he just be kept comfortable. He is unresponsive and does not appear to have any active symptoms. Which of the following orders is the least appropriate?
a) No change in existing orders
b) Discontinue any existing medication or labs and no new orders
c) No change in existing orders but as needed orders for symptoms
d) Discontinue any existing medications and as needed orders for symptoms
e) Discontinue any existing medications and start a morphine infusion

Answer and Discussion
The answer is e. One could support any of the other answers, depending on how one clarifies the goals with the patient's wife. Because he is unresponsive, he may well not have any symptoms so one could wait until/if something developed and provide medication then. It will save the nurse and the patient time and distress if the needs are anticipated and medications already available, rather than having to page if something develops. Starting an infusion in an unresponsive patient, even with family consent, is not proportional to the need and therefore crosses the ethical boundaries of palliative sedation, is not supported by the concept of double effect, and approaches active euthanasia, which is illegal in all states. There is no intractable symptom to address.

4. Mrs. L is a 60-year-old woman with a history of severe osteoarthritis and chronic pain secondary to her osteoarthritis. She was maintained with reasonable comfort on naproxen until recently, when she was diagnosed with congestive heart failure. Her cardiologist stopped the naproxen and advised her that she could not take it again. She is coming to see you for uncontrolled pain. She has been taking eight extra-strength acetaminophen daily and has been using her husband's tramadol 50 mg without any benefit. She rates her pain as 8/10 in her knees and hands and constant, although it gets worse with walking or cooking. Functionally, she is

not able to perform most of the activities that she could while taking the naproxen. Which of the following would be the most appropriate order for her?

a) Propoxyphene/acetaminophen one to two tablets every 4 to 6 hours as needed
b) Celecoxib 200 mg/day
c) Fentanyl patch 25 mcg every 3 days
d) Oxycodone 5 mg every 4 hours as needed, with a plan to convert to sustained-release oxycodone once need is determined
e) Morphine 5 mg liquid every 4 hours, with a plan to convert to sustained-release morphine once need is determined

Answer and Discussion

The answer is e. Propoxyphene has not been shown to be better than placebo and therefore should not be given in this setting. Celecoxib has less gastrointestinal toxicity but is no different in fluid retention than other nonsteroidal anti-inflammatory drugs; therefore, it is contraindicated in congestive heart failure. Fentanyl patches should never be started in opioid-naïve individuals because deaths have been reported. This dose is equivalent to 60 mg of oral morphine in 24 hours. Of the choice of oxycodone or morphine, morphine has a generic; therefore, this should be the first opioid tried. Oxycodone would be a reasonable alternative, although the sustained-release version is the most expensive way to orally manage pain.

5. Mr. R is a 79-year-old gentleman with end-stage lung cancer admitted to home hospice. He is Do Not Resuscitate. He has been quite functional at home on 2/LPM of nasal O$_2$. He had recently returned from a cross-country trip to visit his first great grandchild. He calls the hospice nurse with sudden onset of severe dyspnea and acute anxiety. The nurse calls you for recommendations and also wants to give him morphine for his dyspnea. Which of the following is the most appropriate action?

a) Let her give him as much morphine as needed and keep him comfortable at home.
b) Let her give him 5 mg of oral morphine that may be repeated every 15 minutes × 3 and then arrange an admission to look for a pulmonary embolism.
c) Morphine may decrease his respirations; thus, he may have lorazepam for his anxiety as needed. The nurse should recheck him tomorrow.
d) Send him to the emergency room.
e) Start him on a fentanyl patch 12 mcg/24 hours.

Answer and Discussion

The answer is b. Given his history, the likelihood of a pulmonary embolism is quite high. An admission to hospice does not rule out the evaluation of acute new problems. His goals should be considered in light of

his functional status at the time the new symptom developed. If he was bed bound or did not want to be admitted, then answer a is appropriate. There is evidence to support the role of morphine in cancer dyspnea management (*Cochrane Review*) and also in nonhospice chronic obstructive pulmonary disease (COPD). An Australian study started COPD patients on 20 mg of sustained-release morphine once daily for dyspnea. The worse the COPD, the more benefit they obtained from the medication. No one developed a clinical worsening of their respiratory status even though CO$_2$ was not tested. Because hospice provides inpatient benefits, the care should be given in that setting rather than in an emergency room. Although the fentanyl dose might ultimately be appropriate, at the present time, it will take 12 to 16 hours for the patch to have an effect; therefore, it will not relieve his current distress. Even at the lower dose, starting this in a naïve patient is not recommended.

SUGGESTED READINGS

American College of Physicians–American Society of Internal Medicine End-of-Life Care Consensus Panel. *Ethics Manual*, 4th ed. *Ann Intern Med* 1998;128(7):576–594.

American Geriatrics Society Panel on Chronic Pain in Older Persons. The management of chronic pain in older persons. *J Am Geriatr Soc* 1998;46(5):635–651.

Barry LC, Kasl SV, et al. Psychiatric disorders among bereaved persons: the role of perceived circumstances of death and preparedness for death. *Am J Geriatr Psychiatry* 2002;10(4):447–457.

Bennett MI. Death rattle: an audit of hyoscine (scopolamine) use and review of management. *J Pain Symptom Manage* 1996;12:229–233.

Billings JA. Comfort measures for the terminally ill. Is dehydration painful? *J Am Geriatr Soc* 1985;33(11):808–810.

Billings JA. What is palliative care? *J Palliat Med* 1998;1(1):73–78.

Block SD. Perspectives on care at the close of life: psychological considerations, growth, and transcendence at the end of life: the art of the possible. *JAMA* 2001;285(22):2898–2905.

Boyle DM, Abernathy G, et al. End-of-life confusion in patients with cancer. *Oncol Nurs Forum* 1998;25:1335–1343.

Bozzetti F, Amadori D, et al. Guidelines on artificial nutrition versus hydration in terminal cancer patients. European Association for Palliative Care. *Nutrition* 1996;12(3):163–167.

Braun TC, Hagen NA, et al. Development of a clinical practice guideline for palliative sedation. *J Palliat Med* 2003;6(3):345–350.

Breitbart W, Cohen K. Delirium in the terminally ill. In: Chochinov HM, Breitbart W, eds. *Handbook of Psychiatry in Palliative Medicine.* New York: Oxford University Press, 2000:75–90.

Brett AS, Jersild P. "Inappropriate" treatment near the end of life: conflict between religious convictions and clinical judgment. *Arch Intern Med* 2003;163(14):1645–1649.

Brody H, Campbell ML, et al. Withdrawing intensive life-sustaining treatment—recommendations for compassionate clinical management. *N Engl J Med* 1997;336(9):652–657.

Bruera E, Belzile M, et al. Volume of hydration in terminal cancer patients. *Support Care Cancer* 1996;4(2):147–150.

Buckman R. *How to Break Bad News: A Guide for Health Care Professionals.* Baltimore: Johns Hopkins University Press, 1992.

Cain JM. Practical aspects of hospice care at home. *Best Pract Res Clin Obstet Gynaecol* 2001;15(2):305–311.

Campbell M. *Forgoing Life-Sustaining Therapy: How to Care for the Patient Who Is Near Death.* Aliso Veigo, CA: American Association of Critical Care Nurses, 1998.

Center for Gerontology and Health Care Research, Brown University.

Facts on Dying: Policy Relevant Data on Care at the End of Life. 2004. Available at: www.chcr.brown.edu/dying.

Cherny NI, Portenoy RK. Sedation in the management of refractory symptoms: guidelines for evaluation and treatment. *J Palliat Care* 1994;10(2):31–38.

Cleeland CS, Gonin R, et al. Pain and its treatment in outpatients with metastatic cancer. *N Engl J Med* 1994;330(9):592–596.

Cleeland CS, Gonin R, et al. Pain and treatment of pain in minority patients with cancer. *Ann Intern Med* 1997;127:813–816.

Clever SL, Tulsky JA. Dreaded conversations: moving beyond discomfort in patient–physician communication. *J Gen Intern Med* 2002;17(11):884–885.

Cohen SR, Leis A. What determines the quality of life of terminally ill cancer patients from their own perspective? *J Palliat Care* 2002;18(1):48–58.

Cohen SR, Mount BM. Quality of life in terminal illness: defining and measuring subjective well-being in the dying. *J Palliat Care* 1992;8(3):40–45.

Conill C, Verger E, et al. Symptom prevalence in the last week of life. *J Pain Symptom Manage* 1997;14(6):328–331.

Costantini M, Higginson IJ, et al. Effect of a palliative home care team on hospital admissions among patients with advanced cancer. *Palliat Med* 2003;17(4):315–321.

Council on Ethical and Judicial Affairs, American Medical Association. Decisions near the end of life. *JAMA* 1992;267(16):2229–2233.

Council on Ethical and Judicial Affairs, American Medical Association. Medical futility in end-of-life care. *JAMA* 1999;281(10):937–941.

Council on Scientific Affairs, American Medical Association. Good care of the dying patient. *JAMA* 1996;275(6):474–478.

Covinsky KE, Goldman L, Cook EF, et al. The impact of serious illness on patients' families. SUPPORT Investigators. Study to Understand Prognoses and Preferences for Outcomes and Risks of Treatment. *JAMA* 1994;272(23):1839–1844.

Cowan JD, Palmer TW. Practical guide to palliative sedation. *Curr Oncol Rep* 2002;4(3):242–249.

De Graeff A, Dean M. Palliative sedation therapy in the last weeks of life: a literature review and recommendations for standards. *J Palliat Med* 2007;10(1):67–85.

Dixon S, Fortner J, et al. Barriers, challenges, and opportunities related to the provision of hospice care in assisted-living communities. *Am J Hosp Palliat Care* 2002;19(3):187–192.

Du Pen SL, Du Pen AR, et al. Implementing guidelines for cancer pain management: results of a randomized controlled clinical trial. *J Clin Oncol* 1999;17(1):361–370.

Early BP, Smith ED, et al. The needs and supportive networks of the dying: an assessment instrument and mapping procedure for hospice patients. *Am J Hosp Palliat Care* 2000;17(2):87–96.

Edmonds P, Karlsen S, et al. A comparison of the palliative care needs of patients dying from chronic respiratory diseases and lung cancer. *Palliat Med* 2001;15(4):287–295.

Ellershaw J, Smith C, et al. Care of the dying: setting standards for symptom control in the last 48 hours of life. *J Pain Symptom Manage* 2001;21(1):12–17.

Ellershaw J, Ward C. Care of the dying patient: the last hours or days of life. *BMJ* 2003;326(7379):30–34.

Emanuel LL, von Gunten CF, et al. Education for Physicians on End-of-life Care (EPEC) Curriculum. Chicago: American Medical Association, 1999. Available at: www.ama-assn.org/ama/pub/category/2910.html.

Fainsinger R, Bruera E. The management of dehydration in terminally ill patients. *J Palliat Care* 1994;10(3):55–59.

Fainsinger R, Miller MJ, et al. Symptom control during the last week of life on a palliative care unit. *J Palliat Care* 1991;7(1):5–11.

Fainsinger RL, Bruera E. When to treat dehydration in a terminally ill patient? *Support Care Cancer* 1997;5(3):205–211.

Fallowfield L. Communication with the patient and family in palliative medicine. In: Doyle D, Hanks G, Cherny N, et al., eds. *Oxford Textbook of Palliative Medicine*. Oxford: University Press, 2004:101–107.

Field MJ, Cassel CK, eds. *Approaching Death: Improving Care at the End of Life*. Washington, DC: Institute of Medicine, National Academy Press, 1997.

Flowers B. Palliative care for patients with end-stage heart failure. *Nurs Times* 2003;99(11):30–32.

Foley KM, Carver AC. Palliative care in neurology. *Neurol Clin* 2001;19(4):789–799.

Freeborne N, Lynn J, et al. Insights about dying from the SUPPORT project. The Study to Understand Prognoses and Preferences for Outcomes and Risks of Treatments. *J Am Geriatr Soc* 2000;48(5 Suppl):S199–S205.

Friedman BT, Harwood MK, et al. Barriers and enablers to hospice referrals: an expert overview. *J Palliat Med* 2002;5(1):73–84.

Furst CJ, Doyle D. The terminal phase. In: Doyle D, Hanks G, Cherny N, et al., eds. *Oxford Textbook of Palliative Medicine*. Oxford: Oxford University Press, 2004:1117–1133.

Gage B, Miller SC, Mor V, et al. Synthesis and Analysis of Medicare's Hospice Benefit: Executive Summary and Recommendations. Washington, DC: U.S. Department of Health and Human Services, March 2000. Available at: http://aspe.hhs.gov/daltcp/reports/samhbes.htm.

Goetschius SK. Caring for families: the other patient in palliative care. In: Matzo ML, Sherman DW, eds. *Palliative Care Nursing: Quality Care to the End of Life*. New York: Springer, 2001:245–274.

Goodlin SJ, Winzelberg GS, et al. Death in the hospital. *Arch Intern Med* 1998;158(14):1570–1572.

Greenstreet W. The concept of total pain: a focused patient care study. *Br J Nursing* 2001;10(19):1248–1255.

Grossman SA, Benedetti C, et al. National Comprehensive Cancer Network practice guidelines for cancer pain. *Oncology* 1999;13:33–44.

Hallenbeck J. Terminal sedation: ethical implications in different situations. *J Palliat Med* 2000;3(3):313–320.

Hanson LC, Henderson M. Care of the dying in long-term care settings. *Clin Geriatr Med* 2000;16(2):225–237.

Harris JT, Suresh Kumar K, et al. Intravenous morphine for rapid control of severe cancer pain. *Palliat Med* 2003;17(3):248–256.

Hastings Center. *Guidelines on the Termination of Life-Sustaining Treatment and the Care of the Dying*. Bloomington, IN: Hastings Center, 1987.

Higginson IJ, Sen-Gupta G, et al. *Changing Gear—Guidelines for Managing the Last Days of Life in Adults: The Research Evidence*. London: Working Party on Guidelines in Palliative Care, The National Council for Hospice and Palliative Care Services, 1997.

Hospice and Palliative Nurses Association. *Hospice and Palliative Care Clinical Practice Protocol: Terminal Restlessness*. Pittsburgh, PA: Hospice and Palliative Nurses Association, 1997.

Jansen LA, Sulmasy DP. Proportionality, terminal suffering and the restorative goals of medicine. *Theor Med Bioeth* 2002;23(4–5):321–337.

Jansen LA, Sulmasy DP. Sedation, alimentation, hydration, and equivocation: careful conversation about care at the end of life. *Ann Intern Med* 2002;136(11):845–849.

Jaycox A, Carr DB, et al. New clinical-practice guidelines for the management of pain in patients with cancer. *N Engl J Med* 1994;330(9):651–655.

Jaycox A, Carr DB, et al. *Management of Cancer Pain: Clinical Practice Guideline, No 9*. Rockford, MD: Agency for Health Care Policy and Research Publication No. 94-0592, U.S. Department of Health and Human Services, 1994.

Jennings B, Ryndes T, D'Onofrio C, et al. Access to hospice care: expanding boundaries, overcoming barriers. *Hastings Center Rep* 2003;33(2 Suppl).

Kane RL, Klein SJ, et al. The role of hospice in reducing the impact of bereavement. *J Chronic Dis* 1986;39(9):735–742.

Kayser-Jones J, Schell E, et al. Factors that influence end-of-life care in nursing homes: the physical environment, inadequate staffing, and lack of supervision. *Gerontologist* 2003;43(Spec No 2):76–84.

Keay TJ, Schonwetter RS. The case for hospice care in long-term care environments. *Clin Geriatr Med* 2000;16(2):211–223.

Koenig BA. Cultural diversity in decision-making about care at the end-of-life. *Approaching Death: Improving Care at the End of Life*. 1997:363–382.

Krakauer EL. Responding to intractable terminal suffering. *Ann Intern Med* 2000;133(7):560; discussion 561–562.

Krakauer EL, Penson RT, et al. Sedation for intractable distress of a dying patient: acute palliative care and the principle of double effect. *Oncologist* 2000;4(1):53–62.

Larson DG, Tobin DR. End-of-life conversations: evolving practice and theory. *JAMA* 2000;284(12):1573–1578.

Leland JY. Death and dying: management of patients with end-stage disease. *Clin Geriatr Med* 2000;16(4):875–894.

Lichter I, Hunt E. The last 48 hours of life. *J Palliat Care* 1990;6(4):7–15.

Lo B, Quill T, et al. Discussing palliative care with patients. ACP-ASIM End-of-Life Care Consensus Panel. American College of Physicians–American Society of Internal Medicine. *Ann Intern Med* 1999;130(9):744–749.

McCann RM, Hall WJ, et al. Comfort care for terminally ill patients: the appropriate use of nutrition and hydration. *JAMA* 1994;272(16):1263–1266.

McIver B, Walsh D, Nelson K. The use of chlorpromazine for symptom control in dying cancer patients. *J Pain Symptom Manage* 1994;9(5):334–345.

Milch RA. The dying patient: pain management at the hospice level. *Curr Rev Pain* 2000;4(3):215–218.

Miller SC, Gozalo P, et al. Hospice enrollment and hospitalization of dying nursing home patients. *Am J Med* 2001;111(1):38–44.

Miller SC, Kinzbrunner B, et al. How does the timing of hospice referral influence hospice care in the last days of life? *J Am Geriatr Soc* 2003;51(6):798–806.

Miller SC, Mor V, et al. Does receipt of hospice care in nursing homes improve the management of pain at the end of life? *J Am Geriatr Soc* 2002;50(3):507–515.

Miller SC, Mor V, et al. Hospice enrollment and pain assessment and management in nursing homes. *J Pain Symptom Manage* 2003;26(3):791–799.

Miller SC, Mor V, et al. The role of hospice care in the nursing home setting. *J Palliat Med* 2002;5(2):271–277.

Munley A, Powers CS, et al. Humanizing nursing home environments: the relevance of hospice principles. *Int J Aging Hum Dev* 1982;15(4):263–284.

National Hospice and Palliative Care Organization. Available at: www.nhpco.org/files/public/facts_and_figures_0703.pdf.

Norton SA, Talerico KA. Facilitating end-of-life decision-making: strategies for communicating and assessing. *J Gerontol Nurs* 2000;26(9):6–13.

Novak B, Kolcaba K, et al. Measuring comfort in caregivers and patients during late end-of-life care. *Am J Hosp Palliat Care* 2001;18(3):170–180.

O'Neill J, Fallon M. ABC of palliative care: principles of palliative care and pain control. *BMJ* 1997;315(7111):801–804.

Pantilat SZ. End-of-life care for the hospitalized patient. *Med Clin North Am* 2002;86(4):749–770.

Patrick DL, Curtis JR, et al. Measuring and improving the quality of dying and death. *Ann Intern Med* 2003;139(5 Pt2):410–415.

Pickett M, Yancey D. Symptoms of the dying. In: McCorkle R, Grant R, Frank-Stromborg M, Baird S, eds. *Cancer Nursing: A Comprehensive Textbook.* Philadelphia: WB Saunders, 1998:1157–1182.

Portenoy RK. Cancer pain management. *Semin Oncol* 1993;20(2 Suppl 1):19–35.

Portenoy RK. Pharmacologic management of cancer pain. *Semin Oncol* 1995;22(2 Suppl 3):112–120.

Portenoy RK. The physical examination in cancer pain assessment. *Semin Oncol Nurs* 1997;13(1):25–29.

Portenoy RK. Treatment of temporal variations in chronic cancer pain. *Semin Oncol* 1997;24(5 Suppl 16):S16-7–12.

Portenoy RK, Hagen NA. Breakthrough pain: definition, prevalence and characteristics. *Pain* 1990;41(3):273–281.

Portenoy RK, Lesage P. Management of cancer pain. *Lancet* 1999;353(9165):1695–1700.

Post LF, Dubler NN. Palliative care: a bioethical definition, principles, and clinical guidelines. *Bioeth Forum* 1997;13(3):17–24.

Rabow MW, Hauser JM, et al. Supporting family caregivers at the end of life: "they don't know what they don't know." *JAMA* 2004;291:483–492.

Reynolds K, Henderson M, et al. Needs of the dying in nursing homes. *J Palliat Med* 2002;5(6):895–901.

Rousseau P. Management of symptoms in the actively dying patient. In: Berger AM, Portenoy RK, Weissman DE, eds. *Principles and Practice of Palliative Care and Supportive Oncology.* Philadelphia: Lippincott Williams & Wilkins, 2002:789–798.

Sarhill N, Walsh D, et al. Evaluation and treatment of cancer-related fluid deficits: volume depletion and dehydration. *Support Care Cancer* 2001;9(6):408–419.

Silveira MJ, DiPiero A, et al. Patients' knowledge of options at the end of life: ignorance in the face of death. *JAMA* 2000;284(19):2483–2488.

Smith TJ, Coyne P, et al. high-volume specialist palliative care unit and team may reduce in-hospital end-of-life care costs. *J Palliat Med* 2003;6:699–705.

Steiner N, Bruera E. Methods of hydration in palliative care patients. *J Palliat Care* 1998;14(2):6–13.

Steinhauser KE, Christakis NA, et al. Factors considered important at the end of life by patients, family, physicians, and other care providers. *JAMA* 2000;284(19):2476–2482.

Sullivan AM, Lakoma MD, et al. The status of medical education in end-of-life care. *J Gen Intern Med* 2003;18:685–695.

Sulmasy DP. A biopsychological-spiritual model for the care of patients at the end of life. *Gerontologist* 2002;42(Spec No 3):24–33.

Sulmasy DP, Ury WA, et al. Responding to intractable terminal suffering. *Ann Intern Med* 2000;133(7):560–562; discussion 561–562.

Sykes N, Thorns A. Sedative use in the last week of life and the implications for end-of-life decision making. *Arch Intern Med* 2003;163:341–344.

Teno JM, Clarridge BR, et al. Family perspectives on end-of-life care at the last place of care. *JAMA* 2004;291(1):88–93.

Teno JM, Fisher ES, et al. Medical care inconsistent with patients' treatment goals: association with 1-year Medicare resource use and survival. *J Am Geriatr Soc* 2002;50(3):496–500.

Teno JM, Weitzen S, et al. Persistent pain in nursing home residents. *JAMA* 2001;285(16):2081.

The AM, Hak T, et al. Collusion in doctor–patient communication about imminent death: an ethnographic study. *BMJ* 2000;321(7273):1376–1381.

Thielemann P. Educational needs of home caregivers of terminally ill patients: literature review. *Am J Hosp Palliat Care* 2000;17(4):253–257.

Thorns A. Sedation, the doctrine of double effect and the end of life. *Int J Palliat Nurs* 2002;8(7):341–343.

Thorns A, Sykes N. Opioid use in last week of life and implications for end-of-life decision-making. *Lancet* 2000;356(9227):398–399.

Tierney RM, Horton SM, et al. Relationships between symptom relief, quality of life, and satisfaction with hospice care. *Palliat Med* 1998;12(5):333–344.

Tolle SW, Rosenfeld AG, et al. Oregon's low in-hospital death rates: what determines where people die and satisfaction with decisions on place of death? *Ann Intern Med* 1999;130(8):681–685.

Tolle SW, Tilden VP, et al. Family reports of barriers to optimal care of the dying. *Nurs Res* 2000;49(6):310–317.

Truog RD, Berde CB, et al. Barbiturates in the care of the terminally ill. *N Engl J Med* 1992;27(23):1678–1682.

Truog RD, Cist AF, et al. Recommendations for end-of-life care in the intensive care unit: the Ethics Committee of the Society of Critical Care Medicine. *Crit Care Med* 2001;29(12):2332–2348.

Ventafridda V, Ripamonti C, et al. Symptom prevalence and control during cancer patients' last days of life. *J Palliat Care* 1990;6(3):7–11.

Vig EK, Davenport NA, et al. Good deaths, bad deaths, and preferences for the end of life: a qualitative study of geriatric outpatients. *J Am Geriatr Soc* 2002;50(9):1541–1548.

von Gunten CF. Discussing hospice care. *J Clin Oncol* 2002;20(5):1419–1424.

von Gunten CF, Ferris FD, et al. The patient–physician relationship: ensuring competency in end-of-life care: communication and relational skills. *JAMA* 2000;284(23):3051–3057.

Wein S. Sedation in the imminently dying patient. *Oncology* 2000;14:585–592.

World Health Organization. *Cancer Pain Relief.* Geneva, Switzerland: World Health Organization, 1996.

World Health Organization. Palliative Care. 2002. Available at: www.who.int/hiv/topics/palliative/PalliativeCare/en/.

World Health Organization. *Symptom Relief in Terminal Illness.* Geneva, Switzerland: World Health Organization, 1998.

Yan E, Bruera E. Parenteral hydration of terminally ill cancer patients. *J Palliat Care* 1991;7(3):40–43.

Yedidia MJ, MacGregor B. Confronting the prospect of dying: reports of terminally ill patients. *J Pain Symptom Manage* 2001;22(4):807–819.

Chapter 28

Acute Monoarticular Arthritis

Brian F. Mandell

✋ POINTS TO REMEMBER:

- Septic arthritis may be the initial manifestation of systemic bacterial infection and is associated with a >10% mortality.

- The distinction between crystal-induced and bacterial arthritis cannot be made reliably with studies from peripheral blood.

- Calcium pyrophosphate crystals can cause attacks that totally mimic gout (pseudogout), but they can also cause several other syndromes. Radiographic finding of calcium deposition within menisci and other intra-articular cartilage has been termed *chondrocalcinosis* and may be asymptomatic or associated with inflammatory arthritis.

- Seronegative Lyme disease is extremely uncommon, and this diagnosis should be entertained only with a great deal of caution.

Acute monoarticular arthritis represents a medical urgency because of the possibility of joint infection, which can result in total loss of joint function. In addition, septic arthritis may be the initial manifestation of systemic bacterial infection and is associated with a >10% mortality. The appropriate diagnosis of specific crystal-induced arthritis will direct long-term management decisions. The treatment of crystal-induced arthritis and hyperuricemia should be individualized, taking into consideration medical comorbidities, as well as the anticipated frequency and potential adverse effects of treating acute flares of crystal disease in the future.

ETIOLOGY

In an unpublished series of 64 hospitalized and emergency department patients with acute monoarticular or oligoar-

ticular (less than four involved joints) arthritis, 17% had documented bacterial infection (Fig. 28.1). The significant majority of patients had monosodium urate or calcium pyrophosphate crystal-induced arthritis. It is impossible to distinguish between crystal-induced and septic arthritis on clinical grounds alone. Hence, the possibility of bacterial infectious arthritis dictates the diagnostic approach to the patient with acute monoarticular or oligoarticular arthritis.

DIAGNOSIS

History

A thorough history should be obtained, with a focus on several specific issues. Frequently, patients describe a history of trauma before their presentation with acute joint swelling and pain. A careful discussion regarding the mechanism and severity of injury, as well as the timing in relationship to the presentation with acute arthritis, is mandatory. Often, it can be determined that the history of trauma bears no relationship to the acute arthritis. Joint trauma alone rarely elicits a striking inflammatory articular response. The general history surrounding the onset of the arthritis should be explored. The presence of an acute migratory arthralgia prodrome is consistent with infection, including rheumatic fever, disseminated gonorrhoea, bacteremia, and viral infections. Prolonged systemic features before the onset of arthritis are also consistent with a chronic infection, such as bacterial endocarditis or viral hepatitis. Patients should be questioned about prior episodes of arthritis in the same or different joints. Patients with *Borrelia burgdorferi* infection (Lyme disease), crystal disease, psoriasis, enteropathic arthritis, spondylitis, and, occasionally, other syndromes may have a history of prior episodes of self-limited monoarticular or oligoarticular arthritis. Careful questioning should focus on exposure to intravenous drugs or to sexual contact with partners with such exposure, use of medications, or potential exposure to viral

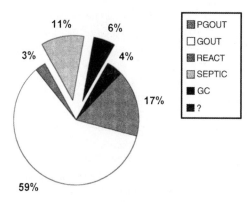

Figure 28.1   Etiology of acute arthritis. GC, gonococcal arthritis; PGOUT, pseudogout; REACT, reactive arthritis; SEPTIC, septic arthritis. Graduate Hospital, Philadelphia: 64 hospitalized patients. *Source:* Mandell BF, unpublished.

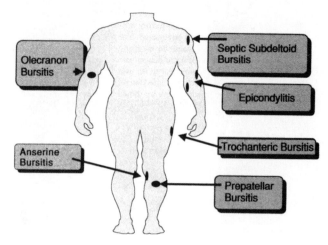

Figure 28.2   Acute soft tissue problems.

hepatitis or HIV infection. Patients living in an area endemic for Lyme disease should be questioned regarding time spent outdoors during the spring, summer, or early autumn months, and a history of any annular rashes.

Physical Examination

A careful physical examination must be undertaken. An entire musculoskeletal screening evaluation should be performed. Although the patient may only complain of single joint pain, physical examination may reveal multiple inflamed joints, coexistent tenosynovitis, or enthesitis. Mucosal surfaces should be carefully examined for the presence of ulcers or inflammation. The conjunctivitis of reactive arthritis (including the subset with what was formerly known as Reiter's syndrome: urethritis, arthritis, and conjunctivitis) is typically mild and asymptomatic. Extremities should be examined for purpura or digital infarcts. Psoriatic lesions should be sought in typical but often unexamined areas (gluteal crease, scalp, behind ears, and umbilicus).

The physical examination must distinguish between bursitis and other soft tissue periarticular pain syndromes and true inflammatory arthritis (Fig. 28.2). Septic bursitis in these areas can be associated with a surrounding erythema or edema and can superficially mimic true joint involvement or cellulitis.

Certain syndromes have a predilection for involving the tendon sheath, as well as the joint structures. Acute tenosynovitis, particularly when accompanying acute arthritis, should prompt a consideration of the diagnosis of infection with *Neisseria gonorrhoeae* or *Haemophilus influenzae*, crystal disease, mycobacterial infection (particularly nontuberculous mycobacteria, such as *Mycobacterium marinum*), and specific fungal infections, such as sporotrichosis. The "sausaging" of digits (dactylitis) suggests the diagnosis of psoriasis, sarcoidosis, spondylitis, or reactive arthritis; however, if in a single digit, soft tissue infection must be considered.

Constitutional symptoms are not sensitive or specific enough to establish the diagnosis of septic arthritis or distinguish infectious from crystal-induced arthritis. A study of 43 patients with documented bacterial arthritis, predominantly due to *Staphylococcus aureus*, revealed the following frequency of systemic features:

- Leukocytosis, 42%
- Temperature >38°C, 41%
- Erythrocyte sedimentation rate (ESR) <30 mm/hour, 24%
- Rigors, 21%

Conversely, a study of documented crystal-induced arthritis found the following:

- Temperature >38°C in 29% of patients with gout (one patient had a maximum temperature of 39.4°C)
- Temperature >38°C in 38% of patients with documented pseudogout
- Temperature >38°C in 50% of patients with polyarticular crystal arthritis

Thus, fever and leukocytosis are neither sensitive nor specific findings in septic arthritis.

Imaging and Laboratory Studies

Initial laboratory and radiographic studies have limited diagnostic value in the setting of acute monoarticular arthritis, and should be kept to a minimum. The laboratory study of choice is synovial fluid analysis. The distinction between crystal-induced and bacterial arthritis cannot be made reliably with studies from peripheral blood. Radiographs are of initial value if significant trauma or osteomyelitis is suspected, but they play no role in the initial distinction of acute crystal-induced versus bacterial arthritis. The presence of chondrocalcinosis does not exclude the possibility of infection as the etiology of the acute arthritis, and the characteristic radiographic findings of septic arthritis take

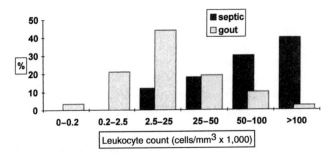

Figure 28.3 Diagnosis of septic arthritis: synovial fluid leukocytosis. *Source:* Reproduced with permission from Krey PR, Bailen DA. Synovial fluid leukocytosis: a study of extremes. *Am J Med* 1979; 67:436–442.

time to develop. Nuclear imaging and MRI do not distinguish crystal-induced from bacterial-induced synovitis.

The measurement of serum urate values is of no diagnostic value in determining the etiology of acute arthritis. The diagnostic test of choice in patients with acute monoarticular arthritis is synovial fluid analysis with cell count, polarized microscopy, and culture (if the fluid is inflammatory: >7,500 white blood cells (WBCs)/mm^3 or with >85% neutrophils). Invariably, patients with infectious or crystal-induced arthritis have synovial fluid leukocytosis with a striking neutrophil predominance (**Fig. 28.3**). The absolute cell count or neutrophil differential count does not reliably distinguish between septic and crystalline arthritis.

The accurate initial diagnosis of monoarticular arthritis rests entirely on the arthrocentesis and a few synovial fluid studies. (A single drop of synovial fluid—as little as that contained in the hub of the needle in an initially presumed "dry tap"—may be sufficient to allow the diagnosis.) The following procedure can be used:

1. Place a single drop of synovial fluid on a glass slide and cover with a coverslip.
2. Perform a wet-preparation microscopic analysis using the 40× objective. Estimate the cell count, one cell per high-power field = ~500 cells/mm^3.
3. Perform polarized microscopy on the same wet preparation to check for crystals.
4. Remove the coverslip, gently heat-fix the fluid, and then perform a Gram stain.

The Gram stain permits a differential cell count of polymorphonuclear neutrophils versus mononuclear cells, as well as staining of bacteria. If the fluid is inflammatory, with >7,500 cells/mm^3, more than 80% neutrophils, and no crystals evident, the fluid should be sent for culture and the patient treated for potential septic arthritis, unless an alternative diagnosis is apparent. Only rarely will a bacterial infection occur with lower cell counts, but even fluids with WBC counts <20,000 are infrequently infected. Infected fluids frequently have synovial fluid WBC counts of <50,000/mm^3. Common conditions, such as uncomplicated osteoarthritis, do not cause inflammatory fluids to

this degree. If the fluid is not inflammatory by these criteria, and no crystals are observed, cultures still should be considered if the patient is febrile or other concerns exist for the possibility of infection, including potential periarticular osteomyelitis. If the fluid is bloody, an evaluation for possible intra-articular injury or synovial tumor should be considered. Intracellular fat droplets suggest the possibility of an intra-articular fracture. Thrombocytopenia, unlike coagulation factor deficiencies, is usually not associated with spontaneous joint hemorrhage. Synovial fluid should be examined promptly, if possible, for the presence of crystals, although if necessary they can be examined the next day.

If prompt analysis is not possible, the fluid should be maintained in a sterile tube in the absence of anticoagulants, pending polarized microscopic evaluation. Alternatively, the fluid can be placed on a glass slide, the coverslip sealed in place with nail polish, and the fluid examined the next day. It should be noted that crystals (especially calcium pyrophosphate) may not be identified on examination as a result of observer inexperience, a limited number of crystals in the fluid, or other undetermined reasons. Hence, if no crystals are initially seen in an inflammatory fluid without etiology, repeat joint aspirations and evaluation of the fluid by polarized microscopy is mandatory. Alizarin stain may help confirm the presence of calcium-containing crystals, although this test is not available uniformly. In immunocompromised patients, it may be of value to save some of the fluid for special studies, including fungal and mycobacterial culture or polymerase chain reaction (PCR) analysis for *Ureaplasma* organisms (in patients with hypogammaglobulinemia). Routinely obtaining cultures for tuberculosis or fungal infection at the time of initial presentation is not warranted. Some reports demonstrate positive bacterial cultures from tissue obtained by synovial biopsy when the fluid culture was negative; however, this procedure is not routinely employed. PCR may occasionally be of value when looking for specific infections.

SPECIFIC ACUTE MONOARTICULAR ARTHRITIS CONDITIONS

Gouty Arthritis

Acute urate crystal arthritis is the most common cause of monoarticular arthritis in adults (**Fig. 28.1**).

Etiology

A review of the natural history of gouty arthritis in older literature reveals that 90% of first attacks are monoarticular, and 60% occur in the first metatarsophalangeal joints (podagra). Approximately 60% of patients may have a recurrence within 1 year; however, 7% may never have another recurrence. Subcutaneous uric acid tophi or radiographic findings of joint damage are rare at the outset of the disease, despite the fact that the synovial tissues are undoubtedly already saturated with uric acid. It is crucial to recognize that attacks of acute gout can be elicited by abrupt changes in serum urate levels, whether up or down. Serum urate may be normal at the time of an attack, but if checked repeatedly, in the absence of hypouricemic therapy, gout patients will almost invariably have serum levels >6.7 mg/dL, the saturation point for urate. Figure 28.4 summarizes serum urate level data at times of an acute gouty attack, demonstrating that patients may have a low, normal, or high serum urate level at the time of an attack.

Pathogenesis

The pathogenesis of an acute gouty attack is reasonably well understood. The cartilage matrix and synovial tissues are saturated with uric acid, a process usually occurring over

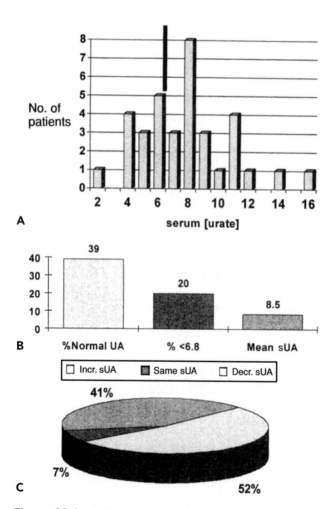

Figure 28.4 A: Serum urate at the time of acute polyarticular gout. **B:** Serum urate at the time of acute articular gout in 59 men with documented gout. **C:** Serum urate at the time of an attack compared with an intercritical period. sUA, serum uric acid; UA, uric acid. *Source:* **A:** Reproduced with permission from Hadler NM, Franck WA, Bress NM, et al. Acute polyarticular gout. *Am J Med* 1974;56:715–716; **B and C:** Reproduced with permission from Schlesinger N, Baker DG, Beutler AM, et al. Serum uric acid during bouts of acute gouty arthritis. *Arthritis Rheum* 1996;39S:348.

years of exposure to elevated levels of urate, above the saturation point (approximately 6.7 mg/dL) in physiological fluids. In some patients, this supersaturation leads to subcutaneous deposits (tophi) or synovial deposits, setting in motion a local granulomatous inflammatory response that invades adjacent bone, causing erosive changes and reactive bone proliferation in these areas. Factors favoring the nucleation of the uric acid crystals into tophi are not well described. Radiographs in long-standing gouty arthritis may demonstrate the presence of erosions, often at sites away from the joint margins, and reactive bone (overhanging edge) in the absence of significant joint space narrowing. This should be distinguished from the joint space narrowing seen in rheumatoid arthritis, which may occur before the onset of significant erosions.

As urate leaches out of the supersaturated synovium and cartilage into the synovial fluid because of a decrease in the serum urate level or microtrauma to the joint, it may crystallize into phlogistic structures. The ability of crystals to induce an inflammatory response can be modified if they are coated with lipoproteins, immunoglobulins, or other proteins present within the synovial fluid. The crystals are phagocytosed by synovial lining cells, neutrophils, or mononuclear cells within the synovial fluid. After phagocytosis, the crystals activate intracellular inflammasomes, and these cells produce several chemokines that can elicit and amplify the inflammatory response. Inflammatory mediators include leukotriene B_4, a crystal-induced protein chemotactic factor (not well defined), interleukin (IL)-8, IL-1, IL-6, tumor necrosis factor, and probably other granule contents and chemokines. Colchicine can suppress the release and synthesis of many of these mediators. Urate crystals activate in neutrophils at least one tyrosine kinase that is sensitive to inhibition by colchicine. Crystals also upregulate the expression of cyclooxygenase-2 in mononuclear cells. Complement and Hageman factor, are activated by urate crystals and may upregulate the inflammatory response, but do not seem to be necessary for the development of the acute inflammatory response in animals. The experimental injection of urate crystals under the skin or into the joints of humans is sufficient to elicit the acute inflammatory response (Fig. 28.5). Urate crystals can be found in the fluid obtained from the asymptomatic joints of patients with a history of gout, despite the absence of significant inflammation. Why the inflammatory response is blunted in this setting is a matter of conjecture, but intriguing in vitro studies suggest that mononuclear cells exposed to crystals mature into macrophages that exhibit a phenotype that is less responsive to crystal-induced activation. In addition, as noted previously, the crystals themselves are modulated during the course of the attack by acquiring a coating of different proteins.

Syndromes of Gouty Arthritis

Several distinct phases occur in the clinical expression of gout. Acute arthritis is often monoarticular, but it may be

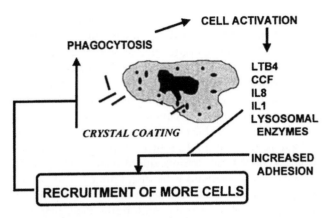

Figure 28.5 Crystal-induced arthritis. CCF, crystal-induced chemotactic factor; IL1, interleukin-1; IL8, interleukin-8; LTB4, leukotriene B4.

oligoarticular or even polyarticular. The initial attack is rarely polyarticular. If untreated, the frequency and severity of attacks tend to increase over time. The attacks tend to last longer and involve additional joints. Initially, there is a predominance of lower extremity joint involvement; however, over time, upper extremity joints may become involved (Fig. 28.6). Case reports describe spine involvement, enthesitis, bursitis, and recurrence in prosthetic joints. Flares may involve osteoarthritic Heberden's nodes of the distal finger joints, causing inflammatory finger nodules. This has been described in postmenopausal, elderly women using thiazide diuretics.

Between attacks (intercritical periods), patients with gout may be totally asymptomatic. Nonetheless, if synovial fluid is obtained at these times, urate crystals may still be found floating in the slightly inflammatory synovial fluid. Chronic treatment with colchicine lowers the WBC counts in these fluids, but fluid crystal number is not likely reduced. Chronic hypouricemic therapy decreases the likelihood of detecting crystals, likely due to the reduced urate burden within the joint, but this may take many months. Saturnine gout occurs in the setting of interstitial renal dis-

ease, historically in patients who have significant lead exposure resulting from ingestion of illicitly distilled liquor.

Attacks of acute gouty arthritis can be precipitated by changes in serum urate levels, either up or down. Documentation of hyperuricemia is *not* equivalent to the diagnosis of acute gouty arthritis in an individual patient. Many patients have hyperuricemia without ever having an attack of gouty arthritis. Both gout and pseudogout attacks are common in the postoperative setting.

There is a growing amount of data that links hyperuricemia as a causative (not simply associated) agent in the development and progression of coronary artery disease, hypertension, metabolic syndrome, and chronic kidney disease. A strong statistical (population-based) association exists, between hyperuricemia and the development of urate nephrolithiasis and gouty arthritis, coronary artery disease, hypertension, and metabolic syndrome. More recently, in one experimental rat model, mild acute hyperuricemia was shown to elicit the development of salt-sensitive hypertension. One small study of adolescents with urate levels >6.0 mg/dL and new-onset "essential" hypertension demonstrated that lowering the urate level also reduced the blood pressure. At present, there are insufficient data to warrant the treatment of asymptomatic hyperuricemia.

Non-Urate Crystalline Arthritis

Not all crystal-induced arthritis is due to uric acid. Calcium pyrophosphate crystals can cause attacks that totally mimic gout (pseudogout), but they can also cause several other syndromes. Radiographic finding of calcium deposition within menisci and other intra-articular cartilage has been termed *chondrocalcinosis* and may be asymptomatic or associated with inflammatory arthritis. Attacks may be infrequent, or a pseudorheumatoid syndrome may develop with a chronic symmetric polyarthritis due to low-grade, crystal-induced inflammation. Some metabolic diseases have been associated with atypical distribution and early onset of osteoarthritis, perhaps owing to the presence of calcium pyrophosphate crystals. The best known of these is hemochromatosis, which causes low-grade inflammation in the wrists and second and third metacarpophalangeal joints with a radiographic picture consistent with osteoarthritis of these joints. Several systemic diseases have been associated with the occurrence of calcium pyrophosphate deposition, including:

- Hyperparathyroidism
- Hypothyroidism
- Hypophosphatasia
- Hypomagnesemia
- Gout
- Amyloidosis
- Prior joint trauma
- Prior joint surgery
- Hemochromatosis

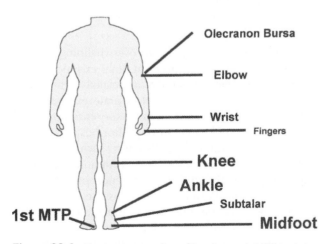

Figure 28.6 Gout: common sites of involvement. MTP, metatarsophalangeal.

Hemochromatosis is emphasized because the gene for hemochromatosis may be present in as many as 10% of the population. Manifestations include a mildly inflammatory osteoarthritislike arthropathy with predominant metacarpophalangeal involvement, with or without chondrocalcinosis. Prominent metacarpophalangeal involvement is not typical of classic osteoarthritis. The arthropathy may precede the recognition of visceral organ iron overload. Unlike the favorable liver and heart response to early initiation of chelation treatment, phlebotomy may not induce a remission of hemochromatosis-related joint symptoms. Nonetheless, recognition of hemochromatosis due to the presence of the unique joint syndrome may preserve organ function by prompting early therapy. Skin pigmentation is due to the deposition of melanin, not iron. Cardiomyopathy, hepatic cirrhosis, and endocrine disturbances, including diabetes mellitus and hypogonadism, are also manifestations of hemochromatosis.

Other crystal-induced arthropathies include (rare) oxalate-induced arthritis in patients on dialysis for treatment of chronic renal insufficiency and arthritis induced by hydroxyapatite crystals. Hydroxyapatite crystals have been associated with a chronic disease known as *Milwaukee shoulder*. This disease tends to affect elderly women, producing severe chronic rotator cuff disease and shoulder effusions composed of an enormous amount of synovial fluid containing few cells and multiple aggregates of apatite crystals. The clinical manifestations include asymptomatic large effusions or severe pain and chronic disability due to shoulder dysfunction. The knees may also be involved similarly.

Treatment of Crystalline Arthritis

Conservative indications for the treatment of hyperuricemia include prophylactic therapy to prevent the tumor lysis syndrome and treatment of recalcitrant gouty arthritis in patients in whom there is significant concern over the use of drugs for acute therapy. Patients who have documented soft tissue tophi or joint erosions owing to uric acid deposits should also be treated with hypouricemic agents. Some clinicians suggest that patients who have had more than one attack of gouty arthritis should be treated with hypouricemic agents because it is implicit in the pathophysiology of an attack that the joint structures are already saturated with uric acid. The concerns with this approach are the potential side effects of hypouricemic therapy, as well as the unpredictability of the course of gouty arthritis in a specific patient. Allopurinol, an inhibitor of xanthine oxidase (the key synthetic enzyme in the uric acid pathway), is generally well tolerated; however, the medication has been associated with life-threatening hypersensitivity reactions and the Stevens-Johnson syndrome. Uricosuric agents, such as probenecid, are well tolerated but are harder to use effectively. For maximal efficacy, patients must ingest significant amounts of fluid and use the probenecid several times daily. Before initiating any therapy to lower the serum urate level, clinicians should be absolutely certain

of the diagnosis of gout, which means synovial fluid analysis should have documented the presence of monosodium urate cystals. Strong consideration should be given to initial simultaneous prophylactic anti-inflammatory therapy using medications such as colchicine or nonsteroidal anti-inflammatory drugs (NSAIDs) because drug-induced hypouricemia frequently precipitates an attack of gout. The frequency at which this occurs is not certain, but may be as high as 30% within 2 months. Hypouricemic therapy should generally not be introduced in the setting of an acute attack, nor should it be discontinued while an attack is under way, due to the belief that abrupt changes in serum urate levels may further prolong the attack or induce another attack.

Abnormally *low* levels of serum urate can be found in select clinical situations, including:

- Syndrome of inappropriate antidiuretic hormone secretion
- High-dose salicylate therapy
- Renal tubular, uric acid wasting diseases (e.g., Wilson's disease, Fanconi's syndrome, genetic dysfunction of the URAT 1 transporter of uric acid)
- Starvation
- Alcohol withdrawal

Hypouricemia also has been described in several other disorders and circumstances:

- Xanthine oxidase deficiency syndromes
- Severe liver disease
- Overhydration
- Total parenteral nutrition
- Following use of iodinated contrast agents

Agents or conditions that induce hyperuricemia include:

- Low-dose aspirin
- Diuretics
- Cyclosporine
- Organic acidosis
- Acute ethanol exposure
- Pyrazinamide
- Ethambutol

Hyperuricemia develops in the overwhelming majority of patients because of insufficient renal excretion rather than overproduction. Disorders associated with the hyperproduction of uric acid (>1 g urate excreted daily while on a normal diet) include hereditary enzymopathies, such as hypoxanthine-guanine phosphoribosyl transferase deficiency, and proliferative disorders, such as psoriasis or Paget's disease of bone. Most commonly, the specific etiology for the inefficient excretion of uric acid is not demonstrable. Polycystic kidney disease, Bartter's syndrome, Down syndrome, starvation, and lead nephropathy have been associated with a reduced excretion of uric acid. Most likely, the reduced excretion is due to the inefficient function of either a voltage-sensitive or anion exchange transporter (URAT 1) in the proximal tubule. These transporters have been identified, and it is possible that functional polymorphisms of one or both genes can explain the inefficient uric acid excretion with resultant hyperuricemia. The necessity of obtaining a 24-hour urine collection in gouty patients to quantify uric acid excretion is arguable, unless the use of a uricosuric agent is being considered. Because the occurrence of stones can be precipitated, uricosurics should be avoided in the minority of patients who "overproduce" and thus excrete large amounts of uric acid. If 24-hour uric acid collections are performed, they should be done at least twice prior to making clinical decisions based on the result because of possible physiological variability in uric acid excretion. Xanthine oxidase inhibition can effectively lower the serum urate level in both overproducers and inefficient excretors. Therapy should be initiated with *low* doses of allopurinol and slowly increased over weeks to achieve the target level of urate (approximately 6 mg/dL). Approximately 50% of patients may require >300 mg daily to reach this target. If this target level of serum urate is not attained, it is unlikely that tophi will be resorbed. Other xanthine oxidase inhibitors and uricase are in clinical development. Although "guidelines" have been published stating that the allopurinol dose must be adjusted in the setting of renal insufficiency, the data to support this recommendation are quite tenuous.

There are many options to treat acute crystal arthritis. Probably any NSAID at a high dose will resolve an acute attack. Aspirin is generally avoided because of its striking effects on urate excretion and the significant side effects associated with high-dose therapy. Concerns over the use of nonselective NSAIDs include renal and platelet dysfunction and gastric toxicity. In addition, NSAIDs are general antipyretics, which in some settings may interfere with clinical observation of a parallel disease process such as postoperative infection. Parenteral use of NSAIDs is no safer than oral use, and (in my opinion) parenteral ketorolac has a poor risk–benefit ratio because it is one of the most gastrotoxic NSAIDs. COX-2-selective NSAIDs are likely as effective as the nonselective NSAIDs when used in high doses, are slightly gastrointestinally safer, and do not affect platelet function. The selective COX-2 inhibitors do, however, share with older NSAIDs the side effects of fluid retention and renal toxicity. Corticosteroid therapy, either oral or parenteral, is quite effective, but should be provided in moderate (not low) doses. Parenteral adrenocorticotropic hormone (ACTH), although it elicits variable cortisol secretion and has more fluid-retentive properties than prednisone, has been suggested by some authors as an extremely effective therapeutic option. ACTH may have anti-inflammatory effects via its interaction with peripheral (nonadrenal) receptors, independent of adrenal stimulation. Concerns about corticosteroid use include:

- Masking signs of infection
- Exacerbation of diabetes

- Decreased wound healing in the postoperative setting (theoretical)
- Diagnostic confusion resulting from the leukocytosis induced by the corticosteroids

Intra-articular corticosteroids are effective; however, in virtually all patients, the possibility of joint infection should be evaluated before intra-articular administration. Colchicine is an effective prophylactic drug and can also be used to treat crystal-induced arthritides, such as gout or pseudogout. The older oral administration regimen of one tablet (0.6 mg) every hour until relief or gastrotoxicity develops (usually diarrhea) is generally unacceptable to patients because the diarrhea occurs at the same time or slightly before clinical relief is obtained. Intravenous colchicine (1- to 2-mg initial dose) is an effective therapy for many patients with acute attacks of crystal disease, but it *can be extremely toxic* if inappropriate doses are used; and is now generally unavailable. Colchicine should not be used in patients with significant hepatic, biliary, or renal disease without a decrease in the dosage (if it is used at all).

In patients who suffer frequent attacks, multiple regimens are potentially of value for prophylaxis. Colchicine, 0.6 to 1.8 mg daily, can be used; diarrhea may limit the dosing. Especially in patients with renal insufficiency, chronic colchicine use can result in a reversible neuromuscular toxicity; this should be regularly monitored by history, examination, and occasional creatine phosphokinase measurement. The dosage must be decreased in this setting. This toxicity syndrome has also been described when statins, macrolide antibiotics, calcium channel blockers, and some other drugs have been prescribed to patients taking daily colchicine.

Daily NSAIDs are not ideal as chronic prophylactic therapy because of their side effect profile. In general, dietary manipulations are not likely to provide an enormous change in the serum urate level; the one exception to this is cautioning patients about intermittent binge ethanol use. In one epidemiologic study, beer and hard liquor ingestion was associated with a greater risk of hyperuricemia and gout (wine was not). High intake of coffee or dairy is associated with lower urate levels. Acute ethanol ingestion causes fluctuations in serum uric acid levels and has been associated with acute gouty attacks.

Gouty Arthritis in Transplantation Patients

Special note should be made of the occurrence of severe gouty arthritis in patients receiving transplanted organs. Cyclosporine is seemingly the risk factor, rather than the transplant itself, at least in part because this drug induces hyperuricemia. The course of gout in transplantation patients is more rapidly progressive than in patients not taking cyclosporine. Tophi develop earlier than expected, and involvement of the joints of the upper extremity and even the axial skeleton frequently occurs. Multiple potential toxicities exist in the treatment of transplantation

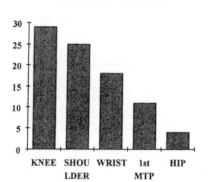

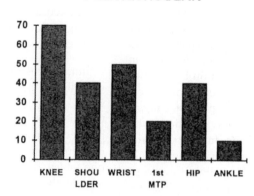

Figure 28.7 Septic arthritis in adults. MTP, metatarsophalangeal. *Source:* Reproduced with permission from Martens PB, Ho G Jr. Septic arthritis in adults: clinical features, outcome, and intensive care requirements. *J Intensive Care Med* 1995;10: 246–252.

patients, including drug interactions between NSAIDs and cyclosporine and between allopurinol and azathioprine. These drug interactions must be closely monitored. The increasing use of mycophenolic acid as a maintenance antirejection therapy simplifies the management of transplant-associated gout.

Septic Arthritis

Bacterial infection is an uncommon (~15%) cause of acute arthritis. Nonetheless, associated morbidity and potential mortality mandate its prompt exclusion as the cause of acute arthritis. The distribution of affected joints is shown in Figure 28.7. Fibrocartilage joints, such as the sternoclavicular, sacroiliac, and acromioclavicular joints, are involved with infections in specific settings. These joints are prone to infection after persistent bacteremia, particularly with gram-negative organisms. Patients with a history of intravenous drug use or intravenous catheters (e.g., total parenteral nutrition, hemodialysis, apheresis) are at particular risk.

Etiology

In most series, staphylococci and streptococci are the most common organisms causing septic arthritis. Disseminated gonococcemia is also a frequent cause of septic arthritis in some populations. The diagnosis of septic arthritis cannot be made with certainty without the culture of synovial fluid. Fever, leukocytosis, rigors, and an elevated ESR are neither specific nor sensitive for the diagnosis of septic arthritis. A positive Gram stain may be seen in only a slight majority of cases of nongonococcal septic arthritis; thus, a negative Gram stain does not exclude the possibility of infection. False-positive Gram stains for bacteria also occur.

Disseminated gonococcal infection produces skin lesions and tenosynovitis more commonly than other infections. The arthritis often follows a syndrome of migratory myalgia and arthralgia. The synovial fluid Gram stain is usually negative in disseminated gonococcal arthritis, and culture is usually negative as well. Why synovial fluid culture results are negative may relate in part to the difficulty in growing the organism, as well as to the pathophysiology by which arthritis can be induced by immune complexes containing gonococcal antigens without live organisms (Fig. 28.8).

Specific Infections and Syndromes

Lyme Disease

Lyme disease results from tick-transmission of the spirochete *B. burgdorferi*. Frequently, there is a history of an initial characteristic rash, erythema chronicum migrans. Erythema chronicum migrans appears as single or multiple

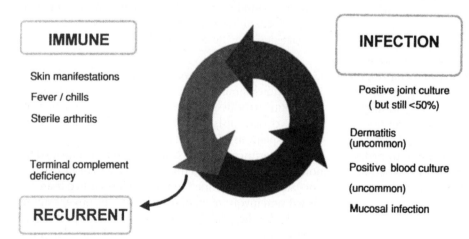

Figure 28.8 Spectrum of disseminated gonococcal infection.

targetlike lesions with central clearing. Studies suggest that the overwhelming majority of patients with Lyme disease have a rash at the onset of their illness. This rash may be associated with a flulike syndrome and symptoms of aseptic meningitis. Fluctuating neurologic syndromes, including facial palsy and radiculitis, may develop shortly thereafter. Cardiac conduction disease, which can fluctuate but may include complete heart block, also occurs. The joint involvement is a monoarticular or oligoarticular, remittent or intermittent, large joint arthritis. It does not cause a symmetric polyarthritis of small joints, as in rheumatoid arthritis. It is associated with inflammatory joint fluid. The provisional diagnosis of Lyme disease must include the following factors:

- Opportunity for exposure to a suitable tick vector
- Clinical pattern of symptoms consistent with described disease manifestations
- Positive enzyme-linked immunosorbent assay (ELISA) supported by a positive Western blot test result (multiple *Borrelia*-associated bands)

Seronegative Lyme arthritis is extremely uncommon, and this diagnosis should be entertained only with a great deal of caution. Fibromyalgia, although described in persons who have had Lyme disease, is not a symptom complex suggestive of active infection and does not warrant antibiotic therapy. Circulating antibodies persist for years, and their presence does not warrant chronic or repeated antibiotic administration.

Culture-Negative and Crystal-Negative Acute Arthritis

If monoarticular arthritis is not initially found to be due to crystals, and if bacterial culture results are negative in the absence of prior antibiotic use, the differential diagnosis should include:

- Gonococcal infection
- Lyme disease (if potential exposure was possible; the absence of a concurrent rash does not exclude this diagnosis)
- Mycobacterial infection
- Fungal infection
- Reactive arthritis
- Tumor
- Periarticular osteomyelitis

Undiagnosed systemic diseases, such as psoriasis or inflammatory bowel disease, can also cause acute or chronic monoarticular arthritis. Periarticular osteomyelitis should also be considered.

Reactive Arthritis

Reactive arthritis is generally a diagnosis of exclusion at the time of first presentation with monoarticular arthritis. The arthritis is presumably reactive to infection elsewhere in the body. The joint fluids are sterile, although some investigators have suggested that specific bacterial antigens, which localize to the synovium and are not successfully cleared, cause the synovitis. Organisms associated with reactive arthritis include *Chlamydia*, *Salmonella*, *Clostridium difficile*, and *Yersinia*. Patients with reactive arthritis may have other features of what formerly was known as "Reiter's syndrome," including mild conjunctivitis or uveitis, allergic or infectious urethritis, balanitis, psoriasiform skin lesions, or oral ulcerations. The pattern of joint involvement is often large joint (knee) with lower extremity predominance; joint fluid may be extremely inflammatory. Sausage digits, enthesitis, and asymmetric sacroiliac involvement may also occur.

Viral Arthritis

Viral infections have also been associated with acute arthritis. Viral arthritis is often associated with a pseudorheumatoid distribution of involved joints. Some forms of viral arthritis (varicella zoster virus, cytomegalovirus, herpes simplex virus type 1, HIV), however, have been associated with monoarticular or oligoarticular arthritis. Rubella-associated arthritis affects females more frequently than males and occurs in 50% to 60% of patients following natural infection, and perhaps in 50% of patients following immunization. In approximately one-third of patients, joint symptoms persist for approximately 1 year.

Parvovirus (fifth disease in children) has been associated with arthritis and arthralgia in adults, usually in a polyarticular pattern without the typical skin eruption that is seen in children. Transient rheumatoid factor may occur in these patients. Parvovirus infection has also been associated with aplastic crises in patients with chronic hemolysis or HIV infection. Hepatitis B and C viruses have been associated with joint symptoms, with or without cryoglobulinemia, which can totally mimic acute rheumatoid arthritis. In one report, an increased frequency of distal finger joint involvement occurred with hepatitis B. The arthritis can be associated with the prodromal phase or in the setting of chronic active hepatitis. It can also be associated with a polyarteritis nodosa syndrome. Hepatitis C–induced arthritis frequently occurs in association with cryoglobulinemia and a high-titer rheumatoid factor; it may be present in patients who have only a minimal elevation in transaminases. HIV infection has been associated with an acute, extremely painful oligoarthritis associated with minimally inflammatory or noninflammatory synovial fluid. Marked hyperesthesia of the joint capsule may be present.

Diagnosis of Septic Arthritis

The diagnosis of gonococcal infection is frequently made by culture from extra-articular sites, predominantly the urogenital tract. It must be noted, however, that the absence of pelvic symptoms (or physical findings) in no way excludes the possibility of disseminated gonococcemia (Fig. 28.9).

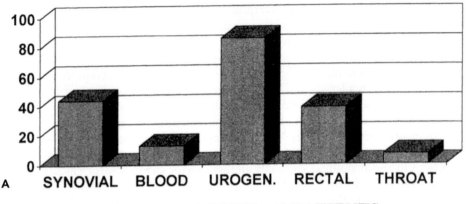

A

BOWMAN GRAY SCH MED: 41 PATIENTS

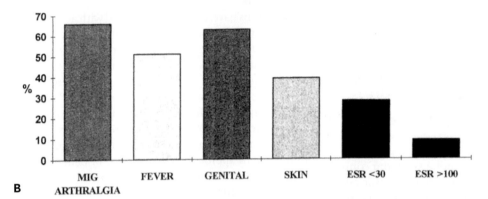

B

Figure 28.9 Positive culture results in patients with gonococcal arthritis. ESR, erythrocyte sedimentation rate; MIG, migratory; UROGEN, urogenital. *Source:* Reproduced with permission from Wise CM, Morris CR, Wasilauskas BL, et al. Gonococcal arthritis in an era of increasing penicillin resistance: presentations and outcomes in 41 recent cases, 1985–1991. *Arch Intern Med* 1994;154: 2690–2695.

The appropriate evaluation of a patient with potential disseminated gonococcemia should include

- Blood and joint fluid cultures
- Cervical cultures (vaginal cultures in postmenopausal women)
- Rectal and pharyngeal cultures

The absence of rectal or pharyngeal symptoms does not obviate the need to obtain samples from these areas for culture. Patients with disseminated gonococcemia may have multiple joints involved. Other bacterial causes of nongonococcal polyarticular infections in patients without underlying rheumatoid arthritis are shown in Figure 28.10. The gold standard for diagnosing septic arthritis is the microbiological identification of an organism in synovial fluid or tissue.

Treatment

The treatment of suspected septic arthritis should not be delayed until culture results are available. If the diagnosis of infection is seriously considered, the involved joint should be treated as a closed-space infection, using parenteral systemic antibiotics and adequate local drainage. The percutaneous drainage of a joint is adequate if it can be performed efficiently. Hip joints are difficult to aspirate, and open drainage is usually used. Until a diagnosis is certain, the percutaneous drainage of an affected joint should be performed daily or as often as necessary to attempt to maintain an effusionfree joint. Successful antibiotic therapy is usually accompanied by a decrease in cell counts; the synovial WBC count generally decreases by 50% each day. Initially, the joint should be splinted for pain control and joint protection; however, as the inflammation resolves over subsequent days, passive and then active physical therapy should be introduced as quickly as possible to preserve joint function. If disseminated gonococcemia is suspected, NSAIDs or other anti-inflammatory drugs should be withheld until the diagnosis is confirmed because a favorable response to antibiotics may be necessary to support the diagnosis of gonorrhea when cultures are negative; a response to NSAID therapy may cause diagnostic confusion. There is no role for intra-articular antibiotics.

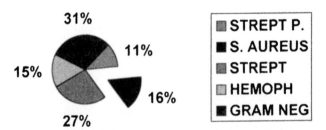

Figure 28.10 Polyarticular infections in patients without rheumatoid arthritis: nongonococcal causative organisms. Polyarticular disease was present in 6% of all infected patients from a selected series. GRAM NEG, gram negative; HEMOPH, *Haemophilus*; STREPT P., *Streptococcus pneumoniae*; STREPT, *Streptococcus*.

At present, no data suggest that any alternative drainage approach (e.g., lavage, arthroscopy, or arthrotomy) is routinely superior to adequate percutaneous drainage in adults. In patients with underlying joint damage (rheumatoid arthritis), a delayed diagnosis, or immunosuppression, however, I frequently employ arthroscopic drainage in the hopes of removing the damaged tissue nidus for recalcitrant infection. Until a diagnosis is confirmed by culture, each aspirated joint fluid sample should be evaluated for the presence of crystals using polarized microscopy because crystals may have been missed on the initial evaluation. Recommended antibiotic regimens vary according to local bacterial resistance profiles and patient demographics. A general empiric antibiotic regimen for treating septic arthritis could include:

- Young healthy patients: treat for gonococcal and staphylococcal infection (methicillin-resistant *Staphylococcus aureus* [MRSA], depending on local community susceptibility profiles).
- Patients with underlying joint disease, prolonged hospitalization, prior antibiotic use, urinary tract infections, or prostate disease: treat for MRSA and gram-negative bacteria.
- Patients with a history of intravenous drug abuse: consider HIV issues, treat for *Pseudomonas* and MRSA.

If Lyme disease is suspected or confirmed and disease stage identified, treatment options include:

- Presence of erythema chronicum migrans: On clinical grounds, treat for 21 to 28 days (do not wait for antibody testing) using doxycycline, 100 twice daily; amoxicillin, 500 three times daily; or erythromycin, 250 to 500 four times daily.
- Stage 2—neurologic/cardiac disease: Treat for 14 to 28 days with intravenous penicillin, 20 million U daily, intravenous ceftriaxone (Rocephin), 1 g every 12 hours, or doxycycline, 100 mg twice daily.

Thirty days of therapy in 38 patients with arthritis caused by Lyme disease produced the following results:

- Doxycycline, 100 twice daily: response in 18 of 20
- Amoxicillin/probenecid, 500 four times daily: response in 16 of 18

Note that although the majority of patients with Lyme arthritis responded to this regimen in less than 1 month, response may take 3 months.

REVIEW EXERCISES

QUESTIONS

1. A 56-year-old man presents to the emergency department with a 2-day history of increasing right wrist pain and associated swelling. He denies a history of prior episodes of arthritis or any antecedent trauma. His only medication is a diuretic for the treatment of hypertension. He was recently hospitalized for a transurethral prostate resection for benign prostatic hypertrophy. His older brother has been diagnosed with gout. The most useful diagnostic tests for this patient include

a) Radiography of the wrist
b) Serum urate level
c) Complete blood cell count with differential and erythrocyte sedimentation rate
d) b and c
e) None is particularly useful

Answer and Discussion

The answer is e. The major differential diagnosis is between acute crystal disease and infection. The only reliable way to distinguish these is by synovial fluid analysis and culture.

2. A 56-year-old man is found to have a serum urate level of 9.4 mg/dL. Clear-cut indications for treatment with allopurinol include

a) A 24-hour urinary uric acid excretion >1,000 mg
b) A creatinine value of 2.6 mg/dL
c) A history of two episodes of documented gouty arthritis in the past 2 years
d) A requirement for chronic hydrochlorothiazide
e) None of the above

Answer and Discussion

The answer is e. Asymptomatic hyperuricemia in general need not be treated. No firm evidence exists that treating hyperuricemia in this range prevents renal disease or other end-organ dysfunction in the absence of any symptoms, laboratory dysfunction, or related problems (e.g., nephrolithiasis).

3. All of the following conditions may be associated with hypouricemia, *except*

a) Syndrome of inappropriate antidiuretic hormone secretion
b) High-dose salicylate therapy
c) Wilson's disease
d) Lactic acidosis
e) Early alcohol withdrawal

Answer and Discussion

The answer is d. Organic acidosis produces mild hyperuricemia, not hypouricemia. The causes of hypouricemia include syndrome of inappropriate antidiuretic hormone secretion, renal tubular disorders, very high-dose aspirin therapy, hydration, and administration of radiocontrast agents.

4. Preoperative medical consultation was requested for a 56-year-old, insulin-dependent, diabetic man with peripheral vascular disease and osteomyelitis and septic arthritis of the fourth toe. Pain, redness, and swelling were noted for 6 weeks and were only minimally responsive to an oral antibiotic. Drainage of pus reportedly had increased over the previous week. Erythrocyte sedimentation rate was 54 mm/hour, and the white blood cell count was 10,500/mm^3. Bone scan was positive in three phases, and radiographs showed periarticular proximal interphalangeal bone erosion with patchy sclerosis and demineralization of the phalanx. As the medical consultant, you recommend

a) Preoperative angiogram, an approach for glucose management, and consideration for spinal anesthesia

b) Percutaneous (needle) bone cultures with the patient off antibiotics, plus the previous preoperative evaluation

c) Culture of a sinus tract for sensitivities and 3 days of preoperative intravenous antibiotics, plus the previous preoperative evaluation

d) Full re-examination of pus, including microscopy, before the previous preoperative evaluation

Answer and Discussion

The answer is d. As the medical consultant, it is worthwhile to review the primary data whenever possible. In this case, examination of the "pus" revealed that the infection was actually a draining uric acid tophus.

5. A 26-year-old African American woman presents with a chief complaint of foot pain. Examination reveals ankle joint arthritis. She is afebrile and otherwise symptom free. She has a documented history of sickle cell anemia. Synovial fluid reveals a white blood cell count of 18,000/mm^3, with 86% neutrophils. No crystals are seen. She is treated with a broad-spectrum antibiotic but experiences only minimal improvement after 3 days. Synovial cultures after 72 hours are negative. The presumptive diagnosis is

a) Gout

b) Salmonella arthritis

c) Avascular necrosis

d) Gonococcal arthritis

e) Reactive arthritis

Answer and Discussion

The answer is d. Seventy-two hours is not always sufficient time to observe a dramatic response to antibiotics. Whereas salmonella or other routine bacterial infections would have been expected to have been recognized in bacterial culture, gonococcus is often not isolated from joint fluid. Gout is more common in sickle cell patients, but the diagnosis of gout should not be made in this setting in the absence of visualized crystals. Avascular necrosis does *not* elicit an inflammatory synovial fluid response.

SUGGESTED READINGS

Cucurull E, Espinoza LR. Gonococcal arthritis. *Rheum Dis Clin North Am* 1998;24:305–321.

Donatto KC. Orthopedic management of septic arthritis. *Rheum Dis Clin North Am* 1998;24:275–286.

George TM, Mandell BF. Gout in the transplant patient. *Clin Rheumatol* 1996;1:328–334.

George TM, Mandell BF. Individualizing the treatment of gout. *Cleve Clin J Med* 1996;63:150–155.

Ho G, DeNuccio M. Gout and pseudogout in the hospitalized patient. *Arch Intern Med* 1993;153:2787–2790.

Johnson RJ, Kivlign SD, Kim YG, et al. Reappraisal of the pathogenesis and consequences of hyperuricemia in hypertension, cardiovascular disease, and renal disease. *Am J Kidney Dis* 1999;33:225–234.

Lin KC, Lin HY, Chai P. The interaction between uric acid level and other risk factors on the development of gout among asymptomatic hyperuricemic men in a prospective study. *J Rheumatol* 2000;27:1501–1505.

Lipkowitz MS, Leal-Pinto E, Rappaport JZ, et al. Functional reconstitution, membrane targeting, genomic structure, and chromosomal localization of a human urate transporter. *J Clin Invest* 2001;107:1103–1115.

Lossos IS, Yossepowitch O, Kandel L, et al. Septic arthritis of the glenohumeral joint. *Medicine (Baltimore)* 1998;77:177–187.

Margaretten ME, Kohlwes J, Moore D, et al. Does this patient have septic arthritis? *JAMA* 2007;297:1478–1488.

Pioro MH, Mandell BF. Septic arthritis. *Rheum Dis Clin North Am* 1997;23:239–258.

Schlapbach P. Bacterial arthritis: are fevers, rigors, leukocytosis, and blood cultures of diagnostic value? *Clin Rheumatol* 1990;9:69–72.

Chapter 29

Osteoarthritis and Polyarticular Arthritis

David E. Blumenthal

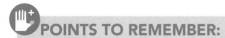

POINTS TO REMEMBER:

- Evidence of osteoarthritis in an unexpected location should prompt a search for the underlying cause.

- Cyclo-oxygenase 2–selective nonsteroidal anti-inflammatory drugs (NSAIDs) are less likely to cause gastric bleeding, but are otherwise not preferable to nonselective NSAIDs.

- Patients receiving therapy with the anti-tumor necrosis factor therapies are at increased risk for the reactivation of latent mycobacterial infections.

- Testing for human leukocyte antigen (HLA)-B27 is seldom clinically useful, however. HLA-B27 is present in 6% to 8% of the population in the United States, and only 1% to 2% of those who carry the HLA-B27 antigen develop ankylosing spondylitis.

The differential diagnosis of musculoskeletal pain is broad. Pain can result from pathology in the articular cartilage, synovium, ligaments, tendons, fibrocartilage, bursae, skeletal muscle, periosteum, bone, peripheral nerves, and nerve roots. This chapter reviews chronic diseases of the articular cartilage and synovium.

OSTEOARTHRITIS

Osteoarthritis (OA) is also known as degenerative arthritis or degenerative joint disease. Some physicians prefer the term osteoarthrosis because inflammation is not a prominent feature of the disease. OA usually begins to appear in midlife and is almost universal in the elderly. The radiographic prevalence of OA in the distal interphalangeal (DIP) joint rises rapidly between ages 40 and 60 years, and reaches a prevalence of about 60% of men and 75% of women by age 75 years.

OA can be further classified into primary OA, which occurs frequently with normal aging, and secondary OA, where another medical condition has caused or accelerated the loss of articular cartilage.

Primary Osteoarthritis

Primary OA occurs in a characteristic distribution. Note that some joints are infrequently affected by primary OA.

Common Site of OA	Uncommon Site of OA
DIP joint	Metacarpal phalangeal
Proximal interphalangeal	(MCP) joint
(PIP) joint	Wrist
First carpometacarpal	Elbow
(CMC) joint	Shoulder (glenohumeral)
Acromioclavicular (AC)	joint
joint	Ankle
Cervical spine	
Lumbar spine	
Hip	
Knee	
First metatarsal phalangeal	
(MTP) joint	

OA is a disease of articular (hyaline) cartilage. With aging, the water content of the cartilage increases, and the content of glycosaminoglycans decreases. The concentrations and activities of matrix metalloproteinases are increased, with a subsequent degradation of collagen and proteoglycans. The cartilage becomes thin, fissured, frayed, and less able to cushion the joint and provide a smooth gliding surface during joint movement. The adjacent bone is exposed to greater forces and reinforces itself by producing osteophytes at the margins of the joint and subchondral sclerosis. Synovial fluid may migrate under pressure through pits in the articular cartilage and result in subchondral cysts. OA is not a simple consequence of "wear

349

and tear" or weight bearing. The ankle is exposed to at least as much weight as the knee, yet it rarely shows signs of OA. Obesity is a risk factor for OA of the knee, and a lesser risk for OA of the hip, but is not a risk factor for OA in other joints.

Patients with OA experience "mechanical" symptoms. The affected joint becomes more painful with use and improves with rest. There may be some stiffness on arising in the morning, but it usually lasts 30 minutes or less. There are no systemic symptoms, and local signs of inflammation are absent. *Gelling*, or a stiffening of the joints during periods of rest, is mild. This history contrasts with that of inflammatory arthritis, as discussed later.

The physical examination reveals bony osteophytes on the margins of the joint. The joint is cool, and the overlying synovium is not usually thickened or inflamed. Crepitus, a sensation of friction within the joint, may be felt with joint motion. The range of motion of the joint is diminished, and angulation deformities may be apparent, especially at the DIPs and PIPs of the fingers, the first MTP, and the knees. A synovial cyst (ganglion) may be seen in the vicinity of the joint, particularly in the fingers.

Radiographs show an asymmetric loss of joint space, subchondral sclerosis, marginal osteophytes, and subchondral cysts.

Secondary Osteoarthritis

Secondary OA is suspected when a joint that is not commonly involved by primary OA shows evidence of OA on physical examination and radiographs. In secondary OA, a primary disorder causes the loss of articular cartilage and the appearance of OA in a joint where it would not ordinarily be expected to occur. Evidence of OA in an unexpected location should prompt a search for the underlying cause. The causes of secondary osteoarthritis include:

- Dysplasia, congenial or acquired
- Trauma
- Osteonecrosis
- Infection
- Chronic inflammation
- Hemarthroses, especially hemophilia
- Metabolic disorders
  - Acromegaly
  - Hemochromatosis
  - Ochronosis
  - Calcium pyrophosphate dihydrate deposition disease (CPPD arthropathy)
- Joint hypermobility
- Mucopolysaccharidoses
- Neuropathy (e.g., neuropathic [Charcot] joint)

Treatment of Osteoarthritis

Pain can be relieved using analgesics. Acetaminophen should be the first analgesic offered to most patients. Some patients report superior pain relief with NSAIDs, which can be considered if acetaminophen is ineffective. Nonselective NSAIDs are more likely to cause adverse effects in the elderly and should be used with caution. COX-2–selective NSAIDs are less likely to cause gastric bleeding, but are otherwise not preferable to nonselective NSAIDs. The nutrient glucosamine may provide pain relief and the possible preservation of articular cartilage. Weight reduction will help OA of the knee and hip. Quadriceps muscle strengthening is beneficial in OA of the knee. An assistive device such as a cane or walker will transfer some of the body weight from the affected lower extremity. Refractory OA of the knee can be treated with viscosupplementation, the intra-articular injection of synthetic hyaluronic acid. If conservative measures fail, an orthopedic surgeon can offer the patient arthrodesis (fusion) or arthroplasty (replacement). Arthrodesis is most useful for the ankle, wrist, spine, and first MTP. Arthroplasty is most useful for the hip, knee, and shoulder.

POLYARTICULAR INFLAMMATORY ARTHRITIS

The hallmark of inflammatory arthritis is inflammation of the synovium. In contrast to the patient with a mechanical joint problem such as OA, the patient with inflammatory arthritis will have "inflammatory symptoms." In addition to joint pain, the patient will complain of morning stiffness that lasts more than 1 hour. The joints feel better with use, and the worst periods are during the night and on arising in the morning. Gelling is prominent. An examination of the joint will reveal warmth, tenderness, joint swelling (a mixture of synovial thickening and joint effusion), loss of function, and, occasionally, erythema. The presence of inflammatory cytokines and other mediators can lead to systemic symptoms, such as fatigue, malaise, weight loss, and fever. The differential diagnosis of polyarticular arthritis is broad, as listed in the following section. The connective tissue diseases, vasculitides, Lyme disease, and varieties of crystal-induced arthritis are reviewed in other chapters.

Differential Diagnosis of Polyarticular Inflammatory Arthritis

The differential diagnoses of polyarticular inflammatory arthritis include:

- Rheumatoid arthritis
- Spondyloarthropathies
- Connective tissue diseases
- Vasculitis
- Polyarticular gout
- Polyarticular CPPD (pseudogout)
- Polymyalgia rheumatica
- Viral arthritis

- Lyme disease
- Sarcoidosis
- Adult-onset Still's disease
- Rheumatic fever
- Serum sickness
- Subacute bacterial endocarditis
- Cryoglobulinemia

RHEUMATOID ARTHRITIS

Rheumatoid arthritis (RA) is the most prevalent chronic inflammatory arthritis, affecting about 1% of the population worldwide. Women are affected two to four times as frequently as men. HLA-DR4 is a risk factor.

Pathophysiology

In RA, an unknown stimulus causes hyperplasia of the resident macrophages and fibroblasts of the synovium and angiogenesis (ingrowth of new blood vessels). The macrophages and fibroblasts secrete inflammatory mediators, including tumor necrosis factor (TNF), interleukin (IL)-1, IL-6, IL-8, prostaglandins, leukotrienes, and nitric oxide. These inflammatory mediators attract B and T lymphocytes into the synovium and neutrophils into the synovial fluid. The synovium becomes an enlarged mass of inflammatory cells and fibroblasts, called *pannus*, that has the potential to damage nearby bone, ligaments, tendons, and articular cartilage. The neutrophils elaborate metalloproteinases, which assist in the degradation of nearby tissues. With time, the articular cartilage thins, ligaments slip, tendons weaken, and the characteristic deformities and disabilities of RA appear.

RA is not merely an articular disease. The inflammation can be accompanied by a variety of extra-articular manifestations, including:

- Rheumatoid nodules
- Interstitial lung disease
- Pleuropericarditis
- Sjögren's syndrome
- Scleritis/episcleritis/corneal melt
- Digital infarcts
- Vasculitis
- Felty's syndrome
- Lower extremity ulcers
- Amyloidosis

Diagnosis

Rheumatoid arthritis is usually a symmetric, polyarticular arthritis, although it may sometimes be asymmetric and oligoarticular early in the course of the disease. Symptoms are those of inflammatory arthritis. The synovium is warm and thickened, and joint effusions are common. With time, characteristic deformities appear, such as swan neck and boutonniere deformities of the fingers, volar subluxation of the carpus, loss of full extension of the elbows and full abduction of the shoulders, valgus angulation at the knees and ankles, and pes planus.

Laboratory testing shows the features of a chronic inflammatory disease. The erythrocyte sedimentation rate (ESR) and C-reactive protein are high, serum albumin is low, and an anemia of chronic disease is often present. The serum rheumatoid factor (RF), an immunoglobin M (IgM) antibody that recognizes immunoglobulin G (IgG) as its antigen, will be present in 75% to 85% of patients. Patients with the serum RF often are called *seropositive*, whereas those who lack RF are called *seronegative*. Seropositive patients generally have a more aggressive arthritis and are at greater risk for the extra-articular manifestations of the disease. A positive RF can be seen in a variety of chronic inflammatory and infectious diseases, and in otherwise healthy elderly patients. RF should not be used as a screening test in low-risk populations and should be interpreted with caution if the history and physical examination are atypical for RA. Antibodies to cyclic citrullinated peptide (anti-CCP) are highly specific for RA (96%–98%), with a sensitivity of about 50%.

Radiographs initially show periarticular osteopenia and soft tissue swelling. As the disease progresses, a symmetric loss of joint space and periarticular erosions appear. The erosions are caused by the synovial pannus invading the periarticular bone.

Treatment

Medications used in RA attempt to decrease the synovial inflammation, and thereby relieve pain, improve joint function, and preserve articular and periarticular tissues. Salicylates and NSAIDs can provide some relief of inflammation and pain, but are seldom sufficient. Selective COX-2 inhibitors may offer less risk of NSAID gastropathy, but they do not appear to be more efficacious than traditional NSAIDs for RA. Corticosteroids, such as prednisone and methylprednisolone, are potent inhibitors of inflammation, but their chronic use can lead to a variety of unacceptable adverse effects, including weight gain, arterial hypertension, glucose intolerance, ocular cataracts, opportunistic infection, and osteoporosis. Intra-articular corticosteroids can provide effective treatment of an injected joint, with fewer systemic effects. Disease-modifying antirheumatic drugs (DMARDs) are used to control the synovial inflammation so that corticosteroid use can be avoided or minimized. The traditional DMARDs are listed as follows. Of these, methotrexate is probably the most efficacious. Potential adverse effects include mucositis, nausea, diarrhea, bone marrow suppression, hepatocellular injury, cirrhosis, pneumonitis, and opportunistic infection. Methotrexate should not be used in patients with hepatic, renal, or bone marrow disease, and should be used with caution in patients with lung disease. Leflunomide is an inhibitor of dihydro-orotate dehydrogenase, an important enzyme in the de novo synthesis of pyrimidines. The efficacy of leflunomide is similar to methotrexate; possible adverse effects include reversible alopecia, rash, diarrhea, and increased hepatic transaminases. Sulfasalazine is often effective, but sulfa allergy and frequent gastrointestinal intolerance limit its usefulness. Hydroxychloroquine is well tolerated and commonly prescribed in combination with other DMARDs, but as a single agent, it will seldom provide adequate control of the synovitis. Clinical studies have demonstrated efficacy for minocycline and cyclosporine, although they are less commonly used in clinical practice. The *biologicals* are proteins administered by subcutaneous injection or intravenous infusion. They are indicated in patients who do not achieve adequate disease control with oral DMARDs. Etanercept, infliximab, and adalimumab are blockers of TNF. Etanercept is a polypeptide comprised of two soluble TNF receptors fused to the Fc portion of IgG. It binds to TNF, thus preventing it from interacting with TNF receptors on the surface of immune cells. The adverse effects of etanercept may include irritation at the site of injection and increased susceptibility to infection. Infliximab and adalimumab are monoclonal antibodies that bind TNF as their antigen. Infliximab is given by intravenous infusion three times during the first 6 weeks, and then every 2 months thereafter. Adalimumab is given by subcutaneous injection every 14 days. Anakinra is a recombinant IL-1 receptor antagonist, which blocks the biological effect of IL-1. It is given daily by subcutaneous injection. Intravenous rituximab is a monoclonal antibody binding to CD 20, a cell surface marker of B cells, leading to B-cell depletion and clinical improvement in rheumatoid synovitis. Intravenous abatacept is a blocker of costimulation antigen-presenting cells and T cells, leading to a reduction in joint inflammation. Single-agent DMARD or biological therapy is often insufficient, and many patients are treated using combinations of antirheumatic drugs. The combinations of methotrexate + sulfasalazine + hydroxychloroquine, methotrexate + leflunomide, and methotrexate + cyclosporine have each been shown to be superior to single DMARD therapy in comparative trials. Biologicals are often used in combination with oral methotrexate or leflunomide. Parenteral gold, oral gold, and penicillamine are seldom used now because so many superior options are available.

Patients receiving therapy with the anti-TNF therapies are at increased risk for the reactivation of latent mycobacterial infections.

Oral DMARDs used to treat RA include:

- Methotrexate (MTX)
- Sulfasalazine (SSZ)
- Hydroxychloroquine (HQ)
- Leflunomide (LF)
- Minocycline
- Cyclosporine (CSA)

Parenteral biologicals used to treat RA include

- Etanercept
- Infliximab
- Adalimumab
- Anakinra
- Rituximab
- Abatacept

Combination therapy used to treat RA include:

- MTX + SSZ + HQ
- MTX + CSA
- MTX + LF
- Biological + MTX or LF

The extra-articular manifestations of RA are often treated with the same immunosuppressive agents used for the synovitis. Vasculitis and vision-threatening eye disease may require treatment with cyclophosphamide. Mechanical pain caused by joint damage is treated with analgesics. Arthrodesis or arthroplasty may be effective in relieving pain in a damaged joint. Surgical synovectomy may provide temporary relief of the synovitis in the surgically treated joint, but it provides no benefit for the other inflamed joints or the systemic features of the disease, and therefore is of limited value.

THE SPONDYLOARTHROPATHIES

The spondyloarthropathies include ankylosing spondylitis, psoriatic arthritis, Reiter's syndrome, and enteropathic arthritis. This group of diseases share several common features:

- Risk of sacroiliitis and spondylitis
- Peripheral arthritis often asymmetric
- Enthesopathy: inflammation of tendon insertions
- Risk of inflammatory eye disease
- Association with HLA-B27

Ankylosing Spondylitis

Ankylosing spondylitis (AS) is most commonly seen in young males (M:F 3:1). The typical patient experiences the onset of inflammatory pain in the low back or buttocks in the late teens or 20s. Onset of symptoms always occurs prior to age 40 years. Inflammation usually begins in the sacroiliac joints and ascends the spine. With time, slender calcifications called *bridging syndesmophytes* extend from one vertebral body to the next, resulting in a fusion of the spine. Peripheral arthritis is seen in about 25% of patients, usually in the hips or shoulders. Patients with AS are at risk to develop inflammation of the aortic root, with resulting aortic insufficiency, iritis/uveitis, and apical pulmonary fibrosis.

Diagnosis

History reveals buttock, back, neck, or peripheral joint pain that has the typical features of an inflammatory process: most severe symptoms in the morning, more than 1 hour of morning stiffness, improvement with increasing activity and worsening with rest, and "gelling" with inactivity. Family history often reveals other affected family members, particularly in male first-degree relatives. Physical examination may reveal a loss of lumbar or cervical lordosis; loss of range of motion in the spine, including an abnormal Schober's test; diminished chest expansion; peripheral arthritis; and evidence of extra-articular manifestations of the disease.

HLA-B27 is a risk factor for developing ankylosing spondylitis, with positive tests in 80% to 98% of Caucasian patients. Testing for HLA-B27 is seldom clinically useful, however. HLA-B27 is present in 6% to 8% of the population in the United States, and only 1% to 2% of those who carry the HLA-B27 antigen develop ankylosing spondylitis. Thus, testing for HLA-B27 in low-risk populations has a low positive predictive value. The test is even less useful in African Americans, in whom only about 50% of patients with AS carry HLA-B27. Other blood tests often show elevated acute phase reactants and anemia of chronic disease.

Plain radiographs show bilateral sacroiliitis, loss of lumbar and cervical lordosis, squaring of vertebral bodies, and bridging syndesmophytes that eventually result in a fusion of the entire spine. In the early stages of the disease, a radionuclide bone scan may show evidence of sacroiliitis or spondylitis before any abnormalities can be appreciated on plain radiographs.

Treatment

NSAIDs are often used to control the stiffness and pain. Sulfasalazine and methotrexate can be used to control peripheral joint synovitis, but they are less effective for the spondylitis. TNF inhibitors can be very effective for both spondylitis and peripheral arthritis. Patients are advised to perform extension exercises and maintain proper posture so that fusion can occur in a functional position.

Psoriatic Arthritis

Psoriatic arthritis can present with a variety of clinical patterns: (a) symmetric, polyarticular, resembling seronegative RA; (b) isolated DIP arthritis; (c) asymmetric, oligoarticular; (d) arthritis mutilans, where the PIPs and DIPs are so severely damaged that the fingers become a "main en lorgnette" or opera glass hand with collapsible digits; and (e) any of the previous patterns, with sacroiliitis or spondylitis. The cutaneous psoriasis need not be severe and is often subtle. An occasional patient may have the typical features of psoriatic arthritis prior to the appearance of the cutaneous disease, which can lead to difficulties with diagnosis.

Diagnosis

Psoriatic arthritis is usually diagnosed on clinical grounds when a patient with evidence of cutaneous psoriasis develops the signs and symptoms of an inflammatory arthritis. Psoriatic arthritis has a number of features that distinguish it from RA. Evidence of the cutaneous disease is usually present: well-demarcated erythematous plaques with superficial scale that bleed on gentle scraping, nail pitting, and onycholysis. The DIPs are commonly involved in psoriatic arthritis, rarely in RA. Enthesopathy occurs in psoriatic arthritis, and the combination of enthesopathy and synovitis leads to dactylitis, also called a "sausage digit." Such diffuse swelling of a digit is characteristic of the spondyloarthropathies and is not seen in RA. Sacroiliitis and spondylitis are not seen in RA, but occur in 20% to 40% of patients with psoriatic arthritis. Psoriatic patients lack serum RF, and the extra-articular manifestations of psoriatic arthritis resemble those of other spondyloarthropathies; psoriatic patients do not develop rheumatoid nodules, vasculitis, or Felty's syndrome. Radiographs in psoriatic arthritis are more likely to show DIP involvement, periostitis, growth of bone at tendon insertions (enthesophytes), and a pencil-in-cup deformity in an interphalangeal joint (the more proximal phalanx is whittled to a point, and the more distal phalanx is flared at its base).

Treatment

Milder cases of psoriatic arthritis can be controlled using NSAIDs. More widespread or destructive arthritis is usually treated using DMARDs, as in RA. Methotrexate, leflunomide, sulfasalazine, etanercept, infliximab, adalimumab, and cyclosporine are all options for more severe disease.

Reiter's Syndrome

Reiter's syndrome occurs when an at-risk individual encounters an antigen, leading to "reactive arthritis" and autoimmune attack on other body tissues. HLA-B27 is present in approximately 80% of affected individuals and appears to be the leading risk factor for the disease. Postvenereal Reiter's occurs after exposure to *Chlamydia trachomatis*. Postdysenteric reactive arthritis occurs after exposure to *Salmonella, Shigella, Campylobacter, Yersinia*, or, occasionally, *Clostridium difficile*. The classic triad consists of arthritis, sterile urethritis, and conjunctivitis, with an onset of symptoms about 2 to 4 weeks after exposure to the microorganism. Affected individuals may develop sacroiliitis and spondylitis; unlike ankylosing spondylitis, the sacroiliitis may be unilateral, and some areas of the spine may be spared. The bridging osteophytes may be more bulky than the delicate syndesmophytes seen in ankylosing spondylitis. The peripheral arthritis is often asymmetric and oligoarticular, with a lower extremity predominance. Of Reiter's patients, 15% to 30% will develop chronic arthritis. Enthesopathy and dactylitis are common, usually presenting as sausage digits, Achilles tendon inflammation, and plantar fasciitis ("lover's heel"). Keratoderma blenorrhagicum is a characteristic skin rash, mainly on the palms and soles, that is indistinguishable from pustular psoriasis in both its appearance and its histopathology. Onycholysis similar to that of psoriasis may be seen, but nail pitting is absent in Reiter's syndrome. Circinate balanitis is an ulcerative lesion of the glans penis. Approximately 20% of Reiter's patients will eventually experience anterior uveitis.

Treatment of Reiter's syndrome is usually with NSAIDs. The disease usually subsides within 6 months, but in 15% to 30% of cases, it may become chronic. The postdysenteric form of the disease is more likely to become chronic. Sulfasalazine and methotrexate can be used for chronic arthritis, and a trial of minocycline or doxycycline may be beneficial for postvenereal forms of the disease. Blockers of TNF may be considered for refractory disease.

Enteropathic Arthritis

Arthritis can occur in association with either ulcerative colitis or Crohn's disease. In patients with inflammatory bowel disease, 10% to 20% will develop nonerosive oligoarticular arthritis of the large joints. Knee involvement is most common, followed by ankles, elbows, shoulders, and wrists. Sacroiliitis and spondylitis occur in about 15% of patients with inflammatory bowel disease. The peripheral joint arthritis often flares in concert with flares of the bowel disease. Activity of the sacroiliitis and spondylitis is usually independent of the bowel disease. The peripheral arthritis is often successfully treated by the same medications used for the bowel disease, which may include corticosteroids, sulfasalazine, methotrexate, azathioprine, or infliximab.

Arthritis may also be seen in association with other bowel disorders, including intestinal bypass, gluten-sensitive enteropathy, Whipple's disease, and collagenous colitis.

POLYMYALGIA RHEUMATICA

Polymyalgia rheumatica (PMR) is a nonerosive arthritis that primarily affects the elderly. The typical patient is a Caucasian woman with a mean age of 70 years. The ratio of women to men is about 2:1. The disease is very rarely seen prior to age 50 years, and is uncommon in African Americans and Asians.

PMR is characterized by stiffness, primarily in the shoulders, upper back, neck, hips, proximal thighs, and low back. Symptoms are usually most severe during the night and on arising in the morning, and the gelling phenomenon is prominent. Fever, weight loss, fatigue, and malaise are common. Some patients will have simultaneous giant cell arteritis and report the headaches, jaw claudication, and scalp tenderness typical of that disease. Arthritis of peripheral joints can occur, but if synovitis of the hands and wrists is a major feature of the illness, then a diagnosis of rheumatoid arthritis may be more appropriate.

The diagnosis is usually made clinically. Laboratory evaluation often shows anemia of chronic disease and an acute phase response, but the ESR can be normal in 20% to 25% of patients. One should keep in mind that the ESR increases with age and that an ESR as high as 40 mm/hour may be normal for a 70-year-old woman.

Occasionally, patients obtain satisfactory relief of symptoms using NSAIDs, but most will require corticosteroids. Prednisone dosed at 10 to 20 mg daily usually provides prompt relief of symptoms. The prednisone dose is then tapered to the lowest effective dose. Disease activity often subsides between 6 months and 5 years after onset, but exacerbations requiring an intensification of therapy are common. Because the typical patient usually has multiple risk factors for osteoporosis prior to instituting corticosteroid therapy, attention should be paid to detecting, treating, and preventing osteoporosis. Patients who cannot taper the prednisone to a dose that is acceptable for long-term use should be considered for steroid-sparing immunosuppressive therapy. The ideal steroid-sparing strategy for PMR has not yet been defined, but a trial of methotrexate may be considered, although trial-based data for its efficacy are mixed.

The practitioner should take care to differentiate PMR from RA because the former diagnosis carries a risk of giant cell arteritis, and the latter diagnosis carries the risk of joint damage if DMARDs are not prescribed. Fibromyalgia is also common in the elderly and has a clinical presentation that can seem quite similar to PMR. Distinguishing between these two conditions is vital because of the risks of chronic corticosteroid therapy in the elderly.

VIRAL ARTHRITIS

True synovitis can be caused by a variety of viruses, including parvovirus B19, acute hepatitis B, chronic hepatitis C, rubella, mumps, and the enteroviruses. With the exception of chronic hepatitis C, viral arthritis is usually self-limited, with resolution of symptoms within 3 months. A positive test for RF is commonly seen in chronic hepatitis C, especially if cryoglobulins are present, which can lead to a mistaken diagnosis of RA.

The diagnosis of viral arthritis is possible if the patient's presentation and exposure history suggest a recent viral illness. Serology can be used to confirm the presence of IgM antibodies or recent seroconversion.

Treatment is supportive. NSAIDs are usually sufficient for relief of symptoms. The arthritis of chronic hepatitis C may respond to treatment of the underlying viral infection with interferon-α or ribavirin.

SARCOID ARTHRITIS

Arthritis is seen in 15% of sarcoidosis patients. It usually occurs in the first 6 months of the illness, and is usually self-limited and nonerosive. Sarcoidosis may present with a triad of acute arthritis, bilateral hilar adenopathy, and erythema nodosum, which is called Lofgren's syndrome.

The acute arthritis can be oligoarticular or polyarticular, but is rarely monarticular. The ankles are almost always involved, followed in frequency by the knees, wrists, and elbows. Treatment with NSAIDs is usually sufficient, and the arthritis usually resolves within 3 to 4 months.

Chronic arthritis is uncommon. When seen, it is usually in patients with skin, lung, or bone involvement who have been ill for at least 6 months. The patient often needs immunosuppressive treatment for involvement of other organ systems. Corticosteroids are the first line of therapy, with methotrexate, cyclosporine, and other cytotoxic medications used as steroid-sparing agents. Blockers of TNF can be considered for refractory disease.

ADULT-ONSET STILL'S DISEASE

The systemic-onset type of juvenile rheumatoid arthritis called Still's disease can also occur in adults. Some patients will give a prior history of Still's disease in childhood. The illness is a systemic, inflammatory, multisystem disease characterized by fever, weight loss, skin rash, pleuropericarditis, hepatosplenomegaly, and lymphadenopathy. The body temperature returns to normal between the once or twice daily fever spikes. The rash is often salmon pink in color and may be evanescent, most notably at times of fever. Polyarticular inflammatory arthritis is common, but the arthritis may not be a prominent feature of the disease.

Laboratory evaluation generally reveals an exuberant acute phase response, with high sedimentation rate, C-reactive protein and platelet count, low albumin, and anemia of chronic disease. The white blood cell count is often >15,000, and increased levels of hepatic enzymes are found in the serum. Serum ferritin may be strikingly elevated. Antinuclear antibodies and RF are negative.

NSAIDs may be effective in some patients, but many require corticosteroids. Methotrexate is an effective steroid-sparing agent. Anakinra can be very effective in refractory cases.

RHEUMATIC FEVER

Rheumatic fever is a late complication of group A streptococcal pharyngitis. It is usually not seen after group A strep infection of other anatomical sites, such as the skin, genital tract, or lung. Certain M serotypes confer a greater likelihood of developing rheumatic fever. Symptoms typically occur 1 to 5 weeks after pharyngeal infection, at a time when throat cultures are negative.

The modified Jones criteria are used to diagnose rheumatic fever in children. A diagnosis of rheumatic fever is considered likely if two major criteria, or one major and two minor, are met, plus evidence of an antecedent streptococcal infection.

The modified Jones criteria include:

- Major criteria
  - Carditis
  - Polyarthritis
  - Chorea
  - Erythema marginatum
  - Subcutaneous nodules
- Minor criteria
  - Arthralgia
  - Fever
  - Increased ESR
  - Increased C-reactive protein
  - Prolonged PR interval

Arthritis is more commonly seen in large joints, is migratory, and not additive. Typically, a joint will be inflamed for less than 1 week and improve, and then the arthritis will appear in another joint. Pain and tenderness are often out of proportion to the observed physical findings. Arthritis improves rapidly after treatment with aspirin or NSAIDs.

Carditis is typically a pancarditis and may present as heart block, a new murmur or evidence of valvular insufficiency, cardiomegaly, congestive heart failure, or pericarditis.

Subcutaneous nodules are similar in appearance and location to rheumatoid nodules, but are often smaller and resolve in 1 to 2 weeks.

Erythema marginatum is a pink to light red rash with a sharp outer border that typically appears on the trunk or proximal extremities and spreads centrifugally with central clearing. The face is usually spared.

A patient can develop sudden, purposeless, involuntary movements, known as *Sydenham's chorea*. These abnormal movements cease when the patient falls asleep. Chorea is often associated with generalized weakness and emotional lability.

Antecedent streptococcal infection is sometimes established by finding prior record of a positive throat culture before the onset of rheumatic fever symptoms. Often, however, the patient has no recollection of a prior pharyngitis, and throat cultures obtained at the time that rheumatic fever is manifest are usually negative. Serologic studies, including antibodies to streptolysin O, hyaluronidase, and DNAse B, can be helpful, especially if more than one of these tests is positive.

The diagnosis in adults can be difficult because chorea and erythema marginatum are rare, and carditis and subcutaneous nodules are less common than in childhood rheumatic fever.

Aspirin or NSAIDs are usually sufficient treatment for acute rheumatic fever. Glucocorticoids may be used for severe carditis. Penicillin or erythromycin is used to eradicate any lingering streptococcal infection.

Patients who have recovered from rheumatic fever may have a recurrence if streptococcal pharyngitis recurs. Repeated bouts of rheumatic carditis can cause additive injury to the heart valves. All patients who have recovered from rheumatic fever should be given antibiotic prophylaxis with either intramuscular benzathine penicillin G, oral penicillin VK, or oral erythromycin. Recommendations vary on the duration of prophylaxis. For most patients, it should be continued until at least age 21 years and for at least 5 years after the last attack of acute rheumatic fever. Some physicians recommend lifelong prophylaxis.

REVIEW EXERCISES

QUESTIONS

1. A 32-year-old man reports pain in the joints and dysuria. The right fourth toe is diffusely swollen, and the right ankle and left knee are warm, with pain on range of motion. The left eye is red. Urinalysis shows 25 to 30 white blood cells/hpf and 1 to 2 red blood cells/hpf. Urine culture and urethral swab for gonococcal infection are both negative. What is the diagnosis?

a) Acute gout
b) Adult-onset Still's disease
c) Reiter's syndrome
d) Polymyalgia rheumatica
e) Acute rheumatic fever

Answer and Discussion

The answer is c. The diffusely swollen toe likely represents a sausage digit, suggesting that the illness is likely to be a spondyloarthropathy. The triad of arthritis, conjunctivitis, and sterile urethritis is diagnostic of Reiter's syndrome. The treating physicians wisely did appropriate cultures to rule out disseminated gonococcal infection, which can also cause arthritis, urethritis, and conjunctivitis.

2. A 67-year-old man complains of gradually worsening knee pain for 5 years. He now can walk only 50 m before stopping due to the pain. Morning stiffness is 20 minutes. The right knee is cool with moderate crepitus, a small effusion, and range of motion from 5 degrees to 90 degrees. On weight bearing, he has a moderate varus deformity. What is your plan?

a) Check baseline hepatic transaminases and start methotrexate.
b) Administer trial of prednisone 20 mg/day for 1 week.
c) Check erythrocyte sedimentation rate and serum rheumatoid factor.
d) Arthrocentesis to rule out gout.
e) Order radiographs and refer to orthopedics.

Answer and Discussion

The answer is e. The history and examination suggest a gradual deterioration of the knee without the signs and symptoms of an inflammatory process. The typical history and physical examination is sufficient to make a diagnosis of osteoarthritis (OA). Because the patient can only walk 50 m at a time and has a marked loss of range of motion of the knee, one can conclude that the OA is rather advanced and the quality of life significantly diminished. Surgery is probably inevitable, and it would be reasonable to proceed with orthopedic consultation.

3. A 35-year-old woman is admitted for dyspnea. On examination, she has decreased breath sounds at the left lung base, and synovial thickening in her metacarpal phalangeals, proximal interphalangeals, wrists, and ankles. The olecranon bursa is diffusely swollen with embedded nodules. Her laboratory results are hemoglobin 11.2, platelets 545K, erythrocyte sedimentation rate 102, C-reactive protein 7.4, antinuclear antibodies + 1:160, and rheumatoid factor 168 (normal 0–20). A chest radiograph shows left pleural effusion. A thoracentesis reveals exudative fluid, pH 7.38, and glucose 24 mg/dL. What is the most likely diagnosis?

a) Systemic lupus erythematosus
b) Bacterial endocarditis with empyema
c) Adult-onset Still's disease
d) Lyme carditis
e) Rheumatoid arthritis

Answer and Discussion

The answer is e. The joint examination suggests a polyarticular inflammatory arthritis. The swollen olecranon bursa with embedded nodules is typical of rheumatoid arthritis (RA). Gout can cause olecranon bursitis with embedded tophi, but polyarticular tophaceous gout would be uncommon in a 35-year-old woman. Evidence suggests an acute phase response, further suggesting the presence of a systemic inflammatory disease. Patients with seropositive RA are at risk for extra-articular manifestations of the disease, including rheumatoid nodules and pleuropericarditis. A positive antinuclear antibodies test is not unusual in RA and does not, by itself, suggest the presence of lupus. The exudative pleural effusion with a low glucose is typical of RA. Although bacterial endocarditis can present as a systemic inflammatory illness with arthritis and a positive rheumatoid factor, the normal pH of the pleural fluid suggests that the low glucose is not caused by an empyema.

4. A 58-year-old diabetic female reports pain with use of the hands. Examination reveals bony enlargement of the metacarpal phalangeal (MCP) joints but no synovial thickening. Laboratory evaluation reveals erythrocyte sedimentation rate of 22 mm/hour. Radiographs reveal joint space narrowing at the MCP and proximal interphalangeal joints with osteophytes on the radial aspect of the metacarpal heads. What is the most likely diagnosis?

a) Primary osteoarthritis
b) Hemochromatosis
c) Rheumatoid arthritis
d) Hepatitis C with cryoglobulinemia
e) Sarcoidosis

Answer and Discussion

The answer is b. The physical examination and radiographs suggest osteoarthritis of the MCP joints, where cartilage loss from aging alone would be unusual. The radiographic findings are typical of hemochromatosis. The diabetes mellitus might be another manifestation of the disease.

5. Which biological therapy depletes peripheral blood and synovial B cells?

a) Rituximab
b) Infliximab
c) Anakinra
d) Etanercept
e) Abatacept

Answer and Discussion

The answer is a. Rituximab is a monoclonal antibody that recognizes CD 20 on the surface of B cells as its antigen. Infusion of rituximab depletes the peripheral blood and synovium of B cells.

SUGGESTED READINGS

Mease P. Current treatment for psoriatic arthritis and other spondyloarthritides. *Rheum Dis Clin North Am* 2006;32(Suppl 1):11–20.

Savage C, St. Clair EW. New therapeutics in rheumatoid arthritis. *Rheum Dis Clin North Am* 2006;32:57–74.

Sun BH, Wu CW, Kalunian KC. New developments in osteoarthritis. *Rheum Dis Clin North Am* 2007;33:135–148.

Unwin B, Williams CM, Gilliland W. Polymyalgia rheumatica and giant cell arteritis. *Am Fam Physician* 2006;74:1547–1554.

Wilson JF. To stop osteoarthritis, fixing cartilage may not be enough. *Ann Intern Med* 2007;7:437–439.

Chapter 30

Systemic Autoimmune Diseases

Abby Abelson

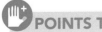

POINTS TO REMEMBER:

- Patients may have systemic lupus erythematous (SLE) with less than 4 of these 11 features because they may present with early disease in two organ systems and supportive serologies, and develop additional features as the disease progresses.

- Coronary artery disease is a leading cause of premature death in SLE. In young women with SLE, the risk of myocardial infarction is increased 50-fold.

- The prior use of systemic corticosteroids has been noted to be a risk factor for the development of scleroderma renal crisis, so steroid use should be minimized in patients with scleroderma.

This chapter focuses on several autoimmune illnesses with diverse multisystem clinical presentations. Specifically, we discuss SLE, antiphospholipid antibody syndrome (APAS), progressive systemic sclerosis (scleroderma), Sjögren's syndrome, and the idiopathic physicians and practitioners in many medical subspecialties. Because early diagnosis and treatment can be lifesaving in the management of these conditions, prompt referral to a rheumatologist should be considered when any of these conditions is suspected.

The clinical history and physical examination are the primary stimuli for diagnosing these complex disorders, which are frequently misdiagnosed. Laboratory work, including specialized serologic tests such as antinuclear antibodies (ANAs), acute phase reactants, and complement, are rarely diagnostic; rather, in most instances, serologies add support to a working diagnosis and provide some information about disease activity.

SYSTEMIC LUPUS ERYTHEMATOSUS

SLE is a complex autoimmune inflammatory disease characterized by the development of a variety of autoantibodies that result in clinical manifestations that can affect multiple organ systems. The multisystem manifestations can potentially result in serious morbidity or even mortality, and the disease presentation and course can be quite variable. Approximately 250,000 people in the United States have SLE, with a prevalence of 30 to 50 per 100,000, and most are women in their childbearing years. The prevalence of the disease ranges from 40 per 100,000 persons in a Northern European population to more than 200 per 100,000 among blacks. Both sexes are affected, although the female-to-male ratio is approximately 8 to 1 during the reproductive years (between ages 15 and 40 years); the ratio normalizes somewhat to 2 to 1 in the older and younger age groups. SLE is characterized by a course of exacerbations and remissions with manifestations, including rashes, arthritis, cytopenias, serositis, nephritis, and neuropsychiatric symptoms.

With current treatment, the life expectancy has improved over the past 50 years from a 50% 4-year survival to the current 15-year survival of 80%. The improvement in SLE survival can be attributed to multiple factors, including treatment with glucocorticoids, mycophenolate mofetil (MMF) and cyclophosphamide, renal dialysis, more effective antihypertensive regimens, improved antibiotic treatments, and early diagnosis. In early disease, morbidity and mortality is attributable to complications of the disease itself, such as renal disease, or to complications of treatment, such as infection. Later in the course of disease, morbidity and mortality are related to cardiovascular disease, osteoporosis, and malignancy.

The pathogenesis of SLE is complex and involves a combination of genetic, environmental, and hormonal factors. Autoantibodies are antibodies that bind to normal constituents. As early as 1967, it was noted that renal pathology from patients with lupus nephritis contained antibodies that bind to native double-stranded DNA. These antibodies to double-stranded DNA are highly specific for SLE because they are present in 70% of patients with SLE and only 0.5% of healthy individuals or patients with other autoimmune diseases. The source of the autoantigens stimulating the production of antibodies in patients with SLE may be apoptotic cells. Patients with lupus exhibit defects in apoptotic cell clearance.

A role for genetics in determining the risk for SLE is suggested by data taken from studies of twins, in which a slightly higher degree of concordance for lupus is observed among monozygotic twins (25%–30%) when compared with dizygotic twins (5%). Furthermore, first-degree relatives of patients with SLE are at a higher risk of developing SLE themselves. A first-degree relative of a patient with SLE is also at higher risk for developing other autoimmune diseases such as rheumatoid arthritis, Sjögren's syndrome, and Hashimoto's thyroiditis.

The role of sex hormones has long been implicated, based on the observation that SLE is more common in women compared with men. The imbalance between the sexes is greatest during the reproductive years, suggesting that estrogen may play some permissive role in the genesis of autoimmunity supported by strong data obtained from animal models in lupus. Environmental triggers also play a role, based on the observation that ultraviolet light can trigger an exacerbation of cutaneous lupus and systemic flares in some individuals. In addition, certain medications cause drug-induced lupus syndromes. Among these are procainamide, hydralazine, isoniazid, methyldopa, chlorpromazine, quinidine, and the anti–tumor necrosis factor agents. The features associated with drug-induced lupus generally remit, however, once the offending agent is removed.

Manifestations of Systemic Lupus Erythematous

SLE can affect virtually any organ system in the body, and the presentation can vary considerably from patient to patient. This can make accurate diagnosis of the patient with SLE a challenge. The American College of Rheumatology has established 11 features of SLE to assist in the identification of patients. A patient is said to have a high likelihood of having SLE if that person exhibits 4 of the 11 features, which include:

- Malar rash
- Discoid rash
- Photosensitivity
- Oral ulcers
- Serositis
- Arthritis
- Renal involvement

- Neurologic involvement
- Hematologic abnormalities
- Positive ANAs
- Evidence of immunologic dysfunction as revealed by false-positive VDRL (Venereal Disease Research Laboratory) test, positive anti–double-stranded DNA antibody, positive anti-Sm (Smith) antibody, or presence of an antiphospholipid antibody

However, patients may have SLE with less than 4 of these 11 features because they may present with early disease in two organ systems and supportive serologies, and develop additional features as the disease progresses. For example, a patient presenting with glomerulonephritis, positive Sm antibodies, and pleuritis as presenting symptoms would clearly require treatment for SLE without waiting for a fourth feature.

The cutaneous manifestations of lupus can be divided into lupus-specific rashes and non–lupus-specific rashes. The lupus-specific rashes include acute cutaneous lupus (malar rash), subacute cutaneous lupus erythematosus, and discoid lupus erythematous. Acute lupus erythematosus presents as a photosensitive malar rash, with erythema over the malar eminences, bridging the nose and sparing the nasolabial folds. Other sun-exposed areas of the face, such as the forehead and chin, may be involved. The lesions are frequently raised due to cutaneous edema. It typically occurs in the setting of a systemic flare of disease and heals without scarring. About 50% of patients with lupus experience a malar rash as part of their syndrome. The rash must be distinguished from other causes of facial erythema, such as rosacea, dermatomyositis, contact dermatitis, seborrheic dermatitis, polymorphous light eruption, and cutaneous sarcoid. Discoid lesions are generally circular, erythematous plaques, with hyperkeratotic scaling, follicular plugging, and an area of central epidermal atrophy. These lesions tend to affect the scalp, face, arms, and upper trunk, and be more chronic. Discoid lupus usually exists by itself in the absence of other systemic features, although 10% of patients with discoid lupus will eventually develop SLE. The discoid lesions tend to heal with scarring. Subacute cutaneous lupus is another photosensitive rash, which might appear as a papulosquamous eruption, psoriasiform eruption, or annular or polycyclic rash, with a predilection for the face, upper trunk, and arms, and usually heals without scarring. Many, but not all, patients with subacute cutaneous lupus harbor antibodies to SSA (Ro) and tend not to have antibodies to double-stranded DNA, Smith, and ribonucleoprotein (RNP).

Many other dermatologic conditions, which are not specific for lupus, may be seen in the patient with lupus. These include livedo reticularis, bullous skin disease, panniculitis, oral ulcers, alopecia, urticaria, purpura, Raynaud's phenomenon, and digital ulcerations.

The musculoskeletal features of lupus include arthralgias, which affect the majority of patients. A subset of patients will experience true arthritis, with joint swelling, synovitis detected by the examining health care worker, and even deformities in the small joints of the hands. The hand deformities of long-standing lupus may have the appearance of those seen in rheumatoid arthritis, with MCP subluxation and swan neck deformities of the fingers. Unlike rheumatoid arthritis, these deformities are generally reducible, and bony erosions on radiographs are unusual in lupus. Avascular necrosis (AVN), particularly of the humeral head, femoral head, tibial plateau, and ankle, occurs in 5% to 10% of patients. Corticosteroid therapy contributes to most cases of AVN, but others may be due to antiphospholipid antibodies, fat emboli, and vasculitis. Pain localized to a single joint with a fairly acute onset, especially in the absence of signs of synovitis disease, should raise concern for AVN. Although a unilateral presentation is typical, AVN is frequently detectable in the contralateral joint by plain radiography or MRI.

Inflammatory muscle disease occurs in 5% to 10% of patients, usually presenting with proximal muscle weakness with an elevated creatine phosphokinase (CPK). Electromyogram (EMG) results vary from being normal to revealing the typical changes of myositis, including spontaneous fibrillations and short-amplitude, polyphasic, short-duration potentials. In the patient with an established diagnosis of lupus, a muscle biopsy is generally unnecessary. Drug-induced myopathy.0 (especially from statins, corticosteroids, or antimalarials) should be considered as an alternative cause of proximal muscle weakness.

About 30% to 40% of patients with lupus develop secondary fibromyalgia during the course of their illness. Features of fibromyalgia syndrome, including fatigue, diffuse myalgias ("pain all over"), and morning stiffness, must be differentiated from symptoms related to lupus. A careful examination of joints (absence of synovial thickening or joint effusions in fibromyalgia) and muscle strength (generally effort related in fibromyalgia, as opposed to proximal weakness in the patient with lupus myositis or steroid myopathy) will help distinguish lupus symptoms from fibromyalgia symptoms. Lab work (erythrocyte sedimentation rate [ESR], dsDNA Ab, and complement levels) may help distinguish symptoms of active lupus from symptoms of active fibromyalgia.

The identification of renal involvement from lupus is especially important because renal disease is a major predictor of morbidity and mortality. The World Health Organization (WHO) has established six classifications of lupus nephritis based on the histopathology of renal biopsy sections as follows:

- WHO IA: normal by all microscopic techniques
- WHO IB: normal by light microscopy with immune complex deposition demonstrated by electron microscopy or immunofluorescence
- WHO II: mesangial disease
- WHO IIIA: focal segmental glomerulonephritis (GN)

- WHO IIIB: focal proliferative GN
- WHO IV: diffuse proliferative GN
- WHO V: membranous GN
- WHO VI: advanced sclerosing nephropathy

Most patients who develop end-stage renal disease requiring dialysis have WHO class III or IV histology, and it is important to identify these patients early and consider the aggressive management of their disease to prevent end-stage renal disease. The International Society of Nephrology/Renal Pathology Society has classified lupus GN. This classification divides diffuse GN into diffuse segmental (IV-S) and diffuse global (IV-G), but the International Society of Nephrology/Renal Pathology Society does not detect pathological or clinical differences among patients with severe lupus glomerulonephritis.

More recently, EULAR (EUropean League Against Rheumatism) has published recommendations (7/07) for the prognosis, diagnosis, monitoring, and treatment of SLE. In patients with proliferative lupus nephritis, glucocorticoids in combination with immunosuppressive agents have been found to limit the progression to end-stage renal disease. Although only cyclophosphamide-based regimens have proven long-term efficacy, other treatment options have been evaluated as a means to avoid the significant long-term toxicities of cyclophosphamide. Mycophenylate Mofetil (MMF) has been shown in short- and medium-term trials to be at least as effective as pulse cyclophosphamide, with a more favorable toxicity profile. Because lupus nephritis frequently flares after remission, close follow-up is recommended with evaluation of the urine sediment, renal function, proteinuria, C3, C4, and dsDNA Ab.

Most patients with WHO class II (mesangial) disease do not require specific treatment of their renal lesion. The optimal strategy for treatment of WHO class V (membranous) disease has not been established. In the patient with WHO class VI, advanced glomerulosclerosis, the risks of immunosuppressive treatment generally outweigh the benefits.

Most patients with lupus exhibit renal involvement on renal biopsies. The 2007 EULAR Task Force for Systemic Lupus Erythematosus treatment recommends that although renal biopsy, urine sediment analysis, and testing for proteinuria and kidney function may independently predict clinical outcome of lupus nephritis treatment, these should be interpreted together. Changes in immunologic tests are limited in their ability to predict response to treatment and should be used only as supplemental information.

Because the treatment of lupus nephritis may be associated with significant side effects, it is desirable to limit the use of these regimens to patients who are likely to benefit from treatment. Recognizing that reversibility is an important factor, the biopsy specimens can be graded according to their "activity" and "chronicity" features. Activity features include those abnormalities that would be expected to be reversible with immunosuppressive therapy, such as

glomerular tuft proliferation, interstitial infiltration, leukocyte infiltrates throughout the glomerulus, cellular crescent formation, karyorrhexis and fibrinoid necrosis, and hyaline thrombi. Other features, such as fibrous crescents, interstitial fibrosis, tubular atrophy, and glomerulosclerosis, are included among the chronicity features that would not be expected to be reversible with treatment and, therefore, portend a poor outcome.

In assessing the patient with possible lupus nephritis, it should be noted that standard office urinalysis is superior to assessment of the blood urea nitrogen (BUN) levels, creatinine levels, or 24-hour protein collection to detect the presence of underlying renal disease. An active sediment is defined by the presence of red blood cell casts or hematuria or pyuria in the absence of infection. The finding of an active sediment should prompt aggressive investigation into the nature of the patient's renal status, including consideration of kidney biopsy.

Other renal manifestations of lupus include interstitial nephritis and renal vein thrombosis. Interstitial nephritis may be associated with tubular dysfunction and acute renal failure. Renal vein thrombosis may occur in the setting of nephrotic syndrome or APAS.

The cardiac manifestations of lupus include pericardial, myocardial, valvular disease, and accelerated atherosclerosis. Pericardial disease is a common early cardiac manifestation, and can range from asymptomatic pericardial rubs, thickening observed in echocardiograms, to acute chest pain syndromes and tamponade. Echocardiographic studies reveal pericardial abnormalities in 11% to 54% of SLE patients.

Libman-Sacks endocarditis is a verrucous nonbacterial endocarditis. The vegetations of various sizes usually form on the ventricular undersurface of the posterior leaflet of the mitral valve, but can extend to the ventricular mural endocardium. The mitral valve is most often affected, but the lesions can occur on any valve. Histologically, proliferating endothelial cells and myocytes are seen, with scattered mononuclear cells and variable degrees of necrosis. Neutrophils are conspicuously absent; their presence raises the question of infectious endocarditis. Libman-Sacks lesions may be too small to be detected in transthoracic echocardiography. Rare complications of valvular disease include embolic phenomena and valvular stenosis or insufficiency.

Myocarditis occurs in patients with SLE, but myocardial dysfunction may also result from accelerated atherosclerosis, renal insufficiency, hypertension, valvular heart disease, or medication toxicity (e.g., hydroxychloroquine).

Coronary artery disease (CAD) is a leading cause of premature death in SLE. In young women with SLE, the risk of myocardial infarction is increased 50-fold. Various mechanisms may be involved in the development of CAD in SLE, including atherosclerosis, coronary arteritis, thrombosis with or without antiphospholipid antibody, corticosteroids, vasospasm, embolization, and hypertension. The role of traditional coronary risk factors such as hypertension, hyperlipidemia, or chronically elevated levels of homocystine may also play a role. However, traditional risk factors do not provide a complete explanation because after adjusting for baseline CAD risk factors (Framingham risk factor estimate), patients with SLE had a 7- to 10-fold increased risk of CAD and stroke with a relative risk of 17 for fatal CAD. At present, recommendations include aggressively minimizing traditional risk factors, such as hypertension and dyslipidemias, that may contribute to atherosclerosis. In addition, because the cumulative dosage and length of glucocorticoid therapy can contribute to the development of atherosclerotic plaque, minimizing steroid exposure may play a role.

The pulmonary manifestations of lupus include alveolar hemorrhage syndrome, which may be heralded by rapidly progressive respiratory insufficiency, associated with declining hemoglobin, diffuse alveolar infiltrates on chest radiograph, and increased $D_L CO$ on pulmonary function tests. Hemoptysis may be present in only half of affected patients. This potentially catastrophic event may occur despite ongoing immunosuppression, raising concerns of infection. Acute lupus pneumonitis presents with dyspnea, alveolar infiltrates on chest radiograph, and, frequently, fever. Pulmonary hypertension and pulmonary embolism may occur in lupus, especially in association with APAS. *Shrinking lung syndrome* is a poorly defined and rare syndrome characterized by dyspnea with diaphragmatic muscle weakness without a true intrinsic pathology of the lungs.

The hematologic manifestations of lupus include leukopenia ($<4,000$ white blood cells/cm^3), lymphopenia ($<1,500$ lymphocytes/cm^3), thrombocytopenia, and anemia. Although Coombs' positive hemolytic anemia occurs, it is far more common for the patient with lupus to have anemia of chronic disease. Chronic use of nonsteroidal therapy can cause iron-deficiency anemia through occult gastrointestinal blood loss. Finally, many patients with lupus are functionally hyposplenic, and consideration of a prophylactic Pneumovax inoculation is appropriate in this patient group.

The neurologic and psychiatric manifestations of lupus are protean (Table 30.1). These include severe catastrophic events such as transverse myelitis, seizures, and stroke, as well as less morbid events such as cranial neuropathy or peripheral neuropathy. Depression is frequently found in lupus patients. A more subtle cognitive abnormality or organic brain syndrome may be seen. Psychosis may occur, sometimes exacerbated by high-dose corticosteroids. Cerebral infarcts and transverse myelitis may result from bland vasculopathy or thrombosis. Less commonly, emboli, hemorrhage, or true small-vessel vasculitis can cause ischemic injury. Possible nonlupus etiologies for these neuropsychiatric manifestations, such as infection or medication-related effects, should be considered. For example, changes in cognitive functioning may be a result of neuropsychiatric lupus, but may also occur in the setting of infection

TABLE 30.1

NEUROLOGIC AND PSYCHIATRIC MANIFESTATIONS OF SYSTEMIC LUPUS ERYTHMATOUS

Central
- Stroke
- Seizures
- Transverse myelitis
- Headache
- Psychosis
- Aseptic meningitis
- Organic brain syndrome
- Demyelinating disease
- Others

Peripheral
- Mononeuritis multiplex
- Acute inflammatory demyelinating polyneuropathy
- Plexopathy
- Others

(central nervous system [CNS] or systemic), electrolyte disturbances, uremia, medication side effects (especially from nonsteroidal anti-inflammatory drugs [NSAIDs], steroids), or primary psychiatric diseases.

Imaging techniques such as CT scanning and MRI can help exclude space-occupying lesions and infarcts, and MRI is superior in assessing acute ischemic injury, such as recent stroke or transverse myelitis. The presence of antiphospholipid antibodies and lupus anticoagulant should be sought in the patient with stroke syndromes, transverse myelitis, or multi-infarct dementia.

Serologic abnormalities are the hallmark of systemic lupus, the most prevalent abnormality being a positive ANA test. The ANA is present in 97% to 100% of patients with lupus. Although ANA is a very sensitive test for detecting patients with lupus, it is lacking in specificity because ANA is found in many other disease states. Positive ANAs are seen in other autoimmune diseases, such as rheumatoid arthritis, Sjögren's syndrome, polymyositis and dermatomyositis, scleroderma, Graves' disease, Hashimoto's thyroiditis, primary biliary cirrhosis, and chronic active hepatitis. Patients with hematologic malignancies may demonstrate a positive ANA. Some patients with certain neurologic disorders, such as myasthenia gravis and multiple sclerosis, exhibit positive ANAs. Relatives of patients with autoimmune disease will not uncommonly demonstrate a positive ANA. Patients exposed to certain drugs, such as procainamide, may develop an asymptomatic positive ANA (or evolve to symptomatic drug-induced lupus). Furthermore, otherwise healthy individuals with no apparent risk factors for developing a positive ANA may have a positive ANA with a prevalence of roughly 5% to 7%, and prevalence increases with age.

Anti–double-stranded DNA antibodies are relatively specific for lupus, especially if they are found in high titer. Anti–single-stranded DNA antibodies are found in both normal controls and lupus patients, and have no diagnostic utility. Of the "extractable nuclear antigens," the presence of antibodies to Smith antigen (Sm) have the greatest specificity for lupus, but the sensitivity of only 30% to 40% hampers their clinical utility when trying to make a diagnosis. The autoantibodies to SSA, SSB, and RNP are seen in a number of autoimmune diseases and are not specific for lupus. The ANA and antibodies to Smith, RNP, SSA, and SSB do not change reliably with disease activity, and longitudinal monitoring is not indicated. The presence of anti-SSA is associated with some SLE clinical subtypes, including patients with subacute cutaneous lupus erythematosus and patients with complement deficiency. Women who have antibodies to SSA or SSB are at increased risk for having a child affected by the congenital or neonatal lupus syndrome, characterized by transient neutropenia, transient skin rash, and complete heart block, which is permanent and requires the insertion of a pacemaker.

Other laboratory studies that may be useful in assessing the patient with lupus include complement levels, particularly C3 and C4. In some, but not all, patients with lupus, the C3 and C4 levels will fall at the time of a flare and return to normal during disease quiescence. Hence, complement levels can help follow disease activity. Another biomarker with clinical utility in following disease activity is the dsDNA Ab because the rise in anti-DNA levels may portend an impending flare, and as the flare resolves, the anti-DNA levels fall again toward their baseline range. Not all lupus patients, however, demonstrate anti–double-stranded DNA antibodies. The ANA, in contrast, does not change significantly between periods of disease activity and quiescence, and repeated measures of the ANA are not indicated in the follow-up of the patient with well-established disease. Acute phase reactants such as ESR and C-reactive protein (CRP) are nonspecific because they may rise with infection, flare of disease, or even malignancy. They may be of use in those patients in whom elevations have been previously correlated with illness or flare, although there may be discordance of the ESR and CRP with flare. These tests may have greatest utility in the management of an individual patient in whom prior flare characteristics (lab profile, etc.) are known.

Treatment of Lupus

The treatment of lupus includes both nonpharmacologic and pharmacologic therapy. Adjunct therapy may include photoprotection with sunscreens and clothing; lifestyle modification with smoking cessation, weight control, and exercise; and other agents such as low-dose ASA, calcium with vitamin D, antiosteoporosis medications, statins, and antihypertensives.

Vigilance for comorbidities in SLE patients is paramount, including infections, atherosclerosis, hypertension, dyslipidemias, diabetes, osteoporosis, avascular necrosis, and malignancy. Appropriate prophylaxis for infections may include influenza vaccine, PCP prophylaxis, and hepatitis and pneumococcal vaccines.

Simple analgesic and low-dose nonsteroidals can be helpful in patients with arthralgias and mild arthritis. Patients with lupus can develop impaired renal function with NSAID therapy and may manifest aseptic meningitis on exposure to ibuprofen and other NSAIDs, although this complication is rare. Hydroxychloroquine (Plaquenil) is a useful agent for the management of the constitutional symptoms, fatigue, dermatologic manifestations, and articular manifestations of the disease. Although it is not indicated as first-line therapy for major organ involvement, data suggest that hydroxychloroquine may help prevent major organ flares in patients who continue to take the drug on a long-term basis.

High-dose glucocorticoids are reserved for serious organ-threatening or life-threatening complications, such as severe hematologic dyscrasias, renal involvement, neurologic involvement, and some cases of refractory serositis. Because of the numerous side effects of long-term steroid use, the minimal effective dose should be used to control the disease process. Methotrexate can be a useful adjunct to treatment of arthritis and myositis, but patients must be closely watched for renal insufficiency because methotrexate is cleared via renal excretion. Cyclophosphamide is reserved for major organ-threatening or life-threatening flares, particularly affecting the CNS or kidneys. The side effects of cyclophosphamide include marrow suppression, hemorrhagic cystitis, stomatitis, hair loss, nausea, vomiting, and increased risk of eventually developing lymphoma, leukemia, and bladder cancer. MMF may be an appropriate alternative to cyclophosphamide in the treatment of lupus nephritis, with less infections or ovarian failure associated with its use. Some patients are treated with short courses of cyclophosphamide for induction therapy for nephritis and are then transitioned to MMF or azathioprine. Newer regimens employing rituximab are also being investigated. For SLE patients with end-stage renal disease, dialysis and transplantation have rates of patient and graft survival that are similar to those observed without diabetes or SLE.

Patients with SLE and neuropsychiatric manifestations believed to be inflammatory in origin, such as optic neuritis, acute confusional state, coma, cranial or peripheral neuropathy, psychosis, or transverse myelitis or myelopathy, may benefit from immunosuppressive treatment after infections have been excluded.

In patients with SLE and antiphospholipid antibodies, low-dose aspirin may be useful in the primary prevention of thrombosis and pregnancy loss. Long-term anticoagulation is effective for secondary prevention of thrombosis in nonpregnant patients with SLE- and APAS-associated thrombosis. Low molecular weight or unfractionated heparin and ASA may reduce the incidence of pregnancy loss in patients with SLE and APAS.

Female patients with SLE do not have lower fertility rates, but pregnancy may increase the risk for flares of the disease.

In patients with lupus nephritis and APAS, there is a higher risk of eclampsia. Women with lupus have a higher risk of miscarriage, stillbirth, prematurity, intrauterine growth restriction, and fetal heart block. Some medications, including MMF, cyclophosphamide, and methotrexate, are contraindicated during pregnancy.

Systemic Lupus versus Drug-Induced Lupus

Drug-induced lupus is a syndrome of lupus-like illness associated with the ingestion of certain medications. The syndrome has been well described with procainamide use and numerous other drugs, including hydralazine, α-methyldopa, isoniazid, quinidine, chlorpropamide, minocycline, and others. Clinical manifestations may include fever, malaise, arthralgias, pleurisy, pericarditis, rashes, and cytopenias. It is unusual to see hypocomplementemia, renal disease, or CNS disease in drug-induced lupus. Positive ANA is required for the firm diagnosis. Antibodies to histone H2b are well described in procainamide-induced lupus; however, antibodies to histone also occur in the majority of systemic lupus patients and therefore do not have a discriminatory value. Anti–double-stranded DNA antibodies are generally not found in drug-induced lupus. The treatment of drug-induced lupus requires recognition of the syndrome and the discontinuation of the offending drug. Most symptoms will resolve with removal of the drug.

ANTIPHOSPHOLIPID ANTIBODY SYNDROME

APAS is a syndrome characterized by recurrent arterial and/or venous thromboses, recurrent fetal loss, and thrombocytopenia in association with sustained elevated titers of antiphospholipid antibodies. The term *antiphospholipid antibodies* actually encompasses a family of antibodies that have in common their in vitro binding to phospholipid or protein-phospholipid complexes. Phospholipids include such molecules as phosphatidylinositol, phosphatidylserine, phosphatidylglycerol, phosphatidylcholine, cardiolipin, and other entities. Some antiphospholipid antibodies are functionally characterized as *lupus anticoagulants*, a doubly troublesome term because the antibodies are not confined to the lupus patient population and are associated with a hypercoagulable state. Historically, however, they were identified because of their ability to induce a prolongation of phospholipid-dependent coagulation assays, including the activated partial thromboplastin time (aPTT), kaolin clot time, dilute Russell viper venom time, and other tests of coagulation that are phospholipid dependent. Refinement of antibody detection techniques led to enzyme-linked immunoabsorbent assays (ELISAs) for specific antibodies to cardiolipin and β-2-glycoprotein-I (β_2GP-I). β_2GP-I is a naturally occurring circulating anticoagulant that has affinity for anionic phospholipids; some investigators believe that antibodies to β_2GP-I are the most pathogenic for APAS. No single assay has 100% sensitivity for APAS, however, and specificity varies as well. Furthermore, evidence is emerging that other members of the coagulation cascade (protein C, protein S, prothrombin, etc.) may be antigenic targets in some patients with APAS.

A recent session of the International Symposium on Antiphospholipid Antibodies recommended that initial testing consist of a lupus anticoagulant assay (usually the aPTT) plus an anticardiolipin ELISA. If these tests are negative or equivocal, then further testing with other coagulation tests (i.e., DRVVT), β_2GP-I ELISA, or assays for other phospholipids can be pursued. When checking the anticardiolipin antibody assay, results are reported in terms of immunoglobulin (Ig) M, IgG, and sometimes IgA units. Clinically, the manifestations of primary or secondary APAS correlate best with moderate to high levels of IgG anticardiolipin antibodies. The significance of IgM or IgA anticardiolipin antibodies is less clear.

The APAS is divided into primary and secondary forms, the latter occurring in patients with systemic lupus. Clinically, the frequencies of thrombotic events, thrombocytopenia, and fetal loss are similar between the two groups. Other less common manifestations of APAS include seizures, Coombs' positive hemolytic anemia, transverse myelitis, pulmonary hypertension, and aortic insufficiency. Livedo reticularis, a blotchy violaceous discoloration of the legs, is not uncommonly seen in this disorder, but may also be seen in patients with cholesterol emboli syndrome and polyarteritis nodosa.

Antiphospholipid antibodies are present in a number of different patient populations, including patients with HIV infection (50%-75%), patients with other autoimmune diseases (rheumatoid arthritis, Sjögren's syndrome, inflammatory myopathy), patients with chronic infectious (syphilis, leishmaniasis, leptospirosis, others), patients taking medications known to cause a drug-induced lupus illness, and even in healthy controls. Patients with drug-induced antiphospholipid antibodies generally do not have clinical manifestations of APAS.

Because this syndrome has only been recognized for 20 years, much is yet to be learned regarding "best treatments" for specific clinical scenarios. Asymptomatic patients who are detected to have antiphospholipid antibody on incidental laboratory evaluation (e.g., preoperative testing reveals an elevated aPTT that fails to correct with mixing and normalizes with the addition of excess phospholipid, thus identifying a lupus anticoagulant) should be placed on daily low-dose (81 mg) aspirin indefinitely, unless contraindications (e.g., allergy) exist, in which case the patient should simply be observed. In the immediate perioperative period, prophylactic heparin can be used instead of aspirin. The recommendation of chronic low-dose aspirin is also offered to the asymptomatic pregnant woman who is known to be anticardiolipin antibody positive. If that patient has an obstetric history suggestive of APAS (prior miscarriage, especially if more than one and especially if occurring at a time other than the first trimester), then treatment may also include low-dose subcutaneous heparin along with low-dose aspirin for the duration of the pregnancy. In persons who have had a clinical event such as a deep vein thrombosis or an arterial thrombosis, full anticoagulation should be employed.

Catastrophic APAS is manifested by widespread thromboses developing rapidly in multiple organ systems, and it is associated with a high mortality rate. The onset is typically abrupt, generally becoming manifest in less than 1 week. No standardized protocols for treatment exist, but aggressive management with steroids, full anticoagulation, and plasmapheresis has been employed.

SCLERODERMA (PROGRESSIVE SYSTEMIC SCLEROSIS)

Scleroderma is a rare disorder, striking 2 to 10 persons per million per year. The female-to-male ratio is less striking than that of lupus, at only 3:1. The onset of disease is generally between ages 30 and 50 years and is typically heralded by Raynaud's phenomenon, with the later development of sclerodactyly and skin thickening and fibrosis over the hands, arms, legs, face, and trunk. As the skin thickening progresses, range of motion is lost in the underlying joints, with secondary muscle atrophy and weakness. Late complications of the musculoskeletal disease include joint contractures, muscle atrophy, and skin ulceration over the contracted joints. Internal organ involvement is common, including pulmonary complications of interstitial lung disease, cardiac arrhythmias due to microscopic areas of ischemia, rapidly progressive renal failure, and gastrointestinal complications of esophageal dysmotility and gut hypomotility.

Limited scleroderma, including CREST (Calcinosis cutis, Raynaud's phenomenon, Esophageal dysmotility, Sclerodactyly, Telangiectasia) syndrome, is characterized by more restricted cutaneous disease, with skin thickening progressing no more proximally than the elbows and knees, but still occurring on the face. Renal involvement and pulmonary fibrosis are much less common in CREST syndrome when compared to diffuse scleroderma. However, patients with CREST must be monitored closely because pulmonary hypertension is more likely. The characteristic autoantibody association is with anticentromere antibody, present in 95% of patients with CREST. In diffuse scleroderma, antibodies to topoisomerase I (anti-Scl-70) are found in about 70% of patients.

The pathogenesis of scleroderma is unclear. It is known that fibroblasts taken from the skin of scleroderma patients continue to produce excessive amounts of type I collagen, the major collagen component of skin, even after several passages in tissue culture. T cells in patients with scleroderma release cytokines such as transforming growth factor-α (TGFα) and interleukin-2 (IL-2) that stimulate fibroblast activity. A role for vascular abnormalities is suggested by the observations that (a) the earliest fibrosis of the skin is seen in perivascular areas; and (b) Raynaud's phenomenon, a vasospastic event, is present at the outset in 95% of patients with scleroderma. Later in the disease, obliteration of the vessel lumen and a net loss of the capillary bed in the affected tissue occur.

Although the cutaneous disease is certainly disabling, the predictor to long-term survival in scleroderma and CREST is the course of major organ involvement. For many years, renal disease was the major determinant of survival, with the majority of early (<2 years) deaths attributable to scleroderma renal crisis. Scleroderma renal crisis is a form of rapidly progressive renal insufficiency that can affect patients with diffuse scleroderma. It tends to occur within the first 4 years of illness, and patients who have rapidly progressive cutaneous disease are at higher risk. The complication is heralded by the sudden onset of severe hypertension, although in 10% of patients with scleroderma renal crisis, the blood pressure can remain in the normal range. A microangiopathic hemolytic anemia and thrombocytopenia in the setting of rising BUN and creatinine levels is the classic clinical picture. The urinalysis is typically bland, with minimal proteinuria and microscopic hematuria; casts are rarely observed. The prior use of systemic corticosteroids has been noted to be a risk factor for the development of scleroderma renal crisis, so steroid use should be minimized in patients with scleroderma. Scleroderma renal crisis was the major cause of mortality in scleroderma until the early 1980s, when angiotensin-converting enzyme (ACE) inhibitors became available. The prompt initiation of ACE inhibitors at the diagnosis of renal crisis is associated with a dramatically enhanced renal and patient survival (<15% at 1 year without ACE inhibitors, 76% at 1 year with ACE inhibitors). Scleroderma renal crisis rarely recurs. Even with appropriate therapy, however, some patients, particularly those who are older than 55 years or present with congestive heart failure (CHF), may still have a poor outcome (permanent dialysis or death).

Cardiac disease in scleroderma arises from microscopic areas of reversible ischemia that may cause the pathological finding of contraction band necrosis. This manifestation can predispose patients to aberrant or delayed conduction, re-entrant arrhythmias, and CHF.

Pulmonary disease has emerged as the major cause of mortality since scleroderma renal crisis has become more manageable. Interstitial inflammation or alveolitis may start early in the disease and lead to interstitial fibrosis with impairment in oxygen transfer and restrictive lung physiology. Pulmonary function testing with $D_L CO$, high-resolution CT scanning, and bronchoalveolar lavage help establish the diagnosis.

Almost the entire gastrointestinal tract is at risk for involvement from scleroderma. Xerostomia is common because many patients have secondary Sjögren's syndrome. Esophageal dysmotility is a prominent feature of diffuse scleroderma and CREST, and it results in reflux esophagitis, esophageal stricture, Barrett's esophagus, or esophageal cancer. Gastric dysmotility is less common but can result in early satiety. Small bowel involvement, from atrophy of smooth muscle fibers, leads to hypomotility, bacterial overgrowth, dilatation, and pseudo-obstruction. Malabsorption and failure to thrive may result from the bacterial overgrowth. Large-mouth diverticula are found at the small or large bowel. Pneumatosis cystoides intestinalis is an unusual complication of scleroderma characterized by multiple air-filled blebs infiltrating the wall of the colon. These are asymptomatic unless rupture occurs, which usually leads to peritonitis.

Treatment for Scleroderma

At present, the treatment of scleroderma is directed toward individual disease manifestations because an effective treatment for the fibroproliferative process has not been established. Raynaud's phenomenon is managed using calcium channel blockers, occasionally α-1-blockers, prostanoids, endothelin antagonists, topical nitrates, or, in severe refractory cases, digital sympathectomy. ACE inhibitors, as mentioned, are organ saving and lifesaving in the treatment of scleroderma renal crisis.

Recent data from the scleroderma lung study did not show benefit with the treatment of patients with scleroderma pulmonary disease using cyclophosphamide.

Treatment regimens for pulmonary hypertension for patients with CREST or generalized scleroderma are similar to those recommended for other causes of pulmonary hypertension. The endothelin-1 antagonist bosentan is approved for the treatment of pulmonary hypertension and has proven efficacious in patients with scleroderma and CREST having this complication.

The gastroesophageal manifestations respond to typical agents for reflux and acid control, and pump inhibitors may be useful. Metoclopramide may be helpful in increasing lower esophageal tone and promoting gastric emptying. Erythromycin may be used as a promotility agent, and rotating antibiotic treatment may be used for treatment of bacterial overgrowth with resultant decrease in symptoms of diarrhea, bloating, and malabsorption. For secondary Sjögren's syndrome, a trial of pilocarpine 5 mg four times a day or treatment with cyclosporine (Restasis) drops can be effective for ocular sicca.

SJÖGREN'S SYNDROME

Sjögren's syndrome is a chronic autoimmune exocrinopathy characterized by the infiltration of exocrine glands (especially salivary and lacrimal glands) by lymphocytes, leading to acinar disruption, scarring, and eventual failure of glandular function. The clinical symptoms that result include the "sicca complex" of dry mouth (xerostomia) and dry eyes (xerophthalmia), often with salivary gland (parotid and/or submandibular gland) enlargement. Patients can develop dryness of the throat (xerotrachea), dry skin, vaginal dryness, and other symptoms from exocrine gland inflammation. Sjögren's syndrome is also characterized by dysregulated B-cell function, with autoantibody production, hypergammaglobulinemia, and increased risk of developing non-Hodgkin B-cell lymphoma.

Sjögren's syndrome is classified as being primary if it is not associated with any other autoimmune disease. Secondary Sjögren's syndrome is frequent, and often unappreciated, in patients with lupus, rheumatoid arthritis, scleroderma, and inflammatory myopathy. Primary Sjögren's syndrome may occur at any age, but the peak age of onset is between 30 and 50 years, with a female predominance (F:M = 9:1).

The extraglandular involvement of primary Sjögren's syndrome reflects the systemic nature of this autoimmune disease. Pulmonary involvement includes interstitial lung disease, alveolitis, xerotrachea, and pseudolymphoma. The gastrointestinal associations include biliary cirrhosis, subclinical pancreatitis, and atrophic gastritis. Vitamin deficiencies and malabsorption may result from the gastric and pancreatic disease. Renal effects include interstitial nephritis with hyposthenuria distal renal tubular acidosis and nephrogenic diabetes insipidus. Patients frequently have arthralgias and sometimes a nonerosive arthritis. One-third experience Raynaud's phenomenon. Autoimmune thyroid disease is present in one-third of patients.

Small- and medium-size vessel vasculitis (similar to polyarteritis nodosa), with manifestations of palpable purpura, ulcerations, gangrene, mononeuritis multiplex, and mesenteric arteritis, may occur. Nervous system involvement can manifest in many ways, including aseptic meningitis, ataxia, transverse myelopathy, optic neuropathy, and stroke syndromes. Patients who experience optic neuropathy or other discrete neurologic events over time might be diagnosed with multiple sclerosis if the other features of Sjögren's are not recognized. Further confusion arises because the spinal fluid in a patient with neurologic manifestations of Sjögren's syndrome, as in SLE, can indeed exhibit evidence of local immunoglobulin synthesis, including oligoclonal bands on agarose gel electrophoresis. MRI scanning in these patients reveals discrete white matter lesions best seen on T_2-weighted images.

Patients with primary Sjögren's syndrome are at a 44-fold increased risk for the development of non-Hodgkin lymphoma, particularly those with lymphadenopathy, splenomegaly, and parotid gland swelling.

The differential diagnosis of salivary gland enlargement is broad, with sicca symptoms occurring in some entities. Infectious causes of salivary gland enlargement include viruses (mumps, Epstein-Barr virus, cytomegalovirus, coxsackie A, HIV, hepatitis C, and influenza), mycobacteria (tuberculosis), fungi (histoplasmosis, actinomycosis), and bacteria (staph, strep). Acute viral and bacterial parotitis is usually painful. Infiltrative disorders, such as sarcoidosis and amyloidosis, may cause painless, gradual parotid swelling. Endocrine disorders, such as diabetes and types II, IV, and V hyperlipidemia, can cause chronic painless salivary gland enlargement with dry mouth. Malnutrition states such as alcoholism, anorexia, and bulimia can lead to salivary gland enlargement, which can develop abruptly with refeeding. Although Sjögren's syndrome may cause bilateral or unilateral salivary gland enlargement, unilateral enlargement should also raise the suspicion of a neoplasm such as lymphoma or primary salivary adenocarcinoma. Laboratories will help differentiate these disorders. In primary Sjögren's syndrome, the ANA is positive in more than 90% of affected patients. The presence of antibodies to SSA (Ro) occurs in about 80% of patients, with antibodies to SSB (La) occurring slightly less frequently at 60% to 70%. Serum protein electrophoresis often shows a diffuse hypergammaglobulinemia, but suppression of IgM levels has been described with the onset of lymphoma. Acute phase reactants are variably elevated, and rheumatoid factor is present in roughly 60%. Schirmer's testing is an objective assessment of tear production, easily performed in the office, in which strips of filter paper are inserted into the unanesthetized eye between the lower lid and the eyeball. After 5 minutes, a minimum of 5 mm of wetting should have occurred. The patient may also undergo ophthalmologic examination using topical staining of the cornea by rose Bengal stain, which allows the appreciation of corneal erosions or abrasions, frequent sequelae of chronic dry eyes. The assessment of salivary gland inflammation is performed via minor salivary gland biopsy from the inner aspect of the lower lip. Infiltration of the glands by focal aggregates of lymphocytes is supportive in establishing a diagnosis of Sjögren's syndrome. A biopsy of the major salivary glands is generally not performed unless a neoplasm is suspected. Parotid gland biopsy carries the risk of facial nerve injury.

The treatment of Sjögren's syndrome is largely symptomatic. For sicca symptomatology, education of the patient and supportive measures are usually sufficient. Patients should be encouraged to use eyedrops on a regular basis (three times a day or more) because they frequently underestimate the degree of drying of the cornea, and use lubricating ointment at bedtime. Oral moisturizers such as artificial saliva are not very palatable, and as a result, patients often suffer from the lack of saliva and its antibacterial properties, leading to rampant dental caries and loss of teeth. Close follow-up with a dental specialist is important. Sialogogues such as pilocarpine are used to stimulate salivary flow. Patients must be informed that it may take 6 weeks or more for the secretagogue action to become appreciable. Contraindications to use of pilocarpine include narrow-angle glaucoma. Hydroxychloroquine (Plaquenil) may be useful in some patients with constitutional and musculoskeletal complaints. For patients who have organ-threatening dysfunction, such as mononeuritis multiplex, CNS disease, or vasculitis, the use of steroids and/or cytotoxics is necessary. The patient with pancreatic insufficiency may benefit from pancreatic enzyme replacement. Whereas many patients carry beverages and hard candy to relieve dry mouth, they should be advised to use sugarless products that do not promote tooth decay.

IDIOPATHIC INFLAMMATORY MYOPATHIES

The idiopathic inflammatory myopathies include seven disorders:

- Polymyositis (PM)
- Dermatomyositis (DM)
- Inclusion body myositis
- Idiopathic inflammatory myopathy associated with malignancy
- Childhood PM/DM
- Amyopathic dermatomyositis
- Overlap syndromes with other collagen vascular diseases

Of these seven, polymyositis and dermatomyositis are the most commonly encountered entities in a general medicine practice, although they are uncommon illnesses with an annual incidence of 2 to 10 new cases per million persons. Mean age of onset is 45 years, and women are affected twice as often as men; however, the genders are equally affected in the pediatric population. These disorders share several clinical features, including gradually progressive proximal muscle weakness that is usually painless. Patients report the subacute onset (3-6 months) of weakness involving the proximal muscle groups such that stair climbing and arising from a squat or seated position become difficult due to hip girdle weakness. Keeping the arms raised to shave or shampoo becomes difficult. Hoarseness and nasal regurgitation reflect pharyngeal muscle involvement. In addition to the complaint of weakness, the patient with dermatomyositis has cutaneous clues to the diagnosis. Periorbital edema and heliotrope rash over the eyelids is typical of dermatomyositis. Gottron's papules, which are flat-topped whitish to violaceous nonpruritic lesions overlying the MCP and PIP joints, are pathognomonic for dermatomyositis. The rash must be distinguished from the erythematous rash that may occur in SLE, which also has a predilection for the dorsum of the hands, but appears on the dorsum of the phalanges and tends to spare the MCP and PIP areas. Vasculitic rashes and Gottron's lesions may appear, particularly on the elbows. More common in children with dermatomyositis than in adults is dystrophic calcification in the soft tissues of the extremities or trunk, a condition known as *calcinosis cutis*. Calcinosis cutis can lead to the breakdown of the overlying skin and secondary infection. Periarticular involvement leads to joint contractures.

TABLE 30.2

DIFFERENTIAL DIAGNOSIS OF INFLAMMATORY MYOPATHY

Drugs/toxins (Table 30.3)
Infection
    Bacterial, mycobacterial, fungal, viral, parasitic, treponemal
Metabolic myopathy
    Glycogen storage diseases
    Carnitine deficiency
    Carnitine palmitoyltransferase deficiency
Endocrinopathy
    Hypothyroidism
    Hyperthyroidism
    Hyperparathyroidism
    Cushing syndrome
    Vitamin D deficiency
Polymyalgia rheumatica
Sarcoidosis
Fibromyalgia
Neuromuscular disorders
    Amyotrophic lateral sclerosis, muscular dystrophy, myasthenia gravis

The *shawl sign* is an erythematous flat rash that occurs in the V of the anterior chest and neck, and drapes across the shoulder girdle posteriorly, like a shawl. Nailfold capillary abnormalities are also frequently seen in dermatomyositis, with capillary loop bushy dilatation and tortuosity. These can be seen with the unaided eye or with the use of the ophthalmoscope and a drop of immersion oil placed on the cuticle area.

The differential diagnosis of idiopathic inflammatory myopathy includes other conditions that might cause a patient to present to his or her physician complaining of "weakness." Such conditions include nonmyopathic processes such as arthritis, CHF, anemia, uremia, and neurologic problems. These are usually easily discerned through careful physical examination and basic laboratory testing. In the patient with true muscular weakness on manual resistive testing, however, one must consider a number of other causes of myopathy (Table 30.2).

The laboratory hallmark of polymyositis and dermatomyositis is a striking elevation of CPK, usually more than 1,000 or even more than 10,000 mg/dL. CPK-MB elevation is also seen, released by regenerating skeletal muscle fibers. Laboratories do not distinguish between CPK-MB of myocardial origin and regenerating skeletal muscle. Cardiac troponin-I, however, does reasonably differentiate between injury of myocardial origin from that of skeletal origin. Less sensitive and specific markers for inflammatory myopathy include aldolase, aspartate aminotransferase (AST), serum glutamic-oxaloacetic transaminase, alanine transaminase (ALT), serum glutamate pyruvate transaminase, and ESR. Aldolase is an enzyme found in the glycolytic pathway, downstream of phosphofructokinase. It is found in muscle fast-twitch fibers, as well as in liver, kidney, brain,

intestines, and fetal tissue. AST and ALT can be elevated into the several hundred range. It is helpful to keep this in mind because many multichannel chemistry batteries, such as the comprehensive metabolic panel, or chemistry screens, such as the SMA-20, do not include CPK as a routine test. In a patient who has elevations of liver function tests (AST and ALT) without an obvious hepatic source, consider checking a CPK and assessing muscle strength.

Laboratory studies more specific for inflammatory myopathy are the relatively myositis-specific autoantibodies that include the members of the antisynthetase family, anti-Jo-1, anti-PL-7, anti-PL-12, and anti-OJ. Anti-Jo-1 antibodies are found in 20% of patients with polymyositis. Other autoantibodies are seen even less frequently. These antibodies are directed against a different amino acid transfer RNA synthetase. Amino acid transfer RNA synthetases are cytoplasmic enzymes that serve as shuttles for specific amino acids in the assembly of proteins. Anti-Jo-1, for example, is directed against histidyl transfer RNA synthetase. The antisynthetase syndrome is characterized by inflammatory myopathy occurring with fever, inflammatory arthritis, interstitial lung disease, Raynaud's phenomenon, and a roughened, fissured rash on the palmar aspect of the fingers/hands (mechanic's hands).

In addition to laboratory testing, the workup of the patient with a suspected inflammatory myopathy often includes neuroelectrodiagnostic studies and muscle biopsy. EMG reveals characteristic abnormalities, including (a) insertional irritability, (b) bizarre polyphasic potentials, (c) absence of full interference pattern on muscle recruitment, and (d) normal nerve conduction studies. One side of the body is examined by EMG, and, based on the results of the test, a muscle from the contralateral side may be

TABLE 30.3

DRUGS/TOXINS ASSOCIATED WITH MYOPATHY

Amiodarone
Chloroquine
Cimetidine
Clofibrate
Colchicine
Corticosteroids
Danazol
Ethanol
Gemfibrozil
HMG-CoA reductase inhibitors
Hydralazine
Ipecac
Ketoconazole
Nicotinic acid
Penicillamine
Procainamide
Rifampin
Vincristine
Zidovudine

biopsied. On histology, the muscle tissue reveals variable degrees of mononuclear cell infiltrate. The histologic features can be patchy; hence, an open muscle biopsy is preferable to needle biopsy. In polymyositis, the lymphocytic infiltrates are present throughout the fascicles, whereas in dermatomyositis they tend to be perifascicular and associated with perifascicular muscle atrophy. A variable degree of myophagocytosis is present, as is centralization of nuclei. Some fibers appear atrophic, and the regeneration of fibers occurs. Special histochemical stains rule out metabolic myopathies, and electron microscopy helps identify inclusion body myositis and other less common entities.

The treatment of the idiopathic inflammatory myopathies starts with corticosteroids, generally prednisone, at a dose of 1 mg/kg/day taken orally in the morning. Treatment at this dose level is continued until after a substantial fall in the CPK occurs. The patient's clinical response in terms of constitutional symptoms and weakness is usually fairly rapid, but lags behind the decrease in CPK. Once a laboratory response is achieved, a very gradual tapering schedule can begin, although it should be noted that by 6 months of therapy, the dose of prednisone is still usually about half the original starting dose. This emphasizes the rather slow pace of the taper that is employed in managing this illness. A rapid taper frequently results in a recurrence of the disease state. Second-line agents, such as methotrexate or azathioprine, can be added when patients require higher doses of steroids than are acceptable. Intravenous immunoglobulin has also been used with success in cases of refractory dermatomyositis. Hydroxychloroquine can be useful for the cutaneous manifestations of dermatomyositis.

It is not uncommon to be faced with the problem of recurrence of proximal muscle weakness after several months of moderate-dose to high-dose prednisone therapy. The question arises as to whether this represents a flare in the patient's underlying disease due to steroid tapering or whether the patient has developed steroid myopathy. Steroid myopathy mimics PM/DM clinically because the proximal muscles are more affected than the distal muscles. Typically, this is a painless weakness similar to the original inflammatory myopathy. Lower extremities such as hip flexors, quadriceps, and hamstrings tend to be affected to a greater degree than the proximal muscle groups in the upper extremities. Unlike a flare of PM/DM, however, CPK and other enzyme levels are normal in steroid myopathy. A muscle biopsy (if required) generally reveals noninflammatory findings. Primarily, steroid myopathy affects type II fibers, those that are fast twitch or glycolytic in energy utilization, unlike PM/DM, which affects both type I and type II muscle fibers. However, type II atrophy may also be seen in postinflammatory states and disuse atrophy, so the finding remains nonspecific. MRI with short inversion time inversion recovery imaging is potentially useful in differentiating muscle edema (caused by active inflammation) from lipomatosis (caused by steroid therapy). If the clinical judgment is that the patient is experiencing a steroid myopathy, then the steroid taper should continue or be accelerated slightly. If, however, the clinical judgment is that the patient's new onset of weakness represents a flare of polymyositis or dermatomyositis, then treatment must be intensified, and a second-line agent must be considered.

An association between inflammatory myopathy and malignancy has been recognized for more than a century. The stronger association appears to be with dermatomyositis in patients older than 40 years of age, but a slight risk is also noted by some authors in patients with polymyositis. The type of malignancy generally reflects the expected malignancies for that patient's age and sex, although non-Hodgkin lymphoma is overrepresented in both sexes, and ovarian cancer is overrepresented in women. No consensus exists on the extent of the "malignancy workup" at time of myositis diagnosis. Certainly, the patient should have a thorough history, physical examination, and baseline laboratory assessment, with age-appropriate cancer screening (e.g., mammography) and follow-up on any abnormalities. Consideration of CT scanning of the chest, abdomen, and pelvis to evaluate the patient for the increased risk of non-Hodgkin lymphoma and ovarian cancer may be appropriate in some settings. In patients with a concurrent malignancy, a recurrence of malignancy is often associated with recurrent myositis.

REVIEW EXERCISES

QUESTIONS

1. A 28-year-old woman presents with a 3-month history of fatigue; patchy hair loss; Raynaud's phenomenon; and joint stiffness, pain, and swelling in the small joints of the hands, wrists, elbows, and knees. Your examination reveals normal vital signs, several shallow oral ulcers, frontal hair loss, and synovitis at the proximal interphalangeals, metacarpal phalangeals, and wrist joints. The most important test to obtain at this point is

a) Anti–double-stranded DNA antibodies
b) Anti–single-stranded DNA antibodies
c) Anti-Smith antibody
d) Microscopic examination of the urinalysis
e) Rheumatoid factor

Answer and Discussion
The answer is d. The finding of an abnormal nuclear antibody, suggesting glomerulonephritis, will dramatically alter therapy.

2. A 48-year-old man has been followed for gradually progressive skin thickening, which began in the hands and spread centrally to now extend to the upper arms, trunk, and face. He has been maintained on calcium channel blockers for Raynaud's phenomenon, although

his borderline low blood pressure has not allowed optimal dosing of the medicine for the vasospasm. He presents for a routine visit with increasing fatigue, some exertional shortness of breath, and a blood pressure of 160/100 mm Hg. Your first action is
a) Arrange for pulmonary function testing to be done.
b) Increase the calcium channel blocker.
c) Order complete blood count (CBC) with peripheral smear and serum creatinine, and institute treatment with an angiotensin-converting enzyme inhibitor.
d) Order CBC with peripheral smear and serum creatinine, and institute treatment with D-penicillamine.

Answer and Discussion
The answer is c. This is scleroderma renal crisis, a true medical emergency.

3. Match the medication with the appropriate side effect association, using each answer once:

Medication
1. Procainamide
2. Penicillamine
3. Pilocarpine
4. Prednisone

Side Effect
a) Avascular necrosis of the femoral head
b) Acute narrow-angle glaucoma
c) Acute-onset pleurisy, fever, and joint pain
d) Myasthenia gravis

Answer
The answer is c, d, b, and a.

4. Match the physical exam finding with the appropriate diagnosis, using each answer once.

1. Rash over dorsum of the phalanges between the metacarpal phalangeals (MCPs) and the proximal interphalangeals (PIPs)
2. Rash over the dorsum of the MCPs and PIPs
3. Tendon friction rubs over the dorsum of the hands
4. Glossitis
a) Diffuse scleroderma
b) Systemic lupus erythematous
c) Sjögren's syndrome
d) Dermatomyositis

Answer
The answer is b, d, a, and c.

5. All of the following statements are true *except*
a) Patients with Sjögren's syndrome are at increased risk for developing Hodgkin lymphoma
b) Patients with dermatomyositis are at increased risk for developing non-Hodgkin lymphoma
c) Patients with Sjögren's syndrome are at increased risk for developing non-Hodgkin lymphoma
d) Patients with lupus who have completed standard treatment for diffuse proliferative glomerulonephritis are at increased risk for developing bladder cancer

Answer
The answer is a.

6. Measures of lupus disease activity include all but
a) Anti–double-stranded DNA antibody levels
b) Antinuclear antibody levels
c) C3 (third component of complement)
d) C4 (fourth component of complement)

Answer and Discussion
The answer is b. The antinuclear antibody does not reliably fluctuate with disease activity.

CASE PRESENTATION

A 39-year-old woman presents to your office with concerns that she may have systemic lupus erythematous (SLE) because her younger sister has been recently diagnosed with the condition by another physician. Your patient describes fatigue, hair loss in the comb but no patchy "bald spots," a weight gain of 20 lb in the past 6 months, and achy joints and muscles. She feels weak and reports shortness of breath with minimal exertion (after climbing one flight of stairs). Her past medical history reveals Hashimoto's thyroiditis diagnosed 6 years ago, and she has been on thyroxine since then, although she has not had follow-up for that condition in more than a year. She also has hypercholesterolemia and takes Pravachol. Her social history reveals cigarette smoking, one pack per day, which she explains helps her defray the stress of her job (she works full time in a family-owned restaurant as the business manager, shopper, and part-time cook). The family history is notable for her father having committed suicide after a long struggle with depression. Her mother has thyroid disease and rheumatoid arthritis; her sister has recently diagnosed SLE, and her twin teenage sons are healthy, but have recently been on a brief detention from school after being caught drinking alcohol on the school premises. On review of systems, she denies Raynaud's phenomenon, hematuria, or pleurisy, but reports occasional painful mouth ulcers, dry mouth and dry eyes, trouble sleeping, and irregular and heavy menses.

Your examination reveals a blood pressure of 135/85 mm Hg and pulse regular at 90 beats/minute, afebrile. Weight is 100 kg. Skin shows mild eczema on the hands, with dry skin. The oral mucosa and hair density on the scalp both appear unremarkable. Eyes are moist, and Schirmer's testing documents 14 mm wetting OU. No enlargement of the thyroid, cervical lymph nodes, or major salivary glands is present. Chest and abdominal examinations are normal. The musculoskeletal exam reveals full strength in the distal muscle groups, but break-away testing proximally, with the patient complaining of soreness in the muscles on manual resistive testing. Tenderness is noted on palpation of the proximal interphalangeals, metacarpal phalangeals, and wrist joints, without distinct synovitis. The articular range of motion is normal throughout, with the patient remarking that the shoulders, neck, and hips feel achy during these maneuvers. The patient has tenderness to soft tissue palpation at 12 tender points.

7. Which of the following statements is true?
a) Stress may be playing a significant role in this patient's presenting complaints.
b) A positive antinuclear antibody test will help establish a diagnosis of system lupus erythematous in this patient.
c) Antibodies to SSA (Ro) and SSB (La) are likely to be present.
d) A normal creatine phosphokinase test would rule out statin-related myopathy.

Answer and Discussion
The answer is a. This patient presents, as many do, with nonspecific complaints and few objective findings. Even the manual resistive testing results are subjective to a degree because they depend on patient effort, which is determined in part by patient pain. The physician must consider a differential diagnosis that includes anemia (from heavy menses), hypothyroidism, statin-induced myopathy (which may occur with a normal creatine phosphokinase test), and fibromyalgia (as suggested by the poor sleep, tender points, and stressful family/social situation). Other etiologies to consider include depression, smoking-related pulmonary disease, idiopathic inflammatory myopathies, and other disorders, the workup for which will be guided by the first battery of test results.

8. The least useful test on this visit would be
a) Thyroid-stimulating hormone
b) Creatine phosphokinase
c) Complete blood count
d) Antinuclear antibody

Answer and Discussion
The answer is d. Although the patient is naturally concerned about systemic lupus erythematous (SLE), she does not display any objective findings that would suggest this illness, and an antinuclear antibody (ANA) test will not be helpful at this time because she might well have a positive ANA related to her Hashimoto's thyroiditis and as a relative of someone with SLE. Likewise, with the lack of objective findings, SSA and SSB autoantibodies are unlikely to be positive.

9. A treatment plan at the end of the first visit (before laboratory data available) would reasonably include which of the following?
a) Addition of prednisone, 5 to 10 mg/day
b) Discontinuation of Pravachol
c) Decrease in thyroxine dose
d) Addition of hydroxychloroquine, 200 mg twice a day

Answer and Discussion
The answer is b. On the initial visit, counseling for stress reduction, smoking cessation, and weight loss would be in order. A Pravachol "drug holiday" would determine whether the myalgias and weakness are related to a statin side effect. There is no immediate indication for corticosteroids or hydroxychloroquine.

SUGGESTED READINGS

Systemic Lupus Erythematosus

Doria A, et al. Cardiac involvement in SLE. *Lupus* 2005;14:683–686.
Mandell BF. Cardiovascular involvement in systemic lupus erythematosus. *Semin Arthritis Rheum* 1987;17:126–141.
Manzi S, et al. Age-specific incidence rates of myocardial infarction and angina in women with SLE. *Am J Epidemiol* 1997;145:400–415.
Rahman A, Isenberg DA. Systemic lupus erythematosus. *N Engl J Med* 2008;358:929–939.
Roman MJ, et al. Prevalence and correlates of accelerated atherosclerosis in SLE. *N Engl J Med* 2003;349:2399–2406.
Santos-Ocampo AS, Mandell BF, Fessler BJ. Alveolar hemorrhage in systemic lupus erythematosus. *Chest* 2000;118:1083–1090.
Schwartz MM. The pathology of lupus nephritis. *Semin Nephrol* 2007;(1):22–34.
Swigris JJ, Fischer A, Gilles J, et al. Pulmonary and thrombotic manifestations of SLE. *Chest* 2008;1333:272–280.

Antiphospholipid Antibody Syndrome

Alarcon-Segovia D, et al. Prophylaxis of the antiphospholipid syndrome: a consensus report. *Lupus* 2003;12:499–503.
Bartholomew JR, Kottke-Marchange K. Monitoring anticoagulation therapy in patients with the lupus anticoagulant. *J Clin Rheumatol* 1998;4:307–311.
Esplin MS. Management of antiphospholipid syndrome during pregnancy. *Clin Obstet Gynecol* 2001;44:20–28.
Pierangeli SS, Gharavi AE, Harris N. Testing for antiphospholipid antibodies: problems and solutions. *Clin Obstet Gynecol* 2001;44:48–57.
Shoenfeld Y. Systemic antiphospholipid syndrome. *Lupus* 2003;12:497–498.
Valesini G, Pittoni V. Treatment of thrombosis associated with immunological risk factors. *Ann Med* 2000;32:41–45.
Vianna JL, Khamashta MA, Ordi-Ros J, et al. Comparison of the primary and secondary antiphospholipid syndrome: a European multicenter study of 114 patients. *Am J Med* 1994;96:3–9.

Scleroderma

Rubin LJ, et al. Bosentan therapy for pulmonary arterial hypertension. *N Engl J Med* 2002;346:896–903.
Steen VD, Costantino JP, Shapiro AP, et al. Outcome of renal crisis in systemic sclerosis: relation to availability of angiotensin converting enzyme (ACE) inhibitors. *Ann Intern Med* 1990;113:352–357.

Tashkin DP, et al. Effects of 1-year treatment with cyclophosphamide on outcomes at 2 years in scleroderma lung disease. *Am J Respir Crit Care Med* 2007;176:1026–1034.

Sjögren's Syndrome

Alexander EL, Malinow K, Lejewski JE, et al. Primary Sjögren's syndrome with central nervous system disease mimicking multiple sclerosis. *Ann Intern Med* 1986;104:323–330.
Davidson BKS, Kelly CA, Griffiths ID. Ten-year follow up of pulmonary function in patients with primary Sjögren's syndrome. *Ann Rheum Dis* 2000;59:709–712.
Johnson R, Haga H, Gordon TP. Current concepts on diagnosis, autoantibodies and therapy in Sjögren's syndrome. *Scand J Rheumatol* 2000;29:341–348.

Idiopathic Inflammatory Myopathy

Bohan A, Peter JB, Bowman RL, et al. A computer-assisted analysis of 153 patients with polymyositis and dermatomyositis. *Medicine* 1977;56:255–286.
Callen JP. Dermatomyositis. *Lancet* 2000;355:53–57.
Dalakas MC. Therapeutic approaches in patients with inflammatory myopathies. *Semin Neurol* 2003;23:199–206.
Hill CL, Zhang Y, Sigurgeirsson B, et al. Frequency of specific cancer types in dermatomyositis and polymyositis: a population-based study. *Lancet* 2001;357:96–100.
Kiely PDW, Bruckner FE, Nisbet JA, et al. Serum skeletal troponin I in inflammatory muscle disease: relation to creatine kinase, CKMB and cardiac troponin I. *Ann Rheum Dis* 2000;59:750–751.
Rendt K. Inflammatory myopathies: narrowing the differential diagnosis. *Cleve Clin J Med* 2001;68:505–519.

Chapter 31

Systemic Vasculitis

Carol A. Langford

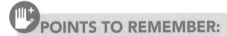

POINTS TO REMEMBER:

- Although some investigators have suggested that antineutrophil cytoplasmic antibodies (ANCA) may be useful to monitor disease activity, they have not been found to be a reliable measure of disease activity, and changes in ANCA level alone should not be used to guide treatment decisions.

- The signs and symptoms of vasculitis are generally nonspecific because they manifest as tissue injury occurring as a result of vascular ischemia or tissue inflammation, regardless of the underlying diagnostic cause.

- The therapy of systemic vasculitis varies, depending on severity, prognosis, and rate of disease progression. Certain types of vasculitis may be self-limiting and merely require careful monitoring, while others necessitate aggressive immunosuppressive treatment.

The term *vasculitis* refers to the presence of blood vessel inflammation. It is a histologic feature that is shared by a heterogeneous group of disorders in which vascular inflammation results in tissue injury and damage. Although the cause of most forms of vasculitis is unknown, the available evidence supports that immune-mediated mechanisms play a critical role in disease pathogenesis. This chapter reviews our current understanding of pathogenesis and classification, and provides a diagnostic and therapeutic approach to the individual vasculitic diseases that are most commonly encountered in internal medicine practice.

ETIOLOGY AND PATHOGENESIS

Prior to the mid-1980s, most theories of the pathogenesis of vasculitis focused on the role of immune complexes (ICs). It has since become apparent that IC deposition in vessels and tissues only explains the initiation of injury in a limited subset of patients. Current evidence suggests several mechanisms through which vascular inflammation may occur:

- IC deposition (vasculitis complicating viral and certain bacterial infections, cryoglobulinemic vasculitis, hypersensitivity vasculitis [HV], Henoch-Schönlein purpura [HSP], or secondary vasculitis occurring in systemic lupus erythematosus [SLE])
- Antibodies that target nonvascular structures: ANCA (including Wegener's granulomatosis [WG], microscopic polyangiitis [MPA], and Churg-Strauss syndrome [CSS])
- Cell-mediated (primarily mononuclear cells, tissue injury, giant cell arteritis [GCA], and Takayasu's arteritis [TAK])
- Combined mechanisms (WG, MPA, CSS)

Immune Complex Deposition

Supportive evidence for circulating IC in certain vasculitic conditions has come from:

- Animal models of IC disease
- Identification of IC in tissues
- Identification of IC in the sera of patients with vasculitis
- Identification of discrete antigens responsible for certain IC disorders

Among the vasculitides, the greatest evidence for IC contributing to vascular injury has come from hepatitis C virus (HCV)–associated cryoglobulinemic vasculitis, the polyarteritis nodosa (PAN)-like vasculitis that has been seen in some patients with hepatitis B virus (HBV), and HV that occurs 7 to 10 days following exposure to a discrete antigen.

Antineutrophil Cytoplasmic Antibodies

ANCA were first identified in 1982 with the use of indirect immunofluorescent (IIF) techniques in a small number of patients with crescentic glomerulonephritis (GN) and vasculitis. Three years later, a Dutch group noted that ANCA were present in a high percentage of patients with WG and were most frequently seen in those patients who had active disease. Since then, presence of ANCA in patients with MPA, CSS, and isolated crescentic GN in which few or no IC are present has also been well documented. For these forms of vasculitis, the presence of ANCA in an appropriate clinical setting has had important implications for diagnosis and may enhance our understanding of pathogenesis.

ANCA are described on the basis of their immunofluorescent pattern and antigenic specificity. By IIF, ANCA can have two main patterns: diffuse cytoplasmic pattern (cANCA) and perinuclear pattern (pANCA).

In patients with vasculitis, the antigen almost always responsible for the cANCA pattern is proteinase-3 (PR-3), a 29-kDa serine protease. The antigen most often associated with the pANCA pattern in vasculitis is the enzyme myeloperoxidase (MPO). MPO and PR-3 are located in the α- or azurophilic granules of granulocytes and the cytosolic granules of monocytes.

Most experts agree that the ANCA test is incomplete if it is only performed by IIF. If IIF is positive, an antigen-specific assay should be performed to determine whether the reaction is to PR-3, MPO, or neither. A large number of conditions, including infections (e.g., endocarditis, sepsis, HIV, malaria, tuberculosis); malignancies; and non-vasculitic, immune dysfunctional diseases (e.g., rheumatoid arthritis, SLE, scleroderma, primary sclerosing cholangitis, ulcerative colitis, Crohn's disease) may be associated with antibody production to leukocyte antigens other than PR-3 or MPO and, rarely, even to PR-3 or MPO. In particular, pANCA reactivity by IIF alone is nonspecific and, in the majority of patients, is owing to antinuclear antibodies (ANAs) or cytoplasmic antigens other than MPO, including lactoferrin, elastase, lysozyme, azurocidin, cathepsin G, and other enzyme antigens. Thus, IIF alone may be falsely positive and clinically misleading.

The strongest association between ANCA and clinical vasculitic disease has been with WG, in which anti-PR-3 cANCA antibodies have been noted in approximately 90% of patients with severe active multisystem disease. Antibodies to MPO are more likely to be found in patients with MPA, and approximately 40% of patients with CSS may have circulating ANCA. Because these diseases share certain characteristics that include small-vessel vasculitis, the potential for pulmonary capillaritis, and a crescentic, necrotizing GN with scant or no IC deposition, some investigators have grouped these together as ANCA-associated vasculitides. The disadvantages of this terminology are that it may overemphasize the role of ANCA in pathogenesis, it fails to recognize the potential for patients to be ANCA negative, and it does not acknowledge the unique aspects of these diseases that may influence diagnosis, treatment, and outcome. For this reason, WG, MPA, and CSS should continue to be viewed as individual disease entities.

Given the moderately high sensitivity ($\sim$70%) and high specificity (>95%), antibodies against PR-3 or MPO can replace the need for biopsy proof of WG or MPA under certain circumstances. These circumstances include a very high pretest probability for the presence of disease (on a clinical basis) and the absence of competing, mimicking diagnoses, especially infection. Although some investigators have suggested that ANCA may be useful to monitor disease activity, it has not been found to be a reliable measure of disease activity, and changes in ANCA level alone should not be used to guide treatment decisions.

At present, it is uncertain whether ANCA are directly pathogenic, although compelling evidence exists from sophisticated animal models and in vitro studies. Laboratory investigation suggests that under certain circumstances, ANCA are capable of binding to activated neutrophils and enhancing the release of their toxic products. MPO and

PR-3 released from neutrophils may bind to endothelial cells and cause injury by a direct action of the enzymes or by binding antibody that is already bound to neutrophils. Whether endothelial cells manufacture and express PR-3 remains a matter of controversy. Arguing against a pathogenic role for ANCA is the absence of this antibody in some patients with WG and the ability for patients to have inactive disease in the presence of high levels of ANCA.

Cellular-Mediated Vascular Injury

GCA and TAK are forms of vasculitis for which there is strong evidence to support cellular-mediated vascular injury. Both diseases involve macrophage and lymphocyte infiltration of the vessel wall. Mononuclear cells access the elastic (aorta and its primary branches) and medium-size muscular arteries (temporal, coronary, distal extremity, etc.) via the vasa vasorum of the adventitia. Evidence from the laboratory has supported that the CD4+ T lymphocyte is the critical cellular player in the vasculitic lesion of GCA, orchestrating macrophage differentiation and inflammation. As the inflammatory process migrates from adventitia, through the media, and toward the primary lumen, the cytokine- and enzyme-mediated destruction of muscle cells and elastic fibers ensues. If the vessel is slow to respond in regard to myointimal proliferation and the formation of fibrotic scar, aneurysm formation may follow. In general, if the aortic root is affected, then aneurysm formation is common. If aortic branch vessel disease occurs, then the result is most often vascular stenosis.

Mixed Mechanisms

It should be appreciated that the pathogenesis of most vasculitic diseases likely represents mixtures of these proposed mechanisms. Among the best examples is WG, in which ANCA may play a role, but for which there is also evidence for macrophage and T-cell (especially Th1-type) injury. In other settings, endothelium may be injured initially by antibody or IC, leading to endothelial activation, secretion of cytokines, or increased display of adhesion molecules; this later becomes the focus for cell-mediated pathological damage. A clearer understanding of the pathological mechanisms involved in these syndromes will facilitate more specific therapies, including biological response modifiers.

CLASSIFICATION

The recognition of different forms of vasculitis has lead to the development of classification schemes to facilitate communication about these diseases and their investigation. Most of these classification systems have been based on the predominant size of vessel being affected as well as on clinical and histologic features. Although vessel size can be useful conceptually, disease may not be limited to one vessel type and often involves multiple-size vascular

beds. These classification and nomenclature schemes continue to be works in progress as our knowledge about these diseases grows.

Two of the most recent classification criteria and nomenclature systems were proposed by the American College of Rheumatology and an international cooperative group convened at the Chapel Hill Consensus conference (Table 31.1). Although these have been useful to ensure the homogeneity of patients for clinical studies, they were not intended and should not be used for the diagnosis of the individual patient. It should also be recognized that these systems were meant to address the most common forms of vasculitic disease and do not include rare, but nevertheless important, forms of primary vasculitis such as primary angiitis of the central nervous system (CNS), Behçet's syndrome, Cogan's syndrome, and many others.

GENERAL PRINCIPLES: CLINICAL PRESENTATION AND DIAGNOSIS

The vasculitic diseases present formidable diagnostic challenges. The signs and symptoms of vasculitis are generally nonspecific because they manifest as tissue injury occurring as a result of vascular ischemia or tissue inflammation, regardless of the underlying diagnostic cause. Certain vasculitic syndromes present greater diagnostic dilemmas than others because of the nature and distribution of their target-organ involvement. For example, when the skin is involved, it is apparent that vasculitis is the underlying process, but a greater challenge is to determine the precise etiology that will guide prognosis and treatment. Systemic vasculitis may also be mimicked by a wide variety of nonvasculitic diseases. Specific warning signs or symptoms of systemic vasculitis include the following:

- Palpable purpuric rash
- Mononeuritis multiplex (foot or wrist drop)
- Digital ischemia
- Pulmonary hemorrhage
- GN

When a careful evaluation for other causes is unrevealing, consideration of vasculitis should also be made in the following settings:

- Fever of unknown origin (FUO) with constitutional symptoms
- Unexplained multisystem disease
- Unexplained inflammatory arthritis
- Unexplained myalgias

Most forms of vasculitis are diagnosed on the basis of having a compatible picture with either histologic confirmation on a tissue biopsy or supportive features by arteriography. The determination of what diagnostic procedure to pursue will be based on the site of organ involvement and the type of vasculitis being considered. These are discussed

TABLE 31.1

NAMES AND DEFINITIONS OF VASCULITIDES ADOPTED BY THE CHAPEL HILL CONSENSUS CONFERENCE ON THE NOMENCLATURE OF SYSTEMIC VASCULITIS

Large-vessel vasculitis

Giant cell (temporal) arteritis	Granulomatous arteritis of the aorta and its major branches, with a predilection for the extracranial branches of the carotid artery. *Often involves the temporal artery. Usually occurs in patients older than 50 years and is often associated with polymyalgia rheumatica.*
Takayasu arteritis	Granulomatous inflammation of the aorta and its major branches. *Usually occurs in patients younger than 50 years.*

Medium-size vessel vasculitis

Polyarteritis nodosa (classic polyarteritis nodosa)	Necrotizing inflammation of medium-size or small arteries without glomerulonephritis or vasculitis in arterioles, capillaries, or venules.
Kawasaki disease	Arteritis involving large, medium-size, and small arteries, and associated with mucocutaneous lymph node syndrome. *Coronary arteries are often involved. Aorta and veins may be involved. Usually occurs in children.*

Small-vessel vasculitis

Wegener's granulomatosis	Granulomatous inflammation involving the respiratory tract, and necrotizing vasculitis affecting small to medium-size vessels (e.g., capillaries, venules, arterioles, arteries). *Necrotizing glomerulonephritis is common.*
Churg-Strauss syndrome	Eosinophil-rich and granulomatous inflammation involving the respiratory tract, and necrotizing vasculitis affecting small to medium-size vessels and associated with asthma and eosinophilia.
Microscopic polyangiitis (microscopic polyarteritis)	Necrotizing vasculitis, with few or no immune deposits, affecting small vessels (i.e., capillaries, venules, or arterioles). *Necrotizing arteritis involving small and medium-size arteries may be present. Necrotizing glomerulonephritis is very common. Pulmonary capillaritis often occurs.*
Henoch-Schönlein purpura	Vasculitis, with IgA-dominant immune deposits, affecting small vessels (i.e., capillaries, venules, or arterioles). *Typically involves skin, gut, and glomeruli, and is associated with arthralgias or arthritis.*
Essential cryoglobulinemic vasculitis	Vasculitis, with cryoglobulin immune deposits, affecting small vessels (i.e., capillaries, venules, or arterioles) and associated with cryoglobulins in serum. *Skin and glomeruli are often involved.*
Cutaneous leukocytoclastic vasculitis	Isolated cutaneous leukocytoclastic angiitis without systemic vasculitis or glomerulonephritis.

From Jennette JC, Falk RJ, Andrassy K, et al. Nomenclature of systemic vasculitis: proposal of an international consensus conference. *Arthritis Rheum* 1994;37:187.

for each individual type of systemic vasculitis in the sections that follow.

SPECIFIC SYSTEMIC VASCULITIDES

Giant Cell Arteritis

GCA (also called temporal arteritis) is the most common primary systemic vasculitis seen in humans. It is a granulomatous vasculitis that affects large and medium-size arteries, particularly cranial branch vessels that originate from the aortic arch. GCA almost exclusively occurs in people older than 50 years, is more common in women, and is rarely seen in African Americans. Classic symptoms of GCA include (Table 31.2):

- Severe headache, often over the temples
- Scalp tenderness
- Transient visual disturbances (amaurosis fugax)
- Blindness
- Jaw or tongue claudication
- Polymyalgia rheumatica (PMR) in 50% of patients
- Large-vessel–related ischemia (arm claudication) or aortic aneurysms (thoracic much greater than abdominal)
- Fever, malaise, or weight loss

The relationship between PMR and GCA is complex. Although pure examples of each are well recognized, 50% of patients with GCA may have symptoms of PMR, and 10% to 20% of patients with isolated PMR may later go on to develop GCA. Increasing evidence indicates that GCA and PMR represent part of a single continuum of vascular inflammatory disease.

The diagnosis of GCA is suggested by compatible clinical features, typically along with an elevation in the erythrocyte sedimentation rate (ESR), which is seen in at least 80% to 90% of patients. The diagnosis of GCA is optimally based on a temporal artery biopsy, although negative biopsies can be seen in 20% to 50% of cases because lesions tend to be patchy in nature. GCA is histologically characterized by granulomatous inflammation of the arterial wall, with destruction of the internal elastic lamina and giant cell formation. If clinical suspicion for GCA is high, glucocorticoid therapy should be started immediately in order to protect vision and not delay pending biopsy results.

Treatment and Outcome of Giant Cell Arteritis

The treatment of GCA consists of high doses of prednisone, 40 to 60 mg/day for ~4 weeks, and then tapers to the lowest dose that maintains freedom from symptoms and suppression of the ESR. Relapses requiring an increase in

TABLE 31.2

CLINICAL MANIFESTATIONS OF GIANT CELL ARTERITIS

Manifestation	% of Patients Affected
Headache	68
Weight loss/anorexia	50
Jaw claudication	45
Fever	42
Malaise/fatigue/weakness	40
Polymyalgia rheumatica	39
Other musculoskeletal pain	30
Transient visual symptoms	16
Synovitis	15
Central nervous system abnormalities	15
Fixed visual symptoms	14
Sore throat	9
Swallowing claudication/dysphagia	8
Tongue claudication	6
Limb claudication	4

From Calamia KT, Hunder GG. Clinical manifestations of giant cell (temporal) arteritis. *Clin Rheum Dis* 1980;6:389–403.

prednisone dose occur in 75% to 90% of patients, and many patients require treatment for more than 4 years. No effective alternative for glucocorticoids has yet been identified. Several recent controlled trials of steroid-sparing agents, such as methotrexate, have yielded mixed results, and infliximab was not found to be effective.

Glucocorticoid toxicity occurs in more than 60% of patients with GCA and results in significant morbidity. Overall, patients with GCA have been found to have a similar rate of survival as compared to those in the general population. Thoracic aortic aneurysms can occur as a late manifestation of disease and represent an important cause of patient mortality from rupture or dissection.

Takayasu's Arteritis

TAK is a large-vessel granulomatous arteritis, primarily affecting the aorta, its main branches, and the pulmonary arteries. TAK occurs predominantly in young women and has a prevalence of ~2.6 cases per 1 million population. Although it has been most often described in Asia, TAK has been described in patients of all races throughout the world. Other than age distribution, little distinguishes TAK from GCA with large-vessel involvement.

The most common presentation of TAK is claudication of the upper extremities. Involvement of the aorta occurs in ~65% of cases and may lead to aneurysm formation (especially the aortic root with aortic regurgitation) or stenosis (especially abdominal aorta). Lightheadedness and, rarely, strokes may be due to disease of the carotid and vertebral arteries. Gastrointestinal (GI) ischemia may result from stenoses and occlusion of the celiac or mesenteric arteries. Coronary artery involvement is uncommon but, when present, is usually due to proximal vessel stenoses. Constitutional and/or musculoskeletal symptoms occur in ~50% of cases.

Hypertension may affect 32% to 93% of patients with TAK and is usually due to renal artery stenosis or occlusion. In some parts of Asia, TAK is the most common cause of childhood hypertension. Because a stenotic lesion may be responsible for a misleading low-extremity cuff blood pressure compared to the central aortic arch pressure, four extremity blood pressure measurements should be routinely performed in all patients with TAK. Occasionally, all extremity pressures are misleading because of bilateral subclavian (or innominate), iliac, and femoral stenoses.

The diagnosis of TAK is typically made by the presence of characteristic stenotic or aneurysmal large-vessel changes in a clinically appropriate setting. There are no diagnostic laboratory features, and, although the ESR is usually elevated, it can be normal in 40% to 80% of patients. Arteriographic imaging of the entire aorta and the origin of its branch vessels should be obtained in all patients suspected to have TAK by catheter-directed dye arteriography, magnetic resonance arteriography (MRA), or CT arteriography. Thorough imaging at diagnosis is essential in order to detect all sites or arterial involvement because this has diagnostic and prognostic importance. Biopsies of the large vessels in TAK are typically obtained only in the setting of vascular bypass surgery and demonstrate histopathological features identical to those of GCA.

Assessment of disease activity remains one of the greatest challenges in TAK, with studies demonstrating active vascular inflammation in 44% of patients who were clinically believed to have quiescent disease. Symptoms can reflect damage rather than ongoing inflammation and ESR and are often not a reliable guide for disease activity. Serial MRA at 6- to 12-month intervals can be used to detect new vascular lesions in new territories, which is considered to be indicative of active disease.

Treatment and Outcome of Takayasu's Arteritis

Glucocorticoids form the foundation of treatment for TAK. Cytotoxic drugs, including methotrexate, may be useful in refractory cases, although up to 25% of patients may continue to have active disease despite therapy. Hypertension must be recognized and controlled if serious morbidity is to be avoided in the forms of hypertensive heart disease, stroke, or renal failure. Severe extremity claudication, severe aortic regurgitation, or coronary artery disease may require surgical therapy. Revascularization through vascular bypass surgery can be effective but is often followed by restenosis. Although angioplasty and vascular stents are less invasive, they are associated with higher rates of restenosis. It is critical to recognize that the effective care of patients with TAK requires a team approach that includes generalists, rheumatologists, and vascular specialists in imaging and surgery if the patient is to have the best possible outcome.

In North American series, the 5-year survival rate of patients with TAK was found to be more than 95%. Mortality rates of up to 35% have been seen in other studies, and morbidity from chronic disease and permanent damage occurs frequently.

Polyarteritis Nodosa

PAN was first described more than 100 years ago by Kussmaul and Maier. As currently defined, PAN is an uncommon disease affecting small and medium-size muscular arteries. PAN does not affect the capillaries and venules, and is not associated with GN or pulmonary hemorrhage. PAN is more common in men than in women (~2:1), and typically presents between the ages of 40 and 60 years, although it can occur at any age.

The clinical features of PAN reflect medium-size vessel disease and include:

- Cardiac, GI, CNS, and peripheral nervous system disease
- Hypertension
- Fever and constitutional symptoms

No laboratory tests are specifically diagnostic for PAN. Elevations in levels of acute phase reactants, including ESR, are typically seen, and an elevated white blood cell count and anemia are frequently present. ANCA (both PR-3 and MPO) are generally absent. The diagnosis of PAN is based on characteristic arteriographic findings or biopsy-proven evidence of vasculitis. Significant debate arises over which is the first test to choose in the process of diagnosing this condition; however, several generalizations can be made:

- Studies or biopsies of clinically normal organs are usually unrewarding. If a biopsy is to be performed, features of disease should be present at that site, whether they are clinical, laboratory, or imaging abnormalities.
- Consider a biopsy of nodular or tender skin lesions, tender muscles, or peripheral nerve in the setting of neuropathy.
- Consider mesenteric and renal arteriography if appropriate signs or symptoms are present (e.g., pain, blood in stools, abnormal hepatic or pancreatic enzymes, new-onset hypertension). Approximately 70% to 80% of patients with PAN will have abnormal arteriograms, with 75% of these patients demonstrating classic multiple microaneurysms.

Most authorities would reserve the term *PAN* for only those patients who do not have a known association with an infection, malignancy, or other primary illness. In the presence of these other systemic diseases, a diagnosis of primary idiopathic PAN cannot be made. Diseases that have been associated with a PAN-like syndrome include:

- HBV and HCV
- HIV infection
- Hairy cell leukemia
- Endocarditis
- Recreational drug abuse
- Connective tissue disease (rheumatoid arthritis, SLE, scleroderma, Sjögren's syndrome, and others)

Treatment and Outcome of Polyarteritis Nodosa

If PAN is left untreated, the 5-year survival rate is 10% to 15%. The introduction of therapy has been reported to increase the 5-year survival rate to 80% or more.

The treatment of PAN generally adheres to the principles of therapy for systemic vasculitis outlined in the final section of this chapter. Patients with life-threatening PAN involving the GI tract, heart, CNS, or kidneys should be treated with prednisone and cyclophosphamide (CYC). Glucocorticoids alone may be indicated for people with limited or non–life-threatening disease. PAN-like disease associated with an underlying viral infection such as HBV, HCV, or HIV requires special considerations on the need for combined therapy to address both inflammatory and viral processes.

Wegener's Granulomatosis

WG is multisystem diseases that is most commonly characterized by clinical involvement of the upper and lower respiratory tract and kidneys, plus the pathological features of necrotizing, granulomatous inflammation with and without vasculitis. Pulmonary and renal disease can vary from being minor and asymptomatic to severe and life threatening. WG is estimated to affect about 3 in 100,000 people and occurs in men and women equally.

The clinical manifestations of WG include (Table 31. 3):

- Upper airways disease such as rhinitis, epistaxis, sinusitis, otitis media, hearing loss, or subglottic stenosis
- Lower respiratory tract symptoms and signs such as cough, hemoptysis, and shortness of breath. Radiographic features may include nodules, cavitating lesions, consolidative infiltrates, or ground-glass infiltrates suggestive of alveolar hemorrhage (Figs. 31.1 and 31.2)
- Renal disease, which occurs in a minority at presentation but is present in the majority over time
- Other target organs such as eyes, ears, skin, CNS or peripheral nervous system, and joints
- Prominent constitutional symptoms

In most instances, the diagnosis of WG is based on the appropriate clinical picture and a compatible biopsy. Characteristic pathological findings include:

- Granuloma formation
- Necrotizing vasculitis
- Tissue necrosis, especially in a "geographic pattern"

Because these features may also be seen in the setting of infection, cultures and special stains for infectious agents should be performed. Sampling error and the patchy nature of the underlying pathology have made the interpretation

TABLE 31.3

CLINICAL FEATURES SEEN IN WEGENER'S GRANULOMATOSIS

Characteristic	Frequency (%)
Upper airways disease	95
Pulmonary disease	
Radiographic nodule/infiltrates	70–85
Alveolar hemorrhage	5–15
Glomerulonephritis	70–80
Arthralgias/arthritis	60–70
Ocular	50–60
Skin	40–50
Nervous system	
Peripheral	40–50
Central	5–10
Cardiac	10–25
Gastrointestinal	<5
Genitourinary	<2
ANCA	
PR-3/cANCA	75–90
MPO/pANCA	5–20

ANCA = antineutrophil cytoplasmic antibodies, MPO = myeloperoxidase, PR-3 = proteinase 3.

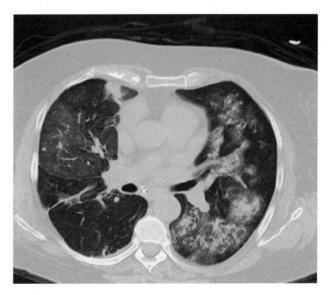

Figure 31.2 Pulmonary hemorrhage in a patient with microscopic polyangiitis. Similar features can be seen in Wegener's granulomatosis.

of biopsy material problematic. Nasal biopsy often shows only nonspecific inflammation or necrosis; however, in approximately 50% of cases, necrotizing vasculitis, granulomatous inflammation, or both can be identified. The highest diagnostic yield comes from open lung biopsy of radiographically abnormal pulmonary parenchyma, which will show characteristic features ~90% of the time. Renal biopsy generally demonstrates a segmental, necrotizing, crescentic GN with few to no IC. These changes are indistinguishable from those found in MPA, CSS, and idiopathic pauci-immune crescentic GN. Percutaneous renal biopsy rarely shows vasculitis outside the glomerulus or granulomas.

The diagnosis of WG has been greatly enhanced by the development of ANCA testing. Antibody detection to PR-3 (i.e., cANCA) can replace the need for tissue confirmation in limited circumstances when the likelihood of disease (the pretest probability) is high. In instances where biopsies are not obtained, meticulous attention must be given to ruling out underlying infection.

Treatment and Outcome of Wegener's Granulomatosis

If untreated, WG in its fully expressed form is uniformly fatal. Current treatment regimens are effective and can induce remission and prolong survival in most patients. Patients with severe active WG should be treated with a combination of high-dose prednisone and daily CYC until remission is achieved in 3 to 6 months. After that time, CYC can be stopped and switched to a less toxic agent such as methotrexate or azathioprine for remission maintenance. Methotrexate may be substituted for CYC as primary therapy in patients who do not have immediately life-threatening disease and who have a serum creatinine level of ≤2.0 mg/dL. Trimethoprim-sulfamethoxazole has been demonstrated to be efficacious in decreasing the rate of upper respiratory flares and may be incorporated into the treatment regimen, especially in those with disease limited to the upper airways. This therapy should not be applied as primary therapy to any patient with features beyond mild upper airway disease and cannot be combined at full strength in patients receiving methotrexate. Disease relapse occurs in more than 50% of patients with WG, and treatment-related toxicity represents an important cause of morbidity.

Microscopic Polyangiitis

MPA refers to a vasculitis that involves small vessels (i.e., capillaries, venules, arterioles, small arteries), with little or

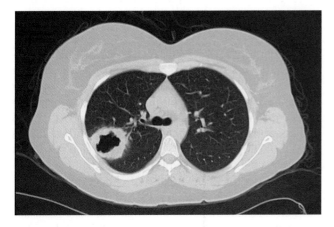

Figure 31.1 Cavitary pulmonary lesion in a patient with Wegener's granulomatosis.

no IC deposition. MPA has a predilection for the lungs, which pathologically display capillaritis without granuloma formation, distinguishing it from WG. MPA is frequently associated with pANCA directed against MPO. Differentiation from WG may be difficult at times when the pathology is not classically abnormal. At times, MPA may resemble PAN because larger vessels may also be involved in MPA.

Characteristics of MPA include the following:

- Nongranulomatous vasculitis involving small and sometimes medium vessels
- Renal involvement common (rapidly progressive GN)
- Pulmonary involvement common (alveolar hemorrhage) (Fig. 31.2)
- ANCA positive in 50% to 80%
- Angiographic abnormalities uncommon (although most cases not studied by angiography)

Treatment and Outcome of Microscopic Polyangiitis

The treatment of MPA should generally follow the principles of therapy outlined for WG. Similar to WG, untreated MPA carries a poor prognosis. Although disease relapses occur in at least 40% of patients with MPA, some evidence suggests that relapse may occur less commonly than in WG.

Churg-Strauss Syndrome

CSS is also known as *allergic angiitis* and *granulomatosis*. CSS was first described in 1951, in a group of patients with necrotizing vasculitis, a history of adult-onset asthma, and striking eosinophilia. CSS is clinically rarer than PAN or WG. In one study from the United Kingdom, the annual incidence was estimated to be 3.1 per 1.0 million population.

CSS is often thought of as having three phases: an allergic phase when rhinitis and asthma are common, an eosinophilic phase, and a vasculitic phase. Although these phases are not seen in all patients, it is not uncommon for vasculitis to be preceded by asthma and/or allergic rhinitis for many years.

CSS is marked by the following features:

- Allergic rhinitis/sinusitis, ~70%
- Asthma (or history of asthma), 100%
- Pulmonary infiltrates, ~70%
- Cardiomyopathy, ~50%
- Peripheral neuropathy, ~65%
- CNS involvement, ~25%, seizures, coma, infarction, confusion, and hydrocephalus
- Myalgias or arthralgias, ~50%
- GN, ~40%

The diagnosis of CSS is typically based on the presence of asthma, eosinophilia, and clinical features of vasculitis. CSS should be suspected in any person with adult-onset asthma who develops palpable purpura or cutaneous infarction, peripheral neuropathy, GI ischemia, cardiomyopathy, or nephritis. The laboratory hallmark of CSS is peripheral eosinophilia, which is generally >1,500 cells/mm^3. ANCA are seen in <40% of patients and are typically an MPO-ANCA. Tissue biopsies can be useful when positive and may demonstrate a small to medium-size vessel disease that may progress to fibrinoid necrosis, infiltration with eosinophils, and granuloma formation.

Treatment and Outcome of Churg-Strauss Syndrome

The initial treatment for CSS is generally high-dose glucocorticoids following the principles of therapy outlined at the end of the chapter. Cytotoxic drugs, such as CYC, are reserved for patients with life-threatening organ system involvement or those with disease refractory to glucocorticoids. In one series of 64 patients with CSS, at a mean period of 7.3 years follow-up, 69% had survived. Cardiac involvement is an important cause of mortality in CSS and should be considered in all affected patients.

Henoch-Schönlein Purpura

HSP is a syndrome characterized by palpable purpura and varying degrees of polyarthralgia, arthritis, myalgia, GI ischemia (including intussusception), and GN. HSP is predominantly a disease of children, although adults may be affected as well. Tissue injury is mediated by immunoglobulin A–containing (less often immunoglobulin G) IC, which can be identified within the tissues, especially the kidney. Biopsies of the skin reveal leukocytoclastic vasculitis and often IgA deposition. In ~60% of cases, patients describe a preceding infection that commonly includes streptococci, mycoplasma pneumonia, *Yersinia*, *Legionella*, *Helicobacter pylori*, Epstein-Barr virus, HBV, varicella, adenovirus, cytomegalovirus, and parvovirus B19. Although a triggering role for infection has been suspected, this has not been definitively proven.

Treatment and Outcome of Henoch-Schönlein Purpura

The treatment of HSP depends on its severity, and mild disease requires essentially no therapy. Glucocorticoids have been found to decrease arthritis and tissue edema, and may lessen the risk of intussusception in children. Although life-threatening visceral disease may require glucocorticoids and possibly even cytotoxic drugs, the use of these agents in controlled trials has not been demonstrated to prevent or improve the course of nephritis in HSP patients.

Relapses occur in up to 30% of patients but are typically cutaneous and of milder severity. Children with HSP have an excellent outcome, although end-stage renal disease can rarely occur. The course of HSP in adults is less clear, although some studies suggest that the disease can be more severe and associated with a higher rate of renal failure.

Cryoglobulinemic Vasculitis

Much progress has been made in the understanding of cryoglobulinemia. Cryoglobulins are characterized on the basis of their content:

- Type I: monoclonal (containing a single immunoglobulin)—most often seen in the presence of lymphoproliferative diseases such as B-cell malignancies
- Type II: mixed (containing a monoclonal and polyclonal immunoglobulin) or monoclonal—often considered to be of unknown or "essential" origin
- Type III: mixed or polyclonal

An important association has been established between HCV infection and type II mixed cryoglobulinemia. This association was based on the following:

- Serologic evidence of exposure to HCV in 90% of cases previously believed to be "essential"
- Evidence of active HCV infection
- Concentration of HCV RNA and antibodies to HCV within the cryoglobulin
- HCV deposition in blood vessels or kidneys

For a long period of time, most cases of type II were believed to be idiopathic. Many studies have now confirmed that HCV RNA is found in the serum and cryoprecipitate in the majority of patients with type II cryoglobulinemia and that HCV represents the most common cause of cryoglobulinemic vasculitis. With the use of molecular techniques (polymerase chain reaction), HCV has been identified and found to be present up to 1,000-fold in the cryoprecipitate.

The signs and symptoms of HCV-associated cryoglobulinemia include:

- Palpable purpura
- Arthralgia
- Weakness
- Peripheral neuropathy
- GN (most frequently membranoproliferative)
- Hepatomegaly and/or splenomegaly
- Skin ulcers

Treatment and Outcome of Cryoglobulinemic Vasculitis

The association of HCV and cryoglobulinemia has provided the rationale for antiviral therapy as is used to treat HCV infection. Current reports evaluating interferon and ribavirin suggest that the majority of patients with HCV associated cryoglobulinemia respond to treatment but with relapse occurring in those patients who do not have a sustained virologic response.

Other therapies that have been used for type II cryoglobulinemia relied on immunosuppression and apheresis although no controlled trials have been undertaken with either of these interventions in the treatment of cryoglobulinemia. In patients with HCV, immunosuppression carries concerns for worsening of the viral process. After a time, a moderate risk exists for the development of lymphoproliferative disease with this condition, and thus alkylating agents (e.g., CYC) should be avoided wherever possible. Most investigators agree that apheresis is useful in controlling many of the acute manifestations, but cryoglobulin levels are quick to rebound after discontinuation of treatment. Other therapies reported to have been palliative include anti-inflammatory drugs, antihistamines, and intravenous immunoglobulin.

The following points should be considered in treating cryoglobulinemic vasculitis:

- Antiviral therapy has been associated with clinical improvement in HCV-associated cryoglobulinemic vasculitis.
- Controlled studies of cytotoxic agents or apheresis have not been conducted.
- Morbidity and mortality are related to the severity of organ involvement.
- A high rate of lymphoproliferative transformation occurs.
- In the presence of active HCV infection, the use of prolonged immunosuppression may have adverse effects on the underlying infectious process.
- HCV-infected patients with symptomatic cryoglobulinemia should be comanaged by a skilled hepatologist and a therapist knowledgeable in the use of immunosuppressive drugs.

Although the overall prognosis for patients with cryoglobulinemia is good, the prognosis depends on the severity of visceral involvement. In most patients with cryoglobulinemic vasculitis, mortality is related to the underlying disease or complications of therapy.

Cutaneous Vasculitis

Cutaneous vasculitis represents the most common vasculitic manifestation encountered in clinical practice. This is typically manifest as palpable purpura and maculopapular lesions, although nodules and ulcerations can also occur. Skin biopsies usually reveal small-vessel (capillaries and venules) inflammation, with leukocytoclasis (nuclear fragmentation).

In more than 70% of cases, cutaneous vasculitis may occur secondary to an underlying disease or trigger. Included among this is the concept of HV, where cutaneous vasculitis occurs following exposure to drugs or serum, or in the setting of recent infection. In HV, strong evidence suggests that most cases have IC deposits in vessels; however, for most cases of cutaneous vasculitis, the pathophysiological mechanisms remain unclear. A wide variety of systemic disorders may also present with cutaneous vasculitis and have occult evidence of involvement of other organ systems or develop the features of other illnesses over time.

The broad differential diagnosis for underlying causes of cutaneous vasculitis include:

- Drug-induced cutaneous vasculitis
- Infection-associated vasculitis
- Malignancy-associated vasculitis
- Primary systemic vasculitis: WG, MPA, CSS, HSP
- Cryoglobulinemia
- Connective tissue–associated vasculitis (SLE, rheumatoid arthritis, Sjögren's syndrome)
- Urticarial hypersensitivity
- Other forms of systemic vasculitis

In the remaining 30% of patients with cutaneous vasculitis, no underlying cause can be found, and this would be considered an idiopathic cutaneous vasculitis.

Treatment and Outcome of Cutaneous Vasculitis

The clinical course of patients with cutaneous vasculitis depends on the underlying cause. In true HV, a pattern of illness usually develops 7 to 10 days after exposure and resolves within a 4- to 6-week period, although recurrences or even chronic disease can develop. The treatment of HV should focus primarily on removal of the inciting antigen. If the antigen is a drug, it should be discontinued, and if an infection is incriminated, it should be treated.

For idiopathic cutaneous vasculitis, there have been no controlled trials, and treatment should be aimed at using the least toxic yet effective approach. Many patients may not require any treatment, whereas patients with more symptomatic disease may require antihistamines, colchicine, dapsone, or glucocorticoids. Cytotoxic drugs should be limited to severe cases with ulceration or where glucocorticoids cannot be effectively tapered. Because of its toxicity, CYC is rarely, if ever, justified for the treatment of cutaneous vasculitis.

PRINCIPLES OF THERAPY FOR SYSTEMIC VASCULITIS

The therapy of systemic vasculitis involves more than just focusing on the vascular inflammatory process. Successful outcomes are highly dependent on meticulous monitoring for complications of therapy as well as careful assessments of disease activity. Regardless of the type of vasculitis being treated, the physician must consider the following:

- Presence or absence of disease activity, which may change during the course of treatment and require adjustment in therapies
- Disease severity—is the disease life or organ threatening?
- Disease-related damage, which is typically permanent and not amenable to treatment directed toward active vasculitis

- Treatment toxicity, for which preventive measures play an important role and which may require new medications, changes in the initial plan, or choices of interventions

Initial Therapy

The therapy of systemic vasculitis varies, depending on severity, prognosis, and rate of disease progression. Certain types of vasculitis may be self-limiting and merely require careful monitoring (HSP, some cases of cutaneous vasculitis). Treatment should always be individualized. General guidelines for the treatment of most forms of severe vasculitis (including PAN, WG, CSS, and MPA) include the initial use of one or more of the following agents:

- Glucocorticoid therapy with prednisone (or its equivalent), 1 mg/kg in the acute phase, with a tapering of dose. Methylprednisolone 1,000 mg daily for 3 days should be considered in fulminant cases.
- CYC 2 mg/kg orally. Higher doses can be used in the first 3 to 4 days of treatment in fulminant circumstances, and dosage reduction should be considered in the setting of renal insufficiency because CYC is renally eliminated. CYC remains the most effective proven therapy for severe vasculitis and although controversial, daily rather than intermittent intravenous administration is recommended.
- For patients with non–life-threatening presentations, methotrexate may be substituted for CYC as primary therapy. The dose is generally 15 mg to start, with titration up to 25 mg/week, depending on intervening toxicity (avoid if serum creatinine >2 mg/dL).

Maintenance Therapy

An advance in the efforts to reduce treatment-related morbidity and mortality is the employment of the so-called "induction-maintenance" approach. This strategy takes advantage of the potency of CYC to induce remission in patients with life-threatening forms of disease, but then reduces the potential for toxicity by limiting duration of CYC exposure. In general, when CYC is initiated, it is continued only for as long as necessary to achieve a remission from all signs of active disease. This generally takes about 3 to 6 months, depending on the individual case. This is then followed by switching to a less toxic agent, such as methotrexate, azathioprine, or mycophenolate mofetil, for the duration of therapy. A number of studies have demonstrated the safety and efficacy of this approach, and most now consider this to be the standard of care.

Treatment Toxicity and Prevention

CYC toxicity may cause or contribute to the following:

- Infections, especially because of profound immunosuppression that occurs with the combination of CYC + glucocorticoids
- Cytopenias—try to avoid severe leukopenia but expect lymphopenia

- Drug-induced cystitis, which is rarely hemorrhagic
- Gonadal dysfunction, sterility
- Bladder cancer
- After extended use, lymphoproliferative and myeloproliferative diseases
- Miscellaneous—nausea, vomiting, rash, hepatitis, and hypersensitivity reactions

The following strategies can be useful to prevent or minimize CYC toxicities:

- Monitoring of the blood counts every 1 to 2 weeks to prevent leucopenia and to maintain the total white blood cells >3,500/mm^3 and absolute neutrophil count >1,500/mm^3
- *Pneumocystis jiroveci* pneumonia prophylaxis, which should be part of any program of immunosuppressive therapy that is likely to produce significant lymphopenia
- Administration of CYC all at once in the morning with a large amount of fluid to minimize bladder toxicity
- Monitoring of the urinalysis for nonglomerular hematuria with cystoscopy, if present

Glucocorticoids have an extensive toxicity profile and are another important cause of morbidity. Osteoporosis represents a preventable toxicity, and all glucocorticoid-treated patients should be placed on a bone protection program to include yearly bone density measurements, calcium, vitamin D, and, where appropriate, consideration of bisphosphonates or other therapies.

REVIEW EXERCISES

QUESTIONS

1. Symptoms and signs that should lead to consideration of an underlying systemic vasculitis include
a) Mononeuritis multiplex
b) Fever of unknown origin
c) Digital ischemia
d) Red blood cell casts in the urine
e) All of the above

Answer and Discussion
The answer is e. The diagnosis of vasculitis begins with clinical suspicion. There are relatively few findings of high diagnostic specificity for systemic vasculitis, but suspicion should mount in the presence of presumptive signs or "red flags" for vasculitis. These include fever of unknown origin with constitutional symptoms; unexplained multisystem organ disease; unexplained inflammatory arthritis; unexplained myalgias; a suspicious rash, in particular palpable purpura; peripheral neuropathies, especially mononeuritis multiplex; unexplained end-organ ischemia, including cardiac, central nervous system, and gastrointestinal; and

glomerulonephritis. Although none of these findings is specific for systemic vasculitis, the presence of any one or more should lead to increasing suspicion of the disease.

2. A 50-year-old man was admitted with a 3-month history of fever, weight loss, abdominal pain, and hypertension. A detailed fever of unknown origin workup was unrevealing. Pertinent physical findings included a blood pressure of 220/120 mm Hg, livedo reticularis on the legs, footdrop on the left, and absent pinprick sensation in the lower legs. Laboratory study results included an erythrocyte sedimentation rate of 100 mm/hour, a creatinine level 2.2 mg/dL, microscopic hematuria, and an aspartate transaminase level of twice normal.

Polyarteritis nodosa is suspected. After consideration of the diagnostic yield and the risks, the logical next step would be
a) Skin biopsy
b) Percutaneous renal biopsy to demonstrate vasculitis of extraglomerular vessels
c) Abdominal angiography
d) Sural nerve biopsy

Answer and Discussion
The answer is d. This patient presents a clinical picture highly suspicious for systemic vasculitis, in particular, polyarteritis nodosa (PAN). Each diagnostic test outlined in the question should be considered in terms of sensitivity, specificity, and risk. A skin biopsy is sensitive but nonspecific because vasculitis of the skin can be caused by so many different conditions. On occasion, a nodular subcutaneous lesion may have characteristic features. Palpable purpura is less specific, and leukocytoclastic vasculitis may occur in many conditions. Percutaneous renal biopsy in this setting is insensitive for demonstrating vasculitis of the extraglomerular vessels and may be risky because PAN can cause microaneurysm formation. Abdominal angiography has increased sensitivity, but in the presence of severe hypertension and azotemia, it carries unacceptable risks. Last, sural nerve biopsy, although somewhat morbid and invasive, has an increasing diagnostic yield (>60%), particularly in the presence of objective neurologic signs and symptoms.

3. The differential diagnosis for the rash shown in Figure 31.1 includes
a) Drug-associated vasculitis
b) Vasculitis with malignancy
c) Henoch-Schönlein purpura
d) Subacute bacterial endocarditis
e) a and b
f) All of the above

Answer and Discussion

The answer is f. The rash shown in Figure 31.3 is palpable purpura. It is highly specific for small-vessel cutaneous vasculitis but is unrevealing of an underlying nosologic diagnosis. Drug-associated vasculitis is an extremely common cause of small-vessel vasculitis. Vasculitis associated with malignancies is most frequently found in the setting of an underlying lymphoproliferative disease. A small-vessel vasculitis such as this would be characteristic. Henoch-Schönlein purpura is characterized not only by such a rash, but also by the presence of abdominal pain and glomerulonephritis. It is most frequently seen in children but may also be seen in adults. Subacute bacterial endocarditis has a variety of extracardiac complications, the majority of which are mediated by immune complexes. A small-vessel vasculitis would not be unusual in subacute bacterial endocarditis, although it is rare for this to be the dominant and presenting finding of the disorder. Many other conditions can be seen with this type of rash, including a variety of connective tissue diseases (e.g., rheumatoid arthritis,

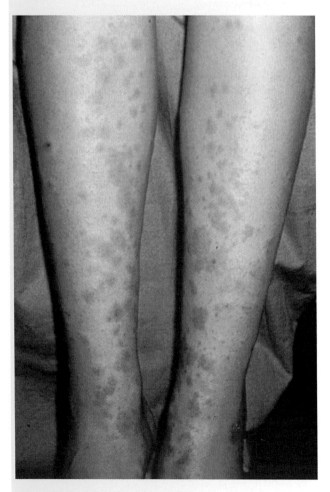

Figure 31.3 Rash. (See Color Fig. 31.3.)

system lupus erythematous), other types of infections, cryoglobulinemia secondary to hepatitis C virus infection, and a variety of miscellaneous systemic diseases.

4. The following is true about the antineutrophil cytoplasmic antibodies (ANCA) test:
a) cANCA representing antibodies to PR-3 is highly correlated with a diagnosis of Wegener's granulomatosis (WG).
b) pANCA by immunofluorescence is sufficient for a diagnosis of WG or microscopic polyangiitis.
c) A rise in ANCA titers alone should prompt an escalation of immunosuppressive therapy.
d) a and b.
e) a, b, and c.

Answer and Discussion

The answer is d. ANCA testing has been a step forward in the diagnostic process for certain forms of systemic vasculitis. The test is generally performed by immunofluorescence, but should also be confirmed by antigen-specific assays. In the majority of cases, an immunofluorescent pattern of cANCA is associated with antibodies to the neutrophil enzyme PR-3. It is highly correlated with the diagnosis of WG, being more than 80% sensitive and more than 95% specific in the presence of active untreated and widespread disease. pANCA by immunofluorescence, however, is not only less sensitive for the diagnosis of WG (present in only a small percentage of cases), but also relatively nonspecific. The pANCA pattern can be mimicked by a variety of antibodies, including ANA. The antibodies of interest in the diagnosis of systemic vasculitis responsible for the pANCA pattern of immunofluorescence are those directed against myeloperoxidase, another neutrophil enzyme. ANCA test results by immunofluorescence should always be confirmed by an antigen-specific assay. Finally, although some studies have suggested that ANCA levels are higher in those patients with active disease, this is not useful at the level of the individual patient. ANCA titers alone are not useful to assess disease activity and should not in and of themselves be used as a justification for the modification of therapy. A clinical evaluation of end-organ damage is still the "gold standard" for determining modifications of therapy.

5. Which of the following statements about cryoglobulinemic vasculitis is correct?
a) The most common clinical finding is a vasculitic rash.
b) If the cryoglobulin is composed only of a monoclonal immunoglobulin, it is generally associated with an underlying malignancy.
c) The most common associated condition is an underlying infection with hepatitis B virus.

d) a and b.

e) a, b, and c.

Answer and Discussion

The answer is d. Cryoglobulinemia and cryo-globulinemic vasculitis result from immunoglob-ulins and other proteins that precipitate from serum at temperatures lower than 37°C. Cryo-globulins are characterized on the basis of their content as type I (monoclonal), type II (mixed or monoclonal), or type III (polyclonal). The vast majority of cases of mixed cryoglobulinemia are associated with underlying hepatitis C virus infection.

Patients with cryoglobulinemia from any underlying cause may have a variety of end-organ manifestations. A small-vessel vasculitis, most often manifesting as pal-pable purpura, is the most frequent finding. Arthralgia and arthritis are also common. With considerable fre-quency, patients also have glomerulonephritis, periph-eral neuropathy, and a variety of other complications.

In questions 6–9, indicate whether each of the follow-ing statements about biopsies and vasculitis is true (T) or false (F).

6. A skin biopsy that reveals small-vessel, leukocytoclastic vasculitis is a reliable measure that disease activity will only involve small vessels elsewhere.

T_____ F_____

Answer and Discussion

False. The presence of leukocytoclastic vasculitis of cap-illaries and postcapillary venules does not preclude the involvement of larger vessels (arteries and veins) in other sites. Although vessel size can be useful concep-tually, disease may not be limited to one vessel type and often involves multiple-size vascular beds. Examples can be seen in Wegener's granulomatosis, microscopic polyangiitis, Behçet's disease, viral-associated vasculi-tides, vasculitis secondary to systemic lupus erythema-tous, and other diseases.

7. Open biopsies of abnormal organs in patients with systemic vasculitis will be diagnostic of vasculitis in more than 90% of cases.

T_____ F_____

Answer and Discussion

False. Vasculitis is a patchy process, and the diagnostic yield will depend on the organ site and the amount of tissue obtained. Skip lesions—the lack of uniform in-volvement of vessels and organs—are responsible for not finding vasculitis in 100% of all biopsies in patients with unequivocal vasculitis. In Wegener's granulomato-sis, upper airways biopsies will have a

positive yield <20% of the time, whereas open lung biopsies of abnormal pulmonary parenchyma may have a yield of as much as 90%.

8. A lung biopsy that reveals necrotizing granulomatous inflammation and vasculitis supports the diagnosis of *only* Wegener's granulomatosis or, if eosinophils are present, Churg-Strauss syndrome.

T_____ F_____

Answer and Discussion

False. These findings may also occur in granulomatous infections such as those due to tuberculosis, atypical mycobacteria, or fungal diseases.

9. Visceral angiography provides diagnostic information that is as revealing as a biopsy of involved organs.

T_____ F_____

Answer and Discussion

False. Angiography is not as specific as histopathol-ogy. Vessels may become stenotic or aneurysmal due to processes other than vasculitis (e.g., Ehlers-Danlos syndrome [type IV], infection, fibromuscular dysplasia, atherosclerosis).

10. Vasculitis associated with hepatitis B or C virus or HIV may have a phenotypic appearance similar to

a) Polyarteritis nodosa

b) Churg-Strauss syndrome

c) Wegener's granulomatosis

d) Giant cell arteritis

Answer and Discussion

The answer is a. The same size vessels may be affected in polyarteritis nodosa (PAN), microscopic polyangiitis (MPA), and viral vasculitides, especially those due to hepatitis and HIV. Thus, the disease phenotypes of PAN and MPA should have viral diagnostic studies as part of their assessment.

SUGGESTED READINGS

Guillevin L, Cohen P, Gayraud M, et al. Churg-Strauss syndrome: clin-ical study and long-term follow-up of 96 patients. *Medicine (Balti-more)* 1999;78(1):26–37.

Hoffman GS, Weyend CM, eds. *Inflammatory Diseases of the Blood Ves-sels.* New York: Marcel Dekker, 2002.

Koening CL, Langford CA. Novel therapeutic strategies for large vessel vasculitis. *Rheum Dis Clin North Am* 2006;32(1):173–186.

Molloy ES, Langford CA. Advances in the treatment of small vessel vasculitis. *Rheum Dis Clin North Am* 2006;32(1):157–172.

Salvarani C, Cantini F, Boiardi L, et al. Polymyalgia rheumatica and giant-cell arteritis. *N Engl J Med* 2002;347(4):261–271.

Specks U. Antineutrophil cytoplasmic antibodies. *Arthritis Rheum* 1998;41:1521–1537.

Vassilopoulos D, Calabrese LH. Hepatitis C virus infection and vas-culitis: implications of antiviral and immunosuppressive therapies. *Arthritis Rheum* 2002;46(3):585–597.

Chapter 32

Selected Musculoskeletal Syndromes

Brian F. Mandell

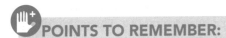POINTS TO REMEMBER:

- When evaluating musculoskeletal pain, eliciting tenderness that does not mimic the patient's pain syndrome is not diagnostic.

- Similar to the situation in the hip, pain surrounding the knee is frequently attributed to osteoarthritis of the knee, especially in the elderly. However, pain in the knee area can be referred from the hip joint, the lumbar spine, and (rarely) the foot in patients with significant pes planus and tightened calf muscles.

- An extremely common cause of regional knee pain, especially in patients with osteoarthritis of the medial compartment of the knee or pes planus, is pain in the area of the pes anserine bursa. Patients with this syndrome frequently complain of pain localized to the medial aspect of the leg slightly below the joint line.

- Acute shoulder pain in the absence of trauma is most frequently caused by rotator cuff disease (periarthritis), rather than true shoulder joint disease.

Musculoskeletal pain is one of the most frequently listed chief complaints of patients seeing general internists. Some of these complaints relate to osteoarthritis or inflammatory joint disease, but the majority are due to soft-tissue musculoskeletal syndromes. Many of these pain syndromes are self-limited or reversible with short-term injection, anti-inflammatory or physical therapy. Clinical recognition of specific syndromes limits the need for expensive diagnostic testing. In particular, recognizing specific syndromes obviates the need for laboratory evaluation or musculoskeletal imaging. As a generality, defined regional pain syndromes or isolated and localized joint pain does not warrant the evaluation of autoimmune serologies.

Although the pathophysiology of many of these syndromes is incompletely understood, accumulated experience permits the clinical diagnosis of discrete syndromes and allows for empiric, therapeutic interventions. Despite the common occurrence of these syndromes, controlled clinical outcome studies have rarely been reported in the medical literature.

HIP GIRDLE SYNDROMES

Pain in the hip region in elderly patients is frequently attributed to hip osteoarthritis. In the elderly, as well as in young patients, however, a focused examination of the painful area may delineate one of several nonarticular pain syndromes. True hip joint discomfort is classically felt by the patient deep to the inguinal crease; swelling or warmth is exceedingly rare in adults. Occasionally, true hip joint pain is felt primarily in the deep gluteal area or radiating down the thigh as far as the knee. Hip joint pain may be elicited by passive range of motion of the hip joint, but is not usually reproduced by palpation. Examination should include:

- Passive internal rotation
- Passive external rotation
- Passive abduction
- Passive flexion
- Passive posterior extension

This last motion, undertaken with the patient lying on his or her abdomen, is frequently neglected. It is uncommon for isolated hip (joint) disease to manifest *only* as lateral hip pain reproducible with pressure over the trochanteric area.

Lateral Hip Pain

The syndrome of lateral hip pain, reproduced with firm pressure to this area, has generally been termed *trochanteric* or *pseudotrochanteric bursitis*. A differential diagnosis of this lateral hip pain syndrome exists, but most commonly it is attributed to trochanteric "bursitis."

Examination of the area is best undertaken with the patient lying on the contralateral side with the upper (symptomatic) leg flexed toward the chest and adducted across the body, with the medial aspect of the upper knee resting on the table. This pulls the tissue overlying the trochanteric area fairly taut, permitting easier examination. The superficial trochanteric bursa directly overlies the trochanteric prominence, and this area should be gently palpated. The deep trochanteric bursa area is proximal and slightly posterior and sits in a deep groove. It can be easily palpated in this position. A reproduction of the patient's pain with pressure in these areas prompts a clinical diagnosis of trochanteric bursitis. When evaluating musculoskeletal pain, eliciting tenderness that does not mimic the patient's pain syndrome is not diagnostic.

This syndrome is exceedingly common and often does not respond to analgesics or nonsteroidal anti-inflammatory drug (NSAID) therapy. It may respond dramatically to local infiltration with lidocaine and a deposit steroid. Injection should be made deep within this tissue area, but not into the periosteum because this provokes extreme and persistent discomfort. As with all steroid injections, the patient should be forewarned about the possibility of infection, as well as atrophy or skin discoloration. The syndrome of trochanteric bursitis is often precipitated by mechanical factors, including primary hip or knee disease, pes planus or other foot disorders, and altered gait because of low back pain or new shoes. Mimics of this syndrome with radiation of pain into the same anatomical area include:

- High lumbar radiculopathy
- Hip abductor muscle strain
- Entrapment neuropathy
- Stress fractures of the femoral neck or pelvis

If the pain is attributable to trochanteric bursitis, the local infiltration of several milliliters of lidocaine or bupivacaine (Marcaine) will provide at least transient, and usually complete, relief of the discomfort. Patients will report that they are able to lie comfortably on this side, which they were not able to do prior to the injection. The inclusion of corticosteroids in the injection provides lasting relief in approximately 70% of patients, perhaps for as long as several months. If a gait disturbance or hip disease is present, the pain will likely return. For isolated trochanteric bursitis, pain relief may be indefinite after a single injection (or, occasionally, several injections). Failure of two (or at most, three) injections to relieve the pain should prompt an aggressive search for other underlying etiologies of the pain, including a generalized myofascial pain syndrome such as fibromyalgia.

The coexistence of trochanteric pain with degenerative disease of the spine or the hip must be noted, although the exact relationship between these conditions is not clear. If pain radiates down the leg from the trochanteric bursa and can be elicited by firm pressure along the fibrous tissue surrounding the muscle bundles (fascia lata), physical therapy directed at stretching this fibrous muscle area should also be provided. Gluteal tendonitis very frequently coexists with trochanteric bursitis, and injection into the tendon sheath area may also be necessary along with physical therapy. The anatomical trochanteric bursa is rarely actually distended with fluid (by imaging), but septic trochanteric bursitis has been reported.

The lasting value of interventional physical modalities, including ultrasonography, transcutaneous electrical nerve stimulation unit application, iontophoresis, or deep heat, has not been clearly established in controlled studies.

Gluteal Pain

Gluteal pain can be caused by strain in the gluteal muscles or a bursitis involving the bursa overlying the ischial prominence and under the gluteal muscles.

Ischial bursitis is best diagnosed with the patient standing and forward flexed at the hips; the area of tenderness can be palpated by firm pressure along the ischial prominence. Gluteal bursitis can be elicited by deep palpation along the gluteal muscles with the muscles pulled taut while the patient is in a lateral position.

Piriform syndrome is a controversial entity, presumably caused by spasms of the piriformis muscle. Patients complain of moderate, severe, or even deep disabling lateral buttock pain. Deep palpation of the piriformis muscle in the lateral upper quadrant of the buttock area, or, more specifically, by rectal wall examination, is considered to be diagnostic. Pain may radiate posteriorly to the upper portion of the thigh. Patients may walk with an antalgic gait. Pain may be elicited with forced internal rotation of the hip against resistance. Treatment, which is also controversial, may include physical therapy or local injection. Acute sacroiliac joint arthritis also can cause buttock pain.

Meralgia Paresthetica

Entrapment of the lateral femoral cutaneous nerve causes the syndrome of meralgia paresthetica. Entrapment usually occurs overlying the superior iliac spine under the inguinal ligament. The clinical syndrome is marked by an area of intense dysesthesia, often with numbness on careful pinprick examination in a patch of skin on the anterior thigh. It can be associated with rapid weight gain, as can be seen in pregnancy, or with use of a tight, constraining belt. Treatment is supportive. No additional evaluation is necessary. It is not associated with systemic disease. It should be remembered, however, that herpes zoster may be heralded by an area of dysesthesia without visible skin lesions.

KNEE PAIN

Similar to the situation in the hip, pain surrounding the knee is frequently attributed to osteoarthritis of the knee, especially in the elderly. However, pain in the knee area can be referred from the hip joint, the lumbar spine, and (rarely) from the foot in patients with significant pes planus and tightened calf muscles.

Examination of the knee should include evaluation for:

- Crepitus
- Synovial thickening, tenderness, or fluid
- Reproduction of pain with pressure and movement of the patella
- Mechanical stability
- Popliteal fullness
- Specific bursitis or tendonitis

An extremely common cause of regional knee pain, especially in patients with osteoarthritis of the medial compartment of the knee or with pes planus, is pain in the area of the pes anserine bursa. Patients with this syndrome frequently complain of pain localized to the medial aspect of the leg slightly below the joint line. Pain is frequently exacerbated by the act of rising from a low chair, walking up steps, and occasionally in bed at night as the two knee areas touch. Patients may describe the need to sleep with a pillow between their legs to avoid the painful pressure of their knees touching. Pain can be elicited by gentle palpation approximately 1 cm below the joint line on the medial aspect of the leg. It is most important to be certain that the pain that is elicited with firm, but not extreme, palpation is the exact pain that the patient experiences; tenderness to palpation alone is not sufficient to make this diagnosis (tenderness is common in normal individuals).

This syndrome frequently does not respond to NSAID therapy, but strikingly responds to local injection. The pain can be debilitating, yet it is often dramatically and immediately relieved by a local infiltration of lidocaine. Corticosteroid is frequently included in the injection mixture.

Prepatellar bursitis is a frequent cause of swelling in the knee area. The area of swelling may appear as a fluctuant mass immediately anterior to the patella. This is frequently a result of direct trauma and is an occupational hazard of patients who work in a kneeling position. The aspiration of the traumatically induced serosanguineous fluid may relieve the discomfort; however, this bursa can be inflamed owing to infection (most frequently, *Staphylococcus aureus*) or gout. Infection is frequently associated with surround-

ing cellulitis and may mimic joint inflammation. The bursa does not communicate with the joint; care should be taken to distinguish this entity from actual arthritis. An attempt at true knee joint aspiration should not be undertaken unnecessarily, especially through an overlying cellulitis. Recurrent bursitis may be relieved by intrabursal steroid injection once infection has been excluded.

ELBOW AREA

The olecranon bursa separates the skin from the olecranon process. Frequently, after minor trauma (e.g., friction or resting of the elbow on a hard surface), the bursa may be distended with sterile, noninflammatory, often serosanguineous fluid. In this case, it may respond to drainage and the injection of a local corticosteroid preparation (once infection has been excluded). The bursa may be involved with urate crystal–induced inflammation or occasionally with infection, similar to the prepatellar bursitis of the knee. Cell counts in septic bursitis are generally much lower than in septic arthritis. Frequently, a surrounding cellulitis is present, with pitting edema of the soft tissue. *S. aureus* is the most common infecting agent.

Specific pain syndromes in the area of the lateral or medial epicondyles of the elbow—tennis and golfer's elbow, respectively—are extremely common. Both pain syndromes are believed to be caused, in part, by frequent and vigorous use of the forearm muscles. Lateral epicondylitis may be reproduced by palpation to the specific area surrounding the lateral epicondyle; however, more specifically, pain can be elicited by resisted, active extension of the middle finger. Pain will radiate specifically to the area of the lateral epicondyle and often to the forearm. Epicondylitis may respond to rest, use of a forearm band, and NSAID therapy. Infiltration of the area with a mixture of lidocaine and a low dose of deposit corticosteroid preparation may be of value in providing more rapid relief, but long-term outcome in most series is identical to treatment with physical therapy alone. Surgical intervention is rarely required. Care must be taken when injecting the medial epicondyle area to avoid the median nerve. Ultrasound high-energy therapy has been shown in some studies to be of benefit. Carpal tunnel syndrome can occasionally cause radiation of discomfort up the forearm toward the elbow region.

THE HAND

Carpal tunnel syndrome, caused by the compression of the median nerve as it travels through the carpal canal, is common. Recognized associations include:

- Diabetes mellitus
- Trauma
- Pregnancy
- Hypothyroidism

- Repetitive palm trauma
- Synovitis of the wrist (most commonly from rheumatoid arthritis)

Association is also recognized with primary and dialysis-related (not secondary) amyloidosis. The development of carpal tunnel syndrome as an overuse (computer) syndrome is debatable. The clinical recognition of the syndrome is by:

- Reproduction of dysesthesias in the appropriate distribution by pressure over the carpal canal (distal to the wrist crease at the base of the palm)
- Elicitation of the symptoms with percussion in the same area by finger or reflex hammer (Tinel's sign)
- Phalen's maneuver

Early in the course of the syndrome, neurologic deficits are not present; however, two-point discrimination and detailed sensory testing over the area of the thumb, index, and middle finger may demonstrate sensory loss. Dysesthesias are occasionally described to occur in all five digits or as extending proximally up the arm. The diagnosis can be confirmed after it has been present for a significant period of time, using nerve conduction testing. In a recent Swedish study, however, 20% of *asymptomatic* volunteers had abnormal conduction of their median nerve compatible with carpal tunnel syndrome.

Initial treatment should include splinting the wrist in a slightly hyperextended, near-neutral position. A local injection of corticosteroid into, or adjacent to, the carpal canal may provide relief but should be performed only by someone with experience and knowledge of the anatomy. Surgical treatment is usually (but not always) curative if nerve damage has not occurred, but large outcome studies are not available. Pregnancy-associated carpal tunnel syndrome may persist for several months post partum, even with the use of a splint.

De Quervain's tenosynovitis, a common cause of pain on the radial aspect of the hand, is frequently described by the patient as thumb or wrist pain. This can occur as a sporadic pain syndrome but is frequently induced by repetitive resisted motion of the thumb. The condition may occur with increased frequency in women caring for a newborn infant. Typical clinical presentation consists of pain overlying the radial styloid, radiating into the thumb and occasionally up the forearm. Visible swelling and erythema may be present over the tendon sheath of the extensor pollicis brevis. Pain can be elicited by resisted abduction of the thumb or by having the patient place the thumb inside a closed fist with gentle movement of the fist by the examiner in an ulnar direction. Pain is elicited over the radial styloid. This syndrome should be distinguished from osteoarthritis of the metacarpophalangeal joint at the base of the thumb. The initial treatment of the tendonitis can be conservative, with use of a custom-made resting thumb splint and NSAID therapy. Some authors have proposed primary infiltration

of the tendon sheath with a corticosteroid-lidocaine mixture. Care should be taken with the injection to avoid the snuffbox area and the radial artery.

Trigger finger can occur owing to the presence of noninflammatory fibrous nodules in the flexor tendon sheath of the palmar tendons. Patients describe the finger(s) as being stuck in a flexed position, with the need to be forcibly extended, eliciting a resultant sharp, painful pop. Frequently, patients may awaken with their finger or thumb "stuck" in a flexed position. Treatment can include passive splinting of the involved finger in an extended position, with or without local infiltration of corticosteroid into the flexor sheath nodule. This should result in the shrinkage of the nodule and less triggering. Progressive fibrosis of the flexor tendons, with contracture and nodularity of the palmar fascia, results in *Dupuytren's contractures.* Most trigger fingers do not evolve into this syndrome. Nonsurgical treatment is usually effective, and surgical intervention is rarely required. Acute severe palmar fasciitis has been rarely associated with carcinoma of the ovary and lung.

SHOULDER AREA

Acute shoulder pain in the absence of trauma is most frequently caused by rotator cuff disease (periarthritis) rather than true shoulder joint disease. Glenohumeral synovitis occurs in the setting of rheumatoid arthritis and polymyalgia rheumatica (mild synovitis and bursitis). Periarthritis can occur in young, active people and in anyone after overuse of the musculature of the shoulder girdle. Pain from periarthritis is frequently described as worsened by specific motions, particularly with extension of the arm. Sharp pain with abduction or full arm motion is termed *impingement* and is often caused by pressure on an inflamed tendon sheath on a bone, osteophyte, or ligamentous structure in the area of the shoulder girdle. Passive joint motion on examination is not as painful as active or resisted motion. Attempts should be made at delineating the specific involved tendon using resistive stressing of the individual tendons of the rotator cuff. The most common form of rotator cuff tendonitis involves the supraspinatus tendon. This can be evaluated by having the patient elevate his arm with the thumb pointed toward the ground; the examiner applies downward pressure, and the patient resists this motion. Pain is usually referred to the deltoid and upper arm region.

Generally, pain with passive motion of the glenohumeral joint within the normal range of motion does not elicit pain in the absence of glenohumeral synovitis. An examination of the shoulder should also routinely include palpation of the acromioclavicular and sternoclavicular joints. Acromioclavicular osteoarthritis can cause pain when the patient reaches across his or her body in the anterior plane or reaches far behind his back, as when putting on a jacket. Cervical radiculitis can also refer to the shoulder area. Posterior pain can be due to a periscapular trigger point or scapulocostal syndrome. Pain from this latter syndrome, reproduced by pressure in a trigger point underneath the medial aspect of the scapula on the chest wall, may radiate down the arm and across the chest. Pain can also be referred to the shoulder area from within the thorax or a subdiaphragmatic, hepatic, or splenic process; in this case, pain is not generally reproduced by active or passive shoulder motion.

The treatment of shoulder periarthritis and rotator cuff tendonitis can be accomplished with a course of NSAID therapy or the injection of corticosteroid and anesthetic into the subacromial space. Injection into the space from the lateral approach through the subacromial bursal area is the safest approach. Physical therapy, with emphasis on range of motion, should be emphasized to avoid the development of adhesive capsulitis (more common in patients with diabetes).

LUMBAR CANAL STENOSIS

Lumbar canal stenosis (spinal stenosis) occurs in the setting of degenerative joint and disc disease. It is characterized by the subacute or, occasionally, acute onset of bilateral leg and back discomfort. The leg discomfort may occur in a pattern of pseudoclaudication of calves or thighs and can mimic vascular ischemia. Because this syndrome occurs in an elderly population, it frequently coexists with the physical findings of peripheral vascular disease. Deep tendon reflexes may be preserved; specific nerve root symptoms are usually not elicited. A clinical clue to distinguish lumbar stenosis from vascular claudication is that pseudoclaudication from the former is often reduced when the patient is bent forward at the waist (i.e., walking while leaning forward on a grocery cart).

Diagnosis is generally made by performing MRI of the lumbar canal and evaluating for vascular occlusion. In the absence of cauda equina syndrome, marked neurologic deficits are not generally appreciated. The pain can be quite limiting to the patient's activity and is frequently associated with lumbar pain.

Conservative treatment is successful in many patients, with the focus on extension-oriented physical therapy. Surgical intervention is an option for patients who fail conservative therapy. Some patients may find the use of subcutaneous calcitonin helpful for the relief of pain, although this should be viewed as experimental therapy.

FIBROMYALGIA

Fibromyalgia is a generalized pain syndrome. It occurs in patients of all ages and seemingly occurs at an increased frequency in patients with underlying systemic disease such as rheumatoid arthritis, systemic lupus erythematosus, multiple sclerosis, and inflammatory bowel disease.

Neurologic complaints of dysesthesia are common; however, objective neurologic abnormalities on physical and electrical examination are absent. No inflammatory markers are present through laboratory testing. Synovitis is notably absent in primary fibromyalgia. Quite frequently, an associated subjective sleep disturbance is reported, with a complaint of not feeling refreshed in the morning. Patients frequently describe multiple awakenings during the night. Mild dryness of eyes or mouth is a frequent complaint. The presence of multiple discrete myofascial tender points on examination is characteristic; the presence of these tender points is required to make an unequivocal diagnosis, but may not be present at the time of every examination. Pressure should be applied to a degree that the fingernail of the examiner is noted to barely blanch with the pressure. Neutral points should also be evaluated. The number of involved tender points and the intensity of tenderness may vary dramatically between different examinations. The tender points are frequently in areas of common myofascial pain syndromes previously described (trochanteric, gluteal, pes anserine); the distinguishing characteristic of the fibromyalgia syndrome is the generalized nature of this pain sensitivity. In the absence of discrete tender points, the diagnosis should be made with trepidation because these features often overlap those of patients having chronic fatigue syndrome. However, these tender points may not be elicited on any given examination day, and, in some patients, tender points are not prominent.

Clinical recognition of this pain syndrome should dramatically limit the need for laboratory testing. Serologic testing has no role in a patient who has no features of specific autoimmune disease (e.g., systemic lupus erythematosus or rheumatoid arthritis). Care should be taken when making this diagnosis, however, to exclude by detailed history and physical examination the presence of an underlying disorder such as hypothyroidism, hypocortisolism, or primary depression. Many patients with fibromyalgia have features of depression with somatization; however, not all patients are clinically depressed.

Treatment is directed at the maintenance of normal activities; reversal of the abnormal sleep cycle (if present) with the use of low doses of soporific tricyclic antidepressants, if not contraindicated; and sparse, judicious use of medications such as cyclobenzaprine (Flexeril), acetaminophen, and NSAIDs. Chronic use of NSAIDs should be discouraged. Narcotics, corticosteroids, and most other chronic pain medications should be avoided. Regular aerobic exercise is believed to be of value in maintaining patient function. Pregabalin has an approved indication for the treatment of the pain of fibromyalgia. Cognitive and stress reduction therapies including mindful meditation can be of significant value in some patients. The distinction between fibromyalgia and chronic fatigue syndrome can be difficult, if not impossible; the conditions are frequently treated in a similar manner.

REVIEW EXERCISES

QUESTIONS

1. A 56-year-old overweight woman with radiographic osteoarthritis of the right knee presents with a chief complaint of increasing, limiting knee pain, most notable when rising from a chair or toilet, while walking up stairs, and in bed at night. Examination reveals valgus deformity with walking, minimal cool-knee effusions, and tenderness to palpation (which mimics the pain) at the medial aspect of the joint, approximately 2 inches distal to the joint line. You suggest

a) Full-dose NSAID trial (patient has been using over-the-counter preparations)
b) Quadriceps-focused strengthening regimen
c) Intra-articular steroid injection
d) Steroid injection of anserine bursa
e) a and b

Answer and Discussion

The answer is d. The pes anserine bursitis should be treated. Patients with osteoarthritis of the knee have many causes of pain. Anserine bursitis is one of the more common nonarticular ones. It is particularly common in overweight patients with valgus deformity. Pain is reproduced by local pressure. It often does not respond to nonsteroidal anti-inflammatory drugs but does respond to local injection. Osteoarthritis is not usually a cause of nocturnal pain in bed; however, patients with anserine bursitis get relief by relieving the pressure of their legs touching by sleeping with a pillow between their knees.

2. A 32-year-old previously healthy secretary complains of recent (3 months) onset of progressive pain in her right arm involving the second and third fingers, forearm, and upper arm. It awakens her from sleep and worsens while driving. It is at times associated with painful tingling. Physical examination reveals normal neck motion, negative Spurling's and Adson's test results, and normal shoulder examination results. Test results of pulses, deep tendon reflexes, pinprick, strength, and elbow are normal. A likely diagnostic test is

a) Nerve conduction of the distal median nerve
b) MRI of the cervical spine
c) Upper extremity angiography
d) Chemical sympathetic block

Answer and Discussion

The answer is a. The patient has carpal tunnel syndrome. Nerve conduction of the median nerve would likely provide the diagnosis. Local provocative testing with Tinel's sign, Phalen's maneuver, or direct compression might also provide suggestive information. Prolonged keyboard typing may be a risk factor. Other tests are not warranted based on the history and examination, which do not suggest radiculopathy, thoracic outlet, or reflex sympathetic dystrophy, or Raynaud's syndrome. Causes include wrist synovitis, hypothyroidism, diabetes mellitus, pregnancy, trauma, primary amyloidosis, acromegaly, and possibly polymyalgia rheumatica.

3. A 64-year-old former construction worker presents with increasing exertional bilateral calf pain and leg tingling. Leg symptoms have been present for 1 year but have worsened during cardiac rehabilitation for his recent myocardial infarction. He could only walk 0.4 mile on the treadmill because of leg pain. He switched to an exercise cycle, on which he could ride for 3 miles. Physical examination demonstrated decreased left distal pulses and a left iliac bruit, with normal foot temperature, color, deep tendon reflexes, pinprick, and strength. The study with high yield for diagnosis is

a) Angiography
b) Abdominal ultrasonography
c) Spinal MRI
d) Electromyography

Answer and Discussion

The answer is c. Although MRI of the spine has limited specificity for diagnosing disc disease and back pain, it is excellent for diagnosing spinal stenosis. This patient has peripheral vascular disease, but the positional aspects of claudication symptoms argue for the presence of neurogenic, not vascular, claudication. Spinal stenosis frequently coexists with peripheral vascular disease, and neurologic examination is often normal for age. Osteoarthritis of the spine is common. Physical therapy is often effective, and surgery may be curative.

4. A 28-year-old woman presents 2 months postpartum, complaining of 4 months of burning pain in her left thigh. She was told of carpal tunnel syndrome during her pregnancy and has been wearing wrist splints, but is now concerned regarding the possibility of multiple sclerosis. Physical examination reveals bilateral wrist Tinel's sign with a positive Phalen's maneuver. The results of hip examination are normal, with negative straight-leg raise. Deep tendon reflexes are preserved. No motor weakness is detected. There is an area approximately the size of a hand with marked dysesthesias to light touch on the anterior lateral left thigh. In addition to clinical diagnosis, a positive test result would include

a) Electromyography of the sacral plexus
b) Tinel's sign over the lateral inguinal ligament
c) Pelvic CT scan
d) Cerebrospinal fluid oligoclonal bands

Answer and Discussion

The answer is b. The patient has meralgia paresthetica caused by entrapment of the lateral femoral cutaneous nerve, which often occurs as it exits through the lateral inguinal ligament. It can be diagnosed clinically and usually requires no workup or treatment. It may accompany weight gain, the wearing of constricting garments, or overtight seat belts. Often self-limiting, it may respond to local steroid injection. A differential diagnosis might include prezoster neuralgia.

5. A 42-year-old woman, with a diagnosis of rheumatoid arthritis for 2 years (fairly well controlled on hydroxychloroquine, nabumetone, and 2.5 mg prednisone daily), 8 months after the birth of a healthy boy, presents for a routine visit complaining of increasing "pain all over." She describes an increase in morning stiffness of her back, neck, and hands; trouble sleeping; and difficulties with painful flares after exposure to any drafts or physical exertion.
The erythrocyte sedimentation rate is 22 mm/hour, and the rheumatoid factor is present in high titer. Joint examination shows multiple tender, nonswollen joints; normal grip strength; bilateral trochanteric bursitis, gluteal tenderness, and costochondritis; and anserine bursitis. The course of action should be to

a) Increase prednisone for 10 days and then taper.
b) Add methotrexate.
c) Add a tricyclic plus physical therapy.
d) b and c.

Answer and Discussion
The answer is c. The patient has fibromyalgia. The diagnosis is most likely secondary fibromyalgia, perhaps precipitated by the stress of a newborn child in the house. The symptoms will not respond to intensified therapy for the rheumatoid arthritis. A detailed examination will likely reveal additional myofascial trigger points. Education is another key element of the therapy.

SUGGESTED READINGS

Anderson BC, Manthey R, Brouns MC. Treatment of Du Quervain's tenosynovitis with corticosteroids: a prospective study of the response to local injection. *Arthritis Rheum* 1991;34:793–798.

Goldenberg DL. Fibromyalgia and chronic fatigue syndrome: are they the same? *J Musculoskelet Med* 1990;7:19–28.

Kang I, Han SW. Anserine bursitis in patients with osteoarthritis of the knee. *South Med J* 2000;93:207–209.

Mandell BF. Avascular necrosis of the femoral head presenting as trochanteric bursitis. *Ann Rheum Dis* 1990;49:730–732.

Pace JB, Nagle D. Piriform syndrome. *West J Med* 1976;124:435–439.

Shbeeb MI, O'Duffy JD, Michet CJ Jr, et al. Evaluation of glucocorticosteroid injection for the treatment of trochanteric bursitis. *J Rheumatol* 1996;23:2104–2106.

Smith DL, McAfee JH, Lucas LM, et al. Treatment of nonseptic olecranon bursitis: a controlled, blinded prospective trial. *Arch Intern Med* 1989;149:2527–2530.

Swezey RL. Pseudo-radiculopathy in subacute trochanteric bursitis of the subgluteus maximus bursa. *Arch Phys Med Rehabil* 1976;57:387–390.

Traycoff RB. "Pseudotrochanteric bursitis": the differential diagnosis of lateral hip pain. *J Rheumatol* 1991;18:1810–1812.

Chapter 33

Venous Thromboembolic Disease

Ossam Khan   Franklin A. Michota

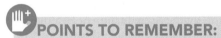

POINTS TO REMEMBER:

- It is estimated that up to 50% of deep vein thromboses (DVTs) are asymptomatic or go undetected.

- In autopsy-based studies, pulmonary embolism (PE) has been identified as the proximate cause or contributor to death in 15% to 30% of all patients.

- Inadequately treated DVT involving the popliteal or more proximal leg veins is associated with a 20% to 50% risk of clinically relevant recurrence and is strongly associated with both symptomatic and fatal PE. In untreated patients, death from PE occurs most frequently within 24 to 48 hours of initial presentation.

- Anticoagulants, such as heparin and low molecular weight heparin (LMWH), may help relieve symptoms related to vessel inflammation, but are probably best reserved for individuals with recurrent superficial vein thrombophlebitis or documented DVT.

- Predictive scoring rules combine patient history and exam elements with objective testing results and are recommended for the most efficient approach to DVT diagnosis.

- Failure to accurately and promptly diagnose DVT and PE can result in excess morbidity and mortality due to postthrombotic syndrome, pulmonary hypertension, and recurrent venous thromboembolic events.

Venous thromboembolic disease is the third most common cardiovascular disease after atherosclerotic heart disease and stroke. It has been estimated that between 500,000 and 2 million venous thromboembolisms (VTEs), including calf vein thrombosis, proximal DVT, and PE, occur annually in the United States alone. It is estimated that up to 50% of DVTs are asymptomatic or go undetected. Antemortem diagnosis may actually be made in less than one-third of patients with suspected PE. In autopsy-based studies, PE has been identified as the proximate cause or contributor to death in 15% to 30% of all patients. In general, VTEs are a major cause of sudden death and in-hospital morbidity and mortality. The extremely high incidence of DVT and PE likely reflects inadequate attention to VTE prophylaxis in high-risk surgical settings and the medically ill patient, in particular.

The spectrum of clinical outcomes secondary to venous thrombosis depends on the extent, location, and setting of the index event. The major clinical consequences of extremity DVT include the postthrombotic syndrome (chronic swelling, stasis dermatitis, stasis ulceration, and venous claudication, all secondary to venous insufficiency) and PE. The major clinical consequences of PE include chronic dyspnea, pulmonary hypertension, pulmonary infarction, and death. DVT restricted to the calf veins uncommonly results in a clinically important PE and is rarely associated with a fatal outcome. In contrast, inadequately treated DVT involving the popliteal or more proximal leg veins is associated with a 20% to 50% risk of clinically relevant recurrence and is strongly associated with both symptomatic and fatal PE. In untreated patients, death from PE occurs most frequently within 24 to 48 hours of initial presentation. All-cause mortality rates in treated patients with PE as high as 11% at 2 weeks and 17% at 3 months have been reported. Even small PE in patients with emphysema, cardiac disease, or lung involvement with malignancy may result in death. Any VTE in a patient with a contraindication to anticoagulation presents a therapeutic challenge and greater likelihood of adverse outcome. In part, for these reasons, calf DVT, proximal DVT, and PE have been considered distinct manifestations of thromboembolic diseases.

This chapter focuses on the diagnostic and therapeutic challenges of the full spectrum of venous thromboembolic disease routinely encountered by the general internist.

SUPERFICIAL THROMBOPHLEBITIS

Thrombosis involving the superficial veins of the lower or upper extremities is often viewed as a common but insignificant form of venous thrombosis and thus neglected by clinicians. Superficial vein thrombophlebitis (SVT) may be at the mild end of the venous thromboembolic disease spectrum with regard to morbidity secondary to limb compromise and PE, but it may be a strong indicator of underlying hypercoagulability or malignancy.

Clinical Presentation and Diagnosis

The diagnosis of SVT is often made on the basis of tenderness, palpable cord, and erythema overlying a superficial vein. SVT is not uncommon in the upper extremities after an indwelling intravenous catheter and in the lower extremities where varicose veins are present. The progression of SVT into the deep venous system has been reported to occur in 7% to 44% of cases. The most common location for the progression from SVT to DVT is at the junction between the greater saphenous vein (a superficial leg vein) and the common femoral vein (a proximal deep leg vein). In patients with SVT, PE in general and symptomatic PE in particular, has been found in 33% and 10% of cases, respectively. The proximity of an SVT to the junction between the involved superficial vein and its connection to the deep venous system does not seem to impact the likelihood of PE. Yet, several reports have described an association between SVT and concomitant DVT.

Treatment

Typically, nonsteroidal anti-inflammatory drugs (NSAIDs) and warm compresses are adequate treatment for SVT symptom control. When the deep system is involved, or symptomatic PE is diagnosed, standard anticoagulant therapy is indicated. Because of the reported high rate of progression from SVT to DVT (3.6% by day 12), many physicians treat SVT with anticoagulants for a variable length of time. Short-term (8–12 days) prophylactic-intensity, fixed-dose LMWH; treatment-intensity, weight-adjusted dose LMWH; and tenoxicam (an NSAID) have been shown to reduce DVT rates compared to placebo. Anticoagulants, such as heparin and LMWH, may help relieve symptoms related to vessel inflammation but are probably best reserved for individuals with recurrent SVT or documented DVT. Serial ultrasound to detect meaningful SVT progression seems

prudent in selected cases, such as those with SVT already present at the saphenofemoral junction. Inherited risk factors for thrombosis are found more commonly in persons with SVT than in controls, but testing has not been shown to warrant an alteration in treatment, impact the rate of progression, or support the need for serial ultrasound. Despite the fact that SVT has been associated with adenocarcinoma, searching for occult cancer with radiographic imaging is not recommended. Age- and gender-appropriate cancer screening is the most reasonable approach.

PREVENTION OF VENOUS THROMBOEMBOLIC DISEASE

The key to proper prophylaxis is the recognition of risk factors for thrombosis. According to the Best Health Care Practice Report by the National Quality Forum (NQF), all hospitalized patients should undergo a formal risk assessment for VTE, and those found to be at risk should receive appropriate prevention strategies. Recently, the NQF and the Joint Commission for the Accreditation of Health Care Organizations released national quality measures for VTE, including prophylaxis measures for hospitalized patients. Computer-based reminders for VTE prophylaxis in at-risk, hospitalized patients have been shown to increase prevention rates and commensurately reduce symptomatic VTE events. Many independent risk factors for VTE have been identified (Table 33.1), and the risk for VTE appears to be cumulative when multiple factors are present. Recent trial evidence confirms that medically ill patients (predominantly those immobilized with cardiopulmonary disease) have a high risk of developing DVT within 14 days of admission in the absence of active prophylaxis. The DVT rate is significantly reduced by the addition of a once-daily, fixed-dose of LMWH (enoxaparin 40 mg or dalteparin 5,000 U) or synthetic heparin pentasaccharide (fondaparinux 2.5 mg), without a concomitant increase in bleeding compared to placebo. Evidence-based guidelines continue to recommend heparin 5,000 U subcutaneously twice or thrice daily based on small placebo controlled trials from the early 1980s. It is unclear whether newer anticoagulants offer an efficacy advantage over standard heparin. Comparison trials have demonstrated the noninferiority of once-daily, fixed-dose LMWH to heparin 5,000 U administered subcutaneously three times a day in heterogeneous medical populations. There are data that LMWH once daily may be superior to heparin dosed three times daily in congestive heart failure patients. Recently, LMWH once daily was shown to have a superior overall net benefit compared to heparin 5,000 U twice daily in ischemic stroke patients. All hospitalized patients should be encouraged to ambulate frequently. Patients already receiving therapeutic-intensity anticoagulation derive no added benefit from the addition of prophylactic-intensity therapy. In patients who cannot receive pharmacologic prophylaxis, thromboembolism

TABLE 33.1
INDEPENDENT RISK FACTORS FOR VENOUS THROMBOEMBOLISM

Age older than 40 years
Restricted mobility
Varicose veins
Myocardial infarction
Congestive heart failure
Stroke
Paralysis
Spinal cord injury
Hyperviscosity syndromes
Polycythemia vera
Severe respiratory disease (pneumonia or chronic obstructive pulmonary disease)
Anesthesia
Surgery
Prior history of deep vein thrombosis (DVT)
Central venous access
Trauma (including hip fracture)
Cancer
Family history of DVT
Inflammatory bowel disease
Nephrotic syndrome
Obesity
Hormone replacement therapy/oral contraception pills
Pregnancy/peripartum period
Sepsis
Nonautologous blood transfusions
Thrombophilia
   Activated protein C resistance from factor V Leiden
   Antithrombin III deficiency
   Protein C or S deficiency
   Homocystinuria
   Antiphospholipid antibody syndrome
   Lupus anticoagulant
   Heparin-induced thrombocytopenia
   Prothrombin gene mutation

TABLE 33.2
WELLS CLINICAL PREDICTION RULE FOR DEEP VEIN THROMBOSIS (DVT)

Clinical Feature	Points
Active cancer (treatment within 6 months, or palliation)	1
Immobilization or paralysis of lower extremity	1
Recently bedridden for more than 3 days or surgery within the past 4 weeks	1
Localized tenderness along distribution of deep veins	1
Entire leg swollen	1
Calf swelling of >3 cm (below tibial tuberosity) as compared to asymptomatic leg	1
Unilateral pitting edema	1
Collateral superficial veins	1
Alternative diagnosis as likely as or more likely than DVT	−2

Pretest probability of DVT: ≥3 points: high risk (75%), 1–2 points: moderate risk (17%), <1 point: low risk (3%).

deterrence stockings and/or pneumatic antiembolism stockings should be used. Retrievable inferior vena caval filters may play a role in preventing PE in very high-risk patients (multisystem trauma) who cannot receive pharmacologic therapy due to risk of bleeding.

ACUTE VENOUS THROMBOEMBOLIC DISEASE

Deep Venous Thrombosis

Clinical Presentation and Diagnosis
DVT can present with limb pain, swelling, redness, warmth, or a palpable cord, or it can be asymptomatic. One should not rule in or rule out DVT based on clinical grounds alone. Predictive scoring rules combine patient history and exam elements with objective testing results and are recommended for the most efficient approach to DVT diagnosis (Table 33.2).

Outpatients, including those who present to the emergency department, should undergo D-dimer testing prior to objective imaging. Increased plasma concentrations of D-dimer reflect thrombus formation and concomitant fibrinolytic cascade activation. Because of its derivation from lysed thrombus and not from circulating fibrinogen, D-dimers have been extensively studied as a VTE diagnostic tool. Monoclonal antibody–based D-dimer assay methodologies differ with regard to ease of use, turnaround time, cost, sensitivity for VTE, and specificity for VTE. Traditional quantitative enzyme-linked immunosorbent assays (ELISAs) and rapid ELISA-derived assays have the best sensitivity and negative predictive value for DVT and PE. Many disparate conditions can lead to an elevation in D-dimer. These conditions may include VTE, myocardial infarction, pneumonia, sepsis, disseminated intravascular coagulation, liver disease, malignancy, surgery, hemorrhage, and trauma. Thus, D-dimer testing may be specific for cross-linked fibrin degradation products, but cross-linked fibrin degradation products are not specific for VTE. To put it simply, a positive D-dimer assay is of limited diagnostic use, whereas a negative test (D-dimer level of <500 ng/mL) with appropriate sensitivity (ELISAs) essentially excludes VTE. The specificity of D-dimer testing is particularly low in the very elderly suspected of having VTE (9% in patients older than 80 years). In cancer patients, who are at high risk for VTE because of the hypercoagulability of malignancy, D-dimer testing may lack sensitivity, specificity, and adequate negative predictive value for VTE exclusion. Therefore, D-dimer testing is best reserved for otherwise healthy outpatients suspected of acute VTE.

For suspected DVT involving the arms or legs, compression ultrasound is the preferred initial imaging test. A diagnosis of acute DVT is based on the inability to completely compress a venous segment. Acute DVT results in dilated, and often thickened, veins filled with uniformly echogenic material. Loss of flow phasicity, direct thrombus visualization, and aberrations on color flow imaging are less validated means of diagnosing DVT. Ultrasonography is noninvasive, rapid, and readily available at most hospitals. It is highly sensitive and specific (>95%) for acute symptomatic DVT and proximal DVT when performed by experienced ultrasonographers. Screening compression ultrasound in asymptomatic patients is less accurate. Another limitation of ultrasound is the inability to diagnose pelvic vein thrombosis. Venography remains the "gold standard" test but is invasive and requires intravenous contrast. MRI is an effective but costly means of diagnosing DVT. Today, computed tomographic venography (CTV) is used to look for DVT in conjunction with CT chest imaging for the evaluation of PE. CTV not only has similar diagnostic accuracy to compression ultrasonography for lower extremity DVT, but also has the ability to assess the pelvic veins. Despite this advantage, CTV should not be used in the evaluation of DVT without signs and symptoms for PE. Significant drawbacks to CTV include radiation exposure and the need for additional intravenous contrast.

Failure to accurately and promptly diagnose DVT and PE can result in excess morbidity and mortality due to postthrombotic syndrome, pulmonary hypertension, and recurrent VTE. Conversely, unnecessary anticoagulation therapy provides risk in the absence of any tangible benefit. Therefore, the proper and timely diagnosis or exclusion of DVT and PE is imperative to ensure optimal patient clinical outcome.

Proximal versus Distal Deep Vein Thrombosis

It is perceived by many that calf DVT is uncommon and of limited clinical significance. This misunderstanding and underappreciation of the morbidity and mortality associated with calf DVT has resulted in a lack of clear consensus on the optimal management strategy for this thrombotic disease. Contemporary clinical studies have revealed that isolated calf DVT may account for as few as 6.2% of all symptomatic acute DVT and as many as 43% of all acute VTE. Studies have also demonstrated that, although calf DVT and proximal DVT may be considered separate diseases at their outset, 15% to 25% of calf DVT propagate and convert into a proximal DVT. Symptomatic and asymptomatic calf DVT appears to propagate with an equal frequency. Such "proximal conversion" renders what was initially a calf DVT just as dangerous as any proximal DVT. Pain, swelling, redness, and increased warmth limited to the calf do not rule out a more proximal DVT. Proximal conversion has been shown to occur within the initial 2 weeks after diagnosis in the majority of cases and warrants treatment accordingly. Current treatment approaches for isolated calf DVT range from identical intensity and duration of anticoagulant therapy, as is used for proximal DVT, to a complete lack of any pharmacologic therapy at all.

Acceptable management, which falls between these extremes, includes serial duplex ultrasound surveillance, with therapy begun only in the event of proximal conversion, and abbreviated courses of standard anticoagulation. Surveillance consists of noninvasive imaging twice weekly for typically no more than 3 weeks (this includes the usual period for proximal conversion). The limitations of serial surveillance, however, include cost, compliance, and convenience. Serial surveillance seems especially prudent in situations such as recent gastrointestinal bleeding, in which the risk of anticoagulation would likely exceed the benefit.

Treatment

Before selecting an approach to DVT management, one must clearly appreciate the goals of therapy. The goals of DVT management include (a) prevention of embolization, (b) prevention of thrombus extension, (c) prevention of early and late recurrence, (d) restoration of venous patency, and (e) prevention of the postthrombotic syndrome. Supportive care alone (i.e., doing nothing) accomplishes none of these goals. The placement of an inferior vena cava (IVC) filter effectively prevents all PE in the short run but probably at the expense of a greater long-term DVT recurrence rate. Intravenous, activated partial thromboplastin time (aPTT)–adjusted, unfractionated heparin and weight-based LMWH effectively prevent embolization, extension, and recurrence. LMWH appears to be slightly but significantly better than standard heparin at restoring venous patency. Catheter-directed fibrinolytic therapy is the most effective means of completely restoring patency but is associated with excessive bleeding and significant cost. Fibrinolysis is best reserved for iliofemoral DVT in the young and those with extensive thrombosis resulting in venous limb gangrene (phlegmasia cerulea dolens).

Several prospective, randomized, controlled trials have demonstrated the equivalent efficacy and safety of intravenous, aPTT-adjusted unfractionated heparin and weight-based LMWH for the treatment of DVT. The major advantage of subcutaneous LMWH is its ability to be self-administered at home without the need for therapeutic monitoring. This translates into a significant reduction in mean hospital length of stay (6.5 days vs. 1.1 days). Patients may be started on LMWH in the hospital and then discharged in an accelerated fashion to continue their conversion to oral warfarin or treated exclusively in the outpatient setting. LMWHs are associated with less osteopenia, less heparin-induced thrombocytopenia, and less nonspecific protein binding than unfractionated heparin. Meta-analyses have demonstrated a survival advantage in those patients with acute DVT who have been treated initially with LMWH versus those treated initially with heparin. This overall survival advantage seems to be derived primarily from a survival advantage imparted on cancer patients with DVT. Of note, the anticoagulant effects of LMWHs are not completely reversed by protamine sulfate. Weight-based fondaparinux (synthetic heparin pentasaccharide) has also been shown to be equivalent to weight-based LMWH (enoxaparin) for the treatment of acute DVT.

Regardless of one's choice of heparin or location of initial therapy, a few key treatment issues must be noted:

- Treatment with intravenous, aPTT-adjusted heparin or weight-based LMWH or fondaparinux should be begun as soon as possible. A delay in achieving a therapeutic intensity of anticoagulation may negatively impact a patient's long-term VTE recurrence rate.
- Weight-based LMWH dosing is the current standard of care. If intravenous heparin is chosen, a weight-based initial dosing of heparin (80 U/kg bolus followed by 18 U/kg/hour) with subsequent dose adjustments based on a standardized nomogram should be used because it allows an aPTT to be reached quickly in the majority of patients.
- Heparin and LMWH therapy must overlap oral warfarin therapy for a minimum of 4 days and, ideally, until a stable target range (2.0-3.0) international normalized ratio (INR) has been achieved.
- The INR, not the prothrombin time or prothrombin time ratio, should be used to monitor warfarin therapy. Monitoring at least every 4 weeks is recommended. More frequent monitoring helps maintain the INR within the target range for a greater amount of time.

Warfarin therapy alone is contraindicated in the setting of acute thrombosis because of the inherent delay in achieving therapeutic anticoagulation and the theoretical transient exacerbation of hypercoagulability caused by a rapid reduction in protein C functional activity. This warfarin-induced paradoxical hypercoagulability may explain warfarin-induced skin necrosis and warfarin-induced limb gangrene in patients with heparin-induced thrombocytopenia. Warfarin therapy can be started as soon as a therapeutic level of heparin or LMWH has been reached. Thus, warfarin can be initiated concomitantly with the first subcutaneous LMWH or fondaparinux dose. Patients on intravenous heparin usually require a 24- to 48-hour delay to ensure a therapeutic aPTT. Bolus dosing of warfarin does not help more quickly achieve a target INR. Initial dosing with 2.5 to 7.5 mg/day (based on patient weight and nutritional status) seems prudent. Because of its teratogenic effects, warfarin therapy is generally contraindicated in pregnancy.

Patients at increased risk for bleeding should probably be treated initially in an inpatient setting. Such patients include those with active bleeding (including occult stool blood), a history of recent surgery and/or neuraxial anesthesia, past gastrointestinal tract bleeding, recent trauma or stroke, concomitant regular NSAID use, thrombocytopenia, and renal insufficiency. Severe renal dysfunction (creatinine clearance of <30 mL/minute) results in a 25% or greater reduction in LMWH clearance and thus results in drug accumulation. Severe renal impairment does not prohibit the use of enoxaparin as long as appropriate dose adjustments are made according to manufacturer guidelines. Unmonitored LMWH therapy may not be suitable for the morbidly obese. Drug doses that are adjusted according to weight are based on higher expected volumes of distribution. This relationship is not known to be linear at the extremes of weight, and patients may receive too much LMWH if dosed on actual body weight. Most reported clinical trials with LMWH have enrolled patients weighing ≤150 kg. LMWHs may be monitored by antifactor Xa activity assays, although this approach has not been studied clinically. Monitored heparin therapy using aPTTs is a reasonable choice for the morbidly obese with acute DVT.

Therapeutic monitoring of LMWH therapy using the antifactor Xa activity assay is not indicated in most patients. An exact therapeutic range has not been carefully determined. Adjusting the dose of LMWH based on such testing may not be superior to simple weight-based dosing in patients who are not at the extremes of weight.

The optimal duration of anticoagulation has been widely studied and debated. For idiopathic DVT, 3 months of therapy is better than 4 weeks, and 6 months is better than 6 weeks. In short, the risk of VTE recurrence is very low as long as therapeutic anticoagulation is continued. Only the 3% to 4% annual risk of major hemorrhage secondary to warfarin prevents physicians from prescribing long-term anticoagulation with abandon. Anticoagulation for 3 to 6 months is generally prescribed for individuals with a first DVT. Situational calf DVT (DVT with a clear precipitant, such as an inflammatory bowel disease flare and prolonged bed rest) can be safely treated for only 6 weeks, assuming the precipitating illness or event has resolved. Recurrent DVT after the completion of a course of anticoagulation usually warrants long-term therapy. Patients with persistent risk factors for thrombosis, such as an antiphospholipid antibody, hyperhomocysteinemia, incurable malignancy, or a deficiency of a natural anticoagulant (protein C, protein S, and antithrombin), usually benefit from long-term therapy.

Idiopathic Deep Vein Thrombosis

Idiopathic distal or proximal DVT may be the initial presentation of occult malignancy, and appropriate history, physical examination, and screening tests should be performed to detect cancer at its earliest stage. The likelihood of being diagnosed with a cancer within 1 year of an idiopathic DVT ranges between 2.5% and 22.6%. Most of these cancers are diagnosed during the index hospitalization for DVT and likely represent the underlying cause of the DVT itself. Thus, not only does cancer promote hypercoagulability and clinical thrombosis, but also idiopathic clinical thrombosis is a harbinger of cancer. A complete medical history, physical examination including digital rectal examination, chest radiograph, and basic laboratory testing are sufficient to uncover the majority of these thrombosis-associated cancers. Abnormal findings warrant further laboratory and imaging studies. Head-to-toe CT scanning is excessive and expensive. With the mounting popularity of outpatient strategies for VTE management, physicians must be sure to not overlook the importance of performing a thorough clinical assessment as a means of diagnosing cancer in its early stages.

With regard to hypercoagulable testing, physicians often focus too much on their ability to find an abnormality and focus too little on how the results of such testing will impact management and help the patient. Testing just to "see what one will find" is not acceptable. The results of testing rarely, if ever, impact acute VTE management. Testing may be best delayed until the patient has completed a course of anticoagulant therapy and has returned to a baseline state of health. A good rule is to obtain testing only if the results will impact at least one of the following:

- Type of anticoagulant therapy
- Intensity of anticoagulant therapy
- Duration of anticoagulant therapy
- Patient prognosis
- Family screening
- Family planning
- Concomitant medication use

Pulmonary Embolism

Clinical Presentation and Diagnosis

PE can present with pleuritic chest pain, dyspnea, palpitations, syncope, cough, dysrhythmias, hemoptysis, or pleural effusion, or it can be asymptomatic (silent PE). As is the case for DVT, one should not rule in or rule out PE based on clinical grounds alone, and PE predictive scoring rules that combine patient history and exam elements with objective testing results are recommended for the most efficient approach to PE diagnosis (Table 33.3).

Prior to the advent of contrast-enhanced, computed tomography pulmonary angiogram (CTPA), the ventilation-perfusion (V/Q) lung scan was the most frequently or-

TABLE 33.3

WELLS CLINICAL PREDICTION RULE FOR PULMONARY EMBOLISM

Clinical Feature	Points
Suspected deep vein thrombosis (DVT)	3
Other diagnosis less likely than pulmonary embolism (PE)	3
Heart rate >100 beats/minute	1.5
Immobilization or surgery within past 4 weeks	1.5
Previous DVT or PE	1.5
Malignancy (active or treated within 6 months)	1
Hemoptysis	1

Pretest probability of PE: >6 points: high risk (78.4%), 2–6 points: moderate risk (27.8%), <2 points: low risk (3.4%).

dered diagnostic test in those with clinically suspected PE. The perfusion study (Q scan) is performed using an intravenous injection of macroaggregated particles of technetium99m-labeled human serum albumin. Any obstruction to arterial flow is viewed as an area of nonperfusion or underperfusion and is termed a perfusion defect. The performance of ventilation scintigraphy (V scan) in individuals with abnormal Q scans helps improve test specificity. A V scan involves the inhalation of a radioactive gas or aerosolized technetium99m that provides an image of all ventilated portions of the lung. Based on the presence and extent of matched (absence of both perfusion and ventilation) and unmatched (absence of perfusion with preserved ventilation) defects, the scan can be interpreted using published criteria as either normal, low probability, indeterminate probability, or high probability for PE. The high negative predictive value of a normal or near-normal scan alone essentially excludes (<5% probability) PE. The high positive predictive value (approximately 90%) of a high-probability scan alone has led most physicians to consider such a scan as diagnostic of PE. A nondiagnostic (indeterminate) scan, one that is interpreted as low or intermediate probability, neither confirms nor refutes the diagnosis of PE and is best interpreted in the context of clinical suspicion and additional testing. For example, in patients in whom a low clinical suspicion for PE exists and who have a low probability scan, PE is unlikely. Other combinations of clinical probability and scan result usually warrant the performance of additional testing before a suitable diagnosis can be achieved. Patients with suspected PE, in whom treatment is withheld on the basis of a low pretest clinical probability and a nondiagnostic scan, have been shown to have a very low (1.7%) 3-month thromboembolic risk as long as lower extremity compression ultrasound does not reveal proximal DVT. The high prevalence of nondiagnostic studies and the failure of many physicians to establish a clinical probability for the likelihood of PE before obtaining and interpreting the scan are significant limitations to its use as a diagnostic tool. In the Prospective Investigation of Pulmonary Embolism Diagnosis (PIOPED) study, 73% of scans were nondiagnostic. This number may be as high as 90% in patients with underlying chronic obstructive pulmonary disease or other underlying pulmonary processes that can result in an abnormal chest radiograph. The scan is an appropriate "first test" to evaluate a patient with suspected PE, if the baseline chest radiograph is normal and there is no history of significant underlying pulmonary disease or history of prior PE.

Today, contrast-enhanced spiral CTPA is replacing the V/Q scan as the initial test of choice for PE diagnosis. With CTPA, PE is diagnosed by identifying a filling defect in the pulmonary arteries. When compared with scintigraphy or pulmonary angiography, the sensitivity and specificity of spiral CT have ranged widely from 53% to 100% and 78% to 100%, respectively. CTPA is best used to identify thrombus within the main pulmonary arteries, lobar pulmonary arteries, and first-order segmental branches of the pulmonary artery. A normal CTPA may not rule out PE and, like V/Q scanning, should be combined with an assessment of clinical probability and other diagnostic tests to arrive at a diagnosis. Whether subsegmental PE is clinically significant and necessary to definitively detect has been debated and is a central issue to consider when choosing a PE diagnostic modality. Data from the PIOPED study suggests that only 6% of PEs is subsegmental. The effects of a subsegmental PE may be negligible in patients with normal cardiopulmonary function. However, subsegmental PE could be disastrous in a patient with decreased cardiopulmonary reserve or severe underlying lung disease. The danger of fatal recurrent PE in patients with an initial subsegmental event is also always present. Two older meta-analyses that evaluated the use of spiral chest CT in the diagnosis of PE suggested that there was insufficient evidence to rely on a negative spiral chest CT scan to justify withholding anticoagulation or to support the insignificance of undetected subsegmental PE. However, the more recent PIOPED II study evaluated the diagnostic accuracy of CTPA combined with clinical suspicion and D-dimer measurement, and achieved positive predictive values similar to that found with V/Q scanning and pulmonary angiography combined with compression ultrasonography in PIOPED. Nonetheless, clinicians should remain cognizant of the potential pitfalls of CTPA. Patients unable to cooperate with breath holding create breathing artifacts that can change the orientation and the diameter of vessels. The presence of hilar lymphadenopathy or other mediastinal soft-tissue mass may mimic the appearance of PE. Any shunt, whether due to a patent foramen ovale or intrapulmonary circulation from pleuroparenchymal disease, or a left-to-right cardiac shunt with prominent bronchopulmonary circulation, may make the CT scan more difficult to accurately interpret. Perhaps the greatest benefit of CTPA is that up to 67% of chest CT scans can lead to or support an alternative diagnosis to explain a patient's presenting symptoms. Therefore, CTPA may be the optimal initial test for PE in undifferentiated patients, particularly those with baseline abnormal chest radiographs. Other factors that may influence the choice between CTPA and V/Q scanning include specific medical contraindications to intravenous contrast use (e.g., contrast allergy or impaired renal function), the lack of local expertise or appropriate equipment in the use of CTPA, personal preferences of the clinicians (e.g., the wish to reduce radiation exposure to patients), or local experience with other imaging modalities.

The role of D-dimers in the evaluation of PE is similar to that of DVT. Testing for D-dimers is highly sensitive for PE, but it is not specific for thrombosis. A negative test essentially rules out thrombosis; a positive test essentially means nothing.

Pulmonary angiography is the historical gold standard for PE diagnosis, to which all other imaging modalities have been compared. PE is diagnosed by the identification of an intraluminal filling defect or arterial cut-off demonstrated in two imaging planes (perpendicular views). Inter-interpreter variability can be high, and the sensitivity for peripheral, subsegmental PE has been questioned. The advantages of pulmonary angiography include the ability to perform adjunctive procedures, such as suction thrombectomy, local catheter-directed thrombolysis, and IVC filter placement, at the same time as the diagnostic procedure. The procedure, however, is invasive and associated with death, major complications, and minor complications in 0.5%, 1%, and 5% of cases, respectively. Pulmonary angiography is most often used as a second- or third-line diagnostic modality. Modern multidetector CT scanners combined with a cooperative patient (minimal breathing artifact) and specialized radiologists have made pulmonary angiography relatively unnecessary for purely diagnostic purposes.

Treatment

In general, acute PE should be treated in the same fashion as acute DVT. It is actually advisable to start anticoagulation at the time of suspected PE even before diagnostic testing has been performed. Weight-based LMWH and fondaparinux have been shown to be safe and effective in patients with acute PE treated in hospital. Outpatient treatment of PE seems reasonable but has not been formally studied to date.

The placement of an IVC filter at the time of PE diagnosis is usually reserved for those with an absolute contraindication to anticoagulation. Many physicians, however, place filters in patients with underlying cardiac or pulmonary disease who are perceived as being at risk for death should they develop a second PE. It is important to note that active bleeding may be a treatable and transient contraindication to anticoagulation. The role of a retrievable IVC filter in this setting has yet to be defined, but may offer an advantage over a permanent filter in that the IVC filter could be removed once anticoagulation was able to be initiated. An IVC filter should not be viewed as an equivalent substitute to anticoagulation in the setting of acute VTE, and it is certainly not an "insurance policy" against subsequent PE. In patients with filters placed because of bleeding, appropriate anticoagulation should begin as soon as the bleeding source has been properly and completely treated. Because of the significant risk of rebleeding, such a patient should have the anticoagulation begun in the hospital. IVC filters, unlike anticoagulation, do not prevent thrombus extension or thrombus recurrence. IVC filters may promote the formation of DVT. Patients with permanent IVC filters have a relative indication for lifelong anticoagulation.

Thrombolysis has been shown to decrease pulmonary artery pressures and clear PE more rapidly than standard anticoagulant therapy. Survival does not appear to be significantly affected, however. Thrombolysis is probably best reserved for the acute treatment of PE patients with significant hemodynamic or respiratory compromise.

Conflicting data exist on whether patients with evidence of right ventricular dysfunction, in particular, benefit from thrombolysis. The obvious major risk of thrombolytic therapy is bleeding.

CHRONIC VENOUS THROMBOEMBOLIC DISEASE

Recurrent Venous Thromboembolism

Choosing the duration of warfarin therapy requires balancing the risks of recurrent and fatal VTE off warfarin therapy against the risks of major and fatal bleeding on warfarin therapy. The rate of recurrent VTE at 1 year following 6 months of oral anticoagulation is approximately 3% to 5%. However, in the setting of unprovoked or idiopathic VTE, the 1-year recurrence rate increases to approximately 10% and, in the setting of cancer, the rate is 20%. The PREVENT (Prevention of Recurrent Venous Thromboembolism) trial compared low-intensity oral warfarin with placebo for the secondary prevention of venous thrombosis, following a standard 6-month course of therapy for an index idiopathic DVT with or without PE. Warfarin with a target INR between 1.5 and 2.0 (low intensity) monitored every 8 weeks resulted in a 64% reduction in thrombosis recurrence rate without a significant difference in major bleeding rate. Subsequently, the ELATE trial investigators concluded that conventional-intensity warfarin therapy (INR 2–3) was more effective than low-intensity therapy (INR 1.5–2.0) because the bleeding rates in their head-to-head comparison were found to be the same. Ultimately, the main message from both studies is that patients with idiopathic VTE benefit from ongoing anticoagulation. However, the intensity that best balances efficacy and safety remain unclear. A summary of recommendations is shown in Table 33.4.

If a patient develops a recurrent VTE in the face of a below-target (<2.0) INR, this may not be a warfarin failure. In this setting, reinstitution of heparin or LMWH until the INR can be properly targeted and regulated is acceptable.

If a lupus anticoagulant is detected, an alternative means of anticoagulation monitoring is indicated. If a persistent and potent prothrombotic state exists, one can either aim for a higher target INR or switch to an alternative anticoagulant. Aiming for an INR in the range of 3.0 to 4.0 is empiric, most likely associated with greater bleeding, and still associated with wide INR fluctuations. Switching to weight-based, treatment-dose LMWH seems justified. IVC filter placement will solely prevent further PE in the short run and will serve as a nidus for subsequent thrombosis in the long run. Fondaparinux may also be an acceptable alternative.

Postthrombotic Syndrome

The postthrombotic syndrome (PTS) develops in up to 50% to 80% of all patients with DVT. This syndrome was once believed to be a late complication of DVT, but it is now known that the majority of cases develop within 2 years of the index acute DVT. Signs and symptoms of PTS include chronic lower extremity swelling, pain, and ulcers. These are believed to develop due to venous hypertension that results from disruption of venous valves from the thrombus itself or from thrombus-associated mediators of inflammation.

Treatment typically focuses on the control of pronounced dependent edema and the tedious healing of venous stasis ulcers. It may take months and thousands of dollars to heal one ulcer, only to have recurrent ulceration within 1 year in approximately one-fourth of cases. Prevention is a must. Many have hoped that the early restoration of venous patency through thrombolytic therapy would translate into less PTS. Clinical trial evidence to this effect is still absent. The only modality shown to significantly reduce the incidence of all degrees of PTS is compression garment therapy. The prescription of fitted, below-knee, 30- to 40-mm Hg graduated compression stockings within weeks of an acute DVT has become an integral part of overall DVT management.

REVIEW EXERCISES

QUESTIONS

1. According to the National Quality Forum, all patients should receive which of the following on admission to the hospital?
a) Screening compression ultrasound of the lower extremities
b) Risk assessment for venous thromboembolism
c) Graded compression stockings
d) D-dimer assay
e) Hypercoagulability testing

Answer and Discussion

The answer is b. In its Best Health Care Practice Report in 2003, the National Quality Forum recommended

---

TABLE 33.4

GUIDELINES FOR DURATION OF ANTICOAGULANT THERAPY FOR VENOUS THROMBOEMBOLISM (VTE)

Risk Factor for VTE	Duration of Treatment (INR 2-3)
Minor transient factor	3 months
Major risk factor	6 months
Unprovoked	Indefinite
Uncontrolled malignancy	Indefinite

INR = international normalized ratio.

that all patients admitted to the hospital undergo a formal risk assessment for venous thromboembolism (VTE), and those found to be at risk should receive appropriate methods of prevention. Ultrasonography and D-dimers should be reserved for patients with signs and symptoms of deep vein thrombosis (DVT) for which a diagnostic evaluation is indicated. Hypercoagulability testing is only indicated in patients with a previous history of idiopathic DVT and in whom a diagnosis would alter long-term management. Graded compression stockings may be used to prevent VTE in low-risk populations. They offer little incremental benefit in patients already receiving pharmacologic prophylaxis.

2. Which of the following statements regarding the diagnosis of deep vein thrombosis is true?
a) Computed tomography venography is the initial diagnostic test of choice.
b) Compression ultrasonography of the lower extremities has the greatest sensitivity in asymptomatic patients.
c) Elevated D-dimers help confirm the diagnosis.
d) MRI is an effective strategy for deep vein thrombosis diagnosis, but it is costly.
e) All the statements are true.

Answer and Discussion
The answer is d. Compression ultrasonography is the initial imaging test of choice, not computed tomography venography. However, compression ultrasonography has the greatest sensitivity in symptomatic patients. D-dimers are best used to help rule out, not rule in, deep vein thrombosis. MRI is an effective diagnostic strategy, but due to cost concerns it is not feasible as an initial choice.

3. For patients being evaluated for pulmonary embolism in the setting of an abnormal baseline chest radiograph, what is the percentage of indeterminate V/Q scans that can be expected?
a) 10%
b) 25%
c) 50%
d) 70%
e) 100%

Answer and Discussion
The answer is d. Ventilation-perfusion (V/Q) scans are reported as normal, low probability, high probability, and indeterminate. In the PIOPED study, 73% of V/Q scans in the setting of an abnormal chest radiograph were indeterminate. Today, contrast-enhanced computed tomography pulmonary angiogram (CTPA) is becoming the initial imaging test of choice for the evaluation of pulmonary embolism. CTPA can lead to or support an alternative diagnosis to explain a pa-

tient's presenting symptoms in two-thirds of patients. V/Q scanning should be used in patients with a normal baseline chest radiograph.

4. Which of the following is not an indication for inferior vena cava filter placement?
a) Acute venous thromboembolism (VTE) with an immediate contraindication to anticoagulation
b) Recurrent VTE in the setting of therapeutic anticoagulation
c) Patients with pulmonary embolism and pulmonary hypertension
d) Prevention of perioperative deep vein thrombosis
e) All of the above

Answer and Discussion
The answer is d. Inferior vena cava (IVC) filters do not prevent deep vein thrombosis (DVT); in fact, they may promote the formation of DVT. IVC filters can prevent pulmonary embolism in perioperative setting, but the use of permanent filters in this setting would inappropriately place patients at risk for future DVT and the postthrombotic syndrome. Retrievable filters offer a potential option for high-risk perioperative patients, but this approach is experimental right now.

5. A 78-year-old man with prostate cancer presents to the emergency department with an acute left superficial femoral deep vein thrombosis. His daughter is a nurse and lives with her father. He is 90 kg, and his creatinine is 3.2 mg/dL. Which of the following is the most appropriate treatment plan?
a) Outpatient enoxaparin 1 mg/kg subcutaneously every 12 hours with a 4-day minimum overlap of warfarin until a stable international normalized ratio (INR) of 2 to 3 is reached
b) Inpatient tinzaparin 175 U/kg subcutaneously daily with a 4-day minimum overlap of warfarin until a stable INR of 2 to 3 is reached
c) Inpatient intravenous activated partial thromboplastin time–adjusted unfractionated heparin with a 5-day minimum overlap of warfarin until a stable INR of 2 to 3 is reached
d) Outpatient fondaparinux 5.0 mg subcutaneously daily for 3 to 6 months before overlapping with warfarin
e) Outpatient enoxaparin 1 mg/kg subcutaneously daily for 3 to 6 months before overlapping with warfarin

Answer and Discussion
The answer is e. This patient has deep vein thrombosis in the setting of active cancer. According to the American College of Chest Physicians, weight-adjusted dose low molecular weight heparin for 3 to 6 months prior to warfarin overlap is the optimal strategy. However,

this patient also has severe renal impairment (creatinine clearance <30 cc/minute); thus, he needs a renal dose adjustment of his enoxaparin. Fondaparinux is contraindicated with a creatinine >2.0 mg/dL.

SUGGESTED READINGS

Büller HR, Agnelli G, et al. Antithrombotic therapy for venous thromboembolic disease: the seventh ACCP conference on antithrombotic and thrombolytic therapy. *Chest* 2004;126(3 Suppl):401S–428S.

Büller HR, Davidson BL, et al. Fondaparinux or enoxaparin for the initial treatment of symptomatic deep venous thrombosis: a randomized trial. *Ann Intern Med* 2004;140(11):867–873.

Deitcher SR, Gomes MPV. Hypercoagulable state testing and malignancy screening following venous thromboembolic events. *Vasc Med* 2003;8:33–46.

Geerts WH, Pineo GF, Heit JA, et al. Prevention of venous thromboembolism: the seventh ACCP conference on antithrombotic and thrombolytic therapy. *Chest* 2004;126(3 Suppl):338S–400S.

Kearon C, Ginsberg JS, et al. Comparison of fixed-dose weight-adjusted unfractionated heparin and low-molecular-weight heparin for acute treatment of venous thromboembolism. *JAMA* 2006;296(8):935–942.

Kearon C, Ginsberg JS, et al. Comparison of low-intensity warfarin therapy with conventional-intensity warfarin therapy for long-term prevention of recurrent venous thromboembolism. *N Engl J Med* 2003;349(7):631–639.

Kucher N, Koo S, Quiroz R, et al. Electronic alerts to prevent venous thromboembolism among hospitalized patients. *N Engl J Med* 2005;352:969–797.

Meignan M, Rosso J, Gauthier H, et al. Systematic lung scans reveal a high frequency of silent pulmonary embolism in patients with proximal deep venous thrombosis. *Arch Intern Med* 2000;160:159–164.

Qaseem A, Snow V, et al. Joint American Academy of Family Physicians/American College of Physicians. Current diagnosis of venous thromboembolism in primary care: a clinical practice guideline from the American Academy of Family Physicians and the American College of Physicians. *Ann Fam Med* 2007;5(1):57–62.

Ridker PM, Goldhaber SZ, Danielson E, et al. Long-term, low-intensity warfarin for the prevention of recurrent venous thromboembolism: a randomized, double-blind, placebo-controlled trial. *N Engl J Med* 2003;348:1425–1434.

Samama MM, Cohen AT, Darmon JY, et al. A comparison of enoxaparin with placebo for the prevention of venous thromboembolism in acutely ill medical patients. Prophylaxis in Medical Patients with Enoxaparin Study Group. *N Engl J Med* 1999;341:793–800.

Simonneau G, Sors H, Charbonnier B, et al. A comparison of low-molecular-weight heparin with unfractionated heparin for acute pulmonary embolism. *N Engl J Med* 1997;337:663–669.

Snow V, Qaseem A, et al. Management of venous thromboembolism: a clinical practice guideline from the American College of Physicians and the American Academy of Family Physicians. *Ann Intern Med* 2007;146(3):204–210.

Chapter 34

Lung Cancer

Joseph G. Parambil   Atul C. Mehta

 POINTS TO REMEMBER:

- In the United States in 2006, 26% of all cancer deaths in women and 31% of all of those in men were caused by lung cancer.

- Lung cancer continues to be the most common fatal malignancy in both genders.

- Histopathologically, bronchogenic carcinoma may be categorized as follows:

- *Non–small-cell lung cancer* (NSCLC), which includes:
  - Adenocarcinoma (30%–35%)
  - Squamous cell carcinoma (30%–32%)
  - Large cell carcinoma (10%)
  - *Small–cell lung cancer* (SCLC) (20%–25%)

- Over the past 30 years, there has been an increased incidence of adenocarcinoma, and this may be attributed to modifications in the histologic classification of lung cancer, increased environmental carcinogens exposure, and increasing incidence of lung cancer detection in women.

■ Adenocarcinoma and large cell carcinoma tend to spread systemically relatively early in their course. Squamous cell carcinoma frequently invades locally prior to systemic spread. SCLC has a very aggressive behavior, with mediastinal and extrathoracic spread at the time of presentation.

■ Surgical resection is the treatment of choice for NSCLC because it offers the best prospect of long-term survival. Unfortunately, only 20% to 33% of patients have resectable disease at the time of diagnosis, and the most commonly performed surgical procedure is lobectomy.

■ Two orally administered tyrosine kinase (TK) inhibitors that specifically target the epidermal growth factor receptor-TK domain, including erlotinib and gefitinib, have been shown to confer a survival advantage for patients with NSCLC, especially in women who never smoked with adenocarcinoma and, particularly, bronchioloalveolar cell carcinoma.

As the leading cause of cancer (Ca) death in the United States, lung Ca continues to be a major health hazard. From 1990 to 2000, lung Ca mortality decreased in men by 1.7%; however, it increased in women by 1%. In the United States in 2006, 26% of all Ca deaths in women and 31% of all of those in men were caused by lung Ca. Although the death rate was expected to have peaked in the 1990s, it will remain high over the next two to three decades.

Lung Ca continues to be the most common fatal malignancy in both genders. The American Cancer Society estimates that 174,770 new cases of lung Ca were diagnosed in 2006, and it is estimated that 162,460 persons died of the disease. The World Health Organization (WHO) estimates that 2 million cases of lung Ca will occur annually worldwide.

ETIOLOGY OF LUNG CANCER

Approximately 90% of all lung Ca is linked to cigarette smoking, the latter being the most important risk factor. The relationship between smoking and lung Ca has been appreciated since the 1950s. In general, smokers have 10 to 25 times the incidence of lung Ca compared with nonsmokers. However, less than 20% of cigarette smokers develop lung Ca, and it may be that other factors do play a role in the disease. When smokers quit, they experience a progressive decline in lung Ca risk that is noticeable 5 years after they stop smoking; after 15 years of abstinence, the risk of developing lung Ca is near that of a lifelong

nonsmoker. Given the inadequate smoking cessation rates with currently available pharmacologic and psychological measures, smoking reduction appears to play a significant risk-modifiable role; among individuals who smoke 15 or more cigarettes per day, smoking reduction by 50% significantly reduces the risk of lung Ca. Cigar and pipe smokers are also at higher risks of developing aerodigestive tract cancers, including lung Ca. The odds of lung Ca are 5.6 and 7.9 in cigar and pipe smokers, respectively, versus nonsmokers.

Many factors are clearly related to a high risk of developing bronchogenic carcinoma:

■ Number of cigarettes smoked
■ Duration in years of smoking
■ Early age at initiation of smoking
■ Depth of inhalation
■ Tar and nicotine content in the cigarettes smoked
■ Use of nonfiltered versus filtered cigarettes

Women who smoke up to half-pack per day have four times the risk for death from lung Ca as nonsmokers; those who smoke one to two packs per day have more than 20 times the risk. Smoking rates among women decreased from 33% in the 1970s to 25% in the 1990s, whereas rates among men declined from 43% to 28% in the same time period. Unfortunately, no decrease in smoking rates has been observed among those 18 to 24 years of age, suggesting that increased advertising and sales promotion by the tobacco industry are successfully reaching this age group. The prevalence of smoking among adolescents has remained unchanged (or even increased slightly) in the past few years. For example, in 2001, 28% of high school seniors had smoked within the previous 3 days. By 2003, the proportion had increased to 30%. Smoking among college students has increased dramatically during the past decade. Of adults ages 18 to 24 years, 45% had used tobacco in the past year, and 33% are current users of tobacco. It has been estimated that every day, 3,000 more young people become regular smokers. A person who has not started smoking as a teenager is unlikely to ever become a smoker. Therefore, it is important that our efforts be directed at preventing young people from starting to smoke.

Second-hand smoking also increases the risk of lung Ca. The effect of passive smoking and lung Ca risk, under conditions of domestic exposure, increases a nonsmoker's low risk by about 30%. The significance of this lies not in the magnitude of the risk for any passive smoker exposed individually, which is quite small, but in the number of excess Ca deaths owing to the frequency of such environmental exposure in the general population. It is estimated that second-hand smoking from spouses of heavy smokers may explain 3,000 to 5,000 lung Ca deaths in the United States every year.

The carcinogenic substances in cigarette smoke are only partially understood. More than 40 carcinogens have been identified in cigarette smoke, including:

- Polycyclic aromatic hydrocarbons
- Nickel
- Vinyl chloride
- Aldehydes
- Catechols
- Peroxides
- Nitrosamines

Evidence suggests that the formation of benzo[a]pyrene causes strong and selective adduct formation at guanine positions in codons 157, 248, and 273 of the *p53* gene. This, in turn, appears to shape the p53 mutational spectrum in lung Ca, providing a direct etiologic link between a chemical carcinogen present in cigarette smoke and human Ca.

Mutations of the *p53* gene are among the most frequent abnormalities occurring in lung Ca. Other significant mutations include those involving the *Rb-1*, *p16*, and *ErbB2* genes. Another frequent mutation is in the *FHIT* gene, which is abnormally spliced in lung Ca, and it has been suggested that this gene is a target of tobacco carcinogens. A host of other genes have been implicated in lung Ca, including N-myc, K-ras, p73, Smad-2, Smad-4, and PTEN, as well as various chromosomal abnormalities, including del(3p) and del(9p). Common polymorphisms of certain genes may help explain why some smokers and passive smokers are more susceptible to lung Ca than others. In particular, the GST-1 null allele is associated with increased risks of lung Ca, especially in women.

The use of filter-tipped, low-tar, and low-nicotine cigarettes does not reduce the risk of lung Ca because smokers increase the number of cigarettes smoked and the depth of inhalation with these cigarettes, thus resulting in an increased nicotine and carcinogen intake. It has also been suggested that the use of menthol cigarettes may increase the relative risk of lung Ca over nonmenthol cigarettes by 1.45 in men; in effect, this suggests that menthol increases the lung Ca-causing effect of cigarette smoking in men.

Other well-documented lung carcinogens include:

- Asbestos
- Ionizing radiation
- Chromium
- Nickel
- Mustard gas
- Vinyl chloride
- Arsenic
- Isopropyl oil
- Hydrocarbons
- Chloroethyl ether

Many of these materials have a carcinogenic effect that is additive or synergistic with cigarette smoke. For example, asbestos exposure in nonsmokers increases the incidence of lung Ca by 3- to 5-fold; in smokers, this risk may be increased 70- to 90-fold.

Radon gas, the decay product of uranium in the earth, has been recognized as a carcinogen for many years. The interaction with cigarette smoking is synergistic. It is estimated that indoor and outdoor radon exposure, in conjunction with past or current cigarette smoking, may explain up to 20,000 lung Ca deaths in the United States, or roughly 5% to 10% of new lung Ca cases. The lifetime risk of a nonsmoker is 1 in 357; if radon was removed from all homes, this risk would decrease to 1 in 492. A lifelong nonsmoker in a home with a high level of radon may have a lifetime lung Ca risk of about 1 in 100; for a pack-a-day smoker, the risk increases to 1 in 14. With the removal of radon from all homes, the pack-a-day smoker's risk would decrease to about 1 in 20.

Less well-established risk factors include:

- Air pollution
- Idiopathic pulmonary fibrosis and pneumoconiosis
- Lung scar from prior mycobacterial or fungal infections
- Genetic determinants (e.g., elevated pulmonary cytochrome P450 enzymes)
- Vitamin A deficiency
- Vitamin E deficiency

PATHOPHYSIOLOGY OF LUNG CANCER

Histopathologically bronchogenic carcinoma may be categorized as follows:

- NSCLC, which includes
  - Adenocarcinoma (30%–35%)
  - Squamous cell carcinoma (30%–32%)
  - Large cell carcinoma (10%)
- SCLC (20%–25%)

These major cell types of lung Ca have been associated with cigarette smoking. Over the past 30 years, there has been an increased incidence of adenocarcinoma, and this may be attributed to modifications in the histologic classification of lung Ca, increased environmental carcinogens exposure, and an increasing incidence of lung Ca detection in women. This increase in lung Ca in women may be due to decreased inherent DNA repair capacities, increased propensity toward *p53* gene mutations, and increased expression of gastrin-releasing peptide in females that stimulates cell proliferation.

Adenocarcinoma forms acinar or glandular structures on histologic examination and usually presents as a solitary peripheral nodule. Bronchioloalveolar cell carcinoma (BAC), an uncommon subtype of adenocarcinoma (3% of all invasive lung malignancies), has unique histologic and clinical presentations. BAC might present as a solitary nodule, multiple diffuse nodules simulating interstitial lung disease, or as lobar consolidation mimicking infectious pneumonia. This carcinoma arises from terminal bronchioloalveolar regions and tends to grow in a lepidic pattern along alveolar walls, rather than invade lung parenchymal structures directly.

Squamous cell carcinomas (SCCs) are composed of flattened or polygonal, stratified, epithelial cells that form intercellular bridges and elaborate keratin. This tumor tends to be central and bulky, usually with an intrabronchial granular or polypoid component that predisposes to luminal obstruction and distal atelectasis. SCC is the cell type most prone to cavitation, although in recent years, a higher incidence of cavitated adenocarcinomas has been reported.

Large cell carcinomas are composed of pleomorphic cells with variably enlarged nuclei and prominent nucleoli with abundant cytoplasm. They do not show squamous or glandular differentiation by light microscopy. The diagnosis of large cell carcinoma might be overestimated because tumors without clear differentiation are often classified as large cell tumors, when in fact they may actually represent adenocarcinomas with poor differentiation. Most of these tumors, similar to adenocarcinoma, are peripheral lesions that are usually unrelated to bronchi except for continuous growth. The metastatic pattern of large cell carcinoma is also similar to adenocarcinoma, with cerebral metastases occurring in half the cases.

SCC, adenocarcinoma, and large cell carcinoma belong to the clinical category of NSCLC. They are separated from SCLC because therapy is different. SCLC was believed to originate from the neuroectoderm, but actually may develop from a common pulmonary stem cell, with secondary differentiation into a cell type with neural characteristics. From the histologic point of view, SCC is a very cellular tumor with scanty cytoplasm and little stroma. SCC expresses many neurohormones that may act locally or may have paraneoplastic systemic effects. Approximately 80% of small cell tumors are central in location and are found mainly submucosally. SCLC is characterized by rapid clinical growth and frequent spread to mediastinal lymph nodes without involving the bronchial tree. Metastatic dissemination on clinical presentation is common in these tumors.

CLINICAL PRESENTATION OF LUNG CANCER

In general, the clinical presentation of lung Ca depends on the cell type. Adenocarcinoma and large cell carcinoma tend to spread systemically relatively early in their course. SCC frequently invades locally prior to systemic spread. SCLC is very aggressive, with mediastinal and extrathoracic spread at the time of presentation. Approximately 15% of all patients are asymptomatic at the time of diagnosis; the tumor is found incidentally as a chest radiographic abnormality. Forty percent of patients present with cough, whereas 70% to 80% develop cough during the course of the disease. A change in the character of the cough in a smoker is a significant clinical manifestation and should trigger the search for a neoplasm. Streaky hemoptysis is present in 60% of patients, while wheezing, dyspnea, stridor, symptoms due to postobstructive pneumonia,

and nonspecific chest pain are occasional presenting symptoms. Bronchorrhea is an uncommon initial presentation of BAC; when it is present (20% of patients), it usually indicates extensive lung involvement.

Other signs and symptoms resulting from local tumor spread include:

- Hoarseness due to involvement of the left recurrent laryngeal nerve, resulting in vocal cord paralysis
- Superior vena cava syndrome secondary to compression or invasion of the superior vena cava
- Pleural effusion owing to direct malignant invasion of the pleural space, mediastinal lymphatic obstruction, or parapneumonic effusion from postobstructive pneumonia
- Esophageal obstruction
- Pericardial involvement with malignant effusion and cardiac tamponade
- Myocardial involvement
- Vertebral invasion

In cases of superior sulcus tumors (Pancoast's tumors), the direct invasion of the apex of the lung causes C7/T2 neuropathy and Horner's syndrome.

Extrathoracic manifestation of lung Ca may be attributable to direct tumor infiltration (metastasis) or to the nonmetastatic paraneoplastic syndromes. Metastatic disease commonly involves:

- Thoracic lymph nodes
- Central nervous system (CNS)
- Liver
- Bone
- Adrenal glands

Bone and CNS involvement are usually symptomatic. SCLC frequently involves the bone marrow (up to 50% of cases) with or without peripheral hematologic abnormalities.

Paraneoplastic syndromes occur in 10% to 15% of patients with lung Ca. Paraneoplastic syndromes are manifestations of malignancies not caused by the direct invasion of the tumor, infection, or side effects of the therapy of the primary tumor. The paraneoplastic syndromes most commonly associated with lung Ca include:

- Hypercalcemia of malignancy
- Syndrome of inappropriate antidiuresis (SIADH)
- Ectopic Cushing's syndrome
- Paraneoplastic neurologic syndromes

The hypercalcemia of malignancy is predominantly associated with SCC, although it may be caused by adenocarcinoma and large cell carcinoma. Present in 15% to 20% of patients with advanced lung Ca, hypercalcemia is caused by the secretion of parathyroid hormone–related peptide in 85% of the cases. This peptide, which has characteristics and functions similar to that of parathyroid hormone, increases osteoclast activity, with resulting increased resorption of bone. The management of hypercalcemia of malignancy in patients with lung Ca includes hydration, inhibition of bone resorption by the administration of bisphosphonates, and treatment of the malignancy. Other treatment options include the use of calcitonin and plicamycin.

The syndrome of inappropriate diuresis is caused by the ectopic secretion of arginine vasopressin, most frequently by SCLC. Atrial natriuretic factor and inappropriate thirst play an important role in the pathogenesis of this syndrome as well. The management of patients with SIADH includes the treatment of SCLC, fluid-water restriction, and use of demeclocycline and fludrocortisone. In severe symptomatic hyponatremia, the use of hypertonic saline and furosemide administration may be needed.

Ectopic Cushing's syndrome is caused by the secretion of proopiomelanocortin, a precursor of adrenocorticotropic hormone. The treatment of the ectopic Cushing's syndrome includes the management of the tumor, as well as administration of adrenal enzyme inhibitors such as ketoconazole, metyrapone, and aminoglutethimide. The administration of the somatostatin analog octreotide has also shown some efficacy. Bilateral adrenalectomy may be considered in selected cases of refractory disease.

Paraneoplastic neurologic syndromes, present in 1% to 3% of patients with lung Ca, are more commonly associated with SCLC. The most common of these is the Lambert-Eaton myasthenic syndrome, an autoimmune disorder of the neuromuscular junction that is characterized by muscle weakness and autonomic dysfunction. Other paraneoplastic syndromes of the neuromuscular junction and muscle include dermatomyositis and acute necrotizing myopathy. Paraneoplastic syndromes can affect the CNS and include paraneoplastic cerebellar degeneration, limbic encephalitis, brainstem encephalitis, Ca-associated retinopathy, paraneoplastic opsoclonus-myoclonus, and stiff person syndrome. Paraneoplastic syndromes can affect the peripheral nervous system as well and include chronic gastrointestinal pseudo-obstruction, sensory neuropathies, sensorimotor neuropathies, and neuromyotonia.

DIAGNOSIS OF LUNG CANCER

Screening

Mass screening of high-risk patients with serial chest radiographs and/or sputum cytology has not shown a favorable impact on survival in patients with lung Ca with no significant improvement in overall survival noted when all patients entered into these studies were analyzed. Consequently, no consensus exists that high-risk patients should undergo yearly chest radiographs or sputum cytology. Nevertheless, for the individual high-risk patient concerned about Ca, it may be reasonable to screen periodically, especially if the patient has multiple risk factors (e.g., a smoker who has been exposed to asbestos and radon). In the pres-

ence of significant chronic obstructive pulmonary disease, a yearly chest radiograph may be helpful.

More recently, low-dose spiral CT has been helpful in the early diagnosis of lung Ca. Low-dose spiral CT is a promising technique that allows the complete imaging of the chest in one breath-hold. Currently, however, no guidelines support the routine screening of patients with low-dose spiral CT, and this technique cannot be recommended for routine practice until further randomized studies clearly demonstrate greater benefit than potential harm.

Diagnostic Studies

Radiography

Most asymptomatic lung Ca are detected on plain chest radiographs (CXRs). However, lesions <5 to 6 mm in diameter are rarely noticed on CXR. Nearly 50% of lung Ca lesions identified on CXR are <4 cm in diameter. In general, the radiographic appearance of a lesion will not distinguish between a benign or malignant process. The radiographic characteristics suggestive of malignancy include lobulation, and margins that are shaggy and ill-defined. Adenocarcinoma usually presents as a peripheral lung lesion and represents 40% of all peripheral lung tumors. BAC presents as a solitary nodule, numerous unilateral or bilateral nodules, or lobar or segmental consolidation.

SCC presents centrally in almost 65% of cases and may cause partial or complete luminal obstruction with radiographic changes of distal atelectasis, postobstructive pneumonia, lung abscess, and mucoid impaction. When SCC presents in a peripheral location, the tumor usually cavitates and may resemble a lung abscess.

Large cell carcinoma is more frequently peripheral (72%) and tends to be sharply defined. The majority of lesions are >4 cm in diameter on presentation.

SCLC is a predominantly central lesion and presents as a hilar mass, which almost never cavitates. Although the primary lesion does not tend to obstruct the central airways, the metastatic adenopathy can cause extrinsic compression of the airways, with subsequent atelectasis or postobstructive pneumonia. SCLC rarely occurs peripherally.

Approximately 30% of all lung Ca presents as a solitary nodule. Solitary pulmonary nodules (SPNs) are characterized by a single lesion up to 3 cm in diameter, surrounded by lung parenchyma. In the United States, the number of SPNs resulting from lung Ca is approximately 55,000 to 111,000 per year. Approximately 40% to 50% of SPNs are malignant. These malignancies are primarily lung Ca, but a small number (10%) are solitary metastatic deposits, and approximately 2% to 3% are carcinoid tumors. Most of the malignant solitary nodules are adeno- and large cell carcinoma. Small cell carcinoma and SCC rarely present as a SPN. Benign nodules are most often infectious granulomas. Other less common benign etiologies include hamartomas and other benign tumors, as well as noninfectious granulomas.

Establishing the etiology of an SPN is a major clinical challenge. The goal in the management of patients with an SPN is to identify malignant nodules that need surgery, while avoiding thoracotomy in those with benign lesions. Absence of growth in the size of the SPN for more than 24 months is often considered a reliable sign of benignity. The presence of characteristic patterns of calcification—such as homogenous, popcorn, laminated, and central calcification—is considered evidence of benignity. If the solitary nodule is noncalcified and the pattern of growth in the preceding 2 years cannot be determined, the probability of Ca based on associated clinical features must be assessed. Important clinical features suggestive of malignancy include:

- Size of the nodule (>3 cm)
- Age of the patient (patients younger than 35 years usually have benign nodules)
- Smoking history
- History of previous malignancy
- Chronic obstructive pulmonary disease (COPD)
- Radiologic characteristics of the edge of the nodule
- Presence or absence of occult calcification determined by CT

The imaging techniques more commonly used in the evaluation of an SPN include CXR and conventional CT. Obtaining previous CXRs is probably the most important diagnostic maneuver in the evaluation of a patient with an SPN. As noted, a lesion that has remained stable in size for more than 2 years is more likely to be benign. Benign nodules, usually of infectious etiology, tend to grow fast (i.e., faster than malignancies), with a doubling time of less than 21 days. Conventional CT allows better visualization of the nodule than does CXR, provides better definition of the margins, and helps detect calcification and the presence of multiple lesions.

In addition to CXR and conventional CT, other imaging techniques that have been used in the assessment of patients with an SPN include contrast-enhancement CT, MRI, and positron emission tomography (PET). For those nodules with indeterminant morphology, intravenous contrast enhancement with helical CT imaging may be a helpful adjunct. Nodular enhancement of >20 Hounsfield units (HU) is a predictive feature of malignancy while contrast enhancement of <15 HU is suggestive of benignity with a sensitivity of 98%, specificity of 73%, and 85% accuracy. MRI has no role in the routine evaluation of the patient with an SPN. The PET scan uses the uptake of 2[F-18]-fluoro-2-deoxy-D-glucose as a marker of hypermetabolism in the malignant tissue. A sensitivity of 96% and specificity of 93% has been reported in patients with indeterminate nodules, but PET scanning has significant limitations and is probably inadequate to evaluate small nodules of ≤1 cm. Contrast-enhancement CT and PET scans may be useful to rule out malignancy in those patients with an SPN who are at low to moderate risk for malignancy. However, if a patient is at high risk for lung Ca, the false-negative rate may remain unacceptable, and in these cases, tissue diagnosis is indicated.

If the noncalcified nodule is still of undetermined etiology after all the previous studies and the probability of Ca is high, then biopsy for tissue diagnosis is a reasonable course of action. If the probability of Ca is high, immediate thoracotomy, has the highest expected utility. In patients with low probability of Ca, however, a "wait and watch" strategy can be proposed.

Tissue Diagnosis

Currently available methods for the tissue diagnosis of suspected lung Ca include:

- Sputum cytology
- Flexible bronchoscopy
- Transthoracic needle aspiration
- Thoracotomy

Other techniques, potentially useful in selected cases, include thoracentesis, pleuroscopy, and mediastinoscopy.

Sputum Cytology

Sputum cytology is occasionally helpful in the diagnosis of central SCC and small cell carcinomas. The results are variable, and the interpretation may be technically difficult. A negative sputum cytology result does not rule out the presence of lung Ca in the appropriate setting.

Bronchoscopy

Flexible bronchoscopy (FB) is helpful in the diagnosis of central airway lesions. In this setting, FB is diagnostic in 90% of the cases. In cases of peripheral lesions (tumor visible on CXR but not on FB), FB has a diagnostic yield of 40% to 80% using transbronchial biopsy, brushings and washings, and biplanar fluoroscopy. This result is significantly lower than the yield in central lesions. The size of the lesion is the best determinant of diagnostic yield in peripheral lesions:

- Lesions <2 cm in diameter: 28% to 30% yield
- Lesions >2 cm in diameter: 64% yield
- Lesions >4 cm in diameter: 80% yield

The complications of FB, which are infrequent (5%), include hemorrhage, pneumothorax, laryngospasm, and transient hypoxemia. However, the yield with FB is significantly improving with advances made in the fields of endobronchial ultrasound and electromagnetic navigation.

Transthoracic Needle Aspiration Biopsy

Transthoracic needle aspiration biopsy has been used to diagnose lung masses and mediastinal lesions. Needle aspiration complements FB in establishing the diagnosis of lung abnormalities. The diagnostic yield of percutaneous transthoracic needle aspiration is >90% for peripheral lesions, but the frequency of complications is increased, reportedly 25% to 30%. Up to 15% of patients require treatment with a chest tube to re-expand the lung. Some of the features associated with lower diagnostic rates are smaller lesion size and central location.

It is important to emphasize that a negative result, unless it establishes a specific benign diagnosis, such as hamartoma, cannot be used to rule out carcinoma. If no clinical contraindication exists, one should proceed to thoracotomy.

Staging

After tissue diagnosis, staging is important to assess the extent of local and distant disease. Accurate staging is crucial in the selection of therapy and for prognostic purposes—the ultimate prognosis of patients with lung Ca depends largely on the stage of disease at the time of the diagnosis. The TNM (*Tumor, Node, Metastasis*) system is used to stage NSCLC. The TNM classification has been revised recently to provide greater specificity for identifying patient groups, and now more accurately reflects survival among homogenous groups:

- Resectable tumors
  - Stage IA (T1N0M0)
  - Stage IB (T2N0M0)
  - Stage IIA (T1N1M0)
  - Stage IIB (T2N1M0)
  - Stage IIB (T3N0M0)
  - Selected stage IIIA (T3N1M0) or (T1–3N2M0)
- Unresectable tumors
  - Stage IIIB (any T, N3, M0)
  - Stage IV (any T, any N, M1)

SCLC is generally not included in the TNM classification because 80% to 90% of tumors have spread beyond the thorax at the time of diagnosis and are in an advanced stage. SCLC has two stages: lmited disease (implies that the tumor is confined within a radiation port) and etensive disease (implies disseminated disease beyond a radiation port).

Clinical staging starts with a careful clinical history and complete physical examination. The history and examination are highly cost-effective staging tools. An examination of the hilar and mediastinal areas is a key step in the staging process; CT scan of the chest is useful in this situation because it offers significant advantages compared with the standard CXR. If the lymph node has a transverse diameter on CT scan of <1 cm, the likelihood of finding metastatic tissue is in the range of 3% to 16%. Nodes that have a diameter of 1 to 2 cm, however, have metastatic disease in 70% of cases and those of >2 cm have a greater chance of being malignant. When a lymph node is enlarged on CT, histologic examination is needed before assuming tumor involvement. Transbronchial needle aspiration, transthoracic needle aspiration, and mediastinoscopy are some of the techniques that have been used to sample mediastinal lymph nodes. Mediastinoscopy remains the standard for the purpose of mediastinal staging in non–small cell carcinoma patients. CT and MRI of the chest are of value in detecting chest wall or pleural involvement in patients with lung Ca. MRI has been found to be helpful, especially for patients who have superior sulcus tumors, for delineating vascular and neural invasion, and for patients with tumor invasion of the pericardium and heart. PET imaging has high sensitivity and specificity for assessing the presence of tumor within mediastinal lymph nodes.

COMPLICATIONS OF LUNG CANCER

The majority of lung cancers metastasize to the liver, CNS, bone, adrenal glands, and supraclavicular lymph nodes. The detection of extrapulmonary metastases begins with a thorough history and physical examination. Suspicious symptoms include weight loss, anorexia, neurologic symptoms, and localized bone pain. Laboratory data, including liver function tests, alkaline phosphatase, and calcium, are necessary and will indicate the need for further workup.

Frequently used screening imaging techniques include CT scan of the chest, which includes the liver and adrenal glands, and PET scan. A screening CT scan of the CNS is probably only justified in patients with adenocarcinoma. Patients with other types of NSCLC do not need a routine CT scan of the head unless there is clinical suspicion of CNS involvement.

In SCLC, extrathoracic staging is particularly important. In these patients, PET scan, and CT scan or MRI of the head is necessary to detect tumor spread. Bone marrow aspiration and biopsy are often used to detect tumor at this site. In patients with obvious metastases, however, examination of the bone marrow is not necessary.

TREATMENT OF LUNG CANCER

Non–Small Cell Lung Cancer

The three major treatment modalities for a patient with NSCLC are surgical resection, radiation therapy, and chemotherapy.

Surgical resection is the treatment of choice because it offers the best prospect of long-term survival. Unfortunately, only 20% to 33% of patients have resectable disease at the time of diagnosis, and the most commonly performed surgical procedure is lobectomy. The overall 5-year survival rate for all stages of surgically resected lung Ca is in the range of 40%:

- Stages IA and IB: 5-year survival of 67% and 57%, respectively
- Stages IIA and IIB: 5-year survival of 55% and 39%, respectively
- Stage IIIA: 5-year survival of 26%

Unfortunately, the majority of patients with NSCLC present with locally advanced (stage IIIB) or metastatic (stage IV) disease that is not curable through surgery and have poor 5-year survival rates of 5% and 1%, respectively. All patients with NSCLC should be evaluated for potential resection as initial therapy. Surgical procedures include pneumonectomy, lobectomy, segmentectomy, wedge resection, and sleeve bronchoplasty. An evaluation of pulmonary reserve must be carried out using pulmonary function tests in patients undergoing resection for lung surgery. A preoperative forced expiratory volume in 1 second (FEV_1) value of >2 L or $>80\%$ of predicted indicates good lung reserve, and the patient may tolerate even pneumonectomy. Patients who have an FEV_1 value $<80\%$ of predicted need a quantitative perfusion scan to predict postoperative lung function. A postoperative predicted FEV_1 of $<40\%$ of normal predicted, postoperative predicted diffusion capacity of $<40\%$, and presence of significant dyspnea suggests the potential for high morbidity and mortality in patients undergoing lung resection.

NSCLCs are relatively unresponsive to chemotherapy. Conversely, radiation therapy is effective in decreasing the size of local tumors in patients with NSCLC and SCLC. Radiation therapy is useful as a palliative measure, especially in patients who have obstruction of airways, compression of vital chest structures by the tumors, pain, or hemoptysis. Radiation therapy may be curative in $<15\%$ of patients with stage I NSCLC.

Abnormalities in several cell signaling pathways have been identified in NSCLC. Tumor growth and progression depends largely on the activity of cell surface membrane receptors that control the intracellular signal transduction pathways regulating proliferation, apoptosis, angiogenesis, adhesion, and motility. One such family of cell surface receptors is the receptor tyrosine kinases (TKs), which include the epidermal growth factor receptor (EGFR); EGFR exists as a monomer on the cell surface, and it must dimerize to activate the TK. Although the TK activity of EGFR is tightly controlled in normal cells, the genes encoding these receptors have escaped from their usual intracellular inhibitory mechanisms in malignant cells through amplification, overexpression, or mutation.

Two orally administered TK inhibitors that specifically target the EGFR-TK domain, including erlotinib and gefitinib, have been shown to confer a survival advantage for patients with NSCLC, especially in women who never smoked with adenocarcinoma, and particularly BAC.

Small Cell Lung Cancer

The treatment of SCLC remains nonsurgical in the vast majority of patients because of the high frequency of metastases at the time of diagnosis. In approximately 80% of cases, SCLC is sensitive to both chemotherapy and radiation therapy. The agents most commonly used for patients with SCLC include:

- Cisplatin and carboplatin
- Etoposide
- Vinorelbine
- Paclitaxel
- Docetaxel
- Gemcitabine
- Irinotecan

The majority of patients with limited disease have a complete response to chemotherapy. Only 15% to 20% of these patients with limited disease survive 3 years, however. Thoracic radiation is used in combination with chemotherapy to control local recurrence in patients with limited disease. Elective cranial irradiation has been used in complete responders to chemotherapy to treat occult brain metastasis but does not prolong survival.

In the uncommon patient with SCLC who presents with an isolated lung nodule, surgical resection is considered the treatment of choice, followed by adjuvant chemotherapy, with a cure rate of up to 50%.

Patients with extensive disease are treated with chemotherapy. The survival rate is 5% at 3 years.

PREVENTION OF LUNG CANCER

The most effective way to prevent lung Ca is to prevent smoking. Every physician has the duty to advise their patients about quitting smoking. Several agents are helpful in smoking cessation. The use of bupropion either alone or in combination with nicotine replacement is associated with a high abstinence rate and with a 20% continuous abstinence rate at 1 year versus 6% in patients given placebo. Other modalities, such as psychotherapy and consultation programs, may be of help as well. Recently varenicline, a partial agonist of nicotinic acetylcholine receptors, demonstrated continuous abstinence of 44% that was significantly higher than with bupropion.

Other modalities of prevention, such as chemotherapy prevention for lung Ca using β-carotene and vitamin A, have not shown significant benefit in reducing the incidence of bronchogenic carcinoma.

REVIEW EXERCISES

QUESTIONS

1. Which one of the following statements is true of lung Ca?
a) The most common histologic type is small cell Ca.
b) It is the second most common Ca in the United States.
c) Ninety percent of lung Ca is due to smoking.
d) Screening has proved beneficial in decreasing mortality from lung Ca.

Answer and Discussion

The answer is c. Lung Ca is the most common cancer in the United States in both men and women. Twenty to 25% are small cell in type, whereas 75% to 80% are non–small cell. Ninety percent of cases are due to smoking. Despite advances in radiologic imaging with low-dose CT and positron emission tomography scanning, screening has not yet proved beneficial in decreasing mortality from lung Ca.

2. Which one of the following is true regarding lung Ca?
a) Bronchioloalveolar carcinomas tend to grow quickly.
b) Five percent of patients with lung Ca develop nonmetastatic paraneoplastic syndromes.
c) Syndrome of inappropriate antidiuresis hormone is associated with hypernatremia.
d) Eighty to 90% of small cell carcinomas have spread beyond the thorax at the time of diagnosis.

Answer and Discussion

The answer is d. Bronchioloalveolar carcinomas tend to grow slowly. Ten to 15% of patients with lung Ca present with or develop complications of nonmetastatic paraneoplastic syndromes. The syndrome of inappropriate diuresis is associated with dehydration and hyponatremia. Eighty to 90% of small cell carcinomas have spread beyond the thorax at the time of diagnosis.

3. Which one of the following statements is true of small cell lung Ca?
a) Surgery is the most important treatment modality.
b) Limited stage disease describes disease less than T2 N1 M0.
c) Approximately 80% of patients respond to chemotherapy.
d) Prophylactic cranial irradiation has been shown to prolong survival.

Answer and Discussion

The answer is c. Small cell lung Ca (SCLC) is considered to be a systemic disease, and thus surgery plays no part in the management of the disease. SCLC is not included in the TNM (*Tumor, Node, Metastasis*) classification and has two stages, limited and extensive. Limited stage disease describes disease confined to one hemithorax that can be included in a reasonable thoracic radiation field. Approximately 80% of patients respond to chemotherapy. Prophylactic cranial irradiation reduces the incidence of brain metastases, but has not been shown to prolong survival.

4. Which one of the following statements is true of surgery for non–small cell lung Ca?
a) Current postoperative mortality rate is approximately 10%.
b) About 60% of patients are suitable for resection at diagnosis.
c) Pneumonectomy is the most commonly performed operation.
d) Surgery offers the best chance of cure.

Answer and Discussion

The answer is d. With currently available modalities in thoracic surgery, postoperative mortality rate is <5%. About 20% to 33% of patients are suitable for resection at the time of diagnosis, and lobectomy is the most commonly performed operation. Surgery offers the best chance of cure for non–small-cell lung Ca.

5. Which one of the following statements is true with regard to the prognosis of non–small cell lung Ca?
a) Stage IIIA disease is associated with 5-year survival rates of almost 40%.
b) Stage IV disease is associated with 5-year survival rates of approximately 10%.
c) Stage IIB disease is associated with 5-year survival rates of 20%.
d) Stage IA disease is associated with 5-year survival rates of nearly 70%.

Answer and Discussion

The answer is d. Stages IA and IB diseases are associated with 5-year survival rates of 67% and 57%, respectively, whereas stages IIA, IIB, and IIIA have 5-year survival rates of 55%, 39%, and 26%, respectively. Advanced stages such as IIIB and IV have poor 5-year survival rates of 5% and 1%, respectively.

SUGGESTED READINGS

Coultas D, Samet J. Occupational lung cancer. *Clin Chest Med* 1992;13:341–354.

Deslauriers J, Gregoire J. Surgical therapy of early non–small-cell lung cancer. *Chest* 2000;65:104–109.

Diagnosis and management of lung cancer: ACCP guidelines. *Chest* 2007;132(3 Suppl).

Gerber R, Mazzone P, Arroliga A. Paraneoplastic syndromes associated with bronchogenic carcinoma. *Clin Chest Med* 2002;23:257–264.

Godtfredsen N, Prescott E, Osler M. Effect of smoking reduction on lung cancer risk. *JAMA* 2005;294:1505–1510.

Gonzales D, Rennard S, Nides M, et al. Varenicline, a $\alpha_4\beta_2$ nicotinic acetylcholine receptor partial agonist vs. sustained-release bupropion and placebo for smoking cessation: a randomized controlled trial. *JAMA* 2006;296:47–55.

Gould M, Maclean C, Kushcner W, et al. Accuracy of positron emission tomography for diagnosis of pulmonary nodules and mass lesions: a metaanalysis. *JAMA* 2001;285:914–924.

Hoffman P, Mauer A, Vokes E. Lung cancer. *Lancet* 2000;355:479–485.

Hurt R, Ebbert J. Preventing lung cancer by stopping smoking. *Clin Chest Med* 2002;23:27–36.

Hyde L, Hyde C. Clinical manifestations of lung cancer. *Chest* 1974;65:299–304.

Jemal A, Siegel R, Ward E, et al. Cancer statistics, 2007. *CA Cancer J Clin* 2007;57:43–66.

Jett J, Midthun D. Screening for lung cancer: current status and future directions. *Chest* 2004;125:158–162.

Johnson B. Management of small cell lung cancer. *Clin Chest Med* 2002;23:225–239.

Jorenby D, Leischow S, Nides M, et al. A controlled trial of sustained release bupropion, a nicotine patch, or both for smoking cessation. *N Engl J Med* 1999;340:685–691.

Mazzone P, Jain P, Arroliga A, et al. Bronchoscopy and needle biopsy techniques for diagnosis and staging of lung cancer. *Clin Chest Med* 2002;23:137–158.

Mountain C. Revisions in the international system for staging lung cancer. *Chest* 1997;111:1710–1717.

Mountain C, Dresler C. Regional lymph node classification for lung cancer staging. *Chest* 1997;111:1718–1723.

Patz E, Swensen S, Herndon J. Estimate of lung cancer mortality from low-dose spiral computed tomography screening trials: implications for current mass screening recommendations. *J Clin Oncol* 2004;22:2202–2226.

Perez-Soler R, Chachoua A, Hammond LA, et al. Determinants of tumor response and survival with erlotinib in patients with non–small-cell lung cancer. *J Clin Oncol* 2004;22:3238–3247.

Rigotti N, Lee J, Wechsler H. US college students' use of tobacco products: results of a national survey. *JAMA* 2000;284:699–705.

Robinson L, Wagner H, Ruckdeschel J. Treatment of stage IIIA non–small cell lung cancer. *Chest* 2003;123:202–220.

Smith-Bilello K, Murin S, Matthay R. Epidemiology, etiology, and prevention of lung cancer. *Clin Chest Med* 2002;23:1–25.

Tan B, Flaherty K, Kazerooni E, et al. The solitary pulmonary nodule. *Chest* 2003;123:89–96.

Thomas L, Doyle L, Edelman M. Lung cancer in women: emerging differences in epidemiology, biology, and therapy. *Chest* 2005;128:370–381.

Thomas R, Weir B, Meyerson M. Genomic approaches to lung cancer. *Clin Cancer Res* 2006;15:4384–4391.

Travis W. Pathology of lung cancer. *Clin Chest Med* 2002;23:65–81.

Travis W, Lubin J, Ries L, et al. United States lung cancer incidence trends. *Cancer* 1996;77:2464–2470.

Williams D, Pairolero P, Davis C, et al. Survival of patients surgically treated for stage I lung cancer. *J Thorac Cardiovasc Surg* 1981;82:70–76.

Wisnivesky J, Henschke C, McGinn T, et al. Prognosis of stage II non–small cell lung cancer according to tumor and nodal status at diagnosis. *Lung Cancer* 2005;49:181–186.

Yoshino I, Maehara Y. Impact of smoking status on the biological behavior of lung cancer. *Surg Today* 2007;37:725–734.

Chapter 35

Obstructive Lung Disease: Asthma and Chronic Obstructive Pulmonary Disease

Loutfi S. Aboussouan

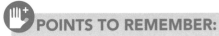

POINTS TO REMEMBER:

- Asthma affects 3% to 5% of the U.S. population.
- Asthma is a chronic, episodic disease of the airways; it has protean manifestations and is best

viewed as a syndrome. Important features of this syndrome include:
- Episodic symptoms
- Airflow obstruction with a reversible component

- Bronchial hyperresponsiveness to a variety of nonspecific and specific stimuli
- Airway inflammation
- A tendency toward atopic and allergic inheritable disease
- Asthma treatment has four key components:
  - Measure lung function both initially and during periodic evaluation, including home peak expiratory flow monitoring.
  - Educate patients in using asthma action plans.
  - Avoid asthma triggers by controlling the environment.
  - Treat the condition pharmacologically.
- An estimated 24 million Americans are afflicted with chronic obstructive pulmonary disease (COPD).
- The Global Initiative for Chronic Obstructive Lung Disease (GOLD) report defines COPD as "a disease state characterized by airflow limitation that is not fully reversible. The airflow limitation is usually both progressive and associated with an abnormal inflammatory response of the lungs to noxious particles or gases."
- Recent studies identify a composite index combining *Body* mass index, airflow *Obstruction*, *Dyspnea*, and *Exercise* capacity (the BODE index), as well as the inspiratory capacity-to-total lung capacity ratio, as better than the forced expiratory volume in 1 second in predicting the risk of death in COPD.
- Severe deficiency of alpha-1 antitrypsin accounts for emphysema in approximately 2% to 3% of adult COPD patients.
- Pulmonary function testing is essential to establish a diagnosis of COPD and its severity.
- The commonly used therapy for stable COPD includes prevention (smoking cessation, annual flu vaccination, and vaccination for pneumococcus), supplemental oxygen if indicated, inhaled bronchodilators, and, in a small subset, theophylline preparations and inhaled or systemic corticosteroids.

Bronchial asthma and COPD represent major causes of morbidity in the United States. Asthma affects 3% to 5% of the U.S. population. An estimated 24 million Americans are afflicted with COPD. Although asthma is not a leading cause of death, it is responsible for approximately 1% of all visits to physicians and results in approximately 500,000 hospital admissions per year. COPD was the fourth leading cause of death in the United States, with approximately 124,000 deaths in 2003. Therefore, both disorders are quite common, pose a significant burden on health care resources, and represent a great measure of human suffering. It is essential for the general internist, as well as the pulmonary subspecialist, to be very familiar with the nuances of management. History, physical examination, and simple ancillary studies (e.g., chest radiograph, spirogram) are usually adequate to establish a diagnosis of asthma or COPD and initiate proper management.

Chronic airflow obstruction is a feature of asthma, chronic bronchitis, emphysema, cystic fibrosis, and other bronchiectatic syndromes. The discussion here is limited to the typical adult patient with asthma and COPD. It is most essential to distinguish patients with bronchial asthma from the usual adult smoker with COPD because the prognosis and emphasis on certain types of management are quite different (e.g., asthma is characterized by exquisite steroid responsiveness).

ASTHMA

Asthma is a chronic, episodic disease of the airways; it has protean manifestations and is best viewed as a syndrome. Important features of this syndrome include:

- Episodic symptoms
- Airflow obstruction with a reversible component
- Bronchial hyperresponsiveness to a variety of nonspecific and specific stimuli
- Airway inflammation
- A tendency toward atopic and allergic inheritable disease

For a patient to be diagnosed with asthma, all of these features need not be present. Although some features overlap between asthma and COPD, it is important to understand the distinctions between these conditions:

- Asthma typically occurs in younger individuals who are nonsmokers.
- The asthmatic's baseline level of functioning, exercise tolerance, and spirometric parameters are usually better preserved between episodes than are those of individuals with COPD.
- The presence of extrinsic triggers, seasonal variability, family history, allergic rhinitis, and positive skin test results or atopy may be helpful in solidifying an initial diagnosis of asthma.
- Physiologically, asthmatics have a normal diffusing capacity, whereas patients with emphysema have a diffusing capacity reduced in proportion to the severity of airflow obstruction.

Etiology

Epidemiology

Data from the Centers for Disease Control and Prevention indicate that 22 million American adults suffer from asthma. The annual rate of asthma mortality, which increased between 1980 and 1995, has decreased more recently, despite the increasing prevalence of the disease. The evolving consensus from a number of retrospective studies is that several risk factors contribute to poor outcomes and fatal asthma:

- Patients with prior serious asthma, requiring emergency room visits or mechanical ventilation, are at the greatest risk.
- Factors that interfere with compliance and access to medical care are important. In the United States, the mortality rate from asthma for African-Americans is three times that for whites.
- Inadequate objective assessment of asthma severity by pulmonary function testing or peak flow measurements appears to be frequently noted in patients who die from asthma.
- Inadequate treatment with either inhaled or systemic corticosteroid is also a frequently described finding.

Therefore, underdiagnosis or underestimation of asthma severity is an important contributing factor in asthma-related fatality. Despite these recent trends, asthma remains a relatively infrequent cause of death.

In the early 1990s, a number of studies suggested a potential role of beta-agonist aerosols in the increasing asthma mortality rate. The hypothesis was that excessive or regularly scheduled use of beta-adrenergic bronchodilators can actually worsen asthma, perhaps contributing to morbidity and mortality. Other studies have indicated that the regular administration of beta-agonist aerosols does not directly cause worse asthma control. Recent studies indicate that polymorphisms for the β-adrenergic receptor gene exist in a subset of patients (perhaps 15%). It is likely that certain variants (i.e., Arg/Arg homozygotes at position 16) do not benefit from chronic beta-agonist administration. If patients require an increasing number of puffs of beta-agonist aerosols, this is usually a marker for the need for more effective anti-inflammatory therapy. Beta-agonist aerosols remain a critical part of the regimen for acute emergency room management of bronchial asthma. For chronic maintenance therapy, it is best to use beta-agonist aerosols on an as-needed basis.

Pathogenesis

In recent years, the central role of airway inflammation in the pathogenesis of asthma has been established. The mechanism by which airway inflammation is related to bronchial reactivity remains unclear. A classic model is that of an allergic asthmatic challenged with an inhaled antigen to which the patient is sensitive. This challenge may result in a biphasic decline in respiratory function. The early asthmatic response may occur within minutes and resolve within 2 hours. The early asthmatic response is believed to be related to the release of preformed mediators (perhaps from mast cells) and is abolished by pretreatment with beta-agonists (but not with corticosteroids). A late asthmatic response usually occurs within 6 to 8 hours and may last for 24 hours or longer. The late asthmatic response is classically associated with airway hyperreactivity and airway inflammatory cell influx; it can be inhibited by pretreatment with corticosteroids (but not beta-agonists). Cromoglycates may block both responses.

The current paradigm is that asthma is not simply bronchospasm but involves a complex cascade of inflammatory events that involves cellular, epithelial, neurogenic, and various biochemical mediators. In addition to the mast cells and eosinophils, the T lymphocyte (TH2) has been added as an important regulator of inflammation. The TH2 lymphocytes appear to mediate allergic inflammation in atopic asthmatics by a cytokine profile that involves interleukin-4 (which directs B lymphocytes to synthesize immunoglobulin E) and interleukin-5 (which is essential for the maturation of eosinophils), along with interleukin-13. Current thinking suggests that asthma is characterized by a TH2 rather than a TH1 response. Other effector cells implicated in asthmatic inflammation include mast cells, eosinophils, epithelial cells, and macrophages. Immunoglobulin E may be an important trigger for activating effector cells. The products of arachidonic acid metabolism have also been implicated in airway inflammation and have been the target of pharmacologic antagonism. Prostaglandins (PGs) are generated by the cyclo-oxygenation of arachidonic acid, and leukotrienes are generated by the lipoxygenation of arachidonic acid. The proinflammatory agents include the leukotrienes, as well as PGD2, PGF2α, and thromboxane. PGE2 and PGI2 (prostacyclin) are believed to be protective and produce bronchodilation.

Research has also focused on airway remodeling, which represents irreversible or permanent changes that may occur over time in asthmatic airways. It is tempting to speculate that long-standing asthma, especially if airway inflammation is not treated or inadequately treated, leads to basement membrane collagen deposition and subepithelial fibrosis. Currently, this remains speculative, and the relationship between airway inflammation and remodeling is unknown, as is how often remodeling occurs and how effectively anti-inflammatory therapy can avoid remodeling.

Clinical Presentation

The history and physical examination are important for several reasons:

- They confirm a diagnosis and exclude mimics, such as upper airway obstruction (UAO) and congestive heart failure.
- They assess the severity of airflow obstruction and the need for admission to a hospital.
- They identify factors that might place a patient at particular risk for poor outcome.

■ They identify comorbid diseases that may complicate the management, such as sinusitis, gastroesophageal reflux, and avoidable external triggers.

The cardinal symptoms of asthma include episodic dyspnea, chest tightness, wheezing, and cough. Some patients may present with atypical symptoms, such as cough alone (cough-equivalent asthma) or only dyspnea on exertion. It is essential to specifically inquire about nocturnal symptoms because this is often ignored.

The most objective indicator of asthma severity is the measurement of airflow obstruction by spirometry or peak expiratory flow. Both the forced expiratory volume in 1 second (FEV_1) and peak expiratory flow yield comparable results. The National Asthma Education Prevention Program (NAEPP), in its Expert Panel Report 3 (updated in 2007), indicates a preference for spirometry over the peak flow meter in the clinician's office. Hyperinflation, the most common finding on a chest radiograph, has no diagnostic or therapeutic value. A chest radiograph should not be obtained unless complications of pneumonia, pneumothorax, or an endobronchial lesion are suspected. The correlation of severity between acute asthma and arterial blood gases is poor. Mild to moderate asthma is typically associated with respiratory alkalosis and mild hypoxemia on the basis of ventilation–perfusion mismatching. Severe hypoxemia is quite uncommon. Normocapnia and hypercapnia imply severe airflow obstruction, with an FEV_1 of usually <25% of predicted. Recent data suggest that hypercapnia in the setting of acute asthma does not necessarily mandate intubation or suggest a poor prognosis.

Numerous parameters from the physical examination and airflow measurement, either separately or as a composite score, have been evaluated to assess the severity of acute asthma and the need for hospital admission. It is true that physical findings such as pulsus paradoxus (inspiratory decline in systolic blood pressure of >12 mm Hg), accessory muscle use including sternocleidomastoid muscle retraction, a respiratory rate of >30 breaths/minute, and a heart rate of >130 beats/minute are generally associated with more severe airflow obstruction. None of these signs alone or in combination, however, is specific or sensitive.

Spirometry in an asthmatic typically shows obstructive airway disease with reduced expiratory flows that improve on administration of bronchodilator therapy (i.e., reduced FEV_1/forced vital capacity [FVC] ratio). Typically, an improvement in either FEV_1 or FVC occurs with the acute administration of an inhaled bronchodilator (12% and 200 mL). The absence of a bronchodilator response, however, by no means excludes asthma. The shape of the flow-volume loop may provide insight into the nature and location of airway obstruction. With disorders that cause UAO, classically, a plateau occurs in either limb of the flow-volume loop during periods of maximal flow. Specifically, the loop shows a flattening of the inspiratory limb with variable extrathoracic UAO, likely caused by a lesion involving the glottic or subglottic area. Flattening of the expiratory limb is seen with variable intrathoracic UAO, such as a mid- or distal tracheal lesion. A fixed UAO produces a boxlike flattening of both inspiratory and expiratory limbs. In patients with atypical chest symptoms of unclear etiology (cough or dyspnea alone), a variety of challenge tests may help identify the presence of airway hyperreactivity. By far, the most commonly used agents are methacholine or histamine, which give comparable results. Exercise, cold air, and isocapnic hyperventilation—other approaches that require complex equipment—have a lower sensitivity. In a patient with known asthma, there is no indication for a challenge procedure. The methacholine challenge test is very sensitive, but it is nonspecific and can occur in a variety of other conditions, including COPD.

Treatment

The NAEPP Expert Panel Report 3 provides an excellent algorithmic framework for the management of bronchial asthma (Tables 35.1 to 35.3). Overall, asthma treatment has four key components:

■ Measure lung function both initially and during periodic evaluation, including home peak expiratory flow monitoring.
■ Educate patients on using asthma action plans.
■ Avoid asthma triggers by controlling the environment.
■ Treat the condition pharmacologically.

In the NAEPP guidelines, severity (which is determined before initiation of long-term control medications) guides the initial treatment of the patient who is not taking long-term control medications (Table 35.1). Subsequent adjustment of medications is based on the monitoring of disease control (Table 35.2). Both severity and control are assessed along the two domains of reduction of impairment and reduction in risk (Tables 35.1 and 35.2).

The goals for reduction of impairment include:

■ Maintain normal activity levels, including exercise, work or school attendance, and athletics.
■ Optimize pulmonary function tests.
■ Prevent chronic and troublesome symptoms including those that disturb sleep.
■ Establish minimal need for rescue medications (up to two times per week).
■ Achieve patient and family satisfaction with asthma care.

The goals for reduction of risk include

■ Prevent exacerbations, emergency room visits, and hospital care.
■ Prevent loss of lung function in adults (and prevent reduced lung growth in children).
■ Avoid adverse effects from asthma medications.

Table 35.2 provides several approaches to the monitoring of disease control, including the use of validated

TABLE 35.1

CLASSIFICATION OF ASTHMA SEVERITY AND INITIATION OF TREATMENT IN AGES ≥12 YEARS AND ADULTS (FOR PATIENTS WHO ARE NOT CURRENTLY TAKING LONG-TERM CONTROL MEDICATIONS)

Components of Severity		Classification of Asthma Severity (≥12 years of age)			
			Persistent		
		Intermittent	Mild	Moderate	Severe
Impairment **Normal FEV$_1$/FVC:**	Symptoms	≤2 days/week	>2 days/week	Daily	Throughout the day
	Nighttime awakenings	≤2 days/month	3–4 ×/month	>1×/week but not nightly	Often 7×/week
8–19 years 85% **20–39 years 80%** **40–59 years 75%** **60–80 years 70%**	SABA use for symptoms control (not prevention of EIB)	≤2 days/week	>2 days/week but not daily	Daily	Several times per day
	Interference with normal activity	None	Minor	Some	Extreme
	Lung function	■ Normal FEV$_1$ between exacerbations ■ FEV$_1$ >80% ■ FEV$_1$/FVC normal	■ FEV$_1$ >80% ■ FEV$_1$/FVC normal	■ FEV$_1$ 60%–80% ■ FEV$_1$/FVC reduced 5%	■ FEV$_1$ <60% ■ FEV$_1$/FVC reduced >5%
Risks	Exacerbations requiring CS	0–1/year	2/year	≥2/year	≥2/year
		Consider severity and interval since last exacerbation. Frequency and severity may fluctuate over time for patients in any severity category. Relative annual risk of exacerbations may be related to FEV$_1$.			
Recommended Steps for Initiating Treatment (See Table 35.3 for details of steps.)		Step 1	Step 2	Step 3 Consider short course of oral corticosteroids.	Step 4 or 5
		In 2 to 6 weeks, evaluate level of asthma control that is achieved, and adjust therapy accordingly.			

CS = corticosteroids, EIB = exercise-induced bronchospasm, FEV$_1$ = forced expiratory volume in 1 second, FVC = forced vital capacity, SABA = short-acting beta-agonist.

questionnaires. The asthma control test, which is one such questionnaire, asks patients to grade five questions related to the symptoms of asthma in the preceding 4 weeks along a 5-point scale from worse to best. The questions are representative of questions from the other questionnaires and include the following:

■ How much of the time did your asthma keep you from getting things done at work, school, or home?
■ How often have you had shortness of breath?
■ How often did your asthma symptoms (wheezing, coughing, shortness of breath, chest tightness, or pain) wake you up at night or earlier than usual in the morning?
■ How often have you used your rescue inhaler or nebulizer medication (e.g., albuterol)?
■ How would you rate your asthma control?

The questionnaires and, more commonly, peak flow monitoring can be used at home for patients to use to self-adjust their medications as part of a pre-established asthma action plan.

Measurements of exhaled nitric oxide may soon become as prevalent as pulmonary function testing for the diagnosis and monitoring of asthma. Exhaled nitric oxide levels have been found to be useful in the diagnosis of asthma, to increase with the severity of asthma, and to correlate with other markers of severity of asthma (e.g., sputum eosinophils). Studies have also shown that treatment of asthma reduces nitric oxide levels and that exhaled nitric oxide can be used to guide therapy of asthma. More widespread use of exhaled nitric oxide may follow once the equipment is more readily available in pulmonary function laboratories, measurement techniques are standardized, and references values are established.

The pharmacologic treatment for asthma can be classified as *symptomatic therapy* ("relievers" or "rescue" medications) using bronchodilators (beta-agonists, theophylline) and *anti-inflammatory therapy* ("controllers") using corticosteroids, chromones that include cromolyn and nedocromil, antileukotrienes, and anti-immunoglobulin E (IgE).

The therapy is further classified as acute versus chronic maintenance therapy. The NAEPP outlines detailed guidelines for stepwise management using these agents (Tables 35.1 to 35.3). For the mildest asthma (intermittent), the

TABLE 35.2

ASSESSING ASTHMA CONTROL AND ADJUSTING THERAPY IN AGES ≥12 YEARS AND ADULTS

Components of Control		Classification of Asthma Control (≥12 Years of Age)		
		Well Controlled	Not Well Controlled	Very Poorly Controlled
Impairment	Symptoms	≤2 days/week	>2 days/week	Throughout the day
	Nighttime awakenings	≤2 ×/month	1–3×/week	≥ 4×/week
	Interference with normal activity	None	Some limitation	Extremely limited
	Short-acting beta 2-agonist use for symptom control (not prevention of EIB)	≤2 days/week	>2 days/week	Several times per day
	FEV$_1$ or peak flow	>80% predicted/ personal best	60%–80% predicted/ personal best	<60% predicted/ personal best
	Validated questionnaires			
	ATAQ	0	1–2	3–4
	ACQ	≤0.75	≥1.5	N/A
	ACT	≥20	16–19	≤15
Risk	Exacerbations requiring oral systemic corticosteroids	0–1/year	≥2/year	≥2/year
	Progressive loss of lung function	Consider severity and interval since last exacerbation. Evaluation requires long-term follow-up care.		
	Treatment-related adverse effects	Medication side effects can vary in intensity from none to very troublesome and worrisome. The level of intensity does not correlate to specific levels of control but should be considered in the overall assessment of risk.		
Recommended action for treatment (See Table 35.3 for details of steps.)		▪ Maintain current step. ▪ Perform regular follow-ups every 1–6 months to maintain control. ▪ Consider step down if well controlled for at least 3 months.	▪ Step up 1 step. ▪ Re-evaluate in 2–6 weeks. ▪ For side effects, consider alternative treatment options.	▪ Consider short course of oral corticosteroids. ▪ Step up 1–2 steps. ▪ Re-evaluate in 2 weeks. ▪ For side effects, consider alternative treatments.

ACQ = Asthma Control Questionnaire, ACT = Asthma Control Test, ATAQ = Asthma Therapy Assessment Questionnaire.

guidelines recommend as-needed use of one to two puffs of a beta-agonist aerosol. Cromolyn may alternatively be used before exposure to a variety of triggers, such as exercise or allergen. For all asthmatics with persistent asthma, the mainstay of maintenance therapy is inhaled corticosteroids with the initial dose based on the assessment of severity and subsequent escalation based on assessment of disease control. Numerous studies have shown that inhaled steroid therapy provides an effective symptomatic control of chronic asthma, as well as the reversal of a number of parameters of airway inflammation.

With the current paradigm of asthma as a chronic inflammatory disorder of the airways, inhaled corticosteroids have assumed the role of first-line therapy for all patients with persistent asthma (mild, moderate, severe). Currently, six specific inhaled corticosteroids are approved in the United States for the maintenance therapy of asthma. The NAEPP report provides a table of comparative-dose, inhaled steroids needed to achieve similar clinical effect. The trend in the use of inhaled steroids has been to use higher and higher doses, especially in the more severe asthmatics.

It is well documented that higher doses of inhaled corticosteroids facilitate a reduction in systemic corticosteroids in severe asthma. However, several meta-analyses demonstrate a flat dose–response relationship such that 80% to 90% of the therapeutic response is reached at daily doses of inhaled corticosteroids equivalent to 200 mcg of fluticasone or 400 mcg budesonide, doses that would be considered low for adults based on the NAEPP guidelines. Accordingly, the addition of long-acting beta-agonists to inhaled corticosteroids is a preferred approach at steps 4 and above of the guidelines, to produce either additive or synergistic effects (Table 35.3). One important caveat is that the SMART study showed a small but statistically significant increase in respiratory-related deaths in patients receiving the long-acting beta-agonist salmeterol. Accordingly, the NAEPP now recommends that the beneficial effects of long-acting beta-agonists be weighed against the uncommon but increased risk for severe exacerbations associated with the daily use of these agents. In practical terms, for a patient whose asthma remains insufficiently controlled with inhaled corticosteroids, the option to increase the inhaled

TABLE 35.3

STEPWISE APPROACH FOR MANAGEMENT OF ASTHMA IN AGES ≥12 YEARS AND ADULTS

Intermittent Asthma	Persistent Asthma: Daily Medication					Assess Control
	Consult with asthma specialist if step 4 care or higher is required. Consider consultation at step 3.					Step up if needed (first check adherence, environmental control, and comorbid conditions). Step down if possible (and asthma is well controlled at least 3 months).
					Step 6 **Preferred:** High-dose ICS + LABA + oral cortico-steroids AND Consider omalizumab for patients who have allergies.	
				Step 5 **Preferred:** High-dose ICS + LABA AND Consider omalizumab for patients who have allergies.		
			Step 4 **Preferred:** Medium-dose ICS + LABA **Alternative:** Medium-dose ICS + either LTRA, theo, or Zileuton			
		Step 3 **Preferred:** Low-dose ICS + LABA OR medium-dose ICS **Alternative:** Low-dose ICS + either LTRA, theo, or Zileuton				
	Step2 **Preferred:** Low-dose ICS **Alternative**: Chromones, LTRA, or theo					
Step 1 **Preferred:** SABA PRN						

Each step: Patient education, environmental control, and management of comorbidities
2–4: Consider subcutaneous allergen immunotherapy for patients who have allergic asthma.

Quick-relief medication is recommended for all patients

ICS = inhaled corticosteroids, LABA = long-acting beta-agonist, LTRA = leukotriene receptor antagonist, PRN = as needed, SABA = short-acting beta-agonist, theo = theophylline.

corticosteroids dose should be given equal weight to the option of adding a long-acting beta-agonist (Table 35.3, step 3).

Combinations of fluticasone and salmeterol, or budesonide and formoterol, are available in single devices. Several recent pivotal studies indicate that the combination product is superior to the individual components in patients with mild and moderately severe chronic asthma. The study by Kavuru et al. is a randomized controlled trial of fluticasone/salmeterol 100/50; administered as a dry powder inhaler, one puff twice a day markedly improved a variety of outcomes, including FEV$_1$ and the probability of having an asthma exacerbation over 12 weeks, compared with each component separately or placebo. The exact molecular mechanism whereby the combination of inhaled steroids and long-acting beta-agonists synergistically improve asthma control is not fully known. Preliminary data indicate that the beta-agonists facilitate the steroid effect, whereas the steroids upregulate the beta-agonist receptors.

Another trend has been the use of inhaled corticosteroids at an earlier stage of asthma. Some data suggest that this might improve the long-term FEV$_1$ by preventing subepithelial fibrosis. Several studies suggest that less frequent dosing, such as once or twice a day, may be equally effective. The less frequent dosing has clearcut benefits in terms of compliance. Some studies have shown a cost advantage to asthma care through the use of inhaled corticosteroids. A case-controlled study indicates that the use of inhaled steroid maintenance therapy (i.e., one canister per month) is associated with lower asthma mortality.

A number of studies have examined the usefulness of inhaled steroids plus other agents, including theophylline and leukotriene antagonists. These studies have strongly indicated that the benefits of combination therapy using these other agents are not as dramatic as with the addition of the long-acting inhaled bronchodilator. These combinations are considered alternative options to management in the NAEPP report (Table 35.3, steps 3 and

4). Recent data suggest that inhaled steroids probably do not cure asthma in the sense that symptoms promptly return if these agents are stopped. These agents clearly reduce airway hyperreactivity. In general, with the use of low-dose inhaled corticosteroid therapy (<1,000 μg/day), systemic complications appear to be negligible. The oral pharyngeal complications of inhaled steroid therapy, such as candidiasis, dysphonia, and hoarseness, are usually mild. The use of a spacer device (or a powder preparation) and routine rinsing of the mouth help minimize these side effects. Data suggest that systemic effects may occur with the use of higher dosages (>1,200 μg/day) of inhaled corticosteroids. Definitely, certain biochemical parameters of the hypothalamic-pituitary-adrenal axis (24-hour urinary free cortisol, morning serum cortisol, and adrenocorticotropic hormone stimulation test) and bone metabolism (serum osteocalcin and urinary hydroxyproline) may be affected. The clinical importance, however, of these effects in terms of bone growth, likelihood for osteoporosis, or fractures is not known.

Data over the past 10 years suggest that the cysteinyl leukotrienes are involved in the pathogenesis of asthma. Three agents that antagonize the leukotriene pathway have been approved for use as maintenance therapy for mild persistent asthma. Zileuton is a synthesis inhibitor that blocks the 5-lipoxygenase enzyme. Zafirlukast and montelukast are selective, competitive receptor antagonists at the LTD4 and LTE4 level. Early clinical trials suggest that these agents have beneficial effects in mild to moderate asthma compared with placebo. The exact place for antileukotrienes in the chronic maintenance therapy for asthma remains to be established. The NAEPP report indicates a possible role for these agents, as an alternative to inhaled corticosteroids, in the initial therapy of mild persistent asthma, or as adjunctive therapy to inhaled steroids in patients with moderate to severe asthma (Table 35.3, steps 2–4). These agents have effects on early and late asthma response. Therefore, they act as a bronchodilator within 1 to 3 hours after administration and as an anti-inflammatory agent having a response over 2 to 4 weeks. The magnitude of increase in FEV_1 at 4 weeks is approximately 14% above that of the placebo. Several published studies directly comparing currently available inhaled corticosteroids with the antileukotrienes indicate that the inhaled steroids have more potent effects, especially in patients with moderate to severe disease. The antileukotrienes facilitate a reduction in the need for inhaled beta-agonists and inhaled corticosteroids, thereby minimizing certain side effects. Also, these oral agents may improve compliance, when compared with the metered-dose inhalers. Antileukotrienes may be particularly beneficial as the drug of choice in a small subset of patients with aspirin-sensitive asthma.

Omalizumab (Xolair), the first selective anti-IgE agent, is a unique humanized monoclonal anti-IgE antibody that binds with high affinity to the receptor-binding site on IgE. Omalizumab binds the free IgE in the serum and reduces the serum level of IgE by more than 95% after a single dose. The rationale for the use of anti-IgE in allergic asthmatic inflammation is that free soluble IgE would not be available to bind to the surface of effector cells and will avoid crosslinking by an allergen and the subsequent downstream release of preformed inflammatory mediators. Omalizumab was approved by the U.S. Food and Drug Administration in 2003 for use in patients with chronic moderate to severe persistent asthma who are symptomatic despite moderate or high doses of inhaled corticosteroids, who are atopic, and whose IgE levels are in the range of 30 to 700 IU/mL (Table 35.3). Several randomized placebo-controlled trials indicate that omalizumab lowers the acute exacerbation rate when added to conventional therapy for chronic asthma. This drug is administered subcutaneously once every 2 or 4 weeks. The dose is determined uniquely by the patient's ideal body weight as well as the serum IgE level. This drug is quite expensive (as most monoclonal antibodies are), and the exact place in long-term asthma management remains to be established. For patients who require frequent inpatient care for asthma, however, this agent appears to be a rational alternative. There is a risk of anaphylaxis in about 0.2% of patients following the administration of omalizumab, even after the second or third dose.

A minority of patients continue to have troublesome asthma symptoms, with frequent exacerbations requiring hospital stays despite maximal conventional therapy. The literature suggests that this is a small subset, perhaps less than 10% to 15% of all asthmatics. The reversible factors that contribute to the subset of steroid-dependent asthma include:

- Patient noncompliance
- Poor self-management strategies by the patient
- Inadequate control of allergen burden at home
- Suboptimal inhaler technique
- Suboptimal pharmacotherapy prescription by the physician

Exciting research has begun into the concept of pharmacogenetics, or the presence of variant genotypes or polymorphisms that modify disease phenotype or response to different classes of drugs. The most widely studied is the β-adrenergic receptor gene, in which more than 15 known variants exist, several of which are associated with poor response to an agonist. Ongoing research explores the relative steroid resistance in a subset of these difficult-to-control asthmatics. Several factors—including steroid metabolism, steroid receptor alternate splice variants, and a variety of intracellular factors—are being studied. It appears that steroid metabolism and steroid receptor polymorphisms are likely to be an explanation in a small minority of patients only. Several polymorphisms also occur in the enzymes involved in leukotriene metabolism. The clinical significance of this burgeoning area of pharmacogenetics to the practicing clinician remains to be established.

The placebo arm of a number of studies has clearly shown that a compulsive traditional management plan, with frequent follow-up (perhaps in an asthma center), can reduce the need for oral steroids by 40% to 50% in steroid-dependent asthma. The literature is replete with numerous studies demonstrating the efficacy of alternative anti-inflammatory therapies that provide a steroid-sparing effect in these individuals. Gold salts, methotrexate, cyclosporine, colchicine, troleandomycin, chloroquine, intravenous gamma-globulin, and dapsone are some of the agents that have been investigated. Overall, no alternative anti-inflammatory agent has been proved to be superior to inhaled corticosteroids in the treatment of asthma, and the use of these therapies should be restricted to clinical trials only.

cough with sputum production, occurring on most days for at least 3 months of the year during at least 2 successive years. Emphysema is anatomically defined as an abnormal permanent enlargement of the air spaces distal to the terminal bronchiole, accompanied by destruction of their walls and without obvious fibrosis.

Several different anatomical types of emphysema occur, the most common being the typical smoking-related centriacinar emphysema. This centriacinar emphysema (synonyms are *centrilobular* or *proximal acinar*) involves the dilatation of the air space between the terminal bronchiole and the first- and second-generation respiratory bronchiole. The other major type of emphysema, panacinar or panlobular emphysema, is usually seen in association with the inherited alpha-1 antitrypsin deficiency.

CHRONIC OBSTRUCTIVE PULMONARY DISEASE

The GOLD report defines COPD as "a disease state characterized by airflow limitation that is not fully reversible. The airflow limitation is usually both progressive and associated with an abnormal inflammatory response of the lungs to noxious particles or gases."

Although most adult patients with COPD exhibit features of both chronic bronchitis and emphysema, neither is included in the current definition of COPD, which highlights instead the importance of airflow limitation on morbidity and mortality. COPD severity is also classified based on the degree of airway obstruction (Table 35.4). Nevertheless, both chronic bronchitis and emphysema remain useful diagnoses from epidemiologic and clinical standpoints. Chronic bronchitis is clinically defined (based on the Ciba Guest Symposium Report of 1959) as chronic

Etiology

Epidemiology, Risk Factors, and Natural History

Overall, smoking is the single most important risk factor for COPD. About 15% to 20% of COPD occurs in never-smokers, however, and only about 20% of ever-smokers develop COPD. Although host factors may explain these findings, current concepts also emphasize the total burden of inhaled particles as an exposure risk factor. In the general nonsmoking population, the FEV_1 percentage predicted follows a unimodal distribution. Among cigarette smokers, the distribution is shifted leftward to lower FEV_1 values. A longitudinal study from East Boston, with a 10-year follow-up, suggested that asymptomatic nonsmoking males showed a prolonged period of either slow growth or plateau phase between ages 23 and 35 years. Age-related decline in lung function began after this period and occurred at a rate of 20 to 30 mL/year. Although most heavy smokers have a slightly reduced FEV_1, only 10% to 15% have a

---

TABLE 35.4

CLASSIFICATION OF COPD SEVERITY (FROM THE GOLD REPORT)

Stage	Characteristics
I: Mild COPD	FEV_1/FVC <70% FEV_1 ≥80% predicted With or without chronic symptoms (cough, sputum production)
II: Moderate COPD	FEV_1/FVC <70% 50% ≤FEV_1 <80% predicted With or without chronic symptoms (cough, sputum production)
III: Severe COPD	FEV_1/FVC <70% 30% ≤FEV_1 ≤50% predicted With or without chronic symptoms (cough, sputum production)
IV: Very severe COPD	FEV_1/FVC <70% FEV_1 <30% predicted or FEV_1 ≤50% predicted plus chronic respiratory failure

COPD = chronic obstructive pulmonary disease, FEV_1 = forced expiratory volume in 1 second, FVC = forced vital capacity, GOLD = Global Initiative for Chronic Obstructive Lung Disease.

significant chronic obstructive airflow limitation (i.e., FEV_1 of <65%). In nonsusceptible smokers, the decline in FEV_1 is similar to that of nonsmokers. In the small subset of susceptible smokers, an accelerated decline in FEV_1 occurs of approximately 70 to 150 mL/year.

The Intermittent Positive-Pressure Breathing Trial Group followed a cohort of 985 patients with established COPD who had a postbronchodilator FEV_1 of approximately 40% for a 3-year period. They noted an average mortality of 23% over the 3-year period and found the postbronchodilator FEV_1 and the patient's age as the most accurate predictors of death. A slightly increased risk is also present with an elevated resting heart rate, untreated hypoxemia, and hypercapnia. More recent studies identify a composite index combining *Body* mass index, airflow *Obstruction*, *Dyspnea*, and *Exercise* capacity (the BODE index), and the inspiratory capacity-to-total lung capacity ratio, as better than the FEV_1 in predicting the risk of death in COPD. Respiratory tract infections do not influence the overall course of the disease. Early evidence suggests that increased baseline airway hyperresponsiveness may imply a better prognosis. This remains controversial and is contrary to the so-called Dutch hypothesis, which holds that in patients with increased bronchodilator responsiveness, an accelerated FEV_1 decline occurs with time. For example, in data from the Lung Health Study, methacholine responsiveness was found to be an important predictor of the progression of airway obstruction in continuing smokers with early COPD.

Pathogenesis

Overwhelming evidence suggests that cigarette smoking is causally related to emphysema. The exact component in smoke that is responsible for this process is unknown. The lung destruction in emphysema is generally explained by the protease–antiprotease hypothesis: It is believed that in a normal nonsmoking individual, a fine balance exists between the elastolytic proteinases and the endogenous agents that inhibit their activity. Specifically, proteinases involved in COPD include those produced by neutrophils (elastase, cathepsin G, and proteinase-3) and macrophages (cathepsins B, L, and S) and various matrix metalloproteinases (MMPs). Alternatively, major antiproteinases providing a screen against the deleterious effects of proteinases include alpha-1 antitrypsin, secretory leukoproteinase inhibitor, and tissue inhibitors of MMPs. It appears that cigarette smoke affects both arms of this balance, thus producing severe lung destruction by a so-called two-hit concept. Components in smoke oxidize alpha-1 antitrypsin as well as directly stimulate neutrophils to produce elastases. Most adult smokers with severe emphysema have serum alpha-1 antitrypsin levels within normal limits. This leads to the notion that additional, poorly understood endogenous antiproteases exist and/or that the protease–antiprotease hypothesis is only one mechanism for the establishment of COPD.

For example, as is apparent from the new definition of COPD, inflammation is now considered a key component of the pathogenesis of emphysema. Important differentiating characteristics from the inflammation found in asthma are outlined in Table 35.5.

A third mechanism in the pathogenesis of COPD is oxidative stress, which can promote cellular dysfunction, damage the extracellular matrix, and unfavorably affect both arms of the proteinase–antiproteinase balance.

Severe deficiency of alpha-1 antitrypsin accounts for emphysema in approximately 2% to 3% of adult COPD patients and should be suspected in those who present with the following features:

- Early-onset emphysema (younger than 50 years)
- Emphysema with minimal smoking history
- Predominantly basilar bullous emphysema
- Family history of emphysema, liver disease, or panniculitis
- Emphysema occurring with liver disease

Notwithstanding these suggestive patterns, current recommendations endorse testing all symptomatic adults for alpha-1 antitrypsin deficiency.

The diagnosis of alpha-1 antitrypsin deficiency is made by measuring the serum alpha-1 antitrypsin level followed

TABLE 35.5

COMPARISON OF INFLAMMATION IN ASTHMA AND COPD (FROM THE GOLD REPORT)

Characteristic	COPD	Asthma
Cells	Neutrophils Large number of macrophages Increase in CD8+ T lymphocytes	Eosinophils Small increase in macrophages Increase in CD4+ Th2 lymphocytes Activation of mast cells
Mediators	LTB4, IL-8, TNFα	LTD4, IL-4, IL-5

COPD = chronic obstructive pulmonary disease, GOLD = Global Initiative for Chronic Obstructive Lung Disease, IL = interleukin, TNFα = tumor necrosis factor-alpha.

by so-called Pi (for protease inhibitor) typing for confirmation. The threshold level for emphysema ($<\sim$50 mg/dL [using nephelometry] or 11 μM) is usually seen only in patients with the Pi*ZZ phenotype (homozygotes). In addition to cigarette smoking and alpha-1 antitrypsin deficiency, there are a number of rare causes for COPD:

- Hypocomplementemic urticarial vasculitis syndrome
- Intravenous methylphenidate (Ritalin) abuse
- Ehlers-Danlos or Marfan's syndrome
- Salla disease
- Alpha-1 antichymotrypsin deficiency
- HIV infection
- Systemic necrotizing vasculitis
- Variant of the gene for tumor necrosis factor-alpha (TNFα)

Clinical Presentation

The cardinal symptoms of COPD include dyspnea and cough, with or without sputum production and wheezing. Symptoms are usually chronic (i.e., of at least 3 to 5 years' duration) and slowly progressive. Patients may give a history of a variable course with occasional acute exacerbations interspersed with periods of stable or slowly progressive illness. The variability in the symptoms is not nearly as dramatic as in young patients with typical asthma, however, in whom the periods between acute exacerbations are quite symptom-free.

Physical examination is tailored to establish whether a patient has an acute exacerbation of her illness and whether a concomitant illness is contributing to symptoms. Although some patients exhibit the classic body habitus of either a "pink puffer" (type A) or a "blue bloater" (type B), most adult patients with COPD exhibit features of both. The lung examination is most remarkable for a decrease in the intensity of breath sounds, prolonged expiratory phase, and occasional scattered wheezes on forced expiration. Rales are usually not present. Heart sounds are often distant and difficult to appreciate. The presence of right ventricular strain or failure can be ascertained by a loud pulmonic component of the second heart sound, a right ventricular heave, elevated neck veins, a pulsatile liver, and edema in the lower extremities. Clubbing of the fingers is not usually present in smoking-related COPD, and its presence should strongly suggest a complicating illness such as lung cancer, pulmonary fibrosis, chronic infection, or liver disease.

Although the chest roentgenogram may offer clues supporting a diagnosis of obstructive airway disease, its primary importance is in excluding important concomitant diseases, such as pulmonary nodules, congestive heart failure, or pulmonary fibrosis. CT scan of the chest shows certain typical features but is not necessary for the diagnosis.

Pulmonary function testing is essential to establish a diagnosis of COPD and its severity (Table 35.4). The typical spirometric abnormalities in COPD consist of a reduction in the FEV_1 and in the ratio of the FEV_1 to the FVC. The single-breath diffusing capacity for carbon monoxide is usually reduced in emphysema and has a good correlation with the extent of anatomic destruction in emphysema.

Many patients with COPD have a significant response to the acute administration of inhaled bronchodilators (an increase in FEV_1 of 12% and 200 mL). Clearly, the presence of bronchodilator response itself is not adequate to distinguish asthma from COPD. Also, a methacholine provocation test result may be positive in more than 60% of patients with COPD, so this also does not distinguish COPD from asthma. There is no indication for this challenge test in patients with known COPD.

Treatment

The management of stable COPD is considered separately from treatment during acute exacerbations. The critical interventions that have been shown to prolong survival and affect the natural history of the underlying disease are oxygen therapy for the chronically hypoxemic patient and perhaps smoking cessation. All other management strategies have less compelling data to suggest long-term measurable benefit, either in terms of survival or other criteria, such as rate of decline in FEV_1. Proposed guidelines from the GOLD report, tailoring the treatment of COPD to stage of disease, are shown in Table 35.6.

The commonly used therapy for stable COPD includes prevention (smoking cessation, annual flu vaccination, and vaccination for pneumococcus), supplemental oxygen if indicated, inhaled bronchodilators, and, in a small subset, theophylline preparations and inhaled or systemic corticosteroids. In a meta-analysis of exercise performance

TABLE 35.6

COPD THERAPY BY STAGE (FROM THE GOLD REPORT)

I: Mild	II: Moderate	III: Severe	IV: Very Severe
Reduce risk factors; administer influenza vaccination; add short-acting bronchodilator when needed.	Add regular treatment with one or more long-acting bronchodilator (when needed); add rehabilitation.	Add inhaled gluco-corticosteroids if repeated exacerbations.	Add long-term O_2 if chronic respiratory failure; consider surgical options.

COPD = chronic obstructive pulmonary disease, GOLD = Global Initiative for Chronic Obstructive Lung Disease.

studies, the overall effect favored pulmonary rehabilitation, with specific benefits including an 11% to 33% increase in maximal work rate, a 9% increase in maximal oxygen consumption, a 38% to 85% increase in exercise endurance time, and increases in 6-minute walk distance by 38 to 96 m. Pulmonary rehabilitation did not improve FEV_1 or survival, however.

The current database showing survival advantage for supplemental oxygen therapy in chronically hypoxemic patients is largely based on two landmark studies: the Nocturnal Oxygen Therapy Trial and the British Medical Research Council Trial. Both studies included patients with severe but stable COPD and resting hypoxemia. The combined results from these studies suggest that continuous oxygen therapy for 24 hours or 12 hours confers a definite survival benefit. Other significant findings included improvement in quality of life and neuropsychiatric function, exercise tolerance, reduction in secondary polycythemia, and reduced pulmonary artery pressure in selected groups of patients. Although the exact mechanism for the survival benefit is unknown, it is probably through improved pulmonary vascular resistance. Patients with a resting room air alveolar oxygen tension of <55 mm Hg or an SpO_2 by pulse oximetry of <88% should be given supplemental oxygen. These criteria should be checked during a period of clinical stability rather than during an acute exacerbation. In patients with alveolar oxygen tension between 55 mm Hg and 59 mm Hg, the additional clinical features of chronic hypoxemia and end-organ damage should be present.

The pharmacotherapy for COPD is mostly used to accomplish symptom control rather than to affect the natural history of the disease (i.e., unlike inhaled steroids in asthma). A stepwise therapy is usually followed, using one or a combination of inhaled bronchodilators, based on disease severity (Table 35.6). The three bronchodilators primarily used and currently available are anticholinergic agents, beta 2-selective adrenergic agents (both short and long-acting), and theophylline preparations.

A variety of studies document the efficacy of each of these agents in the management of stable COPD, either alone or in combination. All three classes of bronchodilators have been shown to produce improvement in symptoms and exercise capacity in COPD, usually without a significant chronic increase in FEV_1. Most symptomatic patients are usually treated with short-acting inhaled beta-agonists (usually albuterol). As in asthma, recent data indicate that the regularly scheduled administration of beta-agonists is not superior to as-needed or on-demand use. It appears that patients with COPD have a significantly increased cholinergic bronchomotor tone.

The human lung has three subtypes of muscarinic cholinergic receptors (M1, M2, and M3). The M2 subtype is postganglionic and is the only type that protects against bronchoconstriction. Both atropine and ipratropium are nonselective and inhibit all three subtypes. A multicenter study suggested that ipratropium showed a bronchodila-

tor effect superior to that of metaproterenol in patients with severe COPD. Over the past 10 years, ipratropium has achieved the status of first-line maintenance therapy for COPD. Results of the Lung Health Study I (prospective evaluation of smoking cessation ± ipratropium over 5 years) were disappointing in that the benefits of ipratropium were modest, occurred during year 1 only, and improvement in lung function was lost within weeks of stopping therapy. It has the advantage of being safe and free of side effects, though recent studies have implicated an increased risk of cardiovascular mortality related to anticholinergic use. It is inconvenient to administer (available only as a metered-dose inhaler and requiring two to six puffs four times a day) and is not as potent because it is nonselective (inhibits M2 receptor as well as M1 and M3). A recently introduced anticholinergic agent, tiotropium bromide (Spiriva, Boehringer-Ingelheim, Inc.,), Ridgefield, CT, is long-acting and may be more potent (has some M1 and M3 selectivity). Several recent studies indicate its superiority over ipratropium. Also, a recent randomized trial suggests that theophylline improves respiratory function and dyspnea in patients with severe COPD.

Numerous studies have examined the role of oral corticosteroid therapy in patients with stable COPD. A meta-analysis by Callahan et al. surveyed 33 original studies of oral corticosteroid use in the literature and selected 15 studies that met some preselected criteria of study quality. Callahan et al. concluded that stable COPD patients receiving steroids have a 20% or greater improvement in baseline FEV_1, approximately 10% more often than similar patients receiving placebo alone. Unfortunately, no satisfactory clinical predictors for response are apparent. In general, steroid use in these patients should be considered as an empirical trial, patient response should be objectively assessed, and benefits should be weighed against the well-known side effects of corticosteroid use. Current guidelines do not recommend the long-term use of corticosteroids in stable COPD due to the risk of skeletal muscle myopathy and other side effects.

Five randomized, large studies have examined the effect of inhaled steroids versus placebo on the annual rate of decline in FEV_1, with a minimum follow-up of 3 years. These studies include the Copenhagen City Lung Study, European Respiratory Society Study on Chronic Obstructive Pulmonary disease trial, Inhaled Steroids in Obstructive Lung Disease study, Lung Health Study II, and the Towards a Revolution in COPD Health (TORCH) study. These studies did not show a beneficial effect for inhaled steroids on lung function decline, except the TORCH study, which showed a small decrease in the rate of lung function decline of uncertain clinical significance. Current evidence and guidelines, however, recommend the use of inhaled corticosteroids to reduce the exacerbation rate and improve the health status in individuals with stage III or IV COPD (FEV_1 <50%) who have repeated exacerbations (e.g., three exacerbations in the preceding 3 years). In the TORCH study, inhaled corticosteroids decreased the rate of exacerbations that required corticosteroids, but did not decrease the rate of exacerbations severe enough to require hospitalization. In at least three randomized trials, the combination of an inhaled corticosteroid with an inhaled long-acting beta 2-agonist improved lung function and dyspnea compared to the individual components. A more recent study by Kardos et al. compared fluticasone/salmeterol to salmeterol, showing that the combination of an inhaled corticosteroid significantly reduced the frequency of moderate and severe exacerbations by 35% and delayed the time to first exacerbation. The TORCH study did not show a decrease in mortality from all deaths in the combination of inhaled fluticasone/salmeterol (hazard ratio 0.83, $p = 0.052$), although adjusted deaths were significantly reduced. One caveat is that the TORCH study and a study by Ernst et al. both show a higher rate of pneumonia in COPD patients taking inhaled corticosteroids.

Mucokinetic agents, such as organic iodides, have not been shown to have objective benefit in COPD. Alpha-1 antitrypsin augmentation therapy is used in nonsmoking younger patients with severe alpha-1 antitrypsin deficiency and associated emphysema. The efficacy of this therapy is unproved, although observational studies show that augmentation therapy decreases the rate of decline of FEV_1, reduces infections, improves survival, and reduces markers of lung inflammation. Human-pooled, plasma-derived alpha-1 antitrypsin is administered by intravenous infusion weekly, biweekly, or monthly. The recommended weekly dose is 60 mg/kg, and the monthly dose is 250 mg/kg. One potentially promising approach for the treatment of COPD is oral phosphodiesterase-4 (PDE4) inhibitors. These agents can improve lung function, although a recent study showed no decrease in exacerbations except for those with very severe COPD and no effect on quality of life.

The two most common causes of COPD exacerbations are infections of the tracheobronchial tree and air pollution, although as many as one-third of exacerbations have no identified cause. Bacteria cause the majority of acute exacerbations. Viruses (in particular, rhinoviruses, although influenza and respiratory syncytial virus are also important) are also a common cause, and a significant percentage of exacerbations are associated with both bacterial and viral infections. Acute exacerbations of COPD are often managed in a hospital setting, using aggressive aerosolized and intravenous pharmacotherapy with the agents discussed previously. Repeated inhaled beta-agonists (either nebulized or by metered-dose inhaler) are preferred over anticholinergics because the onset of action is more rapid. Systemic corticosteroids are usually given during acute exacerbations of COPD (either in the outpatient setting or in the hospital), and good evidence suggests that they accelerate the recovery and restoration of lung function, reduce treatment failure rate, improve subjective dyspnea and symptom scores, and reduce in-hospital days. The maximum benefit from systemic steroids is obtained

during the first 2 weeks of therapy, with no further benefit from more prolonged courses. The efficacy of antibiotic therapy in exacerbations of COPD is a topic of several studies and some controversy. In general, patients with a change in sputum, fever, and new infiltrate are optimal candidates for antibiotics, with the choice of agent directed at local patterns of sensitivity to *Streptococcus pneumoniae*, *Haemophilus influenzae*, and *Moraxella catarrhalis*. *Pseudomonas aeruginosa* may also play a role in severe COPD. There is probably no need for a routine sputum culture. The vast majority of patients with COPD exacerbation can be successfully managed using this therapy alone.

Perhaps 5% to 10% of COPD patients either fail this therapy or initially present with acute respiratory failure requiring intensive care, and perhaps 20% to 60% require ventilatory support, either noninvasively or following intubation and invasive mechanical ventilation. Several randomized controlled trials have shown that, in selected patients, noninvasive positive-pressure ventilation was successful in 80% to 85%, and reduced mortality and hospitalization. Extensive literature documents the intensive care unit (ICU) management of COPD patients; this topic is beyond the scope of this discussion. Previously, the prognosis for patients with acute respiratory failure secondary to COPD exacerbation alone, without complicating illness, was believed to be quite favorable. However, the recovery period can be long, extending over a period of 6 months and even longer in patients who sustain another exacerbation within that time frame. Studies suggest that exacerbation of COPD with admission to an ICU is associated with a hospital mortality rate of 24%. For patients 65 years and older, the 1-year mortality rate is 30% to 59%. In patients with COPD exacerbation and hypercapnia ($PaCO_2$ of ≥ 50 mm Hg), 1- and 2-year mortality rates are 43% and 49%, respectively. An episode of acute respiratory failure caused by an exacerbation of COPD does not appear to significantly alter the overall prognosis of the disease, which is largely dictated by the FEV_1 and age.

Measures that have been shown or proposed to reduce the rate of exacerbations of COPD in some but not all studies include influenza vaccination, inhaled corticosteroids, long-acting beta-agonists, combinations of inhaled corticosteroids and long-acting beta-agonists, long-acting anticholinergic agents, pulmonary rehabilitation, and PDE4 inhibitors.

Surgery for Emphysema

A variety of surgical techniques have been applied to a small subset of patients with advanced or end-stage COPD. Surgical resection of lung tissue in emphysema is "counterintuitive" and is based on the premise that advanced emphysema is characterized by very large, baggy lungs (with hyperinflation and reduced elastic recoil), along with respiratory muscles that are at a mechanical disadvantage because of hyperinflation. A variety of surgeries have been performed, including localized resection or bullectomy for focal giant bullae and lung volume reduction surgery (LVRS) (or bilateral pneumectomy or pneumoplasty). A variety of approaches have been used to perform LVRS, including a thoracoscopic approach using laser resection, median sternotomy using bilateral LVRS, or unilateral LVRS. This procedure has sometimes been used as a bridge during the consideration of lung transplantation. Presently, these techniques should be considered experimental for a small subset of patients who have very advanced emphysema, who remain symptomatic despite maximum medical therapy and oxygen, and whose nonpulmonary medical status is very good. Lung transplantation is an extremely limited surgical option, largely because of the scarcity of donors. This has partly contributed to consideration of alternative surgical procedures such as LVRS.

The physiologic mechanism for the benefit of LVRS in emphysema is probably mediated by increasing the elastic recoil of the lungs and reducing the resting and expiratory lung volumes. This restores the normal outward circumferential force on the airways, thus reducing resistance to expiratory airflow. In addition, improvements probably occur in the configuration of the diaphragm and intercostal muscles and in a greater contribution by the abdominal musculature to total volume. Currently, the selection criteria for LVRS are controversial, but the following features have been proposed to be associated with improved outcome in a systematic review with expert opinion:

- Smoking-related emphysema
- Heterogeneous emphysema on CT (i.e., surgically accessible "target" areas)
- Bilateral LVRS
- Good general fitness/condition
- Thoracic hyperinflation

In addition, in the randomized National Emphysema Treatment Trial Research Group study, survival was improved with LVRS, compared to medical therapy in patients with both predominantly upper-lobe emphysema and low postrehabilitation exercise capacity. Other favorable features include younger than 75 years, FEV_1 between 20% and 40% of predicted, evidence of hyperinflation (residual volume >150%, total lung capacity >100% of predicted), PaO_2 >45 mm Hg, $PaCO_2$ <60 mm Hg, postrehabilitation 6-minute walk >140 m. Selected unfavorable resection criteria include pulmonary hypertension (PA systolic >45 mm Hg, PA mean >35 mm Hg), FEV_1 <20% of predicted, lung diffusion capacity level <20% of predicted, homogeneous emphysema, non–upper lobe predominant emphysema, and high achieved wattage on postrehabilitation cycle ergometry.

Several surgical series using LVRS have indicated short-term improvement of FEV_1 between 50% and 82% at 6 months, along with reduced dyspnea and improved exercise tolerance and quality of life. The procedure does carry significant complications, however, including a 90-day sur-

gical mortality of 5.2% in non–high-risk patients, as compared to 1.5% in medically treated patients, and a mean hospital stay of 7 to 10 days, often due to prolonged air leak (in approximately 40% to 50% of the patients). The few studies with long-term outcomes suggest that, over time, lung volumes return to near preoperative baseline and dyspnea worsens, although the loss of 6-minute walk distance appears to be slower than other functional measures.

Lung transplantation remains an alternative for a few patients with advanced disease who meet the selection criteria noted as follows. Single-lung transplantation has emerged as a transplant procedure of choice for patients with COPD. The American Thoracic Society and European Respiratory Society recommend the following COPD-specific guidelines for the selection of lung transplantation candidates:

- FEV_1 of <25% of predicted (without reversibility), and/or
- Resting, room air $PaCO_2$ of >55 mm Hg, and/or
- Elevated $PaCO_2$ with progressive deterioration requiring long-term oxygen therapy, and/or
- Elevated pulmonary artery pressure with progressive deterioration

REVIEW EXERCISES

QUESTIONS

1. Which of the following is the most important variable to correct in patients with severe chronic obstructive pulmonary disease (either acute or chronic)?
a) $PaCO_2$
b) pH
c) Hypoxemia
d) Pulmonary hypertension
e) Cardiac output

Answer and Discussion

The answer is c. The overriding concern should be to improve tissue oxygen delivery. Although supplemental oxygen may contribute to hypercapnia (mostly by affecting ventilation–perfusion mismatching rather than the suppression of hypoxic drive), correcting hypoxemia (PaO_2 60 mm Hg, SaO_2 of 90%) is critical. The mechanism whereby chronic oxygen improves survival is probably by reducing pulmonary hypertension. The best way to reduce pulmonary artery pressures is to correct hypoxemia.

2. Which one of the following has been shown to increase survival in patients with severe chronic obstructive pulmonary disease?
a) Intensive care unit care and mechanical ventilation
b) Systemic steroids during acute exacerbations
c) Long-term oxygen therapy
d) Smoking cessation
e) Chronic therapy with bronchodilators

Answer and Discussion

The answer is c. All answer choices are reasonable therapies for chronic obstructive pulmonary disease, but only ambulatory home oxygen for more than 12 hours/day has been unequivocally shown to improve survival (in appropriate candidates who have baseline hypoxemia). In the Nocturnal Oxygen Therapy Trial, survival in the continuous oxygen group was 75% versus 54% in the control group at 36 months (oxygen 12 hours/day).

3. All the following regarding asthma therapy are correct, *except*
a) Case-control studies indicate that regular use of inhaled steroids reduces asthma mortality.
b) Chronic maintenance anti-inflammatory is indicated in all patients with persistent asthma.
c) A variety of novel therapies are under development for asthma.
d) Head-to-head studies have proved that inhaled steroids are the best therapy for all patients with asthma.

Answer and Discussion

The answer is d. All agents approved for asthma (cromoglycate, inhaled steroids, antileukotrienes) have shown objective benefit compared with placebo. Limited head-to-head studies do exist, but those available indicate that the magnitude of improvement is higher for inhaled steroids, especially for patients with severe asthma. These agents have the potential for systemic side effects. Therefore, for any given patient, therapy should be individualized.

4. Antileukotrienes may have particular benefit in which subset of asthmatics?
a) Aspirin-sensitive asthma
b) Allergic bronchopulmonary aspergillosis
c) Prednisone-dependent asthma
d) Allergic asthma
e) Occupational asthma

Answer and Discussion

The answer is a. The leukotriene pathway is particularly important in patients with aspirin-induced asthma. Studies show the effectiveness of leukotriene antagonists.

5. Which one of the following statements does not belong with the other choices?
a) Bilateral vocal cord paralysis
b) Postextubation stridor
c) Factitious (or functional) asthma
d) Variable extrathoracic upper airway obstruction
e) Flattening of the expiratory limb of flow–volume loop

Answer and Discussion

The answer is e. With variable extrathoracic upper airway obstruction (i.e., bilateral vocal cord paralysis, postextubation stridor, functional vocal cord adduction), the flow–volume loop would show flattening of the inspiratory limb.

Acknowledgment

The author wants to acknowledge the contributions of Dr. Mani Kavuru to previous editions of this chapter.

SUGGESTED READINGS

Asthma

Broide DH. Molecular and cellular mechanisms of allergic disease. *J Allergy Clin Immunol* 2001;108:S65–S71.

Elias JA, Lee CG, Zheng T, et al. New insights into the pathogenesis of asthma. *J Clin Invest* 2003;111:291–297.

Kavuru M, Melamed J, Gross G, et al. Salmeterol and fluticasone propionate combined in a new powder inhalation device for the treatment of asthma: a randomized, double-blind, placebo-controlled trial. *J Allergy Clin Immunol* 2000;105:1108–1116.

Mannino DM, Homa DM, Akinbami LJ, et al. Surveillance for asthma—United States, 1980–1999. *MMWR Surveill Summ* 2002;51 (SS01):1–13.

National Heart, Lung, and Blood Institute, National Asthma Education and Prevention Program Coordinating Committee. *Expert Panel Report 3 (EPR3): Guidelines for the Diagnosis and Management of Asthma.* Bethesda, MD: National Heart, Lung, and Blood Institute, 2007. (NIH Publication No. 08-4051). Available at: www.nhlbi.nih.gov/guidelines/asthma.

Nelson HS, Weiss ST, Bleecker ER, et al. The Salmeterol Multicenter Asthma Research Trial: a comparison of usual pharmacotherapy for asthma or usual pharmacotherapy plus salmeterol. *Chest* 2006;129:15–26.

Palmer LJ, Silverman ES, Weiss ST, et al. Pharmacogenetics of asthma. *Am J Respir Crit Care Med* 2002;165:861–866.

Reiss TF, Chervinsky P, Dockhorn RJ, et al. Montelukast, a once daily leukotriene receptor antagonist in the treatment of chronic asthma; a multicenter randomized double-blind trial. *Arch Intern Med* 1998;158:1213–1220.

Smith AD, Cowan JO, Brassett KP, et al. Use of exhaled nitric oxide measurements to guide treatment in chronic asthma. *N Engl J Med* 2005;352:2163–2173.

Soler M, Matz J, Townley R, et al. The anti-IgE antibody omalizumab reduces exacerbations and steroid requirement in allergic asthmatics. *Eur Respir J* 2001;18(2):254–261.

Szefler S, Weiss S, Tonascia J, et al. Long-term effects of budesonide or nedocromil in children with asthma. The CAMP Research Group. *N Engl J Med* 2000;343:1054–1063.

Wechsler ME, Lehman E, Lazarus SC, et al. Beta-adrenergic polymorphisms and response to salmeterol. *Am J Respir Crit Care Med* 2006;173:473–474.

Weiss ST. Eat dirt—the hygiene hypothesis and allergic diseases. *N Engl J Med* 2002;347:930–931.

Chronic Obstructive Pulmonary Disease

American Thoracic Society/European Respiratory Society Task Force. *Standards for the Diagnosis and Management of Patients with COPD* (Internet). Version 1.2. New York: American Thoracic Society, 2004 (updated 2005 September 8). Available at: www.thoracic.org/go/copd.

Anthonisen NR, Connett JE, Kiley JP, et al. Effects of smoking intervention and the use of an inhaled anticholinergic bronchodilator on the rate of decline of FEV$_1$: the Lung Health Study. *JAMA* 1994;272:1497–1505.

Callahan CM, Dittus RS, Katz BP. Oral corticosteroid therapy for patients with stable chronic obstructive pulmonary disease: a meta-analysis. *Ann Intern Med* 1991;114:216–223.

Calverley PM, Anderson JA, Celli B, et al. Salmeterol and fluticasone propionate and survival in chronic obstructive pulmonary disease. *N Engl J Med* 2007;356(8):775–789.

Calverley PM, Sanchez-Toril F, McIvor A, et al. Effect of 1-year treatment with roflumilast in severe chronic obstructive pulmonary disease. *Am J Respir Crit Care Med* 2007;176:154–161.

Casaburi R, Briggs DD Jr, Donohue JF, et al. The spirometric efficacy of once-daily dosing with tiotropium in stable COPD: a 13-week multicenter trial. *Chest* 2000;118:1294.

Casanova C, Cote C, de Torres JP, et al. Inspiratory-to-total lung capacity ratio predicts mortality in patients with chronic obstructive pulmonary disease. *Am J Respir Crit Care Med* 2005;171:591–597.

Celli BR, Cote CG, Marin JM, et al. The body-mass index, airflow obstruction, dyspnea, and exercise capacity index in chronic obstructive pulmonary disease. *N Engl J Med* 2004;350:1005–1012.

Connors AF, Dawson NV, Thomas C, et al. Outcomes following acute exacerbation of severe chronic obstructive pulmonary disease. *Am J Respir Crit Care Med* 1996;154:959–967.

Ernst P, Gonzalez AV, Brassard P, et al. Inhaled corticosteroids use in chronic obstructive pulmonary disease and the risk of hospitalization for pneumonia. *Am J Respir Crit Care Med* 2007;176:162–166.

Fein AM, Braman SS, Casaburi R, et al. Lung volume reduction surgery: official statement of the American Thoracic Society. *Am J Respir Crit Care Med* 1996;154:1151.

Fishman A, Martinez F, Naunheim K, et al. A randomized trial comparing lung-volume-reduction surgery with medical therapy for severe emphysema. *N Engl J Med* 2003;348:2059–2073.

Geddes D, Davies M, Koyama H, et al. Effect of lung-volume-reduction surgery in patients with severe emphysema. *N Engl J Med* 2000;343:239.

Global Initiative for Chronic Obstructive Lung Disease Web site: www.goldcopd.com.

Hill NS. Noninvasive ventilation: does it work, for whom, and how? *Am Rev Respir Dis* 1993;147:1050–1055.

International guidelines for the selection of lung transplant candidates. *Am J Respir Crit Care Med* 1998;158:335.

Kardos P, Wencker M, Glaab T, et al. Impact of salmeterol/fluticasone propionate versus salmeterol on exacerbations in severe chronic obstructive pulmonary disease. *Am J Respir Crit Care Med* 2007;175:144–149.

Kotlke TE, Battista RN, DeFriese GH, et al. Attributes of successful smoking cessation interventions in medical practice: a meta analysis of 39 controlled trials. *JAMA* 1988;259:2882–2889.

Lacasse Y, Wong E, Guyatt GH, et al. Meta-analysis of respiratory rehabilitation in chronic obstructive pulmonary disease. *Lancet* 1996;348:1115–1119.

Lung Health Study Research Group. Effect of inhaled triamcinolone on the decline in pulmonary function in chronic obstructive pulmonary disease. *N Engl J Med* 2000;343:1902.

Mannino DM, Gagnon RC, Petty TL, et al. Obstructive lung disease and low lung function in adults in the United States: data from the National Health and Nutrition Examination Survey, 1988–1994. *Arch Intern Med* 2000;160:1683–1689.

Mannino DM, Homa DM, Akinbami LJ, et al. Chronic obstructive lung disease surveillance—United States, 1971–2000. *MMWR Surveill Summ* 2002;51(6):1–16.

Niewoehner DE, Erbland ML, Deupree RH, et al. Effect of systemic glucocorticoids on exacerbations of chronic obstructive pulmonary disease. Department of Veterans Affairs Cooperative Study Group. *N Engl J Med* 1999;340:1941–1947.

Ries AL, Kaplan RM, Limberg TM, et al. Effects of pulmonary rehabilitation on physiologic and psychological outcomes in patients with chronic obstructive pulmonary disease. *Ann Intern Med* 1995;122:823–832.

Rutten-van Molken M, van Doorslaer E, Jansen M, et al. Costs and effects of inhaled corticosteroids and bronchodilators in asthma and COPD. *Am J Respir Crit Care Med* 1995;151:975–982.

Saint S, Bent S, Vittinghoff E, et al. Antibiotics in chronic obstructive pulmonary disease exacerbations: a meta-analysis. *JAMA* 1995;273:957–960.

Sciurba FC, Rogers RM, Keenan RJ, et al. Improvement in pulmonary function and elastic recoil after lung-reduction surgery for diffuse emphysema. *N Engl J Med* 1996;334:1095.

Spencer S, Jones PW, for the Globe Study Group. Time course of recovery of health status following an infective exacerbation of chronic bronchitis. *Thorax* 2003;58:589–593.

Stoller JK, Aboussouan LS. Intravenous augmentation therapy for AAT deficiency: current understanding. *Thorax* 2004;59:708–712.

Tarpy SP, Celli BR. Long-term oxygen therapy. *N Engl J Med* 1995;333:710–714.

Thompson WH, Nielson CP, Carvalho P, et al. Controlled trial of oral prednisone in outpatients with acute COPD exacerbation. *Am J Respir Crit Care Med* 1996;154:407–412.

Weinmann GG, Hyatt R. Evaluation and research in lung volume reduction surgery. *Am J Respir Crit Care Med* 1996;154:1913–1918.

Wilt TJ, Niewoehner D, MacDonald R, et al. Management of stable chronic obstructive pulmonary disease: a systematic review for a clinical practice guideline. *Ann Intern Med* 2007;147:639–653.

Chapter 36

Interstitial Lung Disease

Jeffrey T. Chapman

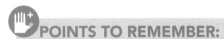

POINTS TO REMEMBER:

- Interstitial lung diseases (ILDs) with known causes are further classified based on specific exposure, association with systemic disease, or association with a known genetic disorder.

- There is considerable variability among the specific diseases in the character and distribution of radiographic abnormalities. However, for most ILDs, the plain chest radiograph will reveal reduced lung volumes with bilateral reticular or reticulonodular opacities.

- The plain radiograph and high-resolution CT in idiopathic pulmonary fibrosis reveal bilateral, peripheral, and basilar predominant disease with reticulonodular infiltrates, often with honeycomb, cystic change.

- A restrictive physiological impairment is the most common finding in ILDs. Both forced expiratory volume in 1 second (FEV_1) and forced vital capacity (FVC) are diminished, and the FEV_1/FVC ratio is preserved or even supranormal.

- Many drugs have been associated with pulmonary complications of various types, including interstitial inflammation and fibrosis, bronchospasm, pulmonary edema, and pleural effusions. Drugs from many different therapeutic classes can cause ILD, including chemotherapeutic agents, antibiotics, antiarrhythmic drugs, and immunosuppressive agents.

- ILD is a well-known complication of several connective tissue diseases. The most commonly implicated disorders are scleroderma, rheumatoid arthritis, Sjögren's syndrome, polymyositis/dermatomyositis, and systemic lupus erythematosus.

The term *interstitial lung disease* (ILD) refers to a broad category of lung diseases rather than a specific disease entity.[1,2] It includes a variety of illnesses with diverse causes, treatments, and prognoses. These disorders are grouped together because of similarities in their clinical presentations, plain chest radiographic appearance, and physiological features.

ORGANIZATION OF THE INTERSTITIAL LUNG DISEASES

Because there are more than 100 separate disorders, it is helpful to group them based on etiology, disease associations, or pathology. An organizational scheme is presented in Figure 36.1. First, the diseases are broken down into those with known causes or associations and those of unknown cause. Diseases with known causes are further classified based on specific exposure, association with systemic disease, or association with a known genetic disorder. These groups are further divided into specific disease entities. Using this organizational scheme, one is able to perform a careful and complete history, develop a focused diagnostic plan, and work toward an accurate diagnosis.

PATHOPHYSIOLOGY

As the name implies, the histologic abnormalities that characterize ILD generally involve the pulmonary interstitium to a greater extent than the alveolar spaces or airways, although exceptions exist. The interstitium is the area between the capillaries and the alveolar space. In the normal state, this space allows close apposition of gas and capillaries with minimal connective tissue matrix, fibroblasts, and inflammatory cells. The interstitium supports the delicate relationship between the alveoli and capillaries, allowing for efficient gas exchange. When responding

425

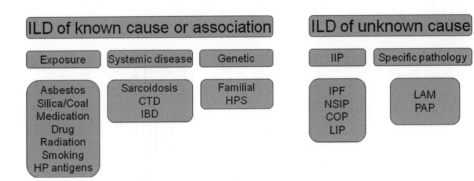

Figure 36.1 Current organization of ILD. COP = cryptogenic organizing pneumonia, CTD = connective tissue disease, IBD = inflammatory bowel disease, ILD = interstitial lung disease, IPF = idiopathic pulmonary fibrosis, HPS = Hermansky-Pudlak syndrome, LAM = lymphangioleiomyomatosis, LIP = lymphocytic interstitial pneumonia, NSIP = nonspecific interstitial pneumonitis, PAP = pulmonary alveolar proteinosis, PLCH = pulmonary Langerhans cell histiocytosis.

to any injury, whether from a specific exposure (e.g., asbestos, nitrofurantoin, or an antigen), an autoimmune-mediated inflammation from a systemic connective tissue disease (e.g., scleroderma, polymyositis, or rheumatoid arthritis), or unknown injury (e.g., idiopathic pulmonary fibrosis [IPF]), the lung must respond to the damage and repair itself. If the exposure persists or if the repair process is imperfect, the lung may be permanently damaged with increased interstitial tissue and scar replacing the normal capillaries, alveoli, and healthy interstitium.

These pathological abnormalities can lead to profound impairment in lung physiology. Gas exchange is impaired owing to ventilation/perfusion mismatch, decreased diffusion across the abnormal interstitium, and shunt. Work of breathing is markedly increased because of decreased lung compliance. Together, these physiological impairments lead to the exercise intolerance seen in all ILDs. Unfortunately, if the initiating injury or abnormal repair from injury is not halted, progressive tissue damage leading to worsening physiological impairment and death can occur.

CHARACTERISTICS OF INTERSTITIAL LUNG DISEASE

Clinical Signs and Symptoms of Interstitial Lung Disease

Many of the ILDs have similar clinical features and are not easily distinguished on examination. Symptoms are generally limited to the respiratory tract, and extrapulmonary symptoms should be heeded as clues to a systemic disorder. Exertional breathlessness (dyspnea) and a nonproductive cough are the most common reasons patients seek medical attention. However, sputum production, hemoptysis, or wheezing can occur and is helpful in classifying the disease. If the patient also has nonrespiratory symptoms, such as myalgia, arthralgia, or sclerodactyly, ILD resulting from underlying connective tissue disease may be present.

Physical Examination

Most patients with ILD have bilateral inspiratory, fine crackles, which are usually most prominent at the lung bases. However, some diseases such as sarcoidosis and lymphangioleiomyomatosis (LAM) may have only decreased breath sounds without adventitious sounds, despite markedly abnormal chest radiographs. Expiratory wheezing is relatively uncommon, and its presence suggests either airway involvement as part of the primary disease process or concomitant airways disease such as emphysema or asthma. Occasionally, wheezing may be a clue to a particular diagnosis, such as sarcoidosis or inflammatory bowel disease–related ILD, which may involve both the airways and the interstitium.

Signs of pulmonary arterial hypertension with right ventricular dysfunction, such as lower-extremity edema or jugular venous distension, may occur late in the course of any ILD and are not helpful in determining the specific ILD.

Examination may also disclose features of underlying connective tissue disease, including sclerodactyly, proximal muscle weakness, joint deformities, or skin rash. Sarcoidosis is suggested by the presence of erythema nodosum or facial skin lesions, whereas chronic intestinal symptoms suggest inflammatory bowel disease–related ILD.

Radiographic Features

There is considerable variability among the specific diseases in the character and distribution of radiographic abnormalities. However, for most ILDs, the plain chest radiograph will reveal reduced lung volumes with bilateral reticular or reticulonodular opacities. The ready availability of high-resolution CT (HRCT) has highlighted significant radiographic differences between diseases that have similar plain chest radiographic patterns.[3] HRCT has the ability to better define the specific characteristics of lung parenchyma seen in each disease, increasing the likelihood of establishing a correct diagnosis.[4]

The plain chest radiograph and HRCT features of IPF are important patterns to recognize because, next to sarcoidosis, IPF is the most common ILD, and IPF images are the prototypical pattern of fibrotic injury response in the lung. The plain radiograph and HRCT in IPF reveal bilateral, peripheral, and basilar predominant disease with reticulonodular infiltrates, often with honeycomb, cystic change. Figure 36.2 shows a plain radiograph with

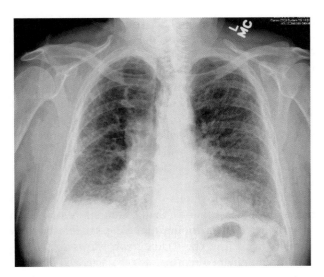

Figure 36.2 Plain chest radiograph of idiopathic pulmonary fibrosis.

bibasilar reticulonodular infiltrates. Note the overall volume loss and poorly demarcated pleural-parenchymal borders along the hemidiaphragms and heart, indicating parenchymal abnormalities extending to the pleura. Figure 36.3 shows an HRCT image of IPF with distortion of the lung architecture and traction bronchiectasis, especially at the lung bases. As predicted by the plain radiograph, the abnormalities are strikingly located in the subpleural and dependent areas of the lung. Ground-glass abnormalities, increased attenuation of the lung tissue without distortion of the underlying blood vessels or bronchi, are absent or minimal in classic IPF. Pleural disease and significant lymphadenopathy are not seen, although up to two-thirds of IPF patients can have mild mediastinal adenopathy.[5] As the burden of disease increases, the chest x-ray examination may reveal multiple, tiny cysts in the most markedly involved regions. This cystic pattern, called honeycombing,

reflects end-stage fibrosis and is a feature of many end-stage ILDs.

In contrast to the fibrotic type of injury, some diseases cause an inflammatory abnormality with a much different radiographic image. In cellular nonspecific interstitial pneumonitis (NSIP), the predominant abnormality is ground glass without distortion of the lung architecture or loss of volume, as seen in Figure 36.4. In addition, the predominant central and mid lung zone location of abnormalities is distinct from IPF. Understanding these two patterns as ends of an extreme, we see how one is able to evaluate other diseases in a similar context.

Physiological Features

Similar to the radiographic findings, there is considerable variability in the physiological abnormalities of the different ILDs. However, a restrictive physiological impairment is the most common finding.[6] Both FEV_1 and FVC are diminished, and the FEV_1/FVC ratio is preserved or even supranormal. Lung volumes are reduced, as is the diffusing capacity of the lung for carbon monoxide (DLCO). This reduction in diffusing capacity reflects both a pathological disturbance of the alveolar–capillary interface and a loss of alveolar units.

Although not commonly pursued, the compliance characteristics of the lungs can be evaluated with an esophageal balloon to measure intrathoracic pressure at various lung volumes. In almost all ILDs, the lungs have reduced compliance and require supranormal transpleural pressures to ventilate. This lack of compliance results in small lung volumes and increased work of breathing.

Less frequently, physiological obstruction may be the pattern seen. This can be the result of the primary disease process (e.g., LAM, pulmonary Langerhans cell histiocytosis [PLCH], sarcoidosis, or inflammatory bowel disease–related ILD) or concomitant emphysema or asthma.[7] If ILD

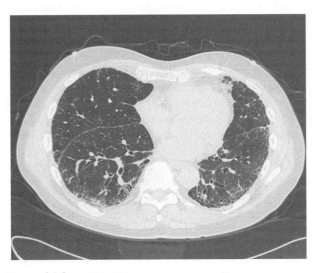

Figure 36.3 HRCT of idiopathic pulmonary fibrosis.

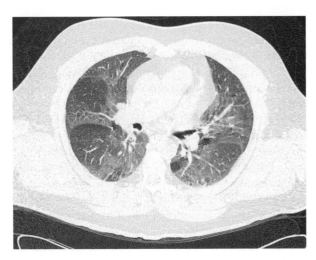

Figure 36.4 HRCT of ground-glass opacity infiltrates as seen in nonspecific interstitial pneumonitis.

develops in a patient with significant emphysema, the opposing physiological effects of the two diseases may result in deceptively normal spirometry and lung volume measurements, as well as apparently normally compliant lungs. However, because both emphysema and ILD result in impaired gas exchange, the DLCO is markedly decreased.

SELECTED SPECIFIC TYPES OF INTERSTITIAL LUNG DISEASE AND THEIR THERAPIES

Exposure-Related Interstitial Lung Disease

Occupational

The three most common types of occupational ILD are asbestosis, chronic silicosis, and coal workers' pneumoconiosis (CWP). Predictable clinical and radiographic abnormalities occur in susceptible patients who have been exposed to asbestos.[8] These abnormalities include pleural changes (plaques, fibrosis, effusions, rounded atelectasis, and mesothelioma) as well as parenchymal scarring and lung cancer. Asbestos exposure alone increases the risk of lung cancer only minimally (1.5–3.0 times). Asbestos exposure *and* cigarette smoking, however, act synergistically to greatly increase the risk of cancer.

Asbestos exposure may also result in benign asbestos pleural effusions (BAPEs) or an entity known as *rounded atelectasis*. BAPEs may be asymptomatic or may be associated with acute chest pain, fever, and dyspnea. Generally, a shorter lag time exists between the initial asbestos exposure and the development of BAPEs (<15 years) than is seen with other manifestations of asbestos exposure. The effusions are characteristically exudative and are often bloody. In a patient with a history of asbestos exposure and a bloody pleural effusion, the major differential diagnostic concern is malignant pleural effusion from a mesothelioma. The clinical course of BAPEs is that of spontaneous resolution, often with recurrences, and treatment is drainage to reduce symptoms. Rounded atelectasis typically presents as a pleural-based parenchymal mass that may be mistaken for carcinoma. The characteristic CT features, however, such as local volume loss, pleural thickening, and the "comet tail" appearance of bronchi and vessels curving into the lesion help distinguish rounded atelectasis from carcinoma.

The term asbestos-related pulmonary disease may be used to encompass these entities, whereas asbestosis is reserved for patients who have evidence of parenchymal fibrosis. Most patients with asbestosis have had considerable asbestos exposure many years before manifestation of the lung disease. Exposure is frequently associated with occupations such as shipbuilding or insulation work. Patients report very slowly progressive dyspnea on exertion[9] and have rales on lung examination. Physiological testing shows restrictive impairment with reduced DLCO. The chest x-ray examination reveals bilateral lower-zone reticulonodular infiltrates similar to those seen in IPF. With an appropriate exposure history, the presence of radiographic pleural plaques or rounded atelectasis indicates asbestos as the cause of the ILD, although neither of these findings is required for establishing the diagnosis.

No medical therapy has been demonstrated to improve or decrease progression of asbestosis. Unfortunately, severe impairment typically occurs 30 to 40 years after exposure, making almost all patients ineligible for lung transplantation because of age. Management of asbestosis is supportive.

Chronic silicosis results from chronic exposure to inhaled silica. Occupations that commonly entail exposure to silica include mining, tunneling, sandblasting, and foundry work. The chest radiograph shows upper lung zone–predominant abnormalities characterized by multiple small nodular opacities in the central lung tissue. These nodules may slowly coalesce into large masses known as progressive massive fibrosis (PMF). Enlargement and eggshell calcification of the hilar lymph nodes is common. Functional and physiological impairment in chronic silicosis is quite variable. Some patients with abnormal chest radiographs report few, if any, symptoms and may have a normal lung examination and pulmonary function testing. Unfortunately, many patients are impaired and have mixed restrictive and obstructive impairment with reduced diffusion capacity. The physiological impairment may remain stable or, if PMF occurs, may progress even in the absence of continued exposure. Symptoms are typically exertional dyspnea and variable mucus production.

It is important to recognize the association of silicosis with lung cancer and active tuberculosis.[10] Patients with silicosis are at increased risk of lung cancer, and the risk is increased when combined with exposure to tobacco smoke, diesel exhaust, or radon gas. Silicosis patients develop active tuberculosis 2- to 30-fold more frequently than coworkers without silicosis. This association is especially important in societies with a high incidence of HIV infection, which markedly increases the risk of silicosis-associated active tuberculosis.

CWP develops as the result of chronic inhalation of coal dust. In the past, it was assumed that silica dust was responsible for the pulmonary disease seen among coal miners because the clinical and radiographic features are quite similar to chronic silicosis. However, it is now recognized that CWP and silicosis are the result of distinct exposures. Simple CWP, characterized by multiple small nodular opacities on the chest x-ray film, is asymptomatic. Cough and shortness of breath do not develop unless the disease progresses to PMF similar to that seen in silicosis.

There are no proven therapies for either silicosis or CWP other than eliminating exposure. In patients with significant obstructive impairment or mucus production, inhaled bronchodilators and corticosteroids may relieve some symptoms. Exacerbations can be frequent and are treated with antibiotics and systemic corticosteroids.

TABLE 36.1

DRUGS ASSOCIATED WITH THE DEVELOPMENT OF INTERSTITIAL LUNG DISEASE

Antibiotics
    Nitrofurantoin
    Sulfasalazine
Antiinflammatory agents
    Aspirin
    Gold
    Penicillamine
    Methotrexate
    Etanercept
    Infliximab
Cardiovascular agents
    Amiodarone
    Tocainide
Chemotherapeutic agents
    Bleomycin
    Mitomycin-C
    Busulfan
    Cyclophosphamide
    Chlorambucil
    Melphalan
    Azathioprine
    Cytosine arabinoside
    Methotrexate
    Carmustine
    Lomustine
    Methyl-CCNU
    Procarbazine
    Zinostatin
    Etoposide
    Vinblastine
    Imatinib
    Flutamide
Drug-induced systemic lupus erythematosus
    Procainamide
    Isoniazid
    Hydralazine
    Hydantoin
    Penicillamine
Illicit drugs
    Heroin
    Methadone
    Propoxyphene
    Talc as an IV contaminant
Miscellaneous agents
    Oxygen
    Drugs inducing pulmonary infiltrate and eosinophilia
        l-tryptophan
    Hydrochlorothiazide
    Radiation

Adapted from Camus P. Drug induced infiltrative lung diseases. In: Schwarz MI, King TE, eds. *Interstitial Lung Disease*, 4th ed. Hamilton, Ontario, Canada: BC Decker, 2003.

Medications, Drugs, and Radiation

Many drugs have been associated with pulmonary complications of various types, including interstitial inflammation and fibrosis, bronchospasm, pulmonary edema, and pleural effusions.[11] Drugs from many different therapeutic classes can cause ILD, including chemotherapeutic agents, antibiotics, antiarrhythmic drugs, and immunosuppressive agents (Table 36.1). There are no distinct physiological, radiographic, or pathological patterns of drug-induced ILD, and the diagnosis is usually made when a patient is exposed to a medication known to result in lung disease, the timing of the exposure is appropriate for the development of the disease, and other causes of ILD have been eliminated. Treatment is avoidance of further exposure and systemic corticosteroids in markedly impaired or declining patients.

Exposure to therapeutic radiation may result in ILD. Patients presenting within 6 months of radiation therapy generally have ground-glass abnormalities believed to represent acute inflammation. The ground-glass abnormalities can occur in both radiation-exposed and unexposed tissue. Short-term systemic corticosteroid treatment can improve lung function. In contrast, dyspnea that develops more than 6 months after therapy typically appears as densely fibrotic tissue within the radiation port. On CT examination, a straight line indicating the margin of radiation is frequently evident, as seen in Figure 36.5. These patients do not improve with corticosteroid therapy, and treatment is supportive.

Hypersensitivity Pneumonitis

Hypersensitivity pneumonitis (HP) is a cell-mediated immune reaction to inhaled antigens in susceptible persons.[12] Patients must be sensitized by an initial exposure, with subsequent re-exposure leading to either acute HP or chronic HP. Patients with acute HP usually present to medical attention with sudden shortness of breath, chest pain, fever, chills, malaise, and a cough that may be productive of purulent sputum. In comparison, patients who are chronically exposed to low levels of inhaled antigens may develop subtle interstitial inflammatory reactions in the lung that do not result in noticeable symptoms for months to years

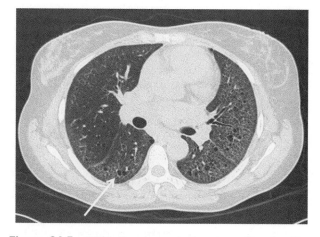

Figure 36.5 HRCT slice demonstrating dense fibrosis with a nonanatomical straight line boundary.

and can present with severe, impairing disease, which can be very difficult to distinguish from IPF.

Common organic antigens known to cause hypersensitivity pneumonitis include bacteria and fungi, which may be found in moldy hay (farmer's lung) or in the home environment, particularly in association with central humidification systems (humidifier lung), indoor hot tubs, and animal proteins (bird fancier's lung). Inorganic antigens from vaporized paints and plastics can also lead to HP. Numerous established antigens are listed in Table 36.2, along with the typical source of exposure and the associated syndrome.

Because the relationship between an exposure and the lung disease may not be obvious, a careful systematic occupational, environmental, and avocational history is critical in evaluating patients with ILD. Elements that strongly suggest a diagnosis of HP are exposure to an appropriate antigen and the correct temporal relationship of symptoms to the exposure. Blood samples may be obtained to determine whether there has been an antibody response to certain antigens associated with HP (serum precipitins); however, the presence of such antibodies is not sufficient to establish the diagnosis of HP because many persons develop antibodies in the absence of disease. Likewise, the absence of detectable antibodies does not rule out the diagnosis of HP because the culprit may be an antigen that is not included in the analysis.

TABLE 36.2

ETIOLOGIES OF HYPERSENSITIVITY PNEUMONITIS

Antigen	Exposure	Syndrome
BACTERIA		
Thermophilic Bacteria		
Saccharopolyspora rectivirgula	Moldy hay	Farmer's lung
Thermoactinomyces vulgaris	Moldy sugarcane	Bagassosis
Thermoactinomyces sacchari	Mushroom compost	Mushroom worker's lung
Thermoactinomyces candidus	Heated water reservoirs	Humidifier lung
		Air conditioner lung
Nonthermophilic Bacteria		
Bacillus subtilis, Bacillus cereus	Water, detergent	Humidifier lung
		Washing powder lung
FUNGI		
Aspergillus sp.	Moldy hay	Farmer's lung
	Water	Ventilation pneumonitis
Aspergillus clavatus	Barley	Malt worker's lung
Penicillium casei, Penicillium roqueforti	Cheese	Cheese washer's lung
Alternaria sp.	Wood pulp	Woodworker's lung
Cryptostroma corticale	Wood bark	Maple bark stripper's lung
Graphium, Aureobasidium pullulans	Wood dust	Sequoiosis
Merulius lacrymans	Rotten wood	Dry rot lung
Penicillium frequentans	Cork dust	Suberosis
Aureobasidium pullulans	Water	Humidifier lung
Cladosporium sp.	Hot-tub mists	Hot tub HP
Trichosporon cutaneum	Damp wood and mats	Japanese summer-type HP
AMOEBAE		
Naegleria gruberi	Contaminated water	Humidifier lung
Acanthamoeba polyphaga	Contaminated water	Humidifier lung
Acanthamoeba castellani	Contaminated water	Humidifier lung
ANIMAL PROTEINS		
Avian proteins	Bird droppings, feathers	Bird breeder's lung
Urine, serum, pelts	Rats, gerbils	Animal handler's lung
CHEMICALS		
Isocyanates, trimellitic anhydride	Paints, resins, plastics	Chemical worker's lung
Copper sulfate	Bordeaux mixture	Vineyard sprayer's lung
Phthalic anhydride	Heated epoxy resin	Epoxy resin lung
Sodium diazobenzene sulfate	Chromatography reagent	Pauli's reagent alveolitis
Pyrethrum	Pesticide	Pyrethrum HP

HP = hypersensitivity pneumonitis.
Adapted from Selman M. Hypersensitivity pneumonitis. In: Schwarz MI, King TE, eds. *Interstitial Lung Disease*, 4th ed. Hamilton: BC Decker, 2003.

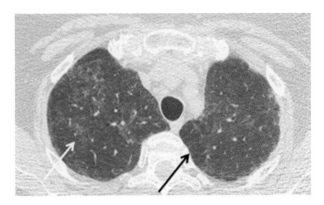

Figure 36.6   HRCT of hypersensitivity pneumonitis demonstrating indistinct centrilobular ground glass (*white arrow*) and air trapping (*black arrow*).

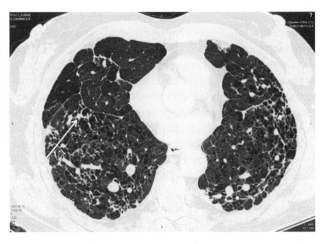

Figure 36.7   HRCT of pulmonary Langerhans cell histiocytosis demonstrating stellate nodule and irregular cyst formation.

Acute or subacute HP often has a characteristic radiographic appearance. The plain chest radiograph can be normal or with minimal bilateral upper and mid lung zone infiltrates. The HRCT images show centrilobular indistinct nodules in the upper and middle lobes with other areas of focal air trapping as seen in **Figure 36.6**. These abnormalities represent the alveolar and bronchiolar location of the immune response to the inhaled antigens.

Specific therapies for HP are strict antigen avoidance and immunosuppression with corticosteroids in patients with symptomatic or physiologically impairing disease. In acute HP, corticosteroids appear to hasten recover, but do not improve ultimate lung function.[13] In chronic HP, patients with fibrosis on CT scan have shorter survival, and it is unknown if long-term immunosuppression is beneficial.[14]

Tobacco-Related Interstitial Lung Disease

Although the association between tobacco use and chronic obstructive pulmonary disease (COPD) is well known, the relationship with ILD is less well appreciated. It is a risk factor for the development of IPF, but not the sole cause. However, the following three types of ILD have a strong association with cigarette smoking: desquamative interstitial pneumonitis (DIP), respiratory bronchiolitis–associated interstitial lung disease (RB-ILD), and PLCH.

Virtually all patients with DIP and RB-ILD are current or former tobacco smokers. HRCT usually demonstrates micronodular central infiltrates in RB-ILD and diffuse ground glass in DIP. Spirometry is variable, with most having significant restriction and variable amounts of obstruction. As with other toxic exposures, complete avoidance of all smoke is important for these patients. In RB-ILD, physiological stabilization and, occasionally, even improvement can occur after abstinence from tobacco. In DIP, the benefits of smoking cessation are unclear. Both groups of patients may benefit from inhaled corticosteroids and bronchodilators, but most patients unfortunately have nonprogressive pulmonary impairment and reduced

exercise tolerance.[15] Chronic immunosuppression is not beneficial in most patients.[16]

PLCH is an ILD found in adult smokers. Patients usually have a significant smoking history and develop cough and progressive dyspnea on exertion. Chest examination is notable for diffuse inspiratory crackles. HRCT demonstrates pathognomonic central, mid lung zone stellate nodules with adjacent thin-walled cysts, as seen in **Figure 36.7**. Pulmonary physiology generally reveals obstructive impairment with a decreased DLCO. The pathological pattern is unique with the hallmark Langerhans histiocytes seen in groups of star-shaped nodules with destruction of adjacent lung tissue. Although PLCH is pathologically similar to childhood LCH, the adult form does not typically involve bone and has not proven to respond to chemotherapy as the childhood form does. The relationship of these two disorders has yet to be defined.

Primary treatment is abstinence from all tobacco exposure, either primary or second hand. In patients with mild or moderate disease, lung function may stabilize after smoking cessation, but some will progressively decline. Stabilization or improvement with oral corticosteroids is described, but overall benefit is unproven. Patients with progressive disease despite avoidance of all smoke exposure can be offered lung transplantation.

Systemic Disease–Associated Interstitial Lung Disease

Connective Tissue Disease

ILD is a well-known complication of several connective tissue diseases.[17] The most commonly implicated disorders are scleroderma, rheumatoid arthritis, Sjögren's syndrome, polymyositis/dermatomyositis, and systemic lupus erythematosus.

In any of these disorders, pulmonary involvement may remain undetected until significant impairment is present because these patients may be inactive as a result of the underlying connective tissue disease. There is generally poor correlation between the severity of the pulmonary and nonpulmonary manifestations of these diseases. In some instances, the lung disease may overshadow or even predate the other symptoms of the underlying disease. When symptoms develop, dyspnea and cough are common. At chest examination, rales, wheezing, or even a pleural rub may be heard because of the varied patterns of lung involvement in these disorders. Physiology is usually restrictive with decreased DLCO but may be obstructive, depending on the anatomical location of the disease, especially with Sjögren's disease.

Unsurprisingly, HRCT findings are variable and range from bronchial thickening to ground-glass abnormalities to reticular and fibrotic changes.[18] The pathological pattern of injury with these diseases is equally diverse and correlates with the HRCT findings. Patterns of lung inflammation are NSIP evidenced by ground glass on HRCT scan and organizing pneumonia (OP) shown by consolidated lung with air bronchograms. Both pathological patterns can improve with aggressive immunosuppression. At the other end of the pathological response spectrum is usual interstitial pneumonitis (UIP), which is associated with reticular opacities and honeycomb cystic fibrosis on HRCT scan that does not generally respond to immunosuppression, although long-term controlled studies are lacking.

Specific treatment of these systemic inflammatory diseases is highly individualized. Patients with evidence of systemic inflammation, an inflammatory pathological pattern such as NSIP or OP, or rapidly progressive symptoms are usually treated with prolonged immunosuppressive agents such as cyclophosphamide, azathioprine, mycophenolate, or tacrolimus.[19,20]

Recent studies have begun to provide evidence-based therapy for these diverse patients. The Scleroderma Lung Study demonstrated that 1 year of oral cyclophosphamide modestly improved lung function compared with a modest decline in the control group.[19] Curiously, those with the highest degree of fibrosis on HRCT improved most, and ground glass or an inflammatory pattern on bronchoalveolar lavage were not predictive of benefit. Unfortunately, after 1 year off immunosuppressive therapy, the cyclophosphamide-treated patients worsened and were indistinguishable from the untreated control group.[21] Many hypothesize that to preserve any lung function gained by cyclophosphamide, continued immunosuppression may be necessary, and mycophenolate is most often used.

Polymyositis-associated interstitial lung disease (PM-ILD) is being increasingly recognized as a common disease entity. Patients usually present with "mechanics' hands" consisting of thickened skin and painful fingertip fissures, and 50% will have Jo-1 antibodies on antinuclear antibody testing. Lung pathology is typically fibrotic NSIP or OP. As would be expected with these inflammatory patterns of injury, patients usually benefit from immunosuppression. Classic treatment is with cyclophosphamide, but tacrolimus is emerging as a salvage agent.

Sarcoidosis

Sarcoidosis is an idiopathic multisystem inflammatory disorder that commonly involves the lung.[22] It is the most common of the ILD in the United States. The tissue inflammation of sarcoidosis has a characteristic pattern in which the inflammatory cells collect in microscopic nodules called granulomas. Unlike IPF, sarcoidosis is more common among young adults than it is among older persons. Sarcoidosis often follows a benign course without symptoms or long-term consequences, and may spontaneously remit.

The most common manifestation of sarcoidosis is asymptomatic hilar adenopathy. Less frequently, the CXR demonstrates parenchymal opacities in the mid lung zone, which may be nodular, reticulonodular, or alveolar. When symptoms occur, cough, chest pain, dyspnea, and wheezing are most common. Pulmonary physiology may be normal, restrictive, obstructive, or mixed with a reduced DLCO. Obstructive impairment may be related to endobronchial granulomatous inflammation or scarring.[23]

Corticosteroids are commonly used in the management of sarcoidosis, but treatment is usually reserved for patients with marked symptoms or physiological impairment attributable to the disease.[24] Other organs that may require corticosteroid therapy include cardiac involvement, uveitis, and central nervous system involvement with cranial nerve abnormalities. Measurement of disease activity remains difficult to ascertain in many patients. Serum angiotensin-converting enzyme levels and gallium scans are not well correlated with disease activity, and their routine use is discouraged. When there is active disease, acutely ill patients are treated with prednisone, and long-term immunosuppression with methotrexate and cyclophosphamide, although infliximab is emerging as a useful agent in some patients.

Interstitial Lung Disease of Unknown Cause

Idiopathic Interstitial Pneumonias

Unfortunately, even after a comprehensive evaluation, many patients with ILD will not have a well-defined specific exposure, a systemic illness, or an underlying genetic cause. Their ILD belongs to either the idiopathic interstitial pneumonia (IIP) group, or to the group consisting of unique pathological patterns as described by surgical lung biopsy.

Idiopathic Pulmonary Fibrosis

IPF is the most common IIP and is defined as a progressive fibrotic lung disease isolated to the lung.[25] The majority of patients are older than 60 years, and it is extremely unusual in persons younger than 40 years. Risk factors for development of IPF include exposure to smoke, metal dust, farming dust, and hairdressing chemicals. Patients present with chronic cough and exertional dyspnea with HRCT demonstrating bibasilar, peripheral reticular abnormalities with focal honeycomb cystic change. Usual interstitial pneumonitis (UIP) is the pathological pattern of injury seen in IPF patients. UIP is characterized by heterogeneous fibrosis most prominent in the peripheral areas, with minimal inflammation. It is important to note that patients other than those with IPF can have UIP on surgical lung biopsy (e.g., connective tissue disease especially rheumatoid arthritis), so this pattern of injury/repair is not unique to IPF.

Patients with an IIP and a classic presentation of age older than 60 years, progressive dyspnea and cough, basilar lung crackles, and HRCT findings of bibasilar, subpleural fibrosis and honeycomb cyst formation may not require a surgical lung biopsy for diagnosis.[26,27] Transbronchial lung biopsies are frequently obtained to eliminate the mimics of IPF, sarcoidosis, and chronic HP. The small biopsies obtained by this route may be able to identify granulomatous inflammation but cannot provide a definitive diagnosis of UIP because this diagnosis requires a piece of tissue much larger than that obtained by transbronchial biopsy.

The majority of patients die of progressive fibrosing lung disease within 4 years of diagnosis. Emerging data show that approximately half of patients will die with gradually progressive disease over several years.[28] However, the other half experience stable lung function or minimal decline for months to years, only to have sudden worsening over a few weeks or months leading to death. Baseline parameters that predict an increased risk of death include severity of dyspnea, severity of restrictive physiological defect, reduced DLCO, pulmonary arterial hypertension, degree of fibrosis on HRCT, and SaO_2 desaturation on exertion.[29] Serial parameters that predict poor survival include worsening dyspnea, FVC, and DLCO.

No medical therapy has proven beneficial for IPF. Recent trials have demonstrated no benefit with interferon-gamma and etanercept. Several medications are currently under investigation, including bosentan, imatinib, and pirfenidone. Immunosuppression with oral corticosteroids and cytotoxic agents such as azathioprine are most commonly used, although they appear to benefit only a minority of patients and are the subject of a current IPF NET trial.[30–32]

Recent studies have highlighted the importance of pulmonary arterial hypertension (PAH) in IPF.[33] Curiously, the degree of PAH does not always correlate with the burden of fibrosis on CT scan or FVC, implying that a vascular process other than obliteration of the capillary bed from fibrosis occurs.[34] Significant PAH is suggested in patients with markedly impaired diffusion capacity but relatively preserved FVC. Again, several PAH agents are under investigation in IPF, but their use outside trials is not recommended.

Nonspecific Interstitial Pneumonia

NSIP is an IIP with diffuse inflammation seen on surgical lung biopsy.[35] These patients are on average 7 to 10 years younger than IPF, but considerable overlap exists. The degree of accompanying interstitial fibrosis is variable between patients. The combination of fibrosis and inflammation (fibrotic NSIP) is most common. Pure cellular NSIP is less common. Patients present with chronic or subacute cough and dyspnea. HRCT demonstrates predominant ground-glass abnormalities in cellular NSIP and both ground-glass and fibrotic changes in fibrotic NSIP. Given that there is significant clinical and radiographic overlap between fibrotic NSIP and IPF, surgical lung biopsy is frequently required to distinguish these two.

The prognosis is much better for NSIP than IPF with most patients surviving 7 to 10 years. Immunosuppression with oral corticosteroids and cytotoxic immunosuppressive agents is the primary therapy. Type and duration of therapy is guided by disease activity and degree of inflammation on biopsy and ground glass on HRCT. Importantly, pathological NSIP is not a unique pattern and can frequently be seen in connective tissue disease or hypersensitivity pneumonitis, and a thorough investigation for these should be undertaken to rule out these alternative diagnoses.

Cryptogenic Organizing Pneumonia

Cryptogenic organizing pneumonia (COP) is the revised nomenclature for bronchiolitis obliterans organizing pneumonia (BOOP). Patients are younger than those with IPF and present with acute or subacute dyspnea and cough. About one-third describe an antecedent viral illness; however, no other risk factors are known. HRCT demonstrates alveolar filling with air bronchograms mimicking acute pneumonia, and the classic COP patient presents after having failed to improve despite several courses of antibiotics. Diagnosis may occasionally require surgical lung biopsy, especially if the clinical and radiographic features are uncertain because small areas of OP can be seen in a variety of inflammatory and fibrotic disorders on transbronchial lung biopsy.

Most patients improve with oral corticosteroids (0.5–1.0 mg/kg for 6–12 weeks). However, many patients will have recrudescence after corticosteroid withdrawal and require long-term immunosuppression with cytotoxic immunosuppressive agents. A minority of patients develops progressive fibrosis despite aggressive immunosuppression and can be offered lung transplantation. Again, OP is not a unique pathological pattern and can frequently be found associated with connective tissue disease; thus, a thorough investigation must be undertaken to eliminate alternative diagnoses.

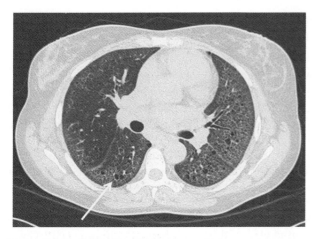

Figure 36.8 HRCT of lymphocytic interstitial pneumonia demonstrating thin-walled cysts with peripheral vessel in the cyst wall (*white arrow*). Also, note the ground-glass opacities, which are suggestive of inflammatory lung injury.

Lymphocytic Interstitial Pneumonia

Lymphocytic interstitial pneumonia (LIP) is a rare disorder of polyclonal lymphocyte aggregates that accumulate diffusely in the interstitium.[36] The diagnosis almost always requires surgical lung biopsy. Patients are typically younger than IPF patients and present with subacute dyspnea and cough. Pulmonary function testing may show a mixed picture, and HRCT typically shows diffuse ground-glass attenuation with variable amounts of fibrosis. Alternatively, some patients' HRCT images demonstrate several 10- to 20-mm peribronchiolar thin-walled cysts with a blood vessel in the wall as seen in Figure 36.8. Most patients respond well to oral corticosteroids, with a minority requiring long-term immunosuppression. LIP is frequently associated with connective tissue diseases, especially Sjögren's disease and in patients with immunodeficiency, and these possibilities should be investigated in all LIP patients.

Interstitial Lung Disease With Distinct Pathology

Lymphangioleiomyomatosis

LAM is a rare disorder of abnormal smooth muscle tissue proliferating around small airways and lymphatic vessels leading to severe obstruction and destruction of alveoli with resultant thin-walled cyst formation.[37] All patients are women, although both males and females with tuberous sclerosis complex can develop lung pathology identical to LAM termed *tuberous sclerosis complex lymphangioleiomyomatosis* (TSC-LAM).

Dyspnea on exertion and an obstructive ventilatory impairment with a reduced DLCO is almost always present, except in very early disease. Disease progression is quite variable, with some women having steadily worsening lung function during midlife, whereas elderly women may experience extremely slow decline over many years. Risk factors for worsening lung function include a significant bronchodilator response and possibly childbearing. Other

important disease manifestations include pneumothorax from a ruptured subpleural cyst, occasionally associated with air travel. Unilateral or, less commonly, bilateral chylothorax is seen in about one-third of patients. This results from lymphatic obstruction by abnormal smooth muscle tissue. Treatment with a low-fat diet or blocking gut fat absorption is usually ineffective, and pleurodesis is required. Importantly, pleurodesis does not preclude subsequent lung transplantation.

Treatment is with inhaled bronchodilators and inhaled corticosteroids. Younger patients may ultimately require lung transplantation. Prior small uncontrolled studies suggested delayed disease progression with progesterone and oophorectomy, but these treatments are unproven, and most experts do not recommend them routinely. Early studies with the immunosuppressant rapamycin, which inhibits LAM in vitro cell proliferation, have been promising and larger trials are underway.

NONSPECIFIC INTERSTITIAL LUNG DISEASE THERAPIES

Oxygen Therapy

As hypoxemia is common in ILD, supplemental oxygen therapy is frequently prescribed, although it has not been studied as extensively as in COPD. Patients with ILD should have arterial oxygen saturation determined at rest and especially during exertion because many patients with only mild disease will desaturate with exertion despite normal saturation at rest. Although studies are limited, supplemental oxygen delivered via nasal cannula can prevent resting hypoxemia and allow greater exertion before desaturation. These benefits improve quality of life and potentially ward off development of pulmonary arterial hypertension, although further studies are needed. We favor continuous rather than pulse delivery because the desaturation with activity seen in most patients is not rectified with pulse therapy. For most patients, liquid oxygen is the best source to provide adequate flow rates. In motivated patients, transtracheal deliver of supplemental oxygen increases the efficiency of delivery and improves cosmesis. However, patients must be chosen carefully because of the need for frequent care and risk of mucous dessication and rare hemorrhage.

Pulmonary Rehabilitation and Exercise Therapy

As with supplemental oxygen therapy, the use of pulmonary rehabilitation in the management of ILD has not been as well studied as it has in obstructive lung disease. Pulmonary rehabilitation is important in building aerobic fitness, maintaining physical activity, and improving quality of life. We encourage our patients to enroll in outpatient pulmonary rehabilitation and to continue maintenance therapy.

Vaccinations and Infection Avoidance

Because many ILD patients are treated with immunosuppressive medications and are at increased risk for the development of infections, patients with ILD should receive a pneumococcal vaccine per Centers for Disease Control and Prevention guidelines and a yearly influenza virus vaccine. In addition, we recommend that patients practice good hand hygiene (e.g., frequent hand washing). We do not recommend use of masks or special antibacterial products. Patients treated with immunosuppressive regimens should receive *Pneumocystis* prophylaxis.

Transplantation

The only therapy shown to prolong life in patients with end-stage, particularly fibrotic ILD is lung transplantation.[38] Transplantation has been performed successfully in the management of most ILDs. Enthusiasm for the procedure is tempered by the significant risk of mortality at 1 year (15%–25%) and 5 years (50%–60%). Furthermore, many patients with ILD are older than the upper age limit of "physiological" age 65 years. In addition, comorbidities such as gastroesophageal reflux disease, especially when associated with the patulous esophagus of scleroderma, preclude lung transplantation owing to the increased risk of chronic rejection and death.

SUMMARY

The entities grouped as ILDs are a diverse group of illnesses of varied causation, treatment, and prognosis. In general, these diseases manifest as chronic, progressive dyspnea on exertion and cough. Findings on examination are often limited to the chest in the form of fine, inspiratory crackles. The most common chest radiograph finding is diffuse reticular or reticulonodular infiltrates with reduced lung volumes. Pulmonary function testing usually reveals restrictive physiology and decreased diffusion capacity; however, other patterns can be seen. Chest CT imaging is an important diagnostic tool, although many patients will still require invasive biopsy to determine a correct diagnosis. Therapy depends on the underlying disease and may consist of immunosuppressive drugs and the avoidance of disease-inducing exposures.

REVIEW EXERCISES

QUESTIONS

1. Which of the following chest radiographic findings is inconsistent with the diagnosis of asbestosis?
a) Presence of pleural plaques
b) Presence of pleural effusion
c) Reticulonodular infiltrates
d) Upper lobe predominance
e) Reduced lung volumes

Answer and Discussion
The answer is d. Asbestosis is characterized by the presence of reticulonodular infiltrates in a lower zone distribution. As the disease progresses, there is often volume loss in the lower lobes. The presence of pleural disease, although not sufficient to make the diagnosis of true asbestosis, may be seen in patients with asbestos exposure and is therefore not inconsistent with the diagnosis of asbestosis.

2. Which one of the following statements regarding idiopathic pulmonary fibrosis (IPF) is incorrect?
a) IPF most commonly affects patients in the sixth and seventh decades of life.
b) There is a familial variety of IPF.
c) The histology of IPF is indistinguishable from that seen in rheumatoid arthritis.
d) Clubbing is a late finding in IPF.
e) Corticosteroids are the only proven effective therapy for IPF.

Answer and Discussion
The answer is e. Answers a through d are all correct. This question is meant to emphasize the fact that although corticosteroid treatment may result in subjective or objective improvements, it has not been proven to improve survival.

3. Which one of the following statements is incorrect?
a) Obtaining an occupational history is imperative before diagnosing a patient with sarcoidosis.
b) An elevated serum angiotensin-converting enzyme level is not diagnostic.
c) Sarcoidosis can involve any organ system.
d) The presence of sarcoid granulomas in the pulmonary parenchyma is an indication for treatment.
e) The most common presentation is an asymptomatic chest radiograph abnormality.

Answer and Discussion
The answer is d. Making a histologic diagnosis of sarcoidosis is not considered sufficient reason to treat with steroids. Commonly accepted indications for treatment include significant symptoms or progressive loss of lung function. Involvement of critical extrapulmonary organs also may prompt treatment.

4. Which one of the following statements is incorrect?
a) Benign asbestos pleural effusion is one of the earliest manifestations of asbestos exposure.
b) Pleural thickening in a patient with asbestos exposure indicates asbestosis.
c) Pleural plaques almost never result in symptoms or physiological impairment.

d) Mesothelioma may develop in patients with brief, low-level exposure to asbestos.

e) Rounded atelectasis is a benign manifestation of asbestos exposure that can be mistaken for a malignancy.

Answer and Discussion

The answer is b. This question is meant to emphasize the fact that the term *asbestosis* should be reserved for patients with evidence of pulmonary parenchymal scarring. Pleural disease does not merit the diagnosis of asbestosis.

5. Which one of the following statements is incorrect?

a) Silicosis shows a predominantly lower zone distribution on the chest radiograph.

b) Progressive massive fibrosis is a complication of silicosis.

c) There is an increased incidence of tuberculosis in patients with silicosis.

d) There is an increased incidence of rheumatoid arthritis and scleroderma in patients with silicosis.

Answer and Discussion

The answer is a. The distribution of abnormalities on the chest radiograph may be helpful in narrowing the differential diagnosis. Silicosis is associated with radiographic changes in the upper lobes.

6. Which one of the following statements is incorrect?

a) Methotrexate pulmonary toxicity may not recur on reinitiation of the drug.

b) Using supplemental oxygen after administration can prevent bleomycin pulmonary toxicity.

c) Radiation pneumonitis may mimic infectious pneumonia (cough, fever, chest pain, dyspnea).

d) Nitrofurantoin pulmonary toxicity may mimic idiopathic pulmonary fibrosis.

e) Pneumonitis owing to amiodarone may appear denser than surrounding soft tissue on a CT scan.

Answer and Discussion

The answer is b. The administration of supplemental oxygen is a risk factor for the development of bleomycin pulmonary toxicity.

7. Which one of the following statements is incorrect?

a) Interstitial lung disease (ILD) is more common in men with rheumatoid arthritis than in women with rheumatoid arthritis.

b) Fifty percent of patients presenting with acute lupus pneumonitis have had no history of lupus.

c) There is a good correlation between the severity of the cutaneous and pulmonary manifestations of scleroderma.

d) Jo-1 antibody is associated with the presence of ILD in patients with polymyositis.

e) ILD associated with Sjögren's syndrome often involves lymphocytic infiltration.

Answer and Discussion

The answer is c. As with many of the connective tissue disease–associated ILDs, there is no real correlation between the severity of the ILD and the extrapulmonary manifestations.

REFERENCES

1. Raghu G, Brown KK. Interstitial lung disease: clinical evaluation and keys to an accurate diagnosis. *Clin Chest Med* 2004;25:409–419, v.
2. King TE Jr. Clinical advances in the diagnosis and therapy of the interstitial lung diseases. *Am J Respir Crit Care Med* 2005;172:268–279.
3. Elliot TL, Lynch DA, Newell JD Jr, et al. High-resolution computed tomography features of nonspecific interstitial pneumonia and usual interstitial pneumonia. *J Comput Assist Tomogr* 2005;29:339–345.
4. Hunninghake GW, Lynch DA, Galvin JR, et al. Radiologic findings are strongly associated with a pathologic diagnosis of usual interstitial pneumonia. *Chest* 2003;124:1215–1223.
5. Souza CA, Muller NL, Lee KS, et al. Idiopathic interstitial pneumonias: prevalence of mediastinal lymph node enlargement in 206 patients. *AJR Am J Roentgenol* 2006;186:995–999.
6. Chetta A, Marangio E, Olivieri D. Pulmonary function testing in interstitial lung diseases. *Respiration* 2004;71:209–213.
7. Cottin V, Nunes H, Brillet PY, et al. Combined pulmonary fibrosis and emphysema: a distinct underrecognised entity. *Eur Respir J* 2005;26:586–593.
8. American Thoracic Society. Diagnosis and initial management of nonmalignant diseases related to asbestos. *Am J Respir Crit Care Med* 2004;170:691–715.
9. Schwartz DA, Davis CS, Merchant JA, et al. Longitudinal changes in lung function among asbestos-exposed workers. *Am J Respir Crit Care Med* 1994;150:1243–1249.
10. Ross MH, Murray J. Occupational respiratory disease in mining. *Occup Med (Lond)* 2004;54:304–310.
11. Camus P, Bonniaud P, Fanton A, et al. Drug-induced and iatrogenic infiltrative lung disease. *Clin Chest Med* 2004;25:479–519, vi.
12. Selman M. Hypersensitivity pneumonitis: a multifaceted deceiving disorder. *Clin Chest Med* 2004;25:531–547, vi.
13. Monkare S. Influence of corticosteroid treatment on the course of farmer's lung. *Eur J Respir Dis* 1983;64:283–293.
14. Vourlekis JS, Schwarz MI, Cherniack RM, et al. The effect of pulmonary fibrosis on survival in patients with hypersensitivity pneumonitis. *Am J Med* 2004;116:662–668.
15. Ryu JH, Myers JL, Capizzi SA, et al. Desquamative interstitial pneumonia and respiratory bronchiolitis–associated interstitial lung disease. *Chest* 2005;127:178–184.
16. Portnoy J, Veraldi KL, Schwarz MI, et al. Respiratory bronchiolitis-interstitial lung disease: long-term outcome. *Chest* 2007;131:664–671.
17. Strange C, Highland KB. Interstitial lung disease in the patient who has connective tissue disease. *Clin Chest Med* 2004;25:549–559, vii.
18. Tanaka N, Newell JD, Brown KK, et al. Collagen vascular disease-related lung disease: high-resolution computed tomography findings based on the pathologic classification. *J Comput Assist Tomogr* 2004;28:351–360.
19. Tashkin DP, Elashoff R, Clements PJ, et al. Cyclophosphamide versus placebo in scleroderma lung disease. *N Engl J Med* 2006;354:2655–2666.
20. Swigris JJ, Olson AL, Fischer A, et al. Mycophenolate mofetil is safe, well tolerated, and preserves lung function in patients with connective tissue disease–related interstitial lung disease. *Chest* 2006;130:30–36.
21. Tashkin DP, Elashoff R, Clements PJ, et al. Effects of 1-year treatment with cyclophosphamide on outcomes at 2 years in

scleroderma lung disease. *Am J Respir Crit Care Med* 2007;176: 1026–1034.

22. Baughman RP. Pulmonary sarcoidosis. *Clin Chest Med* 2004;25: 521–530, vi.

23. Shorr AF, Torrington KG, Hnatiuk OW. Endobronchial involvement and airway hyperreactivity in patients with sarcoidosis. *Chest* 2001;120:881–886.

24. Paramothayan NS, Lasserson TJ, Jones PW. Corticosteroids for pulmonary sarcoidosis. *Cochrane Database Syst Rev* 2005;(2): CD001114.

25. Raghu G, Weycker D, Edelsberg J, et al. Incidence and prevalence of idiopathic pulmonary fibrosis. *Am J Respir Crit Care Med* 2006;174:810–816.

26. Raghu G, Mageto YN, Lockhart D, et al. The accuracy of the clinical diagnosis of new-onset idiopathic pulmonary fibrosis and other interstitial lung disease: a prospective study. *Chest* 1999;116:1168–1174.

27. Hunninghake GW, Zimmerman MB, Schwartz DA, et al. Utility of a lung biopsy for the diagnosis of idiopathic pulmonary fibrosis. *Am J Respir Crit Care Med* 2001;164:193–196.

28. Martinez FJ, Safrin S, Weycker D, et al. The clinical course of patients with idiopathic pulmonary fibrosis. *Ann Intern Med* 2005;142:963–967.

29. Collard HR, King TE Jr, Bartelson BB, et al. Changes in clinical and physiologic variables predict survival in idiopathic pulmonary fibrosis. *Am J Respir Crit Care Med* 2003;168:538–542.

30. Richeldi L, Davies HR, Ferrara G, et al. Corticosteroids for idiopathic pulmonary fibrosis. *Cochrane Database Syst Rev* 2003;(3):CD002880.

31. Davies HR, Richeldi L, Walters EH. Immunomodulatory agents for idiopathic pulmonary fibrosis. *Cochrane Database Syst Rev* 2003;(3):CD003134.

32. Collard HR, Ryu JH, Douglas WW, et al. Combined corticosteroid and cyclophosphamide therapy does not alter survival in idiopathic pulmonary fibrosis. *Chest* 2004;125:216–2174.

33. Nadrous HF, Pellikka PA, Krowka MJ, et al. Pulmonary hypertension in patients with idiopathic pulmonary fibrosis. *Chest* 2005;128:2393–2399.

34. Lettieri CJ, Nathan SD, Barnett SD, et al. Prevalence and outcomes of pulmonary arterial hypertension in advanced idiopathic pulmonary fibrosis. *Chest* 2006;129:746–752.

35. Martinez FJ. Idiopathic interstitial pneumonias: usual interstitial pneumonia versus nonspecific interstitial pneumonia. *Proc Am Thorac Soc* 2006;3:81–95.

36. Cha SI, Fessler MB, Cool CD, et al. Lymphoid interstitial pneumonia: clinical features, associations and prognosis. *Eur Respir J* 2006;28:364–369.

37. Ryu JH, Moss J, Beck GJ, et al. The NHLBI lymphangioleiomyomatosis registry: characteristics of 230 patients at enrollment. *Am J Respir Crit Care Med* 2006;173:105–111.

38. Orens JB, Estenne M, Arcasoy S, et al. International guidelines for the selection of lung transplant candidates: 2006 update—a consensus report from the pulmonary scientific council of the international society for heart and lung transplantation. *J Heart Lung Transplant* 2006;25:745–755.

Chapter 37

Pleural Diseases

Atul C. Mehta   Raed A. Dweik

POINTS TO REMEMBER:

- The standard posteroanterior and lateral chest radiographs remain the most important techniques for the initial diagnosis of pleural effusion.

- A major use of ultrasound is to guide thoracentesis needles into small or loculated pleural effusions, thereby increasing the yield and safety of thoracentesis.

- After obtaining fluid, the first diagnostic step is to classify the effusion as a transudate or an exudate by using the protein and lactate dehydrogenase values of serum and pleural fluid.

- Transudates are formed secondary to elevations in hydrostatic pressure or reductions in colloid osmotic pressure within the systemic or pulmonary circulation. Causes of transudates include
  - Congestive heart failure
  - Nephrotic syndrome
  - Cirrhosis with ascites
  - Peritoneal dialysis

- Atelectasis (early)
- Urinothorax

- In general, no more than 1,000 to 1,500 mL of fluid should be removed at one time. Removal of more fluid risks the development of edema in the underlying lung (*re-expansion pulmonary edema*) or rapid fluid shift from the intravascular space into the pleural space (*postthoracentesis shock*).

A pleural effusion is among the most frequently encountered problems in chest medicine. One estimate places the annual incidence of pleural effusion in the United States at approximately 1 million persons.

An accumulation of pleural fluid is not a specific disease, but rather a reflection of underlying pathology. Pleural effusion may result from many different pulmonary or systemic diseases. The task facing the contemporary clinician is little different from that outlined by Osler in 1892:

"In the diagnosis of pleuritic effusion, the first question is, Does a fluid exudate exist? The second question is, What is its nature?"

DIAGNOSIS OF PLEURAL EFFUSION

Clinical symptoms (dyspnea or pleuritic pain) or signs (diminished breath sounds and dullness to percussion) may suggest the presence of a pleural effusion. Chest radiographic techniques are important in confirming the presence of pleural effusion and in detecting associated abnormalities that may provide important information regarding etiology (Fig. 37.1).

Imaging Studies

Conventional Chest Radiography

The standard posteroanterior and lateral chest radiographs remain the most important techniques for the initial

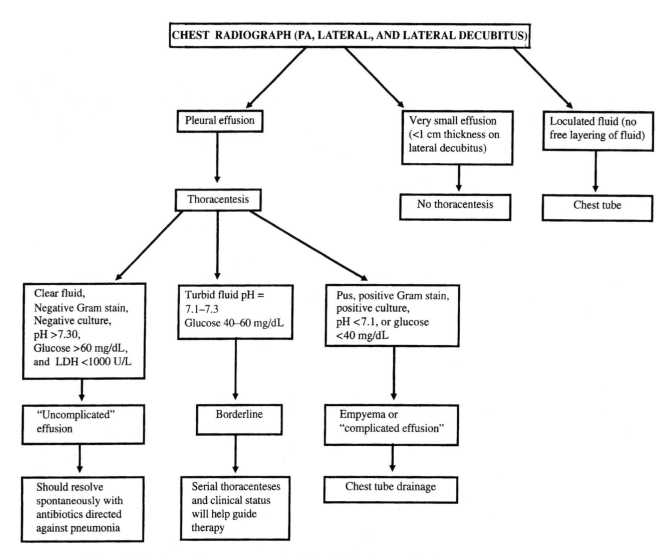

Figure 37.1 Approach to parapneumonic effusion. LDH = lactate dehydrogenase; PA = posteroanterior.

diagnosis of pleural effusion (Fig. 37.1). The distribution of free pleural fluid around the normal lung is influenced primarily by gravity and lung elastic recoil and, to a lesser extent, by *capillary attraction* between the pleural surfaces, which creates the meniscus-shaped upper border. Fluid first gravitates to the inferior portion of the hemithorax and lies between the hemidiaphragm and the inferior surface of the lung. Small fluid collections are best appreciated by an inspection of the posterior costophrenic angle on the lateral radiograph. Larger fluid collections completely obscure the hemidiaphragm on both projections and assume a typical appearance. Most fluid collects around the lateral, anterior, and posterior thoracic wall; less fluid collects along the mediastinal surface of the lung because there is relatively less elastic recoil in this region (the lung is fixed at the hilum and pulmonary ligament).

Occasionally, relatively large pleural effusions may remain confined to the infrapulmonary location (*subpulmonic effusion*). Such effusions may give the radiographic appearance of elevation of the hemidiaphragm. When a subpulmonic effusion occurs on the left side, its presence is suggested by the separation of the *pseudohemidiaphragm* from the gastric bubble. A lateral decubitus roentgenogram is extremely valuable in the detection of subpulmonic effusions.

Lateral decubitus films are also useful in distinguishing *free* pleural fluid from the *loculated* pleural effusion (fluid confined by fibrous pleural adhesions). Pleural effusions might be overlooked on supine or semierect roentgenograms (e.g., portable radiograph obtained in the intensive care unit) because the only abnormality may be a vague increase in radiographic density over the hemithorax.

The lateral decubitus roentgenogram can detect effusions as small as 15 mL. The standard posteroanterior and lateral roentgenogram can detect roughly 250 mL. The "moderate" pleural effusion (1,000 mL) extends upward to approximately one-third or one-half of the hemithorax, typically obscuring the hemidiaphragm.

Other Radiographic Techniques

Ultrasound

Thoracic ultrasound is a rapid and safe technique for defining and localizing pleural fluid. A major advantage over conventional roentgenograms is the ability of ultrasound to differentiate the solid components (e.g., tumor or fibrous peel) from the liquid components of a pleural process. Ultrasound is also valuable in detecting subpulmonic or subphrenic pathology and differentiating these abnormalities (i.e., by evaluating the relationship of radiographic densities to the diaphragm). A major use of ultrasound is to guide thoracentesis needles into small or loculated pleural effusions, thereby increasing the yield and safety of thoracentesis. Portable ultrasound units can be brought to the bedside of extremely ill patients.

Computed Tomography

CT examination of the thorax is a major advance in the evaluation of pleural disease. The cross-sectional tomographic image allows the evaluation of complex situations in which the anatomy cannot be fully assessed by plain films or ultrasound. For instance, CT scans are helpful in distinguishing empyema from lung abscess, in detecting pleural masses (e.g., mesothelioma, plaques), and in outlining loculated fluid collections.

Laboratory Studies

Transudate versus Exudate

Although the history, physical examination, and radiographic studies may provide important clues to the etiology of a pleural effusion, almost all cases should be evaluated through a diagnostic thoracentesis. After obtaining fluid, the first diagnostic step is to classify the effusion as a transudate or an exudate by using the protein and lactate dehydrogenase (LDH) values of serum and pleural fluid (Table 37.1). As described by Light et al., this method is 99% accurate.[1] Previous methods, which used cut-off values for pleural fluid total protein (3.0 g/100 mL) or specific gravity (1.016), are considerably less accurate (60%–90%).

In more recent years, newer criteria have been explored in diagnosing exudative effusions. As outlined in Table 37.2, the more recent criteria use cholesterol levels in the pleural fluid and have a lower threshold for LDH. Although the newer criteria offer no diagnostic improvement over Light et al.'s criteria, they offer the distinct advantage that phlebotomy is not required.[2] These criteria rely on cholesterol levels and on the absolute values of LDH and protein in the pleural fluid rather than on their ratios to the serum values. Furthermore, cholesterol levels in the pleural fluid may be helpful in diuretic-treated congestive heart failure (CHF), a transudate that can be inaccurately classified as an exudate by the traditional Light et al.'s criteria due to high protein levels (3-4 g/dL).

Transudates

Transudates are formed secondary to elevations in hydrostatic pressure or reductions in colloid osmotic pressure

TABLE 37.1

TRANSUDATE AND EXUDATE CLASSIFICATION

	Fluid/ Serum Protein		Fluid/ Serum LDH		Fluid LDH
Transudate	<0.5	and	<0.6	and	<200
Exudate	≥0.5	or	≥0.6	or	≥200

LDH = lactate dehydrogenase.

TABLE 37.2

NEWER CRITERIA FOR CLASSIFICATION OF EXUDATES AND TRANSUDATES

		Criteria				
Test		Pleural/Serum Protein Ratio	Pleural/Serum LDH Ratio	LDH	Sensitivity (%)	Specificity (%)
Light et al.'s	Transudate	≤0.5	≤0.6	≤200 U/L	98	93
	Exudate	>0.5	>0.6	>200 U/L		
Cholesterol	Pleural fluid >60 mg/dL				54	92
	Pleural fluid >43 mg/dL				75	80
	Ratio pleural fluid/serum >0.3				89	81
Albumin	Serum albumin-pleural fluid albumin <1.2 g/dL				87	92

within the systemic or pulmonary circulation. Causes of transudates include:

- CHF
- Nephrotic syndrome
- Cirrhosis with ascites
- Peritoneal dialysis
- Atelectasis (early)
- Urinothorax

Pleuropulmonary disease rarely exists with transudates, which is why the finding is so important. Further analysis of the pleural fluid, or a pleural biopsy, is unlikely to provide positive information and can probably be avoided. A study by Peterman and Speicher[3] supports this approach: 83 transudates were evaluated, with 725 further tests. Only 9 of these follow-up test results were positive, and 7 gave false-positive results.

Nonetheless, it is important to maintain some wariness before dismissing a transudative effusion. The clinician must remain alert to the few instances in which a transudate may be associated with underlying lung disease. Early atelectasis may be associated with a transudate. Also, it is well documented, but often unappreciated, that some patients with malignant pleural effusions have transudative fluids.[4] Most of these patients have concomitant CHF, nephrotic syndrome, or the early stage of mediastinal lymph node involvement with malignancy.

Exudate

Exudative effusions signal the presence of disease involving the lungs or pleura. The following are important or common causes of exudates:

- Malignancy
- Bacterial and fungal infection
- Collagen vascular disease
- Parapneumonic effusion (pleural reaction to pneumonia)
- Pulmonary embolus
- Chylothorax (thoracic duct disruption)
- Uremia
- Asbestos exposure

- Thoracic lymphatic obstruction (e.g., lymphoma, radiation)
- Pancreatitis
- Empyema
- Tuberculosis (TB)
- Viral infections
- Yellow nail syndrome
- Postcardiotomy syndrome
- Subdiaphragmatic abscess
- Esophageal rupture
- Atelectasis (chronic)
- Idiopathic causes

Exudative effusions should not be ignored, and attempts to establish the diagnosis should be undertaken. Additional studies of pleural fluid, such as cell count and differential, cytology, Gram stain, cultures, and glucose, amylase, pH, antinuclear antibodies (ANAs), and complement levels, may help establish the etiology. Pleural biopsy may sometimes help establish the cause of an exudative effusion. Biopsy specimens should be examined histologically (tumor, granuloma) and sent for culture (TB, fungal).

Specific Tests of Pleural Fluid

Glucose

The pleural fluid glucose level of transudates and most exudates is similar to that of serum. There are few causes of a very low pleural fluid glucose (<25 mg/100 mL). Such a finding is seen with rheumatoid disease, TB, empyema, and tumors with extensive pleural involvement. The latter two conditions are usually obvious by the clinical setting or other pleural fluid findings; therefore, a low glucose level may be an important first clue to TB or rheumatoid disease. It has been reported that an intravenous glucose infusion raises the pleural fluid glucose level in TB but not in rheumatoid disease.

Amylase

A high pleural fluid amylase usually indicates pancreatitis or esophageal rupture. Isoenzymes can be used to distinguish pancreatic amylase from salivary gland amylase; however, the clinical setting usually separates these two entities. Also, the fluid pH is low with esophageal rupture and normal in pancreatitis. Approximately 10% of malignant effusions may have elevations of amylase.

pH

The pH of the small amount of pleural fluid present in normal persons is approximately 7.64. A low pleural fluid pH (i.e., <7.30) may be seen with infected parapneumonic effusions, frank empyema, malignancy, collagen vascular disease, TB, esophageal rupture, and urinothorax (the only cause of a low pH transudative effusion). Effusions from other causes almost always have a pH >7.30. It is essential that pleural fluid for pH analysis be aspirated anaerobically and transported on ice. A falsely high pH results if the fluid is exposed to room air, and a falsely low pH results if the fluid is not kept on ice. The pH is stable for 1 to 2 hours at 0°C. The major use of pleural fluid pH is in the management of parapneumonic effusions, as popularized by R. W. Light (see Parapneumonic Effusions section); however, the pH may provide no independent information in this regard beyond that which can be learned by measuring pleural fluid glucose.[5]

Diagnostic Aspects of Certain Exudative Effusions

Collagen Vascular Disease

Systemic lupus erythematosus (SLE) and rheumatoid disease are important causes of pleural effusion. Up to 75% of SLE patients have pleural involvement during the course of their disease. Frequently, the effusion is the only radiographic abnormality in these patients. Lupus effusions are characteristically small to moderate in size but are associated with significant pleuritic pain (pleurisy). Pleuritis may be an important first manifestation of SLE; in approximately 6% of patients, pleural effusion is an isolated first sign, and in an additional 30% of patients, only minor antecedent symptoms are present.

The pleural fluid antinuclear antibody (ANA) titer may be helpful in separating SLE effusions from effusions caused by other etiologies, even in patients with known SLE. A pleural fluid ANA ratio >1:160 or a pleural fluid-to-serum ANA ratio >1.0 indicates lupus pleuritis.[6] Although these criteria appear to be highly specific, they are not highly sensitive (some patients with SLE pleuritis will not fulfill them). The presence of lupus erythematous (LE) cells in pleural effusions is highly specific for SLE or drug-induced lupus, and this finding has been reported to precede the appearance of LE cells or ANAs in serum by several months in some patients; however, the finding of LE cells may not have a high sensitivity. The presence of a speckled staining pattern usually suggests an alternate diagnosis.

Pleural effusions occur in approximately 5% of patients with rheumatoid arthritis. Unlike SLE, the effusions are often asymptomatic, may be quite large, and often persist for many months without change. Interestingly, rheumatoid effusions are more common in men, despite the fact that rheumatoid disease is more common in women. Usually, effusions occur in patients with high serum rheumatoid factor (RF) titers and rheumatoid nodules. Pleural fluid RF titers are not helpful because they may be elevated in pneumonia, TB, malignancy, and SLE. "Silent empyema" is a risk, especially in steroid-treated patients. SLE and rheumatoid effusions may have low complement levels and high levels of immune complexes, but these findings are not completely specific (i.e., they occur with tumors and empyema).

Tuberculosis

The most common form of TB effusion is a "hypersensitivity" reaction that occurs in the postprimary phase of the initial infection. Other evidence of infection is usually lacking. Although these exudates usually resolve spontaneously, approximately 30% of patients develop active disease within 5 years. The diagnosis is difficult and usually requires a pleural biopsy, in which the pleura is examined histologically for granulomas and acid-fast bacilli, and cultured for TB. Pleural fluid analyses (acid-fast bacilli stains and culture) are positive in only 20% to 25% of cases; pleural biopsies increase the yield to 55% to 80%.

Chylothorax

A disruption of the thoracic duct (e.g., by trauma, surgery, or tumor) leads to a chylothorax. A "milky" appearance is characteristic, but occasionally a chronic TB or rheumatoid effusion has this appearance (*pseudochylothorax*). A true chylothorax has a high fat content (>400 mg/100 mL), containing mostly triglycerides. The chylothorax, in contrast, has low fat and high cholesterol levels. A pleural fluid triglyceride level >110 mg/dL indicates a probable chylothorax, whereas a level <50 mg/dL essentially rules out chylothorax. In borderline situations (pleural fluid triglyceride level between 50 and 100 mg/dL), lipoprotein electrophoreses of the pleural fluid is helpful; the finding of chylomicrons in the fluid establishes the diagnosis of chylothorax.

Urinothorax

Urinothorax is a relatively rare disorder in which urine collects in the pleural space because of ipsilateral urinary tract obstruction. The diagnostic triad is transudate, low pH (<7.30), and a pleural fluid-to-serum creatinine ratio >1.0.

Malignancy

Pleural fluid cytology is positive in 60% to 90% of patients with effusion secondary to involvement of the pleura by tumor, except for mesothelioma, in which its sensitivity is only 32%. Remember that bronchogenic cancer may cause effusion owing to atelectasis, pneumonia, or lymphatic obstruction, without involving the pleura. Carcinoembryonic antigen may help differentiate malignant from benign effusions in some cases, but the sensitivity and specificity of this test is not high enough to make it useful in routine evaluation. Mesothelioma appears to be the only cause of an extremely high hyaluronic acid level, although this finding may not be sensitive. In one study, immunocytometry proved helpful in the diagnosis of lymphoma in an idiopathic pleural effusion in which conventional cytologic and histopathological techniques were nondiagnostic.[7]

Asbestosis

The entity of *benign asbestos effusion* is well recognized, and its natural history is better defined. These effusions are often bloody but are otherwise nonspecific exudates. The peak incidence is approximately 10 to 15 years after the onset of asbestos exposure (somewhat earlier than the other pleural complications of asbestos). Approximately one-third of patients are asymptomatic; the remaining cases may have pleuritic discomfort, mild fever, or dyspnea. The effusions persist for a mean of 4 months and then resolve spontaneously in most patients. A variable amount of pleural fibrosis often results. Approximately one-third of patients may have recurrent effusion or persistent pleural pain. Few cases of mesothelioma have occurred in these patients, and usually only after an interval of several years. Thus, benign asbestos pleurisy does not seem to be an indicator for an increased risk of mesothelioma. The diagnosis of benign asbestos pleurisy is by history of asbestos exposure and exclusion of other causes.

Amyloidosis

Amyloidosis can be accompanied by pleural effusion in up to 30% of patients. These effusions are usually transudative and probably most often are caused by CHF; however, one report suggests that amyloid deposition can be found on pleural biopsy specimens in a high percentage of these patients, suggesting that pleural biopsy may be a reasonably sensitive technique in the diagnosis of systemic amyloidosis (8). Furthermore, some patients with pleural amyloidosis have otherwise unexplained exudative effusions, raising the possibility that amyloid deposits may play a causative role in pleural fluid formation.

AIDS

Pleural effusion in hospitalized AIDS patients is not uncommon (27%). Bacterial infection (30%), *Pneumocystis jiroveci* (15%), and TB (8%) are the most common causes. Kaposi's sarcoma and hypoalbuminemia are the most common noninfectious causes.

Pleural Effusions After Coronary Bypass Grafting

Approximately 175,000 patients undergo coronary artery bypass grafting (CABG) each year in the United States. Approximately 50% of these patients develop small pleural effusions in the immediate postoperative period. Most post-CABG effusions are left sided and resolve spontaneously without specific therapy; however, approximately 1% of patients have large pleural effusions (occupying >25% of the hemithorax). These large effusions are usually left sided

TABLE 37.3

DEFINITIVE DIAGNOSES BASED ON PLEURAL FLUID ANALYSIS

Diagnosis	Criteria
Urinothorax	pH <7, *transudate*, pleural/serum creatinine >1.0
Empyema	Pus, positive Gram stain or culture
Malignancy	Positive cytology
Chylothorax	Triglycerides >110 mg/dL, chylomicrons
Tuberculosis, fungal	Positive stains, cultures
Hemothorax	Hematocrit >50% of blood
Peritoneal dialysis	Protein <1 g/dL, glucose 300–400 mg/dL
Esophageal rupture	pH <7, high amylase (salivary)
Lupus pleuritis	Lupus erythmatous cells, pleural/serum antinuclear antibody >1.0

or, if bilateral, the left-side effusion is much larger than the right. In one large study, the following causes were found to contribute to large post-CABG effusions:

- 24% (7/29) CHF
- 7% (2/29) Constrictive pericarditis
- 3% (1/29) Pulmonary embolism
- 66% (19/29) No discernible cause
- 42% (8/19) Bloody
- 58% (11/19) Nonbloody

The bloody pleural effusions post-CABG were probably related to bleeding within the pleural space. These bloody effusions achieved a maximum size within 1 month after CABG, were frequently eosinophilic, had high levels of LDH, and usually resolved after one or two thoracenteses. Nonbloody pleural effusions, in contrast, reached their maximum size more than 1 month after surgery, were mostly lymphocytic, had lower levels of LDH, and were difficult to manage because of recurrence despite multiple thoracentesis, chest tube drainage, and pleurodesis.

Table 37.3 lists some clinical situations in which the pleural fluid analysis can provide a definitive diagnosis of the underlying etiology, whereas Table 37.4 gives examples of the more common scenario, in which the pleural fluid analysis can provide clues to the etiology rather than a definitive diagnosis.

TREATMENT OF PLEURAL EFFUSIONS

Therapeutic Thoracentesis

When a pleural effusion is large enough to cause symptoms (usually dyspnea), and specific therapy of the underlying etiology is ineffective or too slow, a "therapeutic" thoracentesis is indicated. If fluid reaccumulates and symptoms recur, thoracentesis can be repeated two or three times; however, the repetitive removal of large amounts of fluid over a short period is discouraged because of potential

TABLE 37.4	
CLUES FROM PLEURAL FLUID ANALYSIS	
Criteria	Possible Diagnoses
Lymphocytosis (>50%)	Tuberculosis (TB), malignancy
Eosinophilia (>10%)	Air, blood, benign asbestos pleural effusion, drug-induced Churg-Strauss, parasitic/fungal, malignancy
Glucose <60 (or <50% of serum)	TB, esophageal rupture, malignancy
Glucose <30	Empyema, rheumatoid arthritis
High amylase (pleural/serum >1.0, or higher than upper limit (UL) in serum)	Pancreatitis, pseudocyst, pancreatic cancer (10–30× serum level, pancreatic)
	Esophageal rupture (5× serum level, salivary), malignancy, ruptured ectopic pregnancy

complications from protein loss and fluid shifts. More definitive therapy, such as the instillation of a pleural sclerosing agent, is usually indicated when a symptomatic pleural effusion rapidly recurs after a few attempts at drainage using thoracentesis.

In general, no more than 1,000 to 1,500 mL of fluid should be removed at one time. Removal of more fluid risks the development of edema in the underlying lung (*re-expansion pulmonary edema*) or rapid fluid shift from the intravascular space into the pleural space (*postthoracentesis shock*). Both phenomena appear to be related, in part, to creating excessive negative pleural pressures during thoracentesis. If desired, pleural fluid pressures can be measured directly on a periodic basis during thoracentesis by using an Abrams needle connected to a three-way valve and a manometer. Fluid can be safely withdrawn until a pressure of approximately −20 cm water is reached (measured in the eighth or ninth posterior intercostal space). This technique has allowed up to 4 L of effusion to be withdrawn safely at one time. Because removal of 1.0 to 1.5 L is usually enough to provide at least temporary relief of dyspnea, measuring pleural fluid pressures during thoracentesis is generally unnecessary.

Dyspnea secondary to pleural fluid accumulation is probably related more to intrathoracic volume changes than to chemoreceptor input. Even in instances in which thoracentesis provides relief of dyspnea, a temporary decrease in arterial oxygenation often occurs. The magnitude and duration of hypoxia bear a rough correlation to the amount of fluid removed. Hypoxia may last 12 hours or longer. Thus, if a large amount of fluid is removed, or the patient has a low baseline arterial oxygenation level, supplemental nasal oxygen should probably be given for several hours after a thoracentesis.

Transudates

Pleural effusions secondary to heart failure, ascites, or nephrotic syndrome can usually be managed with appropriate medical therapy, such as diuretics and sodium restriction. Acutely, therapeutic thoracentesis allows time for medical management. Rarely, recurrent symptomatic pleural effusions complicate cirrhosis or nephrosis despite optimal medical therapy; doxycycline sclerosis of the pleural cavity (see Pleural Sclerosis section) is usually successful.

Exudates

Parapneumonic Effusions

The management of parapneumonic effusions represents a particular challenge to the clinician. These exudative effusions often accompany bacterial pneumonias, but they usually resolve spontaneously with appropriate antimicrobial therapy of the pneumonia. A minority, probably a subset of those that become infected, progresses to empyema (frank pus in the pleural space) and subsequent loculation and fibrosis of the pleura. Treatment at this late stage may require several tube thoracostomies or even surgical decortication. These complications can usually be prevented by early and complete drainage of the pleural space with a single chest tube; however, the indiscriminate universal application of tube thoracostomy constitutes unnecessary therapy for most patients with parapneumonic effusions. Thus, the task is to intervene with tube thoracostomy selectively, but early enough to be definitive.

All parapneumonic effusions should be evaluated immediately by thoracentesis. An exception may be extremely small parapneumonic effusions (fluid layer seen on lateral decubitus chest film <1 cm thick), which rarely cause complications. The following findings are all indications for complete drainage of the pleural space:

- Presence of *frank pus* (admittedly a loosely defined term)
- Bacteria on Gram stain
- Evidence of loculation (by chest roentgenography)

Thoracentesis may be adequate for complete pleural space drainage in some instances, but tube thoracostomy is usually required. Conversely, effusions that are sterile and not turbid in appearance do not require aggressive intervention; however, many parapneumonic effusions are "borderline," occupying a position between these extremes.

The use of fluid pH level analysis has been advocated as a means of evaluating these borderline effusions. The literature, however, does not support the use of a single "cut-off"

TABLE 37.5

SUGGESTED APPROACH TO CLASSIFICATION AND MANAGEMENT OF PARAPNEUMONIC PLEURAL EFFUSION

	pH	Glucose (mg/dL)	Gram Stain/ Culture	Management
Simple	>7.2	>40	Negative	Antibiotics
Borderline	7–7.2	>40	Negative	Serial thoracentesis
Complicated	<7	<40	Negative	Tube thoracostomy
Empyema	<7	<40	Positive	Tube thoracostomy

pH value as a predictor. Furthermore, misinterpretation is possible if fluid specimens for pH analysis are not kept anaerobic and on ice. Nevertheless, a low pH (<7.0–7.2) usually indicates a fluid with high potential for loculation, whereas a high pH (>7.3) suggests an extremely low risk for complications. In cases that are doubtful, a serial evaluation of the pleural fluid may help guide therapy. All parameters (e.g., appearance, Gram stain, white blood cell count, glucose, protein, LDH, pH) should be evaluated on each thoracentesis. In this setting, a declining pH would argue for tube drainage. Pleural loculation can occur rapidly (i.e., within <24 hours) with certain infections; serial evaluation should not be allowed to delay necessary therapy. At times, two or three thoracenteses should be used in the first day. Finally, it is better to err on the side of early tube drainage rather than risk incomplete drainage of an infected parapneumonic effusion. Table 37.5 gives a suggested approach to the classification and management of parapneumonic effusions.

Malignant Effusions

A variety of malignancies can lead to pleural effusion, usually secondary to direct extension or metastases of the tumor to the pleura. Breast and lung cancers are the most frequent, but many others, including pancreas, colon, esophageal, and ovarian cancers, can also involve the pleura. Lymphomas, in contrast, frequently cause pleural effusion without a direct involvement of the pleura, probably through central obstruction of lymphatics.

The first step in controlling malignant effusions is radiation therapy or systemic chemotherapy, if appropriate for the tumor. With lymphomas, the use of mediastinal radiation (1,400-2,600 rad) is usually effective, even when the chest roentgenogram shows no evidence of central lymph node involvement. Radiation therapy directed to the pleura is usually not appropriate therapy for malignant effusions because of unavoidable exposure of the lung parenchyma. Chemotherapy for carcinomas is usually not effective in controlling malignant effusions, except with some breast, ovarian, or small cell lung cancers.

Needle aspiration is an important early step to assess whether symptoms are relieved by fluid removal and to determine the rate of fluid reaccumulation. Most malignant effusions recur rapidly within 3 or 4 days. Prolonged drainage by tube thoracostomy may be tried but fails in at least 50% of cases.

Pleural Sclerosis

In patients with uncontrolled and symptomatic malignant effusions, pleural symphysis achieved through the instillation of a "sclerosing" agent is indicated. Pleural sclerosis should be attempted only if the lung expands fully after fluid removal. Agents that can be instilled into the pleural cavity to achieve pleural sclerosis include doxycycline, talc slurry, bleomycin, and quinacrine.

We believe these agents work by producing a chemical serositis that heals through fibrosis, rather than through a direct antitumor effect. This is probably true even for most of the antineoplastic agents that have been used. Regardless of what agent is used, proper technique is essential for success. The pleural cavity should be drained completely of fluid to avoid dilution of the sclerosing substance. More important, the visceral and parietal pleura must be approximated closely, obliterating the pleural space, so that fibrotic healing achieves pleural symphysis and thus prevents the recurrence of the effusion.

The ideal sclerosing agent would be readily available at low cost, have a low morbidity and toxicity, and be highly effective. Doxycycline appears to be the agent of first choice. With proper technique, doxycycline sclerosis is 80% to 90% effective:

1. Evacuate the pleural cavity by tube thoracostomy at low suction (approximately 15-20 cm of water).
2. Order a chest radiograph to verify the position of the tube, clearance of pleural fluid, and re-expansion of the lung.
3. Premedicate the patient with a narcotic analgesic 30 to 60 minutes before sclerosis.
4. Instill 15 to 20 mg/kg of doxycycline in 80 mL of saline, combined with 20 mL of 1% lidocaine, into the chest tube.
5. Flush the tube with 20 mL of saline.
6. Clamp the tube (no suction).
7. Place the patient in a prone, supine, right decubitus, left decubitus, and sitting position for 4 to 5 minutes each (20-25 minutes). Repeat each position for 30 minutes each (2.5 hours).
8. Unclamp the tube and connect to low suction.
9. Continue until drainage is <100 to 150 mL/day (this may take 3–5 days).
10. Remove the tube.

Side effects are mild. Approximately one-third of patients have a low-grade febrile response. Chest pain is unpredictable. Sometimes it is absent, and at other times, it is rather severe; however, the pain is self-limited, lasting 30 to 45 minutes. Generally, pain can be prevented by premedication with parenteral narcotics and the concurrent administration of intracavitary lidocaine. Some have advocated giving the intracavitary lidocaine 30 minutes before instilling doxycycline, but this is probably unnecessary. The effectiveness of doxycycline sclerosis is not diminished by peripheral neutropenia because a white cell inflammatory response is not necessary for its action.

Treatment failures are usually related to an inability to approximate the pleural surfaces during doxycycline administration, which may be owing to *atelectasis* (central bronchial obstruction because of tumor) or to a "trapped lung" encased by either a fibrotic visceral pleura or massive tumor involvement. The last circumstance may be suggested when a malignant effusion has an extremely low pH and glucose.

If doxycycline is contraindicated because of allergy or other reasons, bleomycin appears to be a good choice. Although experience with this agent is limited, instillation is well tolerated and often effective. Systemic side effects have not been reported.

Talc is quite effective in producing pleural symphysis. Traditionally, this agent has been introduced as a dry powder abrasive (*talc poudrage*) at open thoracotomy or insufflated through a chest tube. Because even the latter approach is usually done with the patient under general anesthesia, use of talc has been limited; however, a bedside technique using the instillation of a talc saline suspension has been advocated. In this method, 10 g of talc United States Pharmacopeia powder (previously gas sterilized and aerated) is suspended in 250 mL of sterile saline solution. This step can be accomplished using a bulb syringe and sterile plastic cup. The suspension is administered with tube thoracostomy in a manner analogous to doxycycline sclerosis. Because instillation of talc may be painful, narcotic premedication should be given. Talc pleurodesis has rarely been associated with acute pneumonitis and adult respiratory distress syndrome.

Surgical Therapy

Parietal pleurectomy and, if necessary for a trapped lung, decortication of the visceral pleura are both definitive procedures that give a 100% response rate; however, mortality is high (up to 5%–10%) and morbidity may be great (air leaks after decortication). Thus, these procedures should be applied selectively. Surgery should generally be limited to cases in which sclerosis has failed or lung expansion is prevented by thickened pleura. Important considerations before resorting to surgery include:

- Good condition of the underlying lung
- Low tumor burden outside the chest
- Expected long-term survival
- General medical condition good enough for major surgery

When a malignant cause for pleural effusion is discovered at thoracotomy, it is usually appropriate to attempt pleural abrasion, talc poudrage, or pleurectomy at that time.

Chylothorax

The accumulation of chyle in the pleural space is usually secondary to disruption of the thoracic duct by trauma (surgical or nonsurgical) or by malignancy. A congenital form also exists. Most "idiopathic" adult cases are believed to be caused by unrecognized mild trauma. Chylothorax is differentiated from pseudochylothorax by its high triglyceride and low cholesterol content.

Chylothorax may cause dyspnea; other local complications are rare. Chyle is bacteriostatic, and infections rarely occur. Furthermore, chyle does not seem to be highly fibrogenic. The major problem is the nutritive and immunologic cost of the continuous loss of thoracic duct contents. Chyle is high in protein, electrolytes, fat, fat-soluble vitamins, and lymphocytes. Cell-mediated immunity assessed by skin tests and graft survival decreases at 3 to 6 weeks of continuous drainage. Furthermore, the theoretic problem of a permanent loss of T lymphocytes in adults who have little thymic activity is present. Before modern nutritional and surgical therapy, chylothorax had a 50% mortality rate.

The flow within the thoracic duct is highly dependent on diet, especially fat intake. Normal lymph flow is approximately 2.5 L daily (1.38 mL/kg/hour); in starvation, it may decrease to 300 to 500 mL. Dietary manipulation that decreases lymph flow rate is important for the healing of thoracic duct lesions and forms the rationale for conservative therapy. Of note, medium-chain triglycerides (MCTs) are absorbed through the portal venous system, whereas long-chain triglycerides are carried by lymph. Thus, lymph flow is greatly reduced if dietary fat is limited to MCTs.

Conservative Therapy

Initially, two or three thoracenteses are done to assess the reaccumulation rate. If leakage continues, tube thoracostomy drainage should be instituted. Concurrently, oral intake should be limited to an MCT diet (e.g., MCT oil). If necessary, lymph flow is reduced further by using venous hyperalimentation and avoiding oral intake. Of course, this is much less convenient and carries a risk of infection and other complications. Chyle itself should not be reinfused intravenously because of the possibility of venous thrombosis or fatal anaphylaxis.

Pleural sclerosis is usually avoided because it may complicate subsequent surgical therapy if this proves necessary. If a patient is not a surgical candidate, pleural sclerosis may be attempted when dietary manipulation fails.

Surgical Therapy

Surgical therapy consists of ligation of the thoracic duct. Two general approaches are available. The duct can be ligated most easily through a right thoracotomy at the level of T8 to T10, where it usually exists as a single trunk. Alternatively, closure may be attempted directly at the leakage site. Both locating the site (despite the use of dyes to stain the lymph) and sealing the leak may be technically difficult, however. Furthermore, the duct has to be ligated both above and below the leak because of rich anastomotic communications. With either choice, ligation of the thoracic duct has few adverse consequences because lymph reaches the venous system by alternate channels.

Choice of Therapy

The major difficulty is deciding how long to try conservative therapy before resorting to surgery. There is no easy answer; each case must be individualized. A few generalizations may help. Congenital chylothorax in neonates usually responds well to conservative management. With chylothorax owing to malignancies, radiation or systemic chemotherapy may halt chyle leakage in up to two-thirds of lymphomas and in one-half of carcinomas. Furthermore, unless relatively long-term survival is expected, therapy should remain conservative. Traumatic chylothorax eventually ceases spontaneously in approximately 50% of cases; however, it is difficult to predict this outcome. In trauma and other causes of chylothorax, the rate of chyle loss should help guide therapy. If chyle loss is low (i.e., <0.25 mL/kg/hour), a longer trial of conservative therapy will be feasible. If chyle loss is dramatic (>2 mL/kg/hour), conservative therapy will likely be less effective and should be abandoned earlier. As a general rule, it is reasonable to try 1 to 4 weeks of conservative therapy before resorting to surgery.

Effusions of Indeterminate Etiology

The etiology of some pleural effusions remains obscure even after thoracentesis and two or three closed pleural biopsies have been done on separate occasions. A careful general clinical examination, including appropriate laboratory tests (purified protein derivative, ANA, and rheumatoid factor) or radiographs (CT of the thorax), may provide important clues; however, the cause often remains perplexing. At this point, the clinician is faced with a choice of observing the patient or proceeding with thoracoscopy or thoracotomy. A case for taking the conservative approach derives from the fact that many of these effusions (roughly half) resolve spontaneously and no disease is apparent on long-term follow-up; however, that leaves the other half, who have carcinoma, mesothelioma, lymphoma, or other serious diseases.

If the patient looks well and has no fever, pain, or weight loss, careful observation may be warranted. If indications of underlying disease are present, an aggressive diagnostic approach is warranted. Some information in the literature supports the general soundness of this approach. It should be noted, finally, that even a negative exploratory thora-

cotomy does not rule out occult malignancy as a cause for pleural effusion.

Other Effusions

Moderate- or large-size hemothorax should be evaluated promptly and completely. Blood in the pleural space may lead to fibrin deposition, thus causing adhesions and a limitation of lung expansion. Furthermore, as a practical point, tube thoracostomy helps evaluate the rate or recurrence of bleeding. Small hemothoraces usually resolve spontaneously without residua.

The treatment of pleural effusions associated with collagen vascular diseases is directed against the underlying disease. Lupus effusions are usually not large enough to cause symptoms; rather, pain from the pleuritis heralds the process. Appropriate analgesics or anti-inflammatory medications are given. Rheumatoid effusions may present with dyspnea and require therapeutic thoracentesis. Clinically "silent" empyemas may occur in rheumatoid patients on corticosteroids and require tube thoracostomy drainage. Effusions owing to pulmonary thromboembolism or pancreatitis require no specific therapy for the effusion itself.

Tuberculous Effusions

Tuberculous effusions may occur early in the course of the infection, often as part of an otherwise occult process. Such tuberculous pleurisy is usually self-limited, clearing without treatment. Up to one-half of untreated patients, however, subsequently develop active disease elsewhere within 5 years. Thus, antituberculous therapy with an appropriate drug regimen is indicated. Often therapy must be presumptive, pending the results of pleural fluid and biopsy cultures. If the effusion is large and symptomatic, the concurrent use of systemic corticosteroids may have a salutary effect. Tuberculosis may also involve the pleura by direct spread from active disease of lung, lymph nodes, or bone. Frank tuberculous empyema requires chest tube drainage.

Pneumothorax

Pneumothorax, or an accumulation of air in the pleural space, is seen in association with certain lung diseases (see the following list), or it may occur without underlying lung disease (primary pneumothorax). Common causes of secondary pneumothorax include:

- Malignancy
- Infection (e.g., TB, cystic fibrosis, *P. jiroveci* pneumonia)
- Chronic obstructive pulmonary disease and asthma
- Trauma
- Congenital disorders
- Iatrogenic
- Transthoracic needle aspiration
- Subclavian vein puncture
- Thoracentesis
- Transbronchial biopsy

- Pleural biopsy
- Mechanical ventilation
- Aerosolized pentamidine
- Other
- Endometriosis (catamenial pneumothorax)
- Lymphangioleiomyomatosis

Primary spontaneous pneumothorax can occur in otherwise healthy patients with no underlying lung disease. The incidence of primary spontaneous pneumothorax is 9 cases per 100,000 persons per year with a 6:1 male-to-female ratio. The incidence is higher in smokers. Compared with nonsmokers, the relative risk of pneumothorax in men is seven times higher in light smokers (1–12 cigarettes/day), 21 times higher in moderate smokers (13–22 cigarettes/day), and 102 times higher in heavy smokers (>22 cigarettes/day). Table 37.6 lists helpful classifications and definitions for pneumothorax based on an American College of Physicians consensus statement.

Treatment

Simple observation may be all that is needed in patients who have no evidence of tension pneumothorax, are not symptomatic (no dyspnea, no hypoxemia), and in whom the pneumothorax occupies <15% of the hemithorax. The site of the leak usually closes, and the air in the pleural space is gradually absorbed. Supplemental oxygen can enhance the rate of pleural air absorption.

Although simple aspiration may be sufficient in some patients (especially those with primary pneumothorax),

tube thoracostomy is the treatment of choice for most patients with secondary, large, or symptomatic pneumothoraces (Table 37.7). Small-caliber tubes (9 F) can be used for iatrogenic pneumothorax following procedures and for primary spontaneous pneumothorax. Most patients with secondary (other than iatrogenic) or large pneumothoraces require a standard size (28 F) tube thoracostomy for effective treatment.

Patients with recurrent pneumothorax may benefit from pleurodesis. The pneumothorax recurrence rate decreases significantly after pleurodesis compared with the rate for management with chest tube alone (13% vs. 36%, respectively). Video-assisted thoracoscopy should be considered in patients who do not respond to these therapies or who have occupations in which the development of pneumothorax may be dangerous (e.g., airplane pilots or deep sea divers). Because of the association of pneumothorax with smoking, all patients with pneumothorax should be strongly advised to stop smoking.

Tension Pneumothorax

In tension pneumothorax, the pressure of air in the pleural space exceeds ambient pressure throughout the respiratory cycle. Tension pneumothorax may result in acute respiratory failure, hemodynamic compromise, and cardiopulmonary arrest. If tension pneumothorax is suspected, a large-bore needle should be inserted immediately in the affected side to allow for immediate relief of the tension until tube thoracostomy can be performed.

TABLE 37.6

PNEUMOTHORAX CLASSIFICATIONS AND DEFINITIONS

Spontaneous: no antecedent traumatic or iatrogenic cause
Primary spontaneous: no clinically apparent underlying lung abnormalities
Secondary spontaneous: clinically apparent underlying lung disease
Size: determined by distance from lung apex to ipsilateral thoracic cupola at parietal surface as determined by upright standard
  radiograph
- Small pneumothorax: <3 cm apex-to-cupola distance
- Large pneumothorax: >3 cm apex-to-cupola distance
Patient age groups (years)
- Young, 18–40
- Older, >40
Clinical stability
- Stable patient: all of the following present—respiratory rate, <24 breaths/min; heart rate, >60 or <120 beats/min; normal blood
  pressure; room air oxygen saturation, >90%; and patient can speak in whole sentences between breaths
- Unstable patient: any patient not fulfilling the definition of stable
Drainage tube sizes
- Small, 14 F
- Moderate, 16–22 F
- Large, 24–36 F
Simple aspiration: insertion of needle or cannula with removal of pleural air followed by immediate removal of needle or cannula
Sclerosis (pleurodesis) procedure
- Chemical pleurodesis: intrapleural instillation of sclerosing agent through chest tube or percutaneous catheter
- Open or surgical pleurodesis: performed with thoracoscope or through limited or full thoracotomy

Adapted from Colice GL, Curtis A, Deslauriers J, et al., for the American College of Chest Physicians
Parapneumonic Effusions Panel. Medical and surgical treatment of parapneumonic effusions: an evidence-based
guideline. *Chest* 2000;118:1158–1171.

TABLE 37.7
MANAGEMENT OF SPONTANEOUS PNEUMOTHORAX

Primary spontaneous pneumothorax
- Stable patients with small pneumothoraces
- Observe in emergency department for 3–6 hours
- Discharge home if repeat radiography excludes progression
- Follow-up radiograph within 12 hours to 2 days to document resolution

Stable patients with large pneumothoraces

Hospitalize in most instances with insertion of small-bore catheter (14 F) or 16–22 F chest tube

Catheters or tubes may be attached to either a Heimlich valve or a water seal device

If lung fails to re-expand quickly, suction should be applied to water seal device
- Unstable patients with large pneumothoraces
- Hospitalize with insertion of a chest catheter to re-expand lung
- Most patients should be treated with 16–22 F standard chest tube
- 24–28 F standard chest tube may be used if patient requires positive-pressure ventilation

Secondary spontaneous pneumothorax
- All should be hospitalized
- Patients may be observed or treated with a chest tube, depending on the extent of their symptoms and the course of their pneumothorax

Adapted from Colice GL, Curtis A, Deslauriers J, et al., for the American College of Chest Physicians Parapneumonic Effusions Panel. Medical and surgical treatment of parapneumonic effusions: an evidence-based guideline. *Chest* 2000;118:1158–1171.

REVIEW EXERCISES

QUESTIONS

1. A 30-year-old man presents with acute, excruciating, right flank and lower chest pain, nausea, and vomiting. His past medical history is notable for one episode of hematuria 1 year ago. He has a family history of a twin sister with sarcoid. On examination, the patient is in distress with pain, right flank tenderness, and upper-quadrant guarding. Right dullness and pleural rub is present. His chest radiograph shows a moderate right effusion. A kidney and upper bladder film is not obtainable. An analysis of the pleural fluid reveals an amber fluid, with a pH of 6.9; lactate dehydrogenase, 40 IU/dL; protein, 0.5 g/dL; and hemoglobin, +1.

After administration of adequate analgesia, which would be the most appropriate action?
a) Ultrasound of gallbladder and pancreas
b) Ventilation–perfusion scan
c) Closed pleural biopsy
d) Urology consult
e) Upper endoscopy

Answer and Discussion

The answer is d. Urinothorax based on transudate with acidic pH.

2. A 70-year-old man with a history of insulin-dependent diabetes mellitus, alcohol abuse, severe gastroesophageal reflux disease, emphysema, and benign prostatic hyperplasia requiring an indwelling catheter and frequent courses of intravenous antibiotics presents with high-grade fever; congestion; cough productive of thick, yellow, blood-tinged sputum; and right pleuritic chest pain.

On examination, you are presented with an ill-looking man with right upper lung consolidation and right base dullness. His chest radiograph shows right upper lobe alveolar infiltrate with cavity and moderate right effusion. Laboratory findings show leukocytosis with left shift. His arterial blood gas analysis shows pH, 7.32; PCO_2, 52; and arterial oxygenation, 80 on 3 L forced inspiratory oxygen.

His pleural fluid is thick, yellow, and purulent. Laboratory findings are pH, 7.82; glucose, 30 mg/dL; and lactate dehydrogenase, 1,050 IU/dL.

What would be the most appropriate immediate action?
a) Urine culture and sensitivity; replace Foley
b) Continuous broad-spectrum positive/negative intravenous antibiotics
c) Thoracic surgery consult for open thoracostomy
d) Tube thoracostomy
e) Stop antacid, order esophagogastroduodenoscopy

Answer and Discussion

The answer is d. Proteus empyema, urea-splitting property leads to ammonia production and an increased pH.

3. A 60-year-old white man presents with bilateral, vague, nonpleuritic chest pain, and mild shortness of breath; no fever, cough, or night sweats. On history taking, 15 months ago, this patient had right effusion that resolved spontaneously; 5 years ago, he had occasional bilateral wrist pain, treated with aspirin. An annual purified protein derivative test was negative 3 months ago. On examination, you find bibasilar dullness and a hard nodule on the nose. His chest radiograph shows bilateral moderate pleural effusion.

The pleural fluid analysis reveals a white blood cell count of 2,000/mm^3; polymorphonuclear leukocytes, 90%; pH, 7.05; lactate dehydrogenase, 1,000 IU/dL; protein, 4 g/dL; and glucose, 5 mg/dL.

Based on the most likely diagnosis, what would be the most appropriate action?
a) Isoniazid, 300 mg; rifampin, 600 mg; ethambutol, 900 mg daily
b) Prednisone, 40 mg daily
c) Bilateral chest tube placement
d) Intravenous ceftazidime and gentamicin
e) Close observation for spontaneous resolution of fluid

Answer and Discussion

The answer is b. This is rheumatoid effusion.

4. A 30-year-old woman presents with slowly progressing shortness of breath of 6 months' duration. Her past medical history includes pneumothoraces, one on either side, 4 weeks apart 1 year ago.

On examination, she has increased dullness in the left base, right basilar crackles, and small ascites. Her chest radiograph shows hyperinflated lungs, vague interstitial changes, and left effusion. A pleural tap reveals milky white fluid, with triglycerides, 200 mg/dL.

The most likely diagnosis is which of the following?
a) Lymphoma
b) Catamenial pneumothorax
c) Gorham's syndrome
d) Lymphangioleiomyomatosis
e) Histiocytosis X

Answer and Discussion

The answer is d. The chylothorax with interstitial changes in a young woman would suggest lymphangioleiomyomatosis.

5. A 63-year-old man in a wheelchair presents with crippling rheumatoid arthritis. His annual chest radiograph revealed moderate bilateral effusion. No chest pain, cough, or shortness of breath is present.

You review his old radiographs and observe bilateral subpulmonic effusions for 5 years. His purified protein derivative test is negative. His pleural fluid is milky white and shiny; the analysis reveals a white blood cell count of 2,000/mm^3, 90% L; glucose, 16 mg/dL; lactate dehydrogenase, 1,200 IU/dL; triglycerides, 30 mg/dL; cholesterol, 150 mg/dL; and a large amount of cholesterol crystals.

What would be the most appropriate action?
a) Start medium-chain triglyceride diet
b) Lymphangiography

c) Serology for *Wuchereria bancrofti* infestation
d) Bilateral pleuroperitoneal pump
e) Conservative treatment

Answer and Discussion

The answer is e. This is a pseudochylothorax.

6. A 70-year-old man with a history of congestive heart failure, on optimal medication, underwent thoracentesis in the emergency department for large right effusion using a 16-gauge spinal needle (3.5 L of serosanguineous fluid was removed uneventfully). Minutes after the procedure, the patient developed progressive shortness of breath and needed 100% fractional inspired oxygen.

On examination, you observe tachypnea, right lung wheeze, and basilar rales; blood pressure is 100/70 mm Hg, and pulse is 100 beats/minute.

What would be the most appropriate statement regarding the event?
a) Place large-bore chest tube for tension pneumothorax.
b) Transfuse 2 U of pack cells for hemothorax.
c) Administer Lasix, 60 mg intravenously.
d) Intrapleural pressure monitoring could have avoided the event.
e) Check creatine phosphokinase and ventilation/perfusion lung scan.

Answer and Discussion

The answer is d. The patient develops pulmonary edema following drainage of a large volume of a chronic pleural effusion.

7. What is the most important mechanism for the relief of dyspnea after thoracentesis?
a) Arterial oxygen pressure
b) Placebo effect
c) Intrathoracic volume
d) Forced expiratory volume, forced vital capacity
e) Static lung compliance

Answer

The answer is c.

8–13. Match each of the following pleural effusions with the appropriate diagnosis:

	Pleural/ Serum Protein Ratio	Pleural/ Serum LDH Ratio	pH	Glucose (mg/dL)	Triglycerides (mg/dL)
8.	0.1	0.4	6.9	10	0
9.	0.6	0.7	7.4	100	10
10.	0.7	1.2	7.3	93	335
11.	0.4	0.4	7.4	88	30
12.	0.7	5.1	7.2	25	50
13.	0.8	2.2	7.0	50	15

a) Urinothorax
b) Pulmonary embolism
c) Chylothorax
d) Congestive heart failure
e) Rheumatoid effusion
f) Empyema

Answers and Discussions

8. The answer is a. The only transudate with acidic pH.

9. The answer is b. An exudate with a normal pH.

10. The answer is c. High triglyceride (>110 mg/dL) diagnostic of chylothorax.

11. The answer is d. A transudate characteristic of congestive heart failure.

12. The answer is e. An exudate with low pH and extremely low glucose typical of rheumatoid arthritis.

13. The answer is F. Similar to item 12, but pH is much lower, as is seen in empyema.

14–18. Match the following pleural effusions with the appropriate management strategy in a patient with pneumonia:

	Glucose (mg/dL)	pH	LDH (U/L)	Gram Stain	Culture
14.	70	7.30	250	Negative	Negative
15.	55	7.15	1,000	Negative	Negative
16.	35	6.90	1,000	Negative	Negative
17.	30	7.00	1,000	Positive	Pending
18.	30	7.00	1,000	Negative	Positive

a) Simple parapneumonic effusion; treat with appropriate antibiotics
b) Borderline parapneumonic effusion; needs serial thoracentesis in addition to antibiotics
c) Complicated parapneumonic effusion; needs tube thoracostomy in addition to antibiotics
d) Empyema; needs tube thoracostomy in addition to antibiotics

Answers

14. The answer is a.
15. The answer is b.
16. The answer is c.
17. The answer is d.
18. The answer is d.

19. A 35-year-old man who smoked one pack per day for 20 years was diagnosed with AIDS 4 years ago. He is allergic to sulfa and receives aerosolized pentamidine for *Pneumocystis jiroveci* pneumonia prophylaxis. He was doing well until a few days before admission, when he started developing progressive shortness of breath. His respiratory status deteriorated quickly, requiring intubation and mechanical ventilation. The next day, the respiratory therapist called because the patient had developed high airway pressures. This was also associated with a drop in the patient's blood pressure and arterial oxygen saturation. When you examine the patient, you notice decreased air entry on the left side with a deviation of the trachea to the right.

What should you do next?
a) Order chest radiography.
b) Add 10 cm H_2O of positive end-expiratory pressure.
c) Insert a chest tube in the right lung.
d) Insert a large-bore needle in the second intercostal space on the left.
e) Place the patient on his side with the left side down.

Answer and Discussion

The answer is d. The patient has signs of tension pneumothorax on the left.

REFERENCES

1. Light RW, MacGregor MI, Luchsinger PC, et al. Pleural effusions: the diagnostic separation of transudates and exudates. *Ann Intern Med* 1972;77:507–513.
2. Costa M, Quiroga T, Cruz E. Measurement of pleural fluid cholesterol and lactate dehydrogenase. *Chest* 1995;108:1260–1263.
3. Peterman TA, Speicher CE. Evaluating pleural effusions: a two-stage laboratory approach. *JAMA* 1984;252:1051–1053.
4. Sahn SA. Malignant pleural effusions. *Clin Chest Med* 1985;6:113–125.
5. Potts DE, Taryle DA, Sahn SA. The glucose-pH relationship in parapneumonic effusions. *Arch Intern Med* 1978;138:1378–1380.
6. Good JT, King TE, Antony VB, et al. Lupus pleuritis: clinical features and pleural fluid characteristics with special reference to pleural fluid antinuclear antibodies. *Chest* 1983;84:714–718.
7. Kavuru MS, Tubbs R, Miller ML, et al. Immunocytometry in the diagnosis of lymphoma in an idiopathic pleural effusion. *Am Rev Respir Dis* 1992;145:209–211.
8. Kavuru MS, Adamo JP, Ahmad M, et al. Amyloidosis and pleural disease. *Chest* 1990;98:20–23.

SUGGESTED READINGS

General

Diaz-Guzman E, Dweik RA. Diagnosis and management of pleural effusions: a practical approach. *Compr Ther* 2007;33:237-246.
Light RW. *Pleural Diseases*, 5th ed. Philadelphia: Lippincott Williams & Wilkins, 2007:xiii, 427.
Sahn SA. The pleura. *Am Rev Respir Dis* 1988;138:184–234.

Diagnostic Aspects

Heffner JE. Evaluating diagnostic tests in the pleural space: differentiating transudates from exudates as a model. *Clin Chest Med* 1998;19:277–293.
Yataco JC, Dweik RA. Pleural effusions: evaluation and management. *Cleve Clin J Med* 2005;72:854-856, 858, 862-864.

Pleural Biopsy

Mezies R, Charbonneau M. Thoracoscopy for the diagnosis of pleural disease. *Ann Intern Med* 1991;114:271–276.
Poe RH, Israel RH, Utell MJ, et al. Sensitivity, specificity, and predictive values of closed pleural biopsy. *Arch Intern Med* 1984;144:325–328.

Radiographic Evaluation

McLoud TC. CT and MR in pleural disease. *Clin Chest Med* 1998;19:
261–276.

Pugatch RD, Spirn PW. Radiology of the pleura. *Clin Chest Med* 1985;
6:17–32.

Ravin CE. Thoracentesis of loculated pleural effusions using grey scale
ultrasonic guidance. *Chest* 1977;61:666–668.

Parapneumonic Effusions and Empyema

Colice GL, Curtis A, Deslauriers J, et al., for the American College
of Chest Physicians Parapneumonic Effusions Panel. Medical and
surgical treatment of parapneumonic effusions: an evidence-based
guideline. *Chest* 2000;118:1158–1171.

Malignant Effusions

Canto A, Ferrer G, Romagosa V, et al. Lung cancer and pleural effusion:
clinical significance and study of pleural metastatic locations. *Chest*
1985;87:649–652.

Renshaw AA, Dean BR, Antman KH, et al. The role of cytologic evaluation of pleural fluid in the diagnosis of malignant mesothelioma.
Chest 1997;111:106–109.

Sahn SA. Malignancy metastatic to the pleura. *Clin Chest Med* 1998;19:
351–361.

Collagen Vascular Diseases

Halla JT, Schrohenloher RE, Volanakis JE. Immune complexes and
other laboratory features of pleural effusions: a comparison of
rheumatoid arthritis, systemic lupus erythematosus, and other diseases. *Ann Intern Med* 1980;92:748–752.

Hunder GG, McDuffie FC, Hepper NG. Pleural fluid complement in
systemic lupus erythematosus and rheumatoid arthritis. *Ann Intern
Med* 1972;76:357–363.

Pettersson T, Klockars M, Hellstrom P-E. Chemical and immunological features of pleural effusions: comparison between rheumatoid
arthritis and other diseases. *Thorax* 1982;37:354–361.

Asbestos

Epler GR, McLoud TC, Gaensler EA. Prevalence and incidence of benign asbestosis pleural effusion in a working population. *JAMA*
1982;247:617–622.

Nishimura SL, Broaddus VC. Asbestos-induced pleural disease. *Clin
Chest Med* 1998;19:311–329.

Robinson BWS, Musk AW. Benign asbestos pleural effusion: diagnosis
and course. *Thorax* 1981;36:896–900.

Esophageal Rupture

Bellman MH, Rajaratnam HN. Perforation of the esophagus with
amylase-rich pleural effusion. *Br J Dis Chest* 1974;68:18–22.

Dye RA, Laforet EG. Esophageal rupture: diagnosis of pleural fluid pH.
Chest 1974;66:454–456.

Urinothorax

Miller KS, Wooten S, Sahn S. Urinothorax: a cause of low pH transudative pleural effusions. *Am J Med* 1988;85:448–449.

Stark DD, Shaves JG, Baron RL. Biochemical features of urinothorax.
Arch Intern Med 1982;142:1509–1511.

Chylothorax

Teba L, Dedhia HV, Bowen R, et al. Chylothorax review. *Crit Care Med*
1985;13:49–52.

Sassoon CS, Light RW. Chylothorax and pseudochylothorax. *Clin
Chest Med* 1985;6:163–171.

Postcardiac Injury

Light RW, Rogers JT, Cheng D, et al. Large pleural effusions occurring after coronary artery bypass grafting. *Ann Intern Med*
1999;130:891–896.

Stelzner TJ, King TE, Antony VB, et al. The pleuropulmonary manifestations of the postcardiac injury syndrome. *Chest* 1983;84:383–
387.

Indeterminate Effusions

Ansari T, Idell S. Management of undiagnosed persistent pleural effusions. *Clin Chest Med* 1998;19(2):407–417.

Canto A, Rivas J, Saumench J, et al. Points to consider when choosing
a biopsy method in cases of pleurisy of unknown origin. *Chest*
1983;84:176–179.

Ryan CJ, Rodgers RF, Unni KK, et al. The outcome of patients with
pleural effusion of indeterminate cause at thoracotomy. *Mayo Clin
Proc* 1981;56:145–149.

AIDS

Beck JM. Pleural disease in patients with acquired immune deficiency
syndrome. *Clin Chest Med* 1998;19:341–349.

Joseph J, Strange C, Sahn SA. Pleural effusions in hospitalized patients
with AIDS. *Ann Intern Med* 1993;118:856–859.

Pneumothorax

Baumann MH, Strange C, Heffner JE, et al., for the ACCP Pneumothorax Consensus Group. Management of spontaneous pneumothorax: an American College of Chest Physicians Delphi consensus
statement. *Chest* 2001;119:590–602.

Chapter 38

Board Simulation in Critical Care Medicine

Daniel A. Culver   Alejandro C. Arroliga

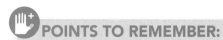

POINTS TO REMEMBER:

- For practical purposes, the diagnosis of acute lung injury (ALI)/acute respiratory distress syndrome (ARDS) requires
  - Ratio of arterial oxygen pressure [PaO_2]:inspired oxygen fraction [FiO_2] <300 (≤200), regardless of the level of applied positive end-expiratory pressure
  - Bilateral pulmonary infiltrates consistent with pulmonary edema
  - No clinical evidence of left atrial hypertension; if pulmonary artery occlusion pressure is measured, it must be ≤18 mm Hg
- The incidence of ARDS has been estimated in the range of 5 to 15 cases per 100,000 per year.
- Patients who survive tend to recover normal or near-normal lung function, although patients with severe ARDS are sometimes left with some degree of restrictive defect.
- The only strategy that has been demonstrated in randomized controlled trials to improve the mortality in ALI/ARDS is the use of low stretch (6 cc/kg predicted body weight tidal volume) ventilation.
- The most common causes of acute shock in the intensive care unit population may be grouped into several categories:
  - *Hypovolemic shock*—commonly due to hemorrhage, external volume loss (e.g., ketoacidosis), or third spacing (e.g., pancreatitis)
  - *Cardiogenic shock*—the most frequent causes include acute myocardial infarction, malignant dysrhythmias, massive pulmonary embolus, acute valvular regurgitation, pericardial tamponade, severe pulmonary arterial hypertension, or non-ischemic cardiomyopathies

- *Distributive shock*—characterized by loss of vascular tone; septic shock is most frequent; other causes include adrenal insufficiency, neurogenic shock, liver cirrhosis, overdoses, and anaphylaxis
- Recent randomized controlled trials of the pulmonary artery catheter in several populations, including ARDS, heart failure, and high-risk surgical patients have failed to demonstrate improved outcomes with its use.
- The strict definition of sepsis requires the presence of three of four systemic inflammatory response criteria, which include
  - Core temperature >38°C or <36°C
  - White blood cell count >12,000 cells/mm³, or <4,000 cells/mm³, or >10% immature (band) forms
  - Heart rate >90 beats/minute
  - Respiratory rate >20 breaths/minute or $PaCO_2$ <32 mm Hg
- Severe sepsis is defined as sepsis with at least one organ failure. Septic shock implies persistence of hypotension despite adequate fluid resuscitation.

This chapter introduces some concepts regarding the pathophysiology and management of some common critical care presentations, including ARDS, sepsis, and management of shock.

ACUTE RESPIRATORY DISTRESS SYNDROME/ACUTE LUNG INJURY

ALI is a clinical syndrome characterized by the presence of increased alveolar-capillary barrier permeability causing pulmonary edema, deficiency of surfactant, and exuberant pulmonary inflammation. These patients have been classified into two groups by severity: those with ALI, in which the patient has moderate to severe hypoxemia (ratio of arterial oxygen pressure [PaO_2]:inspired oxygen fraction [FiO_2] of <300 and >200) and ARDS (PaO_2:FiO_2 ≤200). For practical purposes, the diagnosis of ALI (ARDS) requires:

- PaO_2/FiO_2 <300 (≤200), regardless of the level of applied positive end-expiratory pressure (PEEP)
- Bilateral pulmonary infiltrates consistent with pulmonary edema
- No clinical evidence of left atrial hypertension; if pulmonary artery occlusion pressure is measured, it must be ≤18 mm Hg

It must be recognized that the previous definition is most useful for clinical and epidemiologic research, but that it is only moderately sensitive when compared to autopsy series where pathological findings (diffuse alveolar damage) are consistent with ARDS. In the presence of pulmonary disease, such as pneumonia, the sensitivity is lower than in extrapulmonary disease. The implication is that management strategies in individuals with infiltrates in more than one lobe should mimic those proven useful for ARDS.

Pathophysiology and Etiology

Regardless of the inciting cause, the pathophysiology of ALI includes the loss of alveolar-capillary barrier integrity with leakage of protein-rich exudate (edema) into the alveolar lumen; activation of resident immune cells and emigration into the lung of effector cells, primarily neutrophils; degradation of surfactant, promoting alveolar instability and collapse; and production of multiple proinflammatory cytokines, such as tumor necrosis factor, interleukin (IL)-1, IL-6, and IL-8. In pathological specimens, diffuse alveolar damage is present, with abundant inflammatory cells (neutrophils and macrophages), erythrocytes, hyaline membranes, and proteinaceous edema fluid. These processes cause disruption of the alveolar epithelium. If the stimuli continue, fibroproliferative changes occur, causing progressive lung damage. In patients who survive, the hypoxemia slowly resolves and lung compliance improves. The sequelae of these processes include:

- Loss of pulmonary compliance, thus increasing the work of breathing; the decrease in compliance is due to both the presence of nonaerated (atelectatic) lung and decreased alveolar compliance in aerated but edematous lung regions
- Impairment of gas exchange due to ventilation-perfusion mismatch, shunting, and development of pulmonary hypertension, which occurs in up to 25% of ARDS patients
- Systemic inflammatory responses, which may lead to multisystem organ failure

The incidence of ARDS has been estimated in the range of 5 to 15 cases per 100,000 per year. When ALI is included, the incidence has been estimated to be as high as 79/100,000 per year. Possibly due to underlying risk factors, ALI/ARDS is more common in the elderly. Mortality is also higher in the elderly and increases when there is multisystem organ failure.

The etiology of ARDS is diverse and includes *direct* and *indirect* causes. The most common direct causes are aspiration and infections (pneumonia). The most common indirect causes are sepsis, trauma, and pancreatitis. An increasingly recognized cause is transfusion of blood products, termed *transfusion-related acute lung injury* (TRALI). TRALI should be suspected when new ALI is documented within 6 hours of blood product transfusion.

Prognosis

Some series report survival rates in the range of 50% to 60%. Only a minority (<5%–10%) of the patients die of refractory hypoxemia. In multicenter, controlled clinical trials that exclude subjects with severe pre-existing comorbidities, the rate of survival is approximately 70%. The severity of physiological derangement correlates with the prognosis in patients with ARDS. For example, an elevated alveolar dead space, probably caused by the injury to the pulmonary capillaries, and with obstruction due to thrombosis and inflammation, is associated with an increased risk of dying. It also appears that hospitals with experience caring for larger numbers of ARDS patients (>150/year) exhibit improved survival outcomes. It is important to recognize that the duration of ARDS does not independently influence outcome; thus, persistence of ARDS alone in the absence of other prognostic factors does not represent a rationale for withdrawal of support.

Interestingly, patients who survive tend to recover normal or near-normal lung function, although patients with severe ARDS are sometimes left with some degree of restrictive defect. The pulmonary function abnormalities, however, correlate with a reduction in health-related quality of life. It is important to note that persistent functional disability may be present in a significant percentage of patients who survive ARDS. Up to 50% of the patients were not working 1 year after being discharged from the intensive care unit (ICU), despite improvement in lung function. Many of these patients have significant functional limitation due to muscle wasting and muscle weakness.

Management

In ALI, adequate sedation, nutrition, skin care, attention to details such as optimal fluid and electrolyte management, and adequate prophylaxis for venous thromboembolism and upper gastrointestinal bleeding are essential.

Mechanical ventilation is important in patients with ALI. The objectives of mechanical ventilation are not to normalize arterial blood gas values, but to provide adequate support for oxygenation and acid-base balance, while avoiding further injury that can be induced by mechanical ventilation. The only strategy that has been demonstrated in randomized controlled trials to improve the mortality in ALI/ARDS is the use of low stretch (6 cc/kg predicted body weight [PBW] tidal volume) ventilation. The evidence supporting the use of low stretch ventilation comes from the ARDS Network, which randomized 861 patients with ALI/ARDS to two groups. Patients were ventilated with volume-cycle, assist-control ventilation. One group received conventional mechanical ventilation (tidal volume of 12 cc/kg PBW), and the other group received low tidal volume ventilation (6 cc/kg PBW). The patients assigned to low tidal volume had a 22% relative mortality reduction, from 40% to 31%. Based on this evidence, it is recommended that patients with ARDS be ventilated using low tidal volume, 6 cc/kg of PBW. The use of other ventilator modalities, such as pressure-controlled ventilation or newer adaptive modes, has not been studied adequately enough in this population to demonstrate similar benefits. Several modalities used for severe, refractory ARDS, including extracorporeal membrane oxygenation, delivery of nitric oxide in the ventilator circuit, high-frequency ventilatory modalities, and installation of synthetic surfactant, have all failed to demonstrate survival benefits.

Other recent studies in ALI/ARDS have evaluated use of high levels of positive end-inspiratory pressure (PEEP), corticosteroids for the fibroproliferative phase of ARDS, and prone positioning. These investigations have likewise not demonstrated mortality benefits. The amount of PEEP used should be enough to avoid end-expiratory collapse but not so high that it decreases the venous return and the cardiac output.

The optimal level of hemoglobin in patients with ARDS is not known. The use of a liberal strategy for packed red blood cell transfusion (to keep hemoglobin between 10 and 12 g/dL), however, has not been found to be associated with a better outcome in intubated patients receiving mechanical ventilation when compared with a restrictive red blood cell transfusion strategy that keeps hemoglobin in the range of 7 to 9 g/dL.

Another area of controversy has been the appropriate management of volume status. The presence of excess extravascular lung water in ALI results in decreased pulmonary compliance and impaired oxygenation, and may lead to increased ventilator-induced alveolar injury. Recently, the ARDS Clinical Trials Network conducted a trial of 1,000 patients using an explicit fluid management protocol and a lung-protective ventilator strategy. The subjects were randomized to liberal fluid management (target central venous pressure [CVP] 10–14 mm Hg or pulmonary artery occlusion pressure [PAOP] 14–18 mm Hg) versus a conservative approach (target CVP <4 mm Hg or PAOP <8 mm Hg). There was no difference in the primary endpoint, 60-day mortality. However, patients managed with conservative targets had more ventilatorfree days, earlier discharge from the intensive care unit, and fewer organ failures. On the basis of these findings, present fluid management in ALI patients with adequate urine output and not in shock should include use of diuretics as necessary to target CVP <4 mm Hg or PAOP <8 mm Hg.

Shock and Hemodynamic Monitoring

Definition and General Approach

The syndrome of shock is present when the circulatory system is unable to maintain adequate cellular perfusion. If shock is not reversed, irreversible cellular damage will occur. The majority of patients will require the administration of fluids and/or vasopressor agents. The goal in most situations is to maintain an adequate mean systemic blood pressure, usually 60 to 65 mm Hg; however, other parameters, such as urinary output, skin perfusion, mental status, and heart rate, are very important. Crystalloids and colloids are typically used for volume resuscitation in shock, with the common assumption that colloids may be superior due to their property of enhancing intravascular oncotic pressure. However, studies have not demonstrated a difference in outcome overall between the use of colloids or crystalloids. In several meta-analyses, crystalloid resuscitation has been associated with a lower mortality in trauma patients, and the administration of albumin has been shown not to reduce mortality in patients with hypovolemia, burns, or hypoalbuminemia. The largest study to date randomized 6,997 patients to receive either albumin (4%) or normal saline for intravascular fluid resuscitation. There was no difference in mortality rate, days in the ICU and in the hospital, days on mechanical ventilation, or number of days of renal replacement therapy.

The two vasopressors most frequently used in patients with shock are dopamine and norepinephrine. There have been no trials to date that convincingly demonstrate superiority of either of these pressor agents over the other.

Causes

The most common causes of acute shock in the ICU population may be grouped into several categories:

- *Hypovolemic shock*—commonly due to hemorrhage, external volume loss (e.g., ketoacidosis), or third spacing (e.g., pancreatitis)
- *Cardiogenic shock*—the most frequent causes include acute myocardial infarction, malignant dysrhythmias, massive pulmonary embolus, acute valvular regurgitation, pericardial tamponade, severe pulmonary arterial hypertension, or nonischemic cardiomyopathies
- *Distributive shock*—characterized by loss of vascular tone; septic shock is most frequent; other causes include adrenal insufficiency neurogenic shock, liver cirrhosis, overdoses, and anaphylaxis

In practice, many patients demonstrate more than one of the previously listed shock types simultaneously. For example, distributive shock due to mitochondrial damage may occur in profound gastrointestinal hemorrhage, even after adequate volume resuscitation. Impaired cardiac contractility frequently develops in the later stages of septic shock.

An additional important cause of shock in the ICU occurs when excessive intrathoracic pressure impedes venous return to the right side of the heart. Tension pneumothorax and excessive PEEP (especially unrecognized intrinsic PEEP) are the most common culprits. Tension pneumothorax should be suspected when shock develops in the presence of unilaterally decreased breath sounds, with or without physical examination evidence of tracheal deviation. Intrinsic PEEP (auto-PEEP) generally occurs when expiratory flow limitation (e.g., in severe asthma or COPD exacerbation) prevents the alveoli from emptying adequately during expiration. With cyclic hyperexpansion of the alveoli, a situation develops where intrathoracic pressure is higher than the inferior vena caval pressure throughout the respiratory cycle, and venous return declines. Auto-PEEP can be treated with the use of bronchodilators, adjustment of the ventilator to provide longer expiratory time, and strategies to decrease the breathing frequency such as rate reduction, sedation, and/or paralytics. In extreme cases, it may be necessary to temporarily disconnect the patient from the positive-pressure ventilation to allow return of the end-expiratory alveolar pressure to approach atmospheric pressure.

Diagnosis

In practice, the cause of shock can usually be determined by the history and physical examination. Targeted testing, including blood count, chemistries, cardiac enzymes, and ECG, are useful. An increasingly important adjunct is routine use of echocardiography to guide diagnosis and management of the hypotensive patient. Echocardiography can provide information about the filling and contractile status of both ventricles, the presence of unsuspected valvular or pericardial disease, and development of segmental wall motion abnormalities that may indicate ischemia. An overlooked but accessible and valuable tool for assessing the cause of shock is measurement of the central venous ($ScvO_2$) or the mixed venous oxygen saturation (SvO_2). In normal individuals, the SvO_2 is 65% to 70%, and the SvO_2 obtained from the distal port of a central venous catheter placed in the subclavian or internal jugular vein is usually within 5% to 8% of this value. In the presence of hypovolemic or cardiogenic shock, the saturation should decline progressively as peripheral oxygen extraction is maximized, with humans able to reduce their SvO_2 as low as 20%. In contrast, patients with pure distributive shock will exhibit an inappropriate failure to extract oxygen, and often the measured SvO_2 can be supranormal. In fact, current approaches for sepsis management depend on measurement of $ScvO_2$ to guide therapy.

Hemodynamic Monitoring

The possibility of catheterizing the right ventricle at the bedside and obtaining pressures from the right side of the heart revolutionized critical care medicine. The pulmonary artery catheter (PAC) provides information useful for the management of respiratory and circulatory failure and for the assessment of intravascular volume. Unfortunately, available studies show that a significant proportion of clinicians working in the ICU cannot correctly interpret the data obtained with the catheter or cannot recognize errors in the tracing and in the measurements taken with the catheter. In addition, recent randomized controlled trials of the PAC in several populations, including ARDS, heart failure, and high-risk surgical patients, have failed to demonstrate improved outcomes with its use. The failure to demonstrate improved outcomes may be due to complications associated with its use or errors in the interpretation of the data generated by the catheter. In addition, it is possible that the use of the PAC is a mark of aggressive physician management in the ICU, and this aggressive management is associated with a higher rate of complications and mortality.

A randomized study by the ARDS Network of 1,000 subjects with ALI/ARDS managed with either a central venous catheter or PAC addressed these questions by instituting explicit fluid management and interpretive guidelines, and aggressive quality control of the data obtained from the catheters. In this study, the use of the PAC did not influence the primary end-point (60-day mortality). There were no benefits in the subset with shock at study entry and no improvement in organ failure or time in shock. However, the PAC was associated with a higher rate of complications, especially cardiac dysrhythmias.

Complications that can occur with use of a PAC include:

- Catheter-associated infections
- Insertion complications, such as pneumothorax, arterial puncture, and hematomas
- Cardiac dysrhythmias, including third-degree heart block when there is pre-existing left bundle branch block, or ventricular tachycardia
- Mechanical complications, including cardiac perforation, pulmonary artery rupture, infarction of lung parenchyma, and knotting of the catheter.

Interpretation of Hemodynamic Monitoring

A frequent problem in the reading or interpretation of the data generated with catheterization of the right side of the heart is proper identification of the waveform in the different chambers of the heart. Passage from the right ventricle into the pulmonary artery is evidenced by an increase in the diastolic pressure (the diastolic pressure of the pulmonary artery is higher than the diastolic pressure of the right ventricle). The pulmonary artery waveform has a systolic pressure wave and a diastolic trough. The pulmonary artery waveform also has a dicrotic notch caused by the closure of the pulmonary valve; this can be identified on the terminal part of the systolic pressure wave. To properly assess PAC waveforms, several principles should be considered:

- Measure pressures with a printout that includes ECG monitoring to identify the waveforms
- Measure pressures at end expiration

- Remember to "zero" the transducer to calibrate it to atmospheric pressure
- Assure that the transducer is level with the left atrium
- Avoid "overdamped" or "underdamped" pressure tracings that can occur with kinks, air bubbles, or excessively long tubing

A common use for the PAC is to estimate the left ventricular preload using the pressure measured when the pulmonary artery is occluded with a balloon. Situations that may cause false estimation of the left ventricular end-diastolic volume include decreased ventricular compliance, pulmonary venous disease, increased pleural pressure, catheter tip in a lung region where alveolar pressure exceeds pulmonary venous pressure (i.e., not in West zone 3), mitral stenosis, and left atrial myxoma. Another common use for the PAC is estimation of the cardiac output using either the thermodilution or Fick technique. The thermodilution technique is susceptible to errors when there is tricuspid or pulmonic valve disease, intracardiac shunts, or extremely low cardiac output. The Fick method is less accurate when peripheral oxygen consumption cannot be reliably estimated (e.g., in sepsis).

Sepsis and Septic Shock

Sepsis is a clinical syndrome that is present when systemic inflammation occurs as a result of infection. The strict definition of sepsis requires the presence of three of four systemic inflammatory response criteria, which include:

- Core temperature $>38°C$ or $<36°C$
- White blood cell count $>12,000$ cells/mm^3, or $<4,000$ cells/mm^3, or $>10\%$ immature (band) forms
- Heart rate >90 beats/minute
- Respiratory rate >20 breaths/minute or $PaCO_2$ <32 mm Hg

Severe sepsis is defined as sepsis with at least one organ failure. Septic shock implies persistence of hypotension despite adequate fluid resuscitation. Although infection must be clinically suspected, blood cultures are only positive in approximately 17%, 46%, and 69% of patients with sepsis, severe sepsis, and septic shock, respectively. In clinical trials, the most common sources for sepsis include the lung, abdominopelvic region, urinary tract, soft tissue, and catheter-related infections. However, in nearly one in five patients, the source is still unclear after investigation. Besides infection, other common causes of a septic presentation include severe pancreatitis, burns, and trauma.

Treatment

Management of sepsis can generally be divided into the following goals:

- Identification and treatment of the underlying cause
- Volume resuscitation
- Initiation of catecholamines after or with inadequate response to volume challenge
- Consideration of intravenous corticosteroids
- Evaluation for appropriateness of drotrecogin alpha

Although the source organ is commonly unclear at the time of presentation, it is vital that the clinician carefully evaluate all possible sources. A common cause for poor outcomes is failure to consider multiple sources, such as the presence of an intra-abdominal abscess in an obtunded patient with evidence of a urinary tract infection. Removal of infected foreign bodies, drainage of abscesses, or debridement of soft tissue is at least as important as antibiotics.

In addition to source control, the use of adequate antibiotic regimens in the early management of patients is crucial. In post-hoc analysis of a drug therapy trial, failure to include adequate antibiotics in the initial regimen was associated with an 8% absolute mortality increase (44% vs. 36%); factors independently associated with inadequate regimens included gram-positive infections, polymicrobial infection, presence of *Pseudomonas*, older age, and a known source of infection. Therefore, it is extremely important to consider all possible sources and to have a good working knowledge of local resistance patterns among common organisms. Besides appropriate selection, early administration of antimicrobials has been demonstrated to be an important factor in outcome. In a large cohort study including 2,154 patients, each 1-hour delay from onset of shock to infusion of antibiotics conferred an average of 7.6% increased risk of mortality.

Restoration of adequate intravascular volume is an important initial goal in sepsis. Recent data suggest that a goal-directed approach may improve outcomes. In a study of 263 patients treated in the emergency department setting, management of early septic shock for the first 6 hours using a specific targeted algorithm decreased all-cause mortality from 47% to 31%, compared with a group managed with traditional end-points. The salient features of the early goal-directed therapy (EGDT) approach include using volume infusions to obtain a CVP of 8 to 12 mm Hg, vasopressors titrated to achieve mean arterial pressure (MAP) ≥65 mm Hg, and measurement of $ScvO_2$. In those individuals with $ScvO_2$ $<70\%$ despite adequate CVP and MAP, red blood cell transfusions and/or dobutamine were added. The major differences between traditional management and the protocol-directed group included more aggressive volume resuscitation and higher use of transfusions. The application of EGDT in later stages of septic shock has not been adequately tested to recommend widespread adoption. It is also important to remember that other clinical markers of adequate perfusion should be assessed, including urine output, blood flow in the extremities, and mental status.

The choice of vasopressor agents remains controversial. Animal studies and surrogate outcomes data in humans variably suggest advantages for preferential use of norepinephrine as a first-line catecholamine. However, a recent trial in 330 subjects comparing treatment with norepinephrine plus dobutamine versus epinephrine alone for septic shock was unable to demonstrate any significant outcome difference between agents. The use of vasopressin as a second-line agent has become popular, based on data demonstrating relative vasopressin deficiency in refractory septic shock. However, a beneficial effect of vasopressin on mortality has not been demonstrated. In individuals with substantial tachycardia, phenylephrine, a pure alpha-agonist, may be useful.

The role of corticosteroids in septic shock has been the subject of intense scrutiny recently. By restoring smooth muscle sensitivity to catecholamine effects, corticosteroids may improve outcomes, or at least decrease the time to shock reversal. In a multicenter trial involving 299 patients with refractory septic shock, replacement doses of hydrocortisone (50 mg every 6 hours) and fludrocortisone decreased 28-day mortality from 63% to 53%. The positive effects of the intervention were derived from patients with "relative adrenal insufficiency," a prospectively defined subgroup. For this study, relative adrenal insufficiency was defined as an absolute cortisol increase of ≤9 mcg/dL after administration of 250 mcg cosyntropin. Since publication of these results, several other reports have suggested variously that the free cortisol level is more important, that the stimulation test performance is nonreproducible between institutions and in the same patient, and that a metyrapone test may provide better discriminatory power.

Endothelial function is markedly dysregulated in sepsis, with activation of endogenous pro- and anticoagulants, generation of thrombin, platelet aggregation, further endothelial damage, and resulting release of additional inflammatory mediators. Activated protein C (APC), an important antithrombotic mediator, is deficient due to impaired thrombomodulin-mediated activation. In a randomized, controlled trial of 1,690 subjects (PROWESS trial), treatment with recombinant APC (drotrecogin alpha) led to a 6.1% absolute mortality reduction, from 30.8% to 24.7%. The benefits were entirely derived from patients with more severe sepsis (APACHE II ≥25). The most important side effect of drotrecogin alpha administration is bleeding, with the prevalence around 4% in clinical practice. Of note, a follow-up trial did confirm a lack of mortality benefit in subjects with APACHE II <25 or single-organ failure only. Therefore, use of drotrecogin alpha should be reserved for individuals with APACHE II ≥25 and no excessive bleeding risks. It is most efficacious when used earlier in the severe sepsis syndrome.

REVIEW EXERCISES

QUESTIONS

1. A 44-year-old man with type I diabetes, end-stage renal disease, and diabetic retinopathy develops chest pain and low-grade fever (38.5°C) 5 days after a unilateral below-knee amputation done for a poorly

healing ulcer. He had been recovering in a nursing facility but has missed two dialysis sessions due to low blood pressure and has refused prophylactic subcutaneous heparin. After a 500-mL bolus of saline in the emergency department, he is transferred to the intensive care unit for further management. On examination, he is distressed, with a heart rate 96 beats/minute, respiratory rate 28 breaths/minute, oxygen saturation on room air is 86%, and blood pressure 82/50 mm Hg. The examination is difficult due to his obesity, but does not reveal an obvious cause for his hypotension; the surgical site looks clean and intact, and an indwelling tunneled catheter in his right neck also looks unremarkable. A 12-lead ECG shows nonspecific ST- and T-wave abnormalities but no definite signs of ischemia. A central venous catheter is inserted to guide decision making. Measurement of the a-wave reveals a central venous pressure of 19 mm Hg; the tracing shows preserved waveforms except for loss of the γ descent. Considering the findings of the central venous catheter, which choice most effectively addresses the likely cause of shock in this patient?

a) Start broad-spectrum antibiotics; remove the tunneled catheter; and start fluids, pressor agents, and other modalities for likely septic shock using a "goal-directed therapy" approach.

b) Consult cardiology service for a pericardiocentesis.

c) Resuscitate more aggressively with crystalloids, and consider thrombolytic therapy versus surgical consult for likely massive pulmonary embolus.

d) Urgent coronary angiogram with percutaneous coronary intervention and placement of intra-aortic balloon pump, if needed, in preparation for mitral valve repair.

e) Start dobutamine and prostacyclin for right ventricular failure.

Answer and Discussion

The answer is b. Pericardiocentesis with drainage of effusion leads to cardiac tamponade. Recognition of the right-sided waveforms and their derangements in disease is useful when prioritizing diagnostic tests, when decisions must be made urgently, or when there are conflicting data. It is important to be familiar with expected values for filling pressure (typically 4-8 mm Hg for central venous pressure [CVP]). The differential diagnosis for elevated CVP in the setting of shock includes acute right heart failure (massive pulmonary embolism, right ventricular infarction), pericardial disease, and acute left heart disease (large myocardial infarction, acute mitral regurgitation, acute ventricular septal defect). The finding of an attenuated γ descent is characteristic of cardiac tamponade because there is equalization of pressures between the atria and ventricles, which impairs atrial emptying. In uremic pericarditis, the expected tachycardia may be absent due to autonomic insufficiency; likewise, the ECG may not reveal diffuse ST segment elevations. In the early stages of septic shock, there is usually hypovolemia, so the CVP should be low. Massive pulmonary embolism and acute mitral valve rupture may cause hypotension but should not preferentially affect the y descent.

2. An 18-year-old, 58-kg female asthmatic patient is intubated in the emergency department for respiratory failure from status asthmaticus. Her initial ventilator settings are assist-control mode with a set rate of 18, tidal volume 500 mL, FiO_2 1.0, and positive end-expiratory pressure 5 cm. On arrival to the intensive care unit, she is in shock, with systolic blood pressure of 74 mm Hg. Examination reveals an extremely agitated female with diaphoresis, distended neck veins, and respiratory rate of 36 breaths/minute and SpO_2 88%. Her breath sounds are markedly diminished but equal bilaterally. In addition to aggressive volume resuscitation and ensuring adequate sedation, you should institute which of the following to reverse her hypotension prior to cardiac arrest:
a) Reduce her set rate to 10 breaths/minute.
b) Administer 6 mg of pancuronium IV push.
c) Insert a 16-gauge angiocatheter needle into the second intercostal space bilaterally.
d) Increase the inspiratory flow rate.
e) Administer paralytics, and then remove her from the ventilator for 30 to 60 seconds.

Answer and Discussion
The answer is e. It is important to recognize common complications of mechanical ventilation in patients with severe airways obstruction. Development of intrinsic positive end-expiratory pressure (PEEP) (auto-PEEP, dynamic hyperinflation) is one of the most significant complications. Intrinsic PEEP can result in patient–ventilator dyssynchrony, agitation, difficulty weaning, ventilation/perfusion mismatch, barotrauma, and impairment of right-sided venous return leading to cardiovascular collapse. An important consideration is tension pneumothorax, but typically the patient will exhibit physical examination signs such as tracheal deviation, unilateral decrease of breath sounds, and hyperresonance on percussion. Prevention of intrinsic PEEP is achieved by maximizing alveolar emptying, either by decreasing airways resistance (bronchodilators) or increasing expiratory time. Techniques to increase expiratory time include ensuring a low respiratory rate using sedatives and, if necessary, paralytics, decreasing the inspiratory time by adjusting the flow rate or the I:E ratio, and setting the mandatory rate on the ventilator as low as possible. Hypercapnia is acceptable to achieve this goal. However, none of these techniques

is generally rapid enough to be helpful when hypotension is already established. Temporarily disconnecting the endotracheal tube from the ventilator circuit, and therefore the effects of positive-pressure ventilation, is the quickest way to effectively restore blood pressure.

3. The patient has been stable for 3 days. She is being treated with clarithromycin, ceftriaxone, Solu-Medrol, bronchodilators, and lorazepam. She became agitated overnight and was given haloperidol. Suddenly, she became hypotensive, and her pulse was not palpable. The ECG tracing is shown (ventricular tachycardia) in Figure 38.1. The patient is still hypotensive, her white blood cell count is 15,000/mm^3, and her hemoglobin is 10 g/dL. You will do all of the following, *except*
a) Perform cardioversion-defibrillation.
b) Administer magnesium intravenously.
c) Temporarily disconnect the patient from the ventilator circuit.
d) Correct hypocalcemia, hypokalemia, and alkalosis.

Answer and Discussion
The answer is c. This question highlights an important topic in critical care medicine—drug interactions. An important effect of drug interaction in the critically ill patient is hypotension caused by partial adrenal insufficiency. This drug interaction occurs in patients receiving drugs that can increase the activity of the P450 system (e.g., phenytoin, phenobarbital). When the P450 system is activated, the metabolism of steroids increases, creating a state of partial adrenal insufficiency. This drug interaction should be suspected in patients receiving medication that can increase the metabolism of the P450 system and who present with persistent hypotension in the absence of other etiologies. An increasingly recognized offender is etomidate, a medication commonly used in rapid-sequence intubation, which blocks adrenal steroid production directly.

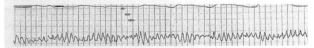

Figure 38.1 The ECG trace in this patient is consistent with a type of ventricular tachycardia called *torsades de pointes*. This type of ventricular tachycardia is characterized by QRS complexes of changing amplitude that appear to twist around an isoelectric line and occur at a rate of 200 to 250 beats/minute. The tachycardia may terminate spontaneously, or it can go to ventricular standstill or a new episode of torsades. Frequently, in the critically ill patient, ventricular fibrillation may supervene. Although several predisposing factors have been cited, the most common predisposing factors in critically ill patients include bradycardia; electrolyte abnormalities; and use of drugs such as cisapride, phenothiazines, and butyrophenones (e.g., haloperidol). The most important aspect of management in this patient is to avoid the arrhythmias by aggressive correction of electrolyte abnormalities, including hypokalemia, hypocalcemia, and hypomagnesemia. It is important to pay attention to drug interactions. In the hemodynamically unstable patient, electric cardioversion is essential.

Macrolides and haloperidol, drugs commonly used in the intensive care unit, are known to increase the QT interval. Patients with underlying ischemic heart disease and electrolyte and acid–base abnormalities are more likely to develop this complication. Phenothiazines, antiarrhythmic medications, tricyclic antidepressants, and antipsychotic agents and cisapride can prolong the QT interval as well.

4. A 34-year-old homeless man is evaluated in the emergency department, where he was brought after being found obtunded. His medical history is remarkable for HIV and polysubstance abuse. Examination reveals an obtunded man with no focal neurologic signs. He is afebrile, with heart rate 104 beats/minute, respiratory rate 22 breaths/minute, and blood pressure 96/68 mm Hg. His sodium is 148 mmol/L, potassium 4.0 mmol/L, chloride 115 mmol/L, bicarbonate 10 mmol/L, blood urea nitrogen 47 mg/dL, creatinine 1.3 mg/dL, and glucose 58 mg/dL. Serum albumin is 2.5 g/dL. Arterial blood gas on room air reveals a pH of 7.12, PCO_2 28 mm Hg, and PaO_2 94 mm Hg. His serum lactate is 2.2 mmol/L. Which of the following is true in your evaluation of this patient?
a) He has an anion gap (AG) metabolic acidosis with appropriate respiratory compensation.
b) He has an AG metabolic acidosis and inappropriate respiratory compensation.
c) He has an AG metabolic acidosis, a metabolic alkalosis, and inappropriate respiratory compensation.
d) He has an AG metabolic acidosis, a non-AG metabolic acidosis, and inappropriate respiratory compensation.
e) He has an AG metabolic acidosis, a non-AG metabolic acidosis, and appropriate respiratory compensation.

Answer and Discussion
The answer is b. Interpretation of arterial blood gas abnormalities is a key skill in critical care medicine. Systematic evaluation of the arterial blood gas results often leads to unsuspected findings, such as triple acid–base disorders or respiratory insufficiency. In this case, use of "Winter's formula" allows assessment of the adequacy of the respiratory response to the primary acidosis:

$$\text{Expected } pCO_2 = ([1.5 \times \text{measured } HCO_3] + 8) \pm 2$$

To evaluate for the presence of two metabolic processes, one must compare the change in AG versus the change in bicarbonate. In the setting of hypoalbuminemia, the expected AG should be reduced by about 2.5 mEq/L for every 1 g/dL decrease in serum albumin, with normal AG in most laboratories ranging from 6 to 12 mEq/L.

Using 12 mEq/L as the AG normal value, in the previous example, the expected AG should be [12 mEq/L − (2.5 × 1.6 g/dL decrease of albumin)] = 8 mEq/L. However, the calculated gap is 23 mEq/L. Thus, the AG has increased by 15 mEq/L over the expected value. Has there been an equivalent (equimolar) change in the bicarbonate level? In this case, the bicarbonate has decreased from 24 mEq/L (normal) to 10 mEq/L = 14 mEq/L. Therefore, all the change in bicarbonate level can be explained by the unmeasured anions. If the change in bicarbonate were more severe than predicted by the change in AG, a superimposed nongapped acidosis would be suspected; if less profound, then a concomitant metabolic alkalosis should be considered.

5. The patient in question 4 is diagnosed with ethylene glycol intoxication, after it is noted that there is an osmolar gap present, and treated with ethanol infusion to competitively prevent metabolism of ethylene glycol to formaldehyde and formic acid. He avoids renal failure; however, on the second day in the intensive care unit, he develops a fever (39.5°C) and hypoxemia. Chest imaging shows bilateral diffuse infiltrates. His hemoglobin is stable at 8.7 g/dL. Over the ensuing 24 hours, he develops refractory hypoxemic respiratory failure, requiring intubation. The most appropriate next step now includes
a) Start ceftriaxone and azithromycin.
b) Start piperacillin-tazobactam, tobramycin, and vancomycin.
c) Start piperacillin-tazobactam, azithromycin, and vancomycin.
d) Start piperacillin-tazobactam and ciprofloxacin.
e) Perform bronchoalveolar lavage to look for infection with *Pneumocystis jiroveci*.

Answer and Discussion
The answer is c. The correct answer depends on recognizing that the likely diagnoses are community acquired pneumonia or aspiration pneumonitis with acute respiratory distress syndrome. The development of pneumonia after 48 hours in the hospital, or within 3 months of a prior hospitalization, classifies as hospital-acquired pneumonia, mandating consideration of antipseudomonal antibiotics as part of the initial therapy. However, in community-acquired pneumonias, there are mitigating factors that may provide indications for more extensive antimicrobial coverage. In patients admitted to the intensive care unit, there is a high likelihood that resistant organisms will be present, including drug-resistant pneumococcus, *Legionella* species, and community-acquired methicillin-resistant *Staphylococcus aureus* (MRSA). Therefore, patients with severe community-acquired pneumonia should be treated

with a combination of a potent antipneumococcal cephalosporin and either an advanced macrolide or quinolone. In patients with risk factors for *Pseudomonas aeruginosa*, including immunosuppression, significant structural lung disease (cystic fibrosis, bronchiectasis, or repeated exacerbations of chronic obstructive pulmonary disease that require frequent glucocorticoid and/or antibiotic use), probable aspiration, or multiple medical comorbidities, an antipseudomonal penicillin should be used. The use of vancomycin in severe community-acquired pneumonia is hotly debated, but should generally be reserved for individuals with gram-positive organisms on sputum examination or risk factors for community-acquired MRSA (recent influenzalike illness, prior antibiotic therapy, end-stage renal disease, or injection drug abuse).

Although this individual may have AIDS, the onset of *Pneumocystis* pneumonia (PCP) is usually subacute. Although the sensitivity of bronchoalveolar lavage for diagnosing PCP is excellent in HIV (97%–99%), it is less sensitive in the non-HIV population.

6. The patient, in his ninth day in the intensive care unit, becomes hypotensive and oliguric. His excreted fraction of sodium is >1, but he is "positive" by 10 L. A pulmonary artery catheter was inserted until a wedge pressure was obtained at 35 cm and was read as 20 mm Hg (Fig. 38.2). Based on the tracing and reading, the senior medical resident on call gave 160 mg of furosemide, and the patient became more hypotensive. What is your next step?

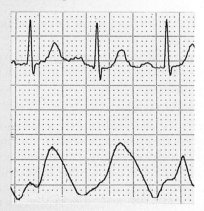

Figure 38.2 A frequent problem in the reading or interpretation of the data generated with catheterization of the right side of the heart is proper identification of the waveform in the different chambers of the heart. In this case, the physician failed to recognize that the catheter never went to the pulmonary artery and stayed in the right ventricle. Passage from the right ventricle into the pulmonary artery is evidenced by an increase in the diastolic pressure (the diastolic pressure of the pulmonary artery is higher than the diastolic pressure of the right ventricle). The pulmonary artery waveform has a systolic pressure wave and a diastolic trough. The pulmonary artery waveform also has a dicrotic notch caused by the closure of the pulmonary valve; this can be identified on the terminal part of the systolic pressure wave.

a) Check hemodynamic readings.
b) Add dobutamine and norepinephrine.
c) Give 320 mg of furosemide and afterload reducer.
d) Increase positive end-expiratory pressure to decrease the preload.

Answer and Discussion

The answer is a. In this case, the clinician failed to recognize that reaching a wedge at 35 cm in an average-size patient is unlikely. The right ventricle should be reached at 30 to 40 cm from the subclavian or internal jugular veins. The pulmonary artery can be reached if the catheter is inserted an additional 10 to 15 cm. The other important information that was not recognized in this case was the fact that the waveform changes when the catheter moves from the right ventricle to the pulmonary artery. The diastolic pressure is higher in the pulmonary artery, and a dicrotic notch due to pulmonary valve closure should be noted in the pulmonary artery waveform.

SUGGESTED READINGS

Annane DP, Vignon A, Renault PE, et al. Norepinephrine plus dobutamine versus epinephrine alone for management of septic shock: a randomised trial. *Lancet* 2007;370(9588):676–684.

Artigas A, Bernard GR, Carlet J, et al. The American-European consensus conference on ARDS, part 2. *Am J Respir Crit Care Med* 1998;157:1332–1347.

Avecillas JF, Freire AX, Arroliga AC. Clinical epidemiology of acute lung injury and acute respiratory distress syndrome: incidence, diagnosis, and outcomes. *Clin Chest Med* 2006;27(4):549–557.

Bernard GR, Artigas A, Brigham KL, et al. The American-European consensus conference on ARDS: definitions, mechanisms, relevant outcomes, and clinical trial coordination. *Am J Respir Crit Care Med* 1994;149:818–824.

Choi PTL, Yip G, Quinonez LG, et al. Crystalloids vs. colloids in fluid resuscitation: a systematic review. *Crit Care Med* 1999;27:200–210.

Coulter TD, Wiedemann HP. Complications of hemodynamic monitoring. *Clin Chest Med* 1999;20:249–267.

Dellinger RP, Levy MM, Carlet JM, et al. Surviving sepsis campaign: international guidelines for management of severe sepsis and septic shock: 2008. *Crit Care Med* 2008;36(1):296–327.

Finfer S, Bellomo R, Boyce N, et al. A comparison of albumin and saline for fluid resuscitation in the intensive care unit. *N Engl J Med* 2004;350(22):2247–2256.

Hebert PC, Blajchman MA, Cook DJ, et al. Do blood transfusions improve outcomes related to mechanical ventilation? *Chest* 2001;119:1850–1857.

Herridge MS, Cheung AM, Tansey CM, et al. One-year outcomes in survivors of the acute respiratory distress syndrome. *N Engl J Med* 2003;348:683–693.

MacArthur RD, Miller M, Albertson T, et al. Adequacy of early empiric antibiotic treatment and survival in severe sepsis: experience from the Monarcs trial. *Clin Infect Dis* 2004;38(2):284–288.

Mandell LA, Wunderink RG, Anzueto A, et al. Infectious Diseases Society of America/American Thoracic Society consensus guidelines on the management of community-acquired pneumonia in adults. *Clin Infect Dis* 2007;44(Suppl 2):S27–S72.

Mughal MM, Culver DA, Minai OA, et al. Auto-positive end-expiratory pressure: mechanisms and treatment. *Cleve Clin J Med* 2005;72(9):801–809.

Orme J Jr, Romney JS, Hopkins RO, et al. Pulmonary function and health-related quality of life in survivors of acute respiratory distress syndrome. *Am J Respir Crit Care Med* 2002;167:690–694.

Rivers E, Nguyen B, Havstad S, et al. Early goal-directed therapy in the treatment of severe sepsis and septic shock. *N Engl J Med* 2001; 345(19):1368–1377.

Romac DR, Albertson TE. Drug interactions in the intensive care unit. *Clin Chest Med* 1999;20:385–399.

Rubenfeld GD, Caldwell E, Peabody E, et al. Incidence and outcomes of acute lung injury. *N Engl J Med* 2005;353(16):1685-1693.

Sandur S, Stoller JK. Pulmonary complications of mechanical ventilation. *Clin Chest Med* 1999;20:223–247.

Task Force of the American College of Critical Care Medicine, Society of Critical Care Medicine. Practice parameters for hemodynamic support of sepsis in adult patients in sepsis. *Crit Care Med* 1999;27:639–660.

Tobin MJ. Advances in mechanical ventilation. *N Engl J Med* 2001; 344:1986–1996.

Ware LB, Matthay MA. The acute respiratory distress syndrome. *N Engl J Med* 2000;342:1334–1349.

Wheeler AP, Bernard GR, Thompson BT, et al. Pulmonary-artery versus central venous catheter to guide treatment of acute lung injury. *N Engl J Med* 2006;354(21):2213–2224.

Wiedemann HP, Matthay MA, Matthay RA. Cardiovascular and pulmonary monitoring in the intensive care unit (I, II). *Chest* 1984;85:537–545, 656–668.

Wiedemann HP, Wheeler AP, Bernard GR, et al. Comparison of two fluid-management strategies in acute lung injury. *N Engl J Med* 2006;354(24):2564–2575.

Chapter 39

Pulmonary Function Tests for the Boards

James K. Stoller

POINTS TO REMEMBER:

- Typical questions on the boards address the following: common features of uncommon diseases, uncommon features of common diseases, disease associations, and knowledge of established treatments.

- Questions on the board examinations are less likely to address straightforward associations, such as common complications of commonly used medications and common medical manifestations of common illnesses.

- Measuring pulmonary function tests can help the astute clinician identify the physiological signature of the pulmonary illness in order to categorize it as restrictive or obstructive and, in so doing, narrow down a specific etiology.

- In addition to the normal flow-volume loop, three characteristic deviations from the normal flow-volume loop suggest various forms of upper airway obstruction.

- The sine qua non of restrictive lung disease is decreased total lung capacity.

- Calculation of the alveolar-arterial oxygen gradient is useful in approaching the differential diagnosis of hypoxemia. Six causes of hypoxemia should be remembered: anatomic shunt, mismatch, diffusion impairment, hypoventilation, inhaling a decreased inspired oxygen fraction, and diffusion-perfusion impairment (e.g., as seen in the hepatopulmonary syndrome).

Typical questions posed in board certification examinations include those addressing the following:

- Common features of uncommon diseases
- Uncommon features of common diseases

- Disease associations, especially those that require integrating knowledge of diagnosis, treatment, and complications of therapy
- Knowledge of established therapies, even if relatively uncommon
- Integration of knowledge (e.g., associating classic disease symptoms with pathological and radiographic manifestations, associating pathological findings with treatments of choice or complications of therapy)

As a general rule, questions posed on this examination are meant to discriminate between the majority of examinees who will pass the examination and a minority (approximately 15%–20% over past years) who will not succeed. The questions are psychometrically validated to achieve this level of discrimination and to serve the goal of a predetermined pass criterion (e.g., 70% correct responses).

Questions on the board examinations are less likely to address straightforward associations, such as common complications of commonly used medications and common medical manifestations of common illnesses. To simulate the way clinicians learn, this chapter presents several matching problems, in which the reader is asked to match the appropriate patient profiles with the best test profile highlighting flow-volume loop patterns, pulmonary function test (PFT) profiles, and arterial blood gas profiles. At the end of the chapter, several other matching questions are offered, meant to enhance the reader's preparedness for the board examination and for clinical practice.

PFTs are a cornerstone of pulmonary practice. Measuring PFTs can help the astute clinician identify the physiologic signature of the pulmonary illness in order to categorize it as restrictive or obstructive and, in so doing, narrow down a specific etiology. Because PFTs are used every day in practice and are important for the internist, questions regarding PFTs are frequently included in the boards and lend themselves to "matching" problems (i.e., associating a clinical picture with a PFT Profile). In this context, this chapter reviews commonly used PFTs—spirometry, flow-volume loops, and arterial blood gases. The chapter presents several sets of matching questions that highlight these PFTs and provide a context in which to help the reader understand these tests and their clinical applications.

In this first block of cases, five cases are presented for your consideration. Each patient has some degree of respiratory distress. Match the patient profiles to the correct patterns of the flow-volume loop shown in Figure 39.1.

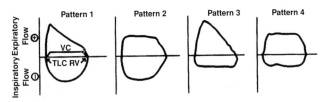

Figure 39.1   Patterns of the flow-volume loop. RV = respiratory volume, TLC = total lung capacity, VC = vital capacity.

Please note that each answer choice can be used once, more than once, or not at all.

CASES 1–5

Patient Information

Patient Profile 1
The patient is a 55-year-old man with history of multiple trauma, acute respiratory distress syndrome, and prolonged intubation.

Patient Profile 2
The patient is a 65-year-old man with long-standing rheumatoid arthritis and cricoarytenoid involvement.

Patient Profile 3
The patient is a 40-year-old woman with painful ears, saddle-nose deformity, and arthralgias.

Patient Profile 4
The patient is a 45-year-old woman with "factitious asthma" presenting as stridor.

Patient Profile 5
The patient is a 30-year-old man with relapsing polychondritis and expiratory wheezing.

QUESTIONS
Match the preceding patient profiles to the correct patterns of the flow-volume loop shown in Figure 39.1.

1. Pattern for Patient 1
2. Pattern for Patient 2
3. Pattern for Patient 3
4. Pattern for Patient 4
5. Pattern for Patient 5

1. What is the flow-volume loop pattern that best matches Patient 1?

Answer and Discussion
The answer is pattern 4. In patient profile 1, the patient is a 55-year-old man with a history of multiple trauma, acute respiratory distress syndrome (ARDS), and prolonged intubation. This is the first case that calls on the reader to recognize an upper airway lesion and to match this with the appropriate pattern of the flow-volume loop. In this first case, the patient described has fixed laryngotracheal obstruction resulting from prolonged intubation complicating ARDS. Overall, the frequency of clinically significant upper airway obstruction following prolonged intubation is 5% to 15%, although controversy still exists regarding whether the risk of laryngeal injury increases as the duration of intubation lengthens. Upper airway obstruction after prolonged intubation may result from several different lesions, including vocal cord stricture (especially at the

posterior glottic chink) and tracheal stenosis, either at the site of the tracheostomy stoma or at the site of the cuff on the endotracheal tube. Because upper airway obstruction complicating prolonged intubation usually consists of granulation tissue, the airway obstruction is usually characterized by *fixed upper airway obstruction*, as demonstrated by pattern 4 in Figure 39.1. This pattern shows flattening of both the expiratory and inspiratory limbs of the flow-volume loop because the obstruction to flow is present both on inspiration and expiration. In contrast, a *variable* or *dynamic* lesion is characterized by floppiness or malacia of the tracheal wall and shows airflow limitation either on inspiration and expiration (but not both), depending on whether the area of malacia is *extrathoracic* or *intrathoracic*. In this terminology, *extrathoracic* denotes a position along the airway cephalad of the thoracic inlet, and *intrathoracic* denotes an airway lesion caudal to the thoracic inlet as far down as the main carina.

Recognizing the patterns of an abnormal flow-volume loop can be helpful in determining the presence and position of upper airway obstruction. In understanding the flow-volume loop, it is important to recognize that *positive flow* (i.e., above the horizontal line) denotes expiration, and *negative flow* (below the horizontal; Fig. 39.1, pattern 1) denotes inspiration.

The flow-volume loop is a different way of graphically presenting the information gathered in a spirogram or volume-time tracing. Specifically, in determining the flow rate (i.e., in liters per second), the slope of the volume-time tracing is determined. The first derivative of volume with respect to time (i.e., dV/dt) represents flow (measured in liters per unit of time). The flow rate or slope of the volume-time tracing then is plotted against the volume (which is on the *vertical axis* of the volume-time tracing) but is transposed to become the *horizontal axis* of a flow-volume loop. Thus, the expiratory limb of the flow-volume loop is an algebraic transformation of the volume-time tracing; however, the inspiratory limb of the flow-volume loop is not depicted on a volume-time tracing (which is confined to expiration). To obtain the inspiratory component of the flow-volume loop, the patient must inspire forcefully from residual volume to total lung capacity. In addition to the normal flow-volume loop (Fig. 39.1, pattern 1), three characteristic deviations from the normal flow-volume loop suggest various forms of upper airway obstruction (Fig. 39.1, patterns 2-4).

Pattern 2 represents *dynamic intrathoracic upper airway obstruction*, pattern 3 represents *dynamic extrathoracic upper airway obstruction*, and pattern 4 represents *fixed upper airway obstruction*. The descriptor "dynamic" denotes that the airway lesion is floppy or malacic, and so the degree of airway blockage will be affected by the transmural pressure gradient (across the airway wall).

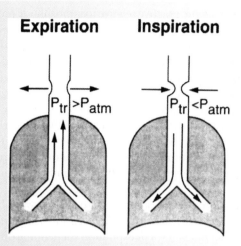

Figure 39.2 Effect of expiration and inspiration on dynamic or nonfixed extrathoracic airway obstruction. **Left:** During forced expiration, intratracheal pressure (P_{tr}) exceeds the pressure around the airway (P_{atm}) or atmospheric pressure, lessening the obstruction. **Right:** During forced inspiration, when pressure around that airway is greater, the obstruction worsens. (From Kryger MH, Bode F, Antic R, et al. Diagnosis of obstruction of the upper and central airways. *Am J Med* 1976;61:85–93, with permission.)

To understand these three variant patterns of the flow-volume loop, one must consider the pressure gradient across the airway walls during inspiration and expiration (Figs. 39.2 and 39.3). During inspiration, intrapleural pressure is negative, so atmospheric gas (considered to have zero pressure, so positive compared with negative pressures generated on inspiration) flows into the lung across a gradient from higher (zero) to lower pressures (negative). The situation reverses during exhalation. During exhalation, as intrapleural pressure

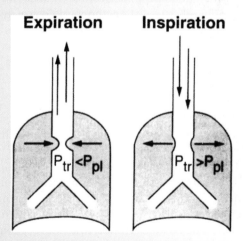

Figure 39.3 Effects of expiration and inspiration on dynamic or nonfixed intrathoracic airway obstruction. **Left:** During forced expiration, pressure exerted around the airway (P_{pl}, or pleural pressure) may exceed intratracheal pressure (P_{tr}), worsening the obstruction. **Right:** During forced inspiration, intratracheal pressure is greater, relieving the obstruction. (From Kryger MH, Bode F, Antic R, et al. Diagnosis of obstruction of the upper and central airways. *Am J Med* 1976;61:85–93, with permission.)

becomes more positive relative to atmospheric pressure, gas leaves the lung and moves to the outside atmosphere, which is now lower in pressure. With this in mind, it stands to reason that any fixed obstruction to airflow in the upper airway will produce a decrease in flows during both inspiration and expiration, causing flow to decrease in both limbs of the flow-volume tracing (Fig. 39.1, pattern 4). Thus, as in the patient profile, flow is decreased during both expiration and inspiration, giving rise to the characteristic flattening of both the inspiratory and expiratory limbs.

In contrast to the situation with fixed airway obstruction, dynamic airflow obstruction affects airflow on either inspiration or expiration (depending on the position of the dynamic airflow obstruction), but not both. To understand more clearly how dynamic airflow obstruction affects the shape of the flow-volume loop, consider the situation in which dynamic airflow obstruction occurs in the extrathoracic upper airway (e.g., cephalad to the thoracic inlet). As shown in Figure 39.1, pattern 3, dynamic extrathoracic upper airway obstruction is characterized by flattening of the inspiratory limb of the flow-volume loop, with preservation of a normal expiratory limb of the loop. Examples of such conditions might include tracheomalacia of the extrathoracic upper airway or vocal cord paralysis. In contrast, dynamic intrathoracic obstruction produces flattening of only the expiratory limb of the flow-volume loop (Fig. 39.1, pattern 3). Examples of conditions that cause dynamic intrathoracic upper airway obstruction include tracheomalacia of the intrathoracic airway or tumors that straddle the main carina. Figures 39.2 and 39.3 graphically review the pathophysiology of dynamic upper airway obstruction.

2. What is the flow-volume loop pattern that best matches Patient 2?

Answer and Discussion
The answer is pattern 4. Patient profile 2 presents a 65-year-old man with long-standing rheumatoid arthritis and cricoarytenoid involvement. The best answer is Figure 39.1, pattern 4, denoting fixed extrathoracic upper airway obstruction. This case demonstrates the consequences of arthritis or ankylosis of the cricoarytenoids, which can cause fixed upper airway obstruction in patients with rheumatoid arthritis. In a series by Lawry et al.,[1] the prevalence of inspiratory difficulty was 29% among 45 patients with rheumatoid arthritis. Notably, the reason for fixed upper airway obstruction (vs. the variable extrathoracic upper airway obstruction that may accompany vocal cord paralysis) in rheumatoid arthritis–related cricoarytenoid involvement is that this is an articulated joint and ankylosis (fixing)

of the joint fixes the vocal cords in an adducted position.

3. What is the flow-volume loop pattern that best matches Patient 3?

Answer and Discussion
The answer is patterns 1, 2, 3, or 4 (i.e., all answers could be correct here). Patient profile 3 is of a 41-year-old woman with painful ears, saddle-nose deformity, and arthralgias. This profile describes the scenario of upper airway involvement in relapsing polychondritis, clinical features of which include recurrent inflammation primarily affecting the nose, respiratory tract, ears, and joints. Notably, 25% of patients with relapsing polychondritis present with respiratory tract complaints, and 50% of patients have respiratory tract symptoms sometime during the course of their illness. Laryngotracheal involvement is responsible for 10% of deaths by pneumonia or by upper airway compromise in patients with relapsing polychondritis. The spectrum of upper airway lesions may include acute inflammation, fibrosis, or dissolution of cartilage and malacia. As a result, the flow-volume loop abnormalities may include fixed upper airway obstruction as well as dynamic intrathoracic or extrathoracic obstruction. As such, the correct answer in this case may be patterns 1, 2, 3, or 4 in Figure 39.1, all of which are possible. In the absence of more defining symptoms, such as inspiratory stridor (which would suggest dynamic extrathoracic upper airway obstruction) or expiratory wheezing (which might favor dynamic intrathoracic upper airway obstruction), she could be normal (hence, answer 1 might be true). In contrast, because relapsing polychondritis can cause tracheomalacia of the intrathoracic or extrathoracic airway or can cause scarring (and hence fixed upper airway obstruction), patterns 2, 3, or 4 could also be correct here. Although the board examination is unlikely to offer a question in which any choice is correct, my purpose here is to emphasize the importance of clarifying the information (e.g., signs and symptoms) that is offered in the stem of the question. Assuming or imputing the presence of signs or symptoms that are not explicitly stated in the text of the stem can cause the inattentive test-taker to be misled.

4. What is the flow-volume loop pattern that best matches Patient 4?

Answer and Discussion
The answer is pattern 3. Patient profile 4 presents a 45-year-old woman with "factitious asthma" presenting as stridor. The correct pattern is 3 in Figure 39.1, characterized by flattening of the inspiratory limb only. The cause of factitious asthma is vocal cord dysfunction. A spectrum of functional vocal cord problems has been observed, including paradoxic inspiratory closure and

paradoxic expiratory closure. As noted, paradoxic inspiratory closure would be more likely to present as stridor and to be characterized by flattening of the inspiratory limb of the flow-volume loop.

5. What is the flow-volume loop pattern that best matches Patient 5?

Answer and Discussion
The answer is pattern 2. Finally, patient profile 5 presents a 30-year-old man with relapsing polychondritis and expiratory wheezing. The correct flow-volume loop abnormality is Figure 39.1, pattern 2. In this case, unlike patient profile 2, the patient's symptoms are explicitly stated and the presence of expiratory wheezing should suggest the presence of intrathoracic upper airway obstruction.

Turning to the interpretation of spirometry, lung volumes, and the diffusing capacity, five more cases are presented for your consideration, again with an invitation to match the patient with the best pulmonary function profile. Each patient has been referred for pulmonary function tests. The challenge is to match each patient to the best pulmonary function profile (Table 39.1), recognizing that each pulmonary function profile answer can be used once, more than once, or not at all. Although the assumption is oversimplified, we assume that values <80% predicted in the PFT profiles are less than normal. (In actual practice, values of the lower limit of normal for each PFT should be provided, and values would be considered low when they fall below the lower limit of normal; we defer this here for the sake of simplicity of presentation.)

TABLE 39.1

PULMONARY FUNCTION TEST RESULTS

FEV$_1$ (% Predicted)	FEV (% Predicted)	FVC (Sit to Supine) (%)	TLC (%)	DLCO (% Predicted)
1. 60	78	19	73	83
2. 50	52	11	65	60
3. 84	91	8	90	90
4. 52	81	12	105	70
5. 45	55	27	70	55

DLCO = diffusing capacity of the lung for carbon monoxide, FEV = forced expiratory volume, FEV$_1$ = forced expiratory volume in 1 second, FVC = forced vital capacity, TLC = total lung capacity.

CASES 6–10

Patient Information

Patient Profile 6
The patient is a 25-year-old man with von Recklinghausen's disease and dyspnea.

Patient Profile 7
The patient is a 62-year-old man 2 days post–coronary artery bypass grafting and short of breath after extubation.

Patient Profile 8
The patient is a 35-year-old obese man with nocturnal cough.

Patient Profile 9
The patient is a 45-year-old woman who has chronic, disabling dyspnea on exertion and has a cirrhotic child.

Patient Profile 10
The patient, a 60-year-old man, smokes one or two packs of cigarettes per day.

QUESTIONS
Match the preceding patient profiles to the correct patterns of the flow-volume loop shown in Figure 39.1.

   6. Results for Patient 6
   7. Results for Patient 7
   8. Results for Patient 8
   9. Results for Patient 9
10. Results for Patient 10

6. What is the pulmonary function test pattern that best matches Patient 6?

Answer and Discussion
The answer is test profile 2. Patient profile 6 presents a 25-year-old with von Recklinghausen's disease and dyspnea. The most appropriate pulmonary function test profile is number 2, demonstrating pulmonary restriction characterized by a total lung capacity of 65% predicted, a proportionate decline in the diffusing capacity (60% predicted), and proportionate decreases in forced expiratory volume in 1 second (FEV$_1$) and forced vital capacity (FVC), such that the FEV$_1$/FVC is preserved. Also, the change in FVC going from sitting to a supine position is normal (i.e., <20%). This pulmonary function profile is characteristic of extrathoracic pulmonary restriction, such as might be seen by the kyphoscoliosis that accompanies von Recklinghausen's disease in up to 20% of patients. Notably, in approximately 5% of affected persons, the kyphoscoliosis is clinically significant. The sine qua non of restrictive lung disease is decreased total lung capacity. In this case, the proportionate decrease in the diffusing capacity suggests extrathoracic disease rather than a parenchymal restrictive lung disease, for example, interstitial lung disease.

7. What is the pulmonary function test pattern that best matches Patient 7?

Answer and Discussion
The answer is test profile 5. Patient profile 7 presents a 62-year-old man 2 days after undergoing coronary artery bypass grafting surgery. He is short of breath after being extubated. The most appropriate pulmonary function test result profile is number 5. As in previous cases, this is a pattern depicting extrathoracic pulmonary restriction with decreased total lung capacity and a roughly proportionately decreased diffusing capacity for carbon monoxide. Unlike Patient 6, the decrease in the FVC on moving from sitting to supine posture exceeds the normal upper boundary of 20%. In this case, the cause is bilateral diaphragmatic paralysis causing an increased decline in the FVC on lying down as the diaphragm is pushed into the chest by the abdominal contents. This case demonstrates the phenomenon of bilaterally damaged phrenic nerves, which may complicate coronary artery bypass grafting surgery (likely as a result of nerve ischemia) in up to 5% of cases. Unilateral diaphragmatic paralysis is more common than bilateral diaphragmatic paralysis, and unilateral paralysis (more commonly on the left than the right) is usually not clinically apparent. When both phrenic nerves are affected, however, the patient exhibits marked orthopnea accompanied by the decline in FVC, as noted already. Thus, this patient's physiological profile is characterized by extrathoracic restriction (due to the effects of recent heart surgery and bilateral diaphragmatic paralysis) and an abnormally increased drop in the FVC going from sitting to supine (due to the bilateral diaphragmatic paralysis).

8. What is the pulmonary function test pattern that best matches Patient 8?

Answer and Discussion
The answer is test profile 1. Patient profile 8 presents a 35-year-old obese man with nocturnal cough. Pulmonary function profile 1 is the best choice and indicates a pattern of airflow obstruction (i.e., a disproportionate decrease in FEV_1 compared with FVC, decreased FEV_1/FVC compared to predicted). In this case, the patient's obesity likely accounts for the mild restrictive lung disease (total lung capacity 73% of predicted, <80% predicted that is considered the lower limit of normal in this problem set). In fact, this case presents combined restrictive and obstructive lung disease, the differential diagnosis of which includes asthma with obesity as well as eosinophilic granuloma of lung (histiocytosis X or Langerhan's cell interstitial lung disease), sarcoidosis, lymphangioleiomyomatosis, and congestive heart failure. In this case, the patient's nocturnal cough is a manifestation of asthma (which may be responsible for cough in up to one-third of patients presenting with cough). In fact, nocturnal symptoms accompany asthma in up to one-third of patients and frequently dominate the clinical presentation.

9. What is the pulmonary function test pattern that best matches Patient 9?

Answer and Discussion
The answer is test profile 4. Patient profile 9 is that of a 45-year-old woman with disabling exertional dyspnea and a cirrhotic child. The case is meant to prompt consideration of severe (e.g., PI*ZZ homozygous) α_1-antitrypsin deficiency. In this regard, the best pulmonary function profile is number 4, demonstrating a pattern of airflow obstruction with a suggestion of alveolar-capillary unit loss demonstrated by the mild decrease in the diffusing capacity. Overall, this pattern suggests lung parenchymal loss consistent with emphysema rather than asthma alone. α_1-Antitrypsin deficiency is an autosomal codominant condition. The major pulmonary manifestation is emphysema, but persons who have the Z allele also may develop cirrhosis and hepatoma, related to inadequate secretion of Z protein from the hepatocyte.

This case also invites consideration of the causes of a decreased diffusing capacity for carbon monoxide. The diffusing capacity is a measurement of gas transfer across the alveolar-capillary units, which may be decreased when there is loss of pulmonary vasculature (e.g., pulmonary vascular disease or lung resection) or loss of lung parenchyma (as may be seen in emphysema or interstitial lung disease). Because uptake of carbon monoxide by erythrocytes requires adequate red blood cells with hemoglobin avid for carbon monoxide, the diffusing capacity will also be decreased in the face of anemia or prior carbon monoxide poisoning (which creates a back pressure that decreases further uptake of carbon monoxide by red blood cells).

Pulmonary features that should lead to consideration of severe α_1-antitrypsin deficiency include emphysema at an early age (e.g., younger than 50 years), emphysema in the absence of antecedent smoking, emphysema with a positive family history of lung or liver disease, and radiographic changes showing basilar hyperlucency (in contrast to the more apical distribution of emphysema changes in "garden variety" emphysema unrelated to α_1-antitrypsin deficiency). α_1-Antitrypsin deficiency is clinically underrecognized, with an estimated 100,000 cases among Americans, <10% of which have been diagnosed. Current guidelines suggest testing with an α_1-antitrypsin serum level for all symptomatic adults with fixed airflow obstruction (i.e., FEV_1/FVC <0.70).

10. What is the pulmonary function test pattern that best matches Patient 10?

Answer and Discussion

The answer is test profile 3 or 4. Patient profile 10 presents a 60-year-old man who smokes one to two packs of cigarettes per day. No lung symptoms (e.g., dyspnea, bronchospasm) are mentioned in the patient description. Pulmonary function profile 3 is considered the best choice, although profile 4 (characteristic of emphysema) would be acceptable if symptoms of obstructive lung disease were offered in the clinical profile. Pulmonary function profile 3 represents normal lung function, emphasizing that although cigarette smoking can cause an accelerated decline in FEV_1, most cigarette smokers escape accelerated airflow obstruction. In fact, "susceptible" smokers with accelerated airflow decline are said to make up approximately 10% to 15% of all smokers. Even in susceptible smokers, cessation of cigarette smoking slows the rate of decline of lung function to that of nonsmokers, although recovery of lost lung function after smoking cessation is uncommon.

The benefits of smoking cessation include a slowing of the rate of decline of lung function, an effect that persists long term in the sustained ex-smoker.

Understanding arterial blood gases is another useful clinical skill and one that is likely to be tested on the board examination. For each of five additional patient vignettes, you are asked to match a room air arterial blood gas profile in Table 39.2. As before, each arterial blood gas profile can be used once, more than once, or not at all.

TABLE 39.2		
ROOM AIR ARTERIAL BLOOD GASES		
PaO₂ (mm Hg)	PaCO₂ (mm Hg)	pH
1. 50	65	7.30
2. 60	60	7.20
3. 50	65	7.37
4. 85	28	7.51
5. 65	35	7.42

$PaCO_2$ = arterial pressure of carbon dioxide, PaO_2 = partial pressure of oxygen in arterial blood

CASES 11–15

Patient Information

Patient Profile 11

The patient is a 70-year-old man with fasciculations and upper motor neuron disease.

Patient Profile 12

The patient is a 50-year-old man with dyspnea and panniculitis.

Patient Profile 13

The patient is a 48-year-old man who is a heavy smoker and experiences acute confusion.

Patient Profile 14

The patient is a 45-year-old woman who has sustained neck trauma.

Patient Profile 15

The patient is a 25-year-old man being seen 3 weeks after a skiing accident and tibial fracture.

QUESTIONS

Match the preceding patient profiles to the correct patterns of the flow-volume loop shown in Figure 39.1.

11. Pattern for Patient 11
12. Pattern for Patient 12
13. Pattern for Patient 13
14. Pattern for Patient 14
15. Pattern for Patient 15

11. Match the room air arterial blood gas profile for Patient 11.

Answer and Discussion

The answer is pattern 3 or 5. Patient profile 11 presents a 70-year-old man with fasciculations and upper motor neuron disease. The clinical scenario is intended to elicit the diagnosis of amyotrophic lateral sclerosis, a degenerative disease of the motor neurons that is slowly progressive and is associated with extrathoracic pulmonary restriction as well as blood gases reflecting hypoventilation or the effect of ventilation/perfusion ratio (V/Q) mismatch. In this instance, the most appropriate blood gas pattern would be profile 3 or 5. Profile 3 represents a pattern of pure hypoventilation (i.e., the alveolar-arterial gradient is normal), which may be seen with neuromuscular disease such as amyotrophic lateral sclerosis. Alternately, patient profile 5 represents hypoxemia with hypocapnia (i.e., chronic respiratory alkalosis). In arterial blood gas profile 5, the alveolar-arterial oxygen gradient is widened, consistent with mismatch or anatomical shunt.

In interpreting room air arterial blood gases, calculation of the alveolar-arterial oxygen gradient is helpful. Table 39.3 presents this calculation. Normal values of the alveolar-arterial oxygen gradient are age dependent, as depicted in Figure 39.4. A useful mnemonic for the mean age-specific alveolar-arterial oxygen gradient is (age/4 + 4), with the upper limit value of the age-specific alveolar-arterial oxygen gradient roughly calculated by the equation (age/4 + 4) + 10 mm Hg.

Calculation of the alveolar-arterial oxygen gradient is useful in approaching the differential diagnosis of

TABLE 39.3

ALVEOLAR-ARTERIAL OXYGEN GRADIENT (AADO₂)

Calculate the alveolar oxygen tension (P_AO_2)
$P_AO_2 = (P_B - 47)FIO_2 - [(PaCO_2)/(\text{resp quotient})]$
P_B = barometric pressure (e.g., 760 mm Hg)
FIO_2 = fraction of inspired oxygen
$PaCO_2$ = arterial CO_2 tension
resp quotient = Respiratory quotient (moles CO_2 produced per mole of O_2 consumed, usually 0.8)
Subtract PaO_2 (arterial oxygen tension)
$AaDO_2 = P_AO_2 - PaO_2$

hypoxemia. Six causes of hypoxemia should be remembered: anatomic shunt, mismatch, diffusion impairment, hypoventilation, inhaling a decreased inspired oxygen fraction, and diffusion-perfusion impairment (e.g., as seen in the hepatopulmonary syndrome). Of these six causes, diffusion-perfusion impairment is uncommon and is confined to patients with hypoxemia caused by the hepatopulmonary syndrome. Hypoxemia relating to inhaling decreased inspired oxygen fractions

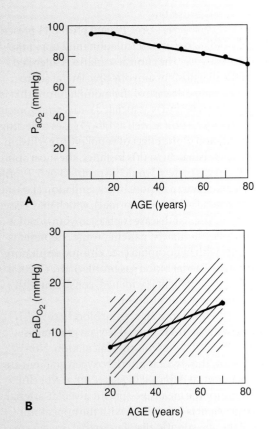

A

B

Figure 39.4 **A:** Variations of arterial oxygen tension with age. **B:** Variations of alveolar-arterial oxygen gradient (A – aDO_2) with age; mean values for A – $aDO_2 = 2.5 \pm 0.21\times$ age; bold line indicates mean values; and shaded area +2 SD. (From Tisi G. *Pulmonary Physiology in Clinical Medicine*. Baltimore: Williams & Wilkins, 1980:78, with permission.)

occurs only when the patient is exposed to high altitude or when a hypoxic gas mixture is breathed at sea level. Among the other four causes of hypoxemia (anatomic shunt, V/Q mismatch, diffusion impairment, and hypoventilation), the age-specific alveolar-arterial oxygen gradient is increased for all causes except hypoventilation, in which the room air alveolar-arterial oxygen gradient is normal. Using a rule-of-thumb equation (Table 39.3) for calculating the room air alveolar-arterial oxygen gradient: 149 – (partial pressure of oxygen in arterial blood [PaO_2] + arterial pressure of carbon dioxide [$PaCO_2$] [1.25]), the alveolar-arterial oxygen gradient in blood gas profile 3 is 149 – (50 + 65[1.25]), or 18 mm Hg, which is normal for a 70-year-old man. Therefore, for a 70-year-old patient, arterial blood gas profile 3 indicates hypoventilation, which might accompany neuromuscular disease such as amyotrophic lateral sclerosis. In contrast, the value of the room air alveolar-room arterial oxygen gradient for blood gas profile 5 is 40 mm Hg, which is elevated even for a 70-year-old man. Such a profile might be seen in neuromuscular disease in which atelectasis is causing V/Q mismatch, resulting in hypoxemia without hypoventilation.

12. Match the room air arterial blood gas profile for Patient 12.

Answer and Discussion
The answer is pattern 5. Patient profile 12 presents a 50-year-old man with dyspnea and panniculitis. The case is meant to suggest α_1-antitrypsin deficiency characterized by panniculitis and emphysema. Arterial blood gas profile 5 is considered the best answer, indicating hypoxemia with chronic respiratory alkalosis on the basis of emphysema and long-standing V/Q mismatch.

13. Match the room air arterial blood gas profile for Patient 13.

Answer and Discussion
The answer is pattern 1. Profile 13 presents a 48-year-old heavy smoker with acute confusion. The history of heavy smoking is meant to suggest severe chronic obstructive lung disease. Such a patient might demonstrate chronic hypoxemia with chronic hypercapnia and compensated respiratory acidosis. The presence of acute confusion, however, suggests an acute worsening of respiratory acidosis, as best demonstrated by the arterial blood gas profile 1.

14. Match the room air arterial blood gas profile for Patient 14.

Answer and Discussion
The answer is pattern 2. Patient profile 14 presents a 45-year-old woman who has had neck trauma. Spinal cord injury above the level of C3, resulting in acute

hypoventilation, should be considered. The expected arterial blood gas profile is that of hypoventilation with acute respiratory acidosis, best represented by arterial blood gas profile 2. In this case, a pH of 7.20 indicates acute respiratory acidosis, and the room air alveolar-arterial oxygen gradient is 14 mm Hg (normal for this patient), again demonstrating hypoventilation.

15. Match the room air arterial blood gas profile for Patient 15.

Answer and Discussion
The answer is profile 4. Patient profile 15 presents a 25-year-old man 3 weeks after a skiing accident and tibial fracture. The clinical setting should suggest the possibility of an acute pulmonary embolism. An acute respiratory alkalosis with a widened alveolar-arterial oxygen gradient would be expected and is best demonstrated by arterial blood gas profile 4. In this case, the alveolar-arterial oxygen gradient is 29 mm Hg, which is above normal for a 25-year-old man. This case serves as a reminder that patients with acute pulmonary emboli may not demonstrate hypoxemia but that the alveolar-arterial oxygen gradient is usually (but not uniformly) elevated.

In summary, these three blocks of matching profiles are intended to provide some applied examples of using common pulmonary function tests, flow-volume loops, spirometry, lung volumes, diffusing capacity for carbon monoxide, and room air arterial blood gases, understanding of which can empower the clinician for practice and for the certification or recertification board examinations.

ASSORTED QUESTIONS REGARDING PULMONARY MEDICINE

In the spirit of simulating the types of questions posed by the board examination, the following sections of this chapter are meant to resemble the type of questions one may see on the certification or recertification examinations.

Recognizing Disease Associations

In the following exercise, the reader is asked to match the lung diseases in the left column with the associated condition or conditions on the right. More than one condition in the right column can be associated with each lung disease on the left, and associating one of the conditions in the right column with the lung disease on the left does not preclude the associated condition from being matched with other lung diseases on the left.

Lung Disease	Associated Condition
PI*ZZ α_1-antitrypsin deficiency	Hepatoma
Intrapulmonary vascular dilatations	Hepatic cirrhosis
	Lymphangioleiomyomatosis
Pulmonary arteriovenous malformation	Ulcerative colitis
Pulmonary hypertension	Hereditary hemorrhagic telangiectasia
Chylous pleural effusion	

1. Which associated condition (or conditions) are associated with PI*ZZ α_1-antitrypsin deficiency?

Answer and Discussion
The answer is both hepatoma and hepatic cirrhosis. Since the early description of α_1-antitrypsin deficiency, hepatic complications were recognized as a feature of PI*ZZ homozygous α_1-antitrypsin deficiency in approximately 12% of affected persons. Postmortem studies suggest that the prevalence of liver disease may be approximately 35%. The spectrum of liver diseases includes cirrhosis, hepatoma, and neonatal jaundice. Indeed, the complications of α_1-antitrypsin deficiency pose a challenge to the internist assessing the patient with idiopathic cirrhosis, although liver complications are far more common in children with α_1-antitrypsin deficiency. In this context, homozygous PI*ZZ α_1-antitrypsin deficiency sometimes causes neonatal jaundice progressing to liver failure, and, as such, α_1-antitrypsin deficiency is the second most common indication for liver transplantation in children. Unlike the mechanism of lung destruction in α_1-antitrypsin deficiency (which is due to unopposed elastolytic activity in the lung interstitium), liver disease seems to result from the intrahepatocyte accumulation of unsecreted Z-type α_1-antitrypsin. The Z mutant form of α_1-antitrypsin is caused by a single amino acid substitution at position 342 of the 394 amino acid glycoprotein that is α_1-antitrypsin. Substitution of a lysine for a glutamic acid residue at position 342 causes abnormal folding as the protein is secreted from the endoplasmic reticulum for glycosylation and packaging at the Golgi apparatus. Abnormal folding allows polymerization within the hepatocyte (a process called *loop-sheet polymerization*), which impairs the normal secretion of the protein from the liver into the bloodstream. As such, liver disease in Z-type α_1-antitrypsin deficiency is more akin to a hepatic inclusion disease (e.g., Gaucher's disease) than it is due to any unopposed proteolytic breakdown of the liver parenchyma. Increasing evidence suggests that PI*ZZ-type persons who develop liver disease have abnormal processing of the unsecreted protein. Current understanding suggests that

persons at risk for liver disease are less able to clear the unsecreted protein than PI*ZZ individuals not destined to develop liver disease, although the pathogenetic mechanism by which the accumulation of intrahepatocyte protein leads to cirrhosis or hepatoma remains unknown.

Although more than 100 alleles for the α_1-antitrypsin protein have been identified, the PI*ZZ homozygous state accounts for 95% of all clinically recognized severe α_1-antitrypsin deficiency. Other rare alleles that can also give rise to liver disease include M_{malton} and S_{iyama}.

Aspects of α_1-antitrypsin deficiency that lend themselves to being tested in the context of a board examination include (a) emphysema with early age of onset or emphysema without concomitant cigarette smoking; (b) emphysema presenting with basilar hyperlucency on the chest radiograph (vs. the more expected clinical changes of emphysema seen with the more common type of α_1-antitrypsin–replete cigarette smoking–related emphysema); (c) the occurrence of liver disease as noted previously, characterized by the presence of inclusion bodies within the hepatocyte (such inclusion bodies stain positively with periodic acid–Schiff and are resistant to digestion by diastase); and (d) the autosomal codominant inheritance pattern of α_1-antitrypsin deficiency.

2. With which associated condition on the right is there an association with intrapulmonary vascular dilatations?

Answer and Discussion

The answer is hepatic cirrhosis. This question asks the examinee to recognize the hepatopulmonary syndrome as a complication of chronic liver disease, usually cirrhosis, of various causes. The hepatopulmonary syndrome is a disease characterized by a widened alveolar-arterial oxygen gradient, often with associated dyspnea or platypnea (breathlessness that develops on upright posture). The physiologic and pathologic hallmark of the hepatopulmonary syndrome is the development of intrapulmonary vascular dilatations, which are sometimes apparent on plain chest radiographs as a "spongy" interstitial pattern of the lung bases. Prevalence estimates suggest that the hepatopulmonary syndrome occurs in up to 40% of patients with chronic liver disease, but it is often subclinical in that it has a relatively small impact on gas exchange or symptoms. However, the hepatopulmonary syndrome can be quite debilitating and can outstrip the symptomatic impact of liver disease on these patients. In such instances, liver transplantation is considered for treatment of the underlying hepatopulmonary syndrome rather than the end-stage liver disease alone. Various series suggest that associated hypoxemia and its symptomatic

consequences can completely reverse following liver transplantation, although predicting this response remains difficult.

Diagnosis of the hepatopulmonary syndrome requires clinical suspicion as well as demonstration of right-to-left intrapulmonary shunt, which is often evaluated using contrast-enhanced echocardiography, using either agitated saline or (less commonly) indocyanine. Visualization of "bubbles" of agitated saline within the left heart chambers is an abnormal finding and demonstrates right-to-left shunt. The timing of the appearance of bubbles in the left heart chambers indicates whether the shunt is *intracardiac* (when bubbles appear within three beats of injection) or *intrapulmonary* (bubbles appear for four to six beats after injection as a result of the need for bubbles to traverse the pulmonary circulation before appearing in the left heart chambers). The so-called bubble echocardiogram is highly sensitive for the presence of the hepatopulmonary syndrome, but it lacks specificity in that many patients lacking clinically significant manifestations of the hepatopulmonary syndrome show evidence of a positive "bubble study."

3. With which associated condition(s) are pulmonary arteriovenous malformations matched?

Answer and Discussion

The answer is hepatic cirrhosis and hereditary hemorrhagic telangiectasia. This question asks the reader to recognize that hereditary hemorrhagic telangiectasia (otherwise known as Osler-Weber-Rendu syndrome) is accompanied by various arteriovenous malformations, including pulmonary arteriovenous malformations in 5% to 15% of affected persons. In addition, hepatic cirrhosis is considered correct because intrapulmonary vascular dilatations, a hallmark feature of hepatopulmonary syndrome, are a type of arteriovenous malformation in the lung.

First recognized by Rendu in 1896, *hereditary hemorrhagic telangiectasia* is an autosomal dominant disease with variable penetrance characterized by the development of vascular abnormalities in various organs. The most common manifestation is epistaxis due to nasal telangiectasia, usually with onset by the age of 21 years. Telangiectasias characterized by small lesions, usually on the lips, tongue, or fingers, are of later onset. The subject of this question is the development of pulmonary arteriovenous malformations, which occur in 5% to 15% of persons with hereditary hemorrhagic telangiectasia. These arteriovenous malformations are often multiple and are located in the lower lobes of the lung. Chest radiographic features include smooth, nodular densities sometimes with "vascular feeder" vessels entering the pulmonary "nodule."

Hypoxemia may result from the concomitant right-to-left shunt, as can platypnea. Several points emphasize the importance of recognizing pulmonary arteriovenous malformations. First, clinical suspicion of a vascular abnormality is important to avoid attempted biopsy, which could be accompanied by serious bleeding. Second, clinical recognition is important because pulmonary arteriovenous malformations allow venous blood to enter the systemic arterial circulation without normal filtration by the lung vasculature. As such, patients with pulmonary arteriovenous malformations complicating the Osler-Weber-Rendu syndrome are at risk for brain abscess. This risk has led to the clinical recommendation that pulmonary arteriovenous malformations should be ablated, either surgically or by embolization. Such embolization therapy can reverse hypoxemia, but it also lessens the risk of brain abscess.

Diagnostic criteria for the hereditary hemorrhagic telangiectasia syndrome include the presence of at least two of the following diagnostic criteria: recurrent epistaxis; telangiectasias outside the nose; autosomal dominant inheritance; or visceral involvement of lung, gastrointestinal tract, or brain. Specifically, the brain and gastrointestinal tract can also be the site of vascular abnormalities predisposing to bleeding or vessel rupture with associated neurologic consequences.

4. With which associated condition is pulmonary hypertension best matched?

Answer and Discussion

The answer is **hepatic cirrhosis.** This question asks the reader to recognize the association between hepatic cirrhosis and pulmonary hypertension, another pulmonary manifestation of chronic liver disease. Unlike the hepatopulmonary syndrome, in which pulmonary vascular resistance is actually decreased (because arteriovenous channels open), pulmonary hypertension complicating hepatic cirrhosis has been called the *portopulmonary hypertension*. Less common than the hepatopulmonary syndrome, portopulmonary hypertension occurs in 3% to 5% of patients with chronic liver disease. The pathophysiology is poorly understood, but the presence of portal hypertension is required, and portopulmonary hypertension has been described in cases of portal hypertension in the absence of substantial parenchymal liver damage (e.g., hepatic vein thrombosis).

The question also invites the reader's understanding of the etiologies of pulmonary hypertension, which can be considered according to an anatomic schema. Starting with the left ventricle, left-sided congestive heart failure or ventricular hypertrophy with a noncompliant left ventricle can cause pulmonary hypertension.

Diseases affecting the mitral valve, including mitral stenosis, mitral regurgitation, and left atrial myxoma, may also contribute to pulmonary hypertension. Diseases of the pulmonary veins, such as pulmonary vein thrombosis (e.g., pulmonary veno-occlusive disease), and diseases encasing the pulmonary veins (e.g., fibrosing mediastinitis, neoplasm) can cause pulmonary hypertension. Diseases of the pulmonary capillaries, such as pulmonary hemangiomatosis, are also a consideration. Diseases causing constriction of the pulmonary arteries, such as hypoxic states with secondary pulmonary vasoconstriction, can cause pulmonary hypertension. Pulmonary thromboembolic disease is an important consideration, as are diseases causing primary vasospasm of the pulmonary arteries. Examples include collagen-vascular diseases, such as scleroderma and systemic lupus erythematosus, HIV infection, diet pills (including the European drug called "aminorex" and dexfenfluramine, which has been withdrawn from the American market), and true "primary," now called idiopathic pulmonary arterial hypertension, which denotes pulmonary arterial pressure elevation in the absence of an alternative explanation. Diseases causing increased flow through the pulmonary artery, such as atrial or ventricular septal defects, can cause pulmonary hypertension and should be considered in the differential diagnosis.

5. With which associated condition(s) is a chylous pleural effusion related?

Answer and Discussion

The answer is **lymphangioleiomyomatosis.** Chylous pleural effusion, as commonly seen in lymphangioleiomyomatosis and other conditions (see following discussion), is characterized by the presence of chyle within the pleural fluid. The source of chyle is the thoracic duct, so a chylous pleural effusion reflects disruption of the thoracic duct or interruption of normal lymph flow.

A defining characteristic of chylothorax is the presence of chyle, most frequently demonstrated by the presence of a triglyceride level >110 mg/dL within the pleural fluid. However, a triglyceride level <50 mg/dL is believed to exclude chylothorax and triglyceride values in between 50–110 mg/dL are equivocal and require validation by demonstrating other elements of chyle, for example, chylomicrons. Chylomicrons can be demonstrated through lipoprotein electrophoresis. A common, but not universal, feature of chylothorax is the milky appearance. Dietary avoidance of complex fats can cause chylothoraces to lack this suggestive feature.

Causes of chylothorax characteristically involve disruption or interruption of normal lymph flow. Neoplasm represents the most common cause, most frequently lymphoma. Surgical or other trauma represents another common etiology, including the possibility of disruption of the thorax duct by placement of a central venous catheter into the right neck. Congenital and idiopathic causes constitute a third broad group, as do miscellaneous causes. Among the miscellaneous causes, pulmonary lymphangioleiomyomatosis figures prominently, along with tuberculosis, sarcoidosis, Behçet's syndrome with superior vena cava obstruction, and Gorham's syndrome, a rare disease of children and young adults characterized by intraosseous development of vascular or lymphatic channels contributing to bone lysis.

Among the known etiologies of chylous pleural effusion, only lymphangioleiomyomatosis appears among the choices given. Hence, this is the preferred answer.

Lymphangioleiomyomatosis is an uncommon condition occurring almost exclusively in women and characterized by proliferation of smooth muscle in the lung interstitium. Common presenting symptoms include dyspnea and pneumothorax, but chylous pleural effusion, chyloptysis (the expectoration of chylous material), and chylous ascites have been described. The presumed mechanism is lymphatic obstruction by the known smooth muscle proliferation. One other testable feature of lymphangioleiomyomatosis is the fairly characteristic appearance of the high-resolution chest CT, showing a reticulonodular interstitial infiltrate characterized by diffuse cystic changes. Although characteristic of lymphangioleiomyomatosis, cysts may also occur in eosinophilic granuloma of lung, a distinction that may require lung biopsy. Finally, patients with lymphangioleiomyomatosis may demonstrate associated renal angiomyolipomas, which are hamartomatous tumors of the kidneys, also seen in association with tuberous sclerosis.

6. A 45-year-old man with known insulin-dependent diabetes mellitus has developed infection causing diabetic ketoacidosis. With this episode, his electrolytes are sodium, 145 mEq/L; chloride, 90 mEq/L; potassium, 5.1 mEq/L; and bicarbonate, 16 mEq/L. His anion gap (delta) is 29. Arterial blood gases are drawn on room air because he is tachypneic. The arterial blood gases show PaO_2 70 mm Hg, $PaCO_2$ 40 mm Hg, and pH 7.28. In addition to his anion gap metabolic acidosis, you are called on to assess whether his respiratory response is appropriate for the clinical condition. Specifically, is this a simple metabolic acidosis? Is he compensating appropriately for the metabolic acidosis?

1. Yes

2. No

Answer and Discussion

The answer is 2. No, the patient has a complex acid–base disorder with an anion gap metabolic acidosis, a respiratory acidosis, and a concomitant antecedent metabolic alkalosis.

The assessment of whether the respiratory response to a metabolic acidosis is appropriate can be aided by using the "Winter's equation." The Winter's equation predicts the PCO_2 for observed serum bicarbonate with the following relationship:

$$PCO_2 = [1.5(HCO_3^-) + 8] \pm 2$$

Specifically, in the current case, the patient's serum bicarbonate is 16 mEq/L, suggesting that an inappropriate respiratory response would be a PCO_2 of $[1.5(16) + 8] \pm 2$, or 30 to 34 mm Hg.

The patient's observed PCO_2 is 40 mm Hg, higher than expected, and indicates a respiratory acidosis on top of the metabolic acidosis. Further assessment of the case indicates the presence of metabolic alkalosis as well. Using the concept of the "delta delta" (as discussed in Chapter 50), we can determine what the patient's serum bicarbonate was before he experienced this metabolic acidosis. Specifically, to have an elevated anion gap of 29 (which exceeds the upper limits of normal [12] by 17), the patient would have had a serum bicarbonate 17 mEq/L higher than the currently observed value of 16 mEq/L, or 33 mEq/L. In other words, to get to the current serum bicarbonate of 16 mEq/L, 17 mEq/L of bicarbonate was eliminated by the patient's current acid load. The serum bicarbonate value of 33 mEq/L at that time suggests a slight metabolic alkalosis before the current illness.

The Winter's equation to determine an appropriately compensated PCO_2 response to a metabolic acidosis is clinically important because it allows the clinician to assess whether the patient may be experiencing respiratory failure. In the current case, although the PCO_2 is 40 mm Hg and is in the normal range, the presence of a respiratory acidosis on top of a metabolic acidosis raises some concern about the possibility of ventilatory failure and would cause the clinician to observe the patient more closely over the short term with regard to worsening hypercapnia.

The Winter's equation was derived from studying a population of patients with metabolic acidosis of various types and performing a regression equation of the observed PCO_2 against the measured serum bicarbonate values. None of these patients had intrinsic pulmonary disease, neuromuscular disease, or other insults that would cause respiratory depression or stimulate respiratory drive (e.g., aspirin overdose, liver disease).

REFERENCE

1. Lawry GV, Finerman, ML, Hanafee WN, et al. Laryngeal involvement in rheumatoid arthritis: a clinical, laryngoscopic, and computerized tomographic study. *Arthritis Rheum* 1984;27:873–882.

SUGGESTED READINGS

Aboussouan LS, Stoller JK. Diagnosis and management of upper airway obstruction. *Clin Chest Med* 1994;15:35–53.
Albert MS, Dell RB, Winters RW. Quantitative displacement of acid-base equilibrium in metabolic acidosis. *Ann Intern Med* 1967;66:312–322.
Kryger MH, Bode F, Antic R, et al. Diagnosis of obstruction of the upper and central airways. *Am J Med* 1976;61:85–93.
Light RW. Chylothorax and pseudochylothorax. In: *Pleural Diseases*, 3rd ed. Baltimore: Williams & Wilkins, 1995:284–295.
McFarlane MJ, Imperiale TF. Use of the alveolar-arterial oxygen gradient in the diagnosis of pulmonary embolism. *Am J Med* 1994;96:57–62.
Miller RD, Hyatt RE. Obstructing lesions of the larynx and trachea: clinical and physiologic characteristics. *Mayo Clin Proc* 1969;44:145–161.
Narins RD, Emmett M. Simple and mixed acid-based disorders: the practical approach. *Medicine* 1980;59:161–187.
Stein PD, Goldhaber SZ, Henry JW. Alveolar-arterial oxygen gradient in the assessment of acute pulmonary embolism. *Chest* 1995;107:139–143.
Stoller JK. Spirometry: a key diagnostic test in pulmonary medicine. *Cleve Clin J Med* 1992;59:75–78.
Stoller JK, Aboussouan LS. Alpha-1 antitrypsin deficiency. *Lancet* 2005;365:2225–2236.

Chapter 40

Thyroid Disorders

Christian Nasr   Charles Faiman

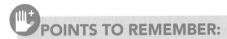

POINTS TO REMEMBER:

- A high T_4 uptake (T_4U) test (or low T_3 resin uptake [T_3RU] test) indicates that thyroid hormone–binding sites are present in excess, which can be caused by
  - Excessive binding protein (see previous discussion)
  - Diminished occupancy (hypothyroidism)
- A low T_4U (or high T_3RU test) indicates that thyroid hormone–binding sites are deficient because of
  - Diminished binding protein (see previous discussion)
  - Excessive occupancy (hyperthyroidism)

Thyroid hormone secretion is regulated by the hypothalamo-pituitary-thyroid axis (Fig. 40.1), which has the following characteristics—secretion of thyrotropin (thyroid-stimulating hormone [TSH]) is regulated by two factors: stimulation by the hypothalamic factor thyrotropin-releasing hormone (TRH) and negative feedback by circulating free thyroid hormones. TRH is also under negative feedback control by circulating free thyroid hormones. The net effect of TSH on thyroid follicular cells is an increase in production of thyroid hormones.

Approximately 25% of the circulating triiodothyronine T_3 is derived from direct secretion by the thyroid gland; the remainder comes from peripheral conversion. Reverse T_3, which is biologically inert, is produced instead of active T_3 in the sick euthyroid state and in the fetus.

Circulating thyroid hormones are mainly bound to proteins:

- Thyroxine-binding globulin (TBG) binds both thyroxine T_4 and T_3.
- Thyroid-binding prealbumin (TBPA, also called *transthyretin*) binds only T_4.
- Albumin binds both T_4 and T_3.
- 99.97% of T_4 and 99.7% of T_3 are bound.

Only free hormones are active.

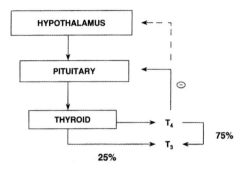

Figure 40.1 Hypothalamo-pituitary-thyroid axis. T_3 = triiodothyronine, T_4 = thyroxine.

TABLE 40.1
FACTORS INHIBITING T_4 TO T_3 CONVERSION
Systemic illness (acute or chronic) Caloric deprivation (fasting, anorexia nervosa, or protein-calorie malnutrition) Surgery Newborn Aging Drugs (glucocorticoids, propranolol [high doses], amiodarone, propylthiouracil) Contrast media (ipodate, iopanoic acid)

T_3 = triiodothyronine, T_4 = thyroxine.

THYROID FUNCTION TESTS

Thyroid function tests include:

- TSH (sensitive/ultrasensitive), the single best indicator of thyroid function
- Total T_4
- T_4U or T_3RU (estimates of binding)
- Free thyroxine index (FTI), adjusted for serum protein binding
- Free T_4 (FT_4)
- Total T_3
- Free T_3

Factors that alter binding or binding capacity result in alterations in total T_4 and total T_3:

- Changes in TBG influence both total T_4 and total T_3 values.
- Changes in TBPA influence total T_4 values only.

The following conditions are associated with TBG excess:

- Pregnancy
- Drug use (estrogen, tamoxifen, raloxifene, heroin, methadone, perphenazine)
- Acute hepatitis
- Chronic active hepatitis
- Acute intermittent porphyria
- Hereditary conditions

The following conditions are associated with TBG deficiency:

- Excess androgens
- Acromegaly
- Hypoproteinemia
- Nephrotic syndrome
- Chronic liver disease
- Glucocorticoids (large doses)
- Hereditary conditions

Measurement of the binding proteins by a T_4U test or T_3RU test and calculation of the FTI help correct for the effect of changes in the binding proteins on thyroid hormone levels. Newer assays of FT_4 are at least equal to the FTI and, in some cases, better. FT_4 by equilibrium dialysis remains the gold standard, but it is too expensive for routine clinical use.

Drugs or conditions (e.g., sick euthyroidism) that interfere with thyroid hormone protein binding are listed in Tables 40.1 to 40.3. Thyroid function tests are readily interpretable in ambulatory patients, but are often not helpful or may be confusing in the hospitalized sick patient.

Tests for Hypothyroidism

Thyroid function tests for diagnosing hypothyroidism include:

- TSH (0.4–4.5 μU/mL, normal); the upper limit of normal remains controversial, with values as low as 2.5 to 3.5 advocated but not generally accepted. TSH >10 to 20 μU/mL is generally diagnostic (caveats: newborn or recovery phase of sick euthyroidism). Values between 4.5 and 10.0 μU/mL are considered borderline and represent subclinical hypothyroidism (may be normal for geriatric population). In these cases, it is recommended to assess for goiter; order T_4, FTI, or FT_4; order thyroid microsomal

TABLE 40.2
EUTHYROID HYPOTHYROXINEMIA
Decreased thyroxine-binding globulin production Severe systemic illness Glucocorticoids Androgens Familial X-linked (many variants) Excessive thyroxine-binding globulin loss Protein-losing enteropathy Nephrosis Jejunoileal bypass Inhibition of protein binding Systemic illness (free fatty acids and tissue factor) Dilantin (in vitro, possibly not in vivo) Salicylates Furosemide Fenclofenac

TABLE 40.3

EUTHYROID HYPERTHYROXINEMIA

Binding protein abnormalities (excess binding to thyroxine-binding globulin, thyroxine-binding prealbumin, or albumin [rare to T_4 antibodies])

Transient hyperthyroxinemia of acute medical or psychiatric illness

Decreased peripheral conversion of T_4 to T_3, especially by propranolol or amiodarone

Amphetamine ingestion

Tissue resistance to thyroid hormone

T_3 = triiodothyronine, T_4 = thyroxine.

---

antibodies (TMAs); and decide on replacement therapy versus observation. Beware that normal (or low) values can be seen with pituitary (secondary) or hypothalamic (tertiary) hypothyroidism.

- FTI or FT_4. These may also be used as primary tests if TSH is deemed unreliable in certain clinical scenarios. These tests are usually less discriminating than TSH.
- T_3 is of no value.
- Radioactive iodine uptake (RAIU) is not indicated and may mislead.
- Consider TMA as a supportive test to diagnose the cause of the hypothyroidism, but this test is generally unnecessary in the presence of a goiter.

Tests for Hyperthyroidism

Thyroid function tests for diagnosing hyperthyroidism include:

- TSH. This is usually suppressed in the range of 0.02 to 0.1 μU/mL (depending on assay sensitivity). When the TSH is 0.1 to 0.4 μU/mL, consider early autonomy, slight overreplacement with levothyroxine, drug effect (e.g., steroids, dopamine), and pregnancy (first trimester).
- FTI or FT_4. Helpful if elevated, particularly if TSH is low.
- T_3 or FT_3 (if TSH suppressed and FTI or FT_4 normal). In this case, consider early hyperthyroidism or ingestion of liothyronine preparations.

Tests for Euthyroid Sick Syndrome (Nonthyroidal Illness)

Thyroid function tests for diagnosing euthyroid sick syndrome include:

- T_4, normal (N), or ↑
- T_4U, ↓, or N
- T_3RU, ↑, or N
- FTI or FT_4, N, or ↓
- T_3, ↓
- Reverse T_3, ↑
- TSH, N, or ↓ (↑ in recovery phase)

In the euthyroid sick syndrome, response to TRH is normal or blunted. TRH testing is of little or no value with the advent of sensitive TSH assays, except as a test for pituitary function (TSH and prolactin reserve). No more vexing problem arises in the interpretation of thyroid function tests than the euthyroid sick syndrome. The information in this chapter is a guide, but it does not represent an absolute interpretation because overlap in test results is common, and confounding factors are frequent. Therefore, clinical acumen is critical. Because isolated TSH deficiency is uncommon (isolated secondary hypothyroidism), it is important to look for other signs of hypopituitarism; however, gonadotropins may also be suppressed during the acute stress and starvation state. The new tests of FT_4 have problems similar to those of FTI in this syndrome. The changes in thyroid function tests reflect the severity of illness.

Mortality is inversely proportional to total T_4 in euthyroid medical intensive care unit patients. T_4 treatment of patients with severe nonthyroidal illness and low T_4 does not help, however, and could possibly harm.

Other Thyroid Tests

Other diagnostic thyroid tests include:

- TMA, also called *thyroid peroxidase* (TPO) antibodies
- Thyroglobulin (Tg) antibodies
- Thyroid receptor antibodies, stimulating (thyroid-stimulating immunoglobulins [TSIs]) and receptor binding
- Tg
- Serum or urinary iodide
- RAIU
- Thyroid scan (RAI or pertechnetate)
- Thyroid ultrasound
- Fine-needle aspiration biopsy

The measurement of serum Tg, the protein that is iodinated to make T_4 and T_3, can reveal either increased or decreased thyroid activity: Elevated Tg levels reflect increased secretory activity by or damage to the thyroid, and low Tg levels indicate a paucity of thyroid tissue or suppressed activity. The test is useful in the diagnosis of thyrotoxicosis factitia. The highest Tg levels are seen in metastatic differentiated nonmedullary thyroid carcinoma; therefore, the test is also useful in monitoring patients with thyroid cancer (see Thyroid Nodules and Cancer section). Beware of artifacts caused by the presence of antithyroglobulin antibodies because these antibodies can make serum Tg determinations difficult or impossible to interpret.

The measurement of serum thyroid antibodies provides additional information on antimicrosomal (peroxidase) and antithyroglobulin, and TSH receptor–stimulating antibodies. Antimicrosomal (peroxidase) antibodies and antithyroglobulin antibodies are occasionally useful in the management of hypothyroidism and in screening for the polyglandular autoimmune syndrome. TSH receptor–stimulating antibodies, the cause of thyrotoxicosis in Graves' disease, may help predict remission of this disease following treatment with antithyroid drugs.

Thyroid scanning and RAIU are less helpful because patients with hypothyroidism can have low, "normal," or high RAIU, and patients with hyperthyroidism can have low, "normal," or high RAIU. The RAIU is clinically useful only in the differential diagnosis of hyperthyroidism, in the calculation of radioiodine dosage, and in concert with a scan in the management of thyroid carcinoma. Note that RAIU gives you a number, whereas a scan gives you a picture.

SCREENING FOR THYROID DYSFUNCTION

Neonatal Screening

Neonatal screening programs, usually based on heel-prick blood TSH assays, are mandatory in most states in the United States and in most developed countries. The prevention of cretinism (1:4,000 live births) is far more cost effective using TSH assays than were the original phenylketonuria screening programs. However, certain caveats exist: the decision to institute and maintain the treatment in neonates with abnormal test results, the need for new strategies to help differentiate the physiological neonatal TSH surge from pathological primary hypothyroidism (not a problem when studies are done on or after 3 days of life), and rare cases of hypothalamic-pituitary hypothyroidism, which can be missed unless a simultaneous T_4 assay is performed.

Adult Screening

Who should be screened? Keep in mind that to screen for a disease assumes that detecting the disease is beneficial to the patient and that screening itself is not harmful to those without the disease. Even in hypothyroidism, in which therapy is easy, the costs of screening a large population are not trivial. Therefore, screening should be performed only in populations with a reasonably high prevalence of thyroid dysfunction, such as women older than 40 years and patients admitted to specialized geriatric units. There is little reason to screen the general population, either in the ambulatory setting or on hospitalization. The issue of the treatment of subclinical thyroid disease is controversial. Data are accumulating, however, to indicate that subclinical thyroid disease is common (5%–10% in population surveys) and is worth delineating from a cost-effectiveness point of view.[1,2] Because undiagnosed hypothyroidism in pregnancy may adversely affect fetal neurologic development, screening for thyroid deficiency during pregnancy may also be warranted.[3]

How should screening be done? High-sensitivity TSH screening is probably the most effective way to screen ambulatory populations because it has superior test characteristics, primary hypothyroidism is the most common form of abnormal thyroid function (far more common than secondary hypothyroidism), and primary hyperthyroidism is far more common than secondary hyperthyroidism.

In outpatients, the sensitivity and specificity of FT_4 and FTI is approximately 90% in the diagnosis of hyperthyroidism, whereas the sensitivity and specificity of the high-sensitivity TSH assay is approximately 99%. The operating characteristics of these tests are far worse in hospitalized patients, in whom the specificity of the TSH assay is particularly low (Table 40.4).

HYPOTHYROIDISM

Hypothyroidism is the clinical disorder that results from insufficient thyroid hormone action.

Etiology

Hypothyroidism is a common disease, more prevalent in women (1%–2% prevalence) than in men (0.1% prevalence). In one large study from England, 25% to 30% of

---

TABLE 40.4

SUMMARY OF RECOMMENDED TESTS FOR THYROID DYSFUNCTION

Condition	Type	Recommended Tests	Additional Tests
Hypothyroidism	Primary	TSH	Thyroid microsomal antibody
	Pituitary/hypothalamic	T_4-FTI or free T_4	Pituitary function (e.g., cortisol)
Hyperthyroidism	Various	TSH	T_4-FTI, free T_4, T_3
		Radioactive iodine uptake scan	
		TSH receptor antibodies	
Sick euthyroid		TSH, free T_4, T_3	Pituitary function
Thyroid cancer	Papillary/follicular	Thyroglobulin, TSH	T_4-FTI, free T_4, T_3
Screening	Neonatal	TSH	T_4
	Adult	TSH	

FTI = free thyroxine index, T_3 = triiodothyronine, T_4 = thyroxine, TSH = thyroid-stimulating hormone.

cases were iatrogenic. Hypothyroidism is particularly common in elderly persons. Congenital hypothyroidism occurs in 1 of every 4,000 newborns. The causes of hypothyroidism can be subdivided into three groupings (common causes are italicized):

- Primary (thyroid cause)
  - Agenesis
  - Destruction of gland
  - Surgical removal
  - *Irradiation* (therapeutic radioactive iodine for thyrotoxicosis or external irradiation therapy for nonthyroid malignant disease of the neck)
  - *Autoimmune disease* (Hashimoto's disease)
  - *Idiopathic atrophy* (possibly after autoimmune disease)
  - Replacement by cancer or other infiltrative process
  - Inhibition of synthesis and release of thyroid hormone
  - Iodine deficiency
  - Excess iodide in susceptible individuals
  - Antithyroid drugs
  - Lithium
  - Inherited enzyme defects
- Transient causes
  - After surgery or therapeutic radioactive iodine
  - Postpartum
  - In the course of thyroiditis
- Secondary to pituitary or hypothalamic disease
- Resistance to thyroid hormones

Clinical Presentation

The clinical presentation of hypothyroidism depends on the pathogenesis: sudden onset (e.g., after thyroidectomy) versus gradual decline (e.g., owing to idiopathic atrophy). In the former, the clinical onset relates to the serum half-life of T_4 (1 week) and occurs in a matter of weeks. In the latter, decreases in thyroid hormone levels may take place over years. In addition, the clinical picture depends on the age of the patient. Because thyroid hormone is essential for brain development, a neonatal onset has different manifestations from an adult onset.

Symptoms of hypothyroidism include:

- Constitutional symptoms (weakness, fatigue, lethargy, and sleepiness)
- Mental slowness
- Cold intolerance
- Muscle aches
- Paresthesias (especially carpal tunnel syndrome)
- Diminished sweating
- Hoarseness
- Weight gain
- Constipation
- Hair loss
- Menstrual dysfunction (usually heavy, frequent menses, rarely amenorrhea, and galactorrhea)

The signs of hypothyroidism include:

- Dry, coarse, cold skin
- Edema of eyelids
- Puffy hands and swelling of feet (myxedema)
- Coarse hair and hair loss
- Thick tongue
- Slow speech
- Hoarse voice
- Slow movements
- Pseudomyotonia (delayed relaxation phase of deep tendon reflexes)
- Sallow, pale complexion

Note that many of these features are common in normal aging.

Myxedema coma represents the end stage of hypothyroidism or the combination of severe hypothyroidism, plus one or more complicating factors. The pathophysiology involves respiratory failure, decreased cardiac output, anemia, hypothermia, hypoglycemia, hyponatremia, and thyroid hormone deficiency. Respiratory dysfunction plays an important role in the development of most cases of myxedema coma. Hypothyroidism affects the respiratory system at all levels, from the respiratory center to peripheral oxygen delivery. Respiratory center depression manifests by impaired responses to hypercapnia and hypoxia and results in hypoventilation and a diminished ability to respond to acute hypoxemia-producing insults.

Diagnosis

In the diagnosis of hypothyroidism, other abnormalities may include increased serum creatine phosphokinase and cholesterol, hyponatremia, and ECG changes (low voltage, bradycardia).

Primary hypothyroidism caused by Hashimoto's thyroiditis may be associated with other autoimmune diseases (e.g., autoimmune adrenal insufficiency, polyglandular autoimmune syndrome).

Two vital questions to answer in making the diagnosis of hypothyroidism are: Is the patient hypothyroid? If the patient is hypothyroid, is the cause primary or secondary? The answer to the latter question has important implications for therapy, as outlined in the preceding section.

Treatment

The treatment of hypothyroidism is two pronged: to administer thyroid hormone and to treat the underlying disease. Secondary and tertiary hypothyroidism (i.e., hypothyroidism attributable to pituitary or hypothalamic insufficiency) often require therapy directed at both the causes and the effects of thyroid hormone deficiency. The causes of primary hypothyroidism (i.e., diseases directly affecting the thyroid gland) do not, as a general rule, require treatment directed at the cause. Rather, the key in treatment is therapy directed toward amelioration of the effects of thyroid hormone deficiency.

The treatment of hypothyroidism is simple: Administer thyroid hormone. Levothyroxine (LT_4) is the preparation of choice. Its advantages include that the patient given T_4 develops a substantial peripheral pool of T_4, which turns over more slowly than does T_3 and provides a buffer against lapses in the ingestion of medication. In addition, the pool of T_4 acts as a continuous source of T_3, thereby maintaining a stable T_3 serum concentration.

When first diagnosed, hypothyroidism is usually of long duration and seldom requires rapid reversal. Therefore, the restoration of a normal metabolic state may be undertaken gradually. The untreated hypothyroid patient is extremely sensitive to small doses of thyroid hormone. In the hypothyroid patient with long-standing hypothyroidism, high-dose T_4 may precipitate a myocardial infarction or congestive heart failure.

In secondary hypothyroidism, it is important to treat adrenal insufficiency, if present, before thyroid replacement.

Conversely, no untoward risk is present in initiating therapy with full replacement doses of LT_4 (estimated at 1.6 μg/kg body weight) in most younger adult patients with hypothyroidism. In the pediatric age group, requirements are considerably higher. Monitoring therapy is best accomplished by means of the high-sensitivity TSH assay, with the aim of restoration to the normal range. Because of the inherent lag of TSH in the system, no dose adjustments based on the TSH value should be made for a minimum 6-week interval. On clinical grounds, however, small dose adjustments working toward total replacement can be made safely at 2-week intervals in elderly patients and in those with a precarious cardiac status.

In hypothalamic-pituitary hypothyroidism, TSH determinations are of no value. Monitoring is best accomplished by using an FTI or FT_4 assay. If hyperthyroxinemia develops, the T_3 radioimmunoassay should be used to determine whether overtreatment has occurred (values should be <130–140 ng/dL; normal, 80–170 ng/dL). Overtreatment may result in accelerated bone mineral loss especially in postmenopausal women.

The following additional considerations should be noted in patients on LT_4 therapy:

- Use the same brand name drug (avoid generics).
- Monitor compliance and dosage requirements at 6- to 12-month intervals.
- Beware of the concomitant use of preparations that may interfere with absorption (soybean, infant formula; soy milk in adults [4], cholestyramine, sucralfate [polyaluminum hydroxide], antacids [aluminum hydroxide], or iron), with metabolism (anticonvulsants [phenytoin or carbamazepine] or rifampin) or with both (proton pump inhibitors). The effects of anticonvulsants are complex; TSH values remain the best guide (except in *hypothalamic-*

pituitary hypothyroidism, where reliance on TSH values is valueless or misleading and T4 and/or T3 estimates can be used).

One study suggests that replacement therapy with combined LT_4 plus LT_3 may be preferable to treatment with LT_4 alone;[5] however, three more recent studies provide strong evidence against this notion.[6–8] Accordingly, this approach is not recommended.

In the past, hypothyroidism has been considered a contraindication for surgery; however, the intraoperative and perioperative risks tend to be minor and can be managed pre-emptively.[9]

HYPERTHYROIDISM

Hyperthyroidism is a common clinical condition.[10]

Etiology

As with most thyroid disorders, hyperthyroidism is much more common in women than in men. A cross-sectional study of autoimmune thyroid disease in an English community revealed a prevalence of established hyperthyroidism of 2% in women and an annual incidence of 3 in 1,000 women. The causes of hyperthyroidism can be subdivided into three groupings:

- Primary thyroid overproduction (RAIU elevated or high normal, unless iodide pool is expanded, such as recent radiocontrast Jod-Basedow [iodide-induced hyperthyroidism]):
  - Graves' disease
  - Toxic multinodular goiter (Plummer's disease)
  - Toxic adenoma (uninodular Plummer's disease)
  - Certain cases of follicular thyroid carcinoma (metastatic)
  - Human chorionic gonadotropin (HCG) mediated
  - Trophoblastic disease
  - Hyperemesis gravidarum
- TSH receptor abnormality (enhanced HCG recognition)
  - Fetal/neonatal
- TSH mediated
  - Pituitary adenoma
  - Pituitary thyroid hormone resistance
  - Iodide excess
  - Intrinsic TSH receptor abnormality
  - Thyroid damage (RAIU low)
  - Subacute (painful, de Quervain's) thyroiditis
  - Painless and postpartum thyroiditis
  - Amiodarone (clinical significance is uncertain)
  - Nonthyroidal disease (RAIU low)
  - Exogenous hormone use (excessive dose; factitious use)
  - Accidental exposure (laced hamburgers)
  - Struma ovarii (extremely rare)

Clinical Presentation

Symptoms of hyperthyroidism include:

- Nervousness
- Fatigue
- Weakness
- Palpitations
- Heat intolerance
- Increased sweating
- Dyspnea
- Hyperdefecation
- Insomnia
- Poor concentration
- Infrequent, scanty menses

Signs of hyperthyroidism include:

- Weight loss
- Proximal myopathy
- Tachycardia, arrhythmias
- Warm, moist skin
- Tremor
- Eye conditions (stare, lid lag, and lid retraction)
- Emotional lability
- Hyperactive deep tendon reflexes
- Radiologic evidence of thymic enlargement in Graves' disease[11]

Thyroid storm, which represents the extreme form of hyperthyroidism, presents with:

- Exaggerated typical signs
- Exaggerated typical symptoms
- Fever
- Changes in neurologic function (delirium)

Diagnosis

A biochemical diagnosis of suppressed TSH and elevated circulating T_4 or T_3 requires an RAIU test (a thyroid scan may also prove useful) to confirm the diagnosis and aid in the treatment plan. Contraindications to the use of RAI in testing or therapy include:

- Pregnancy
- Lactation
- Iodide (nonradioactive) overload
- Intercurrent illness or therapy (which precludes waiting for the test to be done)

A positive thyroid receptor antibody test can be helpful in such situations.

GRAVES' DISEASE

In 1835, Robert Graves published a report of three patients with cardiac palpitations and goiter. One of the three patients also had exophthalmos. This condition is now recognized as the most common cause of noniatrogenic hyperthyroidism in the United States. Three major manifestations of the disease appear:

- Hyperthyroidism with diffuse goiter
- Ophthalmopathy (eye disease)
- Dermopathy (pretibial myxedema)

Several lines of evidence support the role of hereditary factors in the development of Graves' disease in the children and siblings of patients with Graves' disease. The presence of certain human leukocyte antigens is associated with an increased incidence of Graves' disease; in particular, the HLA-DR3 antigen in white persons may confer a fourfold risk for the development of the disease. An increased incidence of other autoimmune disorders (e.g., Hashimoto's thyroiditis, pernicious anemia, myasthenia gravis, Addison's disease) also occurs in patients with Graves' disease and their family members. The disease occurs most frequently between the ages of 20 and 40 years, and it has a marked female sex preponderance (approximately 3–8:1). Therapy may consist of iodine-131 (^{131}I), antithyroid drugs or, rarely, surgery (see following discussion). Symptomatic treatment with beta-blockers is also useful.

Hyperthyroidism With Diffuse Goiter

The thyrotoxicosis and goiter of Graves' disease result from stimulation of the gland by autoantibodies (immunoglobulins of the IgG class). These autoantibodies are polyclonal and are collectively referred to as TSIs. The antigen to which these are directed is the TSH receptor, or a region adjacent to it, on the plasma membrane. The binding of these immunoglobulins to the TSH receptor mimics the action of TSH, stimulating adenyl cyclase and thereby initiating a chain of reactions that leads to thyroid growth, increased vascularity, and hypersecretion of hormone.

Ophthalmopathy

The ophthalmopathy (eye disease) of Graves' disease is probably present to some degree in most patients, although only approximately one-third to one-half of patients has obvious symptoms or signs of eye disease. Symptoms include pain, lacrimation, photophobia, blurred vision, and diplopia.

Signs of ophthalmopathy include periorbital edema, lid edema, lid lag, chemosis, ophthalmoplegia, proptosis, corneal ulcerations, optic neuropathy, and dermopathy. Infiltrative dermopathy (skin disease) occurs in only approximately 1% of patients with Graves' disease. The pretibial myxedema (most common site) is a consequence of the accumulation of acid mucopolysaccharides and lymphocytes, and the presentation is quite variable. The etiology is not known.

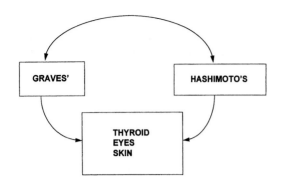

Figure 40.2 Spectrum of autoimmune thyroid disease.

AUTOIMMUNE THYROID DISEASE

Autoimmune thyroid disease can be viewed as a spectrum of diseases in individuals and in their family members (Fig. 40.2). The clinical presentation of the disorder, according to this view, depends on the morphologic state of the gland and the mixture of circulating antibodies at any particular point in time. The antibodies include:

- Microsomal (TMA, TPO)
- Tg
- Thyroid damaging
- Receptor binding (stimulating [TSI], blocking, binding)
- Growth promoting (may be independent from stimulating)

Thus, Graves' disease may "burn out" to become hypothyroidism; receptor-blocking antibodies may result in transient hypothyroidism, giving way to Graves' hyperthyroidism when TSI prevails, and different family members may have different presentations.

TOXIC MULTINODULAR GOITER (PLUMMER'S DISEASE)

Toxic multinodular goiter is a disorder in which hyperthyroidism arises in a multinodular goiter, usually of long-standing duration. The development of this type of goiter probably starts with the appearance of local areas of autonomous thyroid hyperplasia within individual follicles, followed by their continued replication and growth. The process is accompanied by areas of involution, so functional and anatomical heterogeneity (nodules) appears. If the autonomous regions grow and function sufficiently, hyperthyroidism ensues. Because this process is a slow one, the typical age of appearance of hyperthyroidism tends to be older than in Graves' disease, usually past the age of 50 years. Therapy may consist of ^{131}I (high, multiple doses may be required) or, occasionally, surgery; antithyroid drugs may be used, but therapy must be permanent.

TOXIC ADENOMA

Toxic adenoma, considered to be a true benign tumor of the thyroid gland, is a far less common cause of thyrotoxicosis than Graves' disease or toxic multinodular goiter. Adenomatous tissue develops in the thyroid, which secretes thyroid hormone autonomously, without stimulation by TSH or other thyroid stimulators. This condition tends to occur in patients in their 30s and 40s, somewhat younger than those with toxic multinodular goiter. A single palpable nodule is found on physical examination; a radioactive iodine scan reveals uptake of the isotope only in the adenoma, resulting in a "hot" nodule. (The excess circulating thyroid hormone suppresses TSH secretion and the nonautonomous areas of the thyroid gland; therefore, neither takes up iodine nor produces thyroid hormone.) Therapy usually consists of ^{131}I or surgery.

IODIDE-INDUCED THYROTOXICOSIS (JOD-BASEDOW PHENOMENON)

Jod-Basedow phenomenon refers to iodide-induced hyperthyroidism. (*Jod* is German for iodine, and *von Basedow* was one of the early describers of thyrotoxicosis.) This condition occurs most commonly in patients with underlying thyroid disease, who reside in areas of iodide deficiency and who subsequently receive a load of exogenous iodide (e.g., iodide-containing contrast dye). The pathogenesis, although unclear, is believed to be due to an overproduction of thyroid hormone by autonomously functioning thyroid tissue when presented with excess substrate (iodide). This is the only form of thyrotoxicosis in which ongoing overproduction of thyroid hormone by the thyroid gland occurs, associated with a low RAIU. This occurs because the radioactive isotopic iodide is diluted by large quantities of circulating stable iodide; therefore, only a small quantity of the radioisotope is taken up by the gland. Therapy consists of removing the source of iodide. Occasionally, surgery is necessary (especially in amiodarone-induced hyperthyroidism).

SUBACUTE THYROIDITIS (DE QUERVAIN'S, GRANULOMATOUS THYROIDITIS)

Subacute thyroiditis is a painful inflammatory process involving the thyroid gland. It results in an elevation of the serum concentration of thyroid hormone into the thyrotoxic range. A history of viral illness often precedes onset, and a number of different viruses have been shown to be associated. The inflammation in the thyroid gland results in the destruction of the follicular epithelium, with the subsequent discharge of large amounts of preformed thyroid hormone into the circulation. Histologically, infiltration of the interstitial areas by histiocytes and lymphocytes occurs; these often appear to congregate into *giant cells*. The characteristic feature of subacute thyroiditis is a painful, tender, mildly enlarged thyroid gland. Systemic manifestations, such as fever, fatigue, and malaise, are also common. Half of patients experience symptoms of hyperthyroidism. Laboratory abnormalities include an extremely high erythrocyte sedimentation rate (ESR) and an extremely low RAIU (the damaged follicles are unable to concentrate iodine). Moreover, the suppressed TSH resulting from the release of excessive amounts of preformed thyroid hormone (the thyroid gland usually has a month's supply of thyroid hormone stored) leads to inactivity even of the undisrupted thyroid follicles. The course of subacute thyroiditis is self-limited, with complete recovery being the general rule. Therapy is primarily supportive and directed toward relief of symptoms (aspirin and beta-blockers). Occasionally, glucocorticoids are necessary, but relapses may occur when the glucocorticoids are stopped.

PAINLESS THYROIDITIS

Painless thyroiditis is another inflammatory condition of the thyroid in which preformed thyroid hormone is discharged from damaged follicles into the circulation. The association in most patients with high titers of antimicrosomal antibodies suggests an autoimmune pathogenesis. Painless thyroiditis occurs most commonly in postpartum women. The course is quite similar to that of subacute thyroiditis, except for the absence of pain and thyroidal tenderness. The RAIU is similarly low, although the ESR is usually normal. Therapy is primarily supportive.

TREATMENT OF THYROTOXICOSIS

Radioactive Iodine

The administration of ^{131}I results in thyroid damage through two different mechanisms: acute radiation thyroiditis and chronic gradual thyroid atrophy. Acute cell death leads to an inflammatory response, with infiltration by granulocytes and mononuclear cells. The eventual result is a progressive atrophy associated with an obliterative endarteritis and interstitial fibrosis that occurs over a period of years. The usual dose of ^{131}I for the treatment of Graves' disease results in the delivery of 7,000 to 10,000 rad to the thyroid bed. The treatment for toxic multinodular goiter or toxic adenoma generally requires higher doses of [131]I. Therapy with ^{131}I is safe, with the only major side effect being the frequent development of hypothyroidism in patients with Graves' disease. Posttreatment hypothyroidism has been believed to be quite uncommon with toxic multinodular goiter or toxic adenoma.

In the latter two conditions, after destruction of autonomously functioning tissue, follicles that were previously suppressed (and thus did not take up the radioiodine) resume normal function. One study suggests, however, that eventual hypothyroidism may be seen in as many as 30% of ^{131}I-treated solitary toxic adenoma patients.[12] Fears that ^{131}I therapy is a risk factor for thyroid or other neoplasms have proved unfounded. The gonadal radiation exposure following a standard dose of ^{131}I is less than 3 rad (approximately the same as for an intravenous pyelogram or a barium enema) and thus does not pose a risk for an increased incidence of genetic defects in the offspring of treated patients. Because iodine crosses the placenta and is also excreted in breast milk, ^{131}I therapy is absolutely contraindicated in pregnant women or breastfeeding mothers because destruction of the fetal or neonatal thyroid gland may be the consequence. One disadvantage of this form of therapy is that amelioration of the thyrotoxicosis may take up to 3 months or longer. Therefore, for patients who are quite symptomatic, treatment both before and after radioiodine therapy may be necessary using other agents (e.g., antithyroid drugs or beta-blockers).

Radioiodine therapy for Graves' hyperthyroidism has been reported to increase the development or worsen already present ophthalmopathy, when compared with therapy using antithyroid drugs. This worsening of ophthalmopathy is often transient and may be prevented through the use of prednisone.[13] Cigarette smoking, a known risk factor for the development of Graves' ophthalmopathy, appears not only to aggravate the eye risk due to radioiodine therapy, but also to have a negative impact on the treatment of the eye disease through prednisone or orbital radiotherapy.[14] [131]I therapy is not effective in treating conditions in which thyrotoxicosis is not a consequence of overproduction of thyroid hormone by the thyroid gland (e.g., subacute thyroiditis).

Antithyroid Drugs (Propylthiouracil or Methimazole)

The mechanism of action of antithyroid drugs is the inhibition of thyroid hormone biosynthesis through the blocking of iodine oxidation, organification, and iodotyrosine coupling, all reactions that are catalyzed by TPO. An additional mechanism of action, unique to propylthiouracil, is the inhibition of peripheral conversion of T_4 to T_3. This particular effect is useful in patients who are extremely thyrotoxic. In addition to their antithyroid effects, both drugs have immunosuppressive activity and thus may ameliorate the underlying pathogenetic process in Graves' disease. Because these drugs inhibit thyroid autoantibody production, their use in Graves' disease for a 12-month period is associated with long-term remission in approximately 30% to 40% of cases.

These drugs do not alter the underlying pathogenetic process in toxic multinodular goiter or toxic adenoma;

therefore, life-long term therapy is required for these conditions. Some improvement in symptoms is usually apparent after 1 to 2 weeks of therapy and is substantial after 4 to 6 weeks of treatment. This fairly rapid onset of action makes antithyroid drug therapy particularly useful for toxic patients before definitive treatment with ^{131}I or surgery.

Adverse drug reactions occur in as many as 5% to 10% of patients treated with antithyroid medication. The most common side effect is a rash, occurring in 3% to 5% of patients. The most serious side effect, *agranulocytosis* (the complete absence of circulating granulocytes), is seen in 0.5% of patients. It occurs abruptly and, although it is reversible with cessation of the drug, may result in serious illness or even death, especially in older patients. Patients must be cautioned to discontinue the drug and report for a white blood count immediately on the advent of a severe sore throat or fever. Monitoring white blood counts in anticipation is of no value and is not recommended.

Surgery

The surgical removal of abnormally functioning thyroid tissue is usually definitive, although there may be 10% of patients with Graves' disease in whom thyrotoxicosis recurs after subtotal thyroidectomy. The prevalence of postoperative hypothyroidism (up to 40%) and other surgical complications (vocal cord paralysis owing to recurrent laryngeal nerve damage or permanent hypoparathyroidism) makes surgery less than ideal as a form of therapy and rarely the first choice, although in expert hands surgical complications are minimal.

Beta-Blocking Agents

Many of the symptoms and signs of thyrotoxicosis are similar to those of excessive beta-adrenergic stimulation. These manifestations are ameliorated when pharmacologic agents that block the beta-receptor are used (e.g., propranolol). These agents, therefore, are extremely useful in treating some of the symptoms of thyrotoxicosis until definitive therapy of the underlying cause is effective or a transient pathogenetic process resolves (e.g., subacute thyroiditis). Caution must be exercised in patients with a history of asthma or in the presence of cardiac failure.

SUBCLINICAL THYROID DISEASE

This controversial topic was studied in detail by a panel of 13 experts in endocrinology, epidemiology, and preventive services. The consensus guidelines[15] and clinical applications[16] were published in 2004. The major conclusions are quoted verbatim:

> Data supporting associations of subclinical thyroid disease with symptoms or adverse clinical outcomes or benefits of treatment are few. The consequences of subclinical thyroid disease (serum TSH 0.15–0.45 μU/mL or 4.5–10.0 μU/mL)

are minimal, and we recommend against routine treatment of patients with TSH levels in these ranges. There is insufficient evidence to support population-based screening. Aggressive case finding is appropriate in pregnant women, women older than 60 years, and others at risk for thyroid dysfunction.

THYROIDITIS

Acute Suppurative Thyroiditis

Bacterial infection of the thyroid is rare. It presents with pain, fever, and other signs of infection.

Subacute Thyroiditis

Subacute thyroiditis is a cause of thyrotoxicosis (see preceding discussion).

Hashimoto's Thyroiditis

Hashimoto's (lymphocytic) thyroiditis, an autoimmune disorder, is a common cause of *goiter* (enlarged thyroid) and hypothyroidism. It is more frequent in women and may run in families. It is associated with autoimmune disorders involving other endocrine glands, such as Addison's disease (adrenal insufficiency) and insulin-dependent diabetes mellitus, and involving other systems, such as rheumatoid arthritis. The pathogenesis involves cell-mediated immunity. In addition, thyroid autoantibodies against Tg and the microsome TPO enzyme are found, although their significance in vivo is not clear.

In Hashimoto's, the titer of antimicrosomal antibodies is usually >1:400. Pathologically, diffuse lymphocytic infiltration by germinal centers, fibrosis, and obliteration of the thyroid follicles are observed. Abnormalities in thyroid hormone biosynthesis include an organification defect demonstrable by the perchlorate discharge of radioiodine. Abnormal iodoproteins may be released. As long as intact follicles remain, iodine trapping is preserved.

This disorder frequently produces a goiter, and some patients develop hypothyroidism. Some patients with Graves' disease may have histologic features of Hashimoto's thyroiditis, giving rise to the basically meaningless term *Hashitoxicosis* (see Autoimmune Thyroid Disease section).

Painless Thyroiditis

Painless thyroiditis most commonly occurs postpartum. It may have a typical three-phase course—hyperthyroidism, hypothyroidism, and then a return to the euthyroid state—or it can present with hypothyroidism or hyperthyroidism alone. Women with antimicrosomal antibodies are more likely to develop this disease: Some clinicians advocate measuring TMA in pregnancy, especially in the presence of goiter, and monitoring thyroid status routinely in the puerperium. At present, however, no compelling evidence supports such a practice.

DRUGS AND THYROID DYSFUNCTION

Lithium

Lithium causes primary hypothyroidism. Also, lithium therapy has been associated with hyperthyroidism and hypercalcemia, and it can cause nephrogenic diabetes insipidus.

Amiodarone

Amiodarone causes both hypothyroidism and hyperthyroidism. The former is more common in persons with antimicrosomal antibodies. The latter probably has more than one cause: iodine-induced thyrotoxicosis and drug-induced thyroid damage.

The therapy of the hypothyroidism should include cautious thyroid hormone replacement; patients on amiodarone have significant heart disease. Hyperthyroidism therapy may be difficult because antithyroid drugs are often ineffective. The combination of high-dose propylthiouracil and potassium perchlorate (not routinely available) has been effective in some patients. Surgery is sometimes necessary.

THYROID NODULES AND CANCER

Thyroid Nodules

Thyroid nodules occur commonly and may be single or multiple. Most are benign. The major issue for the clinician is to determine which nodules are likely to be malignant and require surgical removal. Most thyroid nodules are "cold" on thyroid scans; thus, scanning is not very helpful.

Those clinical features raising the likelihood of malignancy include:

- Male sex
- Family history (especially of multiple endocrine neoplasia type II, which includes medullary thyroid carcinoma)
- History of radiation treatment to the head and neck, especially in childhood or adolescence
- Hoarseness or vocal cord paralysis
- A single nodule or a dominant nodule in a multinodular gland
- Lymphadenopathy

Diagnostic techniques include:

- Fine-needle biopsy, which is the most cost effective. Various techniques are used. It is crucial to have access to an experienced cytologist.
- Ultrasound, which might reveal additional nodules
- RAIU scan of limited value in the case of nodules
- Chest radiography
- Tg

The best diagnostic approach involves fine-needle aspiration biopsy, which has excellent sensitivity and specificity. There are some limitations, especially in the diagnosis of follicular neoplasms, because cytologic differentiation between adenoma and carcinoma cannot be done with any certainty. Such lesions should be removed.

The therapy of nontoxic nodular thyroid disease is controversial.[17] LT$_4$ suppressive therapy has been used with variable results. Nodules that continue to enlarge despite LT$_4$ therapy, even with negative cytology, merit surgical removal. Compressive symptoms and signs similarly demand surgical attention. The use of radioiodine therapy for symptomatic nontoxic multinodular goiter in Europe has gained little attention in the United States or Canada.

Thyroid Cancer

The major types of thyroid cancer are:

- Primary
  - Papillary
  - Follicular
  - Anaplastic
  - Medullary (sporadic, familial, multiple endocrine neoplasia type II)
  - Hürthle cell
- Mixed
- Secondary
- Lymphoma

Papillary and *follicular cancers*, which tend to be relatively slow growing, account for the vast majority of cases.[18] Papillary cancer tends to metastasize to lymph nodes, whereas follicular cancer tends to have earlier hematogenous spread, primarily to lung and bone.

Anaplastic cancer, which presents with a rapidly growing mass, has a dismal prognosis.

Medullary cancer is a tumor of C cells associated with calcitonin production. It can be sporadic or familial, or occur as part of multiple endocrine neoplasia type II. Family members should be screened.

Thyroid lymphoma appears to be increasing in frequency. It may occur in a gland involved with Hashimoto's thyroiditis.

The treatment of the common cancers (papillary or follicular) usually includes surgery (near total thyroidectomy is recommended, although some centers recommend more conservative surgery), ablative ^{131}I therapy, and LT$_4$ suppression of TSH.[19] Serial serum Tg determinations are of value in monitoring disease eradication or recurrence.

The periodic withdrawal of suppressive LT$_4$ therapy permits endogenous TSH to rise and to stimulate any residual thyroid tissue, as demonstrated by whole body scans or serum Tg determinations. Further therapy with ^{131}I can be administered, within limits, as required. Regrettably, LT$_4$ withdrawal can be associated with unwanted and sometimes serious morbidity. Recombinant human TSH is available for use to identify patients with residual tumor tissue; this agent avoids the need to render patients hypothyroid. To date, the results obtained in identifying residual tumor tissue are less sensitive compared with those following withdrawal of thyroid hormone.

REVIEW EXERCISES

QUESTIONS

1. A patient being screened for intermittent diarrhea has a T_4 (total) value of 19.6 μg/dL (normal, 5.0–10.5). No other features of hyperthyroidism are present; no goiter is present. A T_4U test is elevated at 2.01 (normal, 0.8–1.20), whereas the T_3RU test is subnormal at 15% (normal, 25%–35%). The free thyroxine index is calculated to be 9.8 (normal, 5.0–10.5). What single test would be most helpful in delineating the patient's thyroid status?
a) Thyroid-stimulating hormone
b) Thyroid receptor antibodies
c) Serum T_3
d) Serum FT_4 equilibrium dialysis
e) None of the above

Answer and Discussion
The answer is a. The aim of the question is to help gain understanding of the role of free (nonprotein bound) thyroid hormone in regulating thyroid-stimulating hormone (TSH) secretion. The hypothalamo-pituitary unit "reads" the free hormone level, not the total hormone level, which is subject to changes owing to alterations in protein binding (thyroxine-binding globulin, thyroid-binding prealbumin, albumin, or conditions that may interfere with binding).

In practice, the free thyroxine index can be calculated from total T_4 and an estimate of protein binding (T_4U or T_3RU; T_4U measures binding directly, whereas T_3RU provides an index of unbound hormone). Automated FT_4 assays are replacing these more indirect indices; the gold standard, FT_4 by equilibrium dialysis, is available in some reference laboratories but is rarely needed. Thus, serum TSH in this patient should provide the best indicator of thyroid function status and is independent from thyroid hormone protein–binding abnormalities.

2. The serum thyroid-stimulating hormone test result is 3.0 μU/mL (normal, 0.4–5.5). No drugs or hepatic disease explain the findings. What is the best working diagnosis?
a) Antibodies against circulating T_3
b) Hereditary increase in thyroxine-binding globulin production (X-linked)
c) Hereditary increase in thyroid-binding prealbumin production

d) All of the above
e) None of the above

Answer and Discussion
The answer is b. This question explores thyroid hormone binding in more detail. The major normal thyroid hormone–binding proteins are thyroxine-binding globulin (TBG) and thyroid-binding prealbumin (TBPA). Certain drugs and conditions can alter these levels or binding capacity. Antibodies against T_4 and T_3 rarely occur in patients who have Hashimoto's thyroiditis (haptenic autoantigen). Hereditary increases in TBG (binds both T_4 and T_3) or TBPA (binds T_4 only) occur uncommonly. The increases in thyroid hormone–binding capacity in this patient are reflected by both the T_4U (high) and the T_3RU (low) tests. Antibodies against T_3 would be expected to lower the T_3RU test results, but not affect the T_4U test; increased TBPA levels would result in increased T_4U values, but not affect T_3RU values (because T_3 does not bind to the TBPA ligand).

3. A patient with primary hypothyroidism has been stable (normal thyroid-stimulating hormone [TSH]) on replacement LT_4 (dose, 1.6 μg/kg of body weight) for several years. On annual follow-up, the following laboratory tests are obtained: T_4, 14.1 μg/dL (normal, 5.0–10.5) and TSH, 23.4 μU/mL (normal, 0.4–5.5). She saw a gastroenterologist 6 months previously for nonsteroidal anti-inflammatory drug–related gastritis and takes an iron preparation and occasional antacids. Which is the most likely diagnosis?
a) Malabsorption of LT_4 owing to concomitant use of antacids and iron
b) Progressive loss of endogenous thyroid function
c) Development of thyroid hormone resistance
d) Poor compliance this past year, with attempt to "catch up" with excessive LT_4 intake recently
e) None of the above

Answer and Discussion
The answer is d. This question helps understand the time lag in the hypothalamo-pituitary-thyroid axis. Although TSH secretion may be acutely altered by stress, illness, or drugs, the major regulation is based on the integrated thyroid hormone exposure over the preceding 2 to 5 weeks. Although iron preparations and aluminum-containing compounds can interfere with T_4 absorption, the elevated serum T_4 level argues against this notion. Similarly, a progressive loss of thyroid function would be expected to lead to low or low-normal T_4 values. Although acquired thyroid hormone resistance may occur hypothetically, no clinical descriptions of such disorders exist. The correct answer is not a rare occurrence: Patients often want to please their health care

provider, even if it means not being perfectly honest on occasion.

4. The development of Graves' hyperthyroidism following the presence of Hashimoto's hypothyroidism is best explained by which of the following?

a) The finding of histopathological changes of Hashimoto's thyroiditis in Graves' thyroid glands
b) Graves' hyperthyroidism as a natural phase of Hashimoto's disease
c) That the two disorders are part of the spectrum of autoimmune thyroid disease, the clinical manifestations of which depend on the mixture of circulating polyclonal antibodies and the morphologic state of the gland at a particular point in time
d) All of the above
e) None of the above

Answer and Discussion
The answer is c. This question gains understanding of the concept that the correct answer helps explain this, as well as a number of other clinical conditions (see Autoimmune Thyroid Disease section).

5. You are asked to see a 75-year-old white man who was admitted to the psychiatric ward with a diagnosis of delirium. The history obtained from the wife revealed that he was well until 6 months before admission. He has had a 30-lb weight loss with a poor appetite since then. No history is present of any medication, recent investigations involving radiocontrast media, goiter, or neck discomfort. No family history of thyroid disease is present. On physical examination, he is afebrile; he looks cachectic but is not pigmented; no features of infiltrative eye changes are present; and the thyroid gland is prolapsed, but may be just palpable on swallowing. The pulse rate is irregular at 120 beats/minute. The ECG shows atrial fibrillation. The serum T_4 is 19.7 μg/dL (normal, 5.0–10.5) with a serum thyroid-stimulating hormone <0.02 μU/mL (normal, 0.4–5.5).

The next step in diagnosis is to order

a) Serum T_3
b) 24-Hour radioactive iodine uptake (RAIU)
c) 24-Hour RAIU and scan
d) Thyroid-stimulating antibodies
e) Thyroid microsomal (TPO) antibodies

Answer and Discussion
The answer is c. This question reinforces the clinical presentation of elderly patients with thyrotoxicosis and their management. Although weight loss despite a generous appetite is characteristic in the younger adult, anorexia is not an uncommon finding in the elderly. Cachexia in an "apathetic" patient should be considered. (Concomitant Addison's disease in a pa-

tient with known thyroid autoimmunity is a "distractor" in the current case presentation; the lack of pigmentation was intended to get the reader back on focus.) A cardiac dysrhythmia (usually atrial fibrillation) or congestive heart failure may be the major feature(s). The most common cause of hyperthyroidism in this age group is toxic multinodular goiter (sometimes iodide induced), but the absence of a goiter may be seen in up to 25% of elderly patients (5% in young adults).

Serum T_3 may be of academic interest (and occasionally a higher T_4:T_3 ratio may help discriminate thyroiditis or toxic multinodular goiter from Graves' hyperthyroidism), but it is generally reserved for cases in which total T_4 and FT_4 values are normal. Thyroid-stimulating antibodies are of minor value in ruling out Graves' disease (usually a positive family history is obtained), but this diagnosis can be inferred from an elevated RAIU and diffuse scan order. Thyroid microsomal antibodies are a less expensive but less specific surrogate for Graves' disease. The RAIU is necessary to discriminate thyroid hyperfunction (autonomous nodule[s], receptor antibody, thyroid-stimulating hormone, or human chorionic gonadotropin driven) from subacute or silent thyroiditis, iatrogenic, or factitious causes. (Recent exposure to radiocontrast media or iodine-containing drugs or pregnancy may preclude its use, however.) A scan is of particular value when the clinician is unsure of the size and nature of the thyroid gland.

6. Management of the patient in the preceding question should include all of the following, *except*

a) Beta-blockers
b) Digoxin
c) Coumadin
d) Propylthiouracil
e) Stress doses of glucocorticoids

Answer and Discussion
The answer is e. Beta-blockers and propylthiouracil are helpful as primary therapy for hyperthyroidism in the elderly. Propylthiouracil is initiated only after the diagnosis is confirmed by a radioactive iodine uptake (and scan, if necessary). Radioactive iodine therapy may cause a transient worsening (radiation thyroiditis) of the hyperthyroidism and is often postponed in elderly patients until euthyroidism is attained (and antithyroid medication transiently withdrawn for 2 to 3 days before ^{131}I treatment). Digoxin is helpful in controlling the heart rate in atrial fibrillation. Coumadin is indicated in preventing embolic consequences of atrial fibrillation. The only drug not indicated without more data (the patient was not in "thyroid storm") is the glucocorticoid.

REFERENCES

1. Canaris GJ, Manowitz NR, Mayor G, et al. The Colorado thyroid disease prevalence study. *Arch Intern Med* 2000;160:526–534.
2. Danese MD, Powe NR, Sawin CT, et al. Screening for mild thyroid failure at the periodic health examination: a decision and cost-effectiveness analysis. *JAMA* 1996;276:285–292.
3. Haddow JE, Palomaki GE, Allan WC, et al. Maternal thyroid deficiency during pregnancy and subsequent neuropsychological development of the child. *N Engl J Med* 1999;341:549–555.
4. Bell DSH, Ovalle F. Use of soy protein supplement and resultant need for increased dose of levothyroxine. *Endocr Pract* 2001;7:193–194.
5. Bunevicius R, Kazanavicius G, Zalinkevicius R, et al. Effects of thyroxine as compared with thyroxine plus triiodothyronine in patients with hypothyroidism. *N Engl J Med* 1999;340:424–429.
6. Walsh JP, Shiels L, Lim EM, et al. Combined thyroxine/ liothyronine treatment does not improve well-being, quality of life, or cognitive function compared to thyroxine alone: a randomized controlled trial in patients with primary hypothyroidism. *J Clin Endocrinol Metab* 2003;88:4543–4550.
7. Sawka AM, Gerstein HC, Marriott MJ, et al. Does a combination regimen of thyroxine (T_4) and 3,5,3'–triiodothyronine improve depressive symptoms better than T_4 alone in patients with hypothyroidism? Results of a double-blind, randomized, controlled trial. *J Clin Endocrinol Metab* 2003;88:4551–4555.
8. Clyde PW, Harari AE, Getka EJ, et al. Combined levothyroxine plus liothyronine compared with levothyroxine alone in primary hypothyroidism: a randomized controlled trial. *JAMA* 2003;290:2952–2958.
9. Ladenson PW, Levin AA, Ridgway EC, et al. Complications of surgery in hypothyroid patients. *Am J Med* 1984;77:261–266.
10. Cooper DS. Hyperthyroidism. *Lancet* 2003;362:459–468.
11. Bergman TA, Mariash CN, Oppenheimer JH. Anterior mediastinal mass in a patient with Graves' disease. *J Clin Endocrinol Metab* 1982;55:587–588.
12. Goldstein R, Hart IR. Follow-up of solitary autonomous thyroid nodules treated with ^{131}I. *N Engl J Med* 1983;309:1473–1476.
13. Bartalena L, Marcocci C, Bogazzi F, et al. Relation between therapy for hyperthyroidism and the course of Graves' ophthalmopathy. *N Engl J Med* 1998;338:73–78.
14. Bartalena L, Marcocci C, Tanda ML, et al. Effect of cigarette smoking on treatment outcome of Graves' eye disease in patients receiving radioiodine ablation. *Ann Intern Med* 1998;129:632–635.
15. Surks MI, Ortiz E, Daniels GH, et al. Subclinical thyroid disease: scientific review and guidelines for diagnosis and management. *JAMA* 2004;291:228–238.
16. Col NF, Surks MI, Daniels GH. Subclinical thyroid disease: clinical applications. *JAMA* 2004;291:239–243.
17. Hermus AR, Huysmans DA. Treatment of benign nodular thyroid disease. *N Engl J Med* 1998;338:1438–1447.
18. Schlumberger JM. Papillary and follicular thyroid carcinoma. *N Engl J Med* 1998;338:297–306.
19. American Thyroid Association Guidelines Taskforce. Management guidelines for patients with thyroid nodules and differentiated thyroid Cancer. *Thyroid* 2006;16(2):1–33.

SUGGESTED READINGS

Abalovich M, Amino N, Barbour LA, et al. Management of thyroid dysfunction during pregnancy and postpartum: an Endocrine Society clinical practice guideline. *J Clin Endocrinol Metab* 2007; 92(8 Suppl 1):S1-S47.
Barbot N, Calmettes C, Schuffenecker I, et al. Pentagastrin stimulation test and early diagnosis of medullary thyroid carcinoma using an immunoradiometric assay of calcitonin: comparison with genetic screening in hereditary medullary thyroid carcinoma. *J Clin Endocrinol Metab* 1994;78:114–120.
Borst GC, Eil C, Burman KD. Euthyroid hyperthyroxinemia. *Ann Intern Med* 1983;98:366–378.
Brent GA, Hershman JM. Thyroxine therapy in patients with severe nonthyroidal illnesses and low serum thyroxine concentration. *J Clin Endocrinol Metab* 1986;63:1–8.

Campbell NRC, Hasinoff BB, Stalts H, et al. Ferrous sulfate reduces thyroxine efficacy in patients with hypothyroidism. *Ann Intern Med* 1992;117:1010–1013.
Cavalieri RR, Gerard SK. Unusual types of thyrotoxicosis. *Adv Intern Med* 1991;36:271–286.
Cooper DS. Antithyroid drugs. *N Engl J Med* 1984;311:1353–1362.
Dayan CM. Interpretation of thyroid function tests. *Lancet* 2001; 357:619–624.
De los Santos ET, Starich GH, Mazzaferri EL. Sensitivity, specificity, and cost-effectiveness of the sensitive thyrotropin assay in the diagnosis of thyroid disease in ambulatory patients. *Arch Intern Med* 1989;149:526–532.
DeGroot LJ. Long-term impact of initial and surgical therapy on papillary and follicular thyroid cancer. *Am J Med* 1994;97:499–500.
Docter R, Krenning EP, de Jong M, et al. The sick euthyroid syndrome: changes in thyroid hormone serum parameters and hormone metabolism. *Clin Endocrinol* 1993;39:499–518.
Dolan JG. Hyperthyroidism and hypothyroidism. In: Panzer RJ, Black ER, Griner PF, eds. *Diagnostic Strategies for Common Medical Problems*. Philadelphia: American College of Physicians, 1991;375–384.
Farrar JJ, Toth AD. Iodine-131 treatment of hyperthyroidism: current issues. *Clin Endocrinol* 1991;35:207–212.
Fisher DA. Screening for congenital hypothyroidism. *Trends Endocrinol Metab* 1991;2:129–133.
Garrity JA, Bahn RS. Pathogenesis of Graves' ophthalmopathy: implications for prediction, prevention, and treatment. *Am J Ophthalmol* 2006;142(1):147-153.
Gharib H. Subclinical thyroid dysfunction: a joint statement on management from the American Association of Clinical Endocrinologists, the American Thyroid Association, and the Endocrine Society. *J Clin Endocrinol Metab* 2005;90(1):581-585; discussion 586-587.
Gharib H, Goellner JR. Fine-needle aspiration biopsy of the thyroid: an appraisal. *Ann Intern Med* 1993;118:282–289.
Hamburger JI. The various presentations of thyroiditis: diagnostic considerations. *Ann Intern Med* 1986;104:219–224.
Helfand M, Crapo LM. Monitoring therapy in patients taking levothyroxine. *Ann Intern Med* 1990;113:450–454.
Helfand M, Crapo LM. Screening for thyroid disease. *Ann Intern Med* 1990;112:840–849. (See letters to the editor: *Ann Intern Med* 1990;113:896–897.)
Klein I, Ojamaa K. Thyroid hormone and the cardiovascular system. *N Engl J Med* 2001;344:501–509.
Ladenson PW, Braverman LE, Mazzaferri EL, et al. Comparison of administration of recombinant human thyrotropin with withdrawal of thyroid hormone for radioactive iodine scanning in patients with thyroid carcinoma. *N Engl J Med* 1997;337:888–896.
LeBeau SO, Mandel SJ. Thyroid disorders during pregnancy. *Endocrinol Metab Clin North Am* 2006;35(1):117–136, vii.
Ledger GA, Khosla S, Lindor NM, et al. Genetic testing in the diagnosis and management of multiple endocrine neoplasia type II. *Ann Intern Med* 1995;122:118–124.
Liel Y, Sperber AD, Shang S. Nonspecific intestinal adsorption of levothyroxine by aluminum hydroxide. *Am J Med* 1994;97:363–365.
Lips CJM, Landsvater RM, Hoppener JWM, et al. Clinical screening as compared with DNA analysis in families with multiple endocrine neoplasia type 2A. *N Engl J Med* 1994;331:828–835.
Mandel SJ, Brent GA, Larsen PR. Levothyroxine therapy in patients with thyroid disease. *Ann Intern Med* 1993;119:492–502.
Mandel SJ, Larsen PR, Seeley EW, et al. Increased need for thyroxine during pregnancy in women with primary hypothyroidism. *N Engl J Med* 1990;323:91–95.
March DE, Desai AG, Park CH, et al. Struma ovarii: hyperthyroidism in a postmenopausal woman. *J Nucl Med* 1988;29:263–265.
Mazzaferri EL. Long-term impact of initial surgical and medical therapy on papillary and follicular thyroid cancer. *Am J Med* 1994;97:418–428.
Mazzaferri EL. Management of a solitary thyroid nodule. *N Engl J Med* 1993;328:553–559.
McDougall IR. Graves' disease: current concepts. *Med Clin North Am* 1991;75:79–95.
Mulligan DC, McHenry CR, Kinney W, et al. Amiodarone-induced thyrotoxicosis: clinical presentation and expanded indications for thyroidectomy. *Surgery* 1993;114:1114–1119.

Pineda JD, Lee T, Ain K, et al. Iodine-131 therapy for thyroid cancer patients with elevated thyroglobulin and negative diagnostic scan. *J Clin Endocrinol Metab* 1995;80:1488–1492.

Refetoff S, Lever EG. The value of serum thyroglobulin measurement in clinical practice. *JAMA* 1983;250:2352–2357.

Rosenbaum D, Davies TF. The clinical use of thyroid autoantibodies. *Endocrinologist* 1992;2:55–62.

Schectman JM, Pawlson LG. The cost-effectiveness of three thyroid function testing strategies for suspicion of hypothyroidism in a primary care setting. *J Gen Intern Med* 1990;5:9–15.

Sherman SI, Tielens ET, Ladenson PW. Sucralfate causes malabsorption of L-thyroxine. *Am J Med* 1994;96:531–535.

Slag MF, Morley JE, Elson MK, et al. Hypothyroxinemia in critically ill patients as a predictor of high mortality. *JAMA* 1981;245:43–45.

Stagnaro-Green A. Postpartum thyroiditis: prevalence, etiology, and clinical importance. *Thyroid Today* 1993;16:1–11.

Surks MI, Chopra IJ, Mariash CN, et al. American Thyroid Association guidelines for use of laboratory tests in thyroid disorders. *JAMA* 1990;263:1529–1532.

Surks MI, Sievert R. Drugs and thyroid function. *N Engl J Med* 1995;333:1688–1694.

Surks MI, Smith PJ. Multiple effects of 5,5′-diphenylhydantoin on the thyroid hormone system. *Endocrinol Rev* 1984;5:514–524.

U.S. Preventive Services Task Force. Screening for thyroid disease: recommendation statement. *Am Fam Physician* 2004;69(10):2415–2418.

Van Middlesworth L. Effects of radiation on the thyroid gland. *Adv Intern Med* 1989;34:265–284.

Weetman AP, McGregor AM. Autoimmune thyroid disease: further developments in our understanding. *Endocrinol Rev* 1994;15:788–830.

Weiss RE, Refetoff S. Thyroid hormone resistance. *Annu Rev Med* 1992;43:363–375.

Whitley RJ, et al. Thyroglobulin: a specific serum marker for the management of thyroid carcinoma. *Clin Lab Med* 2004;24(1):29-47.

Wiener JD. A systematic approach to the diagnosis of Plummer's disease (autonomous goitre), with a review of 224 cases. *Neth J Med* 1975;18:218–233.

Woeber KA. Thyrotoxicosis and the heart. *N Engl J Med* 1992;327:94–98.

Wong TK, Hershman JM. Changes in thyroid function in nonthyroidal illness. *Trends Endocrinol Metab* 1992;3:8–11.

Yassa R, Saunders A, Nastase C, et al. Lithium-induced thyroid disorders: a prevalence study. *J Clin Psychiatry* 1988;49:14–16.

Chapter 41

Female Reproductive Disorders

Adi E. Mehta

👋➕ POINTS TO REMEMBER:

■ Androgen excess is one of the most common endocrine disorders in women, affecting 2% to 8% of all women, and is the most common cause of anovulatory infertility.

■ The most common presentation of androgenic disorders in women is with a complaint of hirsutism, possibly with acne, and irregular and infrequent menses.

■ Polycystic ovary syndrome (PCOS) frequently presents as hirsutism (70%–75%), oligomenorrhea (50%), and resulting infertility. Obesity and insulin resistance leading to diabetes may be present (30%–40%).

■ The presence of the Y chromosome in a phenotypic female subject requires the operative removal of the gonads because they are considered precancerous.

Androgen excess is one of the most common endocrine disorders in women, affecting 2% to 8% of all women. It is the most common cause of anovulatory infertility. The clinical manifestations can vary significantly, from dermatologic manifestations such as hirsutism or acne to menstrual irregularities, amenorrhea, and, rarely, virilization. Prognostically, whereas the short-term manifestations are a cosmetic nuisance and can cause great psychologic and emotional distress because of relatively reduced fecundity, the long-term morbidity and mortality are marked and expensive, causing diabetes, dyslipidemia, and cardiovascular disease.

ANDROGENIC DISORDERS

Anatomy and Physiology of Androgenic Sources

The ovaries and adrenal glands are the source of androgens in women. Androgens may be secreted, in small amounts, as biologically active androgens or may serve as precursor compounds for conversion to active androgens in the periphery. Both ovaries and adrenals produce the hormones in response to their tropic hormones—luteinizing hormone (LH) and adrenocorticotropic hormone (ACTH), respectively—but the androgens cannot act as powerful negative-feedback control hormones for the pituitary. Thus, their secretion is not self-controlled.

The major products of adrenal secretion are dehydroepiandrosterone sulfate (DHEAS), dehydroepiandrosterone (DHEA), and androstenedione; the major ovarian secretory product is androstenedione. Approximately half the circulating levels of testosterone in women are secreted from both glandular sources, whereas the rest is made by peripheral conversion of 17-ketosteroids in the liver, skin, and adipose tissue.

Transport in Serum

The bulk of active androgen (and estradiol, E2) is tightly bound in the circulation to sex hormone–binding globulin (SHBG) of hepatic origin. Lesser binding to albumin also occurs. Thus, only small amounts of free (unbound) sex steroids are present. SHBG production by the liver is influenced by the androgen-to-estrogen balance as well as by thyroid hormone. Estrogen and thyroid hormone stimulate SHBG production. Androgen is inhibitory.

Biological Activity of Androgens

The major biologically active androgen in most target tissues is dihydrotestosterone, which is formed by the conversion of testosterone under the influence of 5-α reductase, which is present in the skin and external genitalia. The effect of androgen on target tissues is thought to be mediated by the ratio of free testosterone to free E2 in the circulation. Thus, simple measurements of total testosterone or E2 may be misleading.

The SHBG multiplier effect can be summarized as follows:

- Hepatic SHBG production is influenced by the androgen-to-estrogen status.

- Binding kinetics for testosterone and E2 to this protein are different. (As SHBG concentration falls under an androgenic influence, a greater increment in unbound testosterone occurs, compared with unbound E2.)
- Androgen excess begets androgen excess.

Clinical Presentation of Androgenic Disorders

The most common presentation of androgenic disorders in women is with a complaint of hirsutism, possibly with acne, and irregular and infrequent menses. Obesity is not an uncommon associated finding in such individuals.

Specific Androgenic Disorders

Polycystic Ovary Syndrome

The 1990 National Institutes of Health consensus criteria define *polycystic ovary syndrome* as the invariable presence of chronic oligo-ovulation or anovulation associated with hyperandrogenism (i.e., signs of androgen excess, such as acne, alopecia, or hirsutism, even without clearly elevated serum androgen levels) in the absence of other known causes of androgen excess, such as congenital adrenal hyperplasia, tumor, or hyperprolactinemia. In 2003, the Rotterdam workshop criteria included polycystic ovarian morphology by ultrasound, requiring two of the three criteria for the diagnosis. The contemporary version for the definition was provided by the Androgen Excess Society in 2006, which highlighted clinical or biochemical hyperandrogenism in combination with functional or ultrasonographic abnormalities in ovarian function. Although there may be associated abnormal gonadotropins or abnormal insulin regulation, these do not have to be invariably present to make the diagnosis.

Pathophysiology

The pathophysiology of PCOS is unclear, but numerous theories exist. Most point to the establishment of a vicious cycle of events, possibly initiated by the presence of two phenomena normally occurring in puberty that in the predisposed person sets this cycle in motion: an early increase in LH and androgen levels as well as insulin resistance. Three proposed theories encompass both phenomena:

- The *LH theory* hypothesizes a primary neuroendocrine defect that causes an exaggerated LH pulse frequency in amplitude.
- The *insulin theory* hypothesizes that PCOS is initiated by the familial presence of decreased peripheral insulin sensitivity and resultant hyperinsulinemia, which is further aggravated by the physiological insulin resistance induced by puberty. Such hyperinsulinemia inhibits the production of insulinlike growth factor 1 (IGF-1)–binding protein and SHBG in the liver. This results in an increased concentration of free IGF-1. In the ovary, both insulin and IGF-1, working in synergy with LH, stimulate

thecal androgen production, possibly by stimulating an existing defect in insulin receptor autophosphorylation: Instead of the usual tyrosine phosphorylation, a unique change occurs in the phosphorylation of the insulin receptor by serine, causing it to have an increased basal activity but decreased insulin responsivity. Thus, both the increased insulin levels and the higher androgen levels lower SHBG, thus further increasing free androgens.

- The *ovarian theory* hypothesizes that a genetic defect exists in the ovary, leading to increased steroidogenic activity. Such a defect is characterized by a dysregulation of the ovarian P450 C17 enzyme due to an increased serine phosphorylation, which increases androgen production, especially in the presence of increased levels of LH and insulin.

Predispositions to the development of PCOS include:

- A family history of noninsulin-dependent diabetes mellitus
- Maternal gestational diabetes mellitus
- Borderline adrenal hyperplasia accentuated by the pubertal adrenarche
- Occult hypothyroidism
- Childhood obesity

In the PCOS-predisposed person, LH and androgen levels are higher, whereas in the healthy person, ovulating cycles decrease LH and attenuate the insulin resistance of puberty; in PCOS-predisposed persons, this does not occur. Thus, PCOS is sometimes termed *hyperpuberty*.

Clinical PCOS frequently presents as hirsutism (70%–75%), oligomenorrhea (50%), and resulting infertility. Obesity and insulin resistance leading to diabetes may be present (30%–40%). Biochemically, an elevation of LH values is frequent (up to 75%), and some schools emphasize an elevated LH-to-follicle-stimulating hormone (FSH) ratio (more than 2:1 or 3:1). Androgens, especially ovarian androgens, are elevated, and adrenal androgens (DHEA) may have up to a twofold increase.

Metabolic Consequences
The following summarize the metabolic consequences of PCOS:

- Insulin resistance is present in a large percentage of women with PCOS.
- Insulin resistance can be present in nonobese women with PCOS as well as in obese women with PCOS, although a percentage of lean women with PCOS are not insulin resistant.
- The insulin resistance manifests more peripherally in muscle than in the liver.
- Insulin potentiates LH-stimulated androgen production from the theca and stroma of the ovary.
- The ovary is not resistant to insulin in the face of the peripheral muscle and adipose tissue insulin resistance.

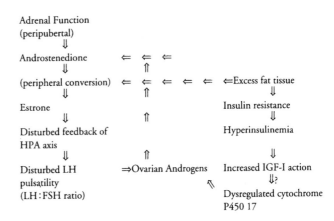

Figure 41.1 The proposed theoretic basis of polycystic ovary syndrome. (FSH, follicle-stimulating hormone; HPA, hypothalamic-pituitary-adrenal; IGF-1, insulinlike growth factor 1; LH, luteinizing hormone.)

- Acanthosis nigricans, a marker of insulin resistance, can be seen but may fade with the reduction of circulating insulin and androgens.
- An increased waist-to-hip ratio is commonly associated with the elevated androgens.

The proposed theoretic basis of PCOS appears in Figure 41.1.

The late consequences of acne, hirsutism, PCOS, and relative subfecundity include:

- Infertility
- Hyperlipidemia
- Hypertension
- Late development of noninsulin-dependent diabetes mellitus
- Increased risk of endometrial and breast cancer
- Cardiovascular disease

These later associations with hyperlipidemia, hypertension, and noninsulin-dependent diabetes mellitus form the metabolic syndrome as defined in the NCEP-ATP III guidelines, which predispose to premature cardiac disease.

Hirsutism
Hirsutism, or excess terminal (sexual) hair in a woman, is characterized by two types of hair:

- Vellus (small diameter, soft texture, and nonmedullated)
- Terminal (large diameter, coarse, medullated), usually found in sex hormone–sensitive skin. This hair is androgen dependent for growth.

Etiology
The causes of hirsutism and virilization include:

- Genetic, racial, atavistic traits (e.g., Mediterranean women)
- Iatrogenic conditions

- Drug side effects
  - Hormones (oral contraceptive pill [OCP], anabolic steroids)
  - Diphenylhydantoin
  - Hexachlorobenzene
  - Diazoxide
  - Cyclosporine
  - Minoxidil (nonsteroidal drugs cause hypertrichosis)
- Adrenal conditions
  - Congenital adrenal hyperplasia (adult-onset variant)
  - Benign and malignant tumors
  - Cushing syndrome
  - Prolactin or growth hormone excess
- Ovarian conditions
  - Idiopathic hirsutism
  - PCOS (Stein-Leventhal)
  - Stromal hyperthecosis (likely a more severe variant of PCOS)
  - Virilizing neoplasms
  - Ovarian steroidogenic block
  - Hermaphroditism
  - Human chorionic gonadotropin (hCG)
  - Peripheral androgen overproduction
  - Obesity
- Other

Diagnosis

In diagnosing hirsutism and virilization, the clinician must attempt to answer several important questions:

Is hirsutism present? Is it because of androgen excess?

Hypertrichosis, which is nonsexual excessive hair growth (i.e., due to ethnic causes, in malnutrition, owing to nonsteroidal drugs), is not associated with virilism. Hirsutism is defined as excessive sexual hair growth (pubic, axillary, abdominal, chest, facial). This hair is coarse and pigmented.

What is the degree of virilism?

Acne and hirsutism are the earliest (and frequently the only) signs of excessive circulating androgen(s).

Anovulation and oligomenorrhea–amenorrhea manifest relatively early in ovarian conditions but tend to appear later in adrenal disorders. Frontal balding, clitoromegaly, low-pitched voice, and increased muscularity indicate marked androgenic stimulation.

What are the points of importance for differential diagnoses?

- Onset
  - Peripubertal (usually benign)
  - Prepubertal or late postpubertal (more ominous)
- Progression
  - Slow or static (benign)
  - Progressive (malignant)
- Family history (positive points to benign)
- Libido enhancement of recent onset (inauspicious)

- Medication use
- Menstrual regularity (uncommon in face of excess androgen)

What is the source of androgen?

- Rule out exogenous sources
- Rule out neoplasia; sudden onset and rapid progression suggest neoplasm (abdominal or pelvic masses)
- High androgen levels (i.e., 17-ketosteroids, DHEAS, testosterone)
- Cushing disease (rare among obese, hirsute women—adult-onset congenital adrenal hyperplasia may be common; produces excess androgen)

Other functional syndromes may have an ovarian or adrenal origin (at present, these cannot be distinguished by dynamic stimulation or suppression tests; indeed, having ruled out organic disease, the definition of the precise source has little practical significance).

Laboratory Tests

Laboratory tests used to diagnosis hirsutism or virilization include:

- Serum DHEAS or urinary (24-hour) 17-ketosteroids (useful to rule out adrenal neoplasms)
- Serum testosterone
  - Into the normal male range (>8 nmol/L) in ovarian (or adrenal) neoplasms
  - Mild to moderately elevated in most cases of PCOS
  - Normal or borderline high (slightly >2 nmol/L) in idiopathic hirsutism
- 17-OH-progesterone (may pick up an occasional adult congenital adrenal hyperplasia case)
- Index of free testosterone or testosterone-to-SHBG ratios where available (often elevated, even when total testosterone levels are normal)
- Other steroids (e.g., androstenedione or metabolites) are of little additional help
  - 5-Androstanediol glucuronide of questionable additional benefit
  - Serum prolactin (elevations may be associated with PCOS)
- Thyroid function tests (hirsutism may be seen in primary hypothyroidism)
- Anatomic studies generally not indicated

Treatment

The treatment regimen for hirsutism includes:

- Treating the organic disease
- Weight loss by diet and exercise in obese women to reduce androgens and insulin
- Medical therapy
  - Glucocorticoids
  - Estrogen and progestin (OCP)
  - Antiandrogens

- Cyproterone acetate and estrogen (OCP)
- Spironolactone
- Flutamide
- Finasteride
- Cimetidine
- Gonadotropic (gonadotropin-releasing hormone [GnRH]) analogs
- Ketoconazole
- Local application of steroids
- Progesterone
- Cyproterone
- Local treatment
  - Shaving
  - Chemical depilatories
  - Wax depilation
  - Bleaching
  - Electrolysis
  - Laser removal of hair
- Ovulation induction (if major complaint is infertility)

The most commonly used insulin sensitizers are metformin and troglitazone. By increasing insulin sensitivity and lowering insulin levels, insulin sensitizers have been shown to reduce androgens and restore menstrual cyclicity or reestablish responsivity to inducers of ovulation. Although earlier therapy for hirsutism—whether of PCOS origin or idiopathic in women not interested in fertility—was an oral contraceptive pill (OCP) containing an antiandrogen, increasing reports now indicate that insulin sensitizer therapy with or without an OCP may be of greater benefit both for the present and for the future in terms of preventing the progression of disease to features of the metabolic syndrome.

Reassurance and support is essential to good outcomes, because treatment requires patience and perseverance; most treatments require 8 to 14 months to achieve a clinical effect.

Amenorrhea

Amenorrhea is the absolute lack of menses for more than 3 months in a woman with previously regular cycles (secondary amenorrhea) or no menses by the age of 16 years (primary amenorrhea).

Diagnosis

It is important to ascertain whether amenorrhea is primary or secondary and whether it is anatomic, owing to hormonal or functional hormone dysregulation, or because of other endocrine or systemic illnesses. The classification breakdown for amenorrhea includes:

- Anatomic
- Primary
  - Congenital uterine absence
  - Cryptomenorrhea
- Secondary
  - Asherman syndrome

- Iatrogenic
- Hysterectomy/oophorectomy
- Chromosomal
  - XO/XO mosaic (Turner syndrome)
  - XY androgen insensitivity
- Hormonal/functional (could be primary but more frequently secondary)
  - Pregnancy
  - Prolactin excess
  - Androgen excess
  - Weight loss
  - Excessive exercise
  - Anorexia nervosa
  - Excessive weight gain
  - Emotional stress
  - Hypopituitarism
  - Ovarian failure
- Other illnesses (usually secondary amenorrhea, occasionally primary)
- Other endocrine diseases
  - Hyperthyroidism/hypothyroidism
  - Adrenal disease
  - Diabetes mellitus
  - Chronic systemic illnesses
  - Crohn disease
  - Ulcerative colitis
  - Rheumatoid arthritis

Laboratory Studies

After ruling out pregnancy as a cause for the amenorrhea, an evaluation of gonadotropin, estrogen, androgen, prolactin, and thyrotropin levels, general chemistry, and a complete blood cell count are usually required. In primary amenorrhea or amenorrhea occurring after only a few irregular cycles in young persons, a karyotype is also indicated.

Treatment

The treatment of amenorrhea is groomed to the patient's requirements and may include simple gonadal steroid replacement; correcting the underlying etiologic disorder, if possible; psychiatric or psychosocial support; and the reestablishment of puberty using exogenous medications or hormones or the newer reproductive technologies. It is important to remember that the presence of the Y chromosome in a phenotypic female subject requires the operative removal of the gonads, as they are considered precancerous.

Premature Ovarian Failure

Growing evidence in the literature indicates that premature ovarian failure (POF) is multifactorial and encompasses a spectrum of clinical presentations, including:

- Permanent hypergonadotropic amenorrhea
- The apparent presence of a prematurely early perimenopausal state

■ A condition waxing and waning from normogonadotropic menstrual cycles
■ Hypergonadotropic amenorrhea

Etiology

The mean age at menopause in North America, 52 years, appears to be unrelated to the age of menarche or to parity, ethnic extraction, nutrition, or environmental factors. Menopause, owing to ovarian failure and the virtual absence of primordial follicles in the ovary, is characterized by low E2 levels, amenorrhea, and sustained elevation of gonadotropin levels. The final cessation of menses may be preceded by 2 to 10 years of progressively irregular cycles with prolonged intermenstrual intervals. During this time, gonadotropins, particularly FSH, may be variably elevated, but E2 levels are usually normal, ovulation is sporadic, and hot flashes are common.

Studies indicate a correlation between the size of the residual follicular stock and the preservation of more normal menstrual function at this stage. Although the primary cause of cessation of menstrual function is no doubt because of the disappearance of ovarian follicles, the nature of pituitary–ovarian interrelationships and a change in the ovarian milieu may help to explain the apparent gonadotropin resistance and relative infertility at this stage.

Because fewer than 2% of women reach menopause before the age of 40 years, this is the currently accepted cutoff for the definition of premature menopause. The etiology of POF is outlined in Table 41.1.

The classification of POF based on the presence or absence of follicles on an ovarian biopsy (at a particular time point) may be overly simplistic because the factors that govern the number of endowed ova, the rate of follicular atresia, the changes in ovarian steroid and peptide hormone production, and the intraovarian milieu as a function of age remain poorly understood.

Autoimmune Oophoritis

Circulating antibodies against some ovarian component (including gonadotropin receptors) define the condition of autoimmune oophoritis in patients presenting with primary or secondary hypoestrogenic, hypergonadotropic amenorrhea and the biopsy-proven presence of ovarian follicles. This occurs in 15% to 40% of such patients. Follicular lymphocytic infiltration, often transient, also may be found in ovarian biopsy specimens, particularly during the early evolution of the condition.

Variables such as the type of antigen used, assay technique, and the time of testing in relationship to disease onset appear to be of critical importance in the detection of this disorder. This concept should not seem surprising in light of identical issues that apply to the prototypic autoimmune glandular disease Hashimoto thyroiditis. In this condition, the antibody mix is heterogenous (organ damaging, antienzyme, growth promoting, receptor agonist, re-

TABLE 41.1
ETIOLOGIC CLASSIFICATION OF PREMATURE OVARIAN FAILURE

Chromosomal
  ■ X-linked: Turner syndrome and variants
  ■ Familial long arm X deletion
  ■ Triple X syndrome
  ■ Autosomal
  ■ Trisomy 13
  ■ Trisomy 18
Enzymatic defects
  ■ 17hydroxylase deficiency
  ■ Galactosemia
Gonadotropin apparatus defects
  ■ Abnormal gonadotropin molecules
  ■ Abnormal gonadotropin receptors
Infection
  ■ Tuberculosis
  ■ Mumps
  ■ Others
Iatrogenic
Surgery
Chemotherapy
Irradiation
Vascular
Torsion/Hemorrhage
Immunologic
Deficiency
Ataxia-telangiectasia
DiGeorge syndrome
Autoimmune diseases
Oophoritis
Idiopathic
  ■ With follicles
  ■ Resistant ovary syndrome
  ■ Afollicular

ceptor blocking); the antibody mix is not fixed in proportion with time (the response varies with the antibody mix and the state of the thyroid gland at a particular time, so transient or permanent hypofunction of the thyroid gland may occur); and the antibodies may disappear after organ death.

The coexistence of autoimmune POF in patients with Addison disease may be as frequent as 25% and may relate to the presence of antibodies directed against the common steroidogenic enzymes shared by the two organs. The association of POF with hypothyroidism is less frequent but more so than in the general population. As with type I diabetes mellitus and Hashimoto thyroiditis, there is an HLA-DR3 locus association with autoimmune oophoritis.

Idiopathic Premature Ovarian Failure and the Resistant Ovary Syndrome

A significant proportion of women with POF, in whom circulating autoantibodies are either not detected or not looked for, and for whom no other cause has been identified, are defined as having idiopathic POF. If ovarian follicles are present, the term *resistant ovary syndrome* has been used to define the condition. The presence or absence of follicles in patients presenting with POF is pivotal, not only for establishing a diagnosis but also in delineating therapeutic options.

Diagnosis

The patient history and physical examination may help to establish the diagnosis of POF. Documentation requires the presence of hypoestrogenemic hypergonadotropism, especially on more than on one occasion. A karyotype is mandatory in primary amenorrhea and can be helpful in secondary amenorrhea as well. Searching for antibodies may be helpful; a positive finding opens up a number of therapeutic options. Testing is generally not available, however, and the procedures have not been standardized.

Establishing the presence or absence of primordial follicles in the ovary is crucial. The gold standard has been a full-thickness biopsy of the ovary to look for primordial follicles. The results are qualitative and presume appropriate representation in the specimen obtained—the major disadvantage of such biopsies. Moreover, the ensuing potential risk of adhesions and mechanical infertility is added to the already e╌╌╌ ╌╌╌╌╌te. Thus, attempts have ╌╌╌╌╌ ╌╌╌╌e transvaginal ultrasound ╌╌╌╌llicles. The data are still ╌╌╌╌ and accuracy of such an ╌╌╌╌

╌╌╌d methods to treat POF ╌╌╌e availability of success-╌╌╌on, and embryo-transfer ╌╌╌biological offspring, the ╌╌╌fferentiate better the het-╌╌╌s is crucial if successful ╌╌╌atment programs are to

╌╌╌rdial follicles, if clearly ╌╌╌cept by donor in vitro ╌╌╌ients with immunologic ╌╌╌imordial follicles might ╌╌╌gh-dose glucocorticoids or plasmapheresis.

Other patients might benefit from megadoses of exogenous gonadotropins or short-term downregulation by estrogen.

Estrogens also may act by ameliorating the autoimmune process. Such regimens have been variably reported to yield successful pregnancies. A more recent approach has been the downregulation by GnRH agonists, followed by attempts at ovulation induction using exogenous gonadotropins.

Overall, the success of therapeutic intervention has been remarkably small, and most schools of thought are that

such attempts are futile. The easy, safe, and highly successful egg donation and in vitro fertilization programs have, therefore, mainly replaced all such endeavors.

MALE ENDOCRINE DISORDERS

Male Hypogonadism

Male hypogonadism is defined as the failure to produce testosterone or sperm.

Etiology

Hypogonadism is usually classified as primary or secondary, according to its cause:

- Primary
  - Genetic disease
  - Klinefelter syndrome
  - Androgen-resistance syndrome
  - Steroidogenic enzyme defects
  - Congenital anorchia
  - Infection
  - Iatrogenic causes
  - Drug side effects
  - Chemotherapy
  - Radiation
  - Vasectomy
  - Toxin exposure (mercury, cadmium)
- Secondary
  - Endocrine disorders
  - Pubertal delay
  - Hypopituitarism
  - Hypothalamic
  - Kallmann syndrome
  - Hyperprolactinemia
  - Adrenal gland dysfunction
  - Thyroid gland dysfunction
  - Systemic illness
  - Malnutrition
  - Weight loss
  - Anorexia nervosa
  - Cancer
  - Drug

Specific Hypogonadism Conditions

Klinefelter Syndrome

Klinefelter syndrome is a chromosomal disorder characterized by the presence of one or two extra X chromosomes, XXY or XXXY. The syndrome occurs in about 1 in 500 male births. The characteristics of the disorder include:

- Presence of variable androgen deficiency
- On average, taller patients, with disproportionate lower segment growth
- Small testes

TABLE 41.2

UNCOMMON TESTICULAR DISORDERS

Testicular Disorder	Association/Cause
Hypogonadotropic hypogonadism	Craniofacial anomalies
Congenital deafness	
Intellectual impairment	
Cerebellar ataxia	
Laurence-Moon-Biedl syndrome	
Prader-Willi syndrome	
Hemochromatosis	
Anorexia nervosa	
Excessive exercise	
Primary hypogonadism	Myotonic dystrophy
Noonan syndrome	
Reifenstein syndrome	
Androgen receptor defects	
Absent vasa deferentia	Cystic fibrosis
Zero motility (cilial defects)	Kartagener syndrome
Varicocele	Renal carcinoma
Renal malformations	
Testicular infarction/Orchitis	Polyarteritis nodosa
Hemophilia	
Sickle cell anemia	
Brucellosis	
Gonorrhea	

- Azoospermia
- Gynecomastia
- Hypergonadotropic hypogonadism

Uncommon Testicular Disorders

Table 41.2 presents uncommon testicular disorders.

Clinical Presentation

Peripubertally, hypogonadism presents as an absence of secondary sex characteristics, including:

- Small testes
- Penis indicating a lack of development
- Eunuchoid proportions (arm span >5 cm longer than height)

Postpubertally, the cardinal features are:

- Decreased libido
- Impotence
- Loss of secondary sexual hair
- Wrinkled skin
- Testicular atrophy
- Little change in penile size

Diagnosis

In laboratory investigation, a check for gonadotropins, prolactin, and testosterone is needed. If the patient is found to be hypogonadotropic with or without hyperprolactinemia, a standard evaluation should be done to rule out hy-pothalamic or pituitary abnormality. If the patient is hypergonadotropic, karyotyping should be done.

Treatment

The treatment of male hypogonadism usually is geared to replacement. In hypogonadotropic persons, fertility may be stimulated by the use of gonadotropins.

Erectile Dysfunction

Erectile dysfunction (ED), formerly termed *impotence*, is the consistent inability to achieve or maintain an erection sufficient for satisfactory sexual activity.

In the United States, ED is estimated to affect as many as 30 million men. The incidence of ED increases with age, but it is not a necessary consequence of aging. It may be significantly underdiagnosed because of a reluctance on the part of patients to discuss the problem with their equally reluctant caregivers.

Simplistically, ED can be organic or psychogenic, although most cases have a combination of the two. Some of the causes of ED include:

- Inflammation
- Mechanical injury
- Psychologic disorders
- Occlusive-vascular disorders
- Traumatic or operative injury
- Endurance-related disorders
- Neurologic disorders
- Chemical exposures
- Endocrine disorders

Up to 35% (in one study) of patients with impotence have an endocrine cause, usually an easy diagnosis to make and relatively easy and gratifying to treat. Common endocrine causes include hypogonadotropic hypogonadism (Kallmann syndrome), hypergonadotropic hypogonadism (Klinefelter syndrome), hyperprolactinemia, and diabetes mellitus.

In hyperprolactinemia, the impotence is thought to develop through two mechanisms:

- A direct feedback of prolactin on the GnRH neurons in the hypothalamus by the ultrashort-loop feedback (the major operative mechanism), whereby GnRH pulsatility, and thus LH pulsatility, is dampened, slowed, and therefore made significantly dysfunctional. Consequently, no stimulation of the testes occurs, and hypogonadotropic hypogonadism ensues.
- A direct effect on the "libidigenous" center by prolactin and a resultant decreased sexual interest and drive. Thus, testosterone supplementation alone is not always or totally effective in restoring libido and potency, and normoprolactinemia usually is required for the full effect of testosterone to be manifested.

Diabetes mellitus is probably the most common cause of impotence. Whereas the patient's age is a factor (i.e., older men are more likely to develop impotence than younger men), the duration of diabetes is also an important variable in the tendency to develop impotence. The longer the duration of diabetes, the higher the incidence of impotence. Etiologically, the impotence of diabetes is caused by the combination of vasculopathy and neuropathy, the relative contribution of each being variable in any one patient. Psychogenic factors may play a significant role early in the disorder: The expectation and fear of failing after one failure commonly worsen the problem initially, and the decreased sensation of orgasm and ejaculation because of neuropathy and retrograde ejaculation takes its toll. Actual hormonal deficiency secondary to diabetes is being reported more frequently; usually, the testosterone level is at the low normal range, and there are reports of improvement of sexual as well as more general symptoms.

Physiology of Erection and Pathophysiology of Erectile Dysfunction

Penile erection occurs because of a series of events that cause a relaxation of the smooth muscle in the corpus cavernosa. Noradrenergic, noncholinergic neurons acting on the endothelial cells generate nitric oxide, which activates guanylate cyclase and fosters the change of guanosine triphosphate to cyclic guanosine monophosphate (cGMP). cGMP causes relaxation and penile erection; however, cGMP is rapidly metabolized by phosphodiesterase-5 (PDE-5) to guanosine monophosphate (GMP), thus relaxation and erection are not maintained. Any agent causing an increase in nitric oxide, and therefore activation to cGMP, or alternatively slowing the breakdown of cGMP by inhibiting PDE-5, causes and maintains penile erection.

Diagnosis

The clinical aspects to be considered in the evaluation of impotence include an evaluation of hormonal function, both by history (libido, hair growth, gynecomastia, previous fertility, and history of alcohol or drug abuse) and by physical examination (hair distribution, body habitus, testes size, prostate size, visual fundi and fields, evidence of other endocrinopathy, and evidence of other illnesses). In the investigation of impotence, in addition to an evaluation of testosterone, gonadotropin, and prolactin levels, it is important to evaluate vascular integrity using Doppler flow studies and neurogenic integrity by the snap gauge test or the more cumbersome nocturnal penile tumescence evaluation. There is no place for an oral glucose tolerance test in the evaluation of impotence. A growing body of evidence shows that the presence of ED is a powerful indicator for the presence of various cardiovascular risk factors and, in fact, may reveal clinically significant but still silent cardiovascular disease in as many as 60% of ED patients. Thus, asking the question may reveal more than just an easily treated, personally embarrassing, awkward situation.

Treatment

The goal of treatment is to find the underlying cause, if possible. Otherwise, testosterone replacement, if needed, can be quite helpful. If no clear cause is found, attempts to induce erection remain the mainstay. Herbal remedies such as ginseng have been tried with low and variable success rates, rarely exceeding 20% to 30%. In the same vein, yohimbine, an α-adrenergic receptor blocker, has had variable and low rates of success (33% in one study). Venous arterial microsurgery is rarely indicated or successful. Penile prostheses have been used with good success, and numerous rigid, semirigid, or inflatable prostheses are available and in use. External mechanical devices, such as vacuum-constrictive pumps, can be used but tend to detract from the spontaneity of the sexual act. The standby therapies with the greatest patient acceptance rates have been transurethral prostaglandin application (alprostadil [MUSE]) and the intracavernosal injection of papaverine or prostaglandin E2. The former was associated with a painful urethritis that limited its use, and the latter suffers from the disadvantage of injections and the lack of spontaneity.

Most recently, the advent of PDE-5 inhibitors (the first of which was sildenafil citrate [Viagra]) has revolutionized the whole picture of ED. Sildenafil is an inhibitor of PDE-5 and therefore allows cGMP to persist and maintain erection. The ease of administration (orally) and the high chance of success (60%–85% in various reports), irrespective of the cause of the ED, have fostered a lot of discussion and "coming out of the closet" of patients with ED. The shorter the duration of ED, the greater the chance of success. Furthermore, because by itself it will not cause erection but is dependent on physical intimacy to induce erection, the spontaneity is better established. Side effects are minimal, consisting of occasional headaches and a temporary blue visual haze at the highest dosage because of blockage of the phosphodiesterase in the retina. Reports of myocardial infarctions occurring while a patient is taking sildenafil are thought to be more likely due to the untoward and unusual resumption of sexual intimacy rather than a direct effect of the drug on the diseased myocardium. Because of the intimate relationship of nitrous oxide to the process of generating cGMP, and the ubiquity of that biochemical mechanism, however, patients taking nitrates may not use PDE-5 inhibitors. These agents also behave like nitrate donors and therefore predispose to severe hypotension if used concurrently. (Using a nitrate spray on the shaft of the penis can cause erection, but it also induces a headache in the partner because of transvaginal absorption of nitrate during intercourse.) In summary, the use of sildenafil has tended to decrease the ancillary testing of ED. Although this may be of economic benefit, it must be stressed that a good history and physical, a marginal hormonal evaluation if indicated, and good hygiene, in terms of the treatment of underlying causes, cannot be replaced by the generalized and thoughtless use of sildenafil.

Gynecomastia

Gynecomastia is defined as palpable glandular tissue below the areola in males. Gynecomastia is caused either by increased estrogen or decreased androgens. Estrogens stimulate breast tissue; androgens inhibit breast tissue. Thus, the ratio of estrogen to androgen determines the degree of stimulation. More important, in the absence of androgens, it requires extremely small concentrations, even below those measurable by conventional assays, to stimulate mammary growth. Estrogen, in men, is derived from the peripheral conversion of precursors like androstenedione and testosterone. LH and hCG stimulate E2 secretion by the testes.

Diagnosis

The evaluation of gynecomastia usually demands a methodologic search to establish the following:

- Presence
- Associations
- Speed of development
- Progression
- Systemic illnesses
- Associated drugs
- Genital abnormalities

Physical Examination

The physical examination must rule out a malignancy with a good detailed examination, including a detailed testicular examination and a mammogram if the index of suspicion is high.

Laboratory Studies

Laboratory evaluation may be unnecessary in asymptomatic, nontender gynecomastia. If the physical evaluation reveals pain, rapid growth, or a large size, laboratory evaluation should include testosterone, LH, hCG, DHEAS, or urinary 17-ketosteroids levels as well as E2, prolactin, thyroid, and liver functions.

Differential Diagnosis

The differential diagnosis of gynecomastia includes:

- Physiological
  - Newborn
  - Pubertal
  - Aging
- Pathological
  - Increased estrogens
  - Tumors (adrenal, testes [Leydig cell tumors], choriocarcinoma)
  - Ectopic gonadotropin
    - Ectopic placental-like hormone
    - Cirrhosis
    - Hyperthyroidism
    - Decreased androgen effect
    - Hypogonadism
    - Klinefelter syndrome
    - Mumps
    - Cytotoxic chemotherapy
    - Irradiation
    - Androgen insensitivity
    - Refeeding
    - Chronic renal failure/dialysis
  - Pharmacologic
    - Estrogens
    - Aromatizable androgens
    - hCG
    - Antiandrogens
    - Psychotropics-phenothiazines
    - Methyldopa
    - Reserpine
    - Spironolactone
    - Cimetidine
    - Ketoconazole
    - Cyproterone
    - Flutamide
    - Estrogenlike agents
    - Digitalis
    - Marijuana
    - Others
    - Central nervous system acting
  - Miscellaneous
    - Idiopathic
    - Pseudogynecomastia (mimics appearance of normal breast)
    - Lipomastia (adipose related)
    - Neoplasm

Among newborns, 60% to 90% have gynecomastia, likely secondary to placental estrogen exposure; this feature regresses over weeks. Among pubertal boys, 50% to 70% have unilateral or bilateral gynecomastia, thought to be secondary to the preponderance of estrogen production over testosterone and the earlier achievement of normal adult values of estrogen; this condition regresses in most cases.

Among elderly men, 4% may have gynecomastia at autopsy, likely secondary to a decrease in testosterone with aging, whereas E2 is still maintained, possibly by increased peripheral conversion.

Tumors, whether producing de novo estrogen or its precursors (adrenal or Leydig cell testicular tumors) or producing hormones such as hCG, which stimulate the testes to produce estrogen, cause gynecomastia.

Gynecomastia in cirrhosis is thought to occur because of two mechanisms: an increased peripheral conversion owing to decreased clearance of androstenedione and an alcohol-mediated suppression of testosterone production by the suppression of the hypothalamic-pituitary-adrenal system.

Hyperthyroidism induces SHBGs, thereby increasing the level of total testosterone and E2. Free testosterone remains normal, but free E2 is increased because of the increased androstenedione available for peripheral conversion.

Gynecomastia associated with hypogonadism is secondary to the increased E2-to-testosterone ratio.

Refeeding seems to induce a "second puberty," and the mechanism of gynecomastia is the same as that seen in pubertal gynecomastia. This is also thought to be one of the factors that cause gynecomastia in chronic renal failure or dialysis.

Treatment

The treatment of gynecomastia is usually to address the underlying cause, if any (which generally helps to resolve the problem), and to reassure the patient if the cause is likely physiological or residual. If no obvious etiology is found, follow-up and observation are all that is indicated. It must be remembered that the resolution of the problem still may leave a mass of fibrous tissue. The treatment regimen may include the following:

- Androgen (testosterone), danazol, or antiestrogens, although medical treatments are not frequently used
- Prevention by radiation before estrogen treatment (has been advocated by a few)
- Surgery and a reduction mammoplasty, which remain the most appropriate treatment of significant, psychologically damaging gynecomastia, although the words of Nuhall are appropriate and bear keeping in mind: "In the absence of pain, rapid change in size, eccentric, or hard breast mass or testicular mass, no further evaluation of gynecomastia in men is necessary."

REVIEW EXERCISES

QUESTIONS

Match the hormone profile, taken in the morning, to the disease in these women with acne and hirsutism:

1. ACTH 22, cortisol 35, DHEAS 5.6, testosterone 75, thyroid-stimulating hormone (TSH) 0.5, T_4 6.4
2. ACTH 22, cortisol 19, DHEAS 3.6, testosterone 72, TSH 3.4, T_4 6.4
3. ACTH <1, cortisol 5, DHEAS 0.9, testosterone 12, TSH 0.6, T_4 6.4
4. ACTH 38, cortisol 14, DHEAS 5.6, testosterone 78, TSH 0.9, T_4 7.3
5. ACTH <5, cortisol 42, DHEAS 9.8, testosterone 112, TSH 0.5, T_4 7.8
6. ACTH 16, cortisol 21, DHEAS 2.5, testosterone 66, TSH 9.8, T_4 6.2

a) Primary hypothyroidism
b) Exogenous steroids
c) Polycystic ovary disease
d) Adrenal carcinoma
e) Congenital adrenal hyperplasia
f) Cushing disease

Answer and Discussion

1. The answer is f. Cushing disease matches the laboratory values of ACTH 22, cortisol 35, DHEAS 5.6, testosterone 75, TSH 0.5, T_4 6.4.
2. The answer is c. Polycystic ovary disease matches the laboratory values of ACTH 22, cortisol 19, DHEAS 3.6, testosterone 72, TSH 3.4, T_4 6.4.
3. The answer is b. Exogenous steroid use matches the laboratory values of ACTH <1, cortisol 5, DHEAS 0.9, testosterone 12, TSH 0.6, T_4 6.4.
4. The answer is e. Congenital adrenal hyperplasia matches the laboratory values of ACTH 38, cortisol 14, DHEAS 5.6, testosterone 78, TSH 0.9, T_4 7.3.
5. The answer is d. Adrenal carcinoma matches the laboratory values of ACTH <5, cortisol 42, DHEAS 9.8, testosterone 112, TSH 0.5, T_4 7.8.
6. The answer is a. Primary hypothyroidism matches the laboratory values of ACTH 16, cortisol 21, DHEAS 2.5, testosterone 66, TSH 9.8, T_4 6.2.

Match the disease scenario with the hormone profile:

7. A 21-year-old woman with primary amenorrhea and no sense of smell
8. A 19-year-old woman with short stature, primary amenorrhea, and a webbed neck
9. A 24-year-old woman with treated schizophrenia, presenting with amenorrhea
10. A 23-year-old with post-OCP amenorrhea
11. A 26-year-old with headaches, visual blurring, and amenorrhea

a) LH <2, FSH <2, prolactin 683
b) LH <2, FSH <2, prolactin 68
c) LH <2.0, FSH <2.0, prolactin 6
d) LH 2.3, FSH 3.1, prolactin 18
e) LH 23, FSH 47, prolactin 8

Answers

7. The answer is c.
8. The answer is e.
9. The answer is b.
10. The answer is d.
11. The answer is a.

Match the hormonal profile to the case presented:

12. A 26-year-old, tall, young man with gynecomastia, microphallus, and small, soft testes (<3 cc)
13. A 24-year-old, tall, young man with widely spread teeth, goiter, skin tags, microphallus, and small, normal-sized testes (6–7 cc)

14. A 19-year-old, tall, young man with bilateral inguinal hernia and an empty scrotum

15. A 25-year-old, tall, young man with a history of pubertal mumps orchitis, a normal-sized penis, and normal testes (8–10 cc)

16. A 22-year-old, tall, young man with microphallus, small testes (4–5 cc), and no sense of smell

a) LH <2, FSH <2, testosterone 25, prolactin 7, growth hormone 11
b) LH <2, FSH 2.3, testosterone 48, prolactin 38, growth hormone 18
c) LH 3.8, FSH 23, testosterone 389, prolactin 7, growth hormone 0.9
d) LH 13.6, FSH 13.8, testosterone 176, prolactin 9, growth hormone 0.6
e) LH 76, FSH 95, testosterone 92, prolactin 12, growth hormone 1.6

Answers
12. The answer is e.
13. The answer is b.
14. The answer is d.
15. The answer is c.
16. The answer is a.

17. Impotence is commonly seen in which of the following?
a) Diabetes mellitus
b) Congenital adrenal hyperplasia
c) Schizophrenia that is well controlled
d) Androgen insensitivity syndrome
e) a and c only
f) b and d only
g) All of the above

Answer
The answer is e.

18. Gynecomastia is commonly seen in which of the following?
a) An XY individual with bilateral inguinal scars and a total lack of secondary sexual hair
b) An XY individual with well-treated and controlled salt-losing congenital adrenal hyperplasia
c) An XY individual with spider nevi, asterixis, and ascites
d) An XY individual who is the "timid" member of a homosexual couple
e) a and c
f) b and d
g) All of the above

Answer
The answer is e.

19. A 27-year-old Italian woman presents for evaluation of hirsutism and a 2-year history of irregular heavy menses. Menarche was at age 13, and her periods were always irregular, except when she was on OCPs (ages 18–24 years). Thelarche and adrenarche were normal. She noted the onset of significant acne at the age of 17 years, for which she was treated with antibiotics and isotretinoin (Accutane). Accutane had to be discontinued because of severe hypertriglyceridemia. At about the same time, she noted the development of hirsutism, which has slowly progressed. She had been trying to become pregnant for the past 3 years.

On examination, her weight is 170 pounds; height is 5 feet, 3 inches. She has hyperpigmentation of the neck and axillary folds; a small goiter; and hirsutism on the chin, upper lip, and side of her face as well as periareolar and periumbilical coarse, dark terminal hair. Her blood pressure is 120/82 mm Hg. Waist-to-hip ratio is 0.95 and no striae. Liver edge is palpable 1 cm below the costal margin.

The differential diagnosis in this case would include
a) Genetic hirsutism
b) Adult-onset congenital adrenal hyperplasia
c) Polycystic ovarian disease
d) Cushing syndrome
e) a, b, and c
f) a and c
g) All of the above

Answer and Discussion
The answer is e. No clinical evidence is given for Cushing disease.

20. In this same case, the appropriate laboratory tests include
a) Serum DHEAS, testosterone, free testosterone
b) Serum TSH, prolactin
c) Serum 17 hydroprogesterone
d) Gonadotropins and E2
e) a, b, and c
f) All of the above laboratory tests

Answer and Discussion
The answer is e. Gonadotropins and E2 are no clinical help.

21. A 26-year-old woman presents for evaluation of amenorrhea of 6 months' duration. She had a normal menarche at age 12 and normal puberty. Her menses had become progressively lighter over the past 2 or 3 years and occurred 4 to 9 weeks apart before amenorrhea. She has been under a significant amount of stress in the past 2 years, completing her medical degree, competing on the university gymnastic team, and experiencing the breakup of a long-term relationship. She has never taken OCPs and has never been pregnant. She denies galactorrhea; has had a 15-pound weight loss; and has no hirsutism, acne, or headache. She was diagnosed with Hashimoto hypothyroidism at age 16, for which she is on LT$_4$ (L-Thyroxine) with a normal serum TSH over the years.

Laboratory examination showed an FSH of 4 IU/L, an LH of 2 IU/L, and a prolactin of 12 mg/mL, with a serum TSH of 10.8 μU/mL, testosterone 42 ng/dL, and DHEAS 3.3 ng/mL. The remaining biochemistry was normal.

Which of the following would *not* be in the differential diagnosis?

a) Functional amenorrhea secondary to stress, weight loss, and exercise
b) Hypothyroidism
c) PCOS
d) POF

Answer and Discussion

The answer is d. Gonadotropins indicate that this is impossible.

22. A 26-year-old man presents with primary infertility. He has been married for 4 years and has been trying to father a child for 3 years. He has no difficulty with sexual function. Past and family history is unremarkable, and he is on no medications and does not smoke, drink, or take any street drugs. He is 6 feet, 2 inches tall (the tallest in his family), weighs 264 pounds, has an arm span of 80 inches, and has a pubis-to-heel length of 39 inches. He has bilateral gynecomastia; a 2.5-inch penis partially embedded in the mons; bilateral small, soft testes; and sparse but present secondary sexual hair growth. His testosterone value is 210 ng/dL (normal, >220 ng/dL), and he is azoospermic.

Your diagnosis is

a) Klinefelter syndrome
b) Congenital hypoorchia
c) Postsubclinical mumps orchitis
d) Kallmann syndrome
e) Pubertal hyperprolactinemia

Answer

The answer is a.

23. In this same case, does the young man with primary infertility, no sexual dysfunction, and azoospermia with small testes but nearly low-normal testosterone need treatment with testosterone?

a) Yes
b) No

Answer and Discussion

The answer is a. The patient needs treatment to stop continued stimulation of the testes, which synthesize E2 and contribute to gynecomastia.

24. A 52-year-old man presents with a complaint of impotence. He reports progressively increasing difficulty, first with maintaining and later with achieving an erection. He is an attorney, married for 24 years, has four children (the youngest age 16 years), and has no verbalized stress. He was found to have hypertension

about 6 years before and suffered a myocardial infarction 4 years earlier. He has been controlled on β-blockers and a thiazide diuretic, has no angina and no arrhythmias, and has well-controlled blood pressure. He has no other symptoms of note. He has a family history of diabetes, hyperlipidemia, hypertension, and heart disease. He does not smoke and only drinks socially.

Examination shows weight 180 pounds; height 5 feet, 9 inches. Blood pressure is 135/84 mm Hg; pulse is 68 beats per minute and regular, with an occasional extra systole. Liver is palpable 1 cm below the costal margin, with a span of 17 cm. No bruits are present. Bilateral lipomastia is noted. Genital examination reveals a normal penis and testicles that measure 4.5 to 3.1 cm bilaterally. A small varicocele is present on the right side. The prostate is mildly enlarged with an intact median groove. Fundi and fields are normal.

The required laboratory evaluation would include which of the following?

a) Gonadotropins, testosterone, thyroid function tests
b) Testosterone, prolactin, TSH
c) Liver, kidney, electrolyte, glucose panel
d) Oral glucose tolerance test
e) a and c
f) b and c
g) b, c, and d

Answer

The answer is f.

25. Which further evaluations are needed for the case in question 25?

a) Snap gauge
b) Nocturnal penile tumescence study
c) Magnetic resonance imaging of the head
d) a and c
e) All of the above
f) None of the above

Answer and Discussion

The answer is a. A snap gauge gives almost the same information as nocturnal penile tumescence evaluation.

26. Which is the treatment option in the case for question 25?

a) T shots
b) Bromocriptine
c) Intravenous injection of papaverine
d) Discontinuation of propranolol (Inderal) and thiazides
e) Penile prosthesis placement
f) Reassurance and support with no treatment

Answer and Discussion

The answer is d. If possible, the propranolol and thiazides should be changed to other medications to determine whether they are contributing to the problem.

SUGGESTED READINGS

Female

Barbieri RL. Hyperandrogenic disorders. *Clin Obstet Gynecol* 1990;33: 640–659.

Barnes R, Rosenfeld RL. The polycystic ovary syndrome: pathogenesis and treatment. *Ann Intern Med* 1989;110:386–399.

Biffignandi P, Massucchetti D, Molinatti GM. Female hirsutism: pathophysiological considerations and therapeutic implications. *Endocr Rev* 1984;5:498–513.

Brodie BL, Wentz AC. Late onset congenital adrenal hyperplasia: a gynecologist's perspective. *Fertil Steril* 1987;48:175–188.

Lobo RA. Hirsutism in polycystic ovary syndrome: current concepts. *Clin Obstet Gynecol* 1991;36:817–826.

McKenna TJ. Pathogenesis and treatment of polycystic ovary syndrome. *N Engl J Med* 1988;318:558–562.

Rittmaster RS, Loriaux DL. Hirsutism. *Ann Intern Med* 1987;106:96–107.

Yen SSC. The polycystic ovary syndrome. *Clin Endocrinol (Oxf)* 1980;12:177–207.

Menstrual Disorders

Dalkin AC, Marshall JC. Medical therapy of hyperprolactinemia. *Endocrinol Metab Clin North Am* 1989;18:259–276.

Reindollar RH, Novak M, Tho SP, et al. Adult-onset amenorrhea: a study of 262 patients. *Am J Obstet Gynecol* 1986;155:531–543.

Premature Ovarian Failure

Mehta AE, Matwijiw L, Lyons EA, et al. Noninvasive diagnosis of resistant ovary syndrome by ultrasonography. *Fertil Steril* 1992;57: 56–61.

Male

Braunstein GD. Gynecomastia. *N Engl J Med* 1993;328:490–495.

Glass AR. Gynecomastia. *Endocrinol Metab Clin North Am* 1994;23:825–827.

Krane RJ, Goldstein L, Saenz De Tejada I. Impotence. *N Engl J Med* 1989;321:1648–1659.

Chapter 42

Diabetes Mellitus: Control and Complications

Robert S. Zimmerman   S. Sethu K. Reddy

POINTS TO REMEMBER:

- Because the methods for measuring glycosylated hemoglobin (HgbA$_{1c}$) are not standardized, it is not recommended for diagnosing diabetes mellitus (DM).

- Intensive insulin therapy in critically ill patients in intensive care units (maintaining glucose between 80–110 mg/dL) versus conventional treatment (insulin infusion of glucose >215 mg/dL with a goal of 180–200 mg/dL) reduced mortality from 8.0% with conventional treatment to 4.6% with intensive treatment.

- The main role of long-acting insulin is to serve as basal insulin in patients using short-acting insulin before each meal.

- Reducing blood pressure with either a β-blocker or an angiotensin-converting enzyme (ACE) inhibitor reduces the risk of *both* microvascular and macrovascular complications and overall mortality.

- It is crucial to always consider causes other than DM in the etiology of any neuropathy.

DM affects more than 7 million people in the United States, and as many as 8 million others may not be aware that they have the disease. DM is a complex metabolic condition with major health and social ramifications. In recent years, many advances have been made that have increased the ability to achieve optimal metabolic control of DM, while a wealth of accumulated data show that improved control delays the long-term complications of the disease.

ETIOLOGY

DM can be broadly classified as follows:

- Type 1: insulin-dependent DM
- Type 2: noninsulin-dependent DM
- Gestational
- Other
  - Pancreatic disease, hormonal disease, drugs
  - Rare genetic forms, insulin-receptor abnormalities
  - Impaired glucose tolerance (IGT)

In North America, most individuals with DM have either type 1 or type 2 DM. Both types involve a tremendous interaction between genetic endowment and environment (Table 42.1).

TABLE 42.1

FEATURES OF TYPE 1 VERSUS TYPE 2 DIABETES MELLITUS

Feature	Type 1	Type 2
Prevalence (%)	0.4	6.6
Annual incidence in United States	15,000	500,000
Ketosis prone	++++	+
Anti–islet cell antibody	+++	−
Anti-GAD antibody	++++	−
Prevalence of other autoimmune conditions	+++	−
Usual age of onset (yr)	<30	>40
Prevalence of obesity	+	++++
Family history	+	++++
HLA linkage	DR3, DR4	−
DQ β-polymorphism	++	−
Insulin secretion	Absent	Abnormal
Insulin resistance	−	+++

The symbols −, +, ++, +++, ++++ indicate relative strength of association with type of diabetes.
GAD, glutamic acid decarboxylase; HLA, human leukocyte antigen.

Type 1 Diabetes Mellitus

A positive correlation appears to exist between the prevalence of type 1 DM and the distance away from the equator. Finland has the highest prevalence, whereas southern European countries have a lower prevalence. Mediterranean countries have an even lower prevalence. It is unknown whether this is related to different genetic backgrounds or environmental factors. No male–female differences are known.

Type 1 DM, predominantly affecting those younger than 30 years, is associated with an absolute insulin deficiency owing to the chronic autoimmune destruction of pancreatic beta cells. These individuals need insulin for survival.

In genetically susceptible individuals, this autoimmune process, which can be detected by the presence of antibodies to various components of β cells (e.g., insulin, glutamic acid decarboxylase, phosphotyrosine, phosphatase), results in the gradual deterioration of insulin production. During this phase (which may last longer than 10 years), no evidence of hyperglycemia may be apparent; at a later time, a critical event such as surgery or a viral illness may result in the acute deterioration of pancreatic function and result in acute severe hyperglycemia.

The presence of a gene(s) within the major histocompatibility complex is essential to the development of type 1 DM. More than 90% of whites with type 1 DM express either HLA-DR3 or HLA-DR4. However, 40% of the nondiabetic population also express one of these alleles. This genetic linkage has been further enhanced by studies showing that 96% of patients with type 1 DM are homozygous for amino acid nonaspartate/nonaspartate at position 57 of the DQ-β chain. Despite such great progress in the understanding of the genetic susceptibility to type 1 DM, the approximately 60% discordance of type 1 DM in identical twins suggests an important role for environmental factors. These environmental factors may be nutritional components such as cow's milk, viral infections, or chemical toxins. Having a first-degree relative with type 1 DM increases the risk of type 1 DM 10-fold. However, type 1 DM will not develop in 95% of these individuals.

Because type 1 DM is an autoimmune disease, its prevention has focused on immune intervention. Various immunosuppressives and immunomodulators have been tested in multicenter trials. Some early studies from Australia and the United States using azathioprine (Imuran) with or without prednisone in subjects with recent-onset type 1 DM were favorable, but further study has been abandoned in favor of safer immunotherapies.

Cyclosporine (Sandimmune) has been evaluated in two large and two small double-blind, placebo-controlled studies as well as in later open studies. In patients with recent-onset type 1 DM, insulinfree remission rates of 18% to 24% at 12 months were observed, but no remissions were evident at 24 months despite continued cyclosporine therapy.

Intensive insulin therapy and oral insulin were thought to possibly preserve pancreatic insulin secretion in new-onset type 1 DM patients. The results of the Diabetes Prevention Trial for type 1 DM did not prove to preserve β-cell function with either intensive insulin therapy or oral insulin. Other potential interventions include induction of tolerance to islet cells by oral antigens (including insulin itself), avoidance of cow's milk in infancy, newer immunomodulatory agents, and free-radical scavengers. No current immunotherapy is close to clinical utility in the prevention of diabetes.

Type 2 Diabetes Mellitus

Type 2 DM accounts for about 85% of the diabetic population. At present, type 2 DM is believed to be the result of many years of insulin resistance, leading to disordered and reduced pancreatic insulin secretion and, in turn, to fasting hyperglycemia. Quite often, weight gain (particularly central obesity), physical inactivity, and a high-fat diet exaggerate the insulin resistance and may accelerate the development of type 2 DM. Individuals with type 2 DM may require insulin therapy for improved control of glucose levels; they are then labeled as "insulin-requiring" type 2 DM. In most Westernized countries, the risk for the development of type 2 DM continues to increase with age, resulting in an approximately 21% prevalence of type 2 DM in people over 60 years of age.

If both parents have type 2 DM, the genetic risk of offspring developing type 2 DM is 50%, whereas the risk declines to 20% if only one parent has type 2 DM. If an identical twin has type 2 DM, the risk is estimated to be more than 90%.

Striking differences occur in the prevalence of type 2 DM among different ethnic groups. For example, Native Americans of the Pima tribe in the southwestern United States have a greater than 30% prevalence of type 2 DM, whereas Americans of European ancestry have approximately a 5% prevalence. Environment, however, is also important in the development of type 2 DM. Within an ethnic group, the prevalence of type 2 DM varies, depending on the presence of obesity, physical inactivity, and dietary composition as well as whether living conditions are urban or rural. Studies of Japanese Americans, aboriginals of North America, Asian immigrants to Europe, Mexican Americans, and natives of the South Pacific have confirmed the importance of these risk factors.

Obesity, particularly central obesity, and elevated insulin-to-glucose ratios have generally been considered to be important risk factors. It should be noted that a family history of type 2 DM also connotes a higher than usual risk for the development of type 2 DM in the obese. Physical activity may also be important. Bjorntorp[1] showed that physically trained insulin-resistant obese subjects could decrease their plasma insulin values by almost 50% without decreasing body fat. Helmrich et al.[2] studied lifestyle habits and health factors in 1962, and again in 1976, in a cohort of 5,990 men. DM developed in 202 men during the 14 years. The incidence of DM was 41% lower in patients doing the highest level of physical activity (>3,500 kcal per week) compared with those doing the lowest level (<500 kcal per week). This effect was independent of other risk factors. A high body mass index (BMI) (>26) was the strongest predictor of type 2 DM. Tuomilehto et al.[3] demonstrated that diet and exercise resulting in 3.5 to 5.5 kg weight loss after 2 years resulted in a 58% decreased incidence of diabetes in patients with IGT. Metformin 850 mg twice daily resulted in a 31% reduction in the development of diabetes in a second group of patients with IGT.[4] Because diabetes prevention is greater with diet and exercise, it is the first line of treatment to prevent diabetes. The American Diabetes Association recommends moderate weight loss (7% weight reduction) coupled with 2.5 hours per week of exercise to prevent diabetes.

Molecular defects in the insulin receptor, glucose transporters, and the insulin gene have been reported in different DM syndromes, but none appears to cause the common form of type 2 DM. Recently, the glucokinase gene, hepatocyte nuclear factors 4-α, 1-α, and 1-β, as well as insulin promoter factor 1 and neurogenic differentiation factor 1, have been associated with different types of maturity-onset DM of the young. The genetic defects in type 2 DM have not been identified.

Secondary Diabetes Mellitus and Diabetes Due to Pancreatic Destruction

Secondary DM may present in individuals with the following conditions:

- Chronic pancreatitis
- Cystic fibrosis
- Hemochromatosis
- Pancreatectomy

Conditions associated with elevated counterregulatory hormones, pheochromocytoma, acromegaly, and Cushing syndrome may also precipitate DM. Drugs may also cause hyperglycemia; these include glucocorticoids, thiazide diuretics, phenytoin (Dilantin), interferon-α, pentamidine (Pentam 300 or Nebupent), diazoxide (Proglycem or Hyperstat I.V.) cyclosporin, tacrolimus, adrenalin, isoproterinol, and nicotinic acid.

COSTS OF DIABETES MELLITUS: MORBIDITY

The prognosis for an individual with type 2 DM may be affected by:

- Inherent background morbidity pattern of the nondiabetic in his or her population
- Competing risks
- Pattern of risk factors
- Quality and quantity of available health care
- Possible differences in etiology of the patient's type 2 DM

TABLE 42.2

INTERPRETATION OF THE ORAL GLUCOSE TOLERANCE TEST

	Normal	Impaired Glucose Tolerance	Diabetes Mellitus	Gestational Diabetes Mellitus (Pregnancy)
Fasting (mg/dL)	<100	<126	≥126	≥95
0.5, 1.0, or 1.5 h postprandial (mg/dL)	—	—	—	≥180
2 h postprandial (mg/dL)	<140	140–199	≥200	≥155
3 h postprandial (mg/dL)	—	—	—	≥140

More than ten studies have documented an excess mortality in type 2 DM; several studies have estimated a 5- to 10-year loss in life expectancy in patients older than 40 years. DM is the leading cause of blindness in adults 25 to 74 years old in Europe and North America. Women appear to be predisposed to retinopathy, and blacks appear to be at more risk than whites. DM also is the leading cause of end-stage renal disease, which also has major implications for a patient's quality of life. DM, which also may have an adverse effect on productivity, leads to a greater use of health care resources. The life expectancy of children with type 1 DM is about 75% of that of nondiabetics. The Edic trial found that cardiovascular event rates (nonfatal myocardial infarction [MI], stroke, or death from cardiovascular cause) decreased from 0.80 per 100 patient-years to 0.38 per 100 patient-years ($p = 0.007$) in intensive treated patients with type 1 DM compared with controls followed for 17 years. Cardiovascular mortality was decreased by two-thirds, although this was not significant. The Accord trial found that in type 2 DM patients at high risk for heart disease, that very tight control (goal, HgbA$_{1c}$ 6%) increased mortality from 11 per 1,000 patient-years to 14 per 1,000 patient-years. This indicates that very tight control should not be a goal in type 2 diabetics with heart disease.

The direct and indirect costs of DM are extremely high. In the United States, it has been estimated that DM care costs more than $100 billion per year, with patients with DM requiring two to three times the cost of health care of individuals without DM.

DIAGNOSIS

Screening

Individuals with the following characteristics should be screened for DM:

- Obesity
- Family history of type 2 DM
- History of gestational DM or giving birth to an infant weighing more than 9 pounds
- Hypertension
- Cardiovascular disease (CVD)
- Belonging to a high-risk ethnic group
- Increasing age (>45 years)

Glucose Testing

Screening should be accomplished using a fasting plasma glucose test. The use of the oral glucose tolerance test (OGTT) is recommended when a patient develops a problem commonly seen in diabetes such as nephropathy, neuropathy, or retinopathy and has normal fasting glucose as well as during pregnancy. The OGTT can also be used in a patient with impaired fasting glucose (IFG) to determine the criteria for diabetes have been met. Because the methods for measuring HgbA$_{1c}$ are not standardized, it is not recommended for diagnosing DM. Screening on a population basis cannot be recommended.

Two fasting plasma glucose levels >126 mg/dL (7 mM) indicate the presence of DM. If the 2-hour postprandial value is >200 mg/dL, the patient is deemed to have DM (Table 42.2). Fasting glucose levels of ≥100 and <126 mg/dL indicate IFG.

Oral Glucose Tolerance Test

The OGTT is a useful tool when used in patients who have fasted for 8 hours (abstaining from caffeine and nicotine) before receiving 75 g of glucose (for adults) or 1.75 g/kg (for children). The total volume of glucose is between 250 and 300 mL and should be ingested over 5 minutes. Patients should not be malnourished and should have eaten at least 150 g of carbohydrate per day for at least 3 days before the test. They should be ambulatory and not acutely ill. The formal OGTT in pregnant women requires a 100-g glucose load and is extended to 3 hours. It should be kept in mind that plasma glucose values are about 15% higher than whole blood glucose values. The following discussion uses plasma glucose values.

During an OGTT, a 2-hour postprandial glucose level between 140 and 200 mg/dL indicates impaired glucose tolerance (IGT). Of patients with IGT, DM will develop in 1% to 5% per year. However, 50% of patients with IGT will have a normal OGTT if repeated in 6 months.

Variables Affecting the Oral Glucose Tolerance Test

The reproducibility of OGTT results is notoriously poor. Several studies have shown that repeat testing of the same individual may result in blood glucose levels that vary by 18 to 27 mg/dL. There is no doubt that this variability is caused by changes in nutritional status, weight, medications, use of caffeine or nicotine, and the normal physiological variability of glucose metabolism. Thus, some investigators advocate that at least two OGTTs are needed to properly classify a patient.

In addition, as one ages, the prevalence of glucose intolerance increases dramatically. In the geriatric population, up to 30% may have DM. Aging is associated with the delayed absorption of glucose but, more important, also with delayed glucose-induced insulin secretion and insulin resistance at the level of the liver and skeletal muscle. The major disturbance appears to be insulin-mediated glucose uptake. It is also worth noting that although the total weight may not change as one ages, the weight distribution may be altered to a central-obesity pattern. Such a pattern has been linked to insulin resistance and related disorders.

Other Potential Uses of the Oral Glucose Tolerance Test

Reactive Hypoglycemia. It has become common practice to perform a 5-hour, prolonged OGTT in patients who have apparent hypoglycemic symptoms postprandially. Several studies have shown significant inconsistencies between symptoms and the presence of hypoglycemia. Other studies have confirmed the inadequacies of the OGTT in the workup of hypoglycemia. A mixed meal tolerance test rather than an OGTT is recommended. The diagnosis is based on blood sugar <50, symptoms of hypoglycemia, and resolution of symptoms with treatment.

Pregnancy. Gestational DM is characterized by a diabetic state first detected during a pregnancy. The prevalence of gestational DM has varied from 0.15% to 12.30%, depending on the study group and the set of diagnostic criteria. The Fourth International Workshop Conference on Gestational Diabetes Mellitus recommends screening all pregnant women with a 50-g OGTT at 24 to 28 weeks. If the 1-hour postload glucose level is >140 mg/dL, then a 3-hour, 100-g OGTT should be performed. This diagnostic algorithm seems to be the most cost-effective in North America. The formal OGTT during pregnancy uses a 100-g glucose load. Two of the three postprandial glucose levels need to be met or exceeded to make the diagnosis of gestational DM (1 hour ≥180, 2 hour ≥155, 3 hour ≥140). In North America, gestational DM has been reported to be associated with a higher frequency of metabolic abnormalities, higher birth weights, and increased morbidity and mortality. In the United States, the relative risk of perinatal mortality of gestational diabetic women compared with that of normal control women was 2.2.

Patients With Apparent Complications of Diabetes. Rarely, patients present with retinopathy, neuropathy, or nephropathy that is suggestive of diabetic complications, but they may have equivocal plasma glucose levels. In such situations, an OGTT can be performed to definitively confirm or refute the diagnosis of DM.

Epidemiologic Research. In the study of the natural history of DM, the OGTT is an invaluable tool. It has been used in many population-based studies to determine the prevalence of DM and associated risk factors.

TREATMENT

Dietary Management

Dietary management is the cornerstone of DM care and should be used in conjunction with exercise to promote a healthy lifestyle. Hopefully, this leads to the maintenance of a lower or ideal body weight; decreased insulin resistance; and improved control of hyperglycemia, dyslipidemia, and hypertension. Individuals with DM should be referred to a registered dietitian for detailed, practical advice. Physicians can help greatly by inquiring about a patient's lifestyle and imparting good nutritional principles. Having three balanced meals per day, enjoying a variety of foods, and spacing meals 4 to 6 hours apart is helpful. Including high-fiber and low-fat items in food choices, as well as moderating the intake of simple sugars, will further the overall goal of reducing the complications of DM. Dietary instructions often depend on the "state" of the patient. The rigor of the lifestyle changes will depend on the following (Table 42.3):

- Age
- Comorbid conditions (e.g., pregnancy or renal failure)
- Activity levels
- Metabolic targets

A maintenance diet is approximately 25 kcal/kg of ideal body weight. The simplest way to calculate the ideal body weight is to use the BMI formula:

$$\text{BMI weight (kg)/height (m)}^2$$

An optimal BMI is <25. A BMI >27 is considered obesity. One kilogram of weight loss is 7,500 to 8,000 kcal; thus, reducing energy intake by 500 to 1,000 kcal per day should result in 0.5 to 1.0 kg of weight loss per week.

Alcohol may be consumed only in moderation, and salt intake should be restricted in patients with hypertension or nephropathy. Artificial sweeteners such as aspartame, cyclamates, and acesulfame potassium may be consumed and are safe in the amounts used in most diets. (Often, patients focus only on the sugar component and do not realize that although they are eating a low-sugar food, they may be ingesting excess fat.) The focus of a diabetic diet has shifted away from pure avoidance of sugars to a more complete, healthy, risk-reduction nutrition plan. The American Diabetic Association's (ADA) dietary recommendation allows a diabetic to ingest up to 10% of daily energy intake from simple carbohydrates.

Currently available is a fat substitute that consists of a sucrose core with six to eight fatty acids (sucrose polyester

TABLE 42.3

SUMMARY OF NUTRITIONAL RECOMMENDATIONS

Nutrient Type	Recommended Intake	Sources
Carbohydrates	50%–55% of total daily energy intake	Mainly complex carbohydrates, high in fiber Bread, cereals, fruits Vegetables Milk Cakes, muffins
Protein	60.8 g/kg of ideal body weight	Meat, fish, poultry Legumes, tofu, cheese, milk
Fat/Cholesterol	Up to 30% of total daily energy intake <10% saturated >10% polyunsaturated >10% monounsaturated	Saturated fat: butter, dairy products, animal fats, margarine — Cholesterol: animal products, egg yolk, organ meats, milk

or olestra), making the molecule too large to be absorbed. Concerns with the use of this product are related to gastrointestinal (GI) side effects and a possible decreased absorption of fat-soluble vitamins. At present, the U.S. Food and Drug Administration (FDA) has approved its use in snack foods only. Used judiciously, this may allow many patients with DM to meet their nutritional goals in fat reduction. Some preliminary evidence suggests that orlistat (Xenical), a drug that impairs fat absorption, may assist in weight loss and improving glycemic levels.

Exercise: Benefits and Risks

The psychosocial, cardiovascular, and metabolic effects of exercise may benefit patients with DM. The benefits of exercise include:

- Improving quality of life and sense of well-being
- Enhancing work capacity
- Ameliorating cardiovascular risk factors such as hypertension and obesity
- Favorably altering the lipid profile
- Reducing serum triglyceride levels
- Raising high-density lipoprotein (HDL) cholesterol levels (To significantly change the HDL cholesterol level, moderate-to-heavy exercise, equivalent to running 4 to 8 miles per day, is required.)
- Achieving ideal body weight (Interestingly, improvements in insulin sensitivity may be evident, independent of the weight loss.)

A myth exists that exercise alone will normalize metabolic control. In type 1 DM, exercise has not been shown to significantly improve glycemic control. It is, however, a useful adjunct to nutritional and pharmacologic therapy. Exercise plays an important role in the management of type 2 DM.

In the fasting state, skeletal muscles obtain energy from fat, whereas in the fed state, glycogen is first consumed, followed by anaerobic glycolysis. This process is most important during a short burst of exercise, but as the exercise continues, anaerobic gluconeogenesis occurs, and glucose uptake rises to almost 20 times the basal rate. With prolonged exercise, free fatty acids become the major substrate for muscle energy production. Insulin levels are usually lower during exercise, allowing more glycogenolysis, but due to enhanced sensitivity during exercise, insulin peripheral glucose uptake is stimulated.

Acute Effect of Excercise

In patients with well-controlled DM, exercise may lower glucose levels because patients are well insulinized and hepatic glucose production is suppressed while muscles take up glucose. Patients with poorly controlled disease, however, are underinsulinized; hepatic glucose production in response to stress hormones is unchecked, and skeletal muscle glucose uptake is diminished. This results in an increase in glucose levels and may even lead to ketosis. Prolonged strenuous exercise (exceeding 80% of maximum capacity) may also lead to the elevation of blood sugars.

Delayed Effect of Exercise

Muscle glycogen stores are depleted after 40 to 60 minutes of moderately intense exercise. After exercise, glucose flux across muscle increases significantly, which may lead to delayed hypoglycemia.

Risks of Exercise

Exercise carries potential risks, as does any therapeutic maneuver. The action of hypoglycemic medications, including sulfonylureas and insulin, may be enhanced through exercise, with resultant hypoglycemia. Because patients with DM are more likely to have heart disease, both symptomatic and asymptomatic, the risk of arrhythmia or ischemic episodes is also increased. In elderly persons, exercise may aggravate degenerative joint disease or more likely lead

TABLE 42.4

TARGETS OF CONTROL

	Goals	Action If:
Premeal glucose (mg/dL)	70–130	<80 or >140
Bedtime glucose (mg/dL)	100–140	<100 or >160
HgbA$_{1c}$ (normal range, 4%–6%)	<7%	>8%
Blood pressure (mm Hg)	<130/80	—
LDL cholesterol (mg/dL)	<100 mg/dL	—

LDL, low-density lipoprotein.

to soft tissue injuries. In patients with active retinopathy, strenuous exercise may precipitate intraocular hemorrhage or retinal detachment and should be avoided. It is important when prescribing exercise that patients are educated on how to avoid hypoglycemia. Screening for cardiac disease should be done in other patients before prescribing exercise. Patients should be prescribed types of exercise that avoid exacerbating preexisting injuries.

Relative Contraindications to Exercise

Before beginning a vigorous aerobic exercise program, patients and physicians must be aware of some relative contraindications:

- Poor metabolic control
- Significant microvascular or macrovascular disease
- Severe peripheral neuropathy
- Hypoglycemic unawareness
- Cardiac autonomic neuropathy

These problems must be corrected before an individualized, safe exercise program can be developed.

Practical Tips

The type of exercise used remains a patient's choice, but an improvement in insulin sensitivity and a reduction in cardiovascular risk are evident after relatively mild training. Although aerobic exercise is preferred, resistance exercise in selected patients is safe and also improves glucose control. Exercise sessions should last for about 20 to 40 minutes, and systolic blood pressure during exercise should be kept to <180 to 200 mm Hg. Patients should exercise at least three times weekly.

Planning and foresight are essential. The ability and willingness to self-monitor blood glucose is crucial as well. In general, it is better to exercise after meals. Blood glucose should be checked before and after exercise, and a source of carbohydrate should readily be available. Dehydration must be avoided. Depending on the time of exercise, a reduction will be necessary in either the intermediate-acting or short-acting insulin. It is preferable to use the abdomen for insulin injections, because absorption of insulin in this area is least affected by exercise.

Standards for Glucose Control

It is necessary to determine whether a patient's blood glucose control is adequate using only dietary and exercise therapy or whether pharmacologic therapy should be initiated. The goal should be a preprandial capillary glucose between 70 and 130 mg/dL. An acceptable HgbA$_{1c}$ target is <7% (normal range, 4%–6%). These criteria also could be used with regard to the later initiation of insulin therapy. In fact, the ADA currently recommends the goals shown in Table 42.4. Outpatient goals are based on the Diabetes Control and Complications Trial,[5] Kumamoto,[6] and the United Kingdom Prospective Diabetes studies[7,8] discussed below.

Intensive insulin therapy in critically ill patients in intensive care units (maintaining glucose between 80–110 mg/dL) versus conventional treatment (insulin infusion of glucose >215 mg/dL with a goal of 180–200 mg/dL) reduced mortality from 8.0% with conventional treatment to 4.6% with intensive treatment.[9] There was increased incidence of glucose <40 mg/dL in the intensive group (39 occurrences vs. 6 occurrences). Recent data in patients undergoing coronary artery bypass graft found that mortality decreased from 14% for patients with average glucose >215 mg/dL to 1% in patients with average glucose <150 mg/dL.[10]

Oral Agents

Sulfonylureas

The sulfonylureas are derived from sulfonamides; thus, about a 15% chance of allergy to a sulfonylurea exists for patients with a history of allergy to sulfonamides. The sulfonylureas chiefly increase insulin secretion in response to glucose by inhibiting potassium efflux from pancreatic β-cells, which results in a depolarization of the cell membrane and releases of insulin. Prolonged therapy leads to increased insulin sensitivity, but the mechanisms for this are poorly understood. It is well known that hyperglycemia exacerbates insulin resistance; conversely, the normalization of glucose levels reduces the degree of insulin resistance. Sulfonylureas are also known to inhibit hepatic glucose production (Table 42.5). Potency is a relative variable and is reflected by the actual dose size of the medication.

TABLE 42.5

SULFONYLUREAS

Sulfonylureas (Milligrams per Day)	Relative Potency	Duration of Action (Hours)	Dose Range (Milligrams per Day)	Risk of Hypoglycemia
Tolbutamide (Orinase)	1	6–10	500–3,000	<1%
Chlorpropamide	6	24–72	100–500	4%–6%
Glyburide	150	18–24	1.25–20.00	4%–6%
Glyburide (extended release)	300	24	12	<4%
Glipizide (Glucotrol)	75	12–24	2.5–40.0	5%
Glipizide (extended release)	150	24	5–20	<4%
Glimepiride (Amaryl)	300	24	1–8	<1.7%

Approximately one-third of patients with type 2 DM initially do not respond to sulfonylureas (primary failure), and of those who respond, 5% to 10% per year have secondary failure. Many primary failures may be caused by using the drugs in inappropriate patients. The characteristics of responders include:

- Age >40 years
- Duration of DM <5 years
- 110% to 160% of ideal body weight
- No previous insulin therapy or good control with <40 U per day
- Fasting plasma glucose level <180 mg/dL

Older obese patients with a mild elevation of blood glucose are ideal candidates for sulfonylureas. Secondary failure to maintain adequate glucose control may be related to decreasing pancreatic function but is often caused by noncompliance with lifestyle changes.

Fewer than 2% of patients taking a sulfonylurea will discontinue therapy because of adverse side effects. A 1% to 3% prevalence of GI side effects exists. As well, <0.1% prevalence of hematologic and dermatologic side effects is possible. Patients should be warned of a possible disulfiramlike reaction if alcohol is ingested. This is observed more frequently with chlorpropamide than with other agents; chlorpropamide may also cause the syndrome of inappropriate antidiuretic hormone secretion with symptomatic hyponatremia.

The risk of severe hypoglycemia is about 0.22 per 1,000 patient-years compared with 100 per 1,000 patient-years for insulin. Prolonged hypoglycemia while using glyburide or chlorpropamide may be caused by the metabolites of these drugs, which also have a hypoglycemic effect. Risk factors for sulfonylurea-induced hypoglycemia include:

- Age >60 years
- Decreased renal function
- Poor nutrition
- Interaction with drugs such as insulin, alcohol, salicylates, phenylbutazone, sulfonamides, warfarin (Coumadin), allopurinol, and β-blockers

Meglitinides

The first clinically useful compound of the meglitinide class of agents, which is derived from benzoic acid, is repaglinide (Prandin). It stimulates the sulfonylurea receptor at a site different from that of the sulfonylurea-binding site and increases glucose-stimulated insulin secretion within 10 minutes. The duration of action is 3 to 4 hours; thus, dosing is three times daily before meals. Doses range from 0.5 to 4.0 mg. There appears to be little risk of severe hypoglycemia. Repaglinide may be used in combination with metformin (Glucophage). Repaglinide is metabolized by the liver into inactive metabolites and thus can be used in patients with renal failure without any concern regarding prolonged hypoglycemia.

Nateglinide is a D-phenylalanine derivative that also binds to the sulfonylurea receptor at a binding site different from that of the sulfonylurea binding site. It increases glucose-stimulated insulin secretion. It is taken before each meal at a dose of 120 mg. Its peak action is at 1 hour, and elimination half-life is 1.5 hours.

Biguanides

The only biguanide available is metformin. It does not bind to plasma proteins and is eliminated solely via the renal route. With a half-life of 2 to 4 hours, metformin, 500 to 1,000 mg, is given with meals up to three times daily, to a maximum dosage of 2,000 mg per day. It does not cause hypoglycemia (it does not work by enhancing pancreatic insulin secretion). It may increase insulin sensitivity or affect glucose metabolism directly. Metformin also can have an anorectic effect, which may be beneficial for obese patients with type 2 DM. As well, it has been shown to lower plasma triglyceride levels.

Metformin may be used as a first-line medication, or it can be combined with a sulfonylurea or insulin. Its chief side effects are GI (up to 20% of patients), but these can be minimized by starting at a low dose and gradually increasing it as tolerance develops. These side effects include dyspepsia, anorexia, diarrhea, and an unpleasant metallic taste. Lactic acidosis potentially is a major side effect; thus, metformin should be avoided in patients with cirrhosis, alcoholism, heart failure, or renal failure. The FDA recommends that patients with creatinine values >1.5 mg/dL (1.4 mg/dL for women) should not take metformin. It should also be avoided in patients with heart failure treated with digoxin or furosemide. It should be held after receiving contrast dye until normal creatinine has been documented and should not be given in the perioperative period due to risk of renal insufficiency and lactic acidosis.

α-Glucosidase Inhibitors

Acarbose (Precose) and miglitol (Glyset) are pseudotetrasaccharides that inhibit α-glucosidases in the brush border of the small intestine. These enzymes are responsible for the digestion of starch, dextrins, maltose, and sucrose into monosaccharides, which can then be absorbed. Acarbose and miglitol reduce postprandial hyperglycemia and are approved for use in patients with type 2 DM. Side effects may include flatulence and diarrhea, but these diminish with continued use of the agents. The α-glucosidase inhibitors can be safely combined with other oral agents. Starting dosage is 25 mg once daily, gradually increased to three times daily; the dosage may be increased to 50 mg three times daily with meals. The expectation is that HgbA$_{1c}$ may be reduced by an absolute level of about 0.75% to 1.00% (normal range, 4%–6%). In patients with higher levels of HgbA$_{1c}$, however, the effect may be greater.

Thiazolidinediones

The thiazolidinediones, a family of compounds known as *insulin sensitizers*, increase insulin sensitivity in fat, skeletal muscle, and liver. They have no effect on insulin secretion. They modestly reduce fasting and postprandial glucose levels in obese patients with type 2 DM. These agents are generally well tolerated. Thiazolidinediones may increase plasma volume in some patients. They should be avoided in those with liver disease and in those with heart failure (class III).

Rosiglitazone (Avandia) may be prescribed at a dose of 4 to 8 mg per day, and pioglitazone (Actos) can be prescribed at a dose of 15 to 45 mg per day. Clinical trials prior to FDA approval showed no increase in hepatotoxicity with rosiglitazone or pioglitazone when compared with a placebo, but the FDA recommends that liver enzymes be checked initially and periodically thereafter because another thiazolidinedione, troglitazone (Rezulin), was associated with a small number of cases of severe hepatic failure. These agents may be used as initial monotherapy or as part of combination therapy. Pioglitazone may be more effective at lowering triglycerides than rosiglitazone.

Dipeptidyl Peptidase-4 Inhibitors

Glucagonlike peptide-1 (GLP-1), secreted by L cells in the ileum, and glucose-dependent insulinotropic polypeptide (GIP), secreted by K cells in the duodenum, are endogenous incretin hormones that are secreted during an oral glucose load and not during intravenous glucose infusion. GLP-1 and GIP-1 increase insulin secretion. GLP-1 inhibits glucagon secretion and decreases gastric emptying. Dipep-tidyl peptidase-4 (DPP-4) breaks down GLP-1 and GIP. Sitagliptin is a DPP-4 inhibitor that increases endogenous GLP-1 and GIP. Sitaglipitin is a new oral hypoglycemic agent that increases insulin in a glucose dependent manner and thus only increases insulin when blood sugars are elevated, so it is not associated with hypoglycemia. As a single agent, sitagliptin is associated with a decrease in HgbA$_{1c}$ of approximately 0.75%.

Exenatide

Exenatide is a 39 amino acid GLP-1 mimetic that increases insulin and decreases glucagon in response to elevated blood glucose. Exenatide decreases gastric emptying and often causes weight loss. It currently is used with two subcutaneous injections daily. It can be associated with GI side effects, including nausea and diarrhea.

Pramlintide

Pramlintide is an amylin mimetic agent. Amylin is a hormone that is cosecreted with insulin from pancreatic B cells. Amylin levels are decreased in patients with diabetes. Pramlintide is given subcutaneously before each meal. This drug decreases postprandial glucose excursions by decreasing gastric emptying, food intake, and postprandial glucagon secretion.

Therapy Using Several Oral Agents

Certainly, no benefit is derived from prescribing two sulfonylureas at the same time, and a greater chance of side effects is possible. A sulfonylurea or repaglinide, however, can be combined with metformin for improved glucose control. No additive effects occur when a sulfonylurea is added to a meglitinide. A thiazolidinedione can be added to all other classes of hypoglycemic agents. The α-glucosidase inhibitors may be combined with any other oral agent.

Sitagliptin can be added to sulfonylureas, metformin, and thiazolidinediones. Another oral agent is normally added if a patient is already taking a maximum dose of the initial oral agent. At this stage in a patient's disease, it would be prudent to advise insulin therapy in the near future. The potential for hypoglycemic episodes increases with the use of multiple medications. Thus, multidrug therapy initially may best be supervised by a specialist.

In a patient already taking a biguanide and sulfonylurea, the addition of a thiozolidinedione may reduce glucose levels by 50 to 75 mg/dL, depending on the severity of baseline hyperglycemia. In patients already on sulfonylureas, these agents could be added but should not replace the sulfonylureas.

Insulin Therapy

The success of insulin therapy depends on the judicious and appropriate use of the variety of available insulins (Table 42.6).

TABLE 42.6

COMMONLY USED INSULIN PREPARATIONS

Type	Onset (Hours)	Peak (Hours)	Duration (Hours)
Rapid			
Insulin lispro	0.25	1	3–4
Insulin aspart			
Insulin glulisine			
Short			
Regular	0.5	2–4	5–7
Intermediate			
NPH	1–2	6–12	14–24
Long			
Detemir	1–2	3–9	17–24
Glargine	1–2	3–9	24

Insulin lispro (Humalog) and insulin aspart (Novolog) have:

- A very rapid dissociation into monomers after subcutaneous injection; thus, they begin to work within 15 minutes
- An action for 3 to 4 hours only
- A half-life apparently unaffected by increases in dose (unlike regular insulin)
- The possibility of combination with other insulin preparations, such as NPH.
- The same potency, unit for unit, as regular insulin but with different onset and duration

Insulin lispro, insulin aspart, and insulin glulisine are short-acting insulins with quick-on and quick-off characteristics. It is easily accepted by patients because of the convenience of not having to take insulin injections 30 to 45 minutes before a meal. Nocturnal hypoglycemic events are less common, and postprandial glucose values are significantly lower than with regular insulin. No increase in antibody response to insulin lispro occurs.

Some modifications with respect to the timing of intermediate-acting insulins in combination with rapid-acting insulins may be required. Insulin lispro, insulin aspart, and insulin glulisine are often used in insulin pump therapy.

Insulin glargine has a duration of 24 hours. It cannot be mixed with other insulins. Insulin detemir is a second long-acting insulin that has been associated with less weight gain and less hypoglycemia than insulin glargine. It may require two injections per day, as it may have a shorter duration of action than insulin glargine at lower doses. The main role of long-acting insulin is to serve as basal insulin in patients using short-acting insulin before each meal. Basal insulin maintains hepatic glycogen stores and avoids increased glycogenolysis during fasting states when prandial insulins are not active.

Special premixed insulin preparations (e.g. 30% regular/70% NPH and 50% regular/50% NPH, 70% NPH 30%

aspart 75% NPH 25% lispro) may be useful for patients who have very stable DM or who might have difficulties with mixing insulins manually. Penlike delivery systems have also increased the convenience and rapidity of learning insulin administration.

The pharmacodynamic profile can be quite variable and can fluctuate by 20% to 30% between individuals and even within the same individual. Factors that decrease or delay the action of insulin injections include:

- Higher dose of insulin
- Higher glucose levels preinjection
- Site of absorption (thigh more than arm more than abdomen)
- Cooler temperature of skin
- Sedentary (vs. exercise)
- Hepatic and renal degradation
- High titers of anti-insulin antibodies (rare)

The side effects of insulin include hypoglycemia and lipohypertrophy. Allergic phenomena include both local and systemic skin reactions and lipoatrophy.

Dosage regimens may start simply and increase in complexity, depending on a patient's target goals and motivation. More intensive regimens require more frequent self-monitoring of blood glucose. Blood glucose monitoring and insulin adjustment guidlines include:

- Morning glucose level reflects the evening intermediate insulin dose.
- Lunch glucose level reflects the morning rapid-/short-acting insulin dose.
- Supper/dinner glucose level reflects the morning intermediate insulin dose.
- Bedtime glucose level reflects the presupper rapid-/short-acting insulin dose.
- Most individuals will require two to four injections per day.

Insulin may be combined with sulfonylureas, metformin, thiazolidenediones or α-glucosidase inhibitors. The most common regimen is the use of bedtime NPH insulin, insulin glargine, or insulin detemir with daytime oral agents.

Initiating Insulin Therapy

Most patients begin insulin therapy with approximately 0.3 to 0.5 U/kg per day. Typically, two-thirds of the insulin is given in the morning and one-third in the evening. If both intermediate- and rapid-acting insulins are needed, typically two-thirds is intermediate and one-third is regular. Insulin regimens include:

- Phase I
  - Morning intermediate only or
  - Bedtime intermediate only or
  - Bedtime insulin detemir or insulin glargine only or
  - Bedtime intermediate plus oral agent during the day

- Phase II
  - Intermediate insulin twice daily (before breakfast and supper) or
  - Intermediate insulin twice daily (before breakfast and at bedtime)
- Phase III
  - Add short-acting insulin before breakfast plus supper
- Phase IV
  - Short-acting insulin before meals plus bedtime intermediate or
  - Short-acting insulin before meals plus bedtime long acting or
  - Insulin pump therapy

COMPLICATIONS

General Mechanisms

The chronic hyperglycemia to which individuals with DM are exposed is paramount in the etiology of diabetic complications. Hyperglycemia may play a role via several mechanisms:

- Nonenzymatic glycosylation of protein structures, leading to altered blood vessel function
- Conversion of glucose to sorbitol via intracellular aldose reductase enzyme, leading to an accumulation of sorbitol, which in turn can have several deleterious effects on cellular function
- Adverse effects on coagulability, platelet function, atherogenic potential of lipoproteins
- Increased susceptibility to free oxygen radical–induced damage

Diabetes Control and Complications Trial

The results of the DCCT, a historic study conducted from 1983 to 1993 and designed to test whether chronic hyperglycemia is related to the development of complications in type 1 DM, clearly demonstrated that intensive treatment delays the onset and progression of long-term complications in patients with type 1 DM without complications or with early complications. More than 1,400 individuals 13 to 39 years of age with type 1 DM were entered into the study, and more than 99% of them completed it. One-half of the subjects were enrolled in a standard treatment program (twice daily insulin injections), whereas the remainder were intensively treated. Intensive therapy included:

- More frequent doses of insulin per day or insulin pump therapy
- Self-adjustment of insulin according to meal content, exercise activity, and glucose levels
- Frequent dietary instructions and monthly clinic visits

The standard treatment group's goals were to remain clinically well and symptom free, whereas the goal of the intensive treatment group was the normalization of blood glucose levels. This regimen required a great deal of commitment from both the volunteer subjects and the diabetes health care teams.

Intensive therapy resulted in an average HgbA$_{1c}$ of 7.2%, whereas standard therapy achieved an average of 9.2%. It reduced clinically meaningful eye changes (three-step changes on a retinopathy scale) by 34% to 76% and the first appearance of any eye changes by 27%. Evidence of kidney complication (defined as albumin excretion rate >300 mg in 24 hours) was reduced by 54% and nerve damage by 60%. Subjects in the intensive treatment group were three times more likely to have severe hypoglycemic reactions and had twice as many hospitalizations due to hypoglycemia. Intensive therapy did not, however, worsen quality of life.

Follow-up of patients in the DCCT was done for an additional 10 years. The mean HgbA$_{1c}$ increased to 8.0% in the intensive group and decreased to 8.2% in the conventional treatment group. Cardiovascular events decreased 42% in the intensive group compared with those in control patients. The relative risk of stroke or death from CVD decreased by 57%.

Patients with the following characteristics may not be good candidates for intensive therapy:

- Inability to comply with intensive treatment
- Age younger than 13 years
- Elderly with established severe complications
- Significant heart disease
- Hypoglycemic unawareness
- Repeated severe hypoglycemia (more than two episodes in the previous 2 years) (relative contraindications)
- End-stage complications

Kumamoto Study

The Kumamoto Study by Okhubo et al.[6] compared the incidence and progression of microvascular complications in 110 Japanese patients with type 2 DM treated with intensive insulin therapy with the incidence and progression of complications in conventionally treated patients with type 2 DM. The intensively treated group had a HgbA$_{1c}$ of 7.1%, whereas the conventionally treated group had a mean HgbA$_{1c}$ of 9.4%. Reductions in the progression of retinopathy and nephropathy, similar to the rates observed in the DCCT, were observed in the intensively treated group. Thus, intensive therapy also appears to be beneficial to patients with type 2 DM.

Wisconsin Epidemiologic Study of Diabetic Retinopathy

The Wisconsin Epidemiologic Study of Diabetic Retinopathy (WESDR) by Klein et al.,[11] a population-based study with a longitudinal follow-up of 2,990 subjects with DM, revealed a significant relationship between baseline HgbA$_{1c}$ and all aspects of retinopathy, microalbuminuria, and gross proteinuria. In both the type 1 and type 2 DM groups, the WESDR showed a similar relationship between HgbA$_{1c}$ and lower extremity amputation as well as all-cause mortality.

United Kingdom Prospective Diabetes Study

The United Kingdom Prospective Diabetes Study (UKPDS),[7,8] begun in 1977, recently reported some initial findings with respect to glucose and blood pressure control and their impact on microvascular and macrovascular complications. More than 4,000 newly diagnosed subjects with type 2 DM were enrolled and randomized to either conventional policy (fasting glucose goal of 270 mg/dL) or intensive policy (fasting glucose goal of 108 mg/dL). Therapeutic choices included sulfonylureas, insulin, or metformin. Subjects were also randomized to either "tight" blood pressure control (150/85 mm Hg) or "less tight" blood pressure control (<180/105 mm Hg) with captopril (Capoten) or atenolol. The clinical implications of the UKPDS include

- Glucose lowering reduces the risk of retinopathy and nephropathy.
- Glucose lowering did not significantly reduce the risk of coronary heart disease (CHD) in the sulfonylurea and insulin groups.
- All glucose-lowering drugs (sulfonylureas, metformin, insulin) have a comparable effect on reducing microvascular diabetic complications. In obese patients, metformin may have a greater benefit in reducing macrovascular diabetic complications. Metformin was the only agent that significantly reduced the risk of CHD in this study.
- Reducing blood pressure with either a β-blocker or an ACE inhibitor reduces the risk of *both* microvascular and macrovascular complications and overall mortality.

Smoking

Despite numerous public strategies to educate people about the hazards of smoking and tobacco consumption, many individuals with DM smoke. In the United States, the 1988 Behavioral Risk Factor Surveillance System reported that the prevalence of smoking in the diabetic population was the same as in the general population. It was also noted that young blacks with DM (18–34 years of age) who had not completed high school had higher rates of smoking than controls.

In view of the overall health of individuals with DM, cigarette smoking is an important cause of increased complications from DM and in DM-associated morbidity and mortality. Several prospective cohort studies lend support to this conclusion. Yudkin[12] calculated that smoking ces-

sation would prolong life by 3 years in a man with DM, whereas aspirin and antihypertensive therapy would prolong life by only 1 year.

Microvascular Complications

Retinopathy

DM is responsible for 8% of cases of blindness in the United States and is the leading cause of blindness in the 20- to 64-year age range. The most common form of retinopathy is nonproliferative (background) retinopathy consisting of microaneurysms, intraretinal hemorrhages, or exudates. Infarction of the nerve layer of the retina may occur, causing cotton-wool exudates. This ischemia is thought to play a role in the eventual proliferation of new, friable vessels from the retina into the vitreous. This latter phase is termed *proliferative retinopathy* and is associated with vitreous hemorrhages, retinal scarring, and potential retinal detachment. An altered expression of various local growth factors within the retina is thought to mediate the vascular changes in the retina. Macular edema is also more prevalent in those with DM and may occur with or without proliferative retinopathy. Patients should be referred to an ophthalmologist at the time of diagnosis of type 2 DM because it is assumed that the disease process has been ongoing, whereas referral to an ophthalmologist should be made 5 years after the diagnosis of type 1 DM if the patient is asymptomatic.

The most important risk factors for retinopathy include:

- Duration of DM
- Glycemic control
- Hypertension

Depending on the stage of retinopathy, management includes the following options:

- Appropriately frequent funduscopic examination (more often during pregnancy)
- Improved control of hyperglycemia and hypertension
- Early laser treatment
- Vitrectomy

Aspirin therapy has no adverse ophthalmic effects.

Nephropathy

Renal failure is a major cause of mortality in patients with DM. In the United States, approximately one in three patients on dialysis has DM. Whereas retinopathy eventually occurs in almost all patients with DM, clinical nephropathy develops in about 40% of patients with type 1 DM and in <20% of those with type 2 DM. The most important risk factors for nephropathy include:

- Duration of DM
- Glycemic control
- Hypertension

- Smoking
- Hypercholesterolemia

Recent prospective studies lend support to the hypothesis that smoking accelerates nephropathy in patients with DM. In a clinic-based prospective study by Chase et al.,[13] the odds ratio for the development of significant albuminuria was 2.2 times higher in smokers than nonsmokers. Most other studies also confirm this finding. Recent interest has focused on the polymorphism of various genes linked to hypertension, such as the ACE gene. Proteinuria, which is 15 times more frequent in diabetics than nondiabetics, worsens the prognosis and is a prognostic factor with respect to renal failure and macrovascular disease.

In 1996, the National Kidney Foundation recommended that all individuals with DM who are 12 to 70 years of age undergo urine testing for albumin at least annually. Ideally, individuals should be metabolically stable. Heavy exercise, urinary tract infection, acute febrile illness, or heart failure may transiently increase urinary albumin excretion. Nonsteroidal anti-inflammatory drugs and ACE inhibitors should be avoided during screening.

A 24-hour or overnight (8–12-hour timed) collection is the most sensitive screening method. Albumin excretion rates >30 mg per 24 hours or >20 mg per minute suggest diabetic nephropathy when confirmed on at least two urine samples. Because timed collections are often impractical, the recommendation of using the albumin-to-creatinine ratio was made. A urinary albumin-to-creatinine ratio of 30 to 300 mg/g indicates the presence of microalbuminuria. Various national guidelines have recommended testing for microalbuminuria at the time of type 2 DM diagnosis and 5 years after the diagnosis of type 1 DM (Table 42.7).

In most circumstances, the blood pressure should be lower than 140/90 mm Hg, but in the presence of microalbuminuria, it should be 130/85 mm Hg or lower. The first measures should be to improve blood glucose control, achieve an optimal body weight and smoking cessation, and follow the proper lifestyle. Subsequently, ACE inhibitors, calcium channel blockers, and α-blockers may be used. In the presence of microalbuminuria, an ACE inhibitor is generally favored. Trials have shown that captopril can reduce the need for dialysis and delay adverse outcomes in type 1 diabetics. Similar effects in type 2 diabetics have recently been shown for several angiotensive receptor blockers.

Neuropathy

Neuropathy, one of the most common complications of DM, can affect the sensory, motor, or autonomic nervous systems. Painful symptoms or paresthesias develop in some patients. For peripheral painful neuropathy, simple analgesics, tricyclic antidepressants, phenytoin, and carbamazepine (Tegretol) have been used, but newer, potentially helpful agents include topical capsaicin (Zostrix), mexiletine (Mexitil), gabapentin (Neurontin), pregabalin (Lyrica), and duloxetine (Cymbalta). Other causes of neuropathy should always be ruled out before DM is assumed to be the cause. Sixty percent of patients with diabetes have neuropathy, and the incidence increases with duration of diabetes. Decreased sensation in the feet can lead to lower extremity ulceration and increased incidence of amputation.

Hypoglycemic unawareness occurs when patients lose the catecholamine response and symptoms of sweats, tachycardia, and tremor associated with hypoglycemia. It is a sign of autonomic dysfunction and is often present in individuals with type 1 DM for more than 15 years. At this point, intensive control of DM is dangerous, and appropriately higher targets for blood glucose control should be set.

Symptoms of postural hypotension are associated with a poor prognosis in patients with DM. Traditionally, norepinephrine bitartrate (Levophed), fludrocortisone (Florinef Acetate), or proamitine have been used. Patients may also respond to low doses of a β-blocker. For associated nocturnal diarrhea, once infectious causes have been ruled out, clonidine (Catapres) or a bile acid sequestrant may be helpful.

TABLE 42.7				
NATURAL HISTORY OF DIABETIC NEPHROPATHY				
Stage	**Renal Pathology**	**Albumin Excretion**	**Glomerular Filtration Rate**	**Management**
Diagnosis	Normal or renal hypertrophy	None	Increased	Improve glucose control
3–15 years	1. Basement membrane thickening	Microalbuminuria (30–300 mg/24 h)	Normal	1. As above
	2. Increased mesangial matrix			2. Monitor and treat hypertension
	3. Glomerulosclerosis			1, 2, and 3. Restrict protein
Incipient nephropathy	Advancing glomerulosclerosis	Macroalbuminuria >1.5 g/24 h	Normal	
Nephrotic syndrome	Progression		Normal or decreased	1, 2, 3, and 4. Diuretic therapy
End-stage renal disease	Loss of tubular function		Progressively decreasing	1, 2, 3, 4, and 5. Manage renal failure

Autonomic dysfunction may affect the GI or genitourinary systems, resulting in constipation, gastroparesis, diabetic diarrhea, erectile dysfunction, or a neurogenic bladder.

It is crucial to always consider causes other than DM in the etiology of any neuropathy.

Macrovascular Complications

Atherosclerotic vascular disease is a major cause of morbidity and mortality in patients with DM. For patients with type 1 DM, more than one-third of mortality is owing to cardiac and cerebrovascular diseases; for patients with type 2 DM, two-thirds of mortality is the result of macrovascular disease. The MRFIT Trial found that over 12 years, diabetic risk of cardiovascular mortality was 3.5 times greater than in nondiabetics.

In the classic Whitehall study, a clearly increased mortality from CHD was observed in glucose-intolerant individuals and in diabetics. Age and blood pressure are the strongest risk factors related to subsequent death from CHD. Cigarette smoking, dyslipidemia, and hyperinsulinemia are also important corisk factors in DM. Other factors associated with the development of macrovascular disease are high fibrinogen levels and the presence of cataracts.

Clinical Presentation

Both the incidence and the extent of atherosclerosis are greater in individuals with DM. Within any artery, the disease also may be diffuse. Although infarct size may not differ from that of nondiabetics, complications after MI occur more frequently in the diabetic population. In a prospective study, Yudkin and Oswald[14] showed that a patient's metabolic control before MI had an impact on early mortality:

- 23% mortality with normal HgbA$_{1c}$
- 33% mortality with HgbA$_{1c}$ of 7.5% to 8.5%
- 63% mortality with HgbA$_{1c}$ >8.5%

A greater late mortality also occurs after MI. These features are no doubt owing to coexisting changes in the hearts of patients with DM (e.g., cardiomyopathy, autonomic neuropathy, and more diffuse atherosclerotic disease).

Women with DM have a higher relative risk for peripheral vascular disease. The Framingham Study reported that the average adjusted incidence of intermittent claudication was 12.6 per 1,000 for diabetic men and 8.4 per 1,000 for diabetic women, compared with 3.3 per 1,000 and 1.3 per 1,000 for nondiabetic men and women, respectively. The relative risk of claudication for diabetic women is 6.5 compared with that found in nondiabetic women and 3.3 for diabetic men compared with that found in nondiabetic men. One potential reason for the absence of protection against atherosclerotic disease in diabetic women is the markedly different lipid profiles evident in these patients.

Quite often, they exhibit elevated triglycerides and lower HDL cholesterol levels.

Coronary Artery Bypass Surgery

Although coronary artery bypass grafting (CABG) is efficacious in diabetics with CHD (criteria are the same for diabetic as for nondiabetic patients), many studies have shown that diabetics will have more associated risk factors, poorer left ventricular function, and a poorer long-term prognosis. The Bypass Angioplasty Revascularization Investigation by Jacobs et al.,[15] involving 1,829 patients needing a first revascularization, reported that the 5-year mortality rate with CABG in a subgroup of 353 drug-treated diabetics was 19% compared with 35% for angioplasty. The 5-year mortality rate for the remaining subjects was 9%. Mortality was not due to acute complications of the procedures.

Compelling evidence exists for the role of hyperglycemia in accelerating atherosclerosis, but well-documented evidence suggests that individuals with IGT but without DM (as defined by national and international guidelines) have much higher rates of CVD. This implies that individuals with IGT of any degree are at increased risk of CVD. In addition, the duration of type 2 DM does not correlate very highly with the incidence of CVD. This latter observation may reflect the lack of early diagnosis of DM in asymptomatic individuals.

The risk of CVD in a particular patient also depends on his or her ethnic origin. For example, diabetics of Japanese origin have a lower prevalence of atherosclerosis when compared with diabetics of Scots origin. On the other hand, Japanese diabetics who have migrated to Hawaii have a higher incidence of CVD than those still living in Japan, underscoring the tremendous interplay between inherited and environmental factors.

Pregnancy

Pregnancy complicated by preexisting DM carries a 10- to 20-fold increased risk of congenital malformations. These include neural tube and cardiac defects. Excellent control after conception leads to a dramatic decrease in complications, but a 2- to 3-fold increase in congenital malformations still remains. It is highly advisable that excellent metabolic control be instituted before pregnancy. Metabolic complications that affect the fetus, such as perinatal death, hypoglycemia, hypocalcemia, respiratory distress syndrome, and jaundice, are reduced in prevalence to levels observed in normal pregnancies. Sufficient animal data demonstrate the toxic effects of ketones on central nervous system development; thus, ketosis should be actively prevented.

The white classification of diabetic pregnancies has been useful in predicting outcomes. Unfavorable variables include:

- Increasing age
- Increasing duration of DM

- Retinopathy
- Nephropathy
- CHD

Gestational DM occurs in approximately 2% to 3% of pregnancies. In North America, screening for DM is recommended for all pregnant women between the 24th and 28th weeks of gestation, according to guidelines outlined in the discussion of OGTT (see above). By definition, a woman with gestational diabetes does not have DM postpartum. No increase in congenital malformations occurs, but there does appear to be an increase in macrosomia and neonatal hypoglycemia. Management is usually with diet, exercise, and insulin (if necessary). Oral agents are not used. Some preliminary evidence suggests that insulin resistance may later develop in the infants of diabetic mothers.

Hypoglycemia

Diabetes-Associated Hypoglycemia

Hypoglycemia associated with DM is often caused by a mismatch of caloric intake to insulin peaks. Physicians must take a careful history, being particularly attentive to the following:

- Late or missed meals
- Exercise
- Excessive insulin or sulfonylurea
- Hypoglycemic unawareness
- Gastroparesis
- Use of alcohol or sedatives
- Renal or hepatic impairment
- Coincidental hypoadrenalism or hypopituitarism

Nondiabetes-Associated Hypoglycemia

The symptoms of nondiabetes-associated hypoglycemia may be either adrenergic or neuroglycopenic, with the adrenergic signs occurring earlier, at glucose levels <50 mg/dL. Clinically, a distinction must be made between fasting and reactive hypoglycemia. Fasting hypoglycemia implies a pathological cause, whereas reactive hypoglycemia tends to be a functional, benign phenomenon.

The gold standard test is the 72-hour fast to measure serial glucose and insulin levels. At the time of hypoglycemia or symptoms, the C-peptide level is also determined. This is critical for ruling out exogenous insulin as a cause. The sulfonylureas may increase C-peptide levels and thus should be screened for in a 24-hour urine test.

The liver is of prime importance in the etiology of hypoglycemia. Thus, growth hormone or cortisol deficiencies, severe malnutrition, excessive alcohol consumption, and liver failure may be associated with reduced hepatic glucose output. The sulfonylureas, quinine, pentamidine, disopyramide (Norpace), or monoamine oxidase inhibitors may increase insulin levels. Rarely, anti-insulin receptor antibody or anti-insulin antibody may be linked to hypoglycemia.

A thorough history and physical examination can rule out many of these causes.

An insulinoma is favored in the presence of fasting symptoms and an insulin-to-glucose ratio >0.3 mU/L/mg/dL; an elevated C-peptide level is very supportive. An insulinoma should be localized preoperatively or intraoperatively using laparoscopic ultrasound of the pancreas. Fewer than 10% of these tumors are multiple and associated with multiple endocrine neoplasia type I syndrome.

REVIEW EXERCISES

QUESTIONS

1. A 55-year-old businessman comes to your office complaining of fatigue. He denies any weight change but has nocturia one or two times a night. His 75-year-old mother is a diabetic; his father died of premature heart disease at 60 years of age. He has a history of hypertension treated with hydrochlorothiazide, 50 mg per day. Physical examination reveals that he is 50% above his ideal body weight; his blood pressure is 135/90 mm Hg but is otherwise unremarkable. Fasting plasma glucose is 120 mg/dL; sodium, 143 mEq/L; potassium, 3.1 mEq/mL; chloride, 100 mEq/L; bicarbonate, 26 mEq/L; blood urea nitrogen (BUN), 12 mg/dL; and creatinine, 1.1 mg/dL. HgbA$_{1c}$ is 6.0% (normal range, 4%–6%).

Which of the following is true?
a) The normal HgbA$_{1c}$ rules out diabetes.
b) An OGTT is not indicated.
c) Risk factors for DM include his family history, obesity, hypertension, and hypokalemia.
d) His hypokalemia need not be corrected before retesting his plasma glucose level.
e) Exercise should be avoided due to his family history of heart disease.

Answer and Discussion

The answer is c. Risk factors for DM include family history, obesity, hypertension, and hypokalemia.

2. The above patient returns to your office 6 months later, having missed several return appointments. Despite following your lifestyle prescription, he continues to be fatigued; has experienced a 10-pound weight loss; and presents with polydipsia, polyuria, and blurred vision. He has been monitoring his capillary blood glucose, and it has consistently been >250 mg/dL. You diagnose DM and examine him more closely.

Which of the following features favors type 1 DM?
a) Presence of vitiligo
b) Obesity and age of 55 years
c) Negative for islet cell antibodies
d) Family history of DM
e) C-peptide levels at upper limit of normal

Answer and Discussion
The answer is a. Vitiligo is an autoimmune condition that is more likely to occur with type 1 DM.

3. The dietitian is on holiday, and you must counsel the patient regarding nutrition. Which of the following recommendations would you *not* make?
a) Avoid all sweet foods.
b) Encourage 50% carbohydrates, <30% fat, and 20% protein.
c) Do not take vanadium or chromium supplements.
d) Increase fiber intake, and decrease amount of saturated fat.
e) Space caloric intake over the whole day.

Answer and Discussion
The answer is a. Some simple sugars are allowed (up to 15% of total calories), provided the overall dietary intake is appropriate.

4. This patient is interested in increasing his physical activity. He wonders how exercise will affect his DM. Which of the following is false?
a) Exercise may acutely increase his blood glucose level.
b) Exercise may acutely decrease his blood glucose level.
c) Exercise may not benefit his glucose control if he has type 2 DM.
d) Exercise may not benefit his glucose control if he has type 1 DM.
e) Exercise will have to be individualized according to his previous habits and the presence of any diabetic complications.

Answer and Discussion
The answer is c. Exercise is very important for controlling type 2 DM.

5. The patient's sister, who is visiting from out of town, is also known to have type 2 DM and hypertension. She is treated with glyburide, 10 mg twice daily, and her fasting blood glucose averages 160 mg/dL, with her HgbA₁c at 8.8%. She seeks your counsel. Physical examination is unremarkable except for moderate obesity. Fasting glucose is 200 mg/dL; BUN, 25 mg/dL; and creatinine, 1.9 mg/dL. Electrolytes and liver enzymes are normal.
Which of the following would be reasonable recommendations in addition to improving her dietary habits and exercise regimen?
a) Discontinue glyburide.
b) Add metformin, 500 mg twice daily after meals.
c) Add acarbose, 25 mg three times daily.
d) Add rosiglitazone, 4 mg daily.

Answer and Discussion
The answer is d. Glyburide should not be discontinued but could be reduced. With an elevated creatinine, metformin should not be prescribed. One should start a patient on acarbose (Precose), slowly and gradually

increasing dosage. Rosiglitazone could be used, starting at 4 mg daily.

6. On a clinic visit 5 years later, the patient in question 1 is noted to have microalbuminuria. Your review indicates he has type 2 DM, a blood pressure of 140/90 mm Hg, and a HgbA₁c of 9.0%. He is being treated with an ACE inhibitor and a maximum dose of glyburide.
Which of the following options would be your management?
a) Intensify the antihypertensive regimen.
b) Intensify glucose control only.
c) Begin insulin-injection therapy.
d) Aim to lower blood pressure and blood glucose.

Answer and Discussion
The answer is d. Both glycemic control and blood pressure control are key factors in the development of diabetic nephropathy.

7. Ten years later, the patient is noted to have orthostatic hypotension. No signs or symptoms of heart failure or respiratory distress are present. Sitting blood pressure is 130/75 mm Hg. He is afebrile.
Which of these is *not* compatible with his presentation?
a) Insomnia
b) Constipation
c) Supine blood pressure of 150/95 mm Hg
d) Gastroparesis
e) Persistent resting sinus tachycardia

Answer and Discussion
The answer is e. All are symptoms and signs of autonomic neuropathy, except insomnia.

REFERENCES

1. Bjorntorp P. New concepts in the relationship obesity—non-insulin dependent diabetes mellitus. *Eur J Med* 1992;1:37–42.
2. Helmrich SP, Ragland DR, Leugn RW, et al. Physical activity and reduced occurrence of NIDDM. *N Engl J Med* 1991;325:147–152.
3. Tuomilehto J, Lindstrom J, Eriksson JG, et al. Prevention of type 2 diabetes mellitus by changes in lifestyle among subjects with impaired glucose tolerance. *N Engl J Med* 2001;344:1343–1350.
4. Diabetes Prevention Trial-Type 1 Diabetes Study Group. Effects of insulin in relatives of patients with type 1 diabetes mellitus. *N Engl J Med* 2002;346:1685–1691.
5. Nathan DM, Cleary PA, Backlund JY, et al.; DCCT/EDIC Study Research Group. Intensive diabetes treatment and cardiovascular disease in patients with type 1 diabetes. *N Engl J Med* 2005;353:2643–2653.
6. Okhubo Y, Kishikawa H, Araki E, et al. Intensive insulin therapy prevents the progression of diabetic microvascular complications in Japanese patients with non-insulin dependent diabetes mellitus: a randomized, prospective 6-year study. *Diabetes Res Clin Pract* 1995;28:103–117.
7. UK Prospective Diabetes Study Group. Intensive blood-glucose control with sulphonylureas or insulin compared with conventional treatment and risk of complications in patients with type 2 diabetes (UKPDS 33). *Lancet* 1998;352:837–853.

8. UK Prospective Diabetes Study Group. Tight blood pressure control and risk of macrovascular and microvascular complications in type 2 diabetes: UKPDS 38. *BMJ* 1998;317:703–713.

9. Van den Berghe G, Wouters P, Weekers F, et al. Intensive insulin therapy in critically ill patients *N Engl J Med* 2001;345:1359–1367.

10. Furnary AP, Gao G, Grunkemeier GL, et al. Continuous insulin infusion reduces mortality in patients with diabetes undergoing coronary artery bypass. *J Thorac Cardiovasc Surg* 2003;123:1007–1021.

11. Klein R, Moss SE, Klein BE, et al. Relation of ocular and systemic factors to survival in diabetes. *Arch Intern Med* 1989;149:266–272.

12. Yudkin JS. How can we best prolong life? Benefits of coronary risk factor reduction in non-diabetic and diabetic subjects. *BMJ* 1993;306:1313–1318.

13. Chase HP, Garg SK, Marshall G, et al. Cigarette smoking increases the risk of albuminuria among subjects with type 1 diabetes. *JAMA* 1991;265:614–617.

14. Yudkin JS, Oswald GA. Determinants of hospital admission and case fatality in diabetic patients with myocardial infarction. *Diabetes Care* 1988;11:351–358.

15. Jacobs AK, Kelsey SF, Brooks MM, et al. Better outcome for women compared with men undergoing coronary revascularization: a report from the bypass angioplasty revascularization investigation. *Circulation* 1998;98:1279–1285.

SUGGESTED READINGS

American Diabetes Association. Standards of medical care in diabetes. *Diabetes Care* 2008;31(SUPPL 1):S12–S54.

Becker K, ed. *Principles and Practice of Endocrinology and Metabolism*, 2nd ed. Philadelphia: JB Lippincott Co, 1995.

Brenner BM, Cooper ME, deZeeuw D, et al. Effects of losartan on renal and cardiovascular outcomes in patients with type 2 diabetes and nephropathy. *N Engl J Med* 2001;345:861–869.

Carel JC, Landais P, Bougneres P. Oral insulin does not prevent type 1 diabetes. *NIDDK* 2003;1–3.

Gerich JE. Oral hypoglycemic agents. *N Engl J Med* 1989;321:1231–1245.

Jarrett RJ. Cardiovascular disease and hypertension in diabetes mellitus. *Diabetes Metab Rev* 1989;5:547.

Kahn SE, Haffner SM, Heise MD, et al. Glycemic durability of rosiglitazone, metformin or glybiride monotherapy. *N Engl J Med* 2006;355:2427–2443.

Kannel WB, McGee DL. Diabetes and cardiovascular risk factors: the Framingham Study. *Circulation* 1979;59:8–13.

Lewis E, Hunsicker LG, Clarke, WR, et al. Renoprotective effect of the angiotensin-receptor antagonist irbesartan in patients with nephropathy due to type 2 diabetes. *N Engl J Med* 2001;345:851–860.

Metzger BE, Coustan DR. Summary and recommendations of the Fourth International Workshop-Conference on Gestational Diabetes Mellitus. The Organizing Committee. *Diabetes Care* 1998;21(suppl 2):B161–B167.

Nauck MA, Meininger G, Sheng D, et al. Efficacy and safety of the dipeptidyl peptidase-4 inhibitor, sitagliptin, compared with the sulfonylurea, glipizide, in patients with type 2 diabetes inadequately controlled on metformin alone: a randomized, double-blind, non-inferiorty trial. *Diabetes Obes Metab* 2007;9(2):194–205.

Nissen SI, Wolski K. Effect of rosiglitizone on risk of myocardial infarction and death from cardiovascular cause. *N Engl J Med* 2007;356:2457–2471.

Parving HH, Lehnert H, Brochner-Mortensen J, et al. The effect of irbesartan on the development of diabetic nephropathy in patients with type 2 diabetes. *N Engl J Med* 2001;345:870–878.

Report of the expert committee on the diagnosis and classification of diabetes mellitus. *Diabetes Care* 1997;20:1183–1197.

Heine RJ, Van Gaal LF, Johns D, et al.; GWAA Study Group. Exenatide versus insulin glargine in patients with suboptimally controlled type 2 diabetes. *Ann Intern Med* 2005;143(8):I30.

Shichiri M, Kishikawa H, Ohkubo Y, et al. Long-term results of the Kumamoto Study on optimal diabetes control in type 2 diabetic patients. *Diabetes Care* 2000;23(supp):B21–B29.

Zinman B. Physiologic replacement of insulin. *N Engl J Med* 1989;321:363–370.

Chapter 43

Adrenal Disorders

S. Sethu K. Reddy   Rossana D. Danese

POINTS TO REMEMBER:

- The most common cause of Addison disease (AD) in adults is autoimmune destruction of the adrenal gland (80%). This often is seen in association with other autoimmune diseases, including Hashimoto thyroiditis, Graves disease, or type I diabetes mellitus.

- Currently, AIDS is the most common cause of infectious adrenal destruction, while the antiphospholipid syndrome (lupus anticoagulant) is increasingly being recognized as a cause of adrenal hemorrhage.

- Hyperkalemia and profound dehydration with orthostatic hypotension are seen only in primary adrenal insufficiency (AI).

- A morning cortisol value <3 μg/dL (assuming normal cortisol-binding globulin) can be sufficient to make the diagnosis of AI; however, the cosyntropin (Cortrosyn) adrenocorticotropic hormone (ACTH) stimulation test is usually required and is the gold standard.

- The recovery of the hypothalamic-pituitary-adrenal (HPA) axis from glucocorticoid suppression generally requires 6 to 12 months.

- Despite an absence of hormone excess, nonfunctional adrenal tumors >4 to 6 cm should be resected owing to an increased risk of malignancy; nonfunctional tumors measuring ≤4 cm can be further evaluated radiographically to determine the likelihood of benign disease.

The adrenal gland consists of the medulla and the cortex. The cortex is further divided into the zona reticularis, the zona fasciculata, and the zona glomerulosa (Fig. 43.1). The medulla produces norepinephrine and epinephrine. The zonae fasciculata and reticularis produce cortisol and androgens (mainly dehydroepiandrosterone sulfate [DHEAS]), whereas zona glomerulosa produces aldosterone. As a result of the absence of 17-hydroxylase in the zonal glomerulosa, cortisol and androgens cannot be produced in that layer.

The zonae reticularis and fasciculata are under the control of ACTH, released by the pituitary gland in response to hypothalamic corticotropin-releasing hormone (CRH). CRH, in turn, is regulated by cortisol negative feedback, stress, and a circadian rhythm. Besides increasing the synthesis of cortisol, ACTH is trophic for the adrenal gland; thus, a lack of ACTH results in atrophy of the zonae fasciculata and reticularis. Although ACTH has some effect on aldosterone production, the zona glomerulosa is predominantly under the control of renin. Understanding the anatomy and physiology of the adrenal gland is crucial to understanding its hypo- and hyperfunction.

ADRENAL INSUFFICIENCY

Etiology

Clinical AI results from hypofunction of the adrenal cortex. This may be due to destruction of the adrenal gland itself (AD or primary AI) or to a lack of ACTH (secondary AI) or CRH. The most common cause of AD in adults is autoimmune destruction of the adrenal gland (80%). This often is seen in association with other autoimmune diseases, including Hashimoto thyroiditis, Graves disease, or type I diabetes mellitus. AI is known as type II autoimmune polyglandular syndrome. (Type I autoimmune polyglandular syndrome, more commonly seen in children, consists of AD, hypoparathyroidism, and mucocutaneous candidiasis.) In addition to the polyglandular syndromes, other clues to the presence of autoimmune AI include:

- Chromosome disorders (Down, Klinefelter, and Turner syndromes)
- Alopecia
- Vitiligo
- Other autoimmune disorders (pernicious anemia, chronic active hepatitis, myasthenia gravis, primary hypogonadism)

517

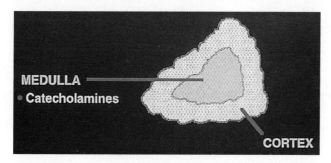

Figure 43.1   The adrenal gland.

In addition to autoimmune disease, other causes of primary AI in adults include:

- Infection (viral, mycobacterial, fungal)
- Hemorrhage/Infarction
- Anticoagulants/Coagulopathy
- Sepsis
- Thrombosis
- Metastatic cancer (breast, lung, gastrointestinal, renal)
- Infiltrative disorders (amyloidosis, sarcoidosis, hemochromatosis)
- Adrenoleukodystrophy/Adrenomyeloneuropathy
  - Affecting young men (X-linked)—abnormal accumulation of very-long-chain fatty acids in adrenal cortex, brain, testes, and liver
- AI and central nervous system (CNS) demyelination

Currently, AIDS is the most common cause of infectious adrenal destruction, while the antiphospholipid syndrome (lupus anticoagulant) is increasingly being recognized as a cause of adrenal hemorrhage.

Secondary AI is a result of adrenal gland atrophy from ACTH deficiency. This most often results from:

- Pituitary corticotroph atrophy owing to previous exogenous glucocorticoid use
- Hypopituitarism
- Isolated ACTH deficiency (usually postpartum)

CLINICAL PRESENTATION

The underlying etiology of AI determines its clinical presentation (Table 43.1). Under the regulation of ACTH, cortisol and adrenal androgens are lost in both primary and secondary AI. Aldosterone production, predominantly regulated by renin, remains intact in secondary AI. Therefore, hyperkalemia and profound dehydration with orthostatic hypotension are seen only in primary AI. Likewise, hyperpigmentation of the skin or mucous membranes (secondary to increased ACTH) is seen only in primary AI. Consequently, the absence of hyperkalemia or hyperpigmentation does not exclude AI.

TABLE 43.1		
ADRENAL INSUFFICIENCY: SIGNS AND SYMPTOMS		
	Primary Adrenal Insufficiency	Secondary Adrenal Insufficiency
Cortisol deficiency	Yes	Yes
Anorexia/Nausea/Vomiting		
Weight loss/Fatigue		
Myalgia/Arthralgia		
Hypotension		
Hyponatremia		
Androgen deficiency	Yes	Yes
Loss of axillary and pubic hair (usually women only)		
Aldosterone deficiency	Yes	No
Hyperkalemia		
Orthostasis		
ACTH excess	Yes	No
Hyperpigmentation		

ACTH, adrenocorticotropic hormone.

In addition to hyponatremia and hyperkalemia, laboratory abnormalities in AI may include

- Hypoglycemia (usually chronic)
- Hypercalcemia
- Eosinophilia
- Lymphocytosis

DIAGNOSIS

The diagnosis of AI is made by demonstrating diminished responsiveness of the HPA axis to stimulation. A morning cortisol value <3 μg/dL (assuming normal cortisol-binding globulin) can be sufficient to make the diagnosis of AI; however, the cosyntropin (Cortrosyn) (ACTH) stimulation test is usually required and is the gold standard:

Time 0 minutes   Baseline cortisol
Cosyntropin, 250 μg
   (intramuscularly or intravenously)
Time 30 or 60 minutes   Cortisol

A rise in the cortisol level to 18 μg/dL is a normal response. If an abnormal response is obtained, an ACTH level then determines primary (high ACTH) versus secondary disease (normal or low ACTH).

In secondary AI, however, the ACTH stimulation test is not always abnormal. Adequate ACTH may be present to prevent adrenal gland atrophy (thereby resulting in a response to the supraphysiological dose of ACTH used in the ACTH stimulation test), but the HPA axis may not be able to respond to stress. In patients with suspected secondary AI and a normal ACTH stimulation test, CRH is available to assess ACTH responsivity. In addition, the insulin tolerance test or the metyrapone test evaluate the integrity of the HPA axis by its response to hypoglycemia or inhibited cortisol synthesis, respectively. Although not widely used yet, some investigators find that a 1-μg ACTH stimulation test may be more sensitive at detecting mild AI.

TREATMENT

The treatment of AI is replacement of the deficient hormones. The following agents may be used in treating AI:

- Hydrocortisone, 30 mg every day
- Prednisone, 7.5 mg every day
- Dexamethasone, 0.75 mg every day

Cortisol, 20 mg in the morning and 10 mg in the evening, or prednisone, 5.0 to 7.5 mg daily, provides dramatic relief of symptoms. To prevent Cushing syndrome, however, the smallest dose needed to control the patient's symptoms should be used. For a minor illness, the glucocorticoid dose should be doubled for as short a time as needed. For a major stress, parenteral hydrocortisone, 200 to 400 mg daily, is given initially and then rapidly tapered. Aldosterone replacement is required in primary AI only; it is given as fludrocortisone (Florinef Acetate), 0.05 to 0.20 mg daily. The dose is adjusted according to the patient's blood pressure and potassium level. Adrenal androgens are not usually replaced, although some recent short-term studies have suggested a variable benefit of replacing with dehydroepiandrosterone (DHEA).

In undiagnosed patients with suspected adrenal crisis, dexamethasone, 2 to 4 mg intravenously or intramuscularly, should be given along with saline and glucose. Dexamethasone does not interfere with the cortisol assay. The ACTH stimulation test should then be done as soon as possible.

In the management of secondary AI caused by previous exogenous steroids, glucocorticoids with short half-lives (usually cortisone) should be given as larger doses in the morning and smaller doses in the evening. The evening doses are gradually tapered, as symptoms permit, to allow overnight hypothalamic-pituitary "desuppression" and a rise in the level of ACTH. This leads to a return of adrenal gland function; when morning cortisol reaches 10 μg/dL, replacement glucocorticoid generally can be discontinued. Stress glucocorticoids, however, should be given until a ACTH stimulation test is normal. The recovery of the HPA axis from glucocorticoid suppression generally requires 6 to 12 months.

HYPOALDOSTERONISM

Hypoaldosteronism results from decreased aldosterone production by the zona glomerulosa of the adrenal cortex. This may be due to deficient renin stimulation or

TABLE 43.2	
ETIOLOGY OF HYPOALDOSTERONISM	
Defective aldosterone secretion	Defective aldosterone stimulation
High renin	Low renin
AI	Renal insufficiency
Critically ill patient syndrome	Diabetes mellitus, pyelonephritis, gout
Heparin	NSAIDs, β-blockers
ACE inhibitors	Autonomic insufficiency AIDS

ACE, angiotensin-converting enzyme; AI, adrenal insufficiency; NSAIDS, nonsteroidal anti-inflammatory drugs.

defective aldosterone production, despite renin stimulation (Table 43.2). In adults, the most common cause of primary hypoaldosteronism is AD. Renal insufficiency (or type IV renal tubular acidosis) is the most common cause of secondary hypoaldosteronism. Children and young adults may have adrenal cortex enzyme deficiencies causing hypoaldosteronism.

The symptoms and signs of mineralocorticoid deficiency include hyperkalemia and metabolic acidosis. Blood pressure may be low, normal, or high. Serum sodium may be normal or low. If necessary, the diagnosis may be established by aldosterone levels that fail to rise with standing or volume depletion with diuretics.

The treatment of hypoaldosteronism involves mineralocorticoid replacement using fludrocortisone, 0.05 to 0.20 mg daily, with dose adjustments based on blood pressure and potassium levels. Patients with hypertension or congestive heart failure are treated with loop diuretics.

LATE-ONSET CONGENITAL ADRENAL HYPERPLASIA

Congenital adrenal hyperplasia (CAH), which is due to deficiency of an enzyme in the cortisol synthesis pathway, occurs in three variant forms:

- Classic CAH
- Simple virilizing CAH
- Late-onset CAH

Late-onset CAH results in a relative cortisol deficiency and increased ACTH levels. Cortisol production is normalized, but at the expense of adrenal hyperplasia and increased androgens. Therefore, late-onset CAH presents with peripubertal (or later) evidence of androgen excess (acne, hirsutism, menstrual irregularities, infertility) and adrenal hyperplasia or nodules. AI is not present.

The most common (relative) enzyme deficiency is 21-hydroxylase, resulting in an accumulation of

17-hydroxyprogesterone (17-OHP). In this case, screening for late-onset CAH may include:

- Random early-morning follicular phase 17-OHP
- Stimulated (by cosyntropin) 17-OHP

Late-onset CAH is best treated with low-dose glucocorticoid to lower ACTH and androgens.

CUSHING SYNDROME

Etiology

Cushing syndrome is a result of glucocorticoid excess. Endogenously, this may be due to increased ACTH secretion by the pituitary gland (Cushing disease) or ectopically or to autonomous cortisol secretion by an adrenal tumor. The most common cause of Cushing syndrome, however, is the exogenous use of glucocorticoids.

Clinical Presentation

The clinical features of Cushing syndrome are listed in Table 43.3. With respect to specificity for Cushing syndrome, thinning of the skin, purple striae, and bruising are the best clinical signs. Hypokalemia, edema, and hyperpigmentation are more commonly seen in ectopic ACTH secretion, in which ACTH and cortisol levels tend to be much higher.

Diagnosis

The diagnosis of Cushing syndrome revolves around the inability to suppress the HPA axis. Two screening tests are employed:

- 24-hour urine collection for free cortisol and creatinine (UFC)

TABLE 43.3

SIGNS AND SYMPTOMS OF CUSHING SYNDROME

Clinical Feature	Approximate Prevalence (%)
Obesity	
General	80–95
Truncal	45–80
Hypertension	75–90
Menstrual disorders	75–95
Osteopenia	75–85
Facial plethora	70–90
Hirsutism	70–80
Impotence/Decreased libido	65–95
Neuropsychiatric symptoms	60–95
Striae	50–70
Glucose intolerance	40–90
Weakness	30–90
Bruising	30–70
Kidney stones	15–20
Headache	10–50

- Overnight dexamethasone suppression test (ODST), in which dexamethasone, 1 mg, is given at 11 pm and a serum cortisol is drawn the following morning (Cortisol <5 μg/dL is a normal (or negative) response.)

The 24-hour UFC is more specific but also is more cumbersome. The value may be elevated in depression, acute illness, and alcoholism. The 1-mg ODST is easy to perform but has several false-positive and false-negative responses. The causes of a false-positive test result include increased cortisol-binding globulin (high circulating estrogen), depression, acute illness, and alcoholism. Drugs that increase the metabolism of dexamethasone (rifampin, phenobarbital, and phenytoin [Dilantin]) may also result in a false-positive response. False-negative tests may be seen in Cushing disease or cyclic intermittent Cushing syndrome.

Differential Diagnosis

If an abnormal result is obtained by either the 24-hour UFC or the 1-mg ODST, the pseudo-Cushing state of alcoholism or endogenous depression should first be sought by a careful history, physical examination, and laboratory evaluation. A repeat UFC during alcohol abstention should be normal. If necessary, the low-dose dexamethasone suppression test (DST) may document true hypercortisolism. Dexamethasone, 0.5 mg orally every 6 hours, is administered for 48 hours, while a 24-hour UFC, including 17-hydroxycorticosteroids (17-OHCS), is collected before and on the second day of dexamethasone. Failure to suppress 24-hour urine 17-OHCS to <4 mg or the UFC to <25 μg suggests pathological hypercortisolism, although pseudo-Cushing states occasionally cannot be suppressed. (Urinary 17-OHCS level is less essential because of the advent of the UFC, but the UFC is not yet as well standardized.) Once true Cushing syndrome has been documented, an ACTH level separates ACTH-dependent from ACTH-independent disease:

- ACTH-dependent hypercortisolism
  - Cushing disease
  - Ectopic ACTH
  - Ectopic CRH
- ACTH-independent hypercortisolism
  - Adrenal adenoma
  - Adrenal carcinoma
  - Nodular adrenal hyperplasia
  - Exogenous glucocorticoids

A low ACTH level prompts computed tomography (CT) of the adrenal to look for a tumor or nodules. A normal or elevated ACTH value suggests Cushing disease or ectopic ACTH production; these can be differentiated using the high-dose (8 mg) ODST. If a morning cortisol level suppresses by 50% in response to 8 mg of dexamethasone the evening before, the diagnosis is presumed to be Cushing disease. The specificity is not 100%, however;

many occult bronchial carcinoid tumors with ACTH secretion can suppress in response to high-dose dexamethasone.

Magnetic resonance imaging (MRI) is not definitive for distinguishing pituitary from nonpituitary tumors, since 50% of Cushing disease patients have occult pituitary adenomas. Furthermore, up to 10% of patients may have false-positive pituitary scans (pituitary "incidentaloma"). Inferior petrosal sinus sampling (enhanced with CRH) may be necessary; an elevated sinus-to-peripheral ACTH gradient suggests Cushing disease.

Treatment

It should be apparent that the diagnostic workup for Cushing syndrome can have many pitfalls. False-positive screening tests, pseudo-Cushing states, modest specificity of the high-dose DST, and pituitary imaging can all lead to an erroneous diagnosis. It is important to correctly diagnose Cushing disease, because the most appropriate treatment is transsphenoidal pituitary adenomectomy performed by an experienced neurosurgeon, although radiation therapy, ketoconazole (Nizoral) or bilateral adrenalectomy may be needed in some cases. Resection or chemotherapy of the underlying tumor is the treatment for adrenal neoplasia and ectopic ACTH production.

HYPERALDOSTERONISM

Excess aldosterone results in hyperaldosteronism with hypertension, hypokalemia, and metabolic alkalosis. This may be associated with Cushing syndrome, particularly in patients with adrenal carcinoma. Isolated primary hyperaldosteronism, marked by an elevated aldosterone level and suppressed plasma renin activity (PRA), accounts for 1% to 2% of patients with hypertension; the presence of spontaneous hypokalemia or a potassium level <3.0 mEq/L on diuretics should prompt an evaluation.

Once hypokalemia is corrected and interfering drugs are discontinued (diuretics, angiotensin-converting enzyme [ACE] inhibitors, and β-blockers), the ratio of aldosterone (ng/dL) to PRA (ng/mL per hour) is a simple screening test. A ratio >20 is quite sensitive but not specific. The saline suppression test confirms the diagnosis. (The test involves a determination of aldosterone and PRA before and after the administration of 2 L of normal saline: Normal patients suppress aldosterone to <5 ng/dL.) A persistently elevated aldosterone-to-PRA ratio after captopril (Capoten) also may be used to confirm the diagnosis.

The next step is to differentiate adrenal adenoma from hyperplasia. An adenoma can be differentiated by CT findings, increased 18-hydroxycorticosterone levels, or bilateral adrenal vein catheterization. Spironolactone (Aldactone), an aldosterone antagonist, is the treatment of choice for patients with hyperplasia, small adenomas, or contraindications to surgery.

OTHER MINERALOCORTICOID EXCESS SYNDROMES

The pathogenesis of several mineralocorticoid excess syndromes has recently been elucidated. Dexamethasone-suppressible hyperaldosteronism is an entity that should be suspected in a young patient with elevated aldosterone, suppressed renin, and an appropriate family history. Through the development of a hybrid gene, the enzyme that catalyzes the final steps of aldosterone synthesis becomes regulated by ACTH. Treatment with dexamethasone suppresses ACTH and subsequently excess aldosterone production.

In patients with suppressed PRA and low aldosterone, a mineralocorticoid other than aldosterone is present. In the syndrome of apparent mineralocorticoid excess, seen in young adults, the mineralocorticoid has been identified as cortisol (which normally has little mineralocorticoid effect). Normally, cortisol is inactivated to cortisone in the renal tubular cell by 11β-hydroxysteroid dehydrogenase. A deficiency of this enzyme allows cortisol to bind to the mineralocorticoid receptor, resulting in hypertension, hypokalemia, and suppressed PRA. Natural licorice (glycyrrhizic acid) is now known to inhibit 11β-hydroxysteroid dehydrogenase, thus explaining licorice-induced hypermineralocorticoidism.

Excess sodium itself serves to suppress PRA and causes hypertension in Liddle syndrome. In this familial syndrome, the constitutive activation of the kidneys' epithelial sodium channel results in increased sodium resorption and potassium excretion, independently of any mineralocorticoid. Spironolactone is therefore ineffective; triamterene (Dyrenium) is the treatment of choice.

PHEOCHROMOCYTOMA

Clinical Presentation

Pheochromocytoma usually arises in the adrenal medulla. It accounts for approximately 0.1% of hypertensive patients. This tumor should be especially suspected in multiple endocrine neoplasia type II (MEN IIA and MEN IIB), in which disease is frequently bilateral:

- MEN IIA
  - Pheochromocytoma
  - Medullary thyroid carcinoma
  - Hyperparathyroidism
- MEN IIB
  - Pheochromocytoma
  - Medullary thyroid carcinoma
  - Mucosal neuromas
  - Marfanoid habitus

The neuroectodermal syndromes also have an increased incidence of pheochromocytoma:

- Neurofibromatosis
- Neurofibromas
- Café au lait spots
- Cerebelloretinal hemangioblastosis
- Renal cell cancer
- Retinal angioma
- CNS hemangioblastoma
- Tuberous sclerosis
- Seizures
- Mental deficiency
- Adenoma sebaceum

The triad of headaches, palpitations, and diaphoresis in the presence of hypertension is classic for pheochromocytoma. Other signs and symptoms include:

- Postural hypotension
- Tachycardia
- Weight loss
- Pallor
- Hyperglycemia
- Anxiety
- Nausea/Vomiting
- Constipation
- Tremulousness

Silent pheochromocytomas are more frequently recognized, presenting as adrenal incidentalomas. Cocaine abuse may be mistaken for pheochromocytoma.

Diagnosis

Screening for pheochromocytoma consists of a 24-hour urine collection for catecholamines and catecholamine metabolites (metanephrines and vanillylmandelic acid). Plasma catecholamines may also be useful; plasma norepinephrine >2,000 pg/mL is specific for pheochromocytoma. Borderline or indeterminate results require further testing. The clonidine (Catapres) suppression test is used to confirm the diagnosis in patients with indeterminate urine or plasma studies. (The test involves the measurement of plasma catecholamines before and 3 hours after clonidine, 0.3 mg, is administered orally: A normal response is a plasma norepinephrine level <500 pg/mL or a 50% decrease from baseline.) The glucagon stimulation test may also be used; an increase in blood pressure and plasma catecholamines strongly suggests pheochromocytoma. The sensitivity of this test is limited, however, and it is potentially dangerous (hypertensive crisis). Chromogranin A, a neuropeptide secreted with the catecholamines, is reasonably sensitive for pheochromocytoma but is of poor specificity; it is elevated with even minor degrees of renal insufficiency and is cosecreted with many hormones.

Once the diagnosis is biochemically established, radiographic localization is indicated. Although CT is the initial choice, MRI may be especially useful because pheochromocytoma can be markedly hyperintense (white) on T2-weighted images. Scanning with iodine-131–labeled metaiodobenzylguanidine (MIBG) is most specific and particularly useful for extra-adrenal (10%) and malignant metastatic tumors (10%). It must be stressed that imaging studies should always follow biochemical confirmation of the disorder.

The treatment of a pheochromocytoma is resection after appropriate operative preparation (volume loading and adrenergic receptor blockade). Calcium channel blockers may also be effective.

INCIDENTALLY DISCOVERED ADRENAL MASS

Incidental adrenal masses are common, detected in approximately 2% of patients having abdominal CT. The differential diagnosis of such masses includes:

- Functioning or nonfunctioning adenoma
- Functioning or nonfunctioning carcinoma
- Pheochromocytoma
- Metastasis from tumors at other sites (especially malignant melanoma, lung, breast, and gastrointestinal cancers)
- Myelolipoma
- Cyst
- Focal enlargement in hyperplastic gland (e.g., Cushing disease, CAH)
- Pseudoadrenal mass arising from nearby organs

Management of an adrenal incidentaloma is controversial; clinical judgment is required. Patients should first be clinically evaluated for evidence of adrenal hormone production (cortisol, androgens, aldosterone, catecholamines). If the tumor appears to be clinically nonfunctional, most endocrinologists still screen biochemically for pheochromocytoma because of the associated morbidity and mortality. Several investigators also recommend dexamethasone suppression testing to exclude preclinical Cushing syndrome. These patients will not have the classic signs or symptoms of hypercortisolism but will have evidence of HPA axis dysfunction, such as loss of diurnal rhythm. The long-term implications of preclinical Cushing syndrome are unknown, and the optimal management is therefore controversial; however, at a minimum, these patients must be identified before adrenal surgery because postoperative AI may develop.

Despite an absence of hormone excess, nonfunctional adrenal tumors >4 to 6 cm should be resected owing to an increased risk of malignancy; nonfunctional tumors measuring ≤4 cm can be further evaluated radiographically to determine the likelihood of benign disease. The attenuation value, obtained from a noncontrast CT scan, is a measure of a tumor's lipid content. A value <10 Hounsfield units (HU) suggests fat density and is specific for adenoma.

Masses of indeterminate attenuation value (10–20 HU) can be further classified by opposed-phase MRI. Masses inconsistent with adenoma by CT or MRI require repeated follow-up with CT to assess growth or fine-needle aspiration (FNA) biopsy.

REVIEW EXERCISES

QUESTIONS

1. A 40-year-old white woman with a history of severe asthma and Hashimoto thyroiditis reports 2 months of fatigue, anorexia, nausea, weight loss, and myalgia. Her examination is remarkable only for a blood pressure of 98/60 mm Hg and a pulse of 98 beats per minute without orthostasis. She shows no hyperpigmentation. Sodium is 130 mEq/L; potassium, 4.5 mEq/L; chloride, 105 mEq/L; and bicarbonate, 24 mEq/L. ACTH stimulation test shows cortisol at 5.8 μg/dL at T 0 minute and 13.2 μg/dL at T 60 minutes.

Which of the following is correct?

a) The most likely cause of her AI is AD.

b) The most likely cause of her AI is prior exogenous corticosteroid use.

c) She does not have AI because her ACTH stimulation test is normal.

d) She will require treatment with prednisone, 7.5 mg daily, and fludrocortisone, 0.1 mg daily.

Answer and Discussion

The answer is b. This case illustrates the differences between primary and secondary AI in clinical presentation and treatment. In secondary AI, the renin–aldosterone axis is intact; therefore, hyperkalemia and metabolic acidosis are not seen, and fludrocortisone is not required for treatment.

2. You are treating a 58-year-old man with hypopituitarism following radiation therapy for craniopharyngioma. He is taking hydrocortisone sodium succinate, 15 mg daily; levothyroxine, 0.15 mg daily; and testosterone injections, 200 mg every 2 weeks. He feels weak and tired. His examination is remarkable only for a blood pressure of 95/58 mm Hg. Sodium is 131 mEq/L; potassium, 4.8 mEq/L; thyroid-stimulating hormone (TSH), 0.23 μIU/mL; and FTI, 9.0 μg/dL.

Which of the following would you do next?

a) Decrease levothyroxine

b) Increase testosterone

c) Add fludrocortisone

d) Increase hydrocortisone

e) Begin desmopressin acetate

Answer and Discussion

The answer is d. This case also illustrates secondary AI and inadequate glucocorticoid replacement. Phys-

iological hydrocortisone replacement is 20 to 30 mg daily. No data suggest the need for desmopressin or increased testosterone. Levothyroxine doses should not be adjusted by the TSH in secondary disease.

3. A 63-year-old woman who you are treating for hypertension, osteoarthritis, gout, and recurrent deep vein thrombosis, and with a 10-year history of type 2 diabetes mellitus, has a potassium level of 6.2 mEq/L at a follow-up appointment. Serum aldosterone is 1.8 ng/dL.

Which of the following is false?

a) A β-blocker and nonsteroidal anti-inflammatory drugs (NSAIDs) may be contributing to the hyperkalemia.

b) An ACE inhibitor may be contributing to the hyperkalemia.

c) Long-term heparin may be contributing to hypoaldosteronism.

d) Prednisone will likely be required as treatment.

Answer and Discussion

The answer is d. This case illustrates several conditions associated with hypoaldosteronism. Although AI can be associated with hypoaldosteronism, no suggestion of AI is present from the history presented, and it is more likely that medications are the cause. A heparin preservative (chlorbutol) can inhibit aldosterone synthesis, whereas NSAIDs (through the inhibition of prostacyclin, a vasodilator and renin secretagogue) and β-blockers suppress renin release.

4. A 37-year-old woman presents to you for evaluation of weight gain and hirsutism of several years duration. Her gynecologist has prescribed an oral contraceptive for oligomenorrhea. She has noted easy bruising but no muscle weakness. On examination, she weighs 240 pounds, with central obesity. Blood pressure is 144/92 mm Hg. She has significant facial hair, mild acne, multiple thin whitish striae on her abdomen, and a small buffalo hump. Her proximal muscle strength is normal. A random glucose level is 183 mg/dL, and potassium is 3.9 mEq/L. Her gynecologist sends you the results of an ODST (morning cortisol of 6.2 μg/dL) and a random ACTH level (25 pg/mL).

Which of the following would you do next?

a) Order MRI of the pituitary.

b) Order CT of the adrenals.

c) Obtain a 24-hour UFC.

d) Perform a high-dose (8 mg) dexamethasone suppression test.

Answer and Discussion

The answer is c. This case illustrates the evaluation of Cushing syndrome. Generally, the 24-hour UFC is the best screening test; the 1-mg ODST is easier to perform but has more false-positive results, including increased cortisol-binding globulin owing to the estrogen in oral contraceptives. Radiographic imaging is not indicated until the diagnosis is established biochemically.

5. A 50-year-old woman on chronic warfarin therapy for a previous pulmonary embolus was recently started on an acetylsalicylic acid (ASA)-containing analgesic for joint pain. She suddenly developed severe abdominal pain, and by the time she was taken to the emergency department, she was partially obtunded, hypotensive, and pale. Hemoglobin was found to be 8 mg/dL.

What would you do next?

a) Check international normalized ratio
b) Do a 1-hour ACTH stimulation test
c) Administer intravenous saline and dexamethasone
d) Do a blood type and match
e) Obtain an abdominal CT

Answer and Discussion

The answer is c. This patient likely has AI from an adrenal hemorrhage through the potentiation of warfarin by ASA. Intravenous fluids and dexamethasone can be lifesaving; then other options can be considered. Dexamethasone does not cross react with cortisol in the radioimmune assay. All choices are reasonable, but answer c should be performed first.

6. A 52-year-old woman is referred to you by her urologist for a 3-cm right adrenal mass detected on abdominal CT. Her weight has been stable, and she has generally felt well. She has not noted hirsutism, acne, proximal myopathy, or easy bruising, but she has felt depressed lately. She also has had diaphoresis and occasional headaches but no palpitations. Her last menstrual period was 6 months earlier. She has a 2-year history of diabetes mellitus that is well controlled by diet. Her last mammogram 8 months earlier was negative, and no breast masses are present. She smokes one pack of cigarettes daily. Blood pressure is 135/85 mm Hg; pulse, 95 beats per minute; and weight, 174 pounds. She has no buffalo hump, supraclavicular fat, or abdominal striae. Proximal muscle strength is normal. Stool is negative for occult blood. Complete blood cell count and chemistry profile are normal.

Which of the following would you do next?

a) Obtain a 24-hour UFC
b) Determine the aldosterone-to-PRA ratio
c) Obtain serum DHEAS and androstenedione levels
d) Obtain a 24-hour urine collection for catecholamines and metanephrines
e) All of the above

Answer and Discussion

The answer is d. This case illustrates the workup of an incidental adrenal mass. Biochemical testing should be influenced by clinical findings. If no evidence of hormone production is apparent through history and physical examination, a biochemical screen-ing for pheochromocytoma should nonetheless be done.

7. A 68-year-old man presents for evaluation of a 2.5-cm adrenal mass. History and physical examination are negative for malignancy and overproduction of any adrenal hormones. A biochemical evaluation for pheochromocytoma is negative. No data are present regarding CT attenuation value, and MRI opposed-phase imaging is not available.

Which of the following would you recommend?

a) Surgery
b) FNA biopsy of the mass
c) Conventional MRI
d) Follow-up CT in 3 to 6 months

Answer and Discussion

The answer is d. Surgery is not recommended for incidental adrenal masses unless they are large (>4 to 6 cm). A FNA biopsy can be diagnostic but should be used only when an immediate answer is needed and an experienced radiologist is available. FNA biopsy can diagnose metastatic disease but cannot always distinguish adrenal carcinoma from adenoma. Conventional MRI cannot distinguish metastasis from adenoma; only opposed-phase imaging (chemical-shift imaging) can do this. When CT or MRI cannot provide a definite diagnosis (metastasis vs. adenoma), follow-up CT is indicated.

SUGGESTED READINGS

Bravo EL. Primary aldosteronism: issues in diagnosis and management. *Endocrinol Metab Clin North Am* 1994;23:271–283.

Byny RL. Withdrawal from glucocorticoid therapy. *N Engl J Med* 1975;1:30–32.

Giordano R, Picu A, Bonelli L, et al. Hypothalamus-pituitary-adrenal axis evaluation in patients with hypothalamo-pituitary disorders: comparison of different provocative tests. *Clin Endocrinol (Oxf)* 2008;68:935–941.

Grinspoon SK, Biller BM. Clinical review 62: laboratory assessment of adrenal insufficiency. *J Clin Endocrinol Metab* 1994;79:923–931.

Gross MD, Shapiro B. Clinical review 50: clinically silent adrenal masses. *J Clin Endocrinol Metab* 1993;77:885–888.

Hamrahian AH, Ioachimescu AG, Remer EM, et al. Clinical utility of noncontrast computed tomography attenuation value (Hounsfield units) to differentiate adrenal adenomas/hyperplasias from nonadenomas: Cleveland Clinic Experience. *J Clin Endocrinol Metab* 2005;90(2):871–877.

Hunt PJ, Gurnell EM, Huppert FA, et al. Improvement in mood and fatigue after dehydroepiandrosterone replacement in Addison's disease in a randomized, double blind trial. *J Clin Endocrinol Metab* 2000;85:4650–4656.

Kong MF, Jeff CW. Eighty-six cases of Addison's disease. *Clin Endocrinol* 1994;41:757–761.

Lovas K, Gebre-Medhin G, Trovik TS, et al. Replacement of dehydroepiandrosterone in adrenal failure: no benefit for subjective health status and sexuality in a 9-month, randomized, parallel group clinical trial. *J Clin Endocrinol Metab* 2003;88:1112–1118.

Miller WL. The adrenal cortex and its disorders. In: Brook CDG, Clayton PE, Rosalind S, eds. *Textbook of Pediatric Endocrinology.* Blackwell Publishing.

Orth DN. Cushing's syndrome. *N Engl J Med* 1995;332:791–803.

Vaughan E Jr. Diseases of the adrenal gland. *Med Clin North Am* 2005;88(2):443–466.

Chapter 44

Pituitary Disorders and Multiple Endocrine Neoplasia Syndromes

S. Sethu K. Reddy   Amir H. Hamrahian

POINTS TO REMEMBER:

- Pituitary tumors may present with either pituitary hypofunction or excess hormone secretion as well as symptoms directly related to the mass effect of the tumor.

- Pituitary adenomas are the most common cause of hypopituitarism. However, other causes, including parasellar diseases, inflammatory disorders, those following pituitary surgery or radiation therapy, and head injury, also must be considered.

- A serum prolactin (PRL) level >100 μg/L is usually indicative of a PRL-producing pituitary tumor.

- Although patients with microprolactinomas can sometimes be followed without therapy, patients with macroprolactinomas must be treated.

- A random growth hormone (GH) level is usually inadequate to establish the diagnosis of acromegaly. Insulinlike growth factor 1 (IGF-1) has a longer plasma half-life than GH and is an excellent initial screening test for those suspected of acromegaly.

- Pituitary apoplexy is an endocrine emergency resulting from a hemorrhagic infarction of the pituitary, usually associated with a preexisting pituitary tumor.

- If pituitary apoplexy is suspected, anterior pituitary insufficiency should be presumed, and the pa-
tient must be treated accordingly. Glucocorticoids, in a dose adequate to the degree of stress and presumptive cerebral edema, are the treatment of choice.

- Sheehan syndrome is the result of an ischemic infarction of the normal pituitary gland, which leads to hypopituitarism secondary to postpartum hemorrhage and hypotension. Patients have a history of failure to lactate postpartum and failure to resume menses.

The pituitary gland consists of the anterior lobe (developed from the Rathke pouch) and the posterior lobe (developed as a diverticulum growing downward from the base of the hypothalamus).

Weighing from 0.5 to 1.0 g, the pituitary sits in the sella turcica, immediately above the sphenoid sinus. It has anterior and posterior bony walls and a bony floor. Superior to the pituitary is a layer of dura (diaphragma sella) and then the optic chiasm, hypothalamus, and third ventricle. Laterally, on each side, is the cavernous sinus, inclusive of the internal carotid artery and cranial nerves III, IV, V_1, V_2, and VI. The optic chiasm may be anterior (15%), above (80%), or behind the sella (5%).

All pituitary hormones are under positive stimulatory effect from the hypothalamus (Table 44.1), except PRL, which is under tonic inhibitory effect through dopamine acting as the main PRL release-inhibiting factor (PIF). For

TABLE 44.1

INTERACTION OF HYPOTHALAMIC REGULATORY HORMONES, PITUITARY HORMONES, AND PERIPHERAL HORMONES FROM TARGET GLANDS

Hypothalamic Hormones	Pituitary Hormones	Target Gland	Feedback Hormone
TRH	TSH	Thyroid	T_4, T_3
GnRH	LH	Gonad	E2, testosterone
GnRH	FSH	Gonad	Inhibin, E2, testosterone
GHRH, SMS	GH	Multiorgans	IGF-1
PIF	PRL	Breast	?
CRH, ADH	ACTH	Adrenal	Cortisol

ACTH, adrenocorticotropic hormone; ADH, antidiuretic hormone; CRH, corticotropin-releasing hormone; E2, estradiol; FSH, follicle-stimulating hormone; GH, growth hormone; GHRH, growth hormone–releasing hormone; IGF-1, insulinlike growth factor 1; LH, luteinizing hormone; GnRH, gonadotropin–releasing hormone; PIF, prolactin release-inhibiting factor; PRL, prolactin; SMS, somatostatin; T_3, triiodothyronine; T_4, thyroxine; TRH, thyrotropin-releasing hormone; TSH, thyroid-stimulating hormone.

the same reason, in the case of any blockage or interruption of hypothalamic-pituitary portal system, all pituitary hormones are decreased, except PRL (which will increase).

Magnetic resonance imaging (MRI) is the best method for visualizing hypothalamic-pituitary anatomy, including the optic chiasm, vascular structures, and tumor extension to cavernous sinuses.

PITUITARY TUMORS

Pituitary tumors may present with either pituitary hypofunction or excess hormone secretion as well as symptoms directly related to the mass effect of the tumor (Table 44.2). Since the advent of computed tomography (CT), microadenomas have been designated arbitrarily as <10 mm in diameter and macroadenomas as ≥10 mm in diameter. They are almost always benign. Pituitary adenomas are rarely associated with parathyroid and pancreatic hyperplasia or neoplasia as part of the multiple endocrine neoplasia

(MEN) type 1 (MEN1) syndrome. Pituitary carcinomas are very rare, but metastases from lung, breast, or renal cell carcinoma may occur.

About 30% of pituitary adenomas are prolactinomas; 15% are GH producing, 10% are adrenocorticotropic hormone (ACTH) producing, 10% are glycoprotein producing, and <1% secrete thyroid-stimulating hormone (TSH). Nonfunctioning pituitary adenomas, or more appropriately named *nonsecretory adenomas*, represent about 25% of pituitary tumors. On morphologic examination, most of these nonsecretory adenomas reveal granules containing glycoprotein hormones or their subunits.

Impingement on the optic chiasm or its branches by a pituitary mass may result in visual field defects, with the most common being bitemporal hemianopsia. A lateral extension of the pituitary tumor to the cavernous sinuses may result in diplopia, ptosis, or altered facial sensation. Among the cranial nerves, third nerve palsy is the most common.

Autopsy studies suggest that up to 20% of normal individuals harbor incidental pituitary tumors, which are

TABLE 44.2

CLINICAL MANIFESTATIONS OF PITUITARY TUMORS

Mass Effects	Endocrine Effects	
	Hyperpituitarism	Hypopituitarism
Headaches	GH: Acromegaly	GH: Short stature in children, increased fat mass, osteoporosis, decreased strength, and quality of life
Chiasmal syndrome	PRL: Hyperprolactinemia	
Cranial nerves III, IV, V_1, V_2, and VI dysfunction	ACTH: Cushing disease; Nelson syndrome	PRL: Failure of postpartum lactation
Obstructive hydrocephalus	LH/FSH: Mostly present with mass effect but may result in gonadal dysfunction	ACTH: Hypocortisolism
		LH or FSH: Hypogonadism
	TSH: Hyperthyroidism	TSH: Hypothyroidism

ACTH, adrenocorticotropic hormone; CSF, cerebrospinal fluid; DI, diabetes insipidus; FSH, follicle-stimulating hormone; GH, growth hormone; LH, luteinizing hormone; PRL, prolactin; SIADH, syndrome of inappropriate secretion of antidiuretic hormone; TSH, thyroid-stimulating hormone.

almost all microadenomas. In such cases, the initial workup should be limited and include serum PRL- and IGF-1–level testing. Other screening tests may be performed depending on clinical features such as obtaining 24-hour urinary free cortisol (UFC) in a patient with clinical features suggestive of Cushing disease. While a follow-up MRI in 1 year in patients with pituitary microadenomas is reasonable to monitor any tumor growth, there is no data to support further imaging studies unless there is a change in clinical symptoms. Patients with pituitary macroadenomas need to be monitored closely by yearly MRI, increasing the duration between imaging studies if tumor size remains stable.

HYPOPITUITARISM

Pituitary adenomas are the most common cause of hypopituitarism. However, other causes, including parasellar diseases, inflammatory disorders, those following pituitary surgery or radiation therapy, and head injury, also must be considered. The usual consequence of pituitary hormone deficiency secondary to a mass effect is in the following order: GH, luteinizing hormone (LH), follicle-stimulating hormone (FSH), TSH, ACTH, and PRL. PRL deficiency is uncommon, except in those with extensive pituitary hemorrhage or infarction. Isolated deficiencies of various anterior pituitary hormones have been described as well.

The symptoms of GH deficiency in adults may include decreased muscle strength and exercise capacity, decreased bone density, and reduced sense of well being (e.g., diminished libido, social isolation). Patients with GH deficiency have increased body fat, particularly intra-abdominally, and decreased lean body mass compared with normal adults. A trial of GH replacement in adults with documented GH deficiency and symptoms, or metabolic abnormalities suggestive of GH deficiency, is indicated. Treatment of GH deficiency has been shown to have a favorable effect on a lipid profile and may result in decreased carotid intima thickness. The most common side effects of GH therapy include fluid retention, carpal tunnel syndrome, and arthralgia. These side effects are usually dose related and improve with dose reduction.

Gonadotropin deficiency may be secondary to a pituitary disorder; hypothalamic deficiency of gonadotropin–releasing hormone (GnRH); or a functional abnormality such as hyperprolactinemia, anorexia nervosa, and severe disease state. In women, gonadotropin deficiency causes infertility and menstrual disorders, including amenorrhea. It is often associated with lack of libido and dyspareunia. In men, hypogonadism is diagnosed less often because decreased libido and impotence may be considered as a function of aging. Hypogonadism is often diagnosed retrospectively when a patient presents with mass effect. Osteopenia is a consequence of long-standing hypogonadism and usually responds to sex steroid hormone replacement therapy.

The symptoms of secondary adrenal insufficiency are similar to primary adrenal insufficiency, with one important difference. Mineralocorticoid secretion is mainly regulated by the renin-angiotensin system, which is preserved in patients with pituitary disorders. Hyperkalemia is thus not a feature of secondary adrenal insufficiency. Symptoms are more chronic in nature and include malaise, loss of energy, anorexia, and hypoglycemia. An acute illness may precipitate vascular collapse and be life threatening if unrecognized.

The symptoms of TSH deficiency are similar to those of primary hypothyroidism, including malaise, leg cramps, lack of energy, and cold intolerance. The degree of hypothyroidism depends on the duration of thyrotropin deficiency. Lactotropin deficiency is associated with lack of lactation in women, such as those with Sheehan syndrome. There is no clearly defined clinical disorder associated with PRL deficiency in men.

PROLACTINOMA

The pituitary content of PRL is approximately 100 μg but can increase 10- to 20-fold during pregnancy and lactation. Although breast tissue is the most important target organ for PRL, PRL receptors have been identified in various tissues, including the liver, kidneys, ovaries, testes, prostate, and seminal vesicles. Any interruption of dopamine transport from the hypothalamus to the pituitary can lead to elevated levels of PRL.

Prolactinomas are the most common secretory pituitary tumors. Observational studies in patients with microprolactinomas indicate that serum PRL concentration or adenoma size increase in only a minority of patients over time. Past estrogen therapy has been suggested as a cause of prolactinoma formation, but careful case-cohort studies have found no evidence that oral contraceptives induce the development of prolactinomas. The clonal analysis of tumor DNA indicates that prolactinomas are monoclonal in origin.

Hyperprolactinemia impairs pulsatile gonadotropin release (LH and FSH), likely through an alteration in hypothalamic GnRH secretion. Women of reproductive age usually present with oligomenorrhea, amenorrhea, galactorrhea, and infertility. Those with long-standing amenorrhea are less likely to have galactorrhea, secondary to long-standing estrogen deficiency. Men and postmenopausal women usually come to medical attention because of mass effect, such as headaches and visual field defects. Many men with hyperprolactinemia do not report any sexual dysfunction, but once treated effectively for hyperprolactinemia, the majority retrospectively complain of decreased libido and erectile dysfunction. Men with long-standing hypogonadism may have decreased beard and body hair, with soft but usually normal-size testes (if hypogonadism starts before completion of puberty, the testes will be small).

TABLE 44.3

DIFFERENTIAL DIAGNOSIS OF HYPERPROLACTINEMIA

Physiological	Pathological	Pharmacologic
Pregnancy	Prolactinoma	Antipsychotic medication
Postpartum	Acromegaly (GH and PRL cosecretion)	Tricyclic antidepressants
Newborn	Pituitary stalk lesion or compression	Some SSRIs, including fluoxetine
Stress	secondary to mass effect	and fluvoxamine
Hypoglycemia	Hypothyroidism	Methyldopa, reserpine, verapamil
Sleep	Renal failure	Metoclopramide
Intercourse	Liver disease	Estrogen, antiandrogens
Nipple stimulation	Chest wall trauma (burn, shingles)	H2 blockers (especially
	Spinal nerves or cord lesions	intravenous preparation)
	Ectopic PRL secretion (very rare)	Opiates, cocaine
		Protease inhibitors

GH, growth hormone; PRL, prolactin; SSRI, selective serotonin reuptake inhibitor.

Patients with microadenomas have a higher frequency of headaches compared with control subjects.

A drug history is a very important part of the initial evaluation of patients with elevated PRL level, because some medications are associated with hyperprolactinemia, and their discontinuation (if possible) will avoid any further and often expensive workup. Other common conditions associated with elevated PRL levels include pregnancy and hypothyroidism (Table 44.3). A serum PRL level >100 μg/L is usually indicative of a PRL-producing pituitary tumor. Conversely, a serum PRL level <100 μg/L in the presence of a large pituitary adenoma is suggestive of stalk compression. The PRL level usually correlates with the size of the tumor.

Bromocriptine mesylate (Parlodel) and cabergoline (Dostinex) are potent inhibitors of PRL secretion and often result in tumor shrinkage. The suppression of PRL secretion through dopamine agonists depends on the number and affinity of dopamine receptors on the lactotroph adenoma. A substantial decrease in the tumor PRL content usually occurs, even when serum PRL levels do not normalize. These medications should be initiated slowly, because side effects often occur at the beginning of treatment. The most common side effects include nausea, headache, dizziness, nasal congestion, and constipation. There has been some report about association of valvular heart disease with high doses of ergot-derived dopamine agonists such as pergolide (withdrawn from the U.S. market in 2007) and cabergoline. While such association with the lower doses of such drugs used for treatment of patients with prolactinoma is unknown, periodic echocardiograms may be a reasonable precaution until further follow-up studies are completed. It may take up to 6 months before testosterone levels increase and normal sexual function is restored in men successfully treated for prolactinomas. PRL appears to have an independent effect in men on libido, because exogenous testosterone works poorly in restoring libido in those who continue to have elevated PRL levels.

Although patients with microprolactinomas can sometimes be followed without therapy, patients with macropro-

lactinomas must be treated. Patients with good response to dopamine agonist therapy may be weaned with no increase in PRL concentration. For this reason, it would be reasonable to try a "drug holiday" after several years of therapy with close follow-up. A prolactin <5 μg/mL during therapy and absence of a pituitary tumor on follow-up imaging study have been associated with increased chance of long-term remission following discontinuation of dopamine agonists.

Medical therapy during pregnancy often stirs debate about the continuation of bromocriptine. Tumor-related complications are seen in <15% of pregnancies and in <5% of women with microadenomas. A sensible approach would be to stop bromocriptine when pregnancy is confirmed and then follow the clinical status with visual field examinations. If any evidence for mass effect presents, bromocriptine may be reinstituted.

Medical therapy with dopamine agonists is the first-line treatment for prolactinoma. Surgery, typically, transsphenoidal resection, is reserved for those who cannot tolerate or do not respond to medical therapy. Even in patients with mass effect, including visual field defects, dopamine agonists are first-line therapy, as a rapid improvement in symptoms is observed in a majority of patients. The main advantage of surgery is the avoidance of chronic medical therapy. Radiation therapy may be considered for patients who poorly tolerate dopamine agonists and who are not likely to be cured by surgery (e.g., tumor invasion of cavernous sinuses).

ACROMEGALY

Acromegaly occurs at a rate of 3 to 4 cases per million per year, with a mean age at diagnosis of 40 years in men and 45 years in women. The GH-secreting tumors tend to be more aggressive in younger patients. Classical clinical features include:

- Coarsening of facial features
- Prominent jaw and frontal sinus

- Broadening of hands and feet
- Hyperhidrosis
- Macroglossia
- Signs of hypopituitarism
- Diabetes mellitus (10%–25%)
- Skin tags
- Hypertension (25%–30%)
- Cardiomyopathy
- Carpal tunnel syndrome
- Sleep apnea

In more than 99% of cases, acromegaly is caused by GH-secreting pituitary tumors, and the rest is usually caused by ectopic growth hormone–releasing hormone (GHRH) and growth hormone secretion. Patients with acromegaly have a three- to fivefold increased mortality rate, with cardiovascular disease (CVD) being the most common cause of death. Somatotroph adenomas appear to be monoclonal in origin. A stimulatory guanosine triphosphate (GTP)-binding protein mutation in a Gsp$_1\alpha$ subunit in GH cells, leading to continuous GH secretion, has been shown to cause acromegaly.

Due to the pulsatile nature of GH secretion, random GH levels can overlap in acromegalic patients and controls. Therefore, a random GH level is usually inadequate to establish the diagnosis. IGF-1 has a longer plasma half-life than GH and is an excellent initial screening test for those suspected of acromegaly. An elevated IGF-1 level in a clinical setting suggestive of acromegaly almost always confirms the diagnosis. The IGF-1 level may be falsely low in patients with poorly controlled diabetes, hypothyroidism, and malnutrition. The IGF-1 may be elevated during the second half of pregnancy and in those with hyperthyroidism. The oral glucose tolerance test remains the gold standard to confirm the diagnosis. Normal individuals suppress their GH level to <1 μg/L within 2 hours following ingestion of a 75-g oral glucose solution.

In the case of ectopic acromegaly, elevated GHRH can be measured in blood to confirm the diagnosis (usually >200 ng/mL). As an exception, patients with hypothalamic GHRH-secreting tumors may have normal GHRH levels, probably secondary to the direct release of GHRH to the hypophyseal portal system. In patients with GH-secreting pituitary adenoma, the GHRH level is low or undetectable.

The early detection of CVD is of particular importance, because CVD is the primary cause of mortality. Patients with acromegaly have an increased risk of colon polyps, with the potential for an increased risk of malignancy. Thus, patients should undergo colonoscopy at diagnosis and then every 3 to 5 years until more data about the frequency of such screening tests are available. It is not clear if more rigorous screening for a variety of cancers, including breast, lung, or prostate cancer, is indicated.

In acromegaly, the primary aims of treatment include relieving symptoms, reducing tumor bulk, normalizing IGF-1 and GH dynamics, and preventing tumor regrowth.

The medical treatment of acromegaly has gained significance as the limitations of radiation therapy have become evident. Current medical therapies for acromegaly include dopamine agonist, somatostatin analogs, and GH receptor antagonist. The normalization of IGF-1 is seen in only 10% to 15% of patients treated with dopamine agonists and is more likely with pituitary tumors cosecreting GH and PRL. Octreotide (a somatostatin analog) and the long-acting preparations (Sandostatin LAR and lanreotide acetate [Somatuline Depot]) lower and normalize IGF-1 in about 90% and 60% of acromegalic patients, respectively. The long-term observations of patients on somatostatin analogs have shown no evidence for tachyphylaxis. Some degree of tumor shrinkage in up to 50% of patients is expected, although in most cases, <50% shrinkage occurs in tumor size. The most common side effects are gastrointestinal, including diarrhea, abdominal pain, and nausea. The gall bladder sludge and cholelithiasis is seen in up to 25% of patients and is mostly asymptomatic. Its long-term management is similar to those with cholelithiasis in the general population, and routine ultrasonographic screening in the absence of symptoms is not indicated.

The GH receptor antagonist pegvisomant has increased affinity to GH receptors compared with native GH and inhibits receptor dimerization, which is necessary for the action of GH. It is administered once daily and is usually reserved for those not responding to other medical therapies. It is very effective with normalization of IGF-1 in up to 95% of patients. Due to its mechanism of action and associated increase in GH during therapy, the tumor size needs to be monitored during therapy. Patients may also develop some reversible liver function abnormalities. For that reason, liver enzymes need to be closely monitored and the drug discontinued if liver enzymes increase to more than three times the upper limit of normal. During therapy with pegvisomant, IGF-1—not serum GH—should be used to monitor therapy.

A surgical approach is the treatment of choice for most patients with acromegaly. Even in those not cured by surgery, tumor debulking usually results in improvement of symptoms and lowering of IGF-1 levels. Radiation therapy almost always induces a decrease in GH level and stabilization of the tumor size, but the cure rate after conventional radiotherapy has been disappointing. Radiosurgery (gamma knife) achieves remission faster, however the rate of hypopituitarism seems to be similar to conventional radiotherapy.

CUSHING DISEASE AND ECTOPIC ACTH SYNDROME

An ACTH-secreting pituitary adenoma is the most common cause of endogenous Cushing syndrome (CS) (65%), with the rest being adrenal (25%) or ectopic (10%) in origin.

The following findings are suggestive of a hypercortisolism state:

- Central obesity
- Muscle wasting with proximal muscle weakness
- Unexplained osteopenia or osteoporosis
- Spontaneous ecchymosis
- Purplish wide striae (>1 cm)
- Hypokalemia
- Serial photographs show change in appearance
- Facial plethora

Other findings that are less helpful in discriminating patients with and without Cushing disease are hypertension, abnormal glucose tolerance, menstrual irregularities, and psychiatric disturbances, including depression. Women with Cushing disease typically have fine facial lanugo hair and may have acne and temporal scalp hair loss secondary to increased adrenal androgen secretion. A 3- to 6-year delay in the diagnosis of patients with Cushing disease is not uncommon.

The screening for CS may be done by midnight salivary cortisol, the 1-mg dexamethasone suppression test (DST), or 24-hour UFC. The 1-mg DST is performed by administration of 1-mg dexamethasone at 11 pm followed by measurement of plasma cortisol at 8 am with a cortisol <1.8 μg/dL as normal response. While the 1-mg DST is an excellent test to rule out CS with <2% false-negative test result, a false-positive rate can be seen in as high as 40% of patients without CS depending on the population being tested. A positive test result needs to be confirmed by 24-hour UFC or salivary cortisol. Values of 24-hour UFC above three to four times upper normal for the assay are usually diagnostic for CS, especially once repeated and confirmed. It is im-

portant to be familiar with assay-specific normative values for their interpretation. Due to the significant overlap between normal individuals and those with Cushing, random serum cortisol has no role in the diagnosis of CS. A 2-day low-dose dexamethasone suppression test (LDDST) or a combination of the LDDST and a corticotropin-releasing hormone (CRH) stimulation test are used in patients with equivocal results or to differentiate CS from those with pseudo-Cushing (Fig. 44.1).

Once the diagnosis of CS has been established, the next step is to find out whether it is ACTH dependent or ACTH independent (Fig. 44.1). Although undetectable or low ACTH levels are consistent with adrenal etiology, low-normal ACTH levels may be seen in both adrenal CS and those with ACTH-secreting pituitary adenoma. The CRH stimulation test may be helpful to differentiate between the two. An increase of ≥50% in the ACTH level following CRH stimulation is suggestive of Cushing disease. Although ACTH levels tend to be higher in those with ectopic CS compared with patients having pituitary disease, considerable overlap occurs. A high-dose (8-mg) dexamethasone suppression test (HDDST) and/or CRH stimulation test may be helpful in differentiating between the two. Patients with Cushing disease suppress their cortisol level more than 80% during the HDDST and have a more than 50% increase in ACTH levels during the CRH stimulation test. The gold standard test to differentiate pituitary Cushing disease from an ectopic ACTH-producing tumor is inferior petrosal sinus sampling. This test should be performed only by an experienced neuroradiologist to localize the source of ACTH secretion and *not* to diagnose CS. Patients with Cushing disease, normal individuals, and those with pseudo-Cushing may have similar inferior petrosal sinus sampling results.

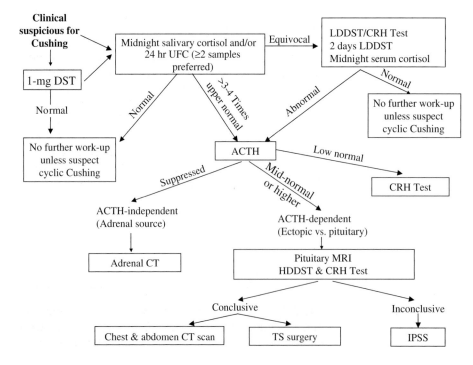

Figure 44.1 Cushing evaluation: workup algorithm. (ACTH, adrenocorticotropic hormone; CRH, corticotropin-releasing hormone; CT, computed tomography; DST, dexamethasone suppression test; HDDST, high-dose dexamethasone suppression test; IPSS, inferior petrosal sinus sampling; LDDST, low-dose dexamethasone suppression test; MRI, magnetic resonance imaging; TS, transsphenoidal; UFC, urinary free cortisol)

Most tumors associated with ectopic ACTH syndrome are carcinomas that have a poor prognosis. These tumors usually present with a rapid-onset syndrome (within 6 months) associated with profound muscle weakness, hyperpigmentation, hypertension, hypokalemia, and edema. Hyperpigmentation is thought to be due to cosecretion of β-melanocyte–stimulating hormone (β-MSH), one of the by-products of ACTH synthesis. Some benign tumors, such as carcinoids or islet cell tumors, have been shown to cause ectopic ACTH syndrome; these are difficult to differentiate from the pituitary causes of CS. This difficulty is exaggerated by radiologic investigations of the sella that are often negative or show a microadenoma, which is incidentally seen in up to 10% of normal individuals.

The surgical (transsphenoidal) removal of ACTH-secreting pituitary tumor is the treatment of choice. The availability of an experienced surgeon is crucial, with an 80% remission rate following surgery. An undetectable postoperative cortisol level without steroid use is considered to be a good marker for long-term cure. Temporary adrenal insufficiency occurs following successful surgery and usually lasts for 3 to 12 months. For those not cured by surgery, other options include a second sellar exploration, medical therapy, and radiation therapy. Patients whose tumor is unresponsive to these therapies may then be offered surgical adrenalectomy. Ectopic ACTH-producing tumors should be resected if possible.

Medical therapy for CS has limited value because of the associated toxicity and gradual decrease in efficacy, however, new agents are being tested in clinical trials. Among available agents, ketoconazole is the most commonly used. During therapy, liver function tests need to be closely monitored. Some reports indicate the efficacy of cabergoline, a dopamine agonist, in at least a subpopulation of patients with CS, which may be worth a trial before initiating ketoconazole. Other medications used include mitotane (Lysodren), aminoglutethimide (Cytadren), and metyrapone (Metopirone).

NONFUNCTIONAL OR GLYCOPROTEIN-SECRETING TUMORS

Nonfunctional or glycoprotein-secreting pituitary tumors are usually clinically silent because they are inefficient in secreting hormones and lack a clinically recognizable syndrome. They usually come to attention because of mass lesion manifestations, including headache and visual field defect. Patients may present with varying degrees of hypopituitarism due to mass effect. Rarely, an FSH-secreting adenoma may cause amenorrhea in a woman, or an LH-secreting adenoma may cause precocious puberty in a boy. The diagnosis is confirmed by the measurement of either intact glycoprotein hormones or their α and β subunits.

The transsphenoidal surgical approach is standard, especially if visual function is abnormal. Radiation therapy is used in those with significant residual tumor or evidence of tumor recurrence. Dopamine agonists, such as bromocriptine and cabergoline, have been used in high doses, but clinical responses (i.e., changes in tumor size or visual symptoms) occur in <10% of patients.

THYROID-STIMULATING HORMONE–SECRETING PITUITARY TUMORS

The clinical picture in patients with TSH-secreting pituitary adenoma includes pituitary mass lesion, hyperthyroidism, and goiter. The most important biochemical feature of TSH-secreting pituitary tumors is the elevation of thyroid hormone levels in the presence of a normal or elevated TSH level. For this reason, any patient presenting with endogenous hyperthyroidism and a normal or elevated TSH should be evaluated further for the presence of a TSH-secreting pituitary adenoma. Elevated serum α subunit favors the diagnosis of a thyrotropic adenoma and against a diagnosis of thyroid hormone resistance syndrome. Octreotide is especially useful in reducing hormone hypersecretion, but its effect on tumor size may be variable. Antithyroid medications may be used to make the patient euthyroid before surgical resection of the tumor is attempted.

LYMPHOCYTIC HYPOPHYSITIS

Lymphocytic hypophysitis is an autoimmune disease that often presents in women during or after pregnancy. The clinical manifestations are secondary to hypopituitarism and adrenal insufficiency or may be caused by a pituitary mass effect. The serum PRL level is elevated in more than half of patients, but it may be decreased. Other autoimmune endocrine disorders, including Hashimoto thyroiditis and Addison disease, have been seen with increased frequency in such patients. Although the diagnosis may be suspected clinically in a pregnant or postpartum woman, a surgical biopsy may be needed to confirm the diagnosis. Isolated ACTH deficiency has been described in some patients, and its presence should alert the physician to the possibility of lymphocytic hypophysitis as an underlying disorder. Some patients recover fully, whereas others may need selective hormone replacement. For this reason, patients must be assessed at regular intervals for the necessity of continued hormone replacement. Serial measurements of plasma ACTH may provide a clue about recovery of ACTH axis.

EMPTY SELLA

The diagnosis of empty sella syndrome is increasingly made owing to the prevalence of CT and MRI. Pituitary fossa enlargement may be secondary to a communication between the pituitary fossa and the subarachnoid space, which causes remodeling and enlargement of the sella. Although a primary empty sella is the result of a congenital diaphragmatic defect, a secondary empty sella may result from previous surgery, irradiation, or infarction of a preexisting tumor. Most patients have no pituitary dysfunction, but a wide spectrum of pituitary deficiencies have been described, especially in those with secondary empty sella. Coexisting tumors may occur. Management usually comprises reassurance and hormone replacement, if necessary.

PITUITARY APOPLEXY

Pituitary apoplexy is an endocrine emergency resulting from a hemorrhagic infarction of the pituitary, usually associated with a preexisting pituitary tumor. A variety of predisposing conditions including bleeding disorders, anticoagulation, diabetes mellitus, pituitary radiation, mechanical ventilation, and trauma have been described. The clinical manifestations of this syndrome are related to the rapid expansion and compression of the pituitary gland and the perisellar structures, leading to hypopituitarism, visual field defects, and cranial nerve palsies. An extravasation of blood or necrotic tissue into the subarachnoid space may cause change in mental status, meningismus, and fever. If pituitary apoplexy is suspected, anterior pituitary insufficiency should be presumed, and the patient must be treated accordingly. Glucocorticoids, in a dose adequate to the degree of stress and presumptive cerebral edema, are the treatment of choice. Any evidence of sudden visual field defects, oculomotor palsies, hypothalamic compression, or coma should lead to immediate surgical decompression. The recovery of a variety of pituitary hormone deficiencies following surgery have been documented, and all patients should be reevaluated for possible recovery of their pituitary hormone axes. A mildly elevated prolactin level prior to surgery predicts a higher chance for recovery of pituitary hormones.

Sheehan syndrome is the result of an ischemic infarction of the normal pituitary gland, which leads to hypopituitarism secondary to postpartum hemorrhage and hypotension. Patients have a history of failure to lactate postpartum, failure to resume menses, cold intolerance, or fatigue. Subclinical central diabetes insipidus (DI) may be present.

MULTIPLE ENDOCRINE NEOPLASIA SYNDROMES

MEN syndromes are rare, but their recognition is crucial because it is important to promptly treat the patient and identify affected family members. MEN syndromes are all inherited as an autosomal dominant trait. It is essential for the treating physician to be alert to the various clinical presentations of MEN syndrome and to use the available molecular DNA testing for diagnostic confirmation.

MEN syndromes include:

- MEN1
- MEN2
- MEN2A
- MEN2B
- Familial medullary thyroid cancer (FMTC)

MEN1 syndrome, which may involve an anterior pituitary tumor, usually manifests in the fourth or fifth decade of life. Its prevalence is about 2 per 100,000. The parathyroid glands (80%–90%), the pancreas (80%), and the pituitary (65%) may be involved. Ninety percent of patients with MEN1 have hypercalcemia by the age of 59 years. Gastrinoma (Zollinger-Ellison syndrome) is the most common pancreatic tumor (70%), followed by insulinoma. Pancreatic tumors may secrete gastrin, insulin, vasoactive intestinal polypeptide (Werner-Morrison syndrome), serotonin, glucagon, somatostatin, pancreatic polypeptide, or GHRH. Carcinoid tumors are also associated with MEN1 and MEN2 syndromes. Hyperparathyroidism is the initial manifestation in the majority of patients. It is estimated that 1% to 2% of all cases of primary hyperparathyroidism are caused by MEN1 syndrome. Pituitary tumors occur in a distribution similar to that of isolated pituitary adenomas.

MEN1 is the result of a mutation at the q13 locus in chromosome 11, resulting in the loss of a tumor suppressor gene. If the q13 locus is lost from both chromosomes 11 (one congential and one acquired), it leads to a homozygous deficiency of the protein *menin*. Clinical management must include genetic counseling, careful gathering of family history, and screening of first-order relatives. Patients with MEN1 are at increased risk of developing thymic carcinoid, which can have an aggressive course. All patients with MEN1 should undergo surveillance CT of the chest periodically.

The clinical spectrum of MEN2A, in order of frequency, includes medullary thyroid cancer, pheochromocytoma, and hyperparathyroidism. Cutaneous lichen amyloidosis has been described in some families and is considered a component of the syndrome. Early diagnosis through screening of family members at risk is essential, because total thyroidectomy can cure or prevent medullary thyroid cancer. MEN2B syndrome consists of medullary thyroid cancer, pheochromocytoma, and multiple mucosal neuromas. FMTC is a variant of MEN2A, in which only a strong predisposition for medullary thyroid cancer exists without the other components of the syndrome. A mutation of the *RET* protooncogene is responsible for the presence of disease in MEN2 syndrome.

POSTERIOR PITUITARY

DI is a syndrome characterized by the chronic excretion of abnormally large volume (>50 mL/kg) of dilute urine.

TABLE 44.4

ETIOLOGIES OF CENTRAL DIABETES INSIPIDUS

Trauma/Postsurgical
Neoplasm: Craniopharyngioma, germinoma, meningioma, leukemia, lymphoma
Metastasis
Granulomatous disease: Histiocytosis, sarcoidosis, tuberculosis
Infectious: Meningitis, encephalitis
Vascular: Aneurysm, Sheehan syndrome
Autoimmune
Familial
Idiopathic

The true prevalence of DI is not known, but it is usually underdiagnosed, since the symptoms and signs are benign and many patients either ignore them or are unaware of them. There are four major types of DI: central (neurogenic) DI, nephrogenic DI, primary polydipsia, and gestational DI. Central DI is secondary to inadequate antidiuretic hormone (ADH) secretion that is insufficient to concentrate the urine. It results from destruction of ADH-producing magnocellular neurons of neurohypophysis and may be caused by a variety of pituitary-hypothalamic lesions (Table 44.4).

DI by itself is usually well tolerated and results in a few symptoms, including polydipsia and polyuria. Nocturia is often the primary reason for which patients seek medical attention. In the majority of patients, DI is not associated with any abnormality on physical examination or routine laboratory evaluation with exception of a low urine osmolality. Overt disturbances in fluid and electrolytes are uncommon unless some other factors such as loss of consciousness interfere with normal compensatory mechanism of polydipsia.

Patients with polydipsia and polyuria should be initially evaluated for uncontrolled diabetes mellitus. Once diabetes mellitus has been excluded, patients should have a 24-hour urinary volume measured during ad libitum fluid intake. DI is diagnosed in those with abnormally high urinary output (>50 mL/kg per day), low urinary osmolality (<300 mOsm/kg), and appropriate creatinine level (14–18 mg/kg body weight). Measurement of spot urine osmolality is usually unreliable to exclude or make the diagnosis of DI, as it may be decreased significantly in an otherwise healthy person who deliberately drinks water and can be increased to normal by fasting in a patient with partial DI. Patients with DI who are conscious usually have sufficient thirst to maintain normal serum sodium despite polyuria. Once diagnosis has been established, the next step is to differentiate the type of DI. A water deprivation test may need to be performed by an experienced endocrinologist to differentiate between different types of partial DI. The posterior pituitary enhances on MRI with gadolinium is a "good assay" of ADH reserve, keeping in mind

that up to 20% of normal individuals do not have a bright spot.

The therapy of choice for central DI is administration of the ADH analogue desmopressin acetate (DDAVP). The drug is available in subcutaneous, oral, and nasal spray formulations. Oral and spray forms of desmopressin usually are started at bedtime and are gradually titrated for desired antidiuretic effect. The duration of response should be determined in each person, as there is a considerable individual variation.

REVIEW EXERCISES

QUESTIONS

1. A 25-year-old shoe salesman reports frontal headaches for 6 months. His free thyroxine (FT_4) level is 0.4 ng/dL μg/dL (normal, 0.7–2.0 ng/dL), and his TSH level is 1.41 mIU/mL (normal, 0.4–5.5 mIU/mL). He also reports some loss of energy, leg cramps, and dry skin.

Which of the following is the most appropriate next step?
a) Start levothyroxine 50 μg every day on empty stomach.
b) Check antimicrosomal antibody.
c) Repeat thyroid function study in 3 months to see if there is any change.
d) Obtain early morning cortisol, testosterone, LH, FSH, PRL, and IGF-1 levels.
e) Utilize thyroid ultrasonography.

Answer and Discussion
The answer is d. The low T_4 along with an inappropriately normal TSH level in an individual who is clinically hypothyroid should prompt a search for hypothalamic-pituitary dysfunction mostly commonly secondary to a pituitary tumor. Treatment of hypothyroidism in a patient with adrenal insufficiency may result in worsening of adrenal insufficiency symptoms due to an increase in metabolism of an already low cortisol level.

2. An MRI of the sella turcica reveals a 2-cm mass. Visual fields appear normal to confrontation, but under Goldmann perimetry, they show bilateral superior-temporal defects. Laboratory findings include normal blood urea nitrogen (BUN), creatinine, and electrolyte levels; a testosterone level of 30 ng/dL (normal, 200–1,000 ng/dL); LH, 2 mIU/mL (normal, 1–7 mIU/mL); FSH, 1.5 IU/mL (normal, 2–10 mIU/mL); morning cortisol, 3.5 μg/dL (normal, 5.0–26.9 μg/dL); and PRL, 400 ng/mL (normal, <15 ng/mL).

Which of the following is false?
a) The patient has secondary hypogonadism.
b) The patient is likely to have cortisol deficiency.
c) The patient's GH reserve is probably normal.
d) The patient has a prolactinoma.

Answer and Discussion

The answer is c. In the presence of pituitary tumors, the pituitary gland sequentially loses the ability to secrete GH, LH, FSH, TSH, and ACTH. This patient has secondary hypogonadism, hypothyroidism, and likely hypoadrenalism. It is almost certain that GH secretion is low. GH deficiency often goes undetected in adults. Because irregular menses often leads to medical investigation, women often present earlier with small prolactinomas.

3. What is the best course of action for the patient in question 2 after adequate replacement with hydrocortisone and thyroid hormone?
a) Emergency transsphenoidal removal of pituitary adenoma
b) Initiation of dopamine agonist therapy
c) Gamma knife surgery
d) Testosterone, 200 mg intramuscularly every 2 weeks

Answer and Discussion

The answer is B. Medical therapy with a dopamine agonist is the first-line therapy for patients with prolactinomas, even in those with visual field defects, because it is very effective and has a rapid onset of action. Most patients, including those with mass effect, report improvement in their symptoms. The recovery of the gonadotropin axis is possible following a decrease in the size of the pituitary adenoma and a normalization of PRL. For this reason, testosterone therapy may be delayed but with close evaluation of patient response to therapy.

Match the following case scenarios with the most compatible laboratory findings (each laboratory result is used only once).
a) Low testosterone, low LH and FSH, and normal PRL (15 ng/mL)
b) Elevated IGF-1 level
c) Normal pituitary function studies
d) Normal T_4 and TSH as well as PRL 50 ng/mL
e) Low testosterone, low LH and FSH, and PRL 250 ng/mL

4. A 25-year-old chronic schizophrenic woman with galactorrhea

Answer and Discussion

The answer is d. This patient likely has drug-induced hyperprolactinemia. Medications such as metoclopramide, haloperidol, tricyclic antidepressants, verapamil, methyldopa, reserpine, and opiates may elevate PRL levels.

5. A 25-year-old man with impotence, galactorrhea, and visual field defect

Answer and Discussion

The answer is e. Men with prolactinomas often present with symptoms related to mass effect. Any pituitary tumor may lead to hypogonadism and gynecomastia, but only hyperprolactinemia leads to galactorrhea.

6. An 18-year-old man with delayed puberty, anosmia, and hypogonadism

Answer and Discussion

The answer is a. The presence of anosmia and hypogonadism is suggestive of a developmental midline defect (Kallmann syndrome). This disorder of hypogonadotropic hypogonadism affects 1 in 10,000 to 60,000 individuals. After suitable priming with LHRH, the pituitary can secrete LH and FSH.

7. A 45-year-old man with worsening diabetes control, coarsening facial features, and skin tags

Answer and Discussion

The answer is b. The measurement of IGF-1 has become a convenient screening test for acromegaly. An elevated IGF-1 level in a clinical setting suggestive of acromegaly almost always confirms the diagnosis. In patients with poorly controlled diabetes and malnutrition, the IGF-1 level may be falsely low. The oral glucose tolerance test remains the gold standard to confirm the diagnosis.

8. A 40-year-old woman with headaches, normal menses, no visual field defect, and a CT head scan suggesting an empty sella

Answer and Discussion

The answer is c. This patient has an empty sella syndrome, which is often associated with normal pituitary function. Occasionally, isolated or multiple hormonal deficiencies may be present.

9. Which of the following tests does not have any role in establishing the diagnosis of CS?
a) Midnight salivary cortisol
b) 24-hour UFC
c) Midnight serum cortisol
d) Random serum cortisol
e) Low-dose DST

Answer and Discussion

The answer is d. Because of the significant overlap between normal individuals and those with CS, random serum cortisol has no role in the diagnosis of CS. All other answers may be used to establish a diagnosis of CS.

10. A 45-year-old white woman with clinical findings suggestive of CS has been found to have two elevated UFCs of 220 and 300 (normal, 2–50 mg/24 hour); her ACTH level is 55 (normal, 5–50 pg/mL), and her pituitary MRI shows a 3-mm adenoma.

Which of the followings is the *best* next course of action?

a) Repeat 24-hour UFC
b) Transsphenoidal surgery
c) LDDST
d) HDDST and/or CRH test
e) Midnight serum cortisol level

Answer and Discussion

The answer is d. The diagnosis of CS has been established in this patient with two significantly elevated 24-hour UFC tests (>4 times the upper normal limit). A slightly elevated ACTH level excludes adrenal origin but may be seen in both Cushing disease and ectopic ACTH-producing tumors. The next step to differentiate between the two is to use the HDDST and/or CRH stimulation test. If the result is not conclusive, inferior petrosal sinus sampling should be done in an experienced center. The presence of a 3-mm pituitary adenoma is suggestive of a pituitary source for ACTH, but it may be a pituitary incidentaloma.

11. Which of the following is *not* seen with increased frequency in patients with newly diagnosed acromegaly?
a) Cholelithiasis
b) Goiter
c) Sleep apnea
d) Galactorrhea
e) Colon polyps

Answer and Discussion

The answer is a. Cholelithiasis is not part of the clinical picture seen in patients with acromegaly caused by excess GH secretion. Although mostly asymptomatic, cholelithiasis and gall bladder sludge may be seen in up to 25% of patients treated with somatostatin analogs.

12. A 65-year-old man with a history of a nonfunctional macroadenoma develops severe retro-orbital headache, nausea, and vomiting with change in mental status. On examination, right third nerve palsy with stiff neck is present. An emergency MRI of the brain shows hemorrhage in the pituitary adenoma, which is enlarged in size.

What is the *best* next course of action?
a) Emergency transsphenoidal surgery
b) Dexamethasone 2 mg intravenously every 6 hours
c) Nitroprusside drip to keep systolic blood pressure between 140 and 160 mm Hg systolic
d) Broad spectrum antibiotic
e) Dopamine agonist

Answer and Discussion

The answer is b. High-dose steroid therapy is the initial step in treating patients with pituitary apoplexy. The glucocorticoids are used for presumptive ACTH deficiency and cerebral edema due to acute mass effect. Patients with altered mental status and neurologic deficits are candidates for surgery once high-dose steroid use has been initiated.

SUGGESTED READINGS

Arnaldi G, Angeli A, Atkinson AB, et al. Diagnosis and complications of Cushing's syndrome: a consensus statement. *J Clin Endocrinol Metab* 2003;88(12):5593–5602.

Aron DC, Howlett TA. Pituitary incidentalomas. *Endocrinol Metab Clin North Am* 2000;29:205–221.

Bjerre P. The empty sella. A reappraisal of etiology and pathogenesis. *Acta Neurol Scand Suppl* 1990;130:1–25.

Bonadonna S, Doga M, Gola M, et al. Diagnosis and treatment of acromegaly and its complications: consensus guidelines. *J Endocrinol Invest* 2005;28(suppl 11):43–47.

Casanueva FF, Molitch ME, Schlechte JA, et al. Guidelines of the Pituitary Society for the diagnosis and management of prolactinomas. *Clin Endocrinol* 2006;65:265–273.

Marx SJ, Simonds W. Hereditary hormone excess: genes, molecular pathways, and syndromes. *Endocr Rev* 2003;26(5):615–661.

Robertson GL. Diabetes insipidus. *Endocrinol Metab Clin North Am* 1995;24:549–572.

Sam S, Molitch ME. The pituitary mass: diagnosis and management. *Rev Endocr Metab Disord* 2005;6(1):55–62.

Schade R, Andersohn F, Suissa S, et al. Dopamine agonists and the risk of cardiac-valve regurgitation. *N Engl J Med* 2007;356:29–38.

Thodou E, Asa SL, Kontogeorgos G, et al. Clinical case seminar: lymphocytic hypophysitis: clinicopathological findings. *J Clin Endocrinol Metab* 1995;80:2302–2311.

Vella A, Young WF. Pituitary apoplexy. *Endocrinologist* 2001;11:282–288.

Verbalis, JG. Disorders of water metabolism. *Res Clin Endocrinol Metab* 2003;17(4):471–503.

Chapter 45

Metabolic Bone Disease and Calcium Disorders

Angelo A. Licata

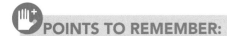

POINTS TO REMEMBER:

- Most patients with hyperparathyroidism are asymptomatic. The detection of abnormalities in serum calcium by routine chemical assays now identifies patients many years before symptoms arise.

- Steroid use in the treatment of hypercalcemia is helpful for specific disorders, such as hypervitaminosis D and myeloma, but it is ineffective in parathyroid disease.

- In simple cases of hypocalcemia and osteomalacia, the dosage may be as small as 50,000 U per week. The most potent vitamin D forms, 25-hydroxyvitamin D (calcifediol) and 1,25-dihydroxyvitamin D (calcitriol), are safer to use but more expensive.

- Osteoporosis has a genetic component; it occurs in families and affects women and men. Of all risk factors discussed in the literature, the most clinically robust is a family history of osteoporosis.

HYPERCALCEMIA

The extent of a patient's symptoms from hypercalcemia depends directly on two major factors: the duration of the hypercalcemic process and the rapidity of its development. The more chronic and slowly progressive the rise in serum calcium, the less likely the patient will be aware of it. If the hypercalcemic process arises rapidly, within weeks to months, symptoms develop that are generally of a neurologic or musculoskeletal nature. The diagnosis of hypercalcemia is separated into two major areas: parathyroid

related and nonparathyroid related; both are discussed in this chapter.

Clinical Presentation

The symptoms of hyperparathyroid hypercalcemia have taken on a vastly different presentation over the last two to three decades:

- Asymptomatic (up to 80%)
- Symptomatic (20%)
- Renal stones (colic), mental status changes, gastritis (ulcers), pancreatitis, constipation, malaise-fatigue-weakness-arthralgia, and bone pain or fractures are some of the symptoms noted in patients. Mild symptoms can be so nonspecific in early disease that a firm diagnosis may be missed.

Most patients with hyperparathyroidism are asymptomatic. The detection of abnormalities in serum calcium by routine chemical assays now identifies patients many years before symptoms arise. Historical descriptions of hyperparathyroidism, however, emphasize symptoms such as osteitis fibrosa cystica (bone pain and arthralgia), renal stone disease, gastric ulcers, pancreatitis, decreased mental status, and weakness.

In patients with other causes of hypercalcemia, the unique presentation of hyperparathyroidism may not be the clinical presentation. An abrupt onset of lethargy, confusion, fatigue, and even outright coma often is the presentation in many patients whose calcium level rises abruptly. In these cases, hypercalcemia occurs so rapidly that problems such as renal stone disease may not have time to develop. Manifestations of bowel dysfunction may be present, however, such as pain or constipation and generalized muscular weakness. Older patients are more likely to be overcome by these symptoms; younger individuals tolerate higher levels of hypercalcemia with fewer symptoms.

Diagnosis

Textbook descriptions of hypercalcemia list extensive causes of this condition:

- Primary hyperparathyroidism
- Cancer (e.g., tumors secreting parathyroid hormone–related protein [PTH-rp] or ectopic vitamin D, bone metastases)
- Endocrine disorders (e.g., thyrotoxicosis, oversecretion of vasoactive intestinal polypeptide, Addison disease, pheochromocytoma)
- Granulomatous diseases
- Drugs (e.g., thiazides, lithium, antiestrogens, vitamins A and D)
- Familial hypocalciuric hypercalcemia
- Parenteral nutrition
- Immobilization
- Milk-alkali syndrome
- Acute and chronic renal insufficiency

A workable approach to this diagnosis separates the causes into two major areas:

- Parathyroid
- Nonparathyroid (hypervitaminosis D [endogenous or exogenous]; malignancy [metastatic or humoral])

The major parathyroid causes of hypercalcemia are related to vitamin D–mediated or malignant processes. Intoxication with exogenous vitamin D is seen because the vitamin is commonly used today to treat osteoporosis. Endogenous hypervitaminosis D usually arises from granulomatous diseases, such as sarcoidosis, but granuloma located in any part of the body may cause this form of hypercalcemia.

Malignant diseases also produce hypercalcemia. Some malignant diseases, such as breast cancer, cause skeletal destruction. Others, such as myeloma and epidermal (squamous) tumors, make chemical (humoral) substances that increase bone metabolism and bone destruction. Myelomas release interleukins and cytokines within the bone marrow from plasma cells, stimulating osteoclastic activity and ultimately bone turnover and calcium loss. Originally, squamous or epidermal tumors were shown to produce PTH-rp. This substance increases bone loss and renal tubular reabsorption of calcium and is distinct from true parathyroid hormone (PTH). Many other types of tumors are known to produce this protein, but they may not all cause hypercalcemia.

Laboratory Study: Parathyroid Hormone Assay

The introduction of the intact-PTH assay, which uses sophisticated chemical techniques, has virtually eliminated those problems noted in the past concerning the differentiation of parathyroid disease from other forms of hypercalcemia (e.g., ectopic) that might be caused by PTH-rp. This new assay clearly differentiates hyperparathyroidism from other disorders. The normal range of PTH is 10 to 65 pg/mL for a serum calcium level of 8.5 to 10.5 mg/dL. Values greater than the normal reference interval in combination with a high calcium value are diagnostic of hyperparathyroidism. In the non-PTH–mediated causes of hypercalcemia, no measurable intact PTH should be present.

Differential Diagnosis

The workup for hypercalcemia can be accomplished simply by using the algorithm shown in Figure 45.1. The level of PTH measured indicates a parathyroid or nonparathyroid problem. Primary hyperparathyroidism is differentiated from other causes by finding a measurable or increased value with an increase of serum calcium. If no measurable hormone is found, vitamin D intoxication or a malignancy probably is present. The serum phosphorus level can sometimes help make the distinction between these processes: When the serum phosphorus level is elevated or high normal, a vitamin D-mediated process is suspected (if renal function is normal). In some cases of metastatic disease to bone, an elevation in serum calcium and phosphorus may be present due to bone destruction, but this should not be a diagnostic difficulty, as the history, physical examination, and radiologic examinations help to identify this problem. When the phosphorus level is low, a humoral agent from a cancer is often suspected—the most common being PTH-rp.

For purposes of board examinations, the algorithm in Figure 45.1 can be quite useful to quickly focus one's thinking, although the algorithm may oversimplify the diagnostic process. Various permutations and combinations of secondary diseases can very well cloud the reality of the diagnosis.

Treatment

The treatment of hypercalcemia is directed toward resolving acute symptoms and instituting the long-term control of the underlying process.

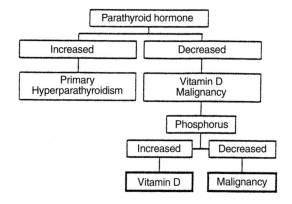

Figure 45.1 Diagnostic algorithm for hypercalcemia.

The treatment of acute symptoms begins with saline hydration to increase the excretion of sodium and calcium in the urine. Adequate hydration is mandatory to avert declining renal function and its secondary reabsorption of calcium. Loop diuretics (furosemide [Lasix]) have been considered first-line therapy in the past, but the use of this therapy is not the major approach taken today. Intravenous doses of a bisphosphonate—pamidronate disodium (Aredia) 60 to 90 mg, etidronate disodium (Didronel) 7.5 mg/kg, or zoledronic acid (Zometa) 4 mg—are used to control the hypercalcemic process; zoledronic acid is the most potent, with pamidronate a close second and etidronate the weakest. Pamidronate and etidronate require infusions over several hours, whereas zoledronic acid can be given as a bolus over a 15 to 30 minute period. The use of a diuretic agent in hypercalcemia may be risky if the patient has not been sufficiently hydrated. Worsening dehydration in the face of diuretic use can actually promote worsening hypercalcemia, renal shutdown, and even death.

Steroid use in the treatment of hypercalcemia is helpful for specific disorders, such as hypervitaminosis D and myeloma, but it is ineffective in parathyroid disease. Injectable calcitonin has been used in the past with some success to control hypercalcemia, but it lacks the prolonged responses seen with the potent bisphosphonate drugs. The dosage range for calcitonin is 7 to 10 U/kg body weight per day. Side effects from the administration of this drug, including nausea and vomiting, limit its usefulness. Nasal spray calcitonin and oral bisphosphonates are not efficacious.

The long-term control of hypercalcemia is directed toward eradicating the underlying disease (Table 45.1). Parathyroid surgery is curative in almost all patients with primary disease. Steroid therapy is *maybe* curative for problems of vitamin D intoxication and certain tumors. Other forms of chemotherapy for cancer may offer long-term control of the hypercalcemic process. For malignancy-related hypercalcemia, however, the weekly or monthly administration of an intravenous bisphosphonate is useful when the underlying disease cannot be completely eradicated. Oral phosphates (e.g., Neutra-Phos) do not work well over the long term; intestinal side effects limit the possible dose and tolerability. Adequate hydration is obviously mandatory. In some cases, added salt in the diet, with a low dose of a loop diuretic, can keep a patient asymptomatic.

HYPOCALCEMIA AND OSTEOMALACIA

Osteomalacia is the hallmark of poor skeletal mineralization owing to hypocalcemia, hypophosphatemia, or both. Symptoms range from subtle and obscure complaints to muscle weakness and overt bone pain on palpation or movement.

Pathophysiology

Overt fractures and pseudofractures are the sign of insufficient mineralization. Osteomalacia due to hypocalcemia and/or hypophosphatemia arises from the following causes:

- Vitamin D deficiency
- Dietary lack
- Deprivation of sunlight
- Malabsorption
- Increased catabolism
- Decreased formation metabolites of vitamin D
- Phosphate depletion
- Renal tubular disorders
- Neoplasm
- Secondary hyperparathyroidism

Endogenous vitamin D arises from the ultraviolet-light irradiation of epidermal cholesterol. A deprivation of sunlight causes vitamin D deficiency, but dietary sources of vitamin D substitute for endogenous forms. In situations in which a dietary lack of this vitamin occurs, or in which abnormalities in the gastrointestinal tract prevent its absorption, a deficiency may arise. Any gastrointestinal disease that alters absorption can lower serum levels of vitamin D. Likewise, increased catabolism of vitamin D produces a relative deficiency of vitamin D. (This occurs when drugs stimulate liver mitochondrial cytochrome P450 and increase the catabolism of vitamin D.) Likewise, renal failure decreases the serum concentration of bioactive vitamin D (1,25-dihydroxyvitamin D).

Phosphorus depletion, an uncommon cause of osteomalacia, may be an isolated finding or may be combined with hypocalcemia. Vitamin D deficiency causes hypophosphatemia and hypocalcemia. Renal tubular disorders cause a primary phosphorus leak or a widespread abnormality, such as that noted in Fanconi syndrome. In either case, the correction of the phosphorus leak is very difficult. Rare mesenchymal tumors also cause osteomalacia because they block production of active vitamin D. The surgical removal of these tumors reverses the process. When severe, secondary hyperparathyroidism also causes hypophosphatemia.

TABLE 45.1

LONG-TERM CONTROL OF HYPERCALCEMIA

Cause	Treatment
Parathyroid disease	Surgery
	No curative medication
Vitamin D related	Steroids
Malignancy	Control of symptoms
	Chemotherapy for underlying tumor
	Steroids

Diagnosis

Laboratory Studies

The primary findings of osteomalacia include:

- Hypocalcemia
- Hypophosphatemia
- Hyperphosphatasia (defined as increased alkaline phosphatase)

On testing, increased total serum alkaline phosphatase is not invariably present in all patients. The degree to which serum alkaline phosphatase is elevated is directly proportional to the underlying changes in bone metabolism. A bone-specific alkaline phosphatase assay is also used but may not be immediately available routinely. New assays for bone collagen fragments in the urine or serum are supplanting the old insensitive assays, such as hydroxyproline. These tests measure the N- or C-telopeptides of α-1 bone collagen. Other tests analyze the urinary pyridinoline or deoxypyridinoline cross links of collagen. These are more sensitive than older urine hydroxyproline tests. Secondary findings include decreased urinary calcium and phosphorus; however, urinary phosphorus increases in cases of renal tubular leak and secondary hyperparathyroidism. Other laboratory findings arise from the underlying diseases.

The laboratory data in osteomalacia can be summarized as follows:

- Primary findings
  - Decreased calcium or phosphorus, or both
  - Variable increase in alkaline phosphatase
- Secondary findings
  - Decreased urinary calcium or phosphorus
  - Increased PTH
  - Other disease-specific changes

Differential Diagnosis

Figure 45.2 contains a useful clinical algorithm with which to establish the general categories of hypocalcemia. The presence of hypocalcemia prompts evaluation for albumin first. Decreased levels of serum albumin cause a corresponding decrease in total serum calcium levels. Every gram of albumin binds 0.8 mg of calcium; hence, a given serum calcium level must first be corrected for serum albumin level. (Serum ionized calcium does not respond to changes in serum albumin.) If the serum albumin level is normal, then the presence of hypocalcemia is real. The ambient phosphorus level thereafter serves to differentiate the causes of hypocalcemia quite nicely. With normal phosphatemia or hypophosphatemia, intestinal disease is probable. Suitable workup is therefore undertaken in that respect. In the presence of increased phosphorus, parathyroid disease or renal disease is the main cause. Serum creatinine differentiates these two possibilities. In renal

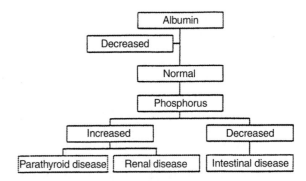

Figure 45.2   Diagnostic algorithm for hypocalcemia.

disease, the level is elevated; in parathyroid disease, it is normal.

Hypoparathyroidism is a very rare phenomenon. Primary hypoparathyroidism—clearly the most rare of the disorders—generally arises early in life. It is associated with either an autoimmune phenomenon of other endocrine glands or embryologic atresia of the parathyroid gland. Secondary hypoparathyroidism is more common. Postoperative hypoparathyroidism may occur after neck surgery for parathyroid, thyroid, or malignant diseases. In some patients, it may develop years after neck surgery. Acute hypoparathyroidism is unusual. Infiltrated diseases of the parathyroid gland are rare. Several subtypes of "apparent" hypoparathyroidism are even more rare. In pseudohypoparathyroidism, for example, the appropriate secretion of PTH is present, but this hormone cannot act because of dysfunction in its target-organ receptor. Another form of apparent hypoparathyroidism arises in intestinal dysfunction and magnesium malabsorption and deficiency. A low magnesium level causes the poor synthesis and secretion of PTH, poor activity of the hormone at its receptor sites, and poor production of vitamin D. True hypoparathyroidism would not cause osteomalacia or bone disease, but in pseudohypoparathyroidism, in which there are defective receptors in the kidneys, one may actually see normal receptors in the bone that respond to PTH, thus causing osteitis.

Treatment

Treatment options for hypocalcemia include:

- Correction of the underlying disease
- Calcium supplementation
- Empiric therapy (i.e., 2-g elemental calcium, tablet or liquid preparations)
- Meal timing
- Vitamin D supplements
- Ergocalciferol (Calciferol)
- Calcifediol (Calderol) (not currently available)
- Calcitriol

It is essential to address first the underlying disease process causing vitamin D and phosphorus abnormalities. Calcium supplementation is used if dietary sources are limited. Dairy products are essential, as they provide 80% of daily calcium needs. The minimum daily requirement for men and premenopausal women is 1,000 mg of elemental calcium. In its absence, calcium supplements are needed. Most supplements are carbonate salt, which provides more calcium per tablet (40% by weight) than other calcium supplements. The carbonate salt may not be absorbed well in patients with achlorhydria. The citrate salt has a theoretic advantage, because it is absorbed more efficiently in all patients regardless of gastric acidity. No data show how effective citrate salts might be in situations in which intestinal dysfunction occurs.

Another consideration is the use of a liquid calcium supplement. Liquids may be more easily absorbed than tablets. In general, generic brands of calcium should be as readily bioavailable as brand names, but this may not always be the situation. Studies have indicated that the dissolution or breakdown of calcium tablets in 1 or 2 ounces of warm (i.e., body temperature) household vinegar is a good sign of the relative bioavailability in the stomach.

Vitamin D supplementation for patients who are vitamin D deficient, or who may need assistance in the absorption of calcium, is the next consideration. The cheaper forms of the vitamin are generally the cholecalciferol or ergocalciferol derivatives, precursors to the 25- and 1,25-hydroxyl derivatives. These vitamins are prescribed in 50,000-U doses per capsule. In profound hypocalcemia from hypoparathyroidism, for example, the number of required daily units may range from 50,000 to 500,000. In simple cases of hypocalcemia and osteomalacia, the dosage may be as small as 50,000 U per week. The most potent vitamin D forms, 25-hydroxyvitamin D (calcifediol) and 1,25-dihydroxyvitamin D (calcitriol), are more expensive, but they are safer to use. If evidence of hypercalcemia exists, the discontinuation of these potent vitamins restores eucalcemia within days. In patients who cannot absorb oral medications, the use of injectable vitamin D is mandatory. Ergocalciferol is generally the vitamin used, but it presently is not available in the United States. An intravenous form of calcitriol is available and is used primarily for dialysis patients. It may be used off label if needed.

OSTEOPOROSIS

Pathophysiology in Women

Osteoporosis is a multifactorial disease that ultimately leads to insufficiency of skeletal strength and increased susceptibility to fracture from relatively minor or nontraumatic causes. It is histologically manifested by thinning, perforation, and breakage of the trabecular plates within the interior of bone, resulting in a subsequent lack of compression strength. The disease is divided into a primary disorder and secondary disorders.

Primary osteoporosis of women occurs from high bone turnover secondary to estrogen deficiency at the time of menopause; later in life, several additional factors aggravate the menopausal bone loss and may cause insufficient osteoblastic activity. Attendant abnormalities include decreased calcium absorption and vitamin D metabolism as well as increased PTH levels. This distinction between menopausal and postmenopausal problems is somewhat artificial, as a blending of pathological processes may occur across all ages.

Secondary causes of osteoporosis run the gamut of many diseases. Material listed in the Suggested Readings section covers these topics in greater depth.

The pathophysiology of osteoporosis can be viewed from four major standpoints:

- Genetic
- Nutritional
- Hormonal
- Lifestyle

Genetic Impact

Osteoporosis has a genetic component; it occurs in families and affects women and men. Of all risk factors discussed in the literature, the most clinically robust is a family history of osteoporosis. This fact alone often pinpoints individuals who have evidence of bone deficiency (osteopenia) without evidence of clinical fracture. Epidemiologic studies clearly indicate that the daughters of individuals with osteoporosis have osteopenia, even in their early years, whereas the daughters of patients without osteoporosis have normal bone mass for age. Racial differences are clearly notable as well. Osteoporosis is present more often in white and Asian American women than in black women when population studies are reviewed. Individual black women can certainly develop this disease either as a primary or secondary problem.

Nutritional Impact

The major nutritional factor involved in osteoporosis is calcium insufficiency. The debate still rages whether calcium is a causal or promoting factor. A deficiency of dairy products in the diet leads to insufficiency of calcium, as these products are the greatest nutrient source of calcium. Most people require 1,000 mg of elemental calcium daily. Postmenopausal women may require more calcium because of a relative inability to efficiently absorb it; the generally recommended dose is 1,500 mg or more.

The effects of calcium on the skeleton are directly related to an individual's age. A degree of bone loss is attributable to the aging process, the exact details of which are not well understood. This degree of loss is small (approximately 0.1% yearly). It tends to arise after 30 years of age. Calcium supplementation is helpful in controlling bone metabolism due to the aging process. Immediately around the time of menopause, however, and for 5 to 10 years afterward, calcium supplementation alone cannot control the turnover of bone. This period is associated with a high degree of bone loss from osteoclastic activity secondary to estrogen deficiency.

The overuse of other substances, such as alcohol and tobacco, has a negative influence on bone metabolism and must be considered in osteoporosis.

Nephrolithiasis does not develop in most individuals when the calcium content in the diet is increased. The body regulates calcium absorption so that hypercalciuria and stone disease generally do not occur. If a preexisting problem with hypercalciuria is present, however, or a patient or family history of renal stones is noted, the patient should be evaluated for hypercalciuria before and, more important, after supplementation is started. A simple test for hypercalciuria can uncover potential problems before they lead to stone disease.

Hormonal Impact

Hormonal factors have long been known to be an associated problem in osteoporosis. With loss of estrogen, postmenopausal women have increased production and activity of osteoclasts and secondarily increased bone turnover and loss. This arises from changes in the ratio of stimulators (receptor-activated nuclear kinase ligand [RANKL]) and inhibitors (osteoprotegerin [OPG]) of osteoclast longevity and function. Estrogen and antiosteoclastic drugs are the most useful treatments for women with osteoporosis at this time because they target osteoclasts, whereas calcium alone is not sufficient. During menopause, bone-loss rates might be 10 to 20 times higher than the rate associated with the aging process.

Pubertal development should also be considered. Estrogen is a major stimulant of bone growth in adolescent girls. Any aberrations in growth at this time will ultimately lead to insufficiency of bone in adult life. Adolescent development directly determines the peak bone mass that each individual will have. The inability to attain this during adolescence leads to a less than maximally calcified adult skeleton.

Lifestyle Impact

An individual's lifestyle and exercise pattern are also intimately related to overall skeletal strength. Increasing muscle mass and strength concurrently strengthens and increases skeletal mass (to a small degree). The dilemma facing clinicians is the amount and types of exercise needed to promote a healthy skeleton. In premenopausal women, especially, too much as well as too little exercise is risky. Too much exercise causes amenorrhea and bone weakening (athletic amenorrhea). Exercise maximizes peak bone mass during adolescence, helps maintain adult bone mass, and attenuates loss because of the aging process.

TABLE 45.2
COMMON SECONDARY CAUSES OF OSTEOPOROSIS IN MEN

Glucocorticoids, alcohol, hypogonadism (45%)
Primary or idiopathic (35%–45%)
Other causes (15%–20%)
   Gastrointestinal
   Hypercalciuria
   Drug side effects (anticonvulsants, glucocorticoids, antigonadotrophins, alcohol, tobacco)
   Hyperparathyroidism
   Neoplasia (monoclonal gammopathy)
   Other endocrine diseases (hypogonadism, hypercortisolism, hyperprolactinemia, acromegaly)
   Metabolic/Genetic (Marfan syndrome, homocystinuria, hypophosphatasia, osteogenesis imperfecta)

Pathophysiology in Men

Many of the causes of primary osteoporosis in women have an analogous cause in men—hypogonadism (testosterone deficiency), poor pubertal development, dietary factors, genetic inheritance, and activity deficiency. The primary form of osteoporosis often arises in men later in life. A large number of men developing this problem before the sixth or seventh decade of life may have secondary causes (Table 45.2). Twenty percent of hip fractures occur in men. Surprisingly, the 1-year mortality for men with these fractures is almost 50%, compared with about 20% for women.

DIAGNOSIS OF OSTEOPOROSIS

The diagnosis of primary osteoporosis in its early asymptomatic stage was a challenge until the introduction of dual-energy x-ray absorptiometry (DXA) scans for the measurement of bone density. An abnormal (i.e., low) bone density, however, is not sufficient to make this diagnosis. Many nonosteoporotic bone problems cause an abnormal density.

Early osteoporosis produces no symptoms; finding it obviously is a challenge. By the time fractures, back pain, height loss, and kyphosis develop, there is little challenge in diagnosing it, as these are the hallmarks of a disease that has gone unchecked for years. Osteopenia noted on radiographs usually indicates a loss of at least 20% to 30% of bone mass, which represents approximately 10 years or more of silent osteoporosis. In most cases of asymptomatic disease, routine health screening blood test results are normal. The new bone markers mentioned earlier do not diagnose osteoporosis; they only indicate an abnormality in bone metabolism.

Bone densitometry results are the single most important factor in the prediction of fracture risk in patients who have osteoporosis. Decreased bone density is a necessary but not sufficient reason for fractures. This testing is performed at the initiation either of a diagnostic workup or of therapy and then repeated 1 or 2 years later to assess the results of therapy. The federal government guidelines provide insurance coverage for testing women over 65 years of age and allow rechecking every 2 years, with limited exceptions. Most insurers follow this protocol. Younger women with significant risks, however, should be checked before this age. The usual considerations for densitometry include the following factors:

- Family history
- Atraumatic fractures
- Steroid use
- Back pain
- Hyperparathyroidism
- Monitoring of therapy
- Decision point for hormone replacement therapy

These measurements focus on the rapid turnover of trabecular bone in the spine or femoral neck, where bone is lost earliest. Bone density measurements at these sites >2.5 standard deviations (SD) below peak mass (commonly called the *young normal value*) identify osteoporosis according to the World Health Organization guidelines. The risk of fracture rises exponentially with a decline in the SD. Values between −1.0 and −2.5 SD below peak bone mass are classified as osteopenic, an intermediate zone that has lower prognostic significance for fracture. Values >−1.0 SD are classified as normal. The chance of fracture with density values in this range is even lower than with values classified as osteopenic. Having said this, however, one must never assume that an absolutely safe, fracturefree density exists. This guideline derives from population data; an individual patient can fracture at any value given the right circumstances.

Treatment

The therapy for primary osteoporosis in women includes:

- Calcium supplementation with or without vitamin D
- Exercise
- Skeletal pharmacologic agents
- Antiresorptives (e.g., estrogen, selective estrogen receptor modulators [SERM], calcitonin, and bisphosphonates—alendronate sodium, risedronate sodium, ibandronate sodium, zoledronic acid)
- Anabolic drugs (PTH 1-34 or teriparatide)

Antiresorptive Therapy

All therapies used until recently are antiresorptive in nature; they work against osteoclasts and reduce bone turnover and loss. Estrogen controls the local production of those bone marrow cytokines (RANKL and OPG) that stimulate osteoclastic bone resorption—thus its use in menopause. SERMs are receptor agonists of estrogen in bone and mimic its activity but are antagonists at other tissue sites. Calcitonin, the first antiosteoclastic drug used in practice, affects osteoclast membrane structure. The bisphosphonates have several actions on osteoclast function: They inhibit osteoclast membrane cholesterol synthesis, increase apoptosis, inhibit the proton pump, and prevent adherence of osteoclasts to the bone surface.

Calcitonin is a drug long recognized for the treatment of osteoporosis. The injectable form has been supplanted by the nasal spray. Both forms yield modest increases in spinal density but not as great as those from estrogen or the bisphosphonates. The average increase is 1% to 3%. No significant increase is seen in hip density.

Bisphosphonate drugs hold a major place in the treatment of osteoporosis. These potent antiresorptives affect osteoclastic function, decrease bone turnover, and increase bone mass to varying degrees. In general, all drugs of the class increase vertebral bone mass 5% to 8% and hip mass 3% to 6%. They all prevent vertebral fractures, but not all show reduction of hip and nonvertebral fractures in studies as yet.

Alendronate (Fosamax), the first approved bisphosphonate, prevents vertebral and hip fractures. Both the daily 10-mg and the weekly 70-mg tablets produce equivalent effects. It is also available with vitamin D_2 as a weekly dose. A weekly 70-mg liquid dose is now available. Lower doses (35 mg weekly) prevent the development or progression of osteoporosis in much the same fashion as does estrogen. Risedronate (Actonel) is approved for the treatment of osteoporosis. It is available as a daily 5-mg tablet, a weekly 35-mg dose, and a monthly 150-mg dose (two 75-mg tablets). It also will increase spinal and hip density to about the same extent as alendronate and inhibit the risk of spine and hip fractures. Its tolerability may be better for patients with gastroesophageal disease.

Ibandronate is a new bisphosphonate available as an oral and an intravenous medication. It originally was available as a daily 2.5-mg dose, then preferentially used as a monthly 150-mg dose, and subsequently as a 3-mg intravenous dose every 3 months.

Zoledronic acid is a recently approved intravenous agent for treatment of osteoporosis. It is administered as a yearly 5-mg dose.

Since the 1950s, estrogen has been recognized as a useful therapy to prevent osteoporosis. In women with an intact uterus, it is combined with a progestin to stop the development of endometrial hyperplasia and reduce the risk of endometrial cancer. The usual daily dose is 0.625 mg of conjugated estrogen or its equivalent. Corresponding doses of progestin are between 2.5 and 5.0 mg. These may be given cyclically or daily. Cyclical use produces menses to varying degrees. Daily combined use prevents it. The influence of the progestin on lipid and cardiovascular function is only beginning to be understood. Women with a prior hysterectomy generally do not use progestin, although some believe it has skeletal benefit. Some women complain of premenstrual symptoms from progestin, which limits its use.

Hormone replacement therapy in the treatment of osteoporosis is now under question as a result of the information from the Women's Health Initiative (WHI). This study was a federally sponsored program to evaluate the effect of estrogen plus progestin (E+P) and estrogen alone (hysterectomized patients) on heart disease and invasive breast cancer. Secondary areas of interest were stroke, pulmonary embolism, colorectal cancer, hip fracture, and death due to other causes.

The E+P arm was stopped prematurely due to an increased incidence of breast cancer as well as an increase in coronary heart disease, stroke, and thromboembolic events. Hip and vertebral fractures declined by about one-third. Colorectal cancer declined 37%. Controversy about the results remains, primarily due to the average age of the patients, the years since menopause, and the possibility that the patients may have had early asymptomatic cardiovascular disease. U.S. Food and Drug Administration (FDA) labeling for combined drug therapy states that the chronic use of conjugated E+P should not be used as primary prevention of cardiovascular disease. Its use should be limited to the short-term treatment of vasomotor symptoms. A risk–benefit analysis for each patient should be discussed to decide on its optimal use.

Estrogen patches are also used to provide replacement therapy. Although they have not been available as long as the oral agents, the patches can prevent osteoporosis. Clinical evidence shows protection from fractures as well. Cessation of estrogen causes bone loss to the degree at which it would have occurred in menopause. Hence, other approaches for long-term therapy are mandatory. Low-dose alendronate and risedronate can prevent osteoporosis. Likewise, the SERM drugs or "antiestrogen" drugs have become a substitute for estrogen.

SERM agents are modeled on the drugs used in the treatment of breast cancer. These agents are estrogen antagonists in the uterus and breasts but are estrogen agonists in the heart, blood vessels, liver (i.e., with regard to lipid profile), and bone. Raloxifene hydrochloride (Evista) is the first such drug available for clinical use. Ongoing studies show favorable effects on skeletal density, vertebral fracture rate, and lipid profile. Menstruation, breast pain, and uterine hyperplasia do not occur. Recent data show a reduction in the incidence of breast cancer. Its daily dosage (60 mg) reduces vertebral fractures about 40% to 50%. Preliminary postmarketing data suggest an effect on nonvertebral fracture reduction, but the original pivotal study did not support this, as the incidence of this type fracture was so low.

Efficacy of Fracture Reduction

A great deal of data exist about fracture reduction. The efficacy of a therapy is based not only on suitable changes in density but also on reduction in fracture rates. The antiresorptive therapies increase vertebral bone mass from about 2% to 8%. They reduce vertebral fractures from 30% to 60%, depending on the study. Calcitonin has the lowest rate of fracture reduction, estrogen and raloxifene an

intermediary rate, and the bisphosphonates the highest rates. Reduction in hip fractures is more tenuous for most drugs, but the bisphosphonates alendronate, risedronate, and zoledronic acid show the advantage. Therapeutic trials of calcitonin and raloxifene do not display the protective effect on hip fractures in the studies performed to date. The WHI study does show that the E+P arm had a significant reduction in hip and vertebral fractures. All studies show that the greatest benefit arises in patients who have had prior fractures.

Therapy for Osteoporosis in Men

The FDA has approved use of alendronate, risedronate, and teriparatide (PTH 1-34, see below) in men. These drugs cover primary or idiopathic problems; however, the secondary causes of osteoporosis are the major issues for younger men. Only after these disorders are treated might it be necessary to resort to the FDA-approved drugs. The appropriate intake of calcium and vitamin D is as important for men as it is for women.

Anabolic Therapy

Teriparatide is the first anabolic-class drug approved for the treatment of osteoporosis in women and men. It is the 1-34 N-terminal fragment of PTH. This type of drug directly affects osteoblastic cells, produces thicker and more plate-like trabeculae, and increases bone volume and connectivity among trabeculae. Paradoxically, this arises because the drug is used as a solitary subcutaneous daily injection. Longer daily exposure to the skeleton, as occurs in primary hyperparathyroidism, promotes activity of osteoclasts and subsequent bone loss. The pivotal study showed a 60% to 65% reduction in new vertebral fractures by 18 months of use and about a 50% to 55% reduction in nonvertebral fractures. No significant long-term effects were noted on serum or urine calcium. The study was originally planned to run for 2 to 3 years, but toxicology concerns in rats prompted suspension of the study at a median 18-month point. In animal studies, rats developed dose-dependent osteosarcoma when given daily doses of the drug, from infancy to old age, at 3 to 60 times the human therapeutic dose. So far, there is one case report of osteosarcoma in a patient out of the hundreds of thousands of patients using the drug. This observation is within the natural occurrence rate of the disorder. Both men and women can use this drug if the prescribing physician feels the patient is at risk for fractures, has failed other therapies, or is intolerant of other therapies. The daily 20-μg injection is delivered from a metered pen device. Other anabolic drugs presently are under study.

PAGET DISEASE OF BONE

Paget disease of bone most often is an incidental finding during routine radiographs taken for other purposes.

It may be present in as many as 3% to 5% of the population older than 50 years. Generally, Paget disease is monostotic, asymptomatic, and discovered incidentally during the workup of other problems. With spread of the disorder, bone deformity and pain may arise. Most commonly, the pelvic, femoral, cranial, and vertebral bones are affected, although any and all bones may be involved.

In the absence of significant clinical findings, most patients do not seek medical care. Only after pain and skeletal deformity arise do most patients seek assistance. Cranial nerves may become involved when skeletal deformity of the cranial vault occurs. More commonly, cranial nerve VIII is affected, although all cranial nerves may be involved in very severe cases. A higher incidence of fractures is seen because the skeletal structure, although appearing more massive, is actually architecturally weaker. Osteosarcoma is an extraordinarily rare complication.

The biochemical evaluation of the disorder usually shows the presence of increased alkaline phosphatase with normal calcium and phosphorus levels. With immobilization, hypercalcemia may arise, although this is not an invariable finding.

The treatment of Paget disease of bone is generally directed toward the control of pain and the underlying pagetic process. Unfortunately, most patients are seen late in the course of the disorder, when anatomic skeletal deformities are beyond treatment with the usual antiresorptive drugs. Calcitonin was the first therapy available to treat this disease. The bisphosphonates are now first-line therapy. Alendronate, risedronate, pamidronate and zoledronic acid are used. Alendronate (40 mg daily) and risedronate (30 mg daily) are given for 3 to 6 months or longer if serum alkaline phosphatase or bone markers of skeletal collagen do not return to normal. The intravenous drugs are pamidronate (30 mg over 4 hours daily for 3 days) and zoledronic acid (5 mg yearly). Any tolerated and effective analgesic may be used to manage pain, although the control of the underlying pagetic process may completely eradicate the pain.

REVIEW EXERCISES

QUESTIONS

1. A 35-year-old man reports a 10-year history of renal stone disease and diffuse arthralgia. He is otherwise healthy and uses no vitamins, minerals, or drugs. Review of systems is normal, but a tibial radiograph shows a lesion at the midshaft. Serum data include a calcium level of 11.8 mg/dL (normal, 8.5–10.5 mg/dL); phosphorus, 2.9 mg/dL (normal, 2.5–4.5 mg/dL); creatinine, 1.0 mg/dL (normal, 0.5–1.3 mg/dL); intact PTH, 87 pg/mL (normal, 10–65 pg/mL); and calcitriol, 52 pg/mL (normal, 13–60 pg/mL).

All of the following are true *except*
a) Treatment with pamidronate is not necessary.

b) Adenomectomy is curative in most cases.
c) Recurrence is unlikely.
d) The chronicity of the problem argues for the presence of a neoplastic disorder.
e) Steroids will not control the problem.

Answer and Discussion

The answer is d. The chronicity of renal stone disease combined with the increased serum calcium, decreased phosphorus, increased PTH, and high-normal calcitriol is typical of hyperparathyroidism. The radiographic finding of a brown tumor or cyst typifies the bone disease (osteitis fibrosa cystica) of hyperparathyroidism. The best treatment is parathyroidectomy. Hyperplasia is an unusual finding.

2. A 53-year-old woman presents with generalized pain, muscle weakness, and weight loss. She uses E+P for menopausal symptoms after surgery for gynecologic cancer, which was also treated with radiation and chemotherapy. She has lost 60 pounds over 3 to 5 years. She has diffuse pain in all bones on examination. Her gait is painful, and her muscles are tender to touch. Baseline laboratory data show a hemoglobin level of 10.3 g/dL; calcium, 5.2 mg/dL; phosphorus, 2.8 mg/dL; albumin, 3.5 g/dL; creatinine, 1 mg/dL; alkaline phosphatase, 226 IU/L; immunoreactive PTH, 206 pg/mL (normal, 10–65 pg/mL); calcitriol, 35 pg/mL (normal, 15–52 pg/mL); and urine calcium, 3 mg per day (normal, 100–300 mg per day).

She is given calcium and vitamin D, and the urine calcium rises to 15 mg daily. She calls and says that she has bruises on her arms and legs.

All of the following are false *except*
a) She has celiac disease.
b) She requires surgery for the hyperparathyroidism.
c) Her serum carotene is likely elevated.
d) Increased oral calcium and vitamin D are the only therapy needed.
e) Increased uncalcified osteoid should be found.

Answer and Discussion

The answer is e. The patient has radiation-induced bowel dysfunction—malabsorption and osteomalacia. Bone will have large amounts of uncalcified osteoid. The secondary hyperparathyroidism is not treated by surgery. Celiac disease is less likely given the clinical facts. Carotene will be low from the poor absorption. More oral therapy is less likely to work in this case. Parenteral treatment is needed.

3. A spinal deformity is noted on the radiograph of a 73-year-old woman who was seen for back pain and a spinal compression fracture. She was previously healthy except for a cholecystectomy. She is a heavy tobacco and perhaps alcohol user and was on a golf outing when the incident occurred. She is being treated with calcium and analgesics. On examination, she is emaciated and has severe pain in the lumbar region. Radiograph of the spine shows an atypical fracture at L2. Laboratory data show a calcium level of 8.6 mg/dL; alkaline phosphatase, 100 IU/L; protein, 6 g/dL; hemoglobin, 10 g/dL; and an erythrocyte sedimentation rate of 100 mm per hour.

Which of the following would you do next?
a) Continue analgesics.
b) Start estrogen and extra calcium.
c) Evaluate the problem further.
d) Start alendronate.
e) Start calcitonin and physical therapy.

Answer and Discussion
The answer is c. When the patient was originally seen, she was quite ill appearing. Her laboratory test results showed anemia and an increased erythrocyte sedimentation rate. Serum calcium level was low normal, and the alkaline phosphatase was high normal. The best response to the question is to evaluate the problem further. None of the answers deals with the critical issue of the abnormal test results. Primary osteoporosis is not associated with any chemical abnormality. An elevated erythrocyte sedimentation rate and anemia are harbingers of other problems. Starting the patient on analgesics to temporize and control some of her discomfort might be reasonable, but clearly, more needs to be done. The use of estrogen and calcium or alendronate or physical therapy and calcitonin is a long-term solution if the problem proves to be primary osteoporosis. In this particular case, the patient's disorder was much more ominous than evident by the atypical compression deformity on the radiograph; the compression deformity was the result of an erosive tumor.

4. A 69-year-old man has had Paget disease of the pelvis for 15 years. He started treatment 5 years ago because of bone pain. He used oral risedronate for 3 to 6 months. The pain diminished, and his serum alkaline phosphatase decreased from 350 IU to 90 IU. The level remained suppressed until a year ago. On routine annual medical examination, his family doctor noted an alkaline phosphatase of 400 IU. The bisphosphonate was restarted, but the level decreased only to 350 IU and slowly increased to 980 IU. At this point, the next consideration would be
a) Switch over to alendronate.
b) Start intravenous zoledronic acid.
c) Order a bone scan.
d) Evaluate him further.

Answer and Discussion
The answer is d. This patient needs further evaluation. He developed metastatic prostate cancer that can mim-

ick the findings of Paget disease. Switching to another oral bisphosphonate drug would not likely be a better therapy. The bone scan was similar in appearance to the original one taken to evaluate Paget disease years previously. Bone x-ray was also taken and could not discriminate the two diseases. Intravenous medicine might be a consideration after the diagnosis is made but not at this point. Prostate examination was suspicious for cancer. The prostate-specific antigen was 20 times the upper reference limit.

5. A 67-year-old woman is evaluated after sustaining an atraumatic hip fracture. She has been using hormone replacement therapy since menopause about 15 years ago and has intermittent episodes of hot flashes. Her spinal T score is –3.0 SD and nonfractured hip T score is –2.9 SD. She has a family history of osteoporosis, uses alcohol rarely, smokes 1 to 2 packs of cigarettes per day, and uses supplemental calcium and vitamin D. Her serum PTH is elevated with a concurrent calcium of 8.5 mg/dL; 25 vitamin D is low, and urine bone turnover marker (NTX) is high. She increases her mineral and vitamin supplements. Two months later, the serum PTH and vitamin D are normal, and the calcium is 9.2 mg/dL. The bone turnover marker has not decreased. Further evaluation found no secondary problems affecting her skeleton. Her family doctor advised that the treatment program be changed. About 6 months later, her turnover marker was normal (in the premenopausal range). What did he do? He told her to
a) Exercise more
b) Change her vitamin brand to something containing strontium
c) Stop smoking
d) Add extra tofu to her diet

Answer and Discussion
The answer is c. This is an interesting real-life case. The high turnover markers indicated that bone metabolism was increased, which increased her risk for fractures. Although the high PTH and low vitamin D might be considered the cause, their improvement with added mineral and vitamin supplements did not alter the turnover marker. Someone using hormone replacement likewise should not have a high marker. Exercise will not measurably improve this degree of turnover. Added dietary strontium will not have a major effect either although pharmacologic doses could. Added dietary tofu would not provide enough estrogenic effect to help. Stopping the use of tobacco is the key issue here. Combustion products of tobacco enhance hormonal catabolism and lower the effective concentration of estrogenic drugs, which the skeleton "sees." Her hot flashes are a clinical sign that the dose of estrogen is not working.

SUGGESTED READINGS

Ariyan CE, Sosa JA. Assessment and management of patients with abnormal calcium. *Crit Care Med* 2004;32(suppl 4):S146–S154.

Blake GM, Fogelman I. Role of dual-energy x-ray absorptiometry in the diagnosis and treatment of osteoporosis. *J Clin Densitom* 2007;10(1):102–110.

Body JJ. Hypercalcemia of malignancy. *Semin Nephrol* 2004;24(1):48–54.

Cremers S, Garnero P. Biochemical markers of bone turnover in the clinical development of drugs for osteoporosis and metastatic bone disease: potential uses and pitfalls. *Drugs* 2006;66(16):2031–2058.

Dickerson RN. Treatment of hypocalcemia in critical illness—part 1. *Nutrition* 23(4):358–361.

Dickerson RN. Treatment of hypocalcemia in critical illness—part 2. *Nutrition* 23(5):436–437.

Ferreira A. Development of renal bone disease. *Eur J Clin Invest* 2006;36(suppl 2):2–12.

Gennari L, Bilezikian JP. Osteoporosis in men. *Endocrinol Metab Clin North Am* 2007;36(2):399–419.

Kamel HK. Update on osteoporosis management in long-term care: focus on bisphosphonates. *J Am Med Dir Assoc* 2007;8(7):434–440.

Keen R. Osteoporosis: strategies for prevention and management. *Best Pract Res Clin Rheumatol* 2007;21(1):109–122.

Langston AL, Ralston SH. Management of Paget's disease of bone. *Rheumatology* 2004;43(8):955–959.

Levine JP. Pharmacologic and nonpharmacologic management of osteoporosis. *Clin Cornerstone* 2006;8(1):40–53.

Lyman D. Undiagnosed vitamin D deficiency in the hospitalized patient. *Am Fam Physician* 2005;71(2):299–304.

Maeda SS, Fortes EM, Oliveira UM, et al. Hypoparathyroidism and pseudohypoparathyroidism. *Arq Bras Endocrinol Metabol* 2006;50(4):664–673.

Ralston SH, Coleman R, Fraser WD, et al. Medical management of hypercalcemia. *Calcif Tissue Int* 2004;74(1):1–11.

Srivastava AK, Vliet EL, Lewiecki EM, et al. Clinical use of serum and urine bone markers in the management of osteoporosis. *Curr Med Res Opin* 2005;21(7):1015–1026.

Turner CH, Robling AG. Mechanisms by which exercise improves bone strength. *J Bone Miner Metab* 2005;23(suppl):16–22.

Whyte MP. Clinical practice. Paget's disease of bone. *N Engl J Med* 2006;355(6):593–600.

Woolf AD. An update on glucocorticoid-induced osteoporosis. *Curr Opin Rheumatol* 2007;19(4):370–375.

Chapter 46

Acute Renal Failure

Joseph V. Nally, Jr.

POINTS TO REMEMBER:

- The therapy for prerenal azotemia is directed at optimizing volume status with isotonic fluids with the expectant improvement in renal function within 48 hours.

- If urinary tract obstruction is a diagnostic consideration, renal ultrasonography is sensitive and specific (90%–95%) in confirming the diagnosis of hydronephrosis.

- The specific diagnosis of acute interstitial nephritis (AIN) as a cause of acute renal failure (ARF) should lead to the discontinuation of possibly offending medications. If the renal insufficiency does not resolve in days to weeks, renal biopsy results may confirm the diagnosis of AIN.

- The oliguric phase usually begins <24 hours after the inciting incident and may last for 1 to 3 weeks.

- The prognosis of acute tubular necrosis (ATN) is dependent on the underlying primary disease that resulted in ARF as well as any complications that arise during the bout of ARF. The mortality rate for patients with ATN may approach 40% to 50%.

- Data suggest that in azotemic patients who require cardiac angiography, a protocol of intravenous hydration and use of a nonionic contrast material appear warranted. Earlier randomized controlled trials have suggested that pretreatment with acetylcysteine might attenuate contrast injury in at-risk patients; however, more recent reviews have called this putative benefit into question.

ARF is a common problem in the contemporary practice of hospital-based medicine. Prospective studies have demonstrated that 2% to 5% of all patients admitted to a general medical-surgical hospital will develop ARF. In selected patients in the intensive care unit (ICU) setting, the incidence may exceed 20%. Marked increases in both morbidity (which prolongs hospitalization) and mortality occur in the patient who develops ARF. The high frequency of occurrence and substantial morbidity and mortality of ARF demand a logical approach to prevention and early diagnosis as well as prompt recognition and management of its complications.

ARF is defined as a rapid decrease in renal function characterized by progressive azotemia (best measured by serum creatinine), which may or may not be accompanied by oliguria. Alternatively, investigators in the critical care medicine arena have defined acute kidney injury (AKI) based on an increase of serum creatinine >0.5 mg/dL and/or a degree of oliguria utilizing the RIFLE criteria.[1] The goal of this multidisciplinary approach is to standardize the definition and staging of AKI and ARF to assist the clinician and clinical investigator in the acquisition of knowledge to improve patient outcomes. Since AKI is an evolving terminology, we will continue to use ARF for the remainder of this text. ARF can be diagnosed with certainty when the patient's prior renal function is known and a decrement is documented. It is important to distinguish the three major causes of ARF: prerenal azotemia, postrenal azotemia or obstruction of the urinary tract, and intrinsic renal disease. Distinguishing among the three basic categories of ARF is a challenging clinical exercise. The importance of differentiating the major causes of ARF must be stressed, because the initial evaluation and management of the ARF patient are tailored to the particular cause. Because the majority of all hospital-acquired ARF is secondary to ATN, special emphasis will be placed on ATN.

PRERENAL AZOTEMIA

Prerenal azotemia is caused by transient renal hypoperfusion that may induce both azotemia and urinary sodium avidity. Prerenal azotemia may be encountered in both the volume-depleted and volume-overloaded patient (Table 46.1). True volume depletion may result from renal or extrarenal losses. In the volume-overloaded patient with edematous states such as cirrhosis, nephrosis, and congestive heart failure, prerenal azotemia may occur because the kidney perceives that the arterial vascular tree is underfilled, resulting in renal hypoperfusion. In addition, prerenal azotemia may occur owing to high-grade bilateral renal artery stenosis.

The pathophysiology of prerenal azotemia relates to the reduction in renal blood flow. Renal hypoperfusion stimulates both the sympathetic nervous system and renin-angiotensin system to cause renal vasoconstriction and

---

TABLE 46.1

PRERENAL ACUTE RENAL FAILURE

A. Cardiac causes: Primary decrease in cardiac output
  1. Acute disorders: Myocardial infarction, trauma, arrhythmias, malignant hypertension, tamponade, acute valvular disease (e.g., endocarditis)
  2. Chronic disorders: Valvular diseases, chronic myocardiopathies (ischemic heart disease, hypertensive heart disease)
  3. Renal artery stenosis (bilateral)
B. Volume depletion
  1. Gastrointestinal losses: Vomiting, diarrhea, fistulas
  2. Renal: Salt-wasting disorders, overdiuresis
C. Redistribution of extracellular fluid
  1. Hypoalbuminemic states: Nephrotic syndrome, advanced liver disease, malnutrition
  2. Physical causes: Peritonitis, burns, crush injury
  3. Peripheral vasodilatation: Sepsis, antihypertensive agents

---

sodium avidity. Furthermore, hypotension is a powerful stimulus to the release of an antidiuretic hormone, which mediates water reabsorption. Hence, urine production is characterized by low volume, decreased concentration of urinary sodium, and increased urinary excretion of creatinine with a high urine osmolality. Results of microscopy of the urinary sediment are usually bland. In essence, prerenal azotemia is "a good kidney looking at a bad world."

The therapy for prerenal azotemia is directed at optimizing volume status with isotonic fluids with the expectant improvement in renal function within 48 hours. In patients with edematous disorders who have prerenal azotemia, special efforts are directed at treating the underlying disease states (i.e., heart failure, cirrhosis) and optimizing systemic hemodynamics and renal perfusion.

POSTRENAL AZOTEMIA

Obstruction of the urinary tract may cause ARF. To be the cause of azotemia, urinary tract obstruction must involve the outflow tract of both normal kidneys unless preexisting renal dysfunction is present, in which case the obstruction may involve only a single kidney. Patients with acute urinary tract obstruction may present with hematuria, flank or abdominal pain, or signs of uremia. A high index of suspicion for urinary tract obstruction should exist for patients with prior abdominal or pelvic surgery, neoplasia, or radiation therapy. Although oliguria or anuria suggests complete obstruction, partial obstruction may exist in the presence of adequate urinary output. The presence of marked oliguria or anuria is a powerful diagnostic clue that suggests urinary tract obstruction, severe ATN with cortical necrosis, or bilateral vascular occlusion. Lesions that may cause obstruction can be either intrinsic or extrinsic to the genitourinary tract (Table 46.2).

TABLE 46.2

POSTRENAL ACUTE RENAL FAILURE

A. Ureteral and pelvic
　1. Intrinsic obstruction
　　(a) Blood clots
　　(b) Stones
　　(c) Sloughed papillae
　　(d) Fungus balls
　2. Extrinsic obstruction
　　(a) Malignancy
　　(b) Retroperitoneal fibrosis
　　(c) Iatrogenic: Inadvertent ligation
B. Bladder
　　(a) Stones
　　(b) Blood clots
　　(c) Prostatic hypertrophy or malignancy
　　(d) Bladder carcinoma
　　　　Neuropathic
C. Urethral
　　(a) Strictures
　　(b) Phimosis

If urinary tract obstruction is a diagnostic consideration, renal ultrasonography is sensitive and specific (90%–95%) in confirming the diagnosis of hydronephrosis. This test may be operator dependent, so the experience of the radiologist is crucial. False-negative test results may be seen with periureteral metastatic disease or retroperitoneal fibrosis. Abdominal computed tomography or retrograde pyelography may be helpful in this circumstance. If urinary tract obstruction is a diagnostic consideration, renal ultrasonography should be performed, as obstruction represents a potentially reversible cause of ARF.

INTRINSIC RENAL DISEASE

The major causes of ARF due to intrinsic renal disease include acute glomerulonephritis, AIN, renal atheroembolic disease (AED), and ATN. Because ATN is by far the most common cause of ARF that develops in the hospital setting, special emphasis will be given to that condition.

Acute Glomerulonephritis

The importance of the urinalysis in the evaluation of patients with ARF cannot be overemphasized: Physicians must develop skill and expertise in interpreting the microscopic findings of urinalysis. In cases of ARF due to intrinsic renal disease, such skills are critical. The presence of proteinuria, hematuria, and red blood cell casts are pathognomonic of glomerulonephritis. The differential diagnosis of rapidly progressive glomerulonephritis is beyond the scope of this review. Evaluation usually includes performance of a renal biopsy as well as a detailed serologic evaluation for the presence of systemic vasculitis, collagen vascular disease, and infectious processes. Specific therapies tailored to the disease entity diagnosed after this thorough evaluation may be lifesaving.

Acute Interstitial Nephritis

The diagnosis of ARF due to AIN also may be suggested on microscopy of the urinalysis by the presence of sterile pyuria, white blood cell casts, and eosinophiluria on Hansel stain. AIN may be secondary to a variety of drugs, including penicillins, methicillin, cephalosporin, nonsteroidal anti-inflammatory drugs, cimetidine, phenytoin, phenobarbital, allopurinol, interferon-alpha, and diuretics. The clinical syndrome may be quite variable, although it is likely to involve an abnormal urinary sediment (proteinuria and pyuria), eosinophilia/eosinophiluria, and fever. Skin rash is seen in approximately 25% of cases. The specific diagnosis of AIN as a cause of ARF should lead to the discontinuation of possibly offending medications. If the renal insufficiency does not resolve in days to weeks, renal biopsy results may confirm the diagnosis of AIN. In selected cases, a trial of steroid therapy may hasten recovery of renal function, yet prospective trials evaluating the efficacy and safety of steroid therapy are lacking.

ACUTE TUBULAR NECROSIS

Incidence and Etiology

Overall, ARF may affect 2% to 5% of patients in a tertiary care hospital, and the incidence of ARF in the surgical or medical ICU may exceed 20% to 30% in selected high-risk patient populations (Table 46.3).

The majority of all hospital-acquired ARF is secondary to ATN. Liano and Pascual[2] in Madrid observed that the causes of ARF in a multicenter tertiary care hospital setting were ATN (45%), ARF superimposed on chronic kidney disease (13%), prerenal disease (21%), urinary tract obstruction (10%), glomerulonephritis and vasculitis (4%), AIN (2%), and AED (1%). Renal hypoperfusion and renal ischemia are the most common causes of ATN, although nephrotoxic insults from various agents are being recognized with increasing frequency. As shown in Table 46.3, the incidence of ARF in the ICU and/or after extensive vascular surgery, such as aortic aneurysm repair or coronary artery bypass grafting, is significant. Because "volume is the primal scream of the kidney," renal ischemia is the leading cause of ARF in this population. Agents (either endogenous or exogenous) that may be toxic to the kidney in any clinical setting are summarized in Tables 46.4 and 46.5.

Table 46.4 lists endogenous nephrotoxic products. Of note, pigment nephropathy may be suspected in the appropriate clinical situation (posttraumatic or atraumatic after intoxications) in which the following discrepancies exist: hematuria by urinary dipstick and the absence of red blood cells on urinary microscopy. The combination of renal hypoperfusion and the nephrotoxic insult of

TABLE 46.3

FREQUENCY OF ACUTE RENAL FAILURE IN DIFFERENT CLINICAL SETTINGS

	Mild Failure (%) (SCr <3 mg/dL)	Severe Failure (%) (SCr >5 mg/dL)
Open heart surgery	5–20	2–5
Abdominal aortic aneurysm resection		
Emergency	30–50	15–25
Elective	5–10	2–5
Severe trauma	10–20	1–5
Neonatal ICU admission	17	6
Aminoglycoside drug administration	5–20	1–2
Admission to general medical-surgical unit	4–10	1–2

ARF, acute renal failure; ICU, intensive care unit; S$_{Cr}$, serum creatinine.

myoglobin or hemoglobin within the proximal tubule may result in ATN. Early recognition of this disorder is crucial, because a forced alkaline diuresis is indicated to minimize nephrotoxicity. Similarly, the tumor lysis syndrome may be suspected in the appropriate clinical setting when marked hyperuricemia and hyperuricosuria as well as crystalluria are recognized. A forced alkaline diuresis may limit nephrotoxicity and is usually recommended prophylactically before an aggressive chemotherapy regimen.

The list of potential exogenous nephrotoxic agents is exhaustive (Table 46.5). Simply stated, when a patient develops ATN while receiving medications, each medication should be reviewed for the possibility of nephrotoxicity. Commonly seen nephrotoxins in the hospitalized patient include:

- Radiographic contrast material
- Antibiotics (especially aminoglycosides and amphotericin B)
- Chemotherapeutic agents (especially cis-platinum and ifosfamide)
- Nonsteroidal anti-inflammatory drugs
- Angiotensin-converting enzyme (ACE) inhibitors and/or angiotensin receptor blockers (ARB)

TABLE 46.4

ACUTE RENAL FAILURE RELATED TO ENDOGENOUS NEPHROTOXIC PRODUCTS

Pigment nephropathy
    Myoglobin
    Hemoglobin[a]
    Methemoglobin[a]
Intrarenal crystal deposition
    Uric acid
    Calcium
    Oxalate
Tumor-specific syndromes
    Tumor lysis syndrome
    Plasma cell dyscrasias (e.g., myeloma kidney)

[a]Questionable direct nephrotoxic effect.

More recently, potential nephrotoxicity of newer agents, such as acyclovir, protease inhibitors, recombinant interleukin-2, interferon, and selected chemotherapeutic agents, is being appreciated.

In the contemporary practice of hospital-based medicine, recognition of ARF in two special patient populations deserves special comment—those with HIV and those who have undergone bone marrow transplantation.

HIV

Patients with HIV may develop ARF due to the same causes as uninfected patients, but protease inhibitors have been associated with the development of ARF. Ritonavir and indinavir (as well as intravenous acyclovir, foscarnet, and sulfadiazine) have been associated with reversible ARF thought to occur secondary to crystalluria and intrarenal obstruction. In addition, patients treated with indinavir may present with renal colic; indinavir renal stones have been associated with urinary tract obstruction.

Bone Marrow Transplantation

ARF may be quite common following bone marrow transplantation, and several nephrologic syndromes may be encountered at various time frames after the procedure has been performed. In the perioperative period, ATN due to tumor lysis syndrome, bone marrow infusion, sepsis, or antibiotics (especially aminoglycoside and amphotericin B) is likely. At days 10 to 16, ARF is commonly attributed to hepatic venoocclusive disease resulting from endothelial cell injury from radiation or chemotherapy. Clinically, the presentation of this entity mimics hepatorenal syndrome. After 4 to 12 months, ARF may be due to hemolytic uremic syndrome, possibly related to cyclosporine A or radiation therapy. Therapies with plasma exchange have been disappointing.

Pathophysiology

Several pathogenic mechanisms have been proposed to account for the abnormalities noted in ARF secondary to

TABLE 46.5

CAUSES OF EXOGENOUS TOXIC ACUTE RENAL FAILURE

Antibiotics
  Aminoglycosides
  Cephalosporin
  Sulfonamide, co-trimoxazole
  Tetracyclines
  Amphotericin B
  Polymyxin, colistin
  Bacitracin
  Pentamidine
  Vancomycin
  Acyclovir
  Foscarnet
Anesthetic agents
  Methoxyflurane
  Enflurane
Contrast media
  Diatrizoate
  Iothalamate
  Bunamiodyl
  Iopanoic acid
Antiulcer regimens
  Cimetidine
  Excess of milk-alkali
Analgesics
  Nonsteroidal anti-inflammatory drugs
Diuretics
  Mercurials
  Ticrynafen
  Others
Chemotherapeutic and immunosuppressive agents
  Cis-platinum
  Carboplatin
  Ifosfamide
  Methotrexate
  Mitomycin
  5-Azacytidine
  Nitrosourea
  Plicamycin
  Cyclosporine A and tacrolimus (FK506)

D-penicillamide
Recombinant interleukin-2
Interferon-alpha or gamma-1-B
HIV protease inhibitors
  Indinavir
  Ritonavir
Organic solvents
  Glycols (ethylene glycol, diethylene glycol)
  Halogenated hydrocarbons (CCl_4, tetra- and trichloroethylene)
  Aromatic hydrocarbons (toluene)
  Aliphatic-aromatic hydrocarbons (Vaseline, kerosene, turpentine, paraphenylene diamine)
Heavy metals
Poisons
  Insecticides (chlordane)
  Herbicides (paraquat, diquat)
  Rodenticides (elemental P)
  Mushrooms
  Snake bites[a]
  Stings[a]
  Bacterial toxins[a]
Chemicals
  Aniline
  Hexol
  Cresol
  Chlorates
  Potassium bromate
Recreational drugs[b]
  Heroin
  Amphetamines
Miscellaneous
  Dextrans
  EDTA
  Radiation
  Silicone
  Epsilon-amino caproic acid[a]
  ACE inhibitors

[a]Direct toxicity or indirect systemic effects (shock, intravascular hemolysis, or coagulation).
[b]Slow onset of renal failure, unless associated with rhabdomyolysis.
EDTA, ethylenediaminetetraacetic acid; ACE, angiotensin-converting enzyme.

ATN.[3] Of note, there are two significant dichotomies regarding the renal physiology and pathology of ATN.

The first dichotomy is a striking reduction in glomerular filtration rate (GFR) in oliguric ARF that is accompanied by a more modest decline in renal plasma flow. This dichotomy of GFR and renal plasma flow reductions suggests a contribution, at least in part, of an intense afferent arteriole vasoconstriction.

The second dichotomy relates to the pathology of ATN. The distribution of the tubular necrosis appears patchy, and the degree of necrosis does not correlate clinically with the level of renal dysfunction. These observations may be reconciled by understanding the pathological location of early ATN. In general, the renal cortex is well perfused and well oxygenated. The corticomedullary junction is much less well oxygenated, however, and oxygen demand and oxygen supply are nearly equal under basal conditions. Following a hypotensive or hypoxic insult, oxygen demand exceeds supply, and ATN develops in the energy-rich, thick ascending limb of Henle in the corticomedullary junction. This imbalance may account for the patchy nature seen pathologically on a renal cross-sectional biopsy sample.

Ischemic and toxic insults may result in identical clinical syndromes associated with azotemia. The pathophysiologic mechanisms postulated for ARF include:

- Tubular back leak of glomerular filtrate
- Tubular obstruction owing to debris or casts
- Vascular theories invoking afferent arteriolar vasoconstriction (i.e., the renin-angiotensin system)
- Diminished permeability of the glomerular basement membrane

Disorders of intracellular adenosine triphosphate and calcium metabolism, membrane and phospholipase abnormalities, abnormalities of tubular cell polarity and cytoskeletal function, and generation of free radical oxygen species and proteases may all be significant in the tubular damage of ATN.[3]

Knowledge of the basic processes involved in the development of ATN is a prerequisite to an understanding of contemporary therapies directed at limiting renal damage and promoting more rapid renal recovery. The sentinel biochemical event in renal ischemia is the depletion of adenosine triphosphate, which is the major energy currency for cellular work. Adenosine triphosphate depletion results in impaired function of the plasma membrane and intracellular adenosine triphosphatases that are vital to normal cell function. As a consequence of these defects, cell swelling and high intracellular levels of calcium result. As the name suggests, ischemic ATN is characterized by renal tubular cell injury. Because obvious necrosis is not a cardinal histopathologic finding in ATN, sublethal injury is important. The sublethal injury to tubular cells leads to aberrations in the cytoskeletal organization of tubular cells with loss of cell polarity.

After sublethal injury, the kidney has a remarkable capacity for repair of the normal structure and function. Renal recovery from ATN is a relatively new concept with great potential for clinical application. Increased mitotic activity and epithelial regeneration are notable features of ATN. Certain aspects of renal recovery duplicate events in renal development. A number of growth factors play a role in recovery. Epidermal growth factor, insulinlike growth factor-1, and hepatocyte growth factor have been shown to limit renal injury and accelerate renal recovery in experimental ischemic ATN, but results in clinical trials have been disappointing to date.

Diagnosis

The tools available to the clinician include:

- A thorough history and physical examination to assess volume status, potential nephrotoxic insults, and evidence of systemic disease
- Urine output
- Urinalysis
- Serum and urine electrolytes
- Radiologic and renal ultrasonography evaluation

The schema for evaluating the patient with ARF is outlined in Table 46.6. The urine output may be a clue to the diagnosis of ARF. The presence of marked oliguria or anuria might suggest urinary tract obstruction, renovascular occlusion, or cortical necrosis. In contrast, nonoliguric ARF is being recognized with increased frequency, and careful

---

TABLE 46.6

DIAGNOSIS OF ACUTE RENAL FAILURE

Step 1: History and Physical Examination		
Prerenal	**Renal**	**Postrenal**
Volume depletion; congestive heart failure; severe liver disease or other edematous states	ATN AIN AGN	Palpable bladder or hydronephrotic kidneys; enlarged prostate; abnormal pelvic examination; large residual bladder urine volume; history of renal calculi

Step 2: Urine Sediment			
Eosinophils	**Red Blood Cell Casts**	**No Abnormalities**	**Renal Tubular Epithelial Cells and "Muddy-brown" Casts**
Suspect AIN	Glomerulonephritis or vasculitis	Suspect prerenal or postrenal azotemia	Suspect ATN

Step 3: Urinary Indices	
U_{Na} <20 mEq/L $U{:}P_{Cr}$ >30 RFI ($U_{Na}/U{:}P_{Cr}$) <1 FE_{Na} <1 U Osm >500 Confirm prerenal azotemia or glomerulonephritis	U_{Na} >40 mEq/L $U{:}P_{Cr}$ <20 $U_{Na}/U{:}P_{Cr}$ >1 U Osm <400 Confirm ATN or obstruction

Step 4: Urinary Output
If urine volume <500 mL/day Correct prerenal or postrenal factors Optional trial of furosemide to convert oliguric to nonoliguric ARF

AIN, acute interstitial nephritis; ARF, acute renal failure; ATN, acute tubular necrosis; FE_{Na}, fractional excretion of sodium; RFI, renal failure index; U_{Na}, urine sodium; U Osm, urine osmolarity; $U{:}P_{Cr}$, Urine:plasma creatinine ratio.

TABLE 46.7

ACUTE RENAL FAILURE URINARY SEDIMENT

Bland or Scant Findings	Granular Casts	Red Blood Cells/ Red Blood Cell Casts	Epithelial and White Blood Cells/ White Blood Cell Casts	Crystalluria
Vasculitides ▪ Preglomerular vasculitis ▪ Hemolytic-uremic syndrome ▪ Scleroderma	*ATN* ▪ Pigmented coarsely granular casts common	*Glomerulonephritis* ▪ RPGN ▪ Small vessel vasculitis	*Eosinophiluria present* ▪ AIN likely	*Uric acid* ▪ Tumor lysis syndrome
Renovascular diseases ▪ Arterial thrombosis or emboli	—	*Interstitial nephritis* ▪ Rarely seen	*Eosinophiluria absent* ▪ AIN still possible	*Calcium oxalate* ▪ Penthrane toxicity ▪ Glycol
▪ Prerenal azotemia ▪ Postrenal azotemia	— —	*ATN* ▪ Rarely seen	*Pyelonephritis* ▪ Severe, with abscesses	

AIN, acute interstitial nephritis; ATN, acute tubular necrosis; RPGN, rapidly progressive glomerulonephritis.

monitoring of serum creatinine in patients at risk is of paramount importance.

Examination of the urinalysis sample is fundamental to the evaluation of the patient with ARF. Simple urinalysis may distinguish the cause of ARF among the various possibilities. The various urinary abnormalities associated with the clinical diagnoses are highlighted in Table 46.7. For example, proteinuria, hematuria, and red blood cell casts are pathognomonic of glomerulonephritis. The classic sediment for ATN includes pigmented (muddy brown) granular casts and renal tubular epithelial cells, which may be seen in nearly 80% of cases of oliguric ARF.

Determination of urinary chemistries may be helpful in determining the etiology of ARF. Urine sodium (U_{Na}), urine creatinine (U_{creat}), and urine osmolality should be measured, and either the fractional excretion of sodium (FE_{Na}) or the renal failure index (RFI) should be calculated, using the following equation:

$$FE_{Na} = \frac{\dfrac{U_{Na}V}{P_{Na}}}{\dfrac{U_{creat}V}{P_{creat}}} \times 100\% \text{ or } RFI = \frac{U_{Na} \times P_{creat}}{U_{creat}}$$

where P_{Na} is plasma sodium, P_{creat} is plasma creatinine, and V is urine volume.

Note that a low FE_{Na} (or RFI) may be associated with either prerenal azotemia or acute glomerulonephritis. These entities could be separated clinically by examination of the urinalysis. Conditions associated with prerenal azotemia would have a bland urinalysis result, whereas proteinuria, red blood cells, and red blood cell casts would be seen with acute glomerulonephritis. Both ATN and obstruction may be associated with an increased FE_{Na} or RFI. Here again, the urinalysis results would be key. ATN would be associated with a classic sediment with pigmented coarsely granular casts; but in obstruction, the urinalysis results are often bland or have isolated hematuria.

Radiologic evaluation in ARF might include renal ultrasonography, plain frontal supine radiography of the abdomen, and retrograde urography. The value of renal ultrasonography in the evaluation of possible urinary tract obstruction was discussed earlier. Such studies as intravenous pyelography or abdominal computed tomography, which use intravenous contrast material, should be avoided because of potential nephrotoxicity.

Stages

The oliguric phase usually begins <24 hours after the inciting incident and may last for 1 to 3 weeks. Urine volume averages 150 to 300 mL per day. The oliguric phase may be prolonged in the elderly. During this phase, the clinician must be alert for the expected complications, with special emphasis on metabolic consequences, gastrointestinal bleeding, and infection.

The diuretic phase is characterized by a progressive increase in urine volume—a harbinger of renal recovery. The serum creatinine may continue to increase for another 24 to 48 hours, however, before it reaches a plateau and decreases. Severe polyuria during this phase is seen less frequently. Careful management during this phase is crucial, because up to 25% of deaths with ARF may occur in this phase, usually related to fluid and electrolyte abnormalities as well as infection. Finally, the recovery phase ensues. Renal function returns to near baseline, but abnormalities of urinary concentration and dilution may persist for weeks or months.

Treatment

During the initial evaluation, it is imperative to search for reversible causes such as volume depletion, obstruction, and vascular occlusion. During the initial stages, a trial of parenteral hydration with isotonic fluids may correct ARF secondary to prerenal causes. In early established oliguric ARF secondary to ATN, a trial of a loop diuretic may be warranted. Pharmacologic intervention to convert oliguric ATN to nonoliguric ATN is a salutary clinical goal. In general, increases in urinary volume make it easier to address problems of volume overload, hyperkalemia, and metabolic acidosis, yet increasing urine output does not always confer benefit on morbidity, dialysis requirements, or mortality.[4,5]

Increases in urine volume also may provide room for supplemental total parenteral nutrition in the critically ill patient. Morbidity, the need for dialysis, and mortality may be less prevalent in the nonoliguric form of ATN. Unfortunately, there are very few prospective, randomized trials that have adequately tested this hypothesis. In particular, the data available for "renal dose" dopamine therapy in oliguric ARF are surprisingly scant and do not confirm clear-cut benefit. If considered, a trial of renal dose dopamine should be used after a clinical challenge of parenteral hydration and a loop diuretic agent. If the treatment is unsuccessful, dopamine should be tapered off within 24 hours. A prospective, randomized trial with atrial natriuretic peptide (ANP) in patients with ATN (oliguric and nonoliguric) has been reported.[6] Overall, there was no established benefit on morbidity and mortality with ANP. In a subset of patients with oliguric ATN, however, clinical improvement was suggested with ANP infusion. A subsequent trial in this select population did not demonstrate clinical benefit. In sum, ANP is not recommended as therapy for ARF.

Once the clinical diagnosis of ATN is made, conservative medical management is in order (Table 46.8). This would include attempts to minimize further renal injury, maintain systolic blood pressure to ensure adequate renovascular perfusion, ensure adequate nutrition, maintain the metabolic balance, and promote recovery of renal function. Optimizing the patient's volume status is imperative, particularly in patients with oliguric ARF. Protein restriction and maintenance of essential amino acids and carbohydrate intake may limit catabolism and help maintain nitrogen balance. Dietary phosphorous and potassium may be restricted. Medications should be adjusted for the level of renal dysfunction.

Dialysis (either hemodialysis or peritoneal dialysis) may be instituted when clinically indicated. The indications for acute dialysis include:

- Volume overload
  Severe hyperkalemia
  Severe, uncorrectable metabolic acidosis
  Pericarditis
  Selected poisonings
  Uremic symptomatology

Intermittent hemodialysis provides a rapid treatment of hyperkalemia and volume overload. Newer dialytic techniques with biocompatible membranes and the use of bicarbonate dialysis and controlled ultrafiltration may allow better treatment tolerance in the hemodynamically unstable patient.[5] However, prospective, controlled trials in patients with ARF treated with different modalities are not available for comparison to offer definitive therapeutic guidelines. A recent trial comparing daily versus every-other-day intermittent hemodialysis suggested a survival benefit for daily therapy.[7]

Prognosis

The prognosis of ATN is dependent on the underlying primary disease that resulted in the ARF as well as any complications that arise during the bout of ARF. The mortality rate for patients with ATN may approach 40% to 50%. During the Madrid trial, the overall mortality rate for all ARF patients was 47% and exceeded 60% in those with ATN (2). This pessimistic outlook has changed little in the past four decades, even with the advent of effective dialysis. Mortality rates remain high today despite effective control of uremia, because we are caring for an older, sicker population with severe concomitant illnesses. Higher mortality rates are seen in elderly patients and in patients with respiratory failure, multiorgan failure with severe forms of oliguric ATN, preexisting chronic diseases, and systemic hypotension. Leading causes of death include bronchopulmonary infections, sepsis, cardiovascular disease, and bleeding disorders. Of patients who survive ATN, nearly half will have a complete recovery of renal function, and a majority of the remainder will have an incomplete recovery (Fig. 46.1). Only approximately 5% to 10% of all ARF patients require chronic maintenance dialysis. In short, with ARF, "you either die or get better."

TABLE 46.8

CHECKLIST OF CONSERVATIVE MEASURES IN THE MANAGEMENT OF ACUTE RENAL FAILURE

Fluid balance
- Carefully monitor intake/output and weights
- Restrict fluids

Electrolytes and acid–base balance
- Prevent and treat hyperkalemia
- Avoid hyponatremia
- Keep serum bicarbonate >15 mEq/L
- Minimize hyperphosphatemia
- Treat hypocalcemia only if symptomatic or if intravenous bicarbonate is required

Uremia and nutrition
- Restrict protein (0.5 g/kg/day), but maintain caloric intake; consider forms of nutritional support
- Maintain carbohydrate intake to at least 100 g/day to minimize ketosis and endogenous protein catabolism

Drugs
- Review all medications
- Stop magnesium-containing medications
- Adjust dosage for renal failure; readjust with improvement of GFR

GFR, glomerular filtration rate.

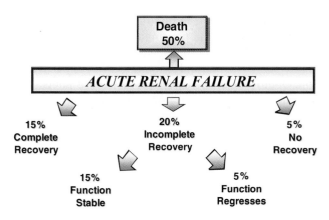

Figure 46.1 Prognosis of acute tubular necrosis.

Prevention

Because the management of ATN is primarily one of conservative care and support, special attention should be focused on the prevention of ARF. Patients at high risk (i.e., patients with preexisting azotemia, the elderly, volume-depleted individuals) warrant careful clinical consideration of the relative risks and benefits of diagnostic or therapeutic interventions that have a potential for nephrotoxicity. This is especially true for patients at risk of undergoing cardiac catheterization or other diagnostic studies requiring intravenous contrast material.

The reader is referred to a comprehensive review that offers a predictive model of contrast-induced ARF and provides a meta-analysis of existing data regarding the prevention of contrast-induced ARF.[8] The authors confirm the beneficial effect of volume expansion on reducing the risk of contrast-induced ARF citing the pioneering studies of Solomon et al.[9] The authors also acknowledge the recent study of isotonic sodium bicarbonate infusions to offer a potential advantage over isotonic saline infusions prior to and after radiocontrast procedures, yet they await confirmatory studies before fully endorsing this approach.[10] This position is also endorsed in a recent review.[11] The current recommendations for volume expansion would be the infusion of isotonic sodium chloride or sodium bicarbonate at a rate of 1 mL/kg per hour for 12 hours before and after radiocontrast administration in high-risk hospitalized patients. An abbreviated regimen of these isotonic fluids (3 mL/kg per hour 1 hour before and 1 mL/kg per hour for 6 hours after) can be administered for patients with urgent procedures.

The comprehensive review also recommends use of nonionic contrast agents at the lowest possible dose to limit potential nephrotoxicity in a patient at risk. Rudnick et al.[12] published a prospective, randomized trial of nearly 1,200 well-hydrated patients undergoing cardiac catheterization to examine the effects of the newer nonionic contrast material. Patients were stratified for the presence or absence of azotemia (serum creatinine ≥ 1.5 mg/dL) or diabetes mellitus. In patients without azotemia (with or without diabetes mellitus), the incidence of contrast-induced renal dysfunction was low (i.e., <1%–2%) with either the ionic or nonionic contrast material. In contrast, in those with preexisting azotemia, a 50% reduction in contrast-associated renal dysfunction was seen when the nonionic material was used.

These data suggest that in azotemic patients who require cardiac angiography, a protocol of intravenous hydration and use of a nonionic contrast material appear warranted. Earlier randomized controlled trials have suggested that pretreatment with acetylcysteine might attenuate contrast injury in at-risk patients; however, more recent reviews have called this putative benefit into question.[13]

REFERENCES

1. Molitoris BA, Levin A, Warnock DG, et al. Improving outcomes of acute kidney injury: report of an initiative. *Nat Clin Pract Nephrol* 2007;3:439–442.
2. Liano F, Pascual J. Epidemiology of acute renal failure: a prospective, multicenter, community-based study. Madrid Acute Renal Failure Study Group. *Kidney Int* 1996;50:811–881.
3. Abuelo JG. Normotensive ischemic acute renal failure. *N Engl J Med* 2007;357:797–805.
4. Mehta RL, Pascula MT, Soroko S, et al. Diuretics, mortality, and nonrecovery of renal function in acute renal failure. *JAMA* 2002;288:2547–2553.
5. Gill N, Nally JV Jr, Fatica RA. Renal failure secondary to acute tubular necrosis: epidemiology, diagnosis, and management. *Chest* 2005;128:2847–2863.
6. Allgren RL, Marbury TC, Rahman SN, et al. Anaritide in acute tubular necrosis. *N Engl J Med* 1997;336:828–871.
7. Schiffl H, Lnag, SM, Fischer R. Daily hemodialysis and the outcome of acute renal failure. *N Engl J Med* 2002;346:305–310.
8. Barrett BJ, Parfrey PS. Preventing nephropathy induced by contrast medium. *N Engl J Med* 2006;354:379–386.
9. Solomon R, Werner C, Mann D, et al. Effects of saline, mannitol, and furosemide to prevent acute decreases in renal function induced by radiocontrast agents. *N Engl J Med* 1994;331:1416–1420.
10. Merten GJ, Burgess WP, Gray LV, et al. Prevention of contrast-induced nephropathy with sodium bicarbonate: a randomized controlled trial. *JAMA* 2004;291:2328–2334.
11. Weisbord SD, Palevsky PM. Prevention of contrast-induced nephropathy with volume expansion. *Clin J Am Soc Nephrol* 2008;3(1):273–280.
12. Rudnick MR, Goldfarb S, Wexler L, et al. Nephrotoxicity of ionic and nonionic contrast media in 1196 patients: a randomized trial. The Iohexol Cooperative Study. *Kidney Int* 1995;47: 254–261.
13. Fishbane S. N-Acetylcysteine in the prevention of contrast-induced nephropathy. *Clin J Am Soc Nephrol* 2007;3:281–287.

Chapter 47

Parenchymal Renal Disease

Gerald B. Appel

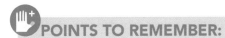

Parenchymal renal diseases affect many millions of persons in the United States and worldwide. In the United States, more than 350,000 persons were in end-stage renal disease (ESRD) programs, largely as a result of renal involvement by parenchymal diseases. One form of glomerular damage alone, diabetic glomerulonephropathy, affects millions of people, with a cost of billions of dollars annually. Worldwide, glomerular disease associated with hepatitis C virus (HCV) and HIV is a major health problem. Fortunately, progress in the diagnosis and treatment of common forms of idiopathic nephrotic syndrome (NS), such as focal glomerulosclerosis and MN, has been striking in the last decade. Table 47.1 shows the incidence of idiopathic NS.

The mechanisms of both glomerular and tubulointerstitial injury are quite varied. In glomerular disease, immune-mediated renal injury is a major initiating pathogenetic mechanism. In diabetic nephropathy and amyloidosis, other mechanisms of damage to the glomerular capillary wall clearly are at work. In tubulointerstitial disease, the primary insult may be immunologic (e.g., drug-induced acute interstitial nephritis [AIN]), toxic-metabolic (e.g., analgesics, oxalate, etc.), or vascular (e.g., sickle cell disease and atheroemboli). The end result is damage to the tubules and interstitial space of the kidney, with eventual renal scarring and fibrosis.

NORMAL GLOMERULUS

Each glomerulus—the basic filtering unit of the kidney—consists of a tuft of anastomosing capillaries formed by the branchings of the afferent arteriole. The millions of glomeruli within each kidney comprise approximately 5% of the kidney's weight and provide 2 m^2 of filtering surface. As well, each glomerulus consists of a combination of cellular elements (endothelial cells, mesangial cells, visceral and parietal epithelial cells) and extracellular matrix (the glomerular basement membrane [GBM] and mesangial matrix). The endothelial cells lining the lumens of the glomerular capillaries have a highly fenestrated cytoplasm attached to the internal aspect of the GBM. These cells possess a variety of histocompatibility antigens, express Fc and C3b receptors that allow the adhesion of macrophages and complement activation, and produce and secrete numerous vasoactive substances (including antihemolytic factor [factor VIII], thrombin receptors, prostacyclin, and heparinlike growth factors). They may contribute to the synthesis and maintenance of the GBM.

TABLE 47.1
INCIDENCE OF IDIOPATHIC NEPHROTIC SYNDROME IN U.S. ADULTS
MCD: 5% FSGS: 20%–25% MN: 25%–30% MPGN: <5% Other proliferative and sclerosing glomerulonephritides: 15%–30%

FSGS, focal segmental glomerulosclerosis; MN, membranous nephropathy; MPGN, membranoproliferative glomerulonephritis.

The mesangium or central stalk region of the glomerulus is composed of both matrix and cells. It is important for mechanical support, transport of molecules out of the capillary loops, and the contractile nature of the glomerular capillaries. The mesangial matrix consists predominantly of type IV collagen, fibronectin, laminin, and proteoglycans. Mesangial cells may proliferate and produce vasoactive substances, including prostaglandins, oxygen radicals, platelet-derived growth factor, and so on.

The GBM is composed of a central dense layer (lamina densa) and more lucent outer and inner layers (lamina rara interna and lamina rara externa). It is chemically composed of type IV collagen and a variety of proteins including entactin, laminin, and fibronectin. The GBM is highly negatively charged and provides both a size- and charge-selective barrier to the passage of circulating macromolecules.

The visceral epithelial cells contain numerous extensions called *foot processes*, which interdigitate with the foot processes of neighboring visceral epithelial cells and are tightly bound to the lamina rara externa of the GBM. The visceral epithelial cells are coated with a highly anionic layer of sialoprotein and are important in the synthesis of many of the components of the GBM. The parietal epithelial cells are simple, flat cells that line the Bowman capsule.

HISTOPATHOLOGICAL TERMS

Understanding renal histopathology requires the knowledge of only a few terms. When dealing with the entire kidney, if all glomeruli are involved, a process is called *diffuse* or *generalized*; if only some glomeruli are involved, the process is called *focal*. When dealing with the individual glomerulus, a process is called *global* if the whole glomerular tuft is involved and *segmental* if only part is involved. The terms *proliferative*, *sclerosing*, and *necrotizing* are often used (e.g., focal and segmental sclerosing glomerulonephritis [GN]; diffuse global proliferative lupus nephritis [LN]). Extracapillary proliferation or crescent formation is caused by the accumulations of macrophages, fibroblasts, proliferating epithelial cells, and fibrin within the Bowman space.

CLINICAL MANIFESTATIONS OF GLOMERULAR DISEASES

Certain laboratory findings common to many glomerular diseases focus the differential diagnosis of unknown parenchymal renal diseases toward a glomerular origin. These include the presence of erythrocyte casts, dysmorphic erythrocytes, or both in the urinary sediment and the presence of large amounts of albumin in the urine. In normal humans, the urinary excretion of albumin is <50 mg daily. Although increases in urinary protein excretion may come from the filtration of abnormal circulating proteins (such as light chains in multiple myeloma) or from the deficient proximal tubular resorption of normally filtered low-molecular-weight proteins (such as β_2-microglobulin), the most common cause of proteinuria—specifically albuminuria—is glomerular injury. In glomerular diseases, protein excretion may range from several hundred milligrams to more than 30 g daily. In some diseases associated with heavy proteinuria, such as minimal-change NS, albumin is the predominant protein found in the urine, and the proteinuria is said to be highly "selective." In other glomerular diseases (such as focal segmental glomerulosclerosis [FSGS] and diabetes), the proteinuria, although still largely composed of albumin, contains many higher-weight molecular proteins as well and is said to be "nonselective" proteinuria. When proteinuria exceeds 3.0 to 3.5 g daily, patients commonly develop hypoalbuminemia, hyperlipidemia, edema, and other manifestations described as NS.

Although a small number of erythrocytes may appear in the urine of normal individuals, urinary excretion of more than 500 to 1,000 erythrocytes/mL defines abnormal hematuria. Although hematuria is common in many glomerular diseases, it is not, of course, specific for glomerular pathology. However, those erythrocytes that pass through gaps in the GBM undergo the osmotic changes imposed as they pass down the tubules and become deformed. These dysmorphic erythrocytes are highly suggestive of glomerular pathology. Likewise, red blood cell casts, which form when erythrocytes pass the glomerular capillary barrier and become enmeshed in a proteinaceous matrix in the tubules, are highly suggestive of glomerular disease.

NEPHROTIC SYNDROME

NS is defined by more than 3.0 to 3.5 g of protein in the urine daily accompanied by hypoalbuminemia, edema, and hyperlipidemia. In clinical practice, many nephrologists refer to "nephrotic range" proteinuria regardless of whether their patients have the other manifestations of the full NS, as the latter are consequences of the proteinuria. Nephrotic proteinuria is always due predominantly to albuminuria.

Hypoalbuminemia is a consequence of urinary protein loss as well as catabolism of filtered albumin by the proximal tubule and the redistribution of albumin within the body. The salt and volume retention in NS may occur through two different major mechanisms. In the classic theory, proteinuria leads to hypoalbuminemia, a low plasma oncotic pressure, and intravascular volume depletion. Subsequent underperfusion of the kidney stimulates the priming of sodium-retentive hormonal systems, such as the renin-angiotensin-aldosterone axis, which causes increased renal sodium and volume retention. In the peripheral capillaries, with normal hydrostatic pressures and decreased oncotic pressure, transcapillary fluid leakage and edema occur. In some patients, however, the intravascular volume has been measured and has been found to be increased along with the suppression of the renin-angiotensin-aldosterone axis. In an animal model of unilateral proteinuria created by the unilateral infusion of the aminonucleoside puromycin, evidence suggests a primary renal sodium retention at a distal nephron site, due to altered responsiveness to atrial natriuretic factor. Here, only the proteinuric kidney retains sodium and volume and at a time when the animal is not yet hypoalbuminemic. Thus, local factors within the kidney may account for the volume retention of NS.

Epidemiologic studies strongly support an increased risk of atherosclerotic complications in conjunction with NS, related in part to the hyperlipidemia of the NS. Most patients have elevated levels of total and low-density-lipoprotein cholesterol, and most have low or normal high-density-lipoprotein cholesterol levels. Levels of lipoprotein(a) are elevated in patients with NS and revert to normal on remission of proteinuria. Antihyperlipidemic medications are effective in favorably altering lipoprotein levels in NS. Aggressive therapy, especially with statins, to lower total cholesterol to <200 mg/dL and low-density-lipoprotein cholesterol to <100 mg/dL has been recommended.

The initial evaluation of the patient with NS includes laboratory tests to define whether the patient has primary, idiopathic NS, or NS due to a secondary cause (e.g., measurement of fasting blood sugar, antinuclear antibodies, serum complement, etc.). Once secondary causes have been excluded, the treatment of the adult nephrotic patient usually requires a renal biopsy to define the pattern of glomerular involvement. In adults, NS is one of the most common conditions requiring renal biopsy. In virtually every study defining the role of the renal biopsy, those patients with heavy proteinuria are most likely to benefit in terms of a change from the prebiopsy diagnosis and in terms of changes in prognosis and therapy.

Minimal-change Disease

Minimal-change disease (MCD), also known as nil disease, is the most common pattern of idiopathic NS in children and comprises approximately 5% of idiopathic NS

in adults. Patients typically present with sudden onset of periorbital and peripheral edema. Severe proteinuria is typical, and values <3.0 g of protein daily are rare. In children, the proteinuria is highly selective, whereas selectivity of the proteinuria is less reliable in adults. Up to 30% of adults with MCD also have hypertension and microscopic hematuria, although active urinary sediment with erythrocyte casts is not found. Many patients have mild to moderate azotemia related to intravascular volume depletion.

In true MCD, histopathology typically reveals no glomerular abnormalities in the light microscopic examination (hence, the "nil" acronym—"*nothing in light microscopy*"). Immunofluorescence (IF) staining and electron microscopy (EM) both show an absence of immune deposits. The GBM is normal, and an effacement or "fusion" of the visceral epithelial foot processes is noted along the entire distribution of every capillary loop.

The course of MCD in both children and adults is often one of relapses and responses to additional treatment. From 90% to 95% of children experience a remission of NS when treated with corticosteroids for 8 weeks. In adults, the response rate is somewhat lower, with 75% to 85% of patients responding to regimens of oral prednisone given daily (60 mg per day) or on alternate days (120 mg every other day). The time to clinical response is slower in adults, and they should not be considered to be steroid resistant until no response has been observed after 16 weeks of treatment. Tapering of the steroid dose should begin 1 to several weeks after complete remission and should continue gradually over 1 to 2 months. Both children and adults are likely to have at least one relapse once steroids have been discontinued. Approximately 50% of children and 30% of adults experience relapse by 1 year, and the number increases with time. Most clinicians treat the first relapse with a regimen similar to the initial treatment regimen. Those patients who experience a third episode, or who become dependent on steroids (i.e., the prednisone dose cannot be decreased beyond a certain level without recurrence of proteinuria), may be successfully treated with other immunosuppressive drugs in a manner similar to treating focal glomerulosclerosis (see below). The response rate is lower among steroid-resistant as opposed to steroid-dependent patients.

Focal Segmental Glomerulosclerosis

Over 20% of adults with idiopathic NS have FSGS. The incidence of FSGS has been dramatically increasing, and it is the most common pattern of idiopathic NS in blacks. FSGS may be either idiopathic or secondary to a number of differing conditions (e.g., heroin nephropathy, HIV nephropathy, sickle cell nephropathy, reflux nephropathy, remnant kidneys, and the healed phase of focal GN, among others). There are a number of genetic forms of FSGS related to abnormal structural proteins or cation channels of the visceral epithelial cell podocytes (e.g., podocin, a-actinin 4, TRPC6).

Patients with idiopathic FSGS typically present with either asymptomatic proteinuria or the full NS. Although NS is present at presentation in two-thirds of adults, protein excretion may vary from <1 g per day to levels as high as 20 to 30 g per day. Proteinuria is nonselective. Hypertension is found in 30% to 50% and microscopic hematuria in 25% to 75% of these patients. The glomerular filtration rate (GFR) is decreased at presentation in 20% to 30% of patients. Complement levels and the results of other serologic tests are normal in FSGS.

The histologic diagnosis of FSGS depends on identifying within only some of the glomeruli (focal) areas of glomerulosclerosis restricted to only some part of the glomerular tufts (segmental lesions). By IF staining, immunoglobulin M (IgM) and C3 are commonly found in the areas of glomerular sclerosis resulting from the entrapment of plasma proteins rather than from true immune complex deposition. By EM, fusion or effacement of the foot processes is found to some extent in all the glomeruli, even those unaffected by areas of segmental sclerosis. No electron-dense immune deposits are present. In biopsy specimens taken early in the course of FSGS, when the GFR is preserved, few glomeruli with segmental sclerosing lesions are present, and almost no global glomerulosclerosis is seen. As renal function declines, repeat biopsy specimens will show many glomeruli with segmental and more global sclerosis.

The course of unresponsive FSGS is usually one of progressive proteinuria and declining GFR. Patients with asymptomatic proteinuria typically develop NS over time. Only a minority of patients experience a spontaneous remission of proteinuria. Eventually, most patients develop ESRD in 5 to 20 years from presentation. Some patients with the collapsing variant (or malignant FSGS) have a more rapid course to ESRD in 2 to 3 years. Idiopathic FSGS may recur in the transplanted kidney and is then manifested by the occurrence of severe proteinuria and NS.

The treatment of FSGS in adults is controversial, with few randomized, controlled trials existing on which to base judgments. In general, patients with a sustained remission of their NS are unlikely to progress to ESRD, whereas those with unremitting NS are likely to progress. Risk factors suggesting a higher rate of progression to renal failure include heavier proteinuria, elevated creatinine levels, presence of interstitial scarring on biopsy specimens, black race, and lack of responsiveness to an initial course of steroids. In older studies, only a small percentage of patients had a remission of proteinuria after treatment with corticosteroids or other immunosuppressives, and the relapse rate after treatment was high. Recent studies using more intensive and especially more prolonged immunosuppressive regimens with steroids or cytotoxics (cyclophosphamide 1–2 mg/kg per day) or both have achieved up to a 60% remission rate, with preservation of long-term renal function. A recent randomized, blinded, controlled trial of cyclosporine (4–6 mg/kg per day for 6 months) versus placebo in patients with steroid-resistant FSGS showed both a higher remission rate with treatment as well as better preservation of renal function after 4 years. Even patients whose disease is unresponsive to cytotoxic agents may show response to this therapy. Some patients, however, experience relapse when the therapy is stopped. Newer therapies include mycophenolate mofetil, tacrolimus, and rituximab.

At present, many clinicians would not use immunosuppressive therapy for patients with subnephrotic levels of proteinuria and little damage apparent on their renal biopsy, treating these patients only with ACE inhibitors or ARBs to reduce proteinuria and its side effects. For FSGS patients with NS and risk of progressive renal failure, a prolonged course of corticosteroids or other immunosuppressive medication would be used in the hope of inducing a remission of the NS and preventing eventual ESRD.

Membranous Nephropathy

MN is the most common pattern of idiopathic nephritic syndrome in white Americans. It typically presents with the onset of heavy proteinuria leading to periorbital and pedal edema. Hypertension and microhematuria are not infrequent findings, but renal function and GFR are usually normal at presentation. MN is the most common pattern of idiopathic NS to be associated with thrombotic events and especially with renal vein thrombosis. The presence of sudden flank pain, deterioration of renal function, or symptoms of pulmonary emboli in a patient with MN should prompt an investigation for renal vein thrombosis. In certain elderly patients with MN, an underlying carcinoma may be the occult cause of the renal lesion.

The course of MN is variable. In general, renal survival is more than 75% at 10 years. A spontaneous remission rate also occurs, which varies from 20% to 30%. The slow progression and spontaneous remission rate have confounded clinical treatment trials. Some trials suggest that short-term corticosteroid therapy leads to preservation of renal function and to remissions of the NS. Other studies have shown no benefit of corticosteroid regimens on the course of MN. A randomized, well-performed, controlled trial of pulse methylprednisolone followed by oral prednisone for 1 month alternating with 1 month of oral chlorambucil, each repeated on alternate months for a total duration of 6 months of treatment, reported a larger number of total remissions and better preservation of renal function. Other recent controlled studies using cytotoxic agents also have shown similar beneficial results. The use of cyclosporine in a double-blind, randomized, controlled trial of patients with steroid-resistant MN also has yielded higher remission rates than placebo. Likewise, mycophenolate mofetil and rituximab have been used successfully in uncontrolled trials of MN.

At present, most clinicians treat only those MN patients who are likely to have the highest rate of progression to renal failure (men, older patients, and especially those with greater degrees of persistent proteinuria). Whether to use corticosteroids, cytotoxic agents, cyclosporine, or a combination of therapies depends on individual patients and the clinician's preference.

ACUTE GLOMERULONEPHRITIS

Immunoglobulin A Nephropathy

IgA nephropathy originally was believed to be an uncommon and benign form of glomerulopathy (Berger disease). It now is recognized as the most frequent form of idiopathic GN worldwide (comprising 15%–40% of primary GN in parts of Europe and Asia) and clearly can progress to ESRD. In geographic areas where renal biopsies commonly are performed for milder urinary findings, a higher incidence of IgA nephropathy is noted. In the United States, some centers report IgA nephropathy to comprise up to 20% of all primary GN. Although men with the disorder outnumber women and the peak occurrence is in the second to third decade of life, IgA nephropathy can occur in patients of both genders and all ages.

The diagnosis of IgA nephropathy is established by finding glomerular IgA deposits either as the dominant or codominant immunoglobulin on IF. In addition to IgA, deposits of C3 and immunoglobulin G (IgG) are common. The light microscopic picture may vary from one of minimal change to mesangial proliferation to crescentic GN. The most common picture is mesangial hypercellularity. By EM, electron-dense deposits are found in the mesangial and paramesangial areas. The pathogenesis of IgA nephropathy is unknown. The predominant antibody is to be composed of polymeric IgA1 originating in the secretory-mucosal system, but the antigen to which it is directed is unknown. Environmental antigens, such as viral or other pathogens, and diet-related antigens have been proposed but remain unproven. Also unknown is which factors subsequent to the deposition of immune complexes containing IgA lead to the inflammatory and sclerosing glomerular features of the disease.

IgA nephropathy often presents with one of two syndromes: asymptomatic microscopically hematuria and/or proteinuria (most common in adults), or episodic gross hematuria after upper respiratory tract infections or exercise (most common in children). The course of IgA nephropathy is variable. Most patients show no decline in GFR over decades, whereas some develop NS, hypertension, and renal failure. Hypertension is present in 20% to 50% of patients. Increased serum IgA levels do not correlate with the course of the disease.

Factors predictive of a poor outcome in IgA nephropathy may include older age at onset; absence of gross hematuria; presence of hypertension; persistent and severe proteinuria; male sex; a reduced GFR and elevated serum creatinine level; and certain histologic features on renal biopsy specimens, including severe proliferation and sclerosis,

severe tubulointerstitial damage, and extracapillary glomerular proliferation (i.e., crescent formation). Renal survival is estimated at 85% at 10 years and 75% at 20 years.

The treatment of IgA nephropathy has included efforts to prevent antigenic stimulation or the entry of environmental stimulants, including the use of broad-spectrum antibiotics (e.g., doxycycline), tonsillectomy, and dietary manipulations to eliminate certain dietary antigens (e.g., gluten). With few exceptions, these attempts have not been successful. The benefits of treatment with glucocorticoids and other immunosuppressives are far from clear for most patients. In one controlled trial of 6 months of corticosteroid therapy in patients with progressive IgA nephropathy, the treated group had improved renal function over 10 years of follow-up. Other efforts at immunosuppression have included combinations of cyclophosphamide and azathioprine, which may have given beneficial effects in only some patients when chronically. Immunosuppressive therapy using cytotoxic agents and pulse methylprednisolone (Solumedrol) has also been used for patients with crescentic lesions. Trials of Ω-fish oils have shown mixed results in IgA nephropathy. In all trials, the use of ACE inhibitors or ARBs has been shown to be beneficial in reducing proteinuria and probably the progression to renal failure. With no clearly proven therapy, many clinicians choose to give only blockers of the renin-angiotensin system (e.g., ACE inhibitors or ARBs) to most patients with IgA nephropathy and reserve other therapy only for those patients at highest risk for progression to renal failure.

Idiopathic Membranoproliferative Glomerulonephritis

Idiopathic membranoproliferative glomerulonephritis (MPGN), or mesangiocapillary GN, is an uncommon glomerular disease that may present in three histologic forms, depending on where the electron-dense deposits are located along the GBM (MPGN types 1, 2, and 3). In series in which biopsies are performed, it comprises only a small percentage of glomerular disease.

By light microscopy, the lesions of types 1, 2, and 3 MPGN look the same and include diffuse mesangial proliferation and exaggeration of the lobular pattern of the glomerular tufts with reduplication of the basement membrane, which results in a double contour or "tram track" appearance. By IF, diffuse granular GBM deposits of C3 and often IgG, IgA, and IgM are present. EM clearly distinguishes the three patterns of MPGN. Type 1 has subendothelial and mesangial deposits. Type 2 has broad, dense, intramembranous deposits along the GBM, Bowman capsule, and tubular basement membranes. Type 3 has subepithelial deposits and intramembranous deposits in addition to subendothelial and mesangial deposits.

The pathogenesis of the idiopathic forms of this type of GN is unknown, but clearly, each differs from the other. By light microscopy, similar patterns of glomerular damage have been seen in association with certain infectious agents (HCV), autoimmune disease (systemic lupus erythematosus [SLE]), and disease of intraglomerular coagulation. Idiopathic MPGN is a rare disease, and many patients with this lesion have SLE or HCV with cryoglobulinemia. Type 2 MPGN, also known as dense deposit disease, has been called an autoimmune disorder, with an autoantibody (an IgG, C3 nephritic factor) directed against C3bBb, the alternate pathway C3 convertase. Because degradation of the enzyme is prevented, increased activation and consumption of complement are noted in dense deposit disease.

Although MPGN may present with asymptomatic microhematuria and proteinuria in some patients, most patients present with NS. Other patients may present with an acute nephritic picture with active urinary sediment, renal insufficiency, and hypertension. The majority of patients have low complement values. Most studies have found similar results for the various patterns of MPGN and have treated them as one disease entity. Attempts to treat MPGN have included the use of corticosteroids and other immunosuppressive medications as well as the use of anticoagulants and antiplatelet agents to minimize glomerular damage from coagulation. No therapy has been conclusively proven to be effective in adults. In children, long-term corticosteroid therapy has led to more remissions of NS and the preservation of renal function.

Rapidly Progressive Glomerulonephritis

Rapidly progressive glomerulonephritis (RPGN) comprises a group of glomerulonephritides that have in common a progression to renal failure in a matter of weeks to months and the presence of extensive extracapillary proliferation (i.e., crescent formation) in a large percentage of the glomeruli. RPGN includes diseases with different etiologies, pathogeneses, and clinical presentations. RPGN has been divided into three patterns, defined by immunologic pathogenesis: type I, characterized by anti-GBM disease; type II, characterized by immune complex deposition (e.g., SLE, poststreptococcal GN, etc.); and type III, characterized by the absence of immune deposits or anti-GBM antibodies (i.e., pauci-immune). Most cases in the latter group fall into the category of antineutrophil cytoplasmic antibody (ANCA)-positive RPGN. In the past, with the exception of those with postinfectious RPGN, prognosis was generally poor regardless of pathogenesis. This prognosis has dramatically changed for many patients.

Anti–Glomerular Basement Membrane Disease
Anti-GBM disease is caused by circulating antibodies that are directed against the noncollagenous domain of type IV collagen and that damage the GBM. This leads to an inflammatory response, breaks in the GBM, and the formation of a proliferative and crescentic GN. If the anti-GBM antibodies cross react with and cause damage to the basement membrane of pulmonary capillaries, the patient develops pulmonary hemorrhage and hemoptysis. The association of anti-GBM antibody–mediated damage to the kidneys and lungs is called *Goodpasture syndrome*. The presentation is a nephritic picture with hypertension, edema, hematuria and active urinary sediment, and reduced renal function. Renal function may deteriorate from normal to dialysis-requiring levels in a matter of days to weeks. Patients with pulmonary involvement may have life-threatening hemoptysis. The course of the disease, once it has progressed to renal failure, is usually one of permanent renal dysfunction. If treatment is started earlier in the course of the disease, patients may regain considerable kidney function.

The pathology shows a proliferative GN, often with severe extracapillary involvement of the Bowman space by crescent formation. By IF study, a linear deposition of immunoglobulin is present along the GBM. EM does not show any electron-dense deposits.

The treatment of type I RPGN mediated by anti-GBM antibodies includes intensive therapy to reduce the production of anti-GBM antibodies using immunosuppressive agents such as cyclophosphamide combined with plasmapheresis to remove circulating anti-GBM antibodies. Therapy is most effective in patients who have less extensive crescent formation and who have a preserved GFR. Some patients with advanced renal failure, however, even those requiring dialysis, have responded to this form of treatment. Rapid, intensive therapy is necessary to prevent irreversible renal damage.

Immune Complex Rapidly Progressive Glomerulonephritis
Type II RPGN, associated with immune complex–mediated damage to the glomeruli, may occur within a spectrum of diseases from primary glomerulopathies, such as IgA nephropathy and MPGN, to secondary GN due to postinfectious GN to SLE. The treatment of IgA nephropathy and MPGN is discussed earlier. Most cases of postinfectious GN resolve with successful treatment of the underlying infection. Here, the potential hazards of immunosuppressive treatment and the limited data available on its benefit should prompt caution in the use of this therapeutic option. The treatment of severe SLE is dealt with in a later section.

Pauci-immune Rapidly Progressive Glomerulonephritis and Vasculitis-associated Rapidly Progressive Glomerulonephritis
Patients with pauci-immune type III RPGN include those with and without evidence of systemic vasculitis. Patients often present with progressive renal failure and a nephritic picture with hematuria, oliguria, and hypertension. Most patients have circulating antibodies directed against neutrophil cytoplasmic antigens (ANCA). Patients who test positive for perinuclear ANCA more often have a clinical picture akin to microscopic polyangiitis (with arthritis, skin involvement with leukocytoclastic angiitis, and

constitutional and systemic signs), whereas those who test positive for C-ANCA are more likely to have granulomatous vasculitic disease associated with the GN (akin to Wegener granulomatosis). Considerable overlap occurs between these groups. As in all RPGN, renal function may deteriorate rapidly. An elevated serum creatinine level and the presence of hypertension are risk factors for poor renal outcome. In some studies of the course of ANCA-associated GN and systemic vasculitis, no difference in renal or patient survival was noted between patients with isolated renal disease and those with systemic involvement. With the use of oral cyclophosphamide in addition to corticosteroids, diseases such as Wegener granulomatosis and microscopic polyangiitis have shown markedly improved survival rates. Plasmapheresis is useful in some patients with severe renal or pulmonary disease. Excellent results includes some patients with true crescentic GN. Successful results have been reported with the use of steroids plus cytotoxic agents, even in oliguric patients and those who are already dialysis dependent. It is clear that pauci-immune RPGN has the most favorable response rate of all patterns of RPGN. It responds well to a number of different immunosuppressive regimens, including pulse steroids and cyclophosphamide given orally or intravenously. The therapeutic regimen of choice and the optimal duration of therapy are being determined in controlled trials.

GLOMERULAR INVOLVEMENT IN SYSTEMIC DISEASES

Diabetes Mellitus

Diabetic nephropathy is the most common cause of ESRD in the United States, comprising 40% to 50% of all new ESRD patients. From 25% to 40% of individuals with either type I or type II diabetes develop nephropathy. The course is characterized initially by glomerular hyperfiltration with a normal serum creatinine level but with microalbuminuria, then by progressively increasing proteinuria and NS and a slow decrease in GFR. Recent evidence supports a similar renal course for those with type I and type II diabetes. The glomerular histopathologic changes in both are similar, with thickening of the GBM, mesangial sclerosis, nodular intercapillary glomerulosclerosis (Kimmelstiel-Wilson nodules), and microaneurysms of the glomerular capillaries.

Recent studies have documented dramatic improvement in altering the progression of diabetic renal disease through a variety of interventions, including control of hyperglycemia and blood pressure as well as the use of ACE inhibitors and angiotensin II receptor blockers. Poor glycemic control is associated with an increased incidence of nephropathy. The Diabetes Control and Complication Trial documented decreased retinopathy and nephropathy in the incidence of fixed microalbuminuria and clinical proteinuria among patients with type I diabetes treated with intensive glucose control. In patients with diabetes, blood pressure control using a variety of antihypertensives leads to decreased proteinuria and a slowing of the rate of GFR decline. In diabetic persons, the use of ACE inhibitors has been shown to reduce microalbuminuria and clinical proteinuria in both proteinuric and nephrotic patients with type I and type II diabetes. In a trial involving more than 400 individuals with type I diabetes with protein excretion >500 mg daily and a serum creatinine level <2.5 mg/dL, the use of captopril three times a day led to amelioration of the decline in GFR compared with that in control patients, despite comparable blood pressure control in the latter group. In a smaller study involving patients with type II diabetes who had milder proteinuria, the group receiving ACE inhibitors had better-preserved renal function and less proteinuria at 5 years follow-up. The use of ARBs also decreases proteinuria in nephrotic diabetic patients. Two large randomized, blinded trials, each enrolling more than 1,500 patients with adult-onset diabetes and proteinuria, have shown less progression to renal failure with use of angiotensin II receptor blockers.

Systemic Lupus Erythematosus

Renal involvement greatly influences the disease course and choice of treatment of lupus patients. The incidence of clinically detectable renal disease varies from 15% to 75% of patients with SLE. Histologic evidence of renal involvement in SLE is found in the vast majority of biopsy specimens when studied by light microscopy, IF, and EM, even in the absence of clinical renal disease. The International Society of Nephrology (ISN) classification of LN has been used successfully for both clinical and research activities. The ISN classes correlate well with the clinical picture of the patients at biopsy and also help to define the clinical course of the patient and provide a guide to therapy (Table 47.2).

Patients with the ISN class I and II biopsy specimens usually have only mild clinical renal disease. They virtually never are nephrotic but may have active serologic findings. They have an excellent long-term prognosis and require no treatment directed at their renal lesions. Patients with ISN class III lesions (focal proliferative LN) have more active sediment changes, increased proteinuria, and often active serologic findings. The lesions may transform or evolve into a class IV pattern. Patients with ISN class IV (diffuse proliferative) LN have the most severe renal involvement, with active sediment, hypertension, heavy proteinuria, frequent NS, and often a reduction of GFR. They have the worst prognosis. Patients with ISN class V (membranous) lesions usually present with NS sometime before fulfilling the American Rheumatism Association criteria for SLE. These patients are typically nephrotic, with inactive serologic findings. Although the short-term prognosis is good, patients can progress to renal failure over many years. ISN class VI includes those patients with an end-stage kidney due to LN.

TABLE 47.2
SERUM COMPLEMENT LEVELS IN GLOMERULAR DISEASES

Diseases with reduced complement levels
   Postinfectious GN (poststreptococcal GN, subacute
      bacterial endocarditis, visceral abscesses)
   SLE
   Cryoglobulinemia
   Idiopathic MPGN
Diseases associated with normal serum complement levels
   Minimal-change NS, focal segmental glomerular sclerosis,
      MN IgA nephropathy, Henoch-Schönlein purpura
   Anti-GBM disease
   Pauci-immune RPGN, polyarteritis nodosa, Wegener
      granulomatosis
   Amyloid, diabetes, and other systemic diseases

GBM, glomerular basement membrane; GN, glomerulonephritis; IgA, immunoglobulin A; MN, membranous nephropathy; MPGN, membranoproliferative glomerulonephritis; NS, nephrotic syndrome; RPGN, rapidly progressive glomerulonephritis; SLE, systemic lupus erythematosus.

In general, all patients with ISN class IV lesions on biopsy deserve vigorous therapy for their LN. Many patients with class III LN (especially those with active necrotizing lesions and large amounts of subendothelial deposits) also would benefit from such therapy. The optimal therapy for patients with class V lesions is less clear. Standard vigorous treatment of severe LN may include a 6-month course of once-monthly intravenous cyclophosphamide (Cytoxan) and intravenous methylprednisolone therapy or other agents such as mycophenolate mofetil, azathioprine, and cyclosporine in various combinations.

Amyloidosis

Amyloidosis is a generic term for a group of diseases in which the extracellular deposition of one of a number of insoluble fibrillar proteins occurs in a characteristic β-pleated sheet configuration. One of the two most common forms of amyloidosis is primary amyloidosis (AL amyloidosis), now called *light chain–associated amyloidosis*, due to a plasma-cell dyscrasia that overproduces a monoclonal immunoglobulin light chain. Of AL amyloid patients, 20% have overt myeloma, whereas 10% to 15% of myeloma patients have AL amyloidosis. AL fibrils are derived from the variable portion of the light chain. Two-thirds to four-fifths of patients with AL amyloid who have a monoclonal protein have overproduction of a λ-light chain. Renal involvement is one of the most common manifestations of AL amyloid, usually presenting as heavy albuminuria and NS.

Secondary amyloidosis (AA amyloidosis) is associated with high circulating levels and the deposition of the serum amyloid A protein (a 12-kd high-density lipoprotein apoprotein synthesized by hepatocytes as an acute-phase reactant in disease states). AA amyloidosis occurs in chronic infections and inflammatory states, including rheumatoid arthritis, ankylosing spondylitis, tuberculosis,

osteomyelitis, and intravenous drug abuse. Renal amyloidosis presents with proteinuria and NS, then progresses to renal insufficiency and renal failure in the majority of cases.

Amyloid deposits are predominantly found within the glomeruli and often appear as amorphous, eosinophilic extracellular nodules. They also may be found deposited in the tubular basement membranes, the interstitium, and the vessels. They stain positively with Congo red and under polarized light display apple-green birefringence. Under EM, amyloid appears as nonbranching rigid fibrils 8 to 10 nm in diameter.

No specific effective therapy is available for renal amyloidosis. In patients with AL amyloidosis, both chemotherapy directed at the abnormal clone of B cells (e.g., melphalan and prednisone) and stem cell transplantation in some patients have been shown to have beneficial results. Dialysis, using either hemodialysis or peritoneal dialysis, and transplantation have been effective in small numbers of patients with primary amyloidosis and ESRD. Recently, bone marrow and renal transplantation has been used to treat these patients as well.

HIV Infection

AIDS affects many millions of persons worldwide and in the United States has caused more than 40,000 deaths. Some cities, like New York City, have reported more than 10,000 cases of AIDS, and up to 500,000 persons in the New York metropolitan area have been reported to be infected with the virus. Many studies have found populations of intravenous drug abusers to have a 60% to 85% carriage rate for HIV. Infection with this virus has been associated with a number of patterns of renal disease, including acute renal failure and a unique form of glomerulopathy now called *HIV nephropathy*.

Acute Renal Failure

The course of disease in patients with acute renal failure and AIDS has been described by a number of investigators. The most common precipitating factors for acute renal failure in all studies have included medications (pentamidine, aminoglycosides, trimethoprim-sulfamethoxazole, nonsteroidal anti-inflammatory drugs [NSAIDs]) and pyrexia and dehydration superimposed on sepsis, hypotension, and respiratory failure. Dialysis support is indicated for the AIDS patient with acute renal failure.

HIV-Associated Nephropathy

Several histologic patterns of glomerulopathy have been seen in patients with HIV infections. However, HIV-associated nephropathy (HIVAN) is a unique pattern of glomerulopathy characterized by heavy proteinuria and a rapid progression to renal failure as well as characteristic ultrasonographic and renal biopsy findings. HIVAN is a better term than AIDS nephropathy, because this glomerulopathy may occur in patients with AIDS or in asymptomatic HIV carriers. Although HIVAN has a prevalence of only 3%

to 7% in unselected autopsy series, it is by far the most common lesion found in HIV-infected patients undergoing renal biopsy. The classic clinical features of HIVAN nephropathy include a higher incidence among blacks, heavy proteinuria (usually with NS), renal insufficiency, and a rapid progression to ESRD with large echogenic kidneys on ultrasonography.

The pathology of HIVAN shows several features distinct from classic FSGS or the older heroin nephropathy. On light microscopy, diffuse global glomerulosclerosis and collapse is common, with striking visceral epithelial cell hypertrophy showing large cytoplasmic vacuoles and resorption droplets. Severe tubulointerstitial changes also occur, with interstitial inflammation, edema, microcystic dilatation of tubules, and severe tubular degenerative changes. On EM, tubuloreticular inclusions are prevalent in the glomerular endothelium.

The optimal treatment of HIVAN remains unclear. At present, highly active antiretroviral therapy is indicated for all patients. Likewise, ACE inhibitors are helpful as long as the potassium and creatinine levels do not rise markedly. The use of any immunosuppressive therapy remains controversial. Dialysis and support seem appropriate for many patients with HIVAN. Whether dialysis support prolongs useful life once AIDS has developed is open to debate.

Hepatitis C Virus Infection

The incidence of HCV infection varies greatly in different geographic locations of the world. In high-risk groups, the incidence is as high as 60% to 90% of persons with hemophilia, 60% to 70% of intravenous drug abusers, and as many as 15% to 25% of certain dialysis populations.

Cryoglobulinemia and Hepatitis C Virus
HCV infection has been associated with arthritis, sicca symptoms, corneal ulcerations, porphyria, autoimmune thyroiditis, and polyarteritis as well as mixed cryoglobulinemia associated with immune complex GN. Cryoglobulinemia refers to circulating immunoglobulins that precipitate on cooling and resolubilize on warming. Cryoglobulinemia is associated with a variety of infections, collagen-vascular disease, and lymphoproliferative diseases. Cryoglobulins have been divided into three major groups: types I, II, and III. In type I cryoglobulinemia, the cryoglobulin is a single monoclonal immunoglobulin, usually without associated antibody activity. This type is found most often in patients with myeloma and Waldenström macroglobulinemia. Types II and III cryoglobulinemia are characterized by mixed cryoglobulins, containing at least two immunoglobulins. In type II, a monoclonal IgM immunoglobulin is directed against polyclonal IgG and has rheumatoid factor activity. In type III, the antiglobulin is polyclonal, with both polyclonal IgG and IgM in most cases. To establish a diagnosis of cryoglobulinemia, the offending cryoglobulins must be demonstrated. The cryoglobulin must be solubilized in a warmed blood sample until the test is run. Hypocomplementemia, especially

of the early components C1q to C4, is a characteristic and often helpful finding.

In the past, no clear etiology was apparent in most cases of mixed cryoglobulinemias, and the name *essential mixed cryoglobulinemia* was appropriate. The systemic manifestations include weakness, malaise, Raynaud phenomenon, arthralgia and arthritis, hepatosplenomegaly presenting with abnormal liver function test results in two-thirds to three-fourths of patients, peripheral neuropathy, and purpuric-vasculitic skin lesions. In up to one-fourth to one-third of patients, an acute nephritic condition with hematuria, hypertension, proteinuria, and acute renal insufficiency develops. Approximately 20% of patients present with NS. In the majority of patients with renal involvement, the disease has a slow, indolent renal course characterized by proteinuria, hypertension, hematuria, and renal insufficiency.

Recent reports have clearly documented HCV as a major cause of cryoglobulin production in many, if not most, patients previously believed to have essential mixed cryoglobulinemia. Antibodies to HCV antigens have been documented in the sera, and HCV RNA and anti-HCV antibodies are enriched in the cryoglobulins of these patients.

Pathogenesis and Pathology
The pathogenesis and pathology of HCV-related cryoglobulin GN and HCV-related membranoproliferative GN is similar.

In cryoglobulinemia, immunoglobulin complexes deposit in the glomeruli, binding complement and inciting a proliferative response. The serum cryoglobulin clearly has been shown to participate in the formation of the glomerular immune complex. Not all patients with HCV infection and GN have detectable cryoglobulins in the serum and the classic histopathology of cryoglobulinemic MPGN. Mesangial proliferative GN (often with IgA deposits), MN, diffuse proliferative GN, a sclerosing GN, and especially MPGN resembling idiopathic type 1 MPGN all have been reported. Although patients with hepatitis B virus infection most commonly have the membranous pattern of glomerulopathy, the MPGN pattern is most common with HCV infection. Patients with HCV and MPGN typically present with proteinuria and often NS. At least 30% to 40% of these patients do not have detectable cryoglobulins. Only one-half of these patients have symptoms suggestive of cryoglobulinemia (purpura, arthritis, etc.). Only 20% have signs of liver disease, but as many as two-thirds have mild elevations of transaminase levels. Once again, total hemolytic complement, and especially C4, is depressed. The pathology of HCV MPGN is similar to that of idiopathic type 1 MPGN in most cases.

Treatment of Hepatitis C Virus–Related Glomerulonephritis
Recent studies involving patients with HCV-related cryoglobulinemic GN have evaluated the use of interferon-α or combined interferon and ribavirin and have shown

improvement of both renal and liver disease. In these studies, treated patients had decreased proteinuria and improved GFR. The number of patients studied so far is small, however. Clinical response often correlates closely with the disappearance of HCV from the blood. Other groups have shown patients to have decreasing proteinuria and normalization of liver function test results but no major improvements in GFR. Relapses after the discontinuance of therapy may occur. In some patients with severe progressive renal disease, immunosuppressive therapy clearly has been used successfully. Rituximab is currently being studied as therapy in HCV GN. The potential benefits of immunosuppressive therapy must be weighed against the potential hazards of activating viral replication.

DRUG-INDUCED ACUTE INTERSTITIAL NEPHRITIS

In recent years, it has become clear that not all AIN is caused by bacterial invasion of the kidney. Among the common types of AIN is drug-induced AIN. The distinct clinical picture, pathology, and clinical course of this form of acute renal failure has been defined especially from the study of patients receiving β-lactam antibiotics of the penicillin or cephalosporin classes.

The renal histology reveals predominantly edema and interstitial infiltrates of mononuclear cells and eosinophils without marked fibrosis and with only patchy tubular damage. In general, glomerular and vascular changes are not prominent. More than 75 medications have been associated with AIN, and the list of offending drugs grows each year.

Penicillin

Despite the numerous implicated drugs, the β-lactam antibiotics—penicillins and cephalosporins—remain among the foremost offenders. All agents of the β-lactam group are capable of producing this lesion. β-Lactam–related AIN occurs in all decades of life. The dosage of the β-lactam antibiotic has usually not been excessive; however, the duration of therapy is often prolonged, with more than three-fourths of patients receiving more than 10 days of therapy and more than one-third receiving more than 20 days of therapy.

The clinical features of penicillin-associated AIN include the hypersensitivity triad of rash (43%), secondary fever (77%), and eosinophilia (80%). Fewer than one-third of patients have the complete triad at diagnosis; yet, the clinician must not wait for this full picture to develop before making a presumptive diagnosis of drug-related AIN. Of the urinary findings, mild proteinuria and pyuria are common but not specific. Nephrotic-range proteinuria and urinary red blood cell casts are rare in this nonglomerular disease and can usually be explained by incidental concomitant glomerular pathology. Hematuria is a cardinal

feature of penicillin-associated AIN; it is present in more than 90% of cases and is macroscopic in one-third. The finding of urinary eosinophiluria on Wright or Hansel stain of the urinary sediment is often present. One recent study suggests eosinophiluria—in which eosinophils comprise more than 5% of the total urinary leukocytes—to be strongly suggestive of AIN. Eosinophiluria has also been noted in RPGN, cystitis, and prostatitis. The majority of patients have nonoliguric renal failure and never have <400 mL of urine volume per day. Positive gallium scanning has been suggested as a screening test to distinguish drug-induced AIN from renal failure due to acute tubular necrosis scan negative).

The histopathology shows patchy tubular damage, interstitial edema, and infiltrates of mononuclear cells and often eosinophils.

Although the pathogenesis of penicillin-associated AIN remains to be defined, good evidence suggests an allergic–immunologic mechanism of renal damage. The small number of patients afflicted despite the extensive use of these drugs; recurrences on rechallenge with another β-lactam drug; the hypersensitivity features of rash, fever, and eosinophilia; and the histopathologic features found in many cases all support an allergic–immunologic mechanism. The first step may be the binding of drug hapten to kidney structural protein, either tubular or interstitial. Subsequently, a humoral response, with the development of antitubular basement membrane antibodies to combined drug hapten and kidney protein, may damage the kidney. In most cases, no evidence suggests such a response (negative IF-staining results, normal serum complement levels lack of circulating antitubular basement membrane or antidrug antibodies), and a cell-mediated cytotoxic reaction may be the cause of ultimate renal damage. However, the pathogenesis may actually be far more complex.

The treatment of penicillin-associated AIN includes prompt discontinuation of the drug and avoidance of rechallenge with other β-lactam agents that may lead to a recrudescence of hypersensitivity symptoms and renal failure. Dialysis and good supportive care are crucial, because the majority of patients recover good renal function. The use of corticosteroids is controversial, but recent studies suggest the use of a short trial in most patients without contraindications. The use of other immunosuppressive agents has been reported only rarely.

Other Medications Producing Acute Interstitial Nephritis

Drug-induced AIN has been well documented in several cases of sulfonamide use—including the antimicrobial combination of trimethoprim-sulfamethoxazole—which can produce this form of renal damage. Rifampin use is associated with a unique pattern of acute renal failure. In more than 60 patients who received either intermittent or discontinuous therapy, on rechallenge with rifampin there occurred the sudden onset of fever, flank pain, hematuria, and acute renal failure. Histopathologic findings range from those of classic AIN to a picture indistinguishable from that of ATN. It is clearly wise to avoid the intermittent or discontinuous use of this drug. The quinolone antibiotics have been well documented to produce AIN. Rarely, diuretics—including the thiazides and chlorthalidone, furosemide, and ticrynafen—have all been well documented to cause AIN. Patients present with the classic hypersensitivity features of rash, fever, and eosinophilia. AIN responds readily to discontinuance of the drug and corticosteroid therapy. Cimetidine, the uricosuric antiplatelet agent sulfinpyrazone, and proton pump inhibitors have all caused AIN.

NSAIDs may produce salt and water retention, decreased renal blood flow and GFR, and hyperkalemia associated with hyporenin hypoaldosteronism, perhaps all due to inhibition of prostaglandins. They also can cause an AIN that presents with a number of unique features. The population developing AIN is usually the older age group (those in their 50s to 80s), despite the fact that many young patients receive these drugs. Patients typically have a prolonged exposure to the drugs (months to years) before developing AIN. The hypersensitivity features of rash, fever, and eosinophilia are rare, as are hematuria and eosinophiluria. Most striking is that AIN caused by NSAIDs has frequently been associated with minimal-change NS. The onset of NS coincides with the onset of ARF from AIN. NS and AIN remit several weeks after discontinuance of the NSAID, regardless of whether steroid therapy is given. Some NSAIDs have been associated with MN.

MEDICATION-INDUCED CHRONIC INTERSTITIAL NEPHRITIS

The use of certain medications has been associated with the development of chronic renal insufficiency and chronic interstitial damage. In general, the relationship between the drug use and the renal lesions often has been more difficult to define than that of drug-induced AIN. This is related in part to the slower disease process, its insidious nature, and to the complexity of the medication regimens of many such patients. Several important groups of medications causing chronic interstitial nephritis include the analgesics phenacetin, acetaminophen, and aspirin; lithium; and the antineoplastic chemotherapeutic agents cisplatin as well as the nitrosourea chemotherapy agents.

Analgesic agents have been used extensively in over-the-counter preparations in recent decades, and concern about their nephrotoxic potential has generated considerable attention and controversy. The incidence of analgesic nephropathy varies greatly among countries and even within regions of one country. In general, those countries with a higher per capita consumption of phenacetin and other analgesic compounds have had a higher incidence

of analgesic nephropathy. Studies have documented analgesic nephropathy as the cause of ESRD in more than 16% of ESRD patients in West Germany, 18% of ESRD patients in Belgium, and 13% of ESRD patients in Australia. In the United States, reports vary from an incidence of >10% in the Southeast to a low of <1% elsewhere. The exact nature of the offending analgesic or combinations of analgesics remains to be defined. Well-controlled study involving more than 600 middle-aged Swiss working women clearly documented a higher incidence of renal insufficiency as well as an increased mortality due to urinary tract disease and cardiovascular disease in a phenacetin-consuming population. A retrospective case-control study in North Carolina also found significantly more renal disease in consumers of analgesics. The risk of renal disease was increased with daily consumption of phenacetin and acetaminophen but not with the daily use of aspirin. This study confirms the risk of renal damage with phenacetin (which has been removed from most analgesic preparations in the United States) but raises the strong possibility that acetaminophen, the major metabolite of phenacetin, is also nephrotoxic.

The characteristic patient who develops analgesic nephropathy is a middle-aged woman (women outnumber men 4:1) with chronic headaches or arthritic problems who has consumed large amounts of compounds containing phenacetin, acetaminophen, or aspirin on a daily basis for many years. The ingestion of at least 1 g or more daily of these analgesics for longer than 2 to 3 years is felt to be the minimum dose-time requirement to produce clinical analgesic nephropathy. Systemic symptoms such as malaise, weight loss, emotional and psychiatric disorders, anemia, and peptic ulcer disease may be related in part to the syndrome of analgesic nephropathy and in part to the population that uses these medications excessively. Diagnosis is often difficult, as most patients do not consider these over-the-counter preparations to be medications. Renal findings may include nocturia and polyuria, sterile pyuria, urinary tract infections, acidification defects, a predisposition to volume depletion, renal colic and hematuria, and hypertension. Renal insufficiency may be present in asymptomatic patients and is often progressive if analgesic consumption is continued. The finding of papillary necrosis on intravenous pyelography, ultrasonography, or computed axial tomography is helpful in establishing the diagnosis.

Lithium salts, which are used widely to treat affective disorders, have been associated with a number of renal abnormalities, most prominently a nephrogenic diabetes insipidus–polyuria syndrome. Although reductions in the GFR and chronic interstitial nephritis have been attributed to lithium use, the relationship is not clearly established. In a composite review of studies covering almost 500 patients receiving lithium, only 15% were found to have a reduced creatinine clearance. Likewise, in a review of studies examining kidney function in more than 500 patients, the GFR was found to be reduced in only 17%. In those patients with a reduced GFR, the reduction was mild, with most patients having GFRs of 60 to 75 mL per minute. Clearly, even the renal dysfunction of these patients cannot all be attributed to lithium use, because psychiatric patient populations not receiving lithium have been noted to have reduced GFRs and chronic changes in renal biopsy specimens when compared with normal subjects. Many studies have also failed to document a positive correlation between the duration of lithium treatment and the reduction in GFR. However, in studies examining a very long duration of treatment (6.5–10 years), a positive correlation has been noted. In some studies, the renal biopsy specimens of lithium-treated patients with normal GFRs have shown focal interstitial fibrotic changes. Overall, the use of lithium for many years is probably associated with some degree of decline in the GFR and interstitial damage. The damage is usually mild to moderate and appears to occur only after the prolonged use of lithium. The contribution to renal disease from other psychotropic medications or from other factors associated with the affective disorders of these patients remains to be defined.

Cis-platinum, an antineoplastic agent widely used to treat a variety of solid tumors, may cause both acute renal failure and, less frequently, chronic renal insufficiency. In those patients suffering from chronic renal damage, interstitial fibrosis and chronic inflammatory changes have been noted on renal biopsy. The nitrosourea compounds methyl-cyclohexylchloroethylnitrosourea and bis-chloroethylnitrosourea can both produce dose-related nephrotoxicity and chronic interstitial nephritis. Renal biopsy specimens from patients experiencing renal damage after receiving these medications have shown severe tubular atrophy, glomerulosclerosis, and interstitial fibrosis with chronic inflammatory infiltrates. In some patients, the chronic tubulointerstitial damage has led to ESRD.

Cyclosporine and tacrolimus, two immunosuppressives widely used in transplantation, can cause acute renal damage as well as chronic tubulointerstitial fibrosis. This is often associated with drug-related microvascular damage to the arterioles of the kidney. These agents can produce a chronic form of tubulointerstitial damage in a bandlike pattern within the kidney, called *striped fibrosis*. This has been seen in both transplant populations and in patients without prior renal disease who are taking this immunosuppressive medicine for autoimmune conditions. It is usually associated with a decreased GFR and renal insufficiency.

SUGGESTED READINGS

Glomerular Disease and Nephrotic Syndrome—General

Appel GB. Improved outcomes in the nephrotic syndrome. *Cleveland Clin J Med* 2006;73:161–167.
Appel GB, Waldman M, Radhakrishnan J. New approaches to the treatment of glomerular disease. *Kidney Int* 2006;70:S45–S50.
Crew JR, Radhakrishnan J, Appel GB. The nephrotic syndrome and its complications. *Clinical Nephrol* 2004;62:245–260.
Orth SR, Ritz E. The nephrotic syndrome. *N Engl J Med* 1998;338:1202–1211.

Minimal-Change and Focal Segmental Glomerulosclerosis

Aggarwal N, Appel GB. Focal segmental glomerulosclerosis in NKF primer on kidney disease 2008. ed. Greenberg A, Falk R.
Pollak M. Inherited podocytopathies: FSGS and nephrotic syndrome from a genetic viewpoint. *J Am Soc Nephrol* 2002;13:3016–3023.
Waldman M, Appel GB. The Course of Adult Minimal Change Disease. *Clinical JASN* 2007;2:445–454.

Membranous Nephropathy

Cattran DC, Appel GB, Hebert L, et al.; North American Nephrotic Syndrome Study Group. Cyclosporine in patients with steroid-resistant membranous nephropathy: a randomized trial. *Kidney Int* 2001;59:1484–1490.
Glassock, RJ. The treatment of idiopathic membranous nephropathy: a dilemma or a conundrum. *Am J Kidney Dis* 2004;44:562–566.
Perna A, Schieppati A, Zamora J, et al. Immunosuppressive therapy for idiopathic membranous nephropathy: a systematic review. *Am J Kidney Dis* 2004;44:385–401.

Immunoglobulin A Nephropathy

Appel GB. To treat or not to treat IgA nephropathy? That is the question! *Clin J Am Soc Nephrol* 2006;1(3):347–348.
Appel GB, Waldman M. The IgA nephropathy treatment dilemma. *Kidney Int* 2006;69:1939–1944.

Membranoproliferative Glomerulonephritis

Appel GB, Cook HT, Hageman G, et al. Membranoproliferative glomerulonephritis type II (dense deposit disease): an update. *J Am Soc Nephrol* 2005;16:1392–1403.

Rapidly Progressive Glomerulonephritis

Hudson BG, Tryggvason K, Sundaramoorthy M, et al. Alport's syndrome, Goodpasture's syndrome, and type IV collagen. *N Engl J Med* 2003;348:2543–2556.
Jennette JC. Rapidly progressive crescentic glomerulonephritis. *Kidney Int* 2003;63:1164–1177.
Levy JB, Turner N, Rees AJ, et al. Long-term outcome of antiglomerular basement membrane antibody disease treated with plasma exchange and immunosuppression. *Ann Intern Med* 2001;134:1033–1042.
Little MA, Pusey CD. Glomerulonephritis due to ANCA associated vasculitis: an update on approaches to management. *Nephrology* 2005;10:368–376.

Hepatitis C Virus

Appel GB. Viral infections and the kidney: HIV, hepatitis B, and hepatitis C. *Cleve Clin J Med* 2007;74:353–360.
Jefferson JA, Johnson R. Treatment of hepatitis C–associated GN. *Semin Nephrol* 2000;20:286–293.

Severe Systemic Lupus Nephritis

Appel GB, Waldman M. Update on the treatment of lupus nephritis. *Kidney Int* 2006;70:1403–1412.

Chan TM, Li FK, Tang CSO, et al. Long-term efficacy of mycophenolate mofetil in patients with diffuse proliferative lupus nephritis. *J Am Soc Nephrol* 2005;16(4):1076–1084.

Ginzler EM, Dooley MA, Aranow C, et al. Mycophenolate mofetil or intravenous cyclophosphamide for lupus nephritis. *N Engl J Med* 2005;353:2219–2228.

Weening J, D'Agati V, Schwartz M, et al. The classification of glomerulonephritis in systemic lupus erythematosus revisited. *J Am Soc Nephrol* 2004;15:241–251.

HIV Nephropathy

Appel GB. Viral infections and the kidney: HIV, hepatitis B, and hepatitis C. *Cleve Clin J Med* 2007;74:353–360.

D'Agati V, Appel GB. HIV infection and the kidney. *J Am Soc Nephrol* 1997;8:138–153.

Szczech LA, Gupta SK, Habash R, et al. The clinical epidemiology and course of the spectrum of renal diseases associated with HIV infection. *Kidney Int* 2004;66:1145–1152.

Amyloidosis and Light Chain Deposition Disease

Dember L, Sanchorawala V, Seldin DC, et al. Effect of dose-intensive melphalan and autologous blood stem-cell transplantation on AL—amyloidosis-associated renal disease. *Ann Intern Med* 2001;134:746–753.

Tubulointerstitial Diseases

Appel GB. The treatment of acute interstitial nephritis: more data at last. *Kidney Int* 2008;73:905–907.

Bhatt P, Appel GB. ACP Med. Chapter on Tubulo-interstitial Diseases. pp 2027–2043, 2006.

Chapter 48

Hallmarks of Essential and Secondary Hypertension

Christopher J. Hebert   *Martin J. Schreiber, Jr.*

POINTS TO REMEMBER:

- Refractory hypertension should prompt investigation for a secondary cause

- A shift in emphasis from diastolic to systolic blood pressure (BP) has occurred over the years as evidence has mounted that reflects the very strong, positive, and causal relationship between systolic BP and cardiovascular risk.

- Patients presenting with blood pressure greater than 180/110 mm Hg should be classified as severe hypertension, hypertensive urgency or hypertensive emergency based on clinical features.

- Primary aldosteronism should be considered in any patient with both refractory hypertension and hypokalemia with inappropriate kaliuresis (24-hour urine potassium >30 mEq); however, not all patients with primary aldosteronism have hypokalemia.

Hypertension is the most common reason for visiting a physician in the United States. Worldwide, it is one of the most important causes of morbidity and mortality.[1] Despite the availability of effective treatments, poor control of BP remains a major public health problem.[2] A solid understanding of the epidemiology, pathophysiology, and treatment of hypertension is essential for any physician involved in the management of this condition.

EPIDEMIOLOGY

Hypertension is currently defined by level of BP and is considered present if the resting BP is consistently ≥ 140/90 mmHg or if antihypertensive medication is needed to maintain BP below this level. If defined in this way, it is the most common modifiable cardiovascular risk factor, affecting approximately 65 million Americans.[3] Individuals who have not developed hypertension by the age of 55 years carry a 90% lifetime risk of developing the condition.[4]

PATHOPHYSIOLOGY

A number of pathophysiological factors have been implicated in the development of hypertension, thus making selective mechanistically based antihypertensive therapy difficult for most patients.[5] In a broad sense, increased sympathetic nervous system activity, autonomic imbalance (increased sympathetic tone, abnormally reduced parasympathetic tone), vascular remodeling, arterial stiffness, and endothelial dysfunction contribute to both the development and maintenance of hypertension. Increased sympathetic activity may stem from alterations in baroreflex and chemoreflex pathways, both peripherally and centrally. The renin-angiotensin system plays a major role in vascular remodeling (the alterations in structure, mechanical properties, and function of small arteries) and critical target organ damage (myocardial fibrosis, renal injury). In addition, arterial stiffness, a primary contributor to increased vascular resistance especially with advancing age, results from continued collagen deposition, smooth muscle hypertrophy, and changes in the elastin media fibers. Whereas intact vascular endothelium is critical to maintaining vascular tone (relaxation and contraction), it is known that multiple insults (decreased nitric oxide synthesis, increased endothelin, estrogen deficiency, high dietary salt intake, diabetes mellitus, tobacco usage, and increased homocysteine) can damage vascular endothelium and are important clinically. These factors or conditions disrupt normal endothelial function and initiate the cascade of cardiovascular events that results in atherosclerosis, thrombosis, and heart failure.

GENETICS OF HYPERTENSION

Hypertension results from a complex interaction of genetic, environmental, and demographic factors. Variations in BP result from the contributions of many different genes (polygenic).[6] In most patients with essential hypertension, genetic profiling is not currently beneficial in the diagnostic evaluation. Exceptions are the occasional cases of secondary hypertension, for which clinical data and biochemical profiling may point to anatomic or functional aberrations, such as abnormal function of the adrenal hormones or abnormal receptor response. Although the majority of cases of essential hypertension are polygenic and characterized by a complex mode of inheritance, rare cases of simple mendelian forms of high BP occur in which a single gene defect may be largely responsible for the hypertensive phenotype. Improved techniques of genetic analysis (i.e., geneticwide linkage analysis) have aided in the search for genes that contribute to the development of hypertension, although uncommon in the general population with elevated BP, and may be more frequent in selective hypertensive populations, particularly in those patients with resistant hypertension. Genome scans have identified regions of specific human chromosomes that influence BP. These regions are called *blood pressure quantitative trait loci* (QTL) (e.g., chromosome 6.2).

From the clinical perspective, a family with a history of hypertension can be a surrogate marker for undefined risk factors shared by the family. Risk factors such as obesity, dyslipidemia, and insulin resistance are predictive of future hypertension. Having a single first-degree relative with hypertension is only a weak predictor of hypertension, whereas a finding of having two or more relatives with hypertension at an early age (before age 55 years) identifies a smaller subset of families who are at much higher risk for the future development of hypertension.[7] Gene-to-drug interactions may explain the heterogeneity of BP responses to different antihypertensive agents. α-Adducin responds best to thiazide diuretics; those with Met235 Thr angiotensinogen respond best to angiotensin-converting enzyme (ACE) inhibitors; and CCB and specific G-protein genes impart a response to beta-blockers and diuretics.[8]

A number of syndromes represent genetic mutations of single-gene forms of hypertension. These include glucocorticoid-remedial hypertension (chimeric gene formation, autosomal dominant), 11-β hydroxylase (mutation in gene encoding), 17-α hydroxylase deficiency, Liddle syndrome (mutation in the sodium channel gene), hypertension exacerbated by pregnancy, syndrome of apparent mineralocorticoid excess, and pseudohypoaldosteronism.[9] Human atrial natriuretic peptide (hANP) is an attractive gene for linking specific population groups to an associated increased risk for hypertension. Polymorphisms of the angiotensinogen gene have been detected in hypertensive patients as well as in the children of hypertensive patients.

Advances in molecular biology and newer techniques make likely the possibility of gene expression profiling being applied to hypertensive research, diagnosis, and treatment selection in the future.[10]

SIGNIFICANCE OF SYSTOLIC, DIASTOLIC, AND PULSE PRESSURE

A shift in emphasis from diastolic to systolic BP has occurred over the years as evidence has mounted that reflects the very strong, positive, and causal relationship between systolic BP and cardiovascular risk. Although both components correlate with risk, systolic pressure is more important, particularly beyond middle age.[10,11] For every 20 mm Hg increase in systolic or 10 mm Hg increase in diastolic BP, there is a doubling of mortality attributable to ischemic heart disease and stroke.[12]

Systolic BP generally increases progressively over a lifetime, even among normotensive individuals. By contrast, diastolic BP increases until approximately 55 years of age and then declines.[13] The pulse pressure is the difference between systolic and diastolic and in older individuals is a marker of large artery stiffness. A growing body of evidence supports pulse pressure as an important predictor of cardiovascular events in patients >65 years of age.[14,15] Furthermore, pulse pressure may be a strong predictor of cardiovascular risk in the presence of compromised left ventricular function with normal or low systolic BP.[16] Situations occur, however, in which increased pulse pressure does not represent arterial stiffness, such as aortic insufficiency, thyrotoxicosis, and fever.

Although pulse pressure is important, it has limitations as a clinical test. For example, it is a rather late manifestation of arterial stiffening. In addition, the inaccuracies of brachial BP measurement are a limitation. Therefore, interest in the measurement of arterial stiffness through aortic pulse wave analysis is growing. For example, applanation tonometry is one method used to measure aortic pulse wave velocity as a marker of arterial stiffness.[17] Such modalities also provide the opportunity to estimate central aortic BP. There is evidence to support the notion that lowering of central aortic BP may be a more important clinical objective than lowering brachial BP.[18] As an indication of the growing importance of arterial stiffness, measurement of pulse wave velocity is now included in the European Society of Hypertension–European Society of Cardiology guidelines.[19]

EVALUATION

A complete history, physical examination, basic serum chemistries analysis, urinalysis, and ECG are recommended for the initial evaluation of a hypertensive patient. The urinalysis is especially important because of the impact that renal disease has on the treatment selection and target goals for BP lowering.

Specific aspects of the patient's history should entail family history, sleep history, nonprescription medication use (nonsteroidal anti-inflammatory drugs, diet pills, decongestants, appetite suppressants, herbal therapy), oral contraceptive pills, and use of alcohol and recreational drugs.

The physical examination should include two or more BP measurements, separated by 2 minutes, with the patient seated. BP should be verified in the contralateral arm, and if there is a discrepancy, the higher value should be considered the better estimate of central aortic pressure (i.e., the BP to which organs are exposed). BP after standing for 2 minutes should be performed in selected patients who may be at risk for orthostatic hypotension, such as the elderly or patients with symptoms suggestive of an orthostatic drop. Measurements of weight, height, and waist circumference should be obtained. A fundoscopic examination should be performed. Special attention should be directed to the presence or absence of carotid bruits or distended neck veins; thyroid enlargement; and examination of the heart, lungs, abdomen, and extremities. As well, examination should include palpation of peripheral pulses, auscultation for abdominal bruits, and evaluation for edema. A neurologic assessment should also be performed.

In most cases, the presence of significant arteriosclerosis of arteriovenous necking on fundoscopic examination indicates that the BP has been elevated for more than 6 months. Arteriolar changes are the most common manifestation of hypertensive retinopathy. The mean ration of arteriolar-to-venular (AV) diameter in nonhypertensive patients is 0.84. AV nicking can be detected where branch retinal arteries cross over the veins. The thickened arteriolar wall compresses the thin-walled vein and causes a tapering or "nicked" appearance.

The physician should always be alert to history of physical examination findings that suggest a secondary cause for the hypertension. Such findings may include an abdominal or flank bruit (renal artery stenosis), central obesity with abdominal striae and buffalo hump (Cushing syndrome), enlarged kidneys (polycystic kidney disease), or diminished pedal pulses and a discrepancy between arm and leg pressures (coarctation of the aorta).

A basic laboratory evaluation should include a urinalysis, complete blood count, blood sodium, potassium, creatinine, uric acid, and fasting glucose and lipids. An ECG should be performed to evaluate for left ventricular hypertrophy as well as evidence of prior myocardial infarction.

Ambulatory BP monitoring may be useful in certain patients, such as those suspected of having white coat hypertension (elevated BP in the office but otherwise normal, masked hypertension (normal in the office but otherwise elevated), or morning hypertension, and to assess for the degree of decrease ("dipping") of BP at night.

CLINICAL APPROACHES

The seventh report of the Joint National Committee on the Prevention, Detection, Evaluation, and Treatment of High Blood Pressure (JNC 7)[20] has provided a framework for the classification and management of hypertension

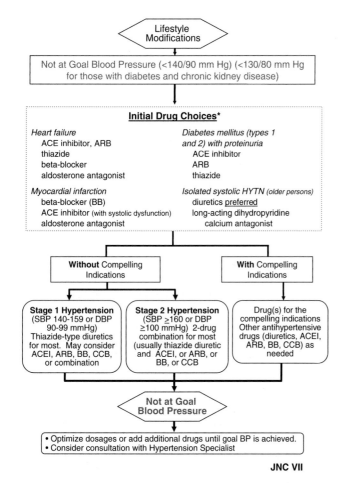

JNC VII

Figure 48.1 Algorithm for the treatment of hypertension (based on randomized controlled trials). (ACE, angiotensin-converting enzyme; ARB, angiotensin II receptor blocker; CCB, calcium channel blocker; HYTN, hypertension.) (Adapted from Abbott KC, Bakris GL. What have we learned from the current trials? *Med Clin North Am* 2004;88:189–207.)

(Fig. 48.1). Hypertension, defined as a sustained BP of 140/90 mm Hg or the requirement of antihypertensive medications, is treated with lifestyle modification and usually medications. Prehypertension, in which the BP is 120 to 139/80 to 89 mg Hg, is generally treated with lifestyle modification, with medication indicated in the presence of diabetes or chronic kidney disease. The feasibility of delaying onset of hypertension with medication has been demonstrated.[21] The impact of such research on guidelines remains to be seen.

Lifestyle changes that have been shown to improve BP include improved diet (decreased salt intake, increased potassium intake, DASH (Dietary Approach to Stop Hypertension)-style eating),[22] weight loss, regular exercise, and moderation in alcohol consumption. In addition, smoking cessation should be top priority.

Regarding pharmacotherapy, two principles that have emerged from the evolving evidence base deserve attention. First, BP control, particularly systolic, is the most important clinical objective and is more important than the

medications used. Staessen et al.[23] have shown that BP difference between treatment arms of the major trials, rather than drug class, largely explains treatment benefit. However, drug selection tailored to the particular patient is still important. Therefore, the second principle, outlined in the JNC 7 guideline, is that certain compelling indications will direct the physician to prescribe specific drug classes.

REFRACTORY HYPERTENSION

Refractory (or resistant) hypertension is defined as the persistence of out-of-office BP levels > 140/90 mm Hg for most patients or > 130/80 mm Hg for those with diabetes mellitus or chronic kidney disease, despite a three-drug regimen that includes a diuretic. Refractory hypertension falls into two categories: apparent resistance and true resistance (Table 48.1).

Refractory hypertension is present in approximately 10% of patients in a primary care setting and in more than 30% of patients seen in subspeciality clinics. Suboptimal therapeutic regimens are the major cause of apparent refractory hypertension[24] (Fig. 48.2). More intensive therapy, with emphasis on the targeted control of volume using diuretic therapy and dietary salt restriction, can achieve the target BP in a significant percentage of patients with apparent resistant hypertension. Some studies have shown that tailoring the regimen to the individual's specific hemodynamic profile has benefit.[25,26]

SECONDARY HYPERTENSION

Refractory hypertension should prompt the consideration of a secondary cause of hypertension. The most important causes of secondary hypertension are listed in Table 48.2 and are discussed next.

TABLE 48.1

CAUSES OF REFRACTORY HYPERTENSION

Apparent Resistance	True Resistance
Suboptimal regimen	Excess plasma volume
Poor adherence to therapy	
White coat hypertension	Associated conditions[a]
Pseudohypertension in the elderly	Medication-related causes[b]
Cuff-related artifact	Secondary hypertension
Prescription errors	

[a]Obesity, insulin resistance, excessive ethanol.
[b]Drug-drug interactions and specific drugs that may produce refractory hypertension include nonsteroidal anti-inflammatory drugs, decongestants, appetite suppressants, corticosteroids, over-the-counter substances (ephedra, ma-huang, bitter orange), cocaine, amphetamines, licorice, chewing tobacco, and multiple prescription medications (tricyclic antidepressants, cyclosporine, tacrolimus, erythropoietin, anabolic steroids, monoamine oxidase inhibitors, oral contraceptives, chlorpromazine.

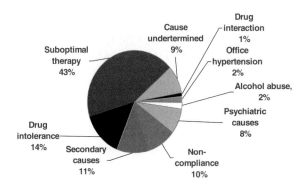

Figure 48.2 Of 436 patients treated at a hypertension clinic, 92 (21%) had refractory hypertension. In 83 patients, a cause was identified, the most frequent being suboptimal therapy. BP was brought under control or improved in 58 patients. (Adapted from Yakovlevitch M, Black HR. Resistant hypertension in a tertiary care clinic. *Arch Intern Med* 1991;151:1786.)

Renal Parenchymal Disease

Hypertension is one of the main contributing factors to progressive renal injury, and lowering BP slows progression. Renal parenchymal disease is a common secondary cause of hypertension, although often not reversible. Renal parenchymal disease is easily detected through serum creatinine and estimate glomerular filtration rate (GFR) as well as urinalysis. Decreased GFR and/or proteinuria and hematuria characterize renal parenchymal disease. ACE inhibitors or angiotensin receptor blockers (ARB) are an important part of the treatment regimen.

Renovascular Disease

Clinical clues to renovascular disease that may be responsible for renovascular hypertension include:

- Abrupt onset of hypertension
- Age younger than 30 or older than 55 years
- Accelerated or malignant hypertension (grade 3 or 4 retinopathy)
- Refractory hypertension
- Diffuse vascular disease
- Systolic/diastolic epigastric bruit

TABLE 48.2

CAUSES OF SECONDARY HYPERTENSION

Renal	Endocrine
Renal artery stenosis	Primary aldosteronism
Renal parenchymal disease	Hypo- or hyperthyroidism
Obstruction	Cushing syndrome
Polycystic kidney disease	Pheochromocytoma
Obstructive sleep apnea	Hypercalcemia
Coarctation of the aorta	Acromegaly
Preeclampsia	Adrenogenital syndrome
Acute intermittent porphyria	Liddle syndrome
	Gordon syndrome

TABLE 48.3

SPECIFICITY AND SENSITIVITY OF SCREENING TESTS FOR RENOVASCULAR HYPERTENSION

Test	Sensitivity (%)	Specificity (%)
Magnetic resonance angiography (MRA)	100	96
Duplex Doppler ultrasonography	69–96	86–90
Spiral computed tomography angiography	98	94
IVP	~75	~85
Captopril renogram	41–93	95
Captopril stimulated PRA	75	89

- Hypertension with unexplained renal insufficiency
- Renal insufficiency induced by ACE inhibitors or ARBs
- Severe hypertension or recurrent "flash" pulmonary edema

A number of specialized tests have been used in the diagnosis of renovascular disease, including duplex Doppler ultrasonography, spiral computed tomography (CT) angiography, and magnetic resonance angiography. These have largely replaced older tests such as intravenous pyelography, plasma renin activity, and captopril renogram. Renal arteriography remains the gold standard for diagnosis. Sensitivity and specificity for these tests are listed in Table 48.3.

Uncontrolled BP and progressive compromise in renal function are the primary indicators for invasive treatment. For younger patients with fibromuscular dysplasia and uncontrolled BP or decreasing renal function, percutaneous transluminal renal angioplasty is the mainstay of therapy, with surgical revascularization as a secondary option. For older patients with atherosclerotic disease, percutaneous transluminal renal angioplasty plus stenting and surgical revascularization and medical therapy are the usual options. Medical therapy includes carefully monitored use of ACE inhibitors or ARBs, usually along with a diuretic as well as other medications (aspirin, statins) as the clinical setting dictates, for cardiovascular risk reduction.

Coarctation of the Aorta

Although coarctation of the aorta may cause left ventricular failure early in life, adults with coarctation are often asymptomatic.[27] As a result, the medical history may be of little help in suggesting the presence of coarctation unless the diagnosis is suspected in association with other congenital malformations, such as bicuspid aortic valve, patent ductus, or ventricular septal defect, and mitral valve abnormalities. The most common location for a coarctation is distal to the left subclavian artery, but it may occasionally involve the origin of the left subclavian artery and may be missed if BP is not checked in both upper extremities and at least one lower extremity. Absent or reduced pulses in the legs together with a BP that is lower in the legs than in the arms are valuable clues to the diagnosis. Systolic BP is elevated disproportionately to the diastolic BP, resulting in wide pulse pressure and bounding pulses proximal to the coarctation. A thrill may be observed in the suprasternal notch together with palpable pulsations or auscultated bruits over the intercostal arteries.

Additional screening studies should include a chest radiograph looking for the "three signs" (proximal aorta, coarctated segment with poststenotic dilation, and indentation of the aortic knob). For diagnosis and localization, echocardiography, magnetic resonance imaging (MRI), or aortography are useful. Management consists of surgical repair or angioplasty.

Endocrine Causes of Secondary Hypertension

Primary aldosteronism is the most common endocrine cause of secondary hypertension. In 70% to 80% of cases, the cause is an aldosterone-producing adenoma. Adrenal hyperplasia, glucocorticoid remedial hypertension, and adrenal carcinoma are other possibilities. The best clues to the presence of primary aldosteronism include hypertension with spontaneous hypokalemia (<3.5 mEq/L), hypertension with provoked hypokalemia (<3.0 mEq/L during diuretic therapy), and hypertension with difficulty maintaining normokalemia despite potassium supplementation.

Primary aldosteronism should be considered in any patient with both refractory hypertension and hypokalemia with inappropriate kaliuresis (24-hour urine potassium >30 mEq); however, not all patients with primary aldosteronism have hypokalemia. Of patients with primary aldosteronism, 7% to 38% have normal serum potassium.[28] Those individuals with hypertension and renal potassium wasting can be differentiated into high-renin and low-renin states (Table 48.4). Usually, the plasma renin activity is <1 ng/mL per hour in mineralocorticoid-excess, low-renin states.

The plasma aldosterone and plasma renin activity together can be used to screen for primary aldosteronism.[29] Ideally, diuretics should be discontinued 1 to 2 weeks prior to the test. In addition, atenolol, ACE inhibitors, ARBs, and aldosterone antagonists can all make interpretation of these tests challenging and are best avoided during the testing period, if possible. A calcium channel blocker and/or alpha antagonist may be used for BP control during this time period. An elevated aldosterone and suppressed renin are suggestive of the disorder. An elevated ratio of aldosterone to renin can be used for screening as well, with the caveat that a very low renin will often lead to a high ratio regardless of the aldosterone level. The most important test to confirm the diagnosis of primary aldosteronism is a 24-hour urine aldosterone level, preferably done during a time of high di-

TABLE 48.4
BIOCHEMICAL CLASSIFICATION OF PATIENTS WITH HYPERTENSION, HYPOKALEMIA, AND RENAL POTASSIUM WASTING (>30 MEQ/24 HR)

High-Renin States	Low-Renin States (<1 ng/mL/hr)
Renovascular disease	Conn syndrome
Malignant hypertension	Bilateral adrenal hyperplasia
Renin-secreting tumors	Glucocorticoid remedial hypertension[a]
	Mineralocorticoid excess syndrome
	Licorice ingestion
	Liddle syndrome[b]

[a]Children, early-onset severe hypertension, history of hemorrhagic stroke; ACTH regulates secretion, and renin-angiotensin system is suppressed. Suppression of ACTH with glucocorticoids decreases aldosterone and cures the hypertension. High 16-hydroxycortisol/18-oxycortisol.
[b]Hypertension, hypokalemia, alkalosis, decreased aldosterone, sodium channel mutation.

etary salt intake (i.e., the patient is instructed to add 1 level teaspoon of table salt per day).

An adrenal CT scan is helpful in differentiating among adrenal adenoma, adrenal hyperplasia, or adrenal carcinoma. Hounsfield units <10 characterize an adenoma, while an adrenal carcinoma is usually large (>5 cm) with Hounsfield units >10. Adrenal hyperplasia is suggested by abnormalities in both glands.

Adrenal vein sampling after the administration of adrenocorticotropic hormone (ACTH) is most useful when no adrenal abnormality exists on CT or MRI or when an asymmetric abnormality is present in both glands. This procedure is technically difficult and should be done in experienced centers. To be certain that the sample is from the adrenal vein, cortisol should be measured and should be approximately the same in each gland and 10-fold higher than peripheral levels.

Surgical removal of an aldosterone-producing adenoma leads to a reduction of BP and restoration of normal potassium in most patients and can be performed laparoscopically. Medical therapy for primary aldosteronism with spironolactone or eplerenone is indicated for patients with bilateral adenomas or bilateral adrenal hyperplasia or in patients who are at high surgical risk or who prefer no surgery.

Combining urinary aldosterone levels with urinary free cortisol can distinguish nonaldosterone mineralocorticoid excess from aldosterone mineralocorticoid excess (Table 48.5). Liddle syndrome is an autosomal dominant disorder resulting in low-normal urinary excretion of aldosterone, increased kaliuresis secondary to increased collecting tubular sodium resorption, and normal urinary free cortisol. The increased sodium resorption in collecting tubules leads to increased potassium secretion and hypokalemia.

TABLE 48.5

COMBINING URINARY ALDOSTERONE LEVELS WITH URINARY CORTISOL RESULTS CAN DISTINGUISH NONALDOSTERONE MINERALOCORTICOID EXCESS FROM ALDOSTERONE MINERALOCORTICOID EXCESS

Urinary aldosterone	Steroid values	Urinary free cortisol		
		Low	Normal	High
	Low-normal	Congenital adrenal hyperplasia	Liddle's syndrome	11 β-OHSD
			Exogenous mineralocorticoids	Cushing's syndrome
				GR
	High		Primary aldosterone	Adrenal cancer
			GRA	Primary aldosteronism with Cushing's

OHSD, hydroxysteroid dehydrogenate deficiency; GR, glucocorticoid remedial; GFR, glucocorticoid remedial aldosteronism.

Patients usually present with hypertension, hypokalemia, and metabolic acidosis at an early age. Amiloride and triamterene have been used to close the sodium channels and correct the defect clinically. Liddle syndrome can be differentiated from congenital adrenal hyperplasia and 11-β hydroxysteroid dehydrogenase deficiency (OHSD) by comparing urinary aldosterone with urinary free cortisol values in addition to the clinical presentation.

11-β OHSD results in the excessive activation of mineralocorticoid receptors (MR) by a steroid dependence on adrenocorticoid receptors by a steroid dependence on ACTH rather than by the conventional mineralocorticoid agonist; there, steroid appears to be cortisol. The MRs in the distal nephron have equal affinity for both aldosterone and cortisol but are normally protected from cortisol by the presence of 11-β dehydrogenase, which inactivates cortisol to cortisone. The structure of aldosterone protects it from the action of 11-β dehydrogenase, allowing the former access to the MR. When this mechanism is defective, either because of congenital 11-β OHSD or enzyme inhibition (e.g., licorice), then intrarenal levels of cortisol increase, and the cortisol causes inappropriate activation of MR. The resulting antinatriuresis and kaliuresis results in hypertension and hypokalemia. The laboratory abnormalities and symptoms are reversed by spironolactone or dexamethasone.

In licorice-induced hypermineralocorticoidism, levels of both aldosterone and plasma renin activity are low. The glycyrrhetinic acid found in black licorice inhibits 11-β dehydrogenase steroid dehydrogenase, thus allowing cortisol to act as the major endogenous mineralocorticoid and binding to MR. Other glycyrrhetinic acid–containing compounds include chewing tobacco, some Asian herbal preparations, and the French beverage Boisson de coco.

Glucocorticoid remedial aldosteronism (GRA) is an autosomal dominant disorder that mimics primary aldosteronism. GFR should be suspected in any patient with a presentation with features of primary aldosterone who also has early age of onset of hypertension (under 21 years) and a family history of early-onset hypertension and stroke. GRA is usually associated with bilateral adrenal hyperplasia. Patients with GRA have ACTH-sensitive aldosterone production occurring in the zona fasciculata rather than in the zona glomerulosa, which is the normal site of production. The isoenzyme produced catalyzes the conversion of deoxycorticosterone to corticosterone and of 18-hydroxycorticosterone to aldosterone. Laboratory testing includes measurement of 18-hydroxycortisol and 18-oxycortisol by a dexamethasone suppression test. Dexamethasone in doses of 2 mg over 24 hours usually results in remission of hypertension and hypokalemia. Genetic testing can detect a chimeric gene responsible for GRA. Regarding treatment, an oral glucocorticoid will suppress ACTH and should correct the metabolic defect and control the hypertension.

Cushing syndrome is suggested by hypertension associated with weight gain, muscle wasting, and easy bruising. Men may experience erectile dysfunction, and women may experience hirsutism and amenorrhea. Physical findings include moon face, central obesity, and abdominal striae.

Laboratory studies in Cushing syndrome may indicate glucose intolerance or frank diabetes and neutrophilia. Pathological fractures are common. A 24-hour urine free cortisol level and dexamethasone suppression test may help to secure the diagnosis. Treatment for Cushing syndrome includes surgical resection of the pituitary or ectopic source of ACTH. Radiation therapy is another option.

Among patients with pheochromocytoma, 80% present with headache, 57% with sweating, 48% with paroxysmal hypertension, 39% with persistent hypertension, and 64% with palpitations. Clinical features suggesting a workup for this condition include:

- Episodic headache, tachycardia, and/or diaphoresis
- Family history of pheochromocytoma or multiple endocrine neoplasia (MEN)
- Unexplained tachy/brady arrhythmias and/or hypertension during intubation or induction anesthesia
- Prolonged hypotension after surgery

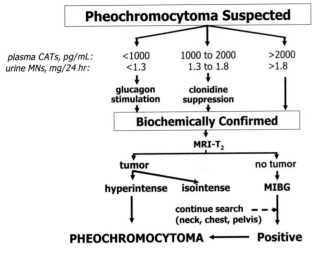

plasma CATs, pg/mL:
urine MNs, mg/24 hr:

Figure 48.3 Pheochromocytoma suspected. (Reproduced with permission from Bravo EL. Pheochromocytoma. *Cardiol Rev* 2002;10:44.)

■ Adverse cardiovascular response to ingestion or inhalation of certain anesthetic agents, glucagons, ACTH, thyrotropin-releasing hormone, antidopaminergic agents, miloxane, phenothiazine, guanethidine, or tricyclic antidepressants

The approach to using plasma catecholamines and urinary metanephrines in the evaluation for pheochromocytoma is illustrated in Figure 48.3. The measurement of fractionated plasma free metanephrines is the best test for familial pheochromocytoma, whereas 24 hour urine metanephrines and catecholamines provide adequate sensitivity and specificity for sporadic pheochromocytoma. A number of drugs interfere with biochemical testing. ACE inhibitors, ARBs, and bromocryptine decrease catecholamine levels, whereas α-1 blockers and β blockers (particularly labetalol) increase catecholamine levels. Phenothiazine, methyldopa, and tricyclic antidepressants have varying effects. When blood specimens are drawn under standardized conditions, a total plasma catecholamine >2,000 pg/mL is diagnostic of pheochromocytoma, whereas a value <500 pg/mL essentially rules it out.

For localization, CT and MRI are equally sensitive (98% and 100%, respectively), and iodine-131 metaiodobenzylguanidine iothalamate is virtually 100% specific but has lower sensitivity (85%). If no tumor is detected by CT or MRI in a highly suspicious setting, then metaiodobenzylguanidine may be used.

A glucagon test is a provocative maneuver that may be employed when the clinical findings are highly suggestive but the BP is normal and plasma catecholamines are between 500 and 1,000 pg/mL. The clonidine suppression test is useful when the plasma catecholamines are between 1,000 and 2,000 pg/mL. Clonidine and other drugs that inhibit central sympathetic outflow will decrease plasma catecholamines in normal or hypertensive subjects but will have little effect on catecholamine secretion in pheochromocytoma. A fall of plasma catecholamines of at least 50% from baseline and below 500 pg/mL is considered normal.

Phenoxybenzamine, a relatively nonspecific, complete, and prolonged α-1 blocker that has traditionally been used perioperatively in the setting of pheochromocytoma, is now often replaced by calcium channel blockers, ARBs, and selective α-1 blockers. The latter drugs are generally effective and lower in side effects.

Thyroid and Parathyroid Disorders

Thyroid dysfunction, along with renovascular hypertension, is a common form of reversible secondary hypertension observed in hypertensive individuals over 60 years of age. Thyrotoxic patients have hyperdynamic hypertension and high cardiac output, seen predominantly as an elevated systolic BP. Conversely, hypothyroid patients have a high prevalence of diastolic BP, which can be an important clue in the elderly, in whom primary diastolic hypertension is rare. A thyroid-stimulating hormone level usually is sufficient for screening.

Most patients with hyperparathyroidism are asymptomatic, and hypercalcemia should suggest the diagnosis. A parathyroid hormone level and phosphorus should be measured in such patients.

TABLE 48.6			
TRIAGE AND APPROACH TO VERY ELEVATED BLOOD PRESSURE			
Intravenous BP	>180/110 mm Hg	>180/110 mm Hg	Often >220/140
Clinical features	Asymptomatic or mild/moderate headache; no acute target organ damage	Severe headache, dyspnea, edema; acute target organ damage usually absent	Chest pain, severe dyspnea, altered mental status, and focal neurologic deficit may be present as well as life-threatening target organ damage
Immediate goal	Lower BP within days	Lower BP within 24–72 hr	Immediate BP reduction; decrease by 15%–25% within 2 hours
Treatment setting	Outpatient	Usually outpatient	Inpatient; ICU
Medications	Long acting, oral	Oral medications with rapid onset of action; occasionally	Intravenous medication

BP, blood pressure; ICU, intensive care unit.

TABLE 48.7

EXAMPLES OF HYPERTENSIVE EMERGENCIES

Acute ischemic or hemorrhagic stroke
Subarachnoid hemorrhage
Acute myocardial ischemia or infarction
Acute heart failure
Acute aortic dissection
Eclampsia
Head trauma
Catecholamine excess states
    β-Blocker or clonidine withdrawal
    Cocaine, PCP use
    Pheochromocytoma crisis
Hemorrhage
    Postsurgical
    Severe epistaxis
    Gross hematuria

PCP, phencyclidine hydrochloride.

HYPERTENSIVE CRISIS

The term *hypertensive crisis* is used to indicate either a hypertensive urgency or emergency. Patients presenting with very high BP—>180/110 mm Hg—should be categorized into one of three mutually exclusive groups (Table 48.6):

- *Severe hypertension:* BP >180/110 mm Hg in the absence of symptoms beyond mild to moderate headache and without evidence of acute target organ damage
- *Hypertensive urgency:* BP >180/110 mm Hg in the presence of significant symptoms such as severe headache or dyspnea but no or only minimal acute target organ damage
- *Hypertensive emergency:* BP very high (often >220/140 mm Hg) with evidence of life-threatening organ dysfunction (Table 48.7)

The history for a patient with very elevated BP should be completed in a timely manner and capture several key pieces of information, including the duration and severity of hypertension and any cormorbid conditions. The relevant symptoms to address include headache, chest pain,

dyspnea, edema, acute fatigue, weakness, epistaxis, seizure, or change in level of consciousness. Direct questioning regarding adherence to antihypertensive medications is necessary as well as recent use of medications such as oral contraceptives, nonsteroidal anti-inflammatory drugs, cyclosporine, stimulant/anorectic agents, and prednisone. The patient should be questioned for use of alcohol as well as illicit drugs, particularly cocaine, amphetamines, and phencyclidine hydrochloride (PCP).

The measurement of BP should be performed with proper technique and in the setting of diminished pedal pulses should include both arms and at least one leg measurement. A fundus examination should be performed to assess for papilledema, hemorrhage, and exudates as well as a careful examination of cardiac, pulmonary, and neurologic function.

In the emergency department setting, expedited testing should include a chemistry panel, creatinine, urinalysis with microscopic examination of sediment, and ECG. A chest radiograph is important if there is a suspicion of heart failure or pulmonary disease. A CT scan of the head is indicated if history or examination suggest a central nervous system disorder.

Goals of Treatment

For patients with only severe hypertension, there is no strong evidence of a benefit to acute lowering of BP, and it may be associated with risk. For example, short-acting nifedipine has been associated with severe hypotension, stroke, acute myocardial infarction, and death and is no longer a part of the management of severe hypertension.[30]

Therefore, management of severe hypertension should include brief office observation (hours), initiation or resumption of oral antihypertensive medication, and arrangement for timely follow-up care.

For patients with hypertensive urgency, trial evidence is lacking, but expert opinion favors judicious acute treatment with an oral agent with rapid onset of action. The short-term goal is to reduce the BP within 24 to 72 hours.

Hypertensive emergency warrants admission to an intensive care unit and treatment with a parenteral agent.

TABLE 48.8

PREFERRED MEDICATIONS FOR HYPERTENSIVE URGENCIES

Agent	Dose	Onset of Action	Comment
Labetalol	200–400 mg orally	30–60 min	Bronchoconstriction, heart block, aggravates heart failure
Clonidine	0.1–0.2 mg orally	30–60 min	Rebound hypertension with abrupt withdrawal
Captopril	12.5–25.0 mg orally	15–60 min	Can precipitate acute renal failure in setting of bilateral renal artery stenosis
Nifedipine, extended release	30 mg orally	20 min	Avoid short-acting oral or sublingual nifedipine due to risk of stroke, acute MI, and/or severe hypotension

MI, myocardial infarction.

TABLE 48.9

PREFERRED MEDICATIONS FOR HYPERTENSIVE EMERGENCIES

Agent	Dose	Onset/Duration of Action (After Discontinuation)	Precautions
Parenteral vasodilators			
Sodium nitroprusside	0.25–10.00 μg/kg/min as IV infusion; maximal dose for 10 min only	Immediate/2–3 min after infusion	Nausea, vomiting, muscle twitching; with prolonged use, may cause thiocyanate intoxication, methemoglobinemia acidosis, cyanide poisoning; bags, bottles, and delivery sets must be light resistant
Glyceral trinitrate	5–100 μg as IV infusion	2–5 min/5–10 min	Headache, tachycardia, vomiting, flushing, methemoglobinemia; requires special delivery systems due to the drug's binding to polyvinyl chloride tubing
Nicardipine	5–15 mg/hr IV infusion	1–5 min/15–30 min, but may exceed 12 hr after prolonged infusion	Tachycardia, nausea, vomiting, headache, increased intracranial pressure, possible protracted hypotension after prolonged infusions
Verapamil	5–10 mg IV; can follow with infusion of 3–25 mg/hr	1–5 min/30–60 min	Heart block (first-, second-, and third degree), especially with concomitant digitalis or β-blockers; bradycardia
Fenoldopam	0.1–0.3 mg/kg/min IV infusion	<5 min/30 min	Headache, tachycardia, flushing, local phlebitis
Hydralazine	10–20 mg as IV bolus or 10–40 mg IM; repeat every 4–6 hr	10 min IV/>1 hr (IV), 20–30 min IM/4–6 hr IM	Tachycardia, headache, vomiting, aggravation of angina pectoris
Enalaprilat	0.625–1.250 mg IV every 6 hr	15–60 min/12–24 hr	Renal failure in patients with bilateral renal artery stenosis; hypotension
Parenteral adrenergic inhibitors			
Labetalol	10–80 mg as IV bolus every 10 min; up to 2 mg/min as IV infusion	5–10 min/2–6 hr	Bronchoconstriction, heart block, orthostatic hypotension
Esmolol	500 μg/kg bolus injection IV or 25–100 μg/kg/min by infusion; may repeat bolus after 5 min or increase infusion rate to 300 μg/kg/min	1–5 min/15–30 min	First-degree heart block, congestive heart failure, asthma
Phentolamine	5–15 mg as IV bolus	1–2 min/10–30 min	Tachycardia, orthostatic hypotension

IM, intramuscular; IV, intravenous.

The short-term goal is to reduce the BP by 15% to 25% within 4 hours. More aggressive reduction may exceed the autoregulatory capacity of the cerebrovascular circulation[31] and therefore elicit hypoperfusion, ischemia, and stroke.

Pharmacotherapy

For severe hypertension, initiation or resumption of long-acting antihypertensive medication is warranted. If immediate reduction of BP is indicated (urgency), medications with rapid onset of action are preferred (Table 48.8). Parenteral agents are indicated for some cases of hypertensive urgency and all cases of hypertensive emergency (Table 48.9).

Prevention

Hypertensive crises are largely preventable. Inadequate treatment of hypertension by the physician, poor adherence to therapy by the patient, and inadequate follow-up care are important areas deserving attention.

REVIEW EXERCISES

QUESTIONS

1. A 70-year-old man presents to the office for a health assessment. Which BP reading would indicate the highest risk for a cardiovascular event?
a) 110/90 mm Hg
b) 120/90 mm Hg
c) 130/70 mm Hg
d) 140/80 mm Hg
e) 150/70 mm Hg

Answer and Discussion

The answer is e. The educational objective is to recognize that systolic BP is more important in determining cardiovascular risk than is diastolic BP, particularly after 55 years of age. The elevated pulse pressure (80 mm Hg) in choice e gives an additional reason that this reading signifies higher risk than any of the other choices.

2. A 50-year-old woman presents with chronic elevation in BP. Which of the following clinical findings is/are suggestive of renovascular hypertension?
a) Systolic/diastolic epigastric bruit
b) Refractory hypertension
c) Gradual onset of hypertension at age 45
d) a and b
e) a, b, and c

Answer and Discussion

The answer is d. The educational objective is to recognize features suggestive of renovascular hypertension. An epigastric bruit with both a systolic and diastolic component is suggestive of renal artery stenosis, which if hemodynamically significant may manifest as renovascular hypertension. This disorder may present as refractory (resistant) hypertension. Abrupt onset of hypertension as well as onset prior to age 30 years or after age 55 years is suggestive of renovascular hypertension. Conversely, gradual onset of hypertension during middle age is typical of essential or primary hypertension.

3. A 60-year-old man is referred by his primary care physician to the emergency department for a severe elevation in BP. He denies any symptoms. The office BP was 206/110 mm Hg, and on presentation to the emergency department, it has now increased to 212/116 mm Hg with a heart rate of 84 beats per minute. He has been prescribed amlodipine, lisinopril, and hydrochlorothiazide in the past but ran out of all medications 1 week prior. Physical examination is unremarkable. Serum creatinine is 1.1; potassium, 4.1; and urinalysis is normal. What is the most appropriate management?
a) Measure 24 hour urine catecholamines and metanephrines
b) Resume the same antihypertensive medications, counsel on the importance of adherence, and schedule a follow-up office appointment with the primary physician
c) Clonidine 0.1 mg orally every 30 to 60 minutes until BP is <180/110 mm Hg, then proceed as described in choice b
d) Prescribe new regimen of minoxidil 5 mg twice daily and arrange follow-up with the primary physician
e) Labetalol intravenously to achieve a 25% reduction in BP within 3 hours, then proceed as in choice b

Answer and Discussion

The answer is b. The educational objective is to identify severe hypertension without crisis and manage appropriately. Acute lowering of BP in this instance has not been shown to be of benefit, and there may be risks attributable to hypotension and hypoperfusion. There are no particular features of pheochromocytoma to warrant measurement of catecholamines and metanephrines. In this case, the cause of the elevated BP is due to stopping medications, and a change in medications is not indicated.

4. You are evaluating a 74-year-old man for secondary causes of hypertension due to a BP of 164/74 mm Hg despite a regimen consisting of chlorthalidone 25 mg daily, amlodipine 10 mg daily, doxazosin 4 mg daily, and metoprolol 100 mg twice daily as well as strict adherence to a low-salt diet. Laboratory testing while on this regimen are as follows:

Serum potassium: 3.5 mEq/L
Serum creatinine: 1.2 mg/dL
Supine plasma renin activity: 0.8 μg/L per hour (0.5–1.8)
Supine plasma aldosterone: 37.1 ng/L (4.5–35.4)
Urinalysis: Normal

Which is the best next step to evaluate for primary aldosteronism?
a) Hold diuretic, advise patient to add 1 teaspoon of salt to the daily diet for 5 days and then collect a 24-hour urine sample for creatinine, sodium, and aldosterone
b) Adrenal CT
c) Adrenal MRI
d) Adrenal vein sampling
e) Iodine-131 metaiodobenzylguanadine iothalamate scan

Answer and Discussion

The answer is a. The educational objective is to recognize that the essential feature of primary aldosteronism is elevated and inappropriate aldosterone. Prior to imaging, it is important to establish whether the mildly elevated aldosterone may be secondary, particularly as a result of dietary salt restriction combined with a diuretic. Although measurement of renin and aldosterone in the blood may be a useful screening test, elevated aldosterone in a 24-hour urine sample during a time of salt loading provides strong evidence for primary aldosteronism. Adrenal vein sampling at this point would present risk and should not be considered prior to demonstrating an elevated and inappropriate aldosterone level.

5. You are performing a routine physical exam on a 30-year-old man. His office BP is 124/70 mm Hg. He has been checking his own BP and has been getting similar values. You should tell him that his current BP falls within the range of
a) Normal
b) Optimal
c) Prehypertension
d) Borderline hypertension
e) Stage 1 hypertension

Answer and Discussion
The answer is c. The educational objective is to be aware of the JNC 7 categories for BP. Prehypertension signifies increased cardiovascular risk as well as risk of developing true hypertension.

6. You are evaluating a 62-year-old woman with a history of missed office visits and erratic behavior. She presents to your office after a brief hospitalization for a hypertensive crisis. Prior to hospitalization, the patient had been prescribed the following regimen for her hypertension:

> Felodipine 10 mg once daily
> Atenolol 50 mg once daily
> Clonidine 0.2 mg twice daily
> Hydrochlorothiazide 25 mg once daily

She presented to the emergency department with headache. BP was 220/126 mm Hg, and heart rate was 120 beats per minute. Weight was 59 kg. She was treated with intravenous labetalol and then discharged on the following regimen:

> Metoprolol 50 mg twice daily
> Hydrochlorothiazide 25 mg daily
> Amlodipine 5 mg daily

In your office today, she reports feeling well. BP is 184/98 mm Hg; heart rate, 84; weight, 85 kg.
On follow-up, you are reviewing results from lab tests performed in the hospital:

> Urine creatinine: 0.8 g/24 hour

> Urine total epinephrine+norepinephrine: 262 μg (26–121 mcg/24 hour)

Among the choices listed, which is the best next step to evaluate further for the possibility of pheochromocytoma?
a) Repeat 24-hour urine

b) Iodine-131 metaiodobenzylguanadine iothalamate scan
c) Adrenal CT
d) Adrenal MRI
e) Clonidine suppression test

Answer and Discussion
The answer is a. The educational objective is to recognize factors that may lead to elevated catecholamine levels in the absence of pheochromocytoma. In this case, the mildly elevated catecholamines may be due to a rebound effect from stopping clonidine; given her history, poor adherence to medications should be strongly suspected. Another possible reason for the elevated catecholamines is a false-positive test due to analytical interference from labetalol. Regardless, pheochromocytoma is not strongly suggested from the above information, and imaging is not warranted prior to biochemical confirmation. Repeat testing for catecholamines as well as metanephrines is in order; consider a clonidine suppression test only if these results are equivocal.

REFERENCES

1. Rodgers A, Ezzati M, Vander Hoorn S, et al. Distribution of major health risks: findings from the Global Burden of Disease study. *PLoS Med* 2004;1(1):e27.
2. Hajjar I, Kotchen TA. Trends in prevalence, awareness, treatment, and control of hypertension in the United States, 1988-2000. *JAMA* 2003;290(2):199–206.
3. Fields LE, Burt VL, Cutler JA, et al. The burden of adult hypertension in the United States 1999 to 2000: a rising tide. *Hypertension* 2004;44(4):398–404.
4. Vasan RS, Beiser A, Seshadri S, et al. Residual lifetime risk for developing hypertension in middle-aged women and men: the Framingham Heart Study. *JAMA* 2002;287(8):1003–1010.
5. Oparil S, Zaman MA, Calhoun DA. Pathogenesis of hypertension. *Ann Intern Med* 2003;139(9):761–776.
6. Cicila GT. Strategy for uncovering complex determinants of hypertension using animal models. *Curr Hypertens Rep* 2000;2(2):217–226.
7. Hunt SC, Hopkins PN, Lalouel J-M. Hypertension. In: King RA, Roubenoff R, Motulsky AG, eds. *The Genetic Basis of Common Diseases*, 2nd ed. New York: Oxford Press, 2002.
8. Turner ST, Schwartz GL, Chapman AB, et al. C825T polymorphism of the G protein beta(3)-subunit and antihypertensive response to a thiazide diuretic. *Hypertension* 2001;37(2 Part 2):739–743.
9. Lifton RP. Molecular genetics of human blood pressure variation. *Science* 1996;272(5262):676–680.
10. Luft FC. Present status of genetic mechanisms in hypertension. *Med Clin North Am* 2004;88(1):vii, 1–18.
11. Beevers DG. Epidemiological, pathophysiological and clinical significance of systolic, diastolic and pulse pressure. *J Hum Hypertens* 2004;18(8):531–533.
12. Lewington S, Clarke R, Qizilbash N, et al.; Prospective Studies Collaboration. Age-specific relevance of usual blood pressure to vascular mortality: a meta-analysis of individual data for one million adults in 61 prospective studies. *Lancet* 2002;360(9349):1903–1913.
13. Burt VL, Cutler JA, Higgins M, et al. Trends in the prevalence, awareness, treatment, and control of hypertension in the adult US population. Data from the health examination surveys, 1960 to 1991. *Hypertension* 1995;26(1):60–69.

14. Staessen JA, Gasowski J, Wang JG, et al. Risks of untreated and treated isolated systolic hypertension in the elderly: meta-analysis of outcome trials. *Lancet* 2000;355(9207):865–872.

15. Vaccarino V, Berkman LF, Krumholz HM. Long-term outcome of myocardial infarction in women and men: a population perspective. *Am J Epidemiol* 2000;152(10):965–973.

16. Mitchell GF, Moye LA, Braunwald E, et al. Sphygmomanometrically determined pulse pressure is a powerful independent predictor of recurrent events after myocardial infarction in patients with impaired left ventricular function. SAVE investigators. *Circulation* 1997;96(12):4254–4260.

17. Laurent S, Cockcroft J, Van Bortel L, et al. Expert consensus document on arterial stiffness: methodological issues and clinical applications. *Eur Heart J* 2006;27(21):2588–2605.

18. Williams B, Lacy PS, Thom SM, et al. Differential impact of blood pressure-lowering drugs on central aortic pressure and clinical outcomes: principal results of the Conduit Artery Function Evaluation (CAFE) study. *Circulation* 2006;113(9):1213–1225.

19. Mancia G, De Backer G, Dominiczak A, et al. 2007 guidelines for the management of arterial hypertension: the Task Force for the Management of Arterial Hypertension of the European Society of Hypertension (ESH) and of the European Society of Cardiology (ESC). *J Hypertens* 2007;25(6):1105–1187.

20. Chobanian AV, Bakris GL, Black HR, et al. Seventh report of the Joint National Committee on Prevention, Detection, Evaluation, and Treatment of High Blood Pressure. *Hypertension* 2003;42(6):1206–1252.

21. Julius S, Nesbitt SD, Egan BM, et al. Feasibility of treating prehypertension with an angiotensin-receptor blocker. *N Engl J Med* 2006;354(16):1685–1697.

22. Appel LJ, Brands MW, Daniels SR, et al. Dietary approaches to prevent and treat hypertension: a scientific statement from the American Heart Association. *Hypertension* 2006;47(2):296–308.

23. Staessen JA, Wang JG, Thijs L. Cardiovascular prevention and blood pressure reduction: a quantitative overview updated until 1 March 2003. *J Hypertens* 2003;21(6):1055–1076.

24. Yakovlevitch M, Black HR. Resistant hypertension in a tertiary care clinic. *Arch Intern Med* 1991;151(9):1786–1792.

25. Taler SJ, Textor SC, Augustine JE. Resistant hypertension: comparing hemodynamic management to specialist care. *Hypertension* 2002;39(5):982–988.

26. Smith RD, Levy P, Ferrario CM; Consideration of Noninvasive Hemodynamic Monitoring to Target Reduction of Blood Pressure Levels Study Group. Value of noninvasive hemodynamics to achieve blood pressure control in hypertensive subjects. *Hypertension* 2006;47(4):771–777.

27. Izzo JL Jr, Black HR, eds. *Hypertension Primer.* Baltimore: Lippincott Williams & Wilkins, 1999.

28. Biglieri EG, Irony I, Kater CE. Identification and implications of new types of mineralocorticoid hypertension. *J Steroid Biochem* 1989;32(1B):199–204.

29. Montori VM, Young WF Jr. Use of plasma aldosterone concentration-to-plasma renin activity ratio as a screening test for primary aldosteronism. A systematic review of the literature. *Endocrinol Metab Clin North Am* 2002;31(3):xi, 619–632.

30. Grossman E, Messerli FH, Grodzicki T, et al. Should a moratorium be placed on sublingual nifedipine capsules given for hypertensive emergencies and pseudoemergencies? *JAMA* 1996;276(16):1328–1331.

31. Strandgaard S, Paulson OB. Cerebral autoregulation. *Stroke* 1984;15(3):413–416.

Chapter 49

Critical Fluid and Electrolytic Abnormalities in Clinical Practice

Marc A. Pohl

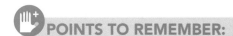

POINTS TO REMEMBER:

- Patients with congestive heart failure, nephrotic syndrome, and decompensated liver disease with ascites are examples of sodium excess states with increased extracellular fluid (ECF) volume, but these patients may have normal, expanded, or contracted plasma volumes.

- The serum sodium concentration in serum is regulated primarily by water balance, not by the total amount of sodium in the body.

- The ECG is frequently, but not always, useful in assessing the magnitude of hyperkalemia: For patients with elevated serum potassium levels in the range of 6.5 to 7.5 mEq/L, electrocardiography typically demonstrates tall, peaked, or tented T waves. Serum potassium levels in the range of 7.5 to 8.0 mEq/L may be associated with loss of T waves or widening of electrocardiographic wave complexes.

- Pinpointing the reason for hypokalemia may be simplified by measuring the 24-hour urinary potassium excretion in conjunction with a simultaneous serum potassium value. Classifying the cause of hypokalemia as either renal or extrarenal guides the differential diagnosis of hypokalemia.

- Severe acute hyponatremia (i.e., hyponatremia developing over 24–48 hours) may be associated with considerable morbidity, including seizures, coma, irreversible neurologic abnormalities, and death. This is most likely to occur with water administration to postoperative patients or in patients with thiazide-induced hyponatremia. Rapid initial treatment is both safe (because the cerebral adaptation is not complete) and may be lifesaving.

- For patients with hyponatremia of unknown duration, overly rapid correction may lead to central pontine myelinolysis, particularly if plasma sodium is increased by more than 25 mEq/L per day, to above 140 mEq/L.

An understanding of fluid and electrolyte abnormalities in clinical practice requires an appreciation of certain pertinent facts:

- The normal distribution of the body fluid compartments and perturbations in the distribution of these compartments
- Recognition of clinical conditions that either contract or expand the individual body fluid compartments
- Differentiation between disturbances of sodium balance and disturbances in water balance
- Identification of the causes of increased or decreased concentrations of sodium and potassium

This chapter discusses the normal and abnormal distribution of the body fluid compartments, clinical conditions associated with sodium excess or depletion, hypokalemia, hyperkalemia, hyponatremia, hypernatremia, and an approach to polyuria.

DISTRIBUTION OF THE BODY FLUID COMPARTMENTS

Total body water (TBW) is approximately 50% to 70% of total body weight. It is generally assumed that females have more fat (hence, less water) than males, and most textbooks indicate that TBW is approximately 60% of body weight for men and 50% of body weight for women. The TBW is subdivided into two major compartments: the intracellular fluid (ICF) compartment and the ECF compartment. The ICF compartment accounts for approximately two-thirds of TBW and the ECF compartment for approximately one-third of TBW. Accordingly, the ICF compartment is approximately 40% of body weight and the ECF compartment approximately 20% of body weight. The ECF compartment is further divided into two subcompartments: the interstitial fluid volume compartment and the plasma volume compartment. The plasma volume compartment accounts for approximately one-fourth of the ECF compartment and therefore represents 5% of body weight. This normal distribution of the body fluid compartments is depicted in Figure 49.1. The transcellular fluid compartment is a minor subdivision of the ECF compartment and includes small volumes such as aqueous humor, cerebral spinal fluid, and synovial fluid.

SODIUM

Approximately 3,500 mEq of sodium is present in the body of a 70-kg man. Approximately one-fifth of this total body sodium is chemically bound in bone and thought to be metabolically unavailable for exchange among the body fluid compartments. The remainder of the total body sodium, approximately 40 mEq/kg of body weight, is biologically active. Most of the total body exchangeable sodium (approximately 2,000 to 2,500 mEq) resides in the

ECF compartment, at a concentration of approximately 135 to 145 mEq/L. Thus, sodium is principally a cation of the ECF compartment.

A relatively small amount of sodium is present within cells (i.e., allocated to the ICF compartment), approximately 5 to 10 mEq/L of intracellular water (in muscle). The great discrepancy between the ECF sodium concentration (135–145 mEq/L) and the ICF sodium concentration (5–10 mEq/L) does not result from an absolute impermeability of cell membranes to sodium. Rather, sodium is continuously diffusing into cells from the ECF and is continuously being extruded to maintain its low intracellular concentration. This extrusion of sodium ions from within the cells to the ECF compartment appears to be a major transport activity of cells. Because this process requires that sodium be transported out of the cell against both an electrical and a chemical concentration gradient, work must be performed in maintaining the ECF position of sodium. The energy for this process derives from the metabolism within cells and is important in preserving cell volume. Impaired cellular metabolism disrupts the active extrusion of sodium from cells, allowing sodium to continually leak into the cell from the ECF, thereby increasing sodium accumulation within the cells. In this setting, chloride also accumulates in the cell, and as a net gain of intracellular solute occurs, cellular swelling ensues. This cellular swelling may have important consequences in clinical conditions of ischemia to kidney tissue cells, heart muscle cells, and brain cells.

Sodium Balance

The normal daily nutritional sodium requirement is met by the average daily diet and is generally in the range of 75 to 250 mEq/day. This variance in daily sodium intake is conditioned by dietary habit and taste in seasoning one's food. Although a small loss of sodium in the form of sweat and desquamated epithelium (12–20 mEq per day) occurs in normal people, for all practical purposes, the urinary sodium excretion is a reflection of the daily dietary sodium intake. Thus, in the steady state, there is no normal value for urinary sodium excretion because the urinary sodium excretion varies directly with the dietary intake of sodium. This concept of sodium balance also holds true for patients receiving chronic diuretic therapy, wherein the 24-hour urinary sodium excretion reflects the dietary sodium intake. A clinical application of sodium balance is the use of the 24-hour urinary sodium excretion in a hypertensive patient who appears to be refractory to antihypertensive drug treatment; such patients frequently ingest large amounts of salt in the diet (and often deny it). Measuring the 24-hour urinary sodium excretion in these patients, whether they are taking diuretics or not, allows the physician to estimate dietary sodium intake accurately.

Because sodium is the major ion in the ECF compartment, the ECF volume is a function of the sodium content in this compartment. External sodium balance is the most

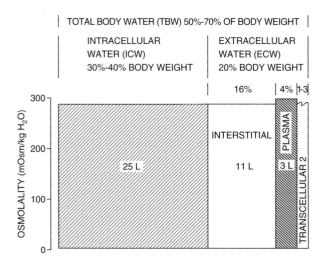

Figure 49.1 Normal distribution of water between ICF and ECF compartments.

important regulator of the ECF volume and hence of the plasma volume. Deficits in total body sodium are clinically reflected by a reduction in the ECF volume, which, if critical enough, leads to serious hemodynamic compromise. Clinical conditions producing ECF volume contraction include gastrointestinal fluid losses (e.g., diarrhea, malfunctioning ileostomy) and excessive diuresis from diuretic usage. Excesses in total body sodium content (sodium excess states) are manifested by an expansion of the ECF compartment, often producing congestion of the central circulation or edema.

Sodium excess states are common in clinical medicine. They may present clinically as an expansion of the interstitial fluid volume compartment, or edema. Increases in the ECF volume compartment may be present with or without a measurable increase in the plasma volume compartment. Primary aldosteronism, oliguric acute renal failure, severe chronic renal failure of any cause, and acute glomerulonephritis are examples of sodium excess states having increased ECF volume and an increase in measured plasma volume. Patients with congestive heart failure, nephrotic syndrome, and decompensated liver disease with ascites are examples of sodium excess states with increased ECF volume, but these patients may have normal, expanded, or contracted plasma volumes. These patients have decreased effective plasma volume (decreased effective arterial blood volume). Other clinical examples of increased ECF volume with decreased or ineffective arterial blood volume include patients with hypothyroidism, preeclampsia, arteriovenous fistulas, and salt and water retention associated with hydralazine and minoxidil therapy. These are all examples of sodium excess states.

Serum Sodium Concentration

The serum sodium concentration is the ratio of the amount of sodium in milliequivalents to body water in liters. The serum sodium concentration in serum is regulated primarily by water balance, not by the total amount of sodium in the body. A low serum sodium concentration (hyponatremia) may be present with deficits in total body sodium (e.g., gastrointestinal fluid losses) or in sodium excess states (e.g., edematous conditions such as ascites and congestive heart failure). A high serum sodium concentration (hypernatremia) may be present with total body sodium deficits (e.g., osmotic diuresis from tube feedings or uncontrolled diabetes mellitus) or with excess total body sodium (e.g., primary aldosteronism).

POTASSIUM

The body of a 70-kg man contains approximately 3,200 mEq of potassium, or approximately 45 to 50 mEq/kg of body weight. In women, because of a smaller body cell mass in proportion to body weight, the normal potassium content is approximately 35 to 40 mEq/kg, or approximately 2,300 to 2,500 mEq of total body potassium. Only a small amount of total body potassium is present in the ECF volume compartment (approximately 70 mEq), at a concentration of 3.5 to 5.0 mEq/L. Most of the total body potassium resides within the cells, where this intracellular potassium forms the major cation of intracellular water, at a concentration of approximately 150 mEq/L. Most of the total body potassium resides within muscle cells. Total body potassium declines with age as body cell mass diminishes. The normal daily dietary potassium requirements are met by an average diet. Daily potassium intake in food is generally in the range of 40 to 100 mEq, almost all of which is excreted in the urine, with a small component excreted in the stool. Accordingly, 24-hour urinary potassium excretion reflects the dietary potassium intake.

The plasma potassium concentration is not a reliable index for estimating total body potassium. Indeed, the serum potassium concentration may be drastically elevated in the presence of marked total body potassium deficits. Several factors affect the distribution of potassium between the ICF and the ECF volume compartments, including ECF pH, ECF osmolality, drugs (e.g., succinylcholine), and cellular catabolic rate or cellular necrosis. Patients with severe hyperglycemia may have concomitant hyperkalemia attributable to the *solvent drag phenomenon*. Metabolic acidosis, with a resulting decrease in blood pH (acidemia), is commonly associated with an elevated serum potassium concentration, reflecting a redistribution of potassium from the ICF to the ECF volume compartment rather than an increase in total body potassium content. Conversely, metabolic alkalosis with an increase in blood pH (alkalemia) is often associated with a low serum potassium concentration, again due to a redistribution of potassium between the ECF and ICF volume compartments. Thus, acidosis is usually associated with hyperkalemia, and alkalosis is usually associated with hypokalemia, and in neither situation is the serum potassium concentration a reflection of the body's potassium content. Conversely, most patients with metabolic acidosis have moderate deficits of total body potassium, and patients with significant metabolic alkalosis have moderate to large total body potassium deficits. A more extensive listing of causes of hyperkalemia is given in Table 49.1.

Concentrations of the serum potassium >7 mEq/L are extremely dangerous, and values of 9 to 12 mEq/L are usually fatal, the cause of death being cardiac arrhythmia or arrest. Hence, severe hyperkalemia is always a medical emergency. The ECG is frequently, but not always, useful in assessing the magnitude of hyperkalemia: For patients with elevated serum potassium levels in the range of 6.5 to 7.5 mEq/L, electrocardiography typically demonstrates tall, peaked, or tented T waves. Serum potassium levels in the range of 7.5 to 8.0 mEq/L may be associated with loss of T waves or widening of electrocardiographic wave complexes. For patients with even more severe

TABLE 49.1

CAUSES OF HYPERKALEMIA

Normal Total Body Potassium	Excessive Total Body Potassium
Pseudohyperkalemia	Excessive intake
Hemolysis of drawn blood	K^+ penicillin (1.7 mEq/10^6 U)
	Salt substitutes (10–14 mEq/g)
Tourniquet-induced ischemia	Stored blood
	Low-salt diet is K^+ rich
High leukocyte count ($>5 \cdot 10^5$ mm^3)	Defects in renin-aldosterone-renal axis
High platelet count ($>7.5 \cdot 10^5$ mm^3)	Renin-substrate deficiency
	Liver failure
Redistributional	Glucocorticoid deficiency
Acidosis (inorganic > organic)	Hyporeninemia
	Aging
Hormonal	ECF expansion
Insulin deficiency	Diabetes mellitus
α-Adrenergic agonists	Interstitial nephritis
β-Adrenergic blockers	Hydronephrosis
Aldosterone deficiency	Drugs and toxins
	NSAIDs
Tissue necrosis	
Familial periodic paralysis	β-Blockers
	α-Agonists
Drugs and toxins	Lead
Digitalis poisoning	Converting enzyme inhibitor
Succinylcholine	Captopril, lisinopril
Arginine, lysine	Aldosterone synthetic defect
Tromethamine	Generalized adrenal failure
Hyperosmolality (in diabetic patients)	Specific synthetic defect
	Idiopathic
	Drugs: Heparin, spironolactone
	Enzyme deficiencies
	Renal aldosterone resistance
	Oliguria, low urinary sodium
	Interstitial nephritis (sickle cell, systemic lupus erythematosus)
	Drugs: Spironolactone
	Hydronephrosis
	Amyloidosis
	Gordon syndrome

ECF, extracellular fluid; K^+, potassium; NSAIDs, nonsteroidal anti-inflammatory drugs.

hyperkalemia (e.g., serum potassium >8.0 mEq/L), electrocardiography demonstrates biphasic electrocardiographic wave complexes, idioventricular rhythm, and terminal sine wave patterns. Treatment options for hyperkalemia are summarized in Table 49.2.

Deficits in total body potassium are often observed in conjunction with a reduced serum potassium concentration (hypokalemia). The normal range for serum potassium in most laboratories is from 3.5 to 5.0 mEq/L. Thus, a serum potassium concentration <3.5 mEq/L is generally regarded as hypokalemic. The more common causes of hypokalemia with a reduction in total body potassium content are due to losses of potassium from the gastrointestinal tract and diarrhea. Occasionally, a very low dietary potassium intake (e.g., anorexia nervosa) may cause significant hypokalemia. Renal losses of potassium, with consequent hypokalemia, are typically seen in patients taking diuretics

TABLE 49.2

TREATMENT OF SEVERE OR MODERATE HYPERKALEMIA

Treatment	Onset	Duration
Calcium infusion	5 min	1–2 hr
Glucose and insulin	15–30 min	1–4 hr
Sodium bicarbonate	15–60 min	1–4 hr
Hypertonic saline	30–60 min	2–6 hr
Cation exchange resins		
Rectal	30–90 min	Indefinite (repeat)
Oral	2–12 hr	Indefinite (repeat)
Dialysis	2–8 hr	Indefinite (repeat)

TABLE 49.3

CAUSES OF HYPOKALEMIA

Gastrointestinal losses
   Vomiting, nasogastric suction, intestinal fistulas
   Diarrhea
   Villous adenoma
   Laxative abuse
Low dietary potassium intake (anorexia nervosa)
Hypomagnesemia
Tumors
   Primary aldosteronism
   Cushing syndrome
   Insulinoma
   Renal losses
   Secondary aldosteronism (cirrhosis, congestive heart failure, accelerated hypertension)
   Alkalosis—metabolic or respiratory
   Diuretics
   Renal tubular acidosis
Familial periodic paralysis

and in patients with renal tubular acidosis, mineralocorticoid excess, and hyperadrenocorticism. A more complete listing of the causes of hypokalemia is given in Table 49.3.

The symptoms of hypokalemia include muscular fatigue, hypotonicity of muscles, paralysis, and, occasionally, apnea in the case of severe hypokalemia affecting the muscles of respiration. Cardiac manifestations of hypokalemia include ectopic atrial, nodal, and ventricular beats as well as tachyarrhythmias. Confusion and agitation may be observed with hypokalemia. Electrocardiography commonly shows diagnostic patterns of hypokalemia when the serum potassium decreases to <2.5 mEq/L; these electrocardiographic changes include wide T waves with flattening or inversion of the T wave, prolonged Q-T interval, and prominent U waves.

Because most causes of hypokalemia are due to gastrointestinal potassium losses, low dietary potassium intake, and renal potassium losses, pinpointing the reason for hypokalemia may be simplified by measuring the 24-hour urinary potassium excretion in conjunction with a simultaneous serum potassium value. Classifying the cause of hypokalemia as either renal or extrarenal guides the differential diagnosis of hypokalemia.

Hypokalemia is not infrequently associated with hypertensive disorders. These hypokalemic/hypertensive conditions may be categorized as being associated with either elevated or depressed plasma renin activity. Renovascular hypertension, malignant hypertension, renin-secreting tumors, and hypertension in association with oral contraceptives are examples of hypokalemia with hypertension and elevated plasma renin activity. Diuretic therapy in patients with essential hypertension also may present with hypokalemia and elevated plasma renin levels. Hypokalemic hypertensive patients with depressed plasma renin activity include patients with primary aldosteronism due to adrenal adenomas or bilateral adrenal hyperplasia, cases of licorice

abuse, and deoxycorticosterone acetate or corticosterone excess states.

In nearly all clinical conditions associated with hypokalemia and total body potassium deficits, the potassium replacement should be in the form of potassium chloride, because in most of these clinical situations, hypokalemia and total body potassium deficit occur in conjunction with metabolic alkalosis, and the administration of chloride is necessary to correct metabolic alkalosis.

CHLORIDE

In a 70-kg man, the total body chloride is approximately 2,000 mEq. Although some chloride is contained within the ICF volume compartment, most of the body chloride resides in the ECF volume compartment at a concentration of 95 to 105 mEq/L. Changes in chloride ion concentration in the plasma generally move in the same direction as the concentration of sodium in the plasma. Thus, hypochloremia (a reduced plasma chloride concentration) usually is seen in conjunction with hyponatremia (e.g., chloride loss from the gastrointestinal tract, as a result of diuretic usage with urinary loss of chloride, and sometimes after administration of adrenal steroids). Hyperchloremia (an increased plasma chloride concentration) usually is seen in combination with hypernatremia; normal anion gap metabolic acidoses (e.g., ureterosigmoidostomies, renal tubular acidosis, diarrhea, mild to moderate chronic renal failure); and iatrogenically, with the excessive administration of ammonium chloride or hydrochloric acid.

BICARBONATE

The bicarbonate (HCO_3^-) concentration of body fluids is usually reported as total serum carbon dioxide or carbon dioxide–combining power. Virtually all total carbon dioxide is dissolved HCO_3^-. Clinically important fluid and electrolyte disturbances include those clinical conditions associated with either a decrease in ECF HCO_3^- concentration (e.g., diarrhea, renal failure) or an increase in ECF HCO_3^- concentration (e.g., vomiting, diuretic usage). Detailed discussions of abnormalities of the plasma HCO_3^- concentration usually occur in the context of describing clinical acid–base disorders, which are reviewed in detail in Chapter 53.

RELATIONSHIP OF PLASMA SODIUM CONCENTRATION TO PLASMA OSMOLALITY

Plasma or serum sodium concentration and plasma or serum osmolality are frequently measured in clinical practice. The plasma osmolality (mOsm/kg) depicts the osmotically active particles in the body fluids relative to the amount of water surrounding those particles. As discussed

TABLE 49.4

ESTABLISHING THE CAUSE OF HYPOKALEMIA

Serum Potassium (mEq/L)	Urinary Potassium (mEq/24 hr)	Cause
≤3.0	>30	Renal
≤3.0	<20	Extrarenal

TABLE 49.5

OSMOTIC AND VOLUME EFFECTS WITH ADDITION OF SODIUM CHLORIDE, WATER, OR ISOTONIC SALINE

	Hypertonic Sodium Chloride	Water	Isotonic Saline
Plasma osmolality	↑	↓	0
Plasma sodium	↑	↓	0
ECF volume	↑	↑	↑
Urine sodium	↑	↑	↑
ICF volume	↓	↑	0

↓, decrease; ↑, increase; ECF, extracellular fluid; ICF, intracellular fluid.
Adapted with permission from Rose BD. *Clinical Physiology of Acid–Base and Electrolyte Disorders*, 4th ed. New York: McGraw-Hill, 1994:224.)

previously, the osmolality across all the body fluid compartments is essentially the same, approximately 280 to 290 mOsm/kg. The relationship of the plasma sodium concentration to the plasma osmolality is depicted in the following equations:

$$P_{osm} = [2P_{Na}] + [glucose/18] + [BUN/2.8]$$

$$Effective\ P_{osm} = 2P_{Na}$$

where P_{osm} is the plasma osmolality, P_{Na} is the plasma sodium concentration, and BUN is the blood urea nitrogen concentration. In patients with normal values for plasma sugar and BUN, the effective estimated plasma osmolality is essentially twice the plasma (or serum) sodium concentration.

In the setting of severe hyperglycemia (e.g., plasma glucose 900 mg/dL), assuming an elevated BUN of 30 mg/dL and a sodium concentration of 132 mEq/L, the calculated plasma osmolality would be approximately 324 mOsm/kg. If the plasma osmolality were actually measured in the laboratory in this example of hyperglycemia, the measured and calculated plasma osmolalities would be similar. Conversely, if an osmotically active particle (not measured by routine laboratory tests—e.g., mannitol) were to reside in the ECF volume compartment, the measured plasma osmolality would be substantially higher than the osmolality calculated by the formula above. This discrepancy between measured and calculated osmolality is known as the osmolal gap. Clinical conditions characterized by a wide osmolal gap (*measured* greater than *calculated* plasma osmolality) include hypermannitolemia, ethylene glycol intoxication, and methanol intoxication. A wide osmolal gap in the setting of severe metabolic acidosis should alert the physician to the likelihood of ethylene glycol or methanol intoxication.

PERTURBATIONS IN THE DISTRIBUTION OF THE BODY FLUID COMPARTMENTS

As depicted in Figure 49.1, the body fluid compartments are divided into the ECF and ICF compartments. Note that the osmolality of the body fluid compartments is the same across all body fluids, approximately 280 mOsm/kg. Sodium is the major ion in the ECF volume compartment and the major contributor to the osmolality of the ECF. Potassium is the major cation in the ICF compartment and with its companion anions, phosphate, and proteins contributes to the osmolality of the ICF. Other osmotically active particles, known as osmolytes, reside primarily in the

ICF; the major intracellular osmolytes are glutamate, glutamine, taurine, and myoinositol. Other organic osmolytes are glycine, alanine, lycine, and betaine. These osmolytes play an important role in the maintenance of cell volume.

Hypertonic states are common in clinical medicine and are characterized by the concentration (i.e., increased osmolality) of the body fluids and a contraction of the ICF compartment. Hyperglycemia, mannitol infusions, and the administration of hypertonic saline are clinical examples of hypertonic states. In these situations, the osmolality of the ECF is acutely increased and water moves out of the ICF (across the semipermeable membrane separating the cells from the ECF) into the ECF compartment. Hyperosmolality of the body fluids ensues, with initial expansion of the ECF and contraction of the ICF. The symptoms of body fluid hypertonicity with associated cell shrinkage include irritability, restlessness, stupor, muscle twitching, hyperreflexia, spasticity, and possibly coma and death. The osmotic demyelinization syndrome that occurs with a too rapid correction of chronic hyponatremia is a clinical example of this pathophysiology. *Hypotonic* states are characterized by dilution of the body fluids (i.e., decreased osmolality), with expansion of the body fluid compartments. Acute water intoxication is an example of a hypotonic state. The clinical consequences of acute hypotonic states include cell swelling; if the brain cells swell too much, cerebral edema and seizures ensue. The effects of administering hypertonic saline, water, and isotonic saline are summarized in Table 49.5.

DEHYDRATION VERSUS VOLUME CONTRACTION

Physicians frequently apply the term *dehydration* to any situation wherein a reduction occurs in the amount of fluid in the body. The previous discussion of the body fluid compartments and appreciating the clinical consequences (described in Table 49.5), however, should draw attention to

TABLE 49.6

VOLUME CONTRACTION VERSUS DEHYDRATION

Loss of 1-L Saline	Type of Change	Loss of 1-L Water
−150 mEq	Change in sodium content	0
−1,000 mL	Change in TBW	−1,000 mL
0	Change in plasma osmolality	+2.5% (7.5 mOsm/L)
−1,000 mL	Change in ECF volume	−333 mL
−250 mL	Change in plasma volume	−83 mL

ECF, extracellular fluid; TBW, total body water.

the difference between loss of water and loss of salt and water from the body fluids. When one loses water from the body (dehydration), the amount of water lost is in proportion to the distribution of that water across all the body fluid compartments—that is, when 1 L of water is lost from the body, such as in profuse sweating, one-third of that water loss comes from the ECF volume compartment, and two-thirds come from the ICF volume compartment. When one loses 1 L of salt and water from the body, as in small intestinal and biliary fluid losses, the patient has essentially lost ECF volume because the concentration of sodium in these gastrointestinal fluids is reasonably close to the concentration of sodium in the ECF volume compartment. Thus, the threat to the central circulation in terms of maintaining blood pressure is formidable when large volumes of salt and water are being lost from the body in comparison with losses of pure water. Loss of water from the body should be referred to as *dehydration*. Loss of salt and water from the body should be termed *extracellular fluid volume contraction* or *volume contraction*.

These concepts are highlighted in Table 49.6, which describes the change in milliliters in the body fluid compartments consequent to the loss of 1 L of normal saline versus the loss of 1 L of water. Greater losses (e.g., 3–4 L) of salt and water would produce reductions in ECF volume and plasma volume, with obvious compromise of the circulation. In treating patients who have undergone body fluid compartment loss from one or more body fluid compartments, it is crucial to recognize the difference between dehydration and volume contraction: Normal saline, not dextrose 5% concentration in water (D_5W), is the treatment for ECF volume contraction. Fluid resuscitation for patients who are truly dehydrated should consist primarily of hypotonic fluids (e.g., D_5W or D_5W with normal saline).

HYPONATREMIA

The range of the serum sodium concentration in most clinical laboratories is 135 to 145 mEq/L. Hyponatremia is present when the serum sodium concentration decreases

to <135 mEq/L. Although total body sodium balance determines the ECF volume, sodium balance per se does not determine the serum sodium concentration. Indeed, a decrease in the serum sodium concentration (hyponatremia) can exist in the face of either an excess or deficit of total body sodium. Patients with cirrhosis and ascites are typically hyponatremic, despite an obvious excess of total body sodium. Patients with profound diarrhea or excessive gastrointestinal fluid losses are often hyponatremic in the face of total body sodium deficit.

Aberrations in the serum sodium concentration usually reflect abnormalities in water balance. For this discussion, hyponatremia indicates a positive water balance (water intake exceeds water excretion). This situation develops when the kidneys fail to excrete water normally in conjunction with continued water intake: A positive water balance ensues, with dilution of the body fluids. With this concept at hand, nearly all types of hyponatremia are dilutional, rendering the term *dilutional hyponatremia* of little differential diagnostic value.

In the normal subject, hyponatremia is prevented by the renal excretion of water excess. The physiological requirements for this elimination of excess water are the following:

- Ability of the hypothalamic osmoregulatory machinery in the brain to inhibit vasopressin (antidiuretic hormone [ADH]) secretion in response to hypoosmolality of the plasma
- Normal intrinsic renal-diluting mechanisms

The relationship between plasma osmolality and plasma ADH is depicted in Figure 49.2. In normal individuals, plasma ADH levels are virtually undetectable when the plasma osmolality falls below 280 mOsm/kg. In most clinical conditions associated with hyponatremia and

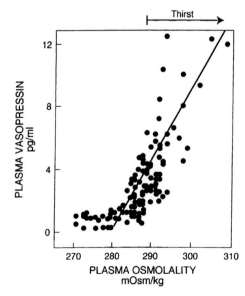

Figure 49.2 Effect of plasma osmolality on plasma ADH and thirst. (Reproduced with permission from Robertson GL, Aycinena P. Neurogenic disorders of osmoregulation. *Am J Med* 1982;72:339.)

reduced plasma osmolality (e.g., plasma osmolality of 260 mOsm/kg), however, plasma ADH levels are elevated, thus promoting the retention of water in the collecting tubules of the kidneys and thereby contributing to a persistent reduction in the plasma sodium concentration. The reason for this increase in ADH despite reduced plasma osmolality is the volume stimulus for ADH release—that is, an actual or perceived reduction (decreased effective arterial blood volume) in plasma volume or a tumor-producing ADH independent of the plasma osmolality. Normal intrinsic renal diluting mechanisms include (a) adequate delivery of salt-containing fluid to the distal diluting sites of the nephron, (b) intact salt transport at the diluting sites in the nephron, and (c) impermeability of the distal nephron to water in the absence of ADH. In most clinical conditions featuring hyponatremia, these normal intrinsic renal-diluting mechanisms are impaired such that the urine is not adequately diluted (urine osmolality is elevated). This results in decreased water excretion and contributes to positive water balance and hyponatremia. Because hyponatremia is prevented in normal subjects by the excretion of water excess (for the reasons described previously), the critical pathophysiological question to ask is, "Why is the excess water not excreted?" If patients with congestive heart failure (frequently hyponatremic) were able to excrete water normally, they would not become hyponatremic. Thus, hyponatremia is a disorder of urinary dilution.

Approach to the Diagnosis of Hyponatremic Syndromes

Excluding causes of pseudohyponatremia, such as hyperlipidemia and hyperproteinemia, is the first step in evaluating the hyponatremic patient. In these two conditions, although the serum sodium concentration may be factitiously low, the sodium concentration of plasma water is normal. With severe hyperlipidemia, the serum will appear lactescent; factitious hyponatremia in conjunction with severe hyperproteinemia is usually observed when the plasma protein concentration is >12 to 15 g/dL. In these two conditions, the plasma sodium concentration is low, but the plasma osmolality is normal.

Hyperglycemia and hypermannitolemia, sometimes categorized as examples of pseudohyponatremia, really produce true hyponatremia. In these situations, water moves from the ICF to the ECF compartment, resulting in a reduction of the serum sodium concentration. In contrast to hyperlipidemia and hyperproteinemia, the low serum sodium concentration associated with hyperglycemia or hypermannitolemia is a true reflection of the ECF sodium concentration. In these latter two conditions, the serum or plasma sodium concentration is low, and the plasma osmolality may be normal or elevated because of the excess sugar or mannitol in the plasma. In other situations of true hyponatremia (to be discussed), the serum osmolality and serum sodium concentration are both depressed.

After excluding factitious hyponatremia, hyperglycemia, and hypermannitolemia, it is worthwhile to consider several causes of hyponatremia related to drugs such as morphine, barbiturates, anesthesia, clofibrate, cyclophosphamide, vincristine, oxytocin, and chlorpropamide. Endocrine disorders, such as adrenal insufficiency, hypopituitarism, and myxedema, may be associated with hyponatremia and also should be excluded. Acute water intoxication in an individual with normal renal function is an extremely rare entity and would be expected to occur only when maximal renal water output (approximately 22 L per day) is exceeded by an unusually large water intake (e.g., psychogenic polydipsia). Most clinical situations of acute water intoxication develop in patients with chronic renal failure and a marked reduction of glomerular filtration rate, because these patients have an inability to maximally dilute their urine and are more susceptible to developing severe hyponatremia after receiving an acute water load (e.g., hypotonic intravenous solutions, psychogenic polydipsia).

With the previously mentioned clinical situations eliminated, a useful approach to the patient with hyponatremia attempts to place the hyponatremic patient into one of three broad categories, based on the history and physical examination:

I. Hyponatremia with hypovolemia (inadequate circulation)
  A. With renal salt retention (urinary sodium concentration <10–15 mEq/L)
    1. Gastrointestinal losses
    2. Profuse sweating
  B. With urinary sodium wasting (urinary sodium >20 mEq/L)
    1. Adrenal insufficiency
    2. Diuretics
    3. Renal salt wasting, as in chronic renal failure or distal renal tubular acidosis
II. Hyponatremia with edema (urinary sodium concentration usually <10 mEq/L)
  A. Congestive heart failure
  B. Hepatic cirrhosis with ascites
  C. Nephrotic syndrome
III. Hyponatremia without evidence of hypovolemia or edema
  A. Syndrome of inappropriate secretion of antidiuretic hormone (SIADH)
  B. Reset osmostat
  C. Drugs (as mentioned previously)

The physical examination easily differentiates patients in category I from patients in category II, and patients who are euvolemic (category III) can usually be differentiated, clinically, from those patients who are either hypovolemic (category I) or edematous (category II). A more complete diagnostic approach to hyponatremia is summarized in Table 49.7.

TABLE 49.7

DIAGNOSTIC APPROACH TO HYPONATREMIA

Step 1: Measure Serum Osmolality

Normal (280–285 mOsm)	Low (<280 mOsm)	Elevated (>.285 mOsm)

1A: Measure blood sugar, lipids, protein
Isotonic hyponatremia
1. Pseudohyponatremia
  Hyperlipidemia
  Hyperproteinemia
2. Isotonic infusions
  Glucose
  Mannitol
  Glycine
	→ → →
	
	→
		Step 1B: Measure blood sugar
		Hypertonic hyponatremia
		1. Hyperglycemia
		2. Hypertonic infusions
		  Glucose
		  Mannitol
		  Glycine

Step 2: Clinically Assess the Extracellular Fluid Volume

Tachycardia, Hypotension, Poor Skin Turgor

Hypovolemic hypotonic hyponatremia

Causes	BUN/Cr	Uric Acid	Urinary Osm	Na
GI losses	↑↑/↑	↑	↑↑	↓↓
Skin losses	↑↑/↑	↑	↑↑	↓↓
Lung losses	↑↑/↑	↑	↑↑	↓↓
Third space	↑↑/↑	↑	↑↑	↓↓
Renal losses				
Diuretics	↑↑/↑	↑	ISO	↑
Renal damage	↑↑/↑↑	↑	ISO	↑
Partial urinary tract obstruction	↑↑/↑	↑	ISO (↓)	↑
Adrenal insufficiency	↑↑	↑	ISO (↓)	↑

Edema

Hypervolemic hypotonic hyponatremia

Causes	BUN/Cr	Uric Acid	Urinary Osm	Na
CHF	↑↑/↑	↑	↑	→
Liver damage	↑↑/↑	↑	↑	→
Nephrosis	(↑↑↑/↑↑)	↑	↑ (ISO ↓↑)	→

Normal Pulse, Blood Pressure, Skin Turgor, No Edema

Isovolemic hypotonic hyponatremia

Causes	BUN/Cr	Uric Acid	Urinary Osm	Na
Water intoxication	↓/↓	↓	↑ (↓)	→
Renal failure	↑↑/↑↑	↑	ISO	→
K+ loss	↑/↑(N)	↑↑	↑	↓
SIADH	↓/↓	↓↓	↑	↑
Reset osmostat	N	N	V	V

BUN/Cr, blood urea nitrogen/creatinine; CHF, congestive heart failure; GI, gastrointestinal; ISO, isotonic; K+, potassium; N, normal; Na, sodium; Osm, osmolality; SIADH, syndrome of inappropriate secretion of antidiuretic hormone; V, variable.

Note: Arrows indicate direction of change. Single and double arrows define the magnitude of change.

Reproduced with permission from Narins RG, Jones ER, Stom MC, et al. Diagnostic strategies in disorders of fluid, electrolyte and acid-base homeostasis. *Am J Med* 1982;72:496–519.

Syndrome of Inappropriate Antidiuretic Hormone

Any discussion of hyponatremia would be incomplete without some comment about SIADH. This relatively rare condition is characterized by:

- Hyponatremia with corresponding hypo-osmolality of the serum and ECFs
- Continued renal excretion of sodium
- Absence of clinical evidence of fluid volume depletion or edema
- Normal renal function
- Normal adrenal and thyroid function
- Osmolality of the urine greater than that appropriate for the concomitant osmolality of the plasma or urine that is less than maximally dilute

Most patients with SIADH have a low or low-normal serum uric acid level.

Disorders in which there is a syndrome probably resulting from inappropriate secretion or aberrant production of ADH (SIADH) include malignant tumors such as carcinoma of the lung, duodenum, and pancreas; central nervous system tuberculosis, purulent bacterial meningitis, acute intermittent porphyria, and subdural hemorrhage; pulmonary disorders, such as tuberculosis, pulmonary abscess, aspergillosis, and viral and bacterial pneumonias; and, finally, idiopathic SIADH. In patients appearing to have idiopathic SIADH, usually a specific underlying cause surfaces eventually.

In treating patients with SIADH, water restriction is critically important. With acute hyponatremia due to SIADH, hypertonic saline, salt tablets, or loop diuretics may be required. The long-term ambulatory management of patients with SIADH has become easier with the use of demeclocycline in dosages from 600 to 900 mg per day. Caution is warranted in using demeclocycline in patients with severe hypoalbuminemia, as acute tubular necrosis may occur.

Treatment

As a general principle, the treatment for hyponatremia depends on the underlying cause:

- If there is contracted ECF volume, the depleted volume should be replenished with sodium and water, usually in the form of normal saline.
- If an edematous state exists, water should be restricted; in most circumstances, both salt and water should be restricted. If congestive heart failure is the reason for the hyponatremia, water restriction, loop diuretics, and cardiotonic measures, such as the use of an angiotensin-converting enzyme (ACE) inhibitor, should alleviate the hyponatremia, especially if cardiac function improves.

- If SIADH is diagnosed, water should be restricted in conjunction with additional treatment recommendations for SIADH as discussed above.

For patients with hypoadrenalism, hypopituitarism, or hypothyroidism, appropriate hormone replacement therapy is required. Patients with adrenal insufficiency who are acutely hyponatremic and volume contracted will initially require the administration of normal saline.

In treating hyponatremia, the physician also must consider the severity of the hyponatremia and the rate of correction of the condition. For patients with moderate hyponatremia (e.g., serum sodium concentration <125–135 mEq/L), one should discontinue the responsible factor (e.g., drug or diuretic), treat the underlying condition (e.g., heart failure), and restrict fluids to allow correction of the hyponatremia through losses of excess water via the skin and mucous membranes and, it is hoped, an increase in renal water excretion. If severe, life-threatening hyponatremia is present (serum sodium concentration <110–115 mEq/L) and especially if obtundation, coma, or seizures exist, (a) enough sodium chloride should be given to increase the serum sodium concentration to approximately 120 mEq/L, (b) isotonic saline or 3% sodium chloride should be administered, (c) a diuretic should be administered and urinary electrolyte losses replaced, and (d) free water should be restricted.

In recent years, much discussion has been generated about the speed (rate) of correction of hyponatremia, the osmotic demyelinization syndrome, and central pontine myelinosis. Several points should be emphasized regarding the rate of correction for severe hyponatremia; severe acute hyponatremia (i.e., hyponatremia developing over 24–48 hours) may be associated with considerable morbidity, including seizures, coma, irreversible neurologic abnormalities, and death. This is most likely to occur with water administration to postoperative patients or in patients with thiazide-induced hyponatremia. Rapid initial treatment is both safe (because the cerebral adaptation is not complete) and may be lifesaving. The plasma sodium concentration should be increased by 1.5 to 2.0 mEq/L per hour for the first 4 to 6 hours but by no more than 20 mEq/L per day. For patients with known chronic hyponatremia (i.e., hyponatremia known to be present for more than 48–72 hours) or for patients with hyponatremia of unknown duration, overly rapid correction may lead to central pontine myelinolysis, particularly if plasma sodium is increased by more than 25 mEq/L per day to above 140 mEq/L. Plasma sodium concentration should be increased in asymptomatic chronic hyponatremic patients at a maximum rate of 0.5 mEq/L per hour. Too rapid correction is most likely to occur with hypertonic saline or after correction of hypovolemia with isotonic saline.

HYPERNATREMIA

Hypernatremia is defined as a serum sodium concentration >145 mEq/L. It may exist in the presence of a decrease or increase in total body sodium. Almost always, hypernatremia is a sign of relative or absolute water deficiency. Because normal osmoregulation and thirst closely fix body fluid osmolality between 280 and 290 mOsm/kg (serum sodium concentration of 135–145 mEq/L), hyperosmolality of the body fluids indicates a deficiency of water. The serum sodium concentration is rarely increased by administration of excess sodium per se, unless an usually large amount of sodium salt is given erroneously.

Hypernatremia is prevented in normal people by the thirst mechanism (Fig. 49.2). A slight increase in plasma osmolality stimulates thirst (at a plasma osmolality of approximately 290 mOsm/kg), which, in turn, increases water intake voluntarily. Obviously, this chain of events does not take place if a person is comatose, does not have access to water, cannot communicate thirst, or if not appropriately administered by paramedical personnel. If the thirst mechanism remains intact and water is available, the osmolality of the body fluids is protected but at the expense of polydipsia and polyuria. Hospitalized patients avoid hyperosmolality of the body fluids from hypernatremia so long as adequate water or dilute intravenous fluids are provided.

The clinical circumstances associated with hypernatremia are:

- Unconscious or confused patients who receive insufficient fluids
- Osmotic diuresis
- Uncontrolled diabetes mellitus
- Tube feedings
- Loss of both thirst and neurohypophyseal function (rare)

- Water-wasting conditions (if not enough water provided)
- True central diabetes insipidus
- Nephrogenic diabetes insipidus (e.g., congenital or lithium toxicity)
- In infants, especially given sodium chloride–containing fluids
- Rapid infusion of hypertonic saline or sodium bicarbonate (unusual)
- Hyperaldosteronism or Cushing syndrome
- Seizures, excessive exercise, rhabdomyolysis
- Osmotic diarrhea

Treatment

The mainstay of treatment for hypernatremia is to provide sufficient water. A reduction of solute intake (e.g., moderate dietary protein restriction) decreases obligatory water losses. For patients with central diabetes insipidus, the most physiological treatment is to administer exogenous vasopressin (ADH), which can be given subcutaneously or intramuscularly or in the form of a lysine-vasopressin nasal spray. Most patients with central diabetes insipidus use desmopressin. Thiazide diuretics in conjunction with a low-salt diet and chlorpropamide are additional nonvasopressin treatment maneuvers that may decrease urine volume in patients with central diabetes insipidus. Thiazides, by producing mild ECF volume contraction, may induce less renal water excretion; chlorpropamide (125–500 mg daily) enhances the action of circulating ADH. Polyuric patients with nephrogenic diabetes insipidus usually do not respond to desmopressin or chlorpropamide. Inducing mild volume contraction with a thiazide diuretic and a low-salt diet, in conjunction with a low-protein diet, may decrease urine volume in these patients. When this condition is due to lithium toxicity, amiloride may be used. Nonsteroidal anti-inflammatory drugs (NSAIDs) may decrease

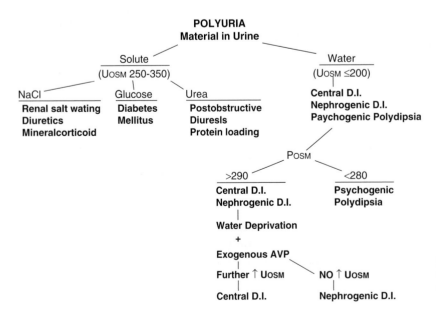

Figure 49.3 Schematic diagram of polyuria. (AVP, arginine vasopressin; D.I., diabetes insipidus; NaCl, sodium chloride; U$_{OSM}$, urine osmolality.)

urine volume in patients with congenital nephrogenic diabetes insipidus or lithium toxicity.

APPROACH TO POLYURIA

Polyuria (daily urine volume >3–4 L) is a relatively common patient complaint. The high urine volume may be driven by excessive fluid intake (oral or intravenous infusion of hypotonic solutions) or may be consequent to a solute diuresis. If the urine is remarkably dilute (i.e., urine osmolality <250 mOsm/kg), a water diuresis is present and attributable to either diabetes insipidus or psychogenic polydipsia. If the urinary osmolality is >300 mOsm/kg, a solute diuresis is the likely basis for the polyuria. A schematic approach to polyuria is given in Figure 49.3. Note that when a water diuresis is diagnosed (urine osmolality <200–250 mOsm/kg), the next diagnostic step is to obtain a plasma osmolality; if in the setting of a water diuresis the plasma osmolality is <280 mOsm/kg, psychogenic polydipsia is likely. If the plasma osmolality is >290 mOsm/kg, diabetes insipidus is the explanation for the water diuresis.

REVIEW EXERCISES

QUESTIONS

1. An internal medical resident ingests 300 mEq of sodium in his diet daily (a "fast-food freak"). His 24-hour urinary sodium excretion, in the chronic steady state, can be expected to be which of the following?
a) 10 mEq per day
b) 100 mEq per day
c) 280 mEq per day
d) 450 mEq per day

Answer and Discussion
The answer is c. In the steady state, the 24-hour urine sodium excretion reflects the dietary sodium intake and vice versa. The ingestion of 300 mEq of sodium in the diet daily should result in a 24-hour urine sodium excretion of approximately 300 mEq. Of the possible answers for this question, 280 mEq per day is the closest to the amount of sodium ingested in the diet.

2. A 70-kg man has profound diarrhea and loses 5 kg in weight. His identical twin (same height and weight) sweats off 5 kg in weight hiking in the desert.
   Answer true or false to each of the following statements.
a) The man with diarrhea has more evidence of arterial volume contraction than the desert hiker.
b) The man with diarrhea has a lower blood pressure than the desert hiker (both started with identical blood pressures).

c) The optimal treatment of the man with diarrhea is with D_5W.
d) The optimal treatment of the desert hiker is with D_5W.

Answer and Discussion
The answers are a, true; b, true; c, false; d, true. The 70-kg man with profuse diarrhea is losing salt and water. The identical twin who sweats off 5 kg in weight is losing essentially water. This water loss comes from TBW—that is, it is lost proportionately to the distribution of water throughout the body fluid compartments. Because the hemodynamic consequences of body fluid losses are greatest when these losses come from the plasma volume or blood volume compartments, the patient with diarrhea loses a substantially larger amount of fluid from his plasma volume than does his identical twin. The man with diarrhea would have more clinical evidence of arterial volume contraction than would the desert hiker and would obviously have a lower blood pressure and more tachycardia than would the desert hiker. Because the man with diarrhea has lost both salt and water from the body, appropriate treatment is normal saline (not D_5W). Treatment of the desert hiker with D_5W is appropriate because he primarily has lost water from the body. More profuse water losses, particularly if accompanied by orthostatic hypotension or orthostatic tachycardia, should be treated initially with normal saline to reverse the compromised arterial volume, followed by appropriate administration of D_5W.

3. A 52-year-old man with a 20-year history of cigarette smoking is admitted to the hospital because of cough and weakness. On admission, his serum electrolytes reveal a serum sodium concentration of 112 mEq/L; potassium, 4.5 mEq/L; chloride, 80 mEq/L; and HCO_3^-, 26 mEq/L. The BUN was 8 mg/dL; serum creatinine, 0.8 mg/dL; and serum uric acid, 3.0 mg/dL.
   These data are most consistent with which of the following?
a) Addison disease
b) Congestive heart failure
c) Cirrhosis with ascites
d) SIADH

Answer and Discussion
The answer is d. The hyponatremia and normal renal function (normal BUN and serum creatinine) in conjunction with a low serum uric acid level all suggest SIADH. The long history of cigarette smoking and cough suggest the possibility of a lung cancer, well known to be associated with SIADH. No evidence of congestive heart failure or cirrhosis with ascites is described on the physical examination. Although the values for sodium, chloride, and potassium concentration are consistent with adrenal insufficiency, one would

expect hyponatremia of this magnitude due to adrenal insufficiency to have clinical and biochemical evidence of ECF volume contraction—that is, a higher BUN, possibly a higher serum creatinine level (depending on the patient's muscle mass), and a higher serum uric acid level.

4. Which one of the following applies best to the pathophysiology of patients with hyponatremia?
a) An inability to concentrate the urine
b) An inability to maximally dilute the urine
c) Congestive heart failure
d) SIADH
e) ECF volume contraction

Answer and Discussion
The answer is b. Patients with hyponatremia become hyponatremic (unless they have pseudohyponatremia) because of an inability to dilute the urine. Patients with congestive heart failure, SIADH, and ECF volume contraction may all demonstrate hyponatremia, and these three conditions share the pathophysiological abnormality of an inability to maximally dilute the urine.

5. A 47-year-old man presents to the emergency room with a serum sodium concentration of 115 mEq/L. Physical examination reveals a supine blood pressure of 120/80 mm Hg and a standing blood pressure of 90/60 mm Hg. The skin turgor is diminished.

Which one of the following is the best treatment for this man's hyponatremia?
a) Restriction of free water
b) Restriction of salt and water
c) Administration of normal saline
d) Treatment of the hyponatremia with demeclocycline

Answer and Discussion
The answer is c. This patient has obvious physical findings of ECF volume contraction (orthostatic hypotension and diminished skin turgor). The proper treatment is to administer ECF (i.e., normal saline). Restriction of salt and water is obviously inappropriate for a patient who requires volume expansion. Although hyponatremic, the restriction of free water would only aggravate the hemodynamic abnormalities present. Consideration of demeclocycline should be reserved for patients with evidence of chronic SIADH, a condition that cannot be diagnosed in the setting of obvious ECF volume contraction.

6. A 57-year-old man with a history of chronic congestive heart failure and a 20-year history of cigarette smoking is admitted with a serum sodium concentration of 120 mEq/L. The serum osmolality is 255 mOsm/kg (normal 280–300 mOsm/kg). The urine osmolality is 460 mOsm/kg. These determinations of serum and urine osmolality are most consistent with which one of the following?
a) Congestive heart failure
b) SIADH
c) Cirrhosis and ascites
d) Severe salt and water depletion
e) All of the above

Answer and Discussion
The answer is e. This patient has hyponatremia and hypo-osmolality of the serum, with evidence of ADH production (i.e., osmolality 460 mOsm/kg). Patients with congestive heart failure, SIADH, ascites, and severe salt and water depletion all may develop hyponatremia with an inability to dilute the urine. ADH levels are increased in all these clinical situations, contributing to an increase in the urine osmolality. The serum and urine osmolality values given are consistent with all the diagnostic possibilities listed.

7. You are called to the surgical intensive care unit to see a 65-year-old white man with known type II diabetes mellitus who is oliguric 24 hours after an abdominal aortic aneurysm resection. Electrolytes reveal a serum sodium concentration of 110 mEq/L; potassium, 5.0 mEq/L; chloride, 75 mEq/L; HCO_3^-, 20 mEq/L; blood sugar, 200 mg/dL; BUN, 45 mg/dL; and plasma osmolality, 410 mOsm/kg.

Answer true or false to the following statements.
a) The measured plasma osmolality is internally consistent with the other reported laboratory test results.
b) The calculated osmolality is approximately 250 mOsm/kg.
c) The discrepancy between the calculated osmolality and the measured plasma osmolality (osmolal gap) could be due to mannitol.
d) If excess mannitol is present in the plasma of this patient, his ICF volume is contracted and the ECF volume is expanded.

Answer and Discussion
The answers are a, false; b, true; c, true; d, true. The calculated osmolality $(2 \cdot serum\ [Na^+]) + (glucose/18) + (BUN/3)$ is 250 mOsm/kg. The measured osmolality of 410 mOsm/kg reported from the chemistry laboratory is significantly greater than the calculated osmolality. Thus, the measured plasma osmolality (410 mOsm/kg) is not internally consistent with the osmolality calculated on the basis of the measured serum sodium concentration, blood sugar, and BUN. The discrepancy between the calculated and measured osmolalities suggests that some other osmotically active particle is residing in the plasma of this patient. This could be mannitol, particularly because some patients receive intraoperative mannitol during resection of an

abdominal aortic aneurysm. Assuming that mannitol is present in the plasma of this patient, he qualifies for the label of *hypertonic state*—the osmolality of the body fluids is increased (410 mOsm/kg), and because the mannitol resides entirely in the ECF compartment, water would come out of the cells, resulting in cell shrinkage. This fluid shift would result in ICF volume contraction and ECF volume expansion.

SUGGESTED READINGS

Anderson RJ, Chung HM, Kluge R, et al. Hyponatremia: a prospective analysis of its epidemiology and the pathogenetic role of vasopressin. *Ann Intern Med* 1985;102:164–168.

Arieff AI, Llach F, Massry SG. Neurological manifestations and morbidity of hyponatremia: correlation with brain water and electrolytes. *Medicine* 1976;55:121–129.

Ashraf N, Locksley R, Arieff AI. Thiazide-induced hyponatremia associated with death or neurologic damage in outpatients. *Am J Med* 1981;70:1163–1168.

Bartter F, Schwartz WB. The syndrome of inappropriate secretion of antidiuretic hormone. *Am J Med* 1967;42:790.

Berl T. Treating hyponatremia—damned if we do and damned if we don't. *Kidney Int* 1990;37:1006–1018.

Berl T, Anderson RJ, McDonald KM, et al. Clinical disorders of water metabolism. *Kidney Int* 1976;10:117–132.

Carrilho F, Bosoh J, Arroyo V, et al. Renal failure associated with demeclocycline in cirrhosis. *Ann Intern Med* 1977;87:195–197.

DeFronzo RA, Thier SO. Pathophysiologic approach to hyponatremia. *Arch Intern Med* 1980;140:897.

Fichman MT, Vorherr H, Kleeman CP, et al. Diuretic-induced hyponatremia. *Ann Intern Med* 1971;75:853.

Forrest JN Jr, Cox M, Hong C, et al. Superiority of demeclocycline over lithium in the treatment of chronic syndrome of inappropriate secretion of antidiuretic hormone. *N Engl J Med* 1978;298: 173–177.

Gullans SR, Verbalis JG. Control of brain volume during hyperosmolar and hypoosmolar conditions. *Ann Rev Med* 1993;44:289–301.

Hantman O, Rosier B, Zohlman R, et al. Rapid correction of hyponatremia in the syndrome of inappropriate secretion of antidiuretic hormone. *Ann Intern Med* 1973;78:870–875.

Harrington JT, Cohen JJ. Clinical disorders of urine concentration and dilution. *Arch Intern Med* 1973;131:810.

Leaf A. The clinical and physiologic significance of the serum sodium concentration (part 1). *N Engl J Med* 1962;267:24–30.

Leaf A. The clinical and physiologic significance of the serum sodium concentration (part 2). *N Engl J Med* 1962;267:77–83.

Leaf A, Cotran R. *Renal Pathophysiology.* New York: Oxford University Press, 1976.

Lee WH, Packer M. Prognostic importance of serum sodium concentration and its modification by converting-enzyme inhibition in patients with severe chronic heart failure. *Circulation* 1986;73:257–267.

Mange K, Matsuura D, Cizman B, et al. Language guiding therapy: the case of dehydration versus volume depletion. *Ann Intern Med* 1997;127:848–853.

Narins RG, Jones ER, Stom MC, et al. Diagnostic strategies in disorders of fluid, electrolyte and acid–base homeostasis. *Am J Med* 1982;72:496–519.

Potassium in Clinical Medicine. Searle & Co. Monograph. Cypress, CA: Medcom Inc., 1973.

Robertson GL, Aycinena P. Neurogenic disorders of osmoregulation. *Am J Med* 1982;72:339–353.

Rose BD. *Clinical Physiology of Acid–Base and Electrolyte Disorders,* 4th ed. New York: McGraw-Hill, 1994:224.

Schrier RW. Pathogenesis of sodium and water retention, high-output and low-output cardiac failure, nephrotic syndrome, cirrhosis, and pregnancy. *N Engl J Med* 1988;319:1065–1072, 1127–1134.

Schrier RW, ed. *Renal and Electrolyte Disorders,* 4th ed. Philadelphia: Lippincott–Raven, 1997.

Sterns RH. Severe symptomatic hyponatremia: treatment and outcome. A study of 64 cases. *Ann Intern Med* 1987;107:656–664.

The Sea Within Us. Searle & Co. Monograph. New York: Science and Medicine Publishing, 1975.

Valtin H, Schafer JA. *Renal Function: Mechanisms Preserving Fluid and Solute Balance in Health,* 3rd ed. Boston: Little, Brown, 1995.

Chapter 50

Acid–Base Disorders

James M. Luther   Julia Breyer-Lewis

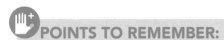
POINTS TO REMEMBER:

- Acidemia and alkalemia are descriptions of the patient's actual blood pH. *Acidosis* and *alkalosis* are descriptions of pathophysiological processes that, if unopposed, may lead to acidemia and alkalemia.

- Compensatory processes may return the ratio of the bicarbonate (HCO_3^-) and the partial pressure of carbon dioxide (PCO_2) back toward normal and thus help to normalize the arterial pH, but with the exception of chronic respiratory alkalosis (>2 weeks), the compensatory response never returns the pH completely to normal.

- In an uncomplicated high anion gap (AG) acidosis, for every 1 mmol rise in the AG, a concomitant fall of 1 mmol should occur in the HCO_3^- concentration. The difference between the patient's AG and a "normal" AG is called the *delta anion gap* (ΔAG).

- With the sole exception of chronic respiratory alkalosis, a normal pH value in the setting of an abnormal HCO_3^- or PCO_2 concentration signifies a mixed disturbance; compensation rarely corrects the pH to normal.

The human body possesses a complex and tightly regulated system to maintain pH within physiological limits. The acidity of body fluids is expressed in terms of the hydrogen ion concentration ($[H^+]$), which normally is 40 nEq/L. $[H^+]$ is expressed in terms of pH, which is by definition the negative $\log_{10}$ of $[H^+]$ (in mol/L). Figure 50.1 shows the relationship between the pH measured in a patient's blood and $[H^+]$, the two most commonly used units for specifying the level of acidity. The figure shows several important points:

- pH and $[H^+]$ are inversely related.
- A normal pH of 7.4 corresponds to $[H^+]$ of 40 nEq/L.
- A reasonably accurate estimate of $[H^+]$ concentration can be made from pH by exploiting the nearly linear relationship between pH and $[H^+]$ between pH 7.0 and 7.5. In

this pH range, $[H^+]$ changes by 1 nEq/L for each 0.01 U change in pH.

Estimating $[H^+]$ is important when performing calculations with acid–base data, particularly to establish the internal validity of the data. To illustrate the pH to $[H^+]$ relationship, given that a normal pH of 7.4 corresponds to a proton concentration of 40 nEq/L, if a patient's pH is 7.2, $[H^+]$ can be quickly estimated as follows:

$$\Delta pH = 7.40 - 7.20 = 0.20 \text{ units}$$
$$\Delta[H^+] = \Delta pH \cdot (1 \cdot nEq/L \cdot per \, 0.01 \, \Delta pH) = \Delta pH \cdot 100$$
$$= 0.2 \cdot 100 = 20 \, nEq/L$$

Therefore, $[H^+]$ at 7.2 = (40 + 20) nEq/L = 60 nEq/L

Another method that relates pH to $[H^+]$ compensates for the true curvilinear relationship between pH and $[H^+]$. Although slightly more complex than the preceding technique, this method is more accurate and works over a broader pH range. This method begins at the point at which pH = 7.40 and $[H^+]$ = 40 nEq/L and proceeds as follows:

- To calculate $[H^+]$ for each 0.1 pH decrement, sequentially multiply 40 nEq/L by 1.25.
- To calculate $[H^+]$ for each 0.1 pH increment, sequentially multiply 40 nEq/L by 0.8.

This relationship appears in Table 50.1.

ACID–BASE TERMINOLOGY

The principal terms in acid–base disorders are defined as:

- *Acidemia*, an increase in $[H^+]$ and a decrease in arterial pH
- *Alkalemia*, a decrease in $[H^+]$ and an increase in arterial pH
- *Acidosis*, a process that acidifies body fluids (i.e., lowers plasma HCO_3^-) and, if unopposed, leads to a fall in pH and acidemia
- *Alkalosis*, a process that alkalinizes body fluids (i.e., raises plasma HCO_3^-) and, if unopposed, leads to an increase in pH and an alkalemia

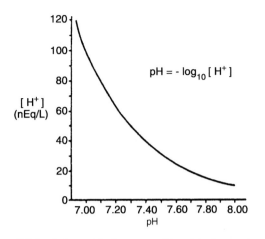

Figure 50.1 Relationship between pH and hydrogen ion concentration (H^+), the two most commonly used units for specifying the level of acidity. (H^+, hydrogen ion concentration.) (Reproduced with permission from Cohen JJ, Kassirer JP. Acid–base chemistry and buffering. In: Kassirer JP, ed. *Acid/Base*. Boston: Little, Brown, 1980:5.)

As serum pH falls below 7.35, a patient is said to be *acidemic*. Conversely, as the pH rises above 7.45, a patient is said to be *alkalemic*. Acidemia and alkalemia are descriptions of the patient's actual blood pH. *Acidosis* and *alkalosis* are descriptions of pathophysiological processes that, if unopposed, may lead to acidemia and alkalemia. In acidosis, the plasma HCO_3^- concentration may be below normal, whereas in alkalosis the plasma HCO_3^- concentration may

TABLE 50.1

RELATIONSHIP BETWEEN pH AND HYDROGEN ION CONCENTRATION

pH	Hydrogen Ion Concentration (nEq/L)
7.80	16
7.75	18
7.70	20
7.65	22
7.60	25
7.55	28
7.50	32
7.45	35
7.40	40
7.35	45
7.30	50
7.25	56
7.20	63
7.15	71
7.10	79
7.05	89
7.00	100
6.95	112
6.90	126
6.85	141
6.80	159

be above normal. For example, if a patient is vomiting, he or she will have a high HCO_3^- (32 mEq/L) and thus an alkalosis, but if at the same time the patient has respiratory failure and a high carbon dioxide (CO_2) pressure (PCO_2 >75 mm Hg), arterial pH actually may be in the acidemic range (e.g., pH 7.25).

THE BODY'S BUFFERS

Despite continuous acid production, the body maintains arterial pH within the narrow range of 7.35 to 7.45. Approximately 15,000 mEq of CO_2 are generated each day by tissue metabolism and are carried by hemoglobin (Hgb)-generated HCO_3^- or Hgb-bound carbamino groups to the lung for excretion as CO_2. Approximately 70 mEq acid per day (~1 mEq/kg per day) are generated as nonvolatile acids (mostly phosphoric and sulfuric acids) and excreted by the kidneys.

Daily acid production can be summarized as:

- 12,000 to 15,000 mEq of volatile acids are produced each day and excreted by the lungs as CO_2.
- 1 mEq/kg of nonvolatile acids are produced each day and excreted by the kidneys.
- pH of body fluids is determined by the acid produced, the buffering capacity, and the ability of the lungs and kidneys to excrete the load.

The latter is a clinically relevant fact. If a patient has renal failure and no longer can excrete the acid that is normally produced, the amount of HCO_3^- needed to buffer the daily acid produced is 1 mEq/kg. If the patient requires more HCO_3^- therapy than 1 mEq/kg to maintain the serum HCO_3^- at any given level, another process, in addition to renal failure, is likely to be contributing to the acidosis.

If an extra base or acid load is introduced, the body reacts with a complex system, composed of buffering and the activation of compensatory mechanisms. As shown in Figure 50.2, if an acid or base load is added, the first defense is extracellular buffering, followed by the intracellular and, more important, skeletal buffering. Skeletal bone represents an enormous reservoir of alkaline salts and serves as the major source for the body's buffer system. As compensation develops, the respiratory system modulates PCO_2, and lastly, the kidneys modulate the plasma HCO_3^- concentration.

Clinical acid–base chemistry is really the chemistry of the body's buffers. Simply stated, a *buffer* is a substance that can either absorb or donate protons to a solution. The most important buffer components in the extracellular fluid at physiologically relevant pH are Hgb, plasma proteins, and HCO_3^-. The principal buffering system for noncarbonic acid in the extracellular fluid is the HCO_3^- buffering system. Because all buffers behave as though they are in functional contact with a common pool of [H^+], the determination of one buffer pair reflects the states of all other buffer

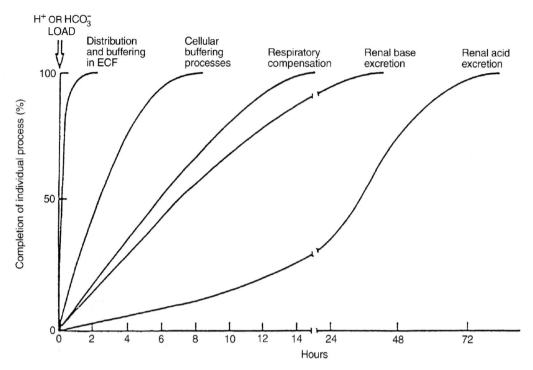

Figure 50.2   Time course for completion of acid–base compensatory mechanisms. (ECF, extracellular fluid; H⁺, hydrogen ion concentration.) (Reproduced with permission from Cogan MG, Rector FC, Seldin DW. Acid–base disorders in the kidney. In: Brenner BM, Rector FC, eds. *The Kidney.* Philadelphia: WB Saunders, 1981:841–907.)

pairs and also of the arterial pH. This relationship, termed the *isohydric principle*, shows that any alteration of $[H^+]$ results in parallel changes in the ratio of each buffer pair within any fluid compartment:

$$HA = H^+ + A^-$$

$$K_a = \frac{[H^+][A^-]}{[HA]}$$

$$[H^+] = \frac{K_1 H_2 CO_3}{HCO_3^-} = \frac{K_2 H_2 PO_4^-}{HPO_4} = \frac{KHgbH^+}{Hgb}$$

Clinically, when we assess a patient's acid–base status, we evaluate the carbonic acid (H_2CO_3)–HCO_3^- system because it can be measured easily. The most abundant extracellular buffer is HCO_3^-. Metabolically produced CO_2 is buffered in the red blood cells and provides the substrate for acid secretion in the kidney.

The PCO_2-HCO_3^- buffer system is reflected in the following formulas:

$$CO_2 \text{ gas} \rightarrow CO_2(\text{dissolved}) + H_2O \leftrightarrow H_2CO_3 + HCO_3^-$$

$$H^+ = \frac{KH_2CO_3}{HCO_3^+}$$

$$pH = pK_a + \frac{(\log[HCO_3^-])}{H_2CO_3}$$

$$[H_2CO_3^-] \sim 0.03 \, (PCO_2) \text{ (solubility coefficient)}$$

The chemical species comprising this buffer system are interrelated:

- Dissolved CO_2 is reversibly hydrated to H_2CO_3 in a slow reaction.
- H_2CO_3 is, therefore, a volatile acid because it is in equilibrium with the gaseous CO_2.
- H_2CO_3 dissociates spontaneously into H^+ and HCO_3^-.
- This equilibrium reaction can be expressed in terms of the Henderson-Hasselbalch equation because the pH equals the pK_a plus the log of the HCO_3^- concentration over the H_2CO_3 concentration.

H_2CO_3 is present in blood in such small quantities that it cannot be measured, but because H_2CO_3 is in equilibrium with the CO_2 in solution, and the dissolved CO_2 depends on the PCO_2 in the arterial blood, the H_2CO_3 term of the equation can be replaced by PCO_2 times the solubility coefficient (0.03). The Henderson-Hasselbalch equation follows:

$$pH = PK_a + \frac{\log[HCO_3^-]}{(0.03)PCO_2} = \frac{\text{kidney}}{\text{lung}} = \frac{\text{metabolic}}{\text{respiratory}}$$

$$7.4 = 6.1 + \frac{\log[24]}{(0.03)(40)}$$

Thus, the pH (i.e., $[H^+]$ of the blood) is determined by the ratio of the serum HCO_3^- concentration to the PCO_2 in the arterial blood. The HCO_3^- concentration is regulated by the kidney. Metabolic processes, such as metabolic acidosis and metabolic alkalosis, affect primarily the HCO_3^-

concentration of the blood. PCO_2 is regulated by ventilation, and respiratory acidosis and alkalosis are reflected in primary changes in the PCO_2.

The Henderson-Hasselbalch equation can be rearranged and simplified to form the following equation:

$$[H^+] = \frac{24 \times PCO_2}{[HCO_3^-]}$$

As noted previously, the $[H^+]$ is calculated from the pH, given that a pH of 7.4 equals an $[H^+]$ of 40 nEq/L and that there is a linear relationship between pH and $[H^+]$ between a pH of 7.1 and 7.5. Also noted, for every 0.01 change in pH, a 1 nEq/L change in $[H^+]$ concentration occurs. The advantage of using this simplified equation is that it facilitates the calculation of one unknown parameter from two known parameters. For example, if the plasma HCO_3^- concentration and the pH are known, the PCO_2 can be calculated. Also, this equation allows the validity of simultaneous laboratory measurements of pH, HCO_3^- concentration, and PCO_2 to be checked. When the reported HCO_3^- concentration and PCO_2 are entered into the right side of the equation, the equation should solve to equal the $[H^+]$ predicted by the arterial pH. If it does not, one of the reported values is wrong. Many an intern has agonized over an acid–base problem without first checking to see whether the numbers are consistent using this equation. Thus, the first step in analyzing acid–base problems is to verify internal consistency of the data.

SIMPLE ACID–BASE DISORDERS

Clinical disorders of acid–base equilibrium are classified according to which of the two variables, PCO_2 or HCO_3^- concentration, is directly affected by the primary pathological process:

- Clinical disorders initiated by a primary change in the HCO_3^- are referred to as *metabolic disorders*.
- Clinical disorders initiated by a change in the PCO_2 are referred to as *respiratory disorders*.

- Decreases in the plasma HCO_3^- result in metabolic acidosis, whereas increases in the plasma HCO_3^- result in metabolic alkalosis.
- *Hypercapnia*, an increase in the PCO_2, results in a respiratory acidosis; *hypocapnia* results in a respiratory alkalosis.

COMPENSATORY RESPONSES

In each of the four primary disturbances shown in Table 50.2, the initiating process not only alters the acid–base equilibrium directly, but it also sets in motion secondary compensatory responses that change the other member of the PCO_2-HCO_3^- pair:

- In metabolic acidosis, the primary disturbance is a decrease in the HCO_3^- level; the body, in an attempt to return the pH or $[H^+]$ to normal, induces a fall in PCO_2 (by means of hyperventilation) so that the ratio approaches normal.
- In metabolic alkalosis, the primary increase in HCO_3^- is compensated for by a decrease in ventilation and an increase in PCO_2.
- In respiratory acidosis, the compensatory response is an increase in the serum HCO_3^- level caused by decreased renal excretion of HCO_3^- and increased renal net acid excretion.
- In respiratory alkalosis, the primary decrease in PCO_2 is compensated by increased renal excretion of HCO_3^- and a resultant fall in serum HCO_3^-.

By remembering the basic principles relating PCO_2 and HCO_3^- to pH or $[H^+]$ and that the body's goal is to maintain a nearly normal pH, all these clinical compensatory responses can be predicted. If only one of these primary processes is present, the patient has a simple acid–base disturbance with an appropriate compensatory response. Conversely, if two or more primary abnormalities are present, the patient is said to have a mixed acid–base disorder. For example, a patient may have a heart attack, become hypotensive, underperfuse his or her organs, and develop a metabolic acidosis as a result of the accumulation of lactic

TABLE 50.2

THE FOUR PRIMARY ACID–BASE DISTURBANCES

Type of Disturbance	Primary Alteration	Compensatory Response	Mechanism of Compensatory Response
Metabolic acidosis	↓ Plasma $[HCO_3^-]$	↓ $PaCO_2$	Hyperventilation
Metabolic alkalosis	↑ Plasma $[HCO_3^-]$	↑ $PaCO_2$	Hypoventilation
Respiratory acidosis	↑ $PaCO_2$	↑ Plasma $[HCO_3^-]$	↑ HCO_3^- reabsorption by the kidney
Respiratory alkalosis	↓ $PaCO_2$	↓ Plasma $[HCO_3^-]$	↓ HCO_3^- reabsorption by the kidney

HCO_3^-; bicarbonate; $PaCO_2$, concentration of carbon dioxide in arterial blood.

acid, but this patient also may have pneumonia, respiratory failure, and a respiratory acidosis. This patient is said to have a mixed acid–base disorder with two primary processes.

The role of compensatory processes can be summarized as:

- These processes may return the ratio of HCO_3^- to PCO_2 back toward normal and thus help normalize the arterial pH.
- Compensation, with one exception (chronic respiratory alkalosis), never returns the pH fully back to normal.
- Compensatory responses require normally functioning lungs and kidneys and take time to occur.
- The lack of compensation in an appropriate interval defines the presence of a second primary disorder.
- The compensatory response creates a second laboratory abnormality.
- The appropriate degree of compensation can be predicted.

Compensatory processes may return the ratio of the HCO_3^- and PCO_2 back toward normal and thus help to normalize the arterial pH, but with the exception of chronic respiratory alkalosis (>2 weeks), the compensatory response never returns the pH completely to normal. For example, if a patient has a metabolic acidosis, and thus a low serum HCO_3^-, the compensatory response of a decrease in the PCO_2 raises the arterial pH. The patient is still acidemic, however; that is, the arterial pH remains below 7.35. The primary process can be determined by looking at the arterial blood gas levels and deciding whether the HCO_3^- or the PCO_2 has moved in the right direction to lead to that change in pH. In our example of simple metabolic acidosis, the patient is acidemic because the fall in the HCO_3^- (the primary process) produces the fall in pH. Although the compensatory fall in PCO_2 increases the pH, it does not return it to normal and is clearly a secondary event. One exception to this rule is chronic respiratory alkalosis for more than 2 weeks: The compensatory fall in HCO_3^- may return the pH to normal. The primary disorder in this setting must be determined by history.

Compensatory responses require normally functioning kidneys and lungs. A patient with significant renal failure cannot develop full metabolic compensation to a primary respiratory disorder. Similarly, a patient on a ventilator whose respiratory rate is mechanically controlled cannot develop a compensatory respiratory response. Compensatory responses take up to 12 to 24 hours to develop fully. Thus, it cannot be said that a patient has failed to compensate if he or she has not yet had time to do so. If an appropriate amount of time has passed and an adequate compensatory response has not developed, this failure defines the presence of a second primary disorder. A clinical example of this situation could be the patient with diabetic ketoacidosis and severe metabolic acidosis who is obtunded. If the arterial blood gas shows a pH of 7.10, PCO_2 of 30,

and HCO_3^- concentration of 9 mEq/L, it can be concluded that the respiratory compensation, although present, is incomplete. Thus, the patient has a mixed acid–base disorder consisting of metabolic and respiratory acidosis.

Finally, the limits of appropriate metabolic compensation (change in HCO_3^-) for any given degree of primary respiratory acidosis or alkalosis, as well as the limits of respiratory compensation (change in PCO_2) for a given degree of primary metabolic acidosis or alkalosis, have been defined. A PCO_2 that lies outside these limits in a patient with a primary metabolic disorder defines a coexistent respiratory disorder. Similarly, an HCO_3^- that lies outside the expected limits of compensation in a patient with a primary respiratory disorder defines a coexistent metabolic disorder. Nomograms such as that shown in Figure 50.3 (which shows 95% confidence limits of compensations for primary "simple" acid–base disturbances) plot the HCO_3^-, pH, and PCO_2 values expected in primary acid–base disorders. Points within the starlike figure are consistent with, but not diagnostic of, a simple acid–base disorder with a single primary disorder and appropriate compensation. Mixed acid–base disorders that include more than one primary acid–base abnormality have values that fall within the starlike figure between two or three contributing acid–base disorders. It should be noted that values falling outside the starlike figure generally predict a mixed disorder, but values that fall within the starlike figure, although usually representing simple disorders, can result from coincidental mixed disturbances. The mild alkalemia shown in the area of pure chronic respiratory acidosis and the nearly consistent hypercapnia with metabolic alkalosis are still somewhat controversial.

One should not rely exclusively on nomograms. Rather, the degree of compensation and its appropriateness can be calculated using equations that predict the expected degree of compensation (Table 50.3). The most useful, and most often used, equation is the expected respiratory compensation in metabolic acidosis. Note that the degree of compensation in respiratory acidosis and alkalosis varies depending on whether the primary process is acute or chronic.

PRIMARY ACID–BASE DISORDERS

Metabolic Acidosis

A summary of the key information concerning metabolic acidosis includes:

- *Definition:* Begins with a fall in serum HCO_3^- due to accumulation of nonvolatile acids
- *Primary defect:* A fall in HCO_3^-; accumulation of metabolic acids is caused by
  - Excess acid production that overwhelms renal capacity for excretion (e.g., diabetic ketoacidosis, lactic acidosis)
  - Loss of alkali, leaving unneutralized acid behind (e.g., diarrhea)

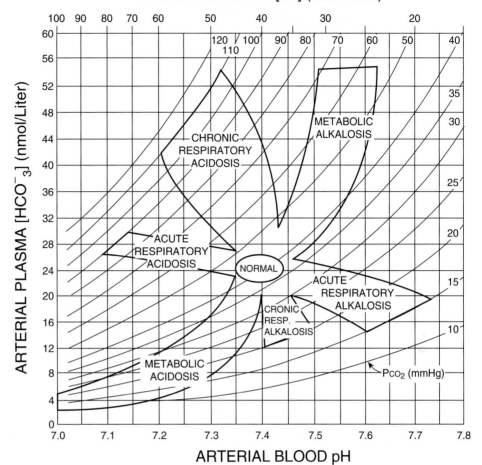

Figure 50.3 Acid–base nomogram. To predict the pH change with changes in the $[HCO_3^-]$ or PCO_2, trace along the diagonal lines for changes in $[HCO_3^-]$ with constant PCO_2; trace along the horizontal lines for changes in PCO_2 with constant $[HCO_3^-]$. (HCO_3^-, bicarbonate; H^+, hydrogen ion concentration.) (Reproduced with permission from Cogan MG, Rector FC Jr, Seldin DW, et al. Acid–base disorders. In: Brenner BM, Rector FC, eds. *The Kidney.* Philadelphia: WB Saunders, 1981:860.)

- Renal excretory failure: normal total acid production in the face of poor renal function (e.g., chronic renal failure of any cause)
- *Compensatory change:*
  - Tissues and red blood cells act to increase serum HCO_3^- by exchanging intracellular Na^+ and K^+ for extracellular H^+, raising serum HCO_3^- and K^+

- *Respiratory alkalosis:* ventilation increases, producing a fall in PCO_2 that brings pH back toward normal.

Before the causes of metabolic acidosis can be discussed further, the AG must be reviewed. Total serum anions include chloride and HCO_3^-, as well as the unmeasured anions (UA^-). Total anions equal the total cations in blood, which include sodium and unmeasured cations (UC^+). The

TABLE 50.3

EXPECTED COMPENSATORY CHANGES IN SIMPLE ACID–BASE DISORDERS

Primary Disorder	Compensatory Change[a]	
	Acute (24 hours)	**Chronic (23 days)**
Metabolic acidosis	$PCO_2 = 1.5\,[HCO_3^-] + 8 \pm 2$	Same
	PCO_2 = Last 2 digits of the pH	
Metabolic alkalosis	$PCO_2 = 40 + 0.6\,(\Delta[HCO_3^-])$	Same
Respiratory acidosis	$\uparrow \Delta[HCO_3^-] = \Delta[HCO_3^-]/10$	$\uparrow \Delta[HCO_3^-] = 3.5 \times \Delta PCO_2/10$
Respiratory alkalosis	$\downarrow \Delta[HCO_3^-] = 2 \times \Delta PCO_2/10$	$\downarrow \Delta[HCO_3^-] = 5 \times \Delta PCO_2/10$

HCO_3^-, bicarbonate; PCO_2, partial pressure of carbon dioxide.
[a]Note that some equations give the answers in terms of the change in the plasma measurement (e.g., $\Delta[HCO_3^-]$, ΔPCO_2), whereas other equations give the absolute value of the measurement (e.g., PCO_2).

TABLE 50.4

CAUSES OF ANION GAP CHANGES

Causes of decreased anion gap	*Causes of increased anion gap*
Increased UC$^+$	Decreased UC$^+$
Increased normally present cation	Hypokalemia
Hyperkalemia	Hypocalcemia
Hypercalcemia	Hypomagnesemia
Hypermagnesemia	Increased UA$^-$
Polyclonal gammopathy	Organic anions
Multiple myeloma (IgG)	Lactate
Retention of abnormal cation	Ketone acids
γ-Globulin	Inorganic anions
Tromethamine (TRIS) buffer	Phosphate
Lithium	Sulfate
Decreased UA$^-$	Proteins
Hypoalbuminemia	Hyperalbuminemia
Laboratory error	Exogenous anions
Systemic error	Salicylate
Hyponatremia due to viscous serum	Formate
Hyperchloremia due to bromide	Nitrate
Random error	Penicillin, carbenicillin, etc.
Falsely decreased serum sodium	Incompletely identified
Falsely increased serum Cl$^-$ or HCO$_3^-$	Paraldehyde poisoning
	Ethylene glycol poisoning
	Methanol poisoning
	Salicylate poisoning
	Uremia
	Hyperosmolar hyperglycemic nonketotic coma
	Laboratory error
	Falsely elevated sodium
	Falsely decreased serum Cl$^-$ or HCO$_3^-$

Cl$^-$, chlorine; HCO$_3^-$, bicarbonate; IgG, immunoglobulin G; UA$^-$, unmeasured anion; UC$^+$, unmeasured cation.

UA$^-$ in healthy persons exceed the UC$^+$, a difference called the *anion gap*, which can be estimated by subtracting the sum of the chloride and HCO$_3^-$ concentrations from the sodium concentration, as shown in the following equations:

$$UA^- + Cl^- + HCO_3^- = Na^+ + UC^+$$
$$AG = UA - UC = Na^+ - (Cl^- + HCO_3^-) = 12$$

In a healthy state, the value is approximately 12 but varies between clinical laboratories. The AG can be increased because of a decrease in UC$^+$, an increase in UA$^-$, or laboratory error in the measurement of Na$^+$, Cl$^-$, or HCO$_3^-$ (Table 50.4). The most common clinical scenario producing a low AG is hypoalbuminemia.

Metabolic acidosis is frequently associated with an increased AG. In fact, metabolic acidoses are categorized clinically by the presence or absence of an abnormally elevated AG. In a high AG acidosis, the proton that titrates HCO$_3^-$ is accompanied by a UA$^-$, resulting in the accumulation of that anion in the blood and a high AG acidosis (Fig. 50.4). If the anion accompanying H$^+$ is chloride, the patient has a metabolic acidosis with a normal AG because the fall in HCO$_3^-$ is matched by an increase in chloride. By definition, this is a hyperchloremic (or non-AG) acidosis. For example, a patient can have a loss of HCO$_3^-$ in the stool due to diarrhea, with an increase in chloride secondary to volume depletion. The result is a normal AG acidosis or hyperchloremic acidosis. Clinically, the AG should be calculated for every patient each time a set of electrolytes is drawn (Fig. 50.5).

The causes of high AG metabolic acidosis include:

- Methanol toxicity
- Uremia
- Ketoacidosis (diabetic or alcoholic)
- Paraldehyde toxicity
- Isoniazid (INH)
- Lactic acidosis

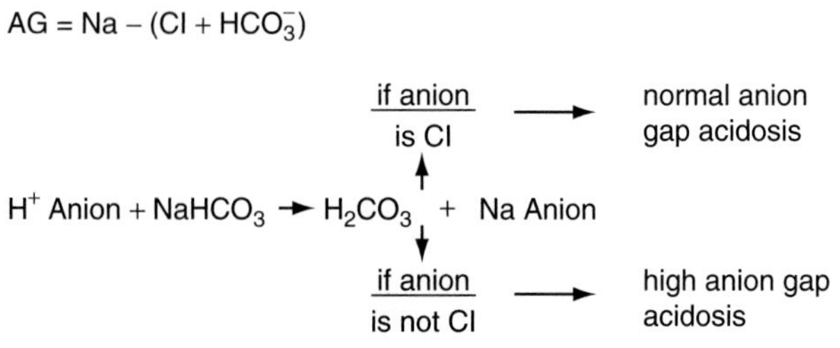

$$AG = Na - (Cl + HCO_3^-)$$

Figure 50.4   Anion gap in metabolic acidosis.

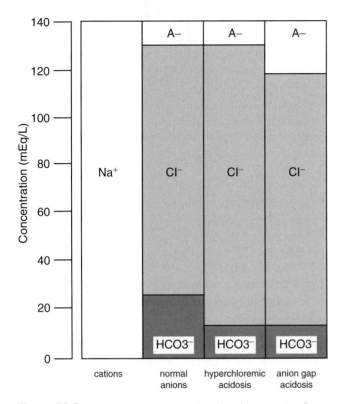

Figure 50.5 The anion gap. (Reproduced with permission from Breyer MD, Jacobson HR. Approach to the patient with metabolic acidosis or metabolic alkalosis. In: Kelley W, ed. *Textbook of Internal Medicine*. Philadelphia: WB Saunders, 1989:923.)

- Ethylene glycol toxicity
- Massive rhabdomyolysis
- Salicylate toxicity

If a patient has an elevated AG, lactic acidosis and ketoacidosis are the most common causes. The serum levels or titers of these organic anions can be measured. Intoxica-

tions with aspirin, antifreeze, methanol, or paraldehyde also can cause an AG acidosis and should be considered (Fig. 50.6), especially in an unconscious patient. Appropriate clinical scenarios should prompt the consideration of poisoning with methanol (blindness), INH (seizures), or ethylene glycol (calcium oxalate crystalluria).

If poisoning is suspected, or the cause of an elevated AG is not immediately apparent, a serum osmolal gap should be determined as a screen for methanol or ethylene glycol intoxication. The osmolal gap is the difference between the *measured* serum osmolality and the *calculated* (or expected) osmolality based on the primary plasma solutes. The osmolal gap is calculated as follows:

$$\text{Calculated osmolality} = \text{Osm}_{calc} = 2 \cdot [\text{Na}^+]$$
$$+ (\text{glucose}/18) + (\text{BUN}/2.8) + (\text{ethanol}/4.6)$$
$$\text{Osmolal gap} = \text{Osm}_{meas} - \text{Osm}_{calc}$$

Note that $[\text{Na}^+]$ is measured in mEq/L, while [glucose], blood urea nitrogen (BUN), and [ethanol] are expressed in mg/dL. The osmolal gap normally is <10 mOsm/L. If the measurement of a specific toxin is available, then its osmotic contribution can be determined by dividing by the appropriate denominator to convert from mg/dL to mosmol/L (ethanol 4.6, methanol 3.2, ethylene glycol 6.2, acetone 5.8, isopropanol 6.0). If the addition of this measurement to the calculated osmolality does not correct the osmolal gap, then an additional substance should be considered. It should be noted that the osmolal gap is insensitive in late presentations of ethylene glycol or methanol ingestion, as these substances are converted into negatively charged metabolites that are accompanied by Na^+. Therefore, it is accounted for by the $2[\text{Na}^+]$ term in the osmolal gap calculation and does not result in an elevation in the osmolal gap.

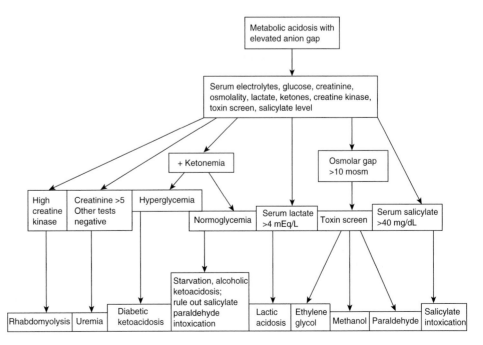

Figure 50.6 Diagnostic algorithm for metabolic acidosis with elevated anion gap. (Reproduced with permission from Breyer MD, Jacobson HR. Approach to the patient with metabolic acidosis or metabolic alkalosis. In: Kelley WN, ed. *Textbook of Internal Medicine*. Philadelphia: WB Saunders, 1989: 926.)

TABLE 50.5

CAUSES OF HYPERCHLOREMIC METABOLIC ACIDOSIS

Hypokalemic
  Proximal renal tubular acidosis, drug induced:
    Acetazolamide, coumarin, mafenide (Sulfamylon)
  Distal renal tubular acidosis
  Posthypocapnea
  Diarrhea
  Ureterosigmoidostomy/Ileal loop
  Pancreatic fistula/Biliary drainage
  Correction phase of diabetic ketoacidosis

Hyperkalemic/Normokalemic
  Type IV renal tubular acidosis:
    Interstitial nephritis, hypoaldosteronism, urinary obstruction
  Hydrochloric acid ingestions/Infusions:
    Hyperalimentation, cholestyramine, $CaCl_2$, NH_4Cl
  Dilutional acidosis

Causes of an elevated osmolal gap include:

- Ethanol
- Diethylene glycol
- Ethylene glycol
- Propylene glycol
- Methanol
- Formaldehyde
- Chronic renal failure (unidentified osmoles)
- Paraldehyde
- Ketoacids (diabetic or alcoholic)
- Lactic acid

Isopropanol and mannitol may also increase the osmolal gap without a concomitant AG acidosis. Severe hyperproteinemia or hyperlipidemia can artificially cause an increase in the osmolal gap by causing pseudohyponatremia.

When a patient has an increased AG, most anions that account for this gap are associated with a single proton. In an uncomplicated high AG acidosis, for every 1 mmol rise in the AG, a concomitant fall of 1 mmol should occur in the HCO_3^- concentration. The difference between the patient's AG and a "normal" AG is called the *delta anion gap*. The ΔAG and ΔHCO_3^- are calculated by the following formulas:

$$\Delta AG = Observed\,AG - Upper\,normal\,AG$$
$$\Delta HCO_3^- = Lower\,normal\,HCO_3^- - Observed\,HCO_3^-$$

For example, a patient with an AG of 20 has a $\Delta AG = 20 - 12 = 8$. The eight UA^- would account for a decrease in the serum HCO_3^- concentration of 8 mmol. When the ΔAG is added back to the $[HCO_3^-]$, this should equal ~24 mEq/L. Any significant deviation from this rule implies the

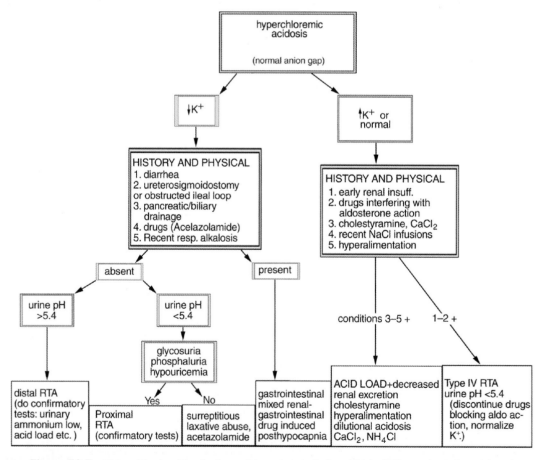

Figure 50.7 Diagnostic algorithm for hyperchloremic metabolic acidosis. (RTA, renal tubular acidosis.)

TABLE 50.6

URINARY CHLORIDE CONCENTRATION IN METABOLIC ALKALOSIS

Less than 20 mEq/L	*Greater than 30 mEq/L*
Vomiting	Primary hyperaldosteronism
Nasogastric suction	Cushing syndrome: Adrenal, ectopic ACTH-producing tumor, pituitary
Chloride wasting diarrhea	Exogenous steroid (licorice, glucocorticoid, carbenoxalone)
Colonic villous adenoma	Adrenal 11- or 17-hydroxylase defects
Diuretic therapy (remote ingestion)	Liddle syndrome
Posthypercapnia	Bartter syndrome
Poorly reabsorbed anions	K^+ and Mg^{2+} deficiency
Glucose refeeding	Milk-alkali syndrome

ACTH, adrenocorticotropic hormone.

existence of a mixed acid–base disorder. When the ΔHCO_3^- is greater than the ΔAG ($\Delta HCO_3^- > \Delta AG$), two possible situations exist if laboratory error is excluded. Most commonly, either a mixed high AG and normal AG acidosis is present, or a mixed high AG acidosis and "chronic" respiratory alkalosis with a compensating hyperchloremic acidosis is present. Conversely, when the AG is greater than the ΔHCO_3^- ($\Delta AG > \Delta HCO_3^-$), a mixed high AG acidosis and primary metabolic alkalosis almost always is present.

The presence of a hyperchloremic or normal AG acidosis suggests a completely different set of diagnoses, including renal tubular acidosis, diarrhea, ileal conduits, and HCl

ingestions (Table 50.5). The diagnostic algorithm appears in Figure 50.7. In patients with a hyperchloremic metabolic acidosis, the urine anion gap (UAG) can be used to distinguish whether the cause of the acidosis is a renal tubular defect or other causes, such as diarrhea. The UAG is calculated as follows:

$$UAG = (Urine\ Na^+ + Urine\ K^+) - (Urine\ Cl^-)$$

Because ammonium is excreted in the urine along with chloride, this index can be used to estimate the concentration of ammonium in the urine in a patient with hyperchloremic metabolic acidosis. A negative UAG

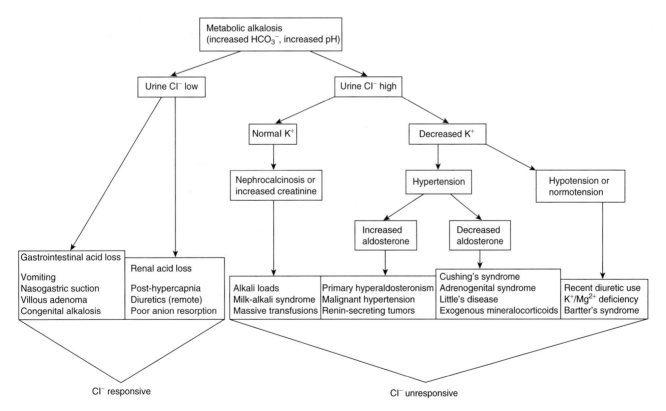

Figure 50.8 Diagnostic algorithm for metabolic alkalosis. (Reproduced with permission from Breyer MD, Jacobson HR. Approach to the patient with metabolic acidosis or metabolic alkalosis. In: Kelley WN, ed. *Textbook of Internal Medicine.* Philadelphia: WB Saunders, 1989:932.)

$(Cl^- > Na^+ + K^+)$ suggests the appropriate excretion of ammonium in the urine with Cl^- and the presence of gastrointestinal loss of HCO_3^-. A positive UAG $(Cl^- < Na^+ + K^+)$ suggests the presence of a renal tubular acidosis with a distal acidification defect and inadequate ammonium excretion in the urine.

Metabolic Alkalosis

A summary of the key information concerning metabolic alkalosis includes:

- *Definition:* A rise in the concentration of serum HCO_3^-
- *Primary defect:* A rise in serum HCO_3^-, with two requirements:
  - New HCO_3^- must be added to the blood from renal or extrarenal sources (the process of generation).
  - The kidney must increase its net resorptive capacity to maintain the higher level of serum $[HCO_3^-]$. The stimuli that increase renal HCO_3^- resorption are high PCO_2, extracellular fluid contraction, Cl^- depletion, steroid excess, and K^+ depletion.

- *Compensatory change:*
  - Tissues and red blood cells act to lower serum HCO_3^- by exchanging intracellular H^+ for extracellular K^+ and Na^+, lowering both serum HCO_3^- and K^+.
  - Alkalosis tends to cause hypoventilation and elevation of PCO_2 (respiratory acidosis). Compensation for alkalosis is more erratic than for acidosis; generally, PCO_2 remains <55 mmHg.

The causes of metabolic alkalosis can be divided into those associated with a high urinary excretion of chloride and those associated with a low excretion of chloride and, therefore, responsive to saline administration (Table 50.6 and Fig. 50.8).

Respiratory Acidosis

A summary of the key information concerning respiratory acidosis includes:

- *Definition:* Decreases pulmonary clearance of CO_2
- *Primary defect:* Increases PCO_2
- *Compensatory change:*
  - In acute syndromes, tissues and red blood cells generate HCO_3^- by taking up H^+ in exchange for Na^+ and K^+. This acts to increase serum HCO_3^- and K^+. In chronic syndromes, renal HCO_3^- synthesis further augments serum HCO_3^-.

TABLE 50.7

CAUSES OF RESPIRATORY ACIDOSIS

Acute
- Airway obstruction: Aspiration of foreign body or vomitus, laryngospasm, generalized bronchospasm, obstructive sleep apnea
- Respiratory center depression: General anesthesia, sedative overdosage, cerebral trauma or infarction, central sleep apnea
- Circulatory catastrophes: Cardiac arrest, severe pulmonary edema
- Neuromuscular defects: High cervical cordotomy, botulism, tetanus, Guillain-Barré syndrome, crisis in myasthenia gravis, familial hypokalemic periodic paralysis, hypokalemic myopathy, drugs of toxic agents (e.g., curare, succinylcholine, aminoglycosides, organophosphorus)
- Restrictive defects: Pneumothorax, hemothorax, flail chest, severe pneumonitis, infant respiratory distress syndrome (hyaline membrane disease), adult respiratory distress syndrome
- Mechanical ventilators

Chronic
- Airway obstruction: Chronic obstructive lung disease (bronchitis, emphysema)
- Respiratory center depression: Chronic sedative depression, primary alveolar hypoventilation (Ondine curse), obesity hypoventilation syndrome (pickwickian syndrome), brain tumor, bulbar poliomyelitis
- Neuromuscular defects: Poliomyelitis, multiple sclerosis, muscular dystrophy, amyotrophic lateral sclerosis, diaphragmatic paralysis, myxedema, myopathic disease (e.g., polymyositis, acid maltase deficiency)
- Restrictive defects: Kyphoscoliosis, spinal arthritis, fibrothorax, hydrothorax interstitial fibrosis, decreased diaphragmatic movement (e.g., ascites), prolonged pneumonitis, obesity

---

TABLE 50.8

CAUSES OF RESPIRATORY ALKALOSIS

Hypoxia
  Decreased inspired oxygen tension
  Ventilation–perfusion inequality
  Hypotension
  Severe anemia

Central nervous system mediated
  Voluntary hyperventilation
  Neurologic disease: Cerebrovascular accident (infarction, hemorrhage), infection (encephalitis, meningitis), trauma, tumor
  Pharmacologic and hormonal stimulation: Salicylates, dinitrophenol, nicotine, xanthines, pressor hormones, pregnancy
  Hepatic failure
  Gram-negative septicemia
  Postmetabolic acidosis
  Anxiety hyperventilation syndrome
  Heat exposure

Pulmonary disease
  Interstitial lung disease
  Pneumonia
  Pulmonary embolism
  Pulmonary edema
  Mechanical overventilation

Reproduced with permission from Cohen JJ, Kassirer JP. Acid–base chemistry and buffering. In: Kassirer JP, ed. *Acid/Base*. Boston: Little, Brown, 1980:361.

TABLE 50.9

SYNDROMES COMMONLY ASSOCIATED WITH MIXED ACID–BASE DISORDERS

Clinical Syndrome	Metabolic Alkalosis	Metabolic Acidosis	Respiratory Alkalosis	Respiratory Acidosis
Cardiopulmonary arrest	T	+	T	+
Severe pulmonary edema		+		+
Ethylene glycol + pulmonary edema		+		+
Methanol + hypoventilation		+		+
Severe hypophosphatemia		+		+
Recent alcohol binge	V	+	+	
Sepsis		+	+	
Severe liver failure	V/D	+	+	
Salicylate intoxication		+	+	
Pregnancy	V		+	
Renal failure	V	+		
Diabetic ketoacidosis	V	+		
Chronic obstructive pulmonary disease	D			+
Severe hypokalemia	+			+
Critically ill patients	V/D	+	+	+

+, syndrome is present; D, diuretics; T, treatment induced; V, vomiting.
Note: Above are some clinical syndromes in which mixed acid–base disturbances are commonly seen. If metabolic alkalosis from vomiting or diuretics is frequently seen in these disorders, this is denoted by "V" or "D." Adapted from Cohen JJ, Kassirer JP. Clinical evaluation of acid–base disorders. In: Cohen JJ, Kassirer JP, ed. *Acid/Base.* Boston: Little, Brown, 1982:405.)

- Acute respiratory acidosis: duration <24 hours; no time for renal compensation. Tissue and red blood cells elevate serum HCO_3^- >4 mEq/L, even with high PCO_2. It is rare to see serum HCO_3^- >31 mEq/L in acute respiratory acidosis.
- Chronic respiratory acidosis: duration >24 hours; serum HCO_3^- rises further as a result of compensatory HCO_3^- synthesis. The elevated PCO_2 stimulates renal tubular H^+ secretion and ammonia production. More acid is excreted; more HCO_3^- is synthesized and returned to the blood (metabolic alkalosis). The high PCO_2 also allows the kidney to reclaim new HCO_3^- when filtered at the glomerulus. Chloride excreted with NH_4^+ acts to lower serum chloride.

The causes of respiratory acidosis are summarized in Table 50.7.

Respiratory Alkalosis

A summary of the key information concerning respiratory alkalosis includes:

- *Definition:* Increased pulmonary clearance of CO_2
- *Primary defect:* Fall in PCO_2
  - *Compensatory change:* Acute respiratory alkalosis; duration <24 hours. No renal compensation acutely. By exchanging intracellular H^+ for extracellular Na^+ and K^+, tissue and red blood cells act to lower HCO_3^-,

which rarely falls below 15 mEq/L, and K^+. Metabolic acid production (lactate) increases slightly.
- Chronic respiratory alkalosis: Chronic alkalosis impairs the kidney's ability to excrete acid. Retained acid further lowers serum HCO_3^- (metabolic acidosis), resulting in more complete compensation. Duration <2 weeks is associated with alkalemia, but longer duration may elicit normal pH. This is the only acid–base disturbance compensation in which pH may return to normal.

The causes of respiratory alkalosis are listed in Table 50.8. Table 50.9 contains common clinical situations in which

TABLE 50.10

DISORDERS OF SERUM CHLORIDE CONCENTRATION

Hyperchloremia
Proportionate increase in chloride and sodium
  Dehydration
Disproportionate increase in chloride compared with sodium
  Hyperchloremic metabolic acidosis
  Renal compensation for primary respiratory alkalosis

Hypochloremia
Proportionate decrease in chloride and sodium
  Overhydration
Disproportionate decrease in chloride compared with sodium
  Metabolic alkalosis
  Renal compensation for primary respiratory acidosis

TABLE 50.11

REPRESENTATIVE EXAMPLES OF MIXED ACID–BASE DISORDERS

Type of Mixed Disorder	Example Number	Illustrative		Laboratory		K⁺ (mEq/L)	Profile		Clinical Circumstance
		pH	PaCO₂ (mm Hg)	HCO₃⁻	Na⁺		Cl	Anion Gap[a]	
Metabolic acidosis and respiratory acidosis	1	7.10	50	15	140	5.0	102	23	Renal failure and hypercapnic respiratory failure
	2	6.99	34	8	141	6.0	105	28	Cardiopulmonary arrest
Metabolic alkalosis and respiratory alkalosis	3	7.69	30	35	134	4.0	84	15	Hepatic failure and nasogastric suction
	4	7.60	40	38	131	3.6	77	16	Congestive heart failure and diuretics
Metabolic alkalosis and respiratory acidosis	5	7.44	55	36	135	3.8	84	15	COPD and diuretics
	6	7.45	48	32	133	4.2	85	16	Adult respiratory distress syndrome and acetate-rich total parenteral nutrition
Metabolic acidosis and respiratory alkalosis	7	7.44	12	8	136	5.5	106	22	Renal failure and Gram-negative septicemia
	8	7.40	15	9	138	4.1	110	19	Salicylate intoxication
Metabolic acidosis and metabolic alkalosis	9	7.43	39	25	132	3.7	84	23	Alcoholic liver disease and diuretics
	10	7.37	35	20	138	4.0	93	25	Diabetic ketoacidosis after NaHCO₃ therapy
Respiratory acidosis	11	7.54	41	34	140	3.8	93	13	COPD under mechanical ventilation
	12	7.68	28	32	137	3.5	91	14	COPD under mechanical ventilation
Respiratory acidosis, metabolic acidosis, and metabolic alkalosis	13	7.38	57	33	134	4.7	77	24	COPD, diuretics, and shock
Respiratory alkalosis, metabolic acidosis, and metabolic alkalosis	14	7.43	25	16	135	3.2	97	22	Congestive heart failure, diuretics, and shock
Hyperchloremic and high AG metabolic acidosis	15	7.12	16	5	137	3.6	114	18	Diabetic ketoacidosis with adequate salt and water balance
Acute or chronic respiratory acidosis	16	7.22	80	32	141	4.3	99	10	COPD and therapy with oxygen-rich mixtures
Acute or chronic respiratory alkalosis	17	7.54	12	10	132	3.2	107	15	Alcoholic liver disease and cerebral bleeding
Acute or chronic respiratory acidosis and metabolic acidosis	18	7.09	65	19	136	3.3	105	12	COPD and diarrhea
Mixed high AG metabolic acidosis and respiratory acidosis	19	7.18	44	16	133	5.7	100	17	Hepatic, renal, and pulmonary failure
Mixed high AG metabolic acidosis and metabolic alkalosis	20	7.36	31	17	132	4.0	89	26	Alcoholic liver disease, vomiting, and lactic acidosis
	21	7.40	40	24	143	5.5	95	24	Diabetic ketoacidosis and lactic acidosis after HCO₃⁻ therapy

AG, anion gap; Cl, chlorine; COPD, chronic obstructive pulmonary disease; HCO₃⁻, bicarbonate; K⁺, potassium; Na⁺, sodium; PaCO₂, concentration of carbon dioxide in arterial blood.

[a]AG is calculated as $[Na^+] - [Cl^-] - [HCO_3^-]$.

more than one primary acid–base problem presents (i.e., a mixed disorder).

MIXED ACID–BASE DISORDERS

A few clues may be helpful in assessing the presence of a mixed acid–base disturbance:

- Normal pH (with the exception of respiratory alkalosis): With the sole exception of chronic respiratory alkalosis, a normal pH value in the setting of an abnormal PCO_2 or HCO_3^- concentration signifies a mixed disturbance; compensation rarely corrects the pH to normal. The more severe the primary disorder, the less effective the compensatory mechanism at returning the pH to normal.
- PCO_2 and HCO_3^- deviating in opposite directions: The PCO_2 and serum HCO_3^- concentration always deviate in the same direction in simple acid–base disorders. If they deviate in opposite directions, a mixed abnormality is present.
- A pH change in the opposite direction for a known primary disorder: A pH change in the opposite direction to that predicted for a known primary disorder signifies a mixed disturbance (e.g., pH is 7.24, while $[HCO_3^-]$ is 30 mEq/L).

The chloride and potassium concentrations also can provide clues to the underlying acid–base disorder. If the chloride concentration changes in proportion to sodium, it reflects a change in hydration (Table 50.10). If chloride changes in excess of serum sodium, however, the cause is an acid–base disorder, with hyperchloremia suggesting an acidosis and hypochloremia suggesting an alkalosis. Similarly, in a general sense, hyperkalemia is associated with acidosis, and hypokalemia is associated with alkalosis.

The approach to the patient with acid–base disorder is summarized as follows:

- Take a careful history: vomiting, diabetes, diarrhea, ingestion of toxin, and sepsis.
- Perform a thorough physical examination: fever, signs of volume depletion, respiratory rate and pattern, blood pressure.
- Determine electrolytes: Na^+, K^+, Cl^-, HCO_3^-.
- Check the internal consistencies of arterial blood gases.
- Determine if the pH is acidemic or alkalemic.
- Determine if the primary disorder is metabolic or respiratory (acidosis or alkalosis).
- Check for adequate compensation.
- Calculate the AG and ΔAG:
  - Note that $\Delta AG = \Delta HCO_3^-$ in a simple disorder.
- Look for clues of mixed disorder (Table 50.11).
- Check nonelectrolyte laboratory results: creatinine (renal failure), glucose (diabetes), hematocrit (volume depletion), ketones, and lactate.

REVIEW EXERCISES

QUESTIONS

1. A 55-year-old white man with type 2 diabetes mellitus and diabetic nephropathy presents to the emergency department for evaluation of malaise and fatigue. He had previously been healthy and recently started on an additional medication to control his diabetes. His laboratory work reveals the following:

Na^+: 140 mEq/L
K^+: 5.5 mEq/L
Cl^-: 104 mEq/L
HCO_3^-: 14 mEq/L
Glucose: 180 mg/dL
BUN: 56 mg/dL
Creatinine: 3.0 mg/dL
Arterial pH: 7.31
PCO_2: 28 mm Hg
Urine ketones: Trace+
Lactate: 10 mEq/L
Serum osmolality: 315 mOsm/L
Urinalysis: No crystals

Which of the following is the most likely scenario?
a) Diabetic ketoacidosis
b) Proximal renal tubular acidosis
c) Metformin-induced lactic acidosis
d) Ethylene glycol intoxication
e) Isopropanol ingestion

Answer and Discussion

The answer is c. The approach to all acid–base questions should involve the following steps:

1. Are the data internally consistent?

$$\text{Predicted } [H^+] \text{ (nEq/L)} = 24 \cdot PCO_2/[HCO_3^-]$$
$$= 24 \cdot 28/14 = 48 \text{ nEq/L}.$$

The pH corresponding to this is ~7.32, which is very close to the measured pH. Thus, the data are internally consistent.

2. Is the primary disturbance acidosis or alkalosis?

The pH is <7.35, therefore the patient is acidemic, and the primary disturbance is an acidosis.

3. Is the primary disturbance metabolic or respiratory?

HCO_3^- is 14 mEq/L, which is consistent with a metabolic acidosis.

PCO_2 is 28, which is consistent with a respiratory alkalosis. We therefore conclude that respiratory response is likely compensatory and that the primary disturbance is a metabolic acidosis.

4. Is the compensation adequate?

For metabolic acidosis, use the Winter formula to estimate the appropriate PCO_2.

Predicted $PCO_2 = 1.5 \cdot [HCO_3^-] + 8\ (\pm 2) = 1.5 \cdot 14 + 8 = 29$.

This is within 2 of the measured PCO_2, so the respiratory compensation is adequate.

5. What is the AG?

The AG is calculated as $Na^+ - (Cl^- + HCO_3^-) = 140 - 118 = 22$. The "normal" AG may vary based on the clinical laboratory, but a typical AG is ~12. Therefore, there is a wide AG metabolic acidosis, which prompts the clinician to consider a different set of diagnoses (Fig. 50.6). Further testing reveals that lactic acidosis is present. Although trace ketones are present, the glucose is only mildly elevated, and diabetic ketoacidosis is less likely given the more impressive elevation of serum lactate. The patient also has renal insufficiency, which would be a risk factor for the development of lactic acidosis during treatment with metformin. Isopropanol ingestion often produces a ketosis but would not cause an elevated AG. Ethylene glycol ingestion could produce a similar scenario (including presence of lactic acidosis), but absence of an osmolar gap or urinary calcium oxalate monohydrate crystals argues against this choice. Detection of lactic acidosis should prompt the clinician to determine the cause such as tissue hypoperfusion, medications (e.g., metformin, linezolid, stavudine, didanosine), or toxins (methanol, ethylene glycol, or salicylate). This case is not consistent with a renal tubular acidosis because of the presence of a wide AG.

6. If there is an AG, calculate the delta AG.

The AG in this case was 22 (normal AG = 12 but may vary by the clinical laboratory), or a ΔAG of 10. If we assume that the ΔAG provides an estimate of the acid load and that 1 mEq/L of acid reduces $[HCO_3^-]$ by 1 mEq/L, then this can be added back to the actual $[HCO_3^-]$ (14 mEq/L) to estimate the starting concentration of $[HCO_3^-]$. In this case, the $[HCO_3^-]$ is estimated to be 24 mEq/L before the acidosis occurred.

2. A 47-year-old woman with advanced amyotrophic lateral sclerosis is evaluated in the clinic. She has recently been stable with no major changes in medical conditions. She is receiving magnesium, potassium, and HCO_3^- supplementation. She has advanced muscle weakness and requires a home mechanical ventilator.

Na^+: 142 mEq/L
K^+: 3.2 mEq/L

Cl^-: 118 mEq/L
HCO_3: 12 mEq/L
Glucose: 96 mg/dL
BUN: 6 mg/dL
Creatinine: 0.2 mg/dL
Arterial pH: 7.49
PCO_2: 16 mm Hg
Urine Na^+: 50 mEq/L
Urine K^+: 20 mEq/L
Urine Cl^-: 10 mEq/L

The single most appropriate treatment for this patient is

a) Increase oral HCO_3^- supplementation
b) Increase oral potassium supplementation
c) Increase magnesium supplementation
d) Increase the respiratory rate (minute ventilation) setting on the ventilator
e) Decrease the respiratory rate (minute ventilation) setting on the ventilator

Answer and Discussion

The answer is e. Follow the same steps as in question 1.

1. The data are internally consistent (calculated H^+ = 32, corresponding to pH ~7.48).
2. Alkalosis.
3. Respiratory alkalosis. There is a metabolic acidosis, which could be compensatory.
4. Compensation is adequate, assuming the process is chronic.

Using the formula for chronic respiratory alkalosis: $\downarrow \Delta[HCO_3^-] = 5 \times \Delta PCO_2/10$, we expect $[HCO_3^-]$ to decrease by 12, which matches the observed change exactly.

5. AG is normal (10).
6. Because the AG is normal, ΔAG cannot be calculated.

Further discussion: If assessment of the $[HCO_3^-]$ were performed without an ABG, it might be concluded that treatment with oral HCO_3^- supplementation would be appropriate. This would lead to further renal HCO_3^- wasting, which would obligate an equal loss of cations (e.g., K^+, Mg^{++}, Ca^{++}) to maintain electroneutrality, further exacerbating the hypokalemia and hypomagnesemia. Although supplementation with oral potassium or magnesium may be warranted, it does not address the underlying problem. In this case, the respiratory set rate was decreased (gradually over a period of weeks), and HCO_3^-, potassium, and magnesium supplementation were gradually tapered. The urinary AG is positive in this case due to renal HCO_3^- loss to compensate for the respiratory alkalosis, but this does not diagnose a renal tubular acidosis, since the primary process is not an acidosis. The very low creatinine provides a clue to the low muscle mass of this patient and may suggest that her metabolic demand and thus need for respiratory excretion of CO_2 may not be as high as a normal patient.

3. A 24-year-old female is brought to the emergency department after a family member found her comatose at home. She had recently told her boyfriend that she would commit suicide if he broke up with her. The following laboratory values were obtained:

> Na^+: 137 mEq/L
> K^+: 3.6 mEq/L
> Cl^-: 100 mEq/L
> HCO_3^-: 16 mEq/L
> Glucose: 96 mg/dL
> BUN: 15 mg/dL
> Creatinine: 0.9 mg/dL
> Arterial pH: 7.39
> PCO_2: 27 mm Hg
> Urine drug screen: Pending
> Serum drug screen: Pending

Which of the following substances would produce this clinical scenario?
a) Oxazepam
b) Aspirin
c) Acetaminophen
d) Methanol
e) Ethylene glycol

Answer and Discussion
The answer is b.

1. Data are internally consistent.
2. Acidosis. The pH is near normal, although both HCO_3^- and PCO_2 clearly are abnormal. The approach to evaluating acidosis is chosen because it is generally simpler and more commonly encountered than for an alkalosis.
3. Metabolic acidosis.
4. For metabolic acidosis, use the Winter formula to estimate the appropriate PCO_2.

   Predicted $PCO_2 = 1.5 \cdot [HCO_3^-] + 8\ (\pm 2) = 1.5 \cdot 16 + 8 = 32$.
   The actual PCO_2 is significantly less than that predicted, so there also is a respiratory alkalosis.

5. The AG is elevated (21).
6. The corrected HCO_3^- is 25, which is normal.

Further discussion: The finding of an elevated AG acidosis with a respiratory alkalosis should prompt a clinician to consider salicylate overdose. Salicylates stimulate central respiratory drive, and respiratory alkalosis is frequently observed in the initial stage of overdose. Salicylates also cause mitochondrial dysfunction and thus accumulation of excess CO_2 and lactic acid. In later stages, the excess CO_2 production overwhelms the abil-

ity to compensate, so absence of respiratory alkalosis may reflect a tenuous respiratory status. It is important to recognize that lactic acidosis is also found in the setting of salicylate overdose and should not dissuade the clinician from evaluating further for salicylate ingestion in the appropriate setting. Sepsis is another important cause of concurrent metabolic acidosis and respiratory alkalosis. Benzodiazepines commonly cause respiratory acidosis in overdose. Acetaminophen may cause high AG acidosis due to accumulation of 5-oxoproline (pyroglutamic acid). Methanol and ethylene glycol may also cause high AG acidosis but do not classically cause a respiratory alkalosis.

5. A 24-year-old man presents to your office with complaints of leg cramps. He denies any other complaints or medical problems and is not taking any medications. The following laboratory values were obtained:

> Na^+: 142 mEq/L
> K^+: 3.2 mEq/L
> Cl^-: 100 mEq/L
> HCO_3^-: 34 mEq/L
> Glucose: 85 mg/dL
> BUN: 25 mg/dL
> Creatinine: 0.9 mg/dL
> Arterial pH: 7.48
> PCO_2: 47 mm Hg

What is the appropriate characterization of this acid–base disorder?
a) Metabolic alkalosis
b) Metabolic alkalosis and respiratory acidosis
c) Metabolic acidosis and respiratory alkalosis
d) Metabolic alkalosis and respiratory alkalosis
e) Metabolic acidosis

Answer and Discussion
The answer is a.

1. The data are internally consistent.
2. Alkalosis.
3. Metabolic.
4. To calculate compensation for metabolic alkalosis:

   Predicted $PCO_2 = 40 + 0.6\ (\Delta[HCO_3^-])$.
   Predicted $PCO_2 = 40 + 0.6\ (10) = 47$.
   Measured PCO_2 is equal to the predicted PCO_2, so this is a simple metabolic alkalosis. Because the compensation is a component of the metabolic alkalosis, it is not necessary to state that the patient has a respiratory acidosis.

5. The AG is normal.

Further discussion: In the absence of an obvious cause of gastrointestinal chloride loss (Fig. 50.8), renal chloride or acid loss is likely. Measuring a urinary chloride would assist in this determination. Additional history is needed in this case, including blood pressure and family history of similar disturbances.

5. A 70-year-old man with recently diagnosed anemia is referred to you for evaluation of acidosis that was detected on routine blood work. He complains of weakness and fatigue but has had no recent illnesses or other chronic medical conditions. The following laboratory values were obtained:

Na^+: 142 mEq/L
K^+: 3.2 mEq/L
Cl^-: 111 mEq/L
HCO_3^-: 18 mEq/L
Phosphorus: 1.9 mg/dL
Glucose: 85 mg/dL
BUN: 25 mg/dL
Creatinine: 1.2 mg/dL
Arterial pH: 7.33
PCO_2: 35 mm Hg
Urine Na^+: 50 mEq/L
Urine K^+: 30 mEq/L
Urine Cl^-: 50 mEq/L
Urinalysis: pH 5.5, specific gravity 1.015, 2+ glucose, negative albumin

The metabolic disturbance is most likely due to
a) Diarrhea
b) Type IV renal tubular acidosis
c) Proximal (type II) renal tubular acidosis
d) Distal (type I) renal tubular acidosis
e) Vomiting

Answer and Discussion
The answer is c.

1. The data are internally consistent.
2. Acidosis.
3. Metabolic.
4. For metabolic acidosis, use the Winter formula to estimate the appropriate PCO_2.

Predicted $PCO_2 = 1.5 \cdot [HCO_3^-] + 8 (\pm 2) = 1.5 \cdot 18 + 8 = 35$.

This is equal to the measured PCO_2, so compensation is adequate.

5. The AG is normal.
6. An additional step to take in the setting of a normal AG acidosis is measurement of the urinary AG. This will help to distinguish between gastrointestinal HCO_3^- loss and renal defects. UAG = (urine Na^+ +

urine K^+) – (urine Cl^-) = 50 + 30 – 50 = +30. The positive urinary AG is indicative of a renal tubular acidosis.

Further discussion: The constellation of a renal tubular acidosis with renal glucosuria (glucose loss in setting of normoglycemia), hypokalemia, and hypophosphatemia suggests global proximal tubular dysfunction (proximal, or type II, renal tubular acidosis). The patient's advanced age and recently diagnosed anemia in this setting further suggests the diagnosis of multiple myeloma as a cause of the renal tubular acidosis.

SUGGESTED READINGS

Adams SL. Alcoholic ketoacidosis. *Emerg Med Clin North Am* 1990;8:749–760.

Adrogue HJ, Wilson H, Boyd AE III, et al. Plasma acid-base patterns in diabetic ketoacidosis. *N Engl J Med* 1982;307:1603–1610.

Adrogue HJ, Madias NE. Management of life-threatening acid-base disorders. First of two parts. *N Engl J Med* 1998;338:26–34.

Adrogue HJ, Madias NE. Management of life-threatening acid-base disorders. Second of two parts. *N Engl J Med* 1998;338:107–111.

Brimioulle S, Kahn RJ. Effects of metabolic alkalosis on pulmonary gas exchange. *Am Rev Respir Dis* 1990;141:1185–1189.

Cooper DJ, Walley KR, Wiggs BR, et al. Bicarbonate does not improve hemodynamics in critically ill patients who have lactic acidosis. A prospective, controlled clinical study. *Ann Intern Med* 1990;112:492–498.

Emmett M, Alpern RJ, Seldin DW. Metabolic acidosis. In: Seldin DW, Giebisch G, eds. *The Kidney: Physiology and Pathophysiology*, 2nd ed., Vols. 1–3. New York: Raven Press, 1992:2759–2836.

Fulop M. Serum potassium in lactic acidosis and ketoacidosis. *N Engl J Med* 1979;300:1087–1089.

Gabow PA, Kaehny WD, Fennessey PV, et al. Diagnostic importance of an increased serum anion gap. *N Engl J Med* 1980;303:854–858.

Jacobson HR, Seldin DW. On the generation, maintenance, and correction of metabolic alkalosis. *Am J Physiol* 1983;245:F425–F432.

Kraut JA, Kurtz I. Toxic alcohol ingestions: clinical features, diagnosis, and management. *Clin J Am Soc Nephrol* 2008;3(1):208–225.

Kraut JA, Madias NE. Serum anion gap: its uses and limitations in clinical medicine. *Clin J Am Soc Nephrol* 2007;2:162–174.

McLaughlin ML, Kassirer JP. Rational treatment of acid-base disorders. *Drugs* 1990;39:841–855.

Mecher C, Rackow EC, Astiz ME, et al. Unaccounted for anion in metabolic acidosis during severe sepsis in humans. *Crit Care Med* 1991;19:705–711.

Narins RG, Cohen JJ. Bicarbonate therapy for organic acidosis: the case for its continued use. *Ann Intern Med* 1987;106:615–618.

Narins RG, Emmett M. Simple and mixed acid-base disorders: a practical approach. *Medicine (Baltimore)* 1980;59:161–187.

Rastegar A. Use of the DeltaAG/Delta. *J Am Soc Nephrol* 2007;18:2429–2431.

Rodriguez SJ. Renal tubular acidosis: the clinical entity. *J Am Soc Nephrol* 2002;13:2160–2170.

Wilson RF, Binkley LE, Sabo FM Jr, et al. Electrolyte and acid-base changes with massive blood transfusions. *Am Surg* 1992;58:535–544.

Wrenn K. The delta (delta) gap: an approach to mixed acid-base disorders. *Ann Emerg Med* 1990;19:1310–1313.

Chapter 51

Liver Disorders

Nizar Zein

✋ POINTS TO REMEMBER:

- Neither blood tests nor scans are able to distinguish benign fatty liver from steatohepatitis before cirrhotic changes become apparent.

- Pegylated interferon α-2a and pegylated interferon α-2b are superior to interferon in producing sustained virologic responses (SVR) and are currently the standard of care for the treatment of chronic hepatitis C virus (HCV).

- Autoantibodies are a nearly universal feature of primary biliary cirrhosis (PBC).

- The mainstay of treatment for ascites is dietary sodium restriction.

- The endoscopic treatment of esophageal varices with band ligation appears superior to injection sclerotherapy.

The recognition of common and uncommon hepatobiliary disorders is a challenge for physicians and surgeons of all specialties. Rote memory will not do. A system of organizing thoughts will go a long way toward making this task manageable. Perhaps the place to begin is a consideration of laboratory tests and how they help to distinguish liver and biliary tract disorders of various etiologies.

SERUM-BASED LIVER TESTS

Readily available tests provide information about the state of the liver, but few are absolutely pathognomonic. Instead, a context-based pattern recognition often is required of the clinician. The first pattern distinction is to determine whether the abnormalities are more suggestive of cholestatic or liver cell injury. *Cholestatic liver disease* refers to impairment of hepatic excretion into the biliary system. This type of blockage may occur at any level. In drug-induced cholestasis (e.g., chlorpromazine or most of the commonly used antibiotics), the defect is at the level of the bile canaliculus (i.e., intrahepatic cholestasis). In cancer of the bile duct (cholangiocarcinoma), the defect is in the large (macroscopically visible) biliary system. In both kinds of blockage, the same pattern is present in serum-based liver function tests. The alkaline phosphatase and γ-glutamyl transpeptidase (GGTP) are elevated to a much greater degree than that of the transaminases (transferases; serum glutamic-oxaloacetic transaminase [SGOT] or aspartate transaminase [AST], serum glutamate-pyruvic transaminase [SGPT] or alanine transaminase [ALT]). The bilirubin level may or may not be elevated, depending on the extent and duration of obstruction. In cholestasis associated with obstruction (stone, cholangiocarcinoma, or biliary stricture), bile ducts proximal to the site of obstruction are typically dilated (seen by imaging such as ultrasound or computed tomography [CT] scan of the liver) compared with intrahepatic cholestasis (such as drug-induced cholestasis), where bile ducts are normal in size.

Special mention must be made of those situations in which an elevation of GGTP is present with a normal bilirubin and normal liver enzymes, including alkaline phosphatase. Current opinion suggests that this problem does not, by itself, call for additional testing. If additional clinically relevant issues point to possible liver disease (e.g., alcohol intake, obesity, etc.), then relevant tests directed by these facts should be considered. In other words, an elevation of GGTP is a frequent finding of little clinical consequence.

When liver disease primarily affects hepatocytes, as in viral hepatitis, alcoholic hepatitis, and many drug-induced problems, a pattern of *liver cell injury* is seen. The transaminases (transferases; SGOT [AST] and SGPT [ALT]) are elevated predominantly. If the hepatocellular process is severe enough to produce an elevation of the prothrombin time (pro time), it will not be corrected by vitamin K. Most often, patients with hepatocyte-centered liver injury do not complain of pruritus, nor do they have xanthelasma or prominent elevations of serum cholesterol.

In fact, most liver and bile duct injuries produce elevations in both the cholestatic and hepatitic tests, so the predominant elevation must be identified. For example, a 10-fold elevation of ALT with a 2-fold elevation of alkaline

TABLE 51.1

ELEVATED BILIRUBIN WITH NORMAL LIVER TEST RESULTS

Condition	Defect	Hints	Sequelae
Unconjugated hyperbilirubinemia			
Gilbert syndrome	Multiple; hepatic uptake of bilirubin defective; bilirubin usually 1.3–3.0 mg/dL, rarely higher	Common; usually apparent in late adolescence or early adulthood. Fasting increases bilirubin further; phenobarbital lowers bilirubin	None
Hemolysis	Increased production of (unconjugated) bilirubin by destruction of red blood cells; bilirubin >8 mg % rules out hemolysis as sole abnormality	Low hemoglobin (occasionally normal if hemolysis is compensated)	Those of underlying disease
Crigler-Najjar syndrome	Diminished or absent ability of liver to conjugate bilirubin	Present at birth or soon after, so will not present as a mystery in an adult; usually high bilirubin (may be >20 mg/dL), kernicterus brain damage usual	Severely debilitating neurologic effects from kernicterus
Conjugated hyperbilirubinemia			
Dubin-Johnson syndrome	Both indirect- and direct-reacting bilirubin present	The liver has black appearance due to pigment deposition; oral cholecystogram does not visualize, raising specter of biliary disease as cause	None
Rotor syndrome	Same as above	Liver not pigmented; otherwise just like Dubin-Johnson syndrome	None

phosphatase would indicate a hepatocellular process; the converse would indicate a bile duct disease.

Jaundice first becomes evident clinically when the bilirubin is elevated, usually to a range of ≥2.5 mg/dL. Lesser elevations usually are not discernible by examination of the sclera and skin. The inherited disorders of bilirubin metabolism should only be considered if other serum-based liver tests are normal. Among these bilirubin metabolism disorders, only Gilbert syndrome is common; it must be differentiated from true liver disease to avoid expensive, invasive, and unnecessary evaluations for liver disease. In a patient with suspected Gilbert syndrome, only two tests are needed. First, the amount of bilirubin present as conjugated and unconjugated direct portions is essential. *Conjugated bilirubin* is measured as direct-reacting bilirubin, and *unconjugated bilirubin* is measured as indirectly reacting bilirubin. In Gilbert syndrome, 90% or more of the bilirubin is indirect reacting. Because hemolysis also results in elevations of indirect-reacting bilirubin, a reticulocyte count helps to exclude a compensated hemolytic anemia (thalassemia minor, spherocytosis, etc.) as a cause for the elevated indirect–reacting bilirubin. The key aspects of syndromes that cause an isolated elevation of bilirubin levels are identified in Table 51.1.

HEPATOCELLULAR DISEASES

Fatty Liver

Fatty liver is one of the most common causes of mild to moderate parenchymal liver test elevations. Benign accumulations of fat may be seen in up to 75% of obese persons

and also may be seen in the nonobese, especially in diabetic persons. Certain drugs (e.g., corticosteroids, estrogens, tamoxifen, amiodarone) may cause fatty liver. Fat also may accumulate in Wilson disease, starvation states, jejunoileal bypass, and in those who consume even moderate amounts of alcohol. Those with elevated serum triglycerides are also at risk. This form of fatty liver is benign, nonprogressive, and requires no specific treatment. Steatohepatitis, a more virulent form of fatty liver, often emerges in the same at-risk population, and the clinical distinction of those with benign fat and those with steatohepatitis is impossible without a liver biopsy. The histologic features of steatohepatitis, in addition to fat accumulation, are a polymorphonuclear inflammatory response that includes the destruction of hepatocytes and the presence of Mallory bodies (identical to those in alcoholic hyaline). Steatohepatitis may progress to cirrhosis in 10% to 50% of patients. Fatty liver or steatohepatitis (termed *nonalcoholic steatohepatitis*) in patients who do not drink alcohol should be suspected in patients with mild to moderate transaminase elevations and whose serologic studies for viral hepatitis, iron overload, and autoimmune disorders are negative. Additional inference regarding the presence of fatty liver can be obtained from hepatic ultrasound (diffusely echogenic) and CT scan (low attenuation compared with spleen and hepatic vasculature). Magnetic resonance imaging (MRI) also may provide information, but cost considerations and its lack of additional utility discourage its use for this condition.

Neither blood tests nor scans are able to distinguish benign fatty liver from steatohepatitis before cirrhotic changes become apparent. Liver biopsy is the best method to assess the presence and relative amount of fat and is required to establish a diagnosis of steatohepatitis. If liver biopsy is contraindicated or is not doable, a presumptive diagnosis and empirical treatment often is recommended. Weight loss in obese patients, the control of elevated triglycerides and diabetes, and the avoidance of alcohol are recommended. Reversal of jejunoileal bypass may be necessary to prevent progressive liver failure. Of several treatment strategies tested in clinical trials, weight loss (at least 5%–10% of total body weight) seems to be the most effective. Weight loss in obese patients with steatohepatitis has shown to be associated with normalization of liver enzymes and improved hepatic histology. Newer studies are targeting insulin resistance as a potential underlying mechanism of fatty liver. Clinical trials assessing the use of insulin-sensitizing agents developed for patients with type 2 diabetes mellitus are currently under way. More data are needed before advocating the routine use of these agents in patients with fatty liver.

Alcohol

In the United States, alcohol is the most common cause of liver cirrhosis. The consumption of large quantities of alcohol over a long period is required before cirrhosis occurs. Similar to patients with nonalcoholic steatohepatitis, fatty accumulation in the liver is considered a precursor lesion in patients with alcoholic liver disease. A reasonable correlation exists between the per capita consumption of alcohol and the prevalence of cirrhosis. Women are more susceptible to the hepatic effects of alcohol. It is estimated that 80 g of alcohol per day in men and 60 g per day in women over the course of approximately 10 to 12 years is required before cirrhosis develops.

Alcohol appears to exert its toxic effect on the liver through the formation of toxic metabolites, induction of enzymes that produce free radicals, and immunologic mechanisms that are activated by free radicals. The parallel and simultaneous enzymatic degradation of alcohol by alcohol dehydrogenase, the microsomal ethanol-oxidizing system within the endoplasmic reticulum, and catalases all convert ethanol to acetaldehyde. This intermediate is toxic; it is rendered nontoxic by a subsequent metabolism to acetate by aldehyde dehydrogenase. Chronic alcohol ingestion induces the microsomal ethanol-oxidizing system enzyme family, which includes cytochrome P450 2E. This enzyme produces hydroxyethyl free radicals that bind to cellular proteins and render some of them immunogenic. Antibodies produced in response to this action may injure the liver further.

A wide spectrum of liver disease is produced by alcohol. Early on, alcohol ingestion results in the accumulation of fat within hepatocytes (fatty liver). Alcoholic steatohepatitis (described previously) produces a clinical syndrome of alcoholic hepatitis. Fibrosis, especially around the central veins, may herald the beginning of the cirrhotic process. When fully developed, Laennec cirrhosis is present. Other coexisting liver diseases such as hepatitis C may hasten the development of cirrhosis in alcoholic persons.

The diagnosis of alcoholic liver disease often is obvious but may be obscure in the well-nourished person who minimizes or denies alcohol ingestion. Cutaneous spider telangiectasias are frequently present. Other stigmata of acute or chronic liver disease may be present, such as jaundice, ascites, edema, encephalopathy, dilated abdominal veins, parotid enlargement, and gynecomastia. These clinical manifestations are often associated with more severe liver diseases, such as those with cirrhosis and portal hypertension.

Blood tests frequently show only modest elevations of the SGOT (AST), almost always <400 IU/L. The SGPT (ALT) is characteristically normal or only slightly elevated; thus, the SGOT-to-SGPT ratio is usually >2. Other abnormal tests often reveal macrocytosis (the B_{12} level is almost invariably elevated, and the folate level may be depressed if the patient has consumed a diet deficient in folate), and the γ-globulin levels are frequently elevated. A liver biopsy is usually not necessary in these cases.

The treatment of severe alcoholic hepatitis is largely supportive. Abstinence, multiple vitamins, and fluids are required. In severely ill hospitalized patients, enteral feeding for several weeks produces a better outcome compared with the use of a standard oral diet. Improved survival, a Child score, liver tests, and a lower incidence of encephalopathy have been described. The use of corticosteroids remains controversial more than 20 years after they were first studied in this condition. Several studies, however, suggest that steroids improve survival for patients with severe alcoholic hepatitis without gastrointestinal bleeding. The definition of severity requires an evaluation of the bilirubin level and the pro time. The so-called *discriminant function value* identifies a group of patients at substantial risk of dying from alcoholic hepatitis.

Discriminant function:

$$4.6(\text{protime} - \text{control[inseconds]}) + (\text{serumbilirubin[mg/dL]}) = 32$$

When severely ill patients with a discriminant function score of ≥ 32 (without gastrointestinal hemorrhage) are given 40 mg of prednisone daily for 28 days, survival is nearly twice as likely. Nutritional therapy appears to benefit patients with moderate malnutrition but not those with severe malnutrition and alcoholic hepatitis. Oxandrolone also may benefit those in whom adequate nutrition can be given. Insufficient evidence is available to recommend propylthiouracil or colchicine in alcoholic liver disease. The treatment of established alcoholic cirrhosis is discussed later.

Viral Hepatitis

Hepatitis may be caused by myriad viruses. Not all are common, and some, especially the herpesviruses, occur in

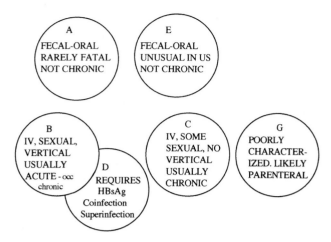

Figure 51.1   Important hepatatrophic viruses. (HBsAg, hepatitis B surface antigen; occ, occasionally; US, United States.)

distinctive clinical settings (e.g., the immunocompromised patient). Those in which the hepatocyte appears to be the major locus of infection (hepatatrophic viruses) are shown in Figure 51.1. Most hepatatrophic viruses also infect other organs, thus providing a potential reservoir for recurrence after antiviral treatment or after liver transplantation. In addition, the extrahepatic manifestations of viral hepatitis may be significant and, from time to time, overshadow the hepatic manifestations. Important extrahepatic manifestations of hepatitis are identified in Table 51.2.

Hepatitis A

Hepatitis A is spread through fecal–oral contamination. The virus usually is not identified in the serum, where it is present only transiently. It is shed in the stool; usually, shedding (and therefore infectivity) has ceased by the time the index case becomes clinically ill. The affected person frequently is not anicteric (jaundiced). The vast majority of cases spontaneously resolve within a few days to weeks. Fewer than 1% result in massive hepatic necrosis and death. The diagnosis can be made by demonstration of antihepatitis A antibodies of the immunoglobulin M (IgM) class. Im-

munoglobulin G (IgG) antibodies denote prior, not acute, infection. No chronic form of hepatitis A or carrier state exists.

Immune globulin provides protection against hepatitis A. Formerly, preexposure prophylaxis was recommended for those who travel internationally to endemic regions, but such persons currently are advised to receive active immunization (see discussion later in this section). Postexposure prophylaxis with immune globulin is recommended for (a) household and sexual contacts under the age of 12 months or over the age of 40 years (for those between 12 months and 40 years, hepatitis A vaccine is preferred); (b) in day care centers (if children in diapers attend) but not to elementary or secondary school contacts unless an outbreak (more than a single case) has been identified; (c) within institutions to contacts only; and (d) in hospitals only if an outbreak occurs. Immune globulin is not recommended for coworkers in offices or factories. Restaurant-exposed persons also may get immune globulin unless the contact was more than 2 weeks previous, in which case no vaccine is recommended. Postexposure prophylaxis is not needed for persons who have been immunized.

In March 1995, the U.S. Food and Drug Administration (FDA) approved an inactivated hepatitis A vaccine. This vaccine is safe and highly immunogenic, at least for those with a normal immune system, and it is likely to provide long-lasting immunity. A protective antibody response to this vaccine is apparent within 2 weeks. Seroconversion rates approaching 100% are seen 1 month after primary vaccination. A booster dose given 6 to 12 months later is recommended. More recently, hepatitis A virus vaccination was incorporated as part of the normal immunization panel for all youngsters, but for those who did not receive the vaccine during childhood, it is only recommended for (a) those at high risk, such as travelers to endemic areas; (b) military personnel; (c) people living in or relocating to areas highly endemic for hepatitis A; (d) residents in a community experiencing an outbreak of hepatitis A; (e) institutionalized children and adults; and (f) children in day care centers.

TABLE 51.2		
EXTRAHEPATIC FEATURES OF VIRAL HEPATITIS		
Hepatitis B	**Hepatitis C**	**Unclassified Hepatitis (Non-A, Non-B, Non-C)**
Serum sickness–like illness	Leukocytoclastic vasculitis	Aplastic anemia
Polyarteritis nodosa	PCT	
Glomerulonephritis (usually membranous)	Glomerulonephritis (usually membranoproliferative)	
	Cryoglobulinemia	
	Autoimmune thyroiditis	
	Sicca syndrome	
	Non-Hodgkin B-cell lymphoma	

PCT, porphyria cutanea tarda.
Reproduced with permission from Brown KE, Tisdale J, Barrett K, et al. Hepatitis-associated aplastic anemia. *N Engl J Med* 1997;336:1059–1064.

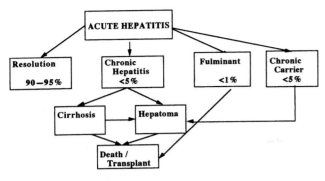

Figure 51.2 The courses of hepatitis B.

Limited data suggest that acute hepatitis A may be particularly devastating to those with chronic liver disease. For this reason, hepatitis A vaccination is recommended for all susceptible persons with chronic liver disease. Detailed recommendations regarding the prevention of hepatitis A after exposure and in international travelers has been published by the 2007 Advisory Committee on Immunization Practices.

Hepatitis B

Viral hepatitis B affects more than 300 million people throughout the world. It is spread by three important routes: parenteral, venereal, and through "vertical transmission." In the United States, parenteral and venereal spread is most common, whereas worldwide, vertical transmission (from mother to offspring) is most common. Clinically, most cases are mild and self-limited. Outcomes for those infected as adults are indicated in Figure 51.2. Chronic disease occurs in a minority of adults infected with hepatitis B virus (HBV). The situation is quite different in children. More than 90% of neonates infected with HBV develop chronic infection. Diagnosis is made easier by the many antigen-antibody systems that have been identified in HBV infections. Distinct genotypes of hepatitis B have been described. It is not yet clear if these genotypes have different biological behavior and respond differently to treatment.

The sequence of antigens and antibodies emergence is available in standard textbooks. A few clinical situations are described:

- *Acute hepatitis B:* Early in the disease, the hepatitis B surface antigen (HBsAg) is present, and possibly hepatitis B e antigen (HBeAg), but no antibodies. If the patient comes to medical attention a little later, both the HBsAg and the HBeAg may have disappeared. The HBsAg will have been replaced by IgM class antihepatitis B core (HB$_c$). The disappearance of HBeAg usually is followed by the emergence of anti-e.
- *Remote resolved infection:* These patients have antihepatitis B surface (HBS) and anti-HB$_c$ in the serum. Many years later, the waxing and waning antibody titers may yield inconstant results for these assays.
- *Chronic hepatitis B:* Found either with disease, such as chronic active hepatitis, or diseasefree (chronic carrier),

this disease has HBsAg and anti-HB$_c$ but no anti-HBS. Hepatitis B carriers have normal liver enzymes and normal liver histology. Elevated liver enzymes and positive HBsAg and anti-HB$_c$ usually denote the presence of chronic hepatitis.

- *Successful immunization status:* The patient has anti-HBS only.

Acute hepatitis B requires only supportive treatment, preferably out of the hospital. Corticosteroids have no established place in the management of either acute or chronic viral hepatitis. Rarely, hepatitis B results in massive hepatic necrosis and should be treated as such (see the Acute Liver Failure section). It may take 6 months or longer before acute hepatitis B resolves.

Interferon-α is useful in many cases of chronic hepatitis B and has received FDA approval for this indication. Five million U of interferon-α given daily for 16 weeks or 10 million U given three times per week seem equally effective. The goal of therapy is to convert the HBeAg-positive patient to HBeAg negative, which usually is accompanied by improved transaminases and improved histology. Interestingly, the elimination of HBeAg often is preceded by a major flare of hepatitis, which can be worrisome and even dangerous to the patient with decompensated cirrhosis. The loss of HBeAg usually implies markedly diminished viral replication, although the HBsAg remains positive. Approximately 35% to 40% of patients have a response to treatment. Treatment successes are durable; few relapses occur in hepatitis B patients. The long-term outlook for those who clear HBeAg positivity with interferon therapy is remarkably improved. Even those with well-compensated cirrhosis appear to benefit from treatment with interferon, if clearance of HBeAg occurs. Such patients have improved aminotransferase levels, experience fewer cirrhotic complications, and live longer than those who do not receive interferon treatment. The successful treatment of hepatitis B with interferon reduces the likelihood of subsequent hepatoma. More recently, a long-acting form of interferon administered once weekly has demonstrated efficacy for the treatment of patients with chronic HBV infection.

Who should be treated with interferon? The HBsAg carrier (normal liver enzymes) probably requires no treatment, because the outcome of this form of hepatitis B seems benign. Historically, Chinese persons, homosexual patients, and those with long-duration disease (i.e., >2 years) have not responded well to treatment. However, more recently, it was reported that the response to interferon in patients with chronic hepatitis B is genotype dependent; those infected with genotype A respond well compared with other genotypes where response is poor. If coinfection with HIV is present, interferon is of unproven value. Those with decompensated cirrhosis tolerate interferon therapy poorly and may have significant worsening of disease while receiving the drug. Those who have none of these features should be considered for therapy if they have had disease for at least 1 year and if they are HBeAg positive.

Nucleoside analogs are active against hepatitis B, and this has created a new opportunity to improve the successful management of hepatitis B. Nucleoside analogs inhibit viral DNA polymerase. Many patients achieve effective blood levels after oral dosing and are relatively free of severe adverse effects; these agents are much less costly than interferon. Most attention has been given to oral lamivudine, which is approved by the FDA for use in hepatitis B. It is remarkably free of side effects, although pancreatitis has been observed in pediatric HIV–infected patients receiving this drug. Resistant strains have emerged, caused by mutations in the YMDD locus of the reverse transcriptase of the DNA polymerase gene, but some evidence suggests that even when this occurs, clinical deterioration is not inevitable. Patients given a dose of 100 mg daily for 1 year had a 72% likelihood of normalization of transaminases and a 16% likelihood of conversion from HBeAg positive to negative. They also had a 56% likelihood of improved histology scores (all results were statistically superior to those given placebo). The limitations of lamivudine include the need for indefinite therapy. Available evidence suggests a rapid reemergence of active viral replication when the drug is stopped. Also, viral mutations (emergence of genotypic mutations in the YMDD locus) occur in approximately 14% of treated patients in the first year. Several more effective nucleosides analoges have been developed and approved by the FDA for the treatment of hepatitis B. These newer agents aree associated with a much smaller likelihood for emergence of resistant strains. Examples include adefovir (Hepsera), entecavir (Baraclude), and telbivudine (Tyzeka). The concept of combining these agents to improve antiviral activity and decrease resistance is gaining more acceptance.

Prophylaxis against hepatitis B is possible for most. In April 1991, the Centers for Disease Control and Prevention (CDC) endorsed universal hepatitis B immunization for young children in the United States. Immunization can be started after birth, just before the infant leaves the hospital, and repeated in 1 to 2 months and again at 6 to 18 months of age. Alternatively, the first injection can be given at 1 to 2 months of age, repeated at 4 months, and finally repeated at 6 to 18 months. The hepatitis B vaccine can be given concomitantly with diphtheria, tetanus, and pertussis; *Haemophilus influenzae* type b conjugate; measles-mumps-rubella; and oral polio vaccine. Some children will escape immunization, and a "catch-up" program for adolescents (at age 13 years) is recommended. Recommendations for postexposure prophylaxis are indicated in Table 51.3.

Hepatitis C

HCV, an RNA virus with similarities to flaviviruses, from which they are, however, distinct, chronically infects 2.7 million Americans; it is estimated that cirrhosis will develop in 20% of those infected. Risk factors (shown in Table 51.4)

for hepatitis C include blood transfusions before 1992, illicit intravenous drug use, and health care workers in contact with blood and blood products. The risk of contracting hepatitis C after a blood transfusion in the United States has diminished from approximately 1 in 10 in the 1980s to a current estimate of 1 case per 100,000 U of blood. A small risk is assumed by sexual partners and household contacts of affected persons. The risk for hemodialysis patients is independent of blood transfusions and is related instead to the total duration of dialysis treatment. Intranasal cocaine use has been recognized as a risk factor. In 40% of infected persons, none of these risks appears to be present. Low socioeconomic status has been invoked to explain this large group with acute hepatitis C without apparent conventional risks. Without further definition, this category appears to serve as a surrogate for a specific risk or risks yet to be identified. The vertical transmission of HCV from mother to infant occurs in approximately 6% of mothers whose serum is positive to HCV RNA. The risk seems proportionate to the titer of circulating virus in the mother.

Approximately 5% of medical personnel suffering accidental needlestick injuries from needles contaminated with blood from HCV-positive persons develop acute hepatitis C, which is usually subclinical or self-limited and transient. No specific postexposure action can be taken to reduce the likelihood of infection in the health care worker. Recommendations, therefore, are not entirely comforting to the exposed person. Nevertheless, the CDC, in collaboration with the Hospital Infection Control Practices Advisory Committee, recommends the following policies:

- For the source, baseline testing for antibody to hepatitis C (anti-HCV)
- For the person exposed to an anti-HCV–positive source, baseline and follow-up (e.g., 6-month) testing for anti-HCV and serum alanine aminotransferase activity
- Confirmation by supplemental anti-HCV testing of all anti-HCV results by enzyme immunoassay. Supplemental testing is often recombinant immunoblot antibody testing, but it could be the determination of HCV through the detection of HCV RNA using polymerase chain reaction (PCR)
- Recommendation against postexposure administration of immune globulin or antiviral agents, such as interferons
- Education of health care workers about the risk for and prevention of blood-borne infections

Clinical Course

Hepatitis C has an incubation period of 14 days to 6 months. Acute infection produces a mild undistinguished illness in most persons. It is much more likely than hepatitis B to become chronic (85%). Recent evidence indicates that resolution with permanent elimination of viremia occurs

TABLE 51.3

GUIDELINES FOR POSTEXPOSURE PROPHYLAXIS[a] OF PERSONS WITH NONOCCUPATIONAL EXPOSURES[b] TO BLOOD OR BODY FLUIDS THAT CONTAIN BLOOD, BY EXPOSURE TYPE AND VACCINATION STATUS

Exposure	Treatment	
	Unvaccinated Person[c]	Previously Vaccinated Person[d]
HBsAg[e]-positive source		
Percutaneous (e.g., bite or needlestick) or mucosal exposure to HBsAg-positive blood or body fluids	Administer hepatitis B vaccine series and hepatitis B immune globulin (HBIG)	Administer hepatitis B vaccine booster dose
Sex or needle-sharing contact of an HBsAg-positive person	Administer hepatitis B vaccine series and HBIG	Administer hepatitis B vaccine booster dose
Victim of sexual assault/abuse by a perpetrator who is HBsAg positive	Administer hepatitis B vaccine series and HBIG	Administer hepatitis B vaccine booster dose
Source with unknown HBsAg status		
Victim of sexual assault/abuse by a perpetrator with unknown HBsAg status	Administer hepatitis B vaccine series	No treatment
Percutaneous (e.g., bite or needlestick) or mucosal exposure to potentially infectious blood or body fluids from a source with unknown HBsAg status	Administer hepatitis B vaccine series	No treatment
Sex or needle-sharing contact of person with unknown HBsAg status	Administer hepatitis B vaccine series	No treatment

HBIG, hepatitis B immune globulin; HBsAg, hepatitis B surface antigen.
[a]When indicated immunoprophylaxis should be initiated as soon as possible, preferably within 24 hours. Studies are limited on the maximum interval after exposure during which postexposure prophylaxis is effective, but the interval is unlikely to exceed 7 days for percutaneous exposures or 14 days for sexual exposures. The hepatitis B vaccine series should be completed.
[b]These guidelines apply to nonoccupational exposures. Guidelines for management of occupational exposures have been published separately (1) and also can be used for management of nonoccupational exposures if feasible.
[c]A person who is in the process of being vaccinated but who has not completed the vaccine series should complete the series and receive treatment as indicated.
[d]A person who has written documentation of a complete hepatitis B vaccine series and who did not receive postvaccination testing.
[e]Hepatitis B surface antigen.

in a small minority of cases (12%), although in another 12%, persistently normal transaminases were present despite viremia. More than three-fourths of patients developed chronic liver disease.

Over the course of several decades, hepatitis C may cause cirrhosis, which sometimes decompensates. Increasing evidence suggests that alcoholic liver disease in the presence of hepatitis C results in higher mean aminotransferase levels and mean histologic activity and progression to advanced

TABLE 51.4

TRANSMISSION OF HEPATITIS C VIRUS

Shared blood
Intravenous drug abuse
Blood transfusion before 1992
Body piercing
Tattoo
Sexual transmission (only in association with high-risk sexual behavior)
Intranasal cocaine
Unknown

cirrhosis. Daily alcohol consumption, even in low amounts (<50 g per day), has been shown to have an additive effect in the risk of symptomatic cirrhosis, and high alcohol intakes (>125 g per day) have a multiplicative effect. Hepatitis C increasingly is recognized as a risk factor for liver cancer and currently is believed to be the most common cause of hepatocellular carcinoma in the United States.

Several extrahepatic manifestations of hepatitis C may overshadow hepatic involvement. The glomerular protein leak in membranoproliferative glomerulonephritis may improve if the hepatitis C is treated successfully using interferon. Porphyria cutanea tarda (PCT), as a result of reduced activity of the enzyme uroporphyrinogen decarboxylase, may be either inherited as an autosomal dominant trait or acquired. Hepatic dysfunction is nearly always seen in PCT, and anti-HCV antibodies are present in four of five patients with acquired PCT but not in patients with familial PCT. The many clinical paths that this infection can take are indicated in Figure 51.3. Other extrahepatic manifestations associated with HCV include cryoglobulinemia and its associated vasculitis, type 2 diabetes mellitus, and lymphoproliferative disorders.

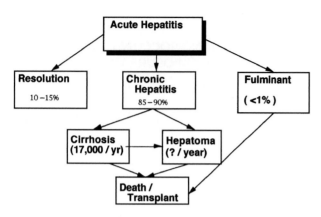

Figure 51.3 Hepatitis C.

Diagnosis

Suspicion of hepatitis C relies on the right epidemiologic background, as described previously, and the presence of otherwise unexplained liver test abnormalities. Laboratory testing confirms the diagnosis. Enzyme-linked immunosorbent assay (ELISA) detects anti-C antibodies. This test is quite sensitive, but false-positive results occasionally occur. Confirmatory antibody tests based on recombinant immunoblot antibody testing are widely used. A confirmation of a positive ELISA anti-HCV should be sought in any case, especially if treatment with interferon is being contemplated. The direct measurement of virologic activity is readily available. The detection of HCV RNA using PCR represents a powerful clinical tool. An easy interpretative guide to the tests most often used to detect hepatitis C is provided in Table 51.5.

Based on the nucleotide sequence of HCV, several distinct genotypes of HCV are recognized. Great geographic diversity exists with respect to the dominant genotype seen. It has been speculated that different genotypes might influence the severity of disease. Increasing evidence suggests that certain genotypes (especially type 1b) are more likely to produce chronic active hepatitis and cirrhosis. Chronic hepatitis C may progress to cirrhosis even with only a mod-

est elevation of transaminases. Currently, the most important observations about HCV genotypes are:

- Genotype 1 predominates in North America.
- Genotypes 2 and 3 are more amenable to treatment than genotypes 1 and 4.
- Six months of treatment suffices for genotypes 2 and 3; 12 months suffices for genotypes 1 and 4.

Treatment

The goals of therapy are multiple: reduction in symptoms, improvement in liver tests and liver histology, prevention of development of cirrhosis or cirrhotic decompensation, and reduction in risk for the development of hepatoma. Whether viral eradication is required to achieve each of these goals remains unproven. Certain lifestyle modifications should take precedence over attempts at viral elimination. Complete alcohol abstinence is thought by most to be essential, as is the cessation of illicit drug use and other high-risk behaviors.

Antiviral treatment usually uses multiple drugs, including interferon. In the past 5 years, a combination of pegylated interferon alpha (2a or 2b) plus ribavirin was established as the treatment of choice for treating patients with chronic HCV infection.

By convention, hepatitis C patients are divided into three categories:

- Treatment naive (never treated)
- Treatment relapser (disappearance of viral RNA during therapy with reappearance after interferon therapy has been stopped)
- Treatment nonresponder (no virologic clearance during treatment)

Treatment-naive patients and treatment relapsers have a much higher likelihood of response to therapy than those who have failed a previous course of interferon.

The current primary endpoint of antiviral therapeutic trials is viral elimination that persists for at least 6 months after therapy is ended (SVR). The absence of circulating

TABLE 51.5		
INTERPRETATION OF HEPATITIS C TEST RESULTS		
Anti–Hepatitis C Virus	**Hepatitis C Virus RNA (Polymerase Chain Reaction)**	**Interpretation**
Negative	Negative	No infection
Positive	Positive	Infection present
Negative	Positive	Infection present: early infection or immunocompromised host
Positive	Negative	Several possibilities: Resolved infection False-positive antibody Passively acquired antibody Chronic infection, low-level viremia

virus 6 months after stopping treatment correlates well with absence of virus for the next several years. Long-term follow-up in those successfully treated with interferon is encouraging. Those who sustain a durable response (negative serum HCV RNA 6 months after the cessation of therapy) are highly likely to remain HCV RNA negative for up to 13 years, and possibly forever. The risk of subsequent hepatoma development appears to be favorably influenced by interferon therapy, both for sustained responders and for responders and relapsers.

Landmark publications comparing monotherapy (interferon) with a combination of interferon and ribavirin indicate a substantial benefit from two-drug therapy in those who can tolerate it. Pegylated interferons (interferon bound to polyethylene glycol) provide for once-weekly dosing. Pegylated interferon α-2a and α-2b are superior to interferon in producing SVR and are currently the standard of care for the treatment of chronic HCV. Two studies demonstrate that those who achieve an initial response to interferon and then relapse are good candidates for re-treatment. Forty-eight weeks on consensus interferon results in a 50% sustained response rate. Alternatively, the combination of interferon and ribavirin for 24 weeks results in a comparable rate of durable virologic response. Several host and viral factors have been identified as predictors of optimal response, including younger age, HCV genotypes 2 or 3, and low pretreatment viral count (Table 51.6).

The large group of treatment nonresponders is probably best left untreated for now, except in research protocols.

The side effects of hepatitis C antiviral therapy are myriad. Interferons frequently (>50%) induce flulike symptoms consisting of one or more of the following: headache, fatigue and asthenia, myalgias, fevers, and rigors. Less often seen (13%–20%) are gastrointestinal symptoms such as anorexia, nausea, and diarrhea. Psychiatric symptoms, either insomnia or depression, may be seen as well as respiratory symptoms, dermatologic problems, and the flare-up of putative autoimmune and inflammatory diseases such as psoriasis, inflammatory bowel disease, and so forth. Thyroid abnormalities, both hypothy-

roidism and hyperthyroidism, are frequent enough that most recommend a thyroid-stimulating hormone test before treatment and 3 months after interferon has been started.

When ribavirin is added to interferon therapy, additional important side effects must be borne in mind. Ribavirin is teratogenic in experimental animals. It is mandatory that effective birth control be in place for both men and women receiving ribavirin, both during and for several months after the cessation of therapy. If pregnancy is a possibility, women should have a negative pregnancy test before starting therapy. Ribavirin accumulates in red blood cells and produces hemolysis (average hemoglobin drop in the first month is 2 g/dL), which may be brisk, resulting in hemoglobin values of <10 g/dL in 10% of patients. This may have dire consequences in patients with ischemic heart disease. Close monitoring of hemoglobin levels early in the course of therapy is mandatory.

Hepatitis D

Hepatitis D (delta virus), discovered in Italy in 1977, is seen throughout the world. It is more prevalent in other countries than in the United States. Because hepatitis D is a defective RNA virus that can exist only in the presence of hepatitis B, it appears to be a virus infecting a virus. Evidence of delta hepatitis is not found unless the patient is HBsAg positive. The diagnosis of delta hepatitis can be made by detecting hepatitis D antigen in the serum. Two forms of infection may occur. When hepatitis B and delta coinfect the liver simultaneously, the illness produced is more severe than usual hepatitis B. A biphasic peak of SGPT may occur. Fulminant disease may occur, although the patient usually recovers. When delta hepatitis superinfects a liver infected with hepatitis B, a severe, sometimes fatal, disease flare-up occurs. Chronic delta hepatitis may respond to high-dose interferon. Nine million U three times weekly for 48 weeks results in normalization of transaminases in 71% of cases, and most responders lose evidence of circulating hepatitis D virus RNA activity. Although more likely to recrudesce than hepatitis B, approximately half of treated patients continue to have normal transaminases 6 months after treatment is stopped. Despite normal enzymes, many have a reemergence of hepatitis D virus RNA activity once treatment is stopped.

Autoimmune Chronic Hepatitis

Autoimmune chronic hepatitis is one of many liver diseases that produce a prominent elevation of transaminases (transferases) and a histologic response within the liver termed *chronic hepatitis*. Autoimmune type hepatitis predominates in women. Transaminases are markedly elevated; progression to cirrhosis and death within just a few months or years may occur unless treatment is given. Fatigue, malaise, change in menstruation patterns (often amenorrhea), and prominent extrahepatic effects such as arthritis and arthralgias may be present, in which case

---

TABLE 51.6

STRATIFICATION OF HEPATITIS C VIRUS TREATMENT CANDIDATES

Optimal	Questionable
Female	Active drug or alcohol use
Young	Decompensated cirrhosis
Nonobese	Comorbidity
Low viral count	Failed previous treatment
No severe fibrosis or cirrhosis	HIV coinfected
Genotype 2 or 3	Immunocompromised
Treatment naive	Normal liver tests

Note: Most candidates are in neither group.

TABLE 51.7

CLASSIFICATION OF AUTOIMMUNE HEPATITIS BY TYPE OF AUTOANTIBODY

Disease	Antinuclear Antibodies	Liver-kidney Microsomal Antibodies	Soluble Liver Antigens	Smooth Muscle Antibodies
Classic (type 1) Autoimmune	+	–	–	+
Anti-LKM1	–	+(1)	–	–
Anti-LKM2	–	+(2)	–	–
Soluble liver antigens	–	–	+	±
Smooth muscle antibodies	–	–	–	+

LKM, liver-kidney microsomal antibodies.

confusion with rheumatoid arthritis or systemic lupus erythematosus may occur. A number of autoantibodies are present, including antinuclear antibody, rheumatoid factor, lupus erythematosus cell phenomena, and false biological tests for syphilis. The globulin fraction of protein often is elevated markedly. The smooth muscle antibody test is present in up to 75% of patients and is a hallmark of the disease, although it also may be present (usually in low titer) in other diseases.

Several additional autoantibodies have been described, which has allowed the subdivision of autoimmune chronic hepatitis based on the types of autoantibodies present (Table 51.7). Such classification schemes are of little practical importance currently, except to highlight that many patients with autoimmune chronic hepatitis test negative for antinuclear antibody and smooth muscle antibody and thus might be thought to have other disorders.

Liver-kidney microsomal antibodies (anti-LKM) have, in some studies, been linked to hepatitis C infection. Some have claimed that hepatitis C triggers this form of disease. More recent studies cast doubt on this putative association. Anti-LKM type 2 primarily affects children and tends to be more severe.

The major histocompatability complex affects autoimmune chronic active hepatitis. Human leukocyte antigens (HLA) A1, B8, and DR3 occur more frequently in younger patients with severe disease activity. Such patients are also more likely to relapse after treatment and require liver transplantation. HLA-DR4 also is associated with autoimmune chronic hepatitis and usually is seen in adult women with higher than usual transaminases; these women are more likely to have additional organs affected by autoimmune diseases and are more likely to respond to corticosteroid therapy. These observations do not imply that HLA typing is needed in the evaluation and management of chronic active hepatitis in clinical practice.

The treatment of severe cases (transaminase values 7–10 times the upper limit of normal) through the use of prednisone is highly effective in controlling disease and is lifesaving.

Azathioprine is frequently added to allow a reduction of the prednisone dose to more acceptable levels. Ordinarily, treatment with azathioprine is given for 6 to 12 months before any attempt is made to wean. Retreatment is frequently necessary, and close follow-up is mandatory to identify recrudescence of disease activity after therapy is stopped. Many patients require lifelong treatment to maintain control.

It is important to distinguish autoimmune chronic hepatitis from hepatitis C. As noted, some patients with the former condition test positive for anti-HCV, especially through ELISA testing. Some patients with chronic C hepatitis have autoantibodies in the serum, usually in low titer. The importance of making the distinction is more than academic, because the treatment of autoimmune chronic active hepatitis with interferon may make the disease much worse. If substantial doubt about the diagnosis remains after careful evaluation, a trial of treatment with corticosteroids should precede the administration of interferon. Confusion should be present infrequently if the differences between these entities are borne in mind.

CHOLESTATIC LIVER DISEASES

Two important causes of cholestatic liver disease are PBC and primary sclerosing cholangitis (PSC). Whereas a superficial resemblance exists between these disorders, the clinical presentations are usually quite different, and laboratory tests show different patterns (Table 51.8). Autoantibodies are much more likely in PBC.

Primary Biliary Cirrhosis

A disease of the interlobular bile ducts, PBC is a chronic disease that is most likely to afflict women older than 30 years. PBC represents a prototypical cholestatic liver disease. Its etiology is poorly understood, but it shares many features with other diseases characterized as autoimmune. Prominent among these are the presence of autoantibodies

TABLE 51.8

CLINICAL COMPARISON OF CHOLESTATIC DISEASES: PRIMARY BILIARY CIRRHOSIS VERSUS PRIMARY SCLEROSING CHOLANGITIS

Marker	Primary Biliary Cirrhosis ($n = 258$)	Primary Sclerosing Cholangitis ($n = 70$)
IgM (mg/dL)	620	70
Antimitochondrial antibodies	96%	4%
Smooth muscle antibody	66%	9%
Rheumatoid factor	70%	2%
Inflammatory bowel disease	0.04%	70.00%

IgM, immunoglobulin M.
Note: Not helpful: ALT, alkaline phosphate, bilirubin, albumin, γ-globulin, pro time, urine, and hepatic copper.
Reproduced with permission from Dickson ER. American Association for the Study of Liver Diseases, 1991 course.

and the tendency of the disease to involve multiple organs, especially the thyroid, and to exist within Sjögren syndrome, Raynaud syndrome, and occasionally CREST syndrome (i.e., *c*alcinosis, *R*aynaud phenomenon, *e*sophageal dysfunction, *s*clerodactyly, *t*elangiectasia). A regular feature is the presence of antimitochondrial antibodies, discussed later. Th-1 class CD4+ T cells predominate in the inflammatory reaction. Most cases are discovered when blood testing done for other reasons reveals abnormal liver test results. Others are discovered during the evaluation of symptoms common in PBC, especially fatigue, pruritus, and skin xanthoma. Metabolic bone disease, especially osteoporosis, is common. The progressive insult to interlobular bile ducts produces a characteristic evolution of bile duct damage, eventuating in the disappearance of most interlobular bile ducts. Thus, it is one of a number of acquired diseases that have been classified as *vanishing bile duct* disorders (Table 51.9).

Immune cholangitis (sometimes termed *autoimmune cholangiopathy* or *autoimmune cholangitis*) appears to represent a trivial variant of PBC—it comprises cases of PBC in which the antimitochondrial antibody is negative. Idiopathic adulthood ductopenia probably refers to this same entity. No evidence has been found for a different etiology, clinical course, or response to therapy. A more difficult diagnostic problem is the patient with labora-

tory and histologic evidence of both parenchymal disease (markedly elevated transaminases and inflammatory infiltrate in the hepatic parenchyma) and cholestatic disease (high alkaline phosphatase and significant bile duct injury). These patients have features of both autoimmune chronic active hepatitis and PBC and represent an overlap syndrome. These persons often respond dramatically to corticosteroids.

Natural History

PBC requires 10 to 20 years to display its natural evolution. Among asymptomatic patients, only 50% develop symptomatic disease over 10 years of observation. Not surprisingly, the histologic pattern progresses as the disease progresses (Table 51.10). Some studies have demonstrated a lack of excess mortality, even after 11 years in asymptomatic patients, although the experience of others suggests excess mortality beginning after 4 or 5 years in this group. Even among initially symptomatic patients, the 4-year survival exceeds 90%. This long disease duration is important in judging the results of clinical therapeutic trials. The Child-Pugh score is an excellent way to predict survival in patients with PBC (Fig. 51.4).

Much has been made of disease-specific predictive scores that claim to be more accurate in predicting outcome. One has won widespread acceptance in clinical research

TABLE 51.9

ACQUIRED VANISHING BILE DUCT SYNDROMES

Major Differential	Also Consider	To Be Complete
PBC	Liver allograft rejection	Histiocytosis X
PSC	Graft-versus-host	Mucoviscidosis
Autoimmune cholangiopathy?	Hepatic sarcoidosis	Septicemia
Idiopathic adulthood ductopenia?	Immunodeficiency and viral	
	Drug-induced and toxic	

PBC, primary biliary cirrhosis; PSC, primary sclerosing cholangitis.
Reproduced with permission from Desmet VJ. Vanishing bile duct disorders. In: Boyer JL, Ockner RK, eds. *Progress in Liver Diseases*, Vol. X. Philadelphia: WB Saunders, 1992:89.

TABLE 51.10

HISTOLOGIC STAGES OF PRIMARY BILIARY CIRRHOSIS

Stage	Key Finding	Additional Findings
1	Mononuclear inflammatory cells around bile ductule in portal areas; some can be seen infiltrating the basement membrane; referred to as *florid duct lesion*	Inflammation in entire portal area, sometimes spilling out into parenchyma; granulomas variably found
2	Bile duct proliferation	Features of earlier stage may be present
3	Fibrosis but not cirrhosis; bile ducts may be difficult to identify	Features of earlier stages may be present
4	Cirrhosis; marked diminution in number of bile ducts; inflammation minimal	Features of earlier stages may be present

circles. Some have found this scoring system awkward to use in clinical practice. We have found that the Child-Pugh score is a simpler yet excellent tool for predicting the likelihood of survival in PBC. The Child B patient with PBC is reaching the end stage of disease and should be considered for liver transplantation when appropriate. Newer tests, such as soluble intercellular adhesion molecule 1, type III procollagen aminoterminal peptide, and hyaluronic acid levels, appear to correlate with the stage of disease but are not routinely available and have not been extensively validated.

Laboratory Findings

The level of alkaline phosphatase is irrelevant in defining the severity of disease or the extent of liver injury, a point of some importance when judging the effects of therapy discussed later. In early-stage disease, tests of liver synthetic function are normal, including serum albumin and pro time. Also normal is the serum bilirubin. When these tests are deranged, late-stage disease (i.e., cirrhosis) is present.

Autoantibodies are a nearly universal feature of PBC. The antimitochondrial autoantibody is seen most regularly (usually with titers >160) and is present in more than 90% of cases. Mitochondria are surrounded by an inner and outer membrane. Multiple antigens are expressed by these membranes; at least 9 (M1 to M9) have been characterized. The presence of antibody directed against the M2 antigen (expressed by the inner membrane) is highly specific for PBC, whereas antibodies against M4 are frequently

seen in the chronic active hepatitis overlap syndrome. Evidence suggests that the mitochondrial oxodehydrogenase enzymes are targeted by these antibodies. Even though antigens also are expressed by mitochondria from cells in nonhepatic organs, some investigators believe that antibodies to mitochondrial antigens are responsible for the bile duct injury in PBC. Factors in favor of this association include:

- The highly directed response of the autoantibody
- The absence of such antibodies in other obstructive biliary tract disorders
- The characteristic constellation of T cells and immune complexes seen around the involved bile duct
- The similarity of the lesion of PBC with graft-versus-host disease

This topic has been reviewed. Other possibly important factors include the aberrant expression of class II major histocompatibility complex and the activation of the complement system.

Diagnostic Workup When Primary Biliary Cirrhosis Is Suspected

The diagnosis of PBC usually is straightforward. A middle-aged woman with elevated cholestatic liver enzymes who is taking no medication, has no pain, and has no previous biliary tract surgery and no signs or symptoms of inflammatory bowel disease needs little diagnostic testing. An antimitochondrial antibody in high titer all but establishes the diagnosis in such patients. Most often, an ultrasound examination (or other noninvasive imaging procedure such as a CT scan) of the liver and biliary tract is done, although in an otherwise straightforward case, the value of these tests is minimal.

A liver biopsy is valuable both in confirming the diagnosis and in establishing the stage of disease. The liver biopsy in PBC is highly characteristic. It should not be surprising that the features vary, depending on the stage of disease at which the biopsy was obtained. The most commonly used pathology staging scale used in the United States over the past 15 years was developed by Ludwig et al. When considering only biopsy features, a number of conditions may be confused with PBC, but in clinical practice, confusion

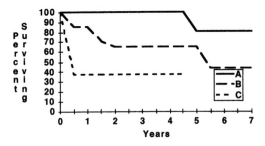

Figure 51.4 Survival probability in primary biliary cirrhosis using the Child-Pugh score at presentation. Pairwise comparison: A versus B, *p* = 0.14; A versus C, *p* < 0.001; B versus C, *p* = 0.005.

should not be frequent. Only the PBC–chronic active hepatitis overlap syndrome is likely to create difficulty for the experienced histopathologist. PSC may bear a superficial resemblance to PBC clinically, biochemically, and histologically, but most often the pathology is sufficiently distinguished that confusion is reduced rather than increased by reviewing the histologic features.

If any reason to suspect PSC is present, cholangiography must be done. However, when in doubt, the biliary anatomy should be defined. Cholangiography usually is necessary when any element of pain or previous or current biliary stone disease is present and if any signs or symptoms of inflammatory bowel disease are evident. Men with apparent PBC, and most patients in whom the antimitochondrial antibody is negative, require cholangiography to exclude PSC.

The extrahepatic manifestations of PBC require attention and occasionally may overshadow the hepatic disease. Some features can be traced to the malabsorption of fat-soluble vitamins, although most patients with PBC have normal serum levels of vitamin A, 25-hydroxy vitamin D, 1,25-dihydroxy vitamin D, prothrombin, and vitamin E levels.

Premature osteoporosis and, occasionally in late-stage disease, osteomalacia may be seen. Bone pain, compression spine fractures, and other pathological bone fractures may be the consequence of PBC-related osteoporosis and occur in up to 20% of affected persons. Malabsorption of vitamin D is one cause; although, as mentioned, only a minority of patients have documented low levels of 25-OH vitamin D. Hepatic biotransformation to 1,25-dihydroxy vitamin D appears to be intact in PBC patients. Despite (usually) normal absorption and biotransformation, bone biopsies in PBC show decreased osteoblastic and increased osteoclastic activity. Most discouraging is the observation of continued rapid bone loss in PBC patients given adequate replacement with calcium and vitamin D.

Treatment

The treatment for PBC may be divided into *supportive* and *specific* regimens. Surprisingly, few controlled clinical trials have been done to establish the use of most supportive therapy (Table 51.11). It is possible to overburden with polypharmacy a patient with a disease that is causing no difficulty. Treatment should be tailored to the patient; most require little supportive therapy. Short-term studies support the regular use of calcium and vitamin D as a means of improving vertebral bone density. One retrospective study suggests that hormone replacement therapy in postmenopausal women with PBC has resulted in lower rates of osteoporosis than in women who have not received hormone replacement therapy. Drugs that have an antiresorptive effect (e.g., calcitonin) appear not to be of value in preventing bone disease; drugs with a similar mode of action, such as bisphosphonates, require further study in this regard. A small 2-year study comparing the cyclic use

TABLE 51.11
SUPPORTIVE THERAPY IN PRIMARY BILIARY CIRRHOSIS
Bone disease prevention
Calcium
Vitamin D
Hormone replacement therapy in postmenopausal women
? Bisphosphonates
Pruritus
Level 1: Skin lubrication
Level 2: Antihistamines (e.g., Benadryl)
Cholestyramine
Level 3: Rifampin
Opioid antagonists (nalmefene, naloxone)?
Night blindness
Vitamin A
Diarrhea (malabsorption)
Level 1: Low-fat diet
Vitamin supplements (A, D, E, K)
Level 2: Medium-chain triglyceride oil

of a bisphosphonate (400 mg etidronate orally for 2 weeks followed by a 13-week "rest") and sodium fluoride (50 mg per day) in women with PBC indicated the possible benefit of bisphosphonate administration. Etidronate-treated women had essentially no change in bone densitometry in the lumbar spine compared with a modest loss in density seen in those who received fluoride. New spontaneous bone fractures were seen only in the fluoride-treated group.

Pruritus is frequent in PBC and may be severe and debilitating. The cause is incompletely understood. Early studies incriminated an accumulation of bile acids in the skin; further research has cast considerable doubt on skin bile acids as an important cause of pruritus. Many treatments are available; none is ideal. Endogenous opiate agonists (e.g., enkephalins) accumulate in cholestatic syndromes, and some investigators have wondered whether pruritus is caused by increased opiate agonist availability at opiate receptor sites in the brain. In less severe cases, simple measures such as skin lubrication sometimes augmented by the use of antihistamines suffice; this may be particularly valuable at bedtime. More severe cases do not respond to antihistamines, however, and cholestyramine, an anion-exchange resin, is generally effective. Its putative mechanism of action is the binding of bile (which contains the pruritogenic substance). It must be taken at a suitable interval from other medications because binding of medication to the resin will result in decreased absorption.

Rifampin has many complex effects on hepatocytes, including the induction of microsomal enzyme activity and stimulation of hepatic bile acid synthesis. When rifampin was given to patients with PBC in a placebo-controlled crossover study design, mean pruritus scores decreased significantly while the patients were on rifampin but not on placebo. However, there was no beneficial effect on liver tests. In another short-term (1-week) crossover study, rifampin was effective in relieving pruritus. Some of these patients were entered into a longer open-label study lasting 18 months. One patient developed an allergic reaction (rash, eosinophilia, facial edema) and was dropped from the study. Of 18 patients treated, 17 sustained complete relief and 1 had partial relief of itching. Compared with phenobarbitone in a 14-day crossover study of 22 patients, 19 had relief of itching using rifampin compared with 8 using phenobarbitone. Other studies support an antipruritic effect of this agent. The relevance of these findings to the pruritus in PSC is likely but has not been proved.

No therapy is known to reverse PBC in the native liver. A great deal of interest has been shown in drugs that appear to have some biological effect against some of the more obvious manifestations of the disease. Colchicine, prednisolone, ursodiol, cyclosporine, and tacrolimus (FK506) all have been shown to have some activity. Methotrexate has its champions, but controlled clinical trials have demonstrated a lack of efficacy. Preliminary studies indicate, moreover, that methotrexate, when used in conjunction with ursodiol, appears to provide no advantage. Because of its toxicity, the use of this agent for PBC outside of research protocols should be considered with exceptional care. Liver transplantation is available as salvage for patients with advanced stages of PBC. Ursodiol and liver transplantation are the most widely embraced therapies at this time.

Ursodiol has a number of properties that may lead to a beneficial effect in PBC. It affords a cell membrane–stabilizing effect and also may have mild immunomodulating properties. A reduced expression of major histocompatability complex class I molecules is seen on hepatocyte membranes in the presence of ursodiol. The first report of the beneficial effect of ursodiol in PBC indicated that this agent improved liver tests and symptoms. Ursodiol has been given to hundreds of patients with PBC in randomized placebo-controlled trials.

The most consistent findings of studies of ursodiol in PBC are those that show an effect on the serum levels used as markers for disease presence (but not severity). Ursodiol regularly reduces the levels of alkaline phosphatase, ALT, and GGTP. It also has an effect on serum bilirubin level and serum albumin, which more closely reflect disease stage. Some studies have demonstrated a beneficial effect on liver histology. These beneficial effects are easiest to demonstrate in stage 1 and stage 2 disease. More recent data confirm the use of ursodiol (13–15 mg/kg daily) in patients with PBC slows development of complications, delays the need for liver transplantation, and offers an overall survival advantage.

When the results from three multicenter trials using comparable doses of ursodiol (13–15 mg/kg daily) are combined (553 evaluable patients), a benefit of ursodiol on survival of 31% was apparent after up to 4 years of therapy, which also may decrease the manifestations of portal hypertension. Patients who received active treatment also had marked improvement in serum markers of disease.

No improvement was seen in metabolic bone disease or fatigue, and a variable effect on pruritus was observed. The beneficial effects were observed even in stage 3 and 4 disease.

Therapy is lifelong. Side effects rarely limit the use of ursodiol. A few develop diarrhea, and occasionally a patient has worsening of pruritus.

Of course, the PBC patient with advanced cirrhosis may develop features of decompensation (ascites, gastrointestinal bleeding, portosystemic encephalopathy). These are handled in the same manner as with other causes of cirrhosis, which are discussed later. Liver transplantation for advanced PBC is highly successful. Although controlled clinical trials comparing liver transplantation and medical therapy have not been performed, survival comparisons of transplantation with the "natural history" have been estimated using the Cox regression model. An apparent advantage of liver transplantation is apparent as early as 6 months after surgery, and this survival benefit is maintained for at least 5 years. The outcome of liver transplantation is better than for many other diseases. The disease affecting the native liver has been shown to recur in many diseases for which liver transplantation is performed. Indeed, some evidence has shown that PBC may recur in approximately 10% of transplant recipients. This area is controversial because the histology of rejection shares some features of PBC. In our transplant program, 30 patients received a graft because of PBC; many have had a recurrence of antimitochondrial antibody, but only one has had a clinical course and serial liver histology consistent with recurrent PBC. In the remainder, recognizable PBC has not emerged. Whether this freedom from recurrence reflects the effects of immunosuppression or other factors is unknown.

The timing of referral for transplantation is always difficult because of the complex interplay of disease progression and the long interval between the approval for transplantation and the operation, which frequently exceeds 1 year. Child B patients with PBC are significantly more likely to die than Child A, and Child C patients are more likely to die than either A or B patients. Once a patient with PBC falls into the Child B range, liver transplantation should be given serious consideration.

Primary Sclerosing Cholangitis

PSC is a chronic hepatobiliary disease of unknown cause that is characterized by diffuse or multifocal fibrosing inflammatory changes in the bile ducts. It is seen most often in association with inflammatory bowel disease. Some have suggested a common pathogenesis. Patients with PSC have circulating immune complexes. An increase in the T-cell helper-to-suppressor ratio has been shown. The increased autoreactivity of T lymphocytes after activation in the autologous mixed lymphocyte reaction also occurs. All these observations suggest the role of a disordered immune system in the pathogenesis of PSC.

PSC is characterized by disease progression and excessive mortality. Although some investigators have suggested that PSC is a relatively indolent disorder, most experiences with this disorder are considerably less benign. It is apparent that regardless of liver stage or clinical status, the disease is progressive. Our experience indicates a 9-year survival of 49%. In one therapeutic trial, 80% of patients showed evidence of disease progression (as assessed by the development of ascites, esophageal varices, increase in bilirubin, progression of histologic stage, referral for liver transplantation, or death within a 3-year study period).

Diagnosis requires cholangiography, although a strong inferential case can be made clinically, especially in those patients with inflammatory bowel disease and a markedly elevated alkaline phosphatase level. The cholangiogram reveals a ratty, irregular biliary tree produced by the fibrosing process. Between the narrowed segments, the biliary tree may be either normal in caliber or even dilated. The process most often is diffuse, but sometimes it is limited to the intrahepatic or extrahepatic biliary tree. The most important differential diagnosis in the cholangiogram is between PSC and cholangiocarcinoma. The more limited the extent of the biliary abnormality, the more concern exists that cancer is present. So many variations and permutations are possible that certain differentiation often is not possible. Cholangiocarcinoma, although usually focal, may be diffuse. Moreover, cholangiocarcinoma may complicate sclerosing cholangitis, usually in patients older than 60 years. Men are more commonly afflicted. Patients present most often with signs or symptoms or laboratory abnormalities suggesting complete or partial biliary tract obstruction.

There is no proven therapy for PSC. Hope that ursodiol may modulate the liver damage in PSC in a manner analogous to its effect in PBC has not been borne out. Important differences in biliary bile acid composition in these disorders may, in part, explain ursodiol's lack of effect in PSC. Virtually no lithocholate was seen in the serum of patients with PSC before or after treatment with ursodiol, and no change in the urinary lithocholate levels was seen after treatment.

Liver transplantation for PSC with or without inflammatory bowel disease may be lifesaving. The PSC patient with cirrhotic complications can anticipate a 1- and 3-year survival rate after liver transplantation of 90% and 89%, respectively. Timing is crucial, particularly in light of the long waiting period required for a donor organ. As in PBC, once a PSC patient is classified as Child B, it is time to consider referral to a transplant center.

INHERITED LIVER DISEASES

The three liver diseases to be considered here are Wilson disease, hemochromatosis, and α_1-antitrypsin (A1AT) deficiency. In particular, persons with the first two disorders must be identified because of the potential for lifesav-

ing treatment. Genetic counseling and screening of family members are also important. Wilson disease may present with either brain or liver disease or occasionally both. It is a disease of abnormal copper metabolism, inherited as autosomal recessive, and it should be suspected in any young person with chronic or severe acute liver disease. It is rare for Wilson disease to manifest for the first time after the age of 40 years. The serum ceruloplasmin is depressed in 95% of persons, which is helpful because ceruloplasmin is an acute-phase reactant and therefore is elevated in most forms of liver disease. A low-normal or clearly low ceruloplasmin level in the setting of liver disease should be considered Wilson disease until proven otherwise. Other causes for a low level include the healthy heterozygote state and fulminant or end-stage liver disease. Kayser-Fleischer rings (brown pigmented rings around the edge of the cornea) should be present if neurologic signs and symptoms are observed, but these may be absent if only the liver is involved. A slit-lamp examination is required to see all but the most florid Kayser-Fleischer rings. In questionable cases, a liver biopsy with quantitative copper determination usually clarifies the diagnosis. Hepatic copper values >250 $\mu g/g$ are virtually diagnostic of untreated Wilson disease. Lesser degrees of hepatic copper elevation may be seen in chronic hepatitis and in chronic cholestatic liver diseases (such as PBC). Copper-chelating drugs are used to treat Wilson disease. The drug of first choice is D-penicillamine, but trientine may be used if D-penicillamine is poorly tolerated. Oral zinc therapy competes with copper absorption and may be used for maintenance therapy in the decoppered patients.

Hereditary hemochromatosis (genetic hemochromatosis, idiopathic hemochromatosis), a heterogeneous group of disorders, is characterized by excessive iron deposition in many organs, including, importantly, the liver. Other targets for excess iron include the pancreas (diabetes may result), heart (conduction disturbances, heart failure), joints (arthritis), gonads (impotence), and skin (darkening). The constellation of bronze skin, diabetes, heart disease, and liver disease describes the fully developed case. To prevent end-organ damage, this disease should be suspected in any patient with chronic liver disease, especially those who manifest injury in one or more other organ systems. Iron may accumulate due to genetic predisposition or to chronic iron overload, such as that which occurs in the multiply transfused patient and chronic anemias (e.g., thalassemia), and it is associated with certain conditions such as PCT.

Hereditary hemochromatosis, a relatively common disorder inherited as an autosomal recessive trait carried on the short arm of chromosome 6 in close association to the HLA-A3 locus, results in a failure of feedback inhibition of intestinal iron absorption. The most common form is inherited as an autosomal recessive trait. The homozygous presence of either of two different genes may result in iron accumulation. It has been estimated that as many as 1 in 250 white persons carries both genes necessary for expression of the disease, an estimate that appears to overstate the frequency with which it is recognized clinically. The precise genetic defect for many cases of hereditary hemochromatosis has been identified, and a clinically important laboratory diagnostic test (hemochromatosis DNA PCR) has revolutionized the approach to identifying those affected. The so-called *HFE* gene is located on chromosome 6, near the locus for the *HLA-A* gene. Two mutations have been described. Most (69%–100%) cases of clinically typical hereditary hemochromatosis have a missense mutation (C282Y) often termed the "major mutation" that causes cysteine to be substituted for tyrosine at the 282 amino acid protein product of the gene. Another mutation on the *HFE* gene at the H63D locus (the "minor mutation"), which results in the substitution of aspartic acid for histidine at position 63, may be present in those with hereditary hemochromatosis. The presence of homozygous H63D may result in iron overload, but the clinical expression (rate and frequency) appears less than when homozygote C282Y defect is present. Finally, a compound heterozygote (one gene containing C282Y and the other H63D) also may result in iron overload.

A laboratory diagnosis of hemochromatosis is important. The diagnosis should be suspected in the following situations:

- Any adult with liver disease, especially men
- Transferrin saturation ≥55%
- Ferritin elevations (>200 μg/L in premenopausal women; >300 μg/L in men and postmenopausal women)

Confirmation of the diagnosis requires a demonstration of increased hepatic iron by liver biopsy. The value of the biopsy is twofold: It provides information about the degree of fibrosis and cirrhosis present, which is vital in predicting the risk of subsequent development of hepatoma, and it provides an assessment of iron stores. The quantitative assessment of hepatic iron is considered superior to semiquantitative staining of liver specimens. The hepatic iron index is calculated as follows:

$$\text{Hepatic iron index} = \frac{\text{Hepatic iron concentration}}{(\mu \text{ mol/g dry weight})}{\text{Patient's age in years}}$$

A hepatic iron index level <1.9 is normal; values >1.9 are seen in hemochromatosis. Interest has been rekindled in assessing hepatic iron through the evaluation of iron stains of liver biopsy material, and this is a satisfactory alternative to quantitative iron determination. Bone marrow iron stores are not adequate to assess total body iron stores; indeed, cases of hemochromatosis with absent stainable bone marrow iron have been reported. The treatment of idiopathic hemochromatosis requires phlebotomy on a weekly basis until iron deficiency is depleted, with maintenance phlebotomies every 1 to 3 months thereafter.

The physician who makes the diagnosis of hemochromatosis in a patient has a responsibility to inform the patient that the disease is inherited and to urge that patient to ensure that all siblings and offspring are informed and screened. Those older than 25 years should be screened because the likelihood of demonstrating excess iron in children and young adults, even in the presence of homozygosity, is low. Of course, genetic testing for C282Y and H63D can be done at any age, although no clear guidelines have been made as to what is the most appropriate screening test (serum iron indices vs. genetic testing) to use in first-degree relatives of patients with hemochromatosis.

In the event that cirrhosis is present, the patient with hemochromatosis must be in a regular surveillance program for hepatoma. Semiannual α-fetoprotein determinations and ultrasound examinations are suggested.

α_1-Antitrypsin Deficiency

A1AT deficiency is the most common cause of persistent jaundice in newborn infants, although it may also present in childhood with prominent pulmonary disease or, less often, with pediatric liver disease. Some cases do not manifest until adulthood. Unexplained liver dysfunction or complications of cirrhosis may be due to A1AT deficiency. It is important to note that A1AT deficiency dose not cause acute liver disease such as acute hepatatitis; rather, patients may present with chronic nonspecific elevation of liver tests or with complications of cirrhosis if not diagnosed at an earlier time point. Many different genetic forms exist, and the protease inhibitor test most often is used to differentiate these. The normal protease inhibitor type is MM. Those with a double Z allele (protease inhibitor ZZ) are most likely to suffer from the disease. Controversy surrounds the association of a single Z allele (e.g., protease inhibitor MZ) and liver disease. Current published evidence and a review of Cleveland Clinic experience suggest that the isolated presence of a single Z allele poses an increased risk for cirrhosis and liver failure. No definitive treatment is available for this disease; liver transplantation should be considered if the stigmata of end-stage cirrhosis develop.

CIRRHOSIS

Cirrhosis is the final outcome of all types of chronic liver injuries whether caused by alcohol, a virus, a medication, or due to an autoimmune or genetic process. The outcome for cirrhotic patients depends on the degree of functional impairment in the liver and the amount of decompensation present. Originally developed to predict survival after portacaval shunt surgery, the Child-Pugh classification (Table 51.12) has been useful in predicting survival in the untreated cirrhotic patient. Only five features (all easily measurable) are needed.

TABLE 51.12

PUGH-MODIFIED CHILD-TURCOTTE CLASSIFICATIONS

	A (1 Point)	B (2 Points)	C (3 Points)
Bilirubin	<2 mg/dL	2–3 mg/dL	>3 mg/dL
Albumin	>3.5 g/dL	2.8–3.5 g/dL	<2.8 g/dL
Ascites	None	Easily controlled	Poorly controlled
Neurologic	No PSE	Mild PSE	Refractory PSE
INR	<1.7	1.7–2.3	>2.3

INR, international normalized ratio; PSE, portosystemic encephalopathy.
Note: For each of five items, a score of 1, 2, or 3 is assigned. The total score is the sum of these items. Child A = 57; B = 810; C = 11 or more.

Cirrhosis may produce no symptoms or signs. When cirrhosis becomes decompensated, it manifests as one or more of the following:

- Ascites and edema
- Gastrointestinal bleeding
- Encephalopathy

Ascites

Ascites occurs because the kidney behaves as if it were receiving an inadequate blood flow. Low urine volume, low urine sodium concentration (often 10 mEq/L), and an activated renin-angiotensin-aldosterone (RAA) system are typical, resulting in sodium and water retention. When the imbalance between sodium intake and excretion goes on long enough, expansion of the intravascular and then extravascular space occurs, which eventually causes edema and or ascites. Atrial natriuretic factor (ANF) often is elevated in patients with cirrhotic ascites. Such elevations probably serve to protect against further volume expansion in early cirrhosis. A complete understanding of sodium retention in cirrhosis has been elusive, but the pathophysiology has been investigated extensively.

Sodium Retention

The vascular, hemodynamic, and humoral characteristics in the cirrhotic patient are dynamic, with fairly subtle early changes and more explicit and numerous abnormalities in decompensated cirrhosis. In a study of 12 cirrhotic patients with diuretic-resistant tense ascites, all had normal or nearly normal serum creatinine (0.85 mg/dL ± 0.2). At the same time, they were mildly hyponatremic (135 mEq/L ± 4). Yet, all had avid sodium retention (urine [Na^+] 5 mEq/L), and urine volume was only 445 mL/24 hours. It is clear that urinary sodium excretion is impaired. However, this study, like most others, takes a "snapshot" late in the course of a long disease process. In order to know more about the evolution of the renal defect in cirrhosis, there is a need to look at the patient, or an experimental animal, much earlier. A direct correlation exists between renal sodium retention and liver function, as measured by the clearance of antipyrine, caffeine, and chocolate, but no relationship is apparent between sodium retention and degree of portosystemic shunting.

Levy et al. have done some of the most elegant experiments in a dog model of cirrhosis and ascites. Using dimethylnitrosamine to create cirrhosis, he studied the blood volume, renal, humoral, and autonomic nervous system changes over time. Before dimethylnitrosamine, not surprisingly, urinary sodium excretion matched sodium intake (i.e., homeostasis was demonstrated). As cirrhosis developed and portal pressure began to rise, but well before ascites formed, progressive impairment of renal sodium excretion resulted in a positive sodium balance and increased intravascular volume. In humans with alcoholic cirrhosis, plasma volume was expanded whether or not ascites was present. A positive correlation was found between plasma volume and wedged hepatic venous pressure (a reflection of portal pressure). Splanchnic plasma volume did not contract during the formation of ascites, nor did it expand when ascites was mobilized. Thus, in both humans and experimental animals with cirrhosis, plasma volume is expanded. The signal initiating inappropriate sodium retention remains elusive, but most investigators believe that arterial underfilling from cirrhosis activates a yet unidentified intrahepatic low-pressure baroreceptor and signals the kidney to conserve sodium.

Renin-Angiotensin-Aldosterone

In healthy humans, the volume, distribution, and composition of extracellular fluid vary within a narrow range. Among the neurohumoral regulators of renal sodium handling, the RAA system plays an important role. In cirrhosis, the equilibrium of this feedback loop frequently is severely disturbed. In cirrhotic preascitic rats, early abnormalities can be detected. For example, urinary aldosterone levels rise before ascites forms, and these levels are temporally related to sodium retention. In other animal experiments, however, sodium retention predated the activation of the RAA system. In humans with cirrhosis, a good correlation exists between plasma aldosterone levels and urinary sodium excretion, except that the system appears "downregulated" in cirrhotics with ascites. For any given level of aldosterone, cirrhotic patients with ascites excrete less sodium than either cirrhotic patients without ascites or healthy subjects. The inhibition of the RAA system by drugs has had a mixed result in increasing natriuresis in cirrhotic ascites. This area of study has not been easy, because drugs that affect the RAA system often have independent effects on the vascular system and renal glomerular blood flow. The greatest support for an important role for the RAA system is the effectiveness of the aldosterone-blocking agent spironolactone in cirrhotic ascites. In such a setting, this agent is superior to furosemide in producing natriuresis. Nevertheless, other drugs that interfere with the RAA system (e.g., captopril, saralasin, β-blockers) do not seem to be effective agents in cirrhosis, although captopril added to diuretic therapy may be effective in some patients with refractory ascites. In summary, the RAA system plays an important but not an exclusive role in the perpetuation of renal sodium retention once it is activated, probably through other factors. The central role in aldosterone antagonism using spironolactone in the treatment of ascites is well accepted.

Other Perturbations

Sympathetic nervous system abnormalities are the rule in cirrhotic patients and appear to play a role in the renal response to this condition. The circulating levels of norepinephrine, the principal neurotransmitter of the adrenergic nervous system, are taken as a measure of sympathetic discharge. Levels are higher in patients with more advanced cirrhosis and higher still in the hepatorenal syndrome. Adrenergic blockade with agents such as clonidine does result in reduced norepinephrine levels; however, as noted, its effect in reducing perfusing pressure overshadows any beneficial effect of norepinephrine, and enhanced sodium excretion does not occur. It is possible that the observed increases in sympathetic activity seen in cirrhosis represent a defense against other changes rather than important pathophysiological events. ANF, a cardiac hormone with powerful vasodilator and natriuretic properties, is often elevated in patients with cirrhotic ascites. Such elevations probably serve to protect against further volume expansion in early cirrhosis. This suggests that either ANF is elevated as a normal response to sodium retention or that a blunted renal response to ANF is present in cirrhosis. Like the sympathetic nervous system, the exact importance of ANF in the pathogenesis of ascites remains obscure.

Ascitic Fluid Analysis

Cirrhotic ascites is similar to serum, except it contains less protein. The serum albumin–ascitic fluid albumin gradient (SAAG) is usually >1.1. This ratio is calculated by subtracting the albumin concentration of ascites from that of serum (albumin ser minus albumin asc). Cardiac ascites will have a similarly high gradient. The SAAG has been established as a clinical valuable test with high specificity to differentiate ascites due to portal hypertension (cirrhosis, Budd-Chiari syndrome, or right heart failure) from other causes of ascites. Low gradients (<1.1) suggest a noncirrhotic (and a noncardiac) cause for ascites, such as malignancy or infection. This test is considered a routine part of the evaluation of ascitic fluid and has largely replaced the exudate–transudate distinction that was based on a consideration of total protein concentration in the ascitic fluid. Although ascites is usually not a threat, it becomes so when infection occurs. Spontaneous bacterial peritonitis (SBP) usually is the result of aerobic gut-derived gram-negative bacteria (*Escherichia coli* and *Klebsiella*), although it may be caused by gram-positive bacteria such as *Streptococcus pneumoniae* (Table 51.13). It usually is not polymicrobial, and anerobes are distinctly unusual. In SBP, the ascitic fluid cell count almost always reveals a polymorphonuclear count >250/mm^3 (considered the gold standard test for the diagnosis of SBP). Interestingly, infected ascites usually maintains an albumen gradient >1. Cultures are most likely to be positive if 10 mL of fluid is poured into a blood culture bottle at the patient's bedside.

The treatment of infected ascites requires systemic antibiotics. Because the kidney of a cirrhotic patient is particularly susceptible to toxicity from aminoglycosides, the use of these agents plus ampicillin has generally given way to the use of a third-generation cephalosporin such as cefotaxime. Five days of treatment are adequate in most cases. Costs are an increasingly important part of medical decision making. The dosage of cefotaxime needed to control infection is lower in cirrhotic patients, in part because of decreased hepatic metabolism. Two grams every 12 hours, instead of every 6 hours, results in satisfactory peak and trough levels and controls infection. Important endpoints of the treatment of SBP with cefotaxime are infection

---

TABLE 51.13

TYPICAL ORGANISMS THAT CAUSE SPONTANEOUS BACTERIAL PERITONITIS

Gram Negative	Percent (%)	Gram Positive	Percent (%)
Escherichia coli	37.0	Pneumococcus	12.0
Klebsiella pneumoniae	17.0	*Streptococcus viridans*	8.5
Enterobacter	6.4	γ-Hemolytic streptococcus	4.3
Other	5.0	Enterococcus	3.2
Other group D streptococci	1.1	Other	5.0

resolution and mortality. The pretreatment predictors of treatment failure are:

- Higher levels of band neutrophils in peripheral blood
- Hospital acquisition of SBP
- Higher blood urea nitrogen
- Higher ALT

Pretreatment predictors of in-hospital mortality are:

- High blood urea nitrogen
- High ALT
- Hospital acquisition of SBP
- Older age
- Child-Pugh score
- Ileus

The prevention of SBP is possible. Both primary prevention (for those with no history of SBP) and secondary prevention studies are available. Quinolone antibiotics are effective, although they are poorly absorbed from the gastrointestinal tract. They are effective in reducing bacterial counts in the gut and the urinary tract, two reservoirs for organisms commonly seen in SBP. For the typical cirrhotic patient with ascites, norfloxacin, 400 mg twice daily, is a simple and effective regimen. The reports of a rapid emergence of resistant organisms have not translated (yet) into a reduced effectiveness in using this strategy to reduce episodes of SBP in cirrhotic patients with ascites. Other agents also appear to be effective in SBP prophylaxis. Sulfamethoxazole-trimethoprim (800 mg/160 mg) (one double-strength tablet Monday through Friday) reduced by 87% the number of episodes of SBP over a median 90-day follow-up period.

When should antibiotic prophylaxis be given to cirrhotic patients with ascites? Based on available evidence for those particularly at risk, it seems prudent to consider prophylaxis for those with one or more of the following risk factors:

- Previous history of SBP
- Ascitic fluid protein concentration <1 g/dL
- Acute upper gastrointestinal bleeding

Treatment of Cirrhotic Ascites

Bed rest is unquestionably helpful in controlling ascites, but seldom is this treatment practical, except in the sickest patients. The effect of posture on renal sodium handling has been elucidated: In an upright posture, the renin-angiotensin system is activated, sympathetic tone increased, and glomerular filtration decreased. The mainstay of treatment for ascites is dietary sodium restriction. A 2-g sodium diet often is prescribed. When this is insufficient, diuretics are used. Spironolactone is the agent of first choice. An initial dose of 100 mg daily is often selected. Dose escalation up to 400 mg daily is possible. In men, painful gynecomastia frequently prevents such a high dose. Proximal tubule or loop diuretics then are added, most fre-

quently a thiazide or furosemide. Diuretics have frequent side effects that regularly cause intravascular volume depletion, electrolyte abnormalities, and a reduction in renal function. These problems are particularly likely to occur if more than 500 to 1,000 mL/24 hours of excess fluid is mobilized.

Paracentesis represents an increasingly popular method of controlling large amounts of ascites and is perhaps the most physiological treatment, given the central role of volume expansion in cirrhotic ascites. The removal of large volumes (even total paracentesis) appears safer than diuretic therapy. The patient so treated is simultaneously begun on a salt-restricted diet and diuretics to minimize the reaccumulation of ascites and to reduce the need for repeated paracentesis. Many hepatology units provide intravenous albumin infusions (e.g., 8 g/L of ascites removed), but the value of this expensive replacement therapy has not been established unequivocally. Whereas transient changes are seen in cardiac output, pulmonary wedge pressure, and central venous pressure, along with activation of the renin-angiotensin system when ascites is removed without providing intravenous colloid, the clinical relevance of these observations remains speculative. One drawback of repeated large-volume removal is protein depletion. Although not much of a clinical problem, the reduction in ascitic fluid opsonic activity raises the theoretic problem of susceptibility to infection; this was not borne out, however, in a carefully controlled clinical trial designed to compare the relative risks of large-volume paracentesis compared with diuretic therapy for cirrhotic ascites.

Peritoneovenous shunting for refractory ascites has been used for 20 years, with mixed results. There seems to be variable success in keeping these shunts patent over an extended period. When they remain patent, rapid natriuresis is observed. Infection, disseminated intravascular coagulation, and clotting are problems described with these shunts. Approximately 50% are occluded within 24 months of placement. Consistent with high early patency rates followed by failures, when peritoneovenous shunting was compared with large-volume paracentesis, early and total rehospitalizations were fewer in the shunted group; total time in the hospital during follow-up, total complication rates, and survival rates were similar in both groups.

Early studies using percutaneous transjugular intrahepatic portosystemic shunts (TIPS) have suggested that they represent an effective way to manage refractory ascites. A reduction in ascites and a reduced need for diuretics or paracentesis have been demonstrated, as have an increase in fractional sodium excretion and decreased plasma renin, aldosterone, and norepinephrine. It appears that the size of the shunt created is more critical for ascites control than for bleeding control. Portosystemic encephalopathy may occur, usually within the first 3 months. Clinical manifestations often recede, even when the TIPS remain patent and the arterial ammonia levels remain elevated, suggesting a role of cerebral adaptation.

After a few months, TIPS tend to occlude in many patients and require repeated balloon angioplasty to restore patency and function. The author considers TIPS for refractory ascites as a bridge to liver transplantation. Hospitalized Child C cirrhotic patients whose refractory ascites is treated using TIPS do not survive hospitalization unless they undergo transplantation. Longer-term studies are needed before deciding that this is a satisfactory long-term treatment.

The 1- and 3-year survival rates after the first development of ascites are 50% and 20%, respectively. These rates compare unfavorably with survival after transplantation. Accordingly, the emergence of conspicuous ascites should at least prompt an inquiry into whether or not liver transplantation should be undertaken in the patient.

Hepatic hydrothorax is the accumulation of pleural effusions, most often right sided, in the setting of cirrhotic ascites. Often, ascites becomes less of a problem as fluid accumulates within the pleural space. Defects within the diaphragm are most often the culprit. Symptomatic hepatic hydrothorax represents a difficult management problem that often occurs toward the latest stages of cirrhosis. Treatment through salt restriction and diuretics or large-volume paracentesis is seldom successful. Repeated thoracentesis is usually poorly tolerated because of the required frequency. Both pleurodesis and TIPS have been used with variable results, although results of TIPS for the management of hepatic hydrothorax are encouraging. Most patients with this complication die of end-stage liver failure within a few months unless they undergo transplantation.

Portal Hypertensive Bleeding

Gastrointestinal bleeding occurs frequently in patients with portal hypertension. Detailed practice guidelines have been published. The pathogenesis of cirrhotic hypertension is complex. Figure 51.5 indicates the major vessels of interest in portal hypertension, and Figure 51.6 shows the major pertubations. In humans, portal pressure is measured somewhat indirectly, because the portal vein is not readily

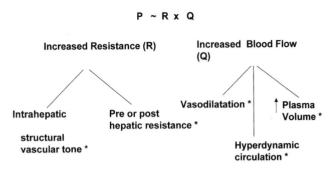

Figure 51.6 Factors contributing to increased portal pressure. (*, potentially reversible.)

accessible for cannulation. The wedge pressure in the hepatic vein is measured, and from this measurement is subtracted the free hepatic vein pressure (or the inferior vena cava pressure); the result is termed the *portal-hepatic vein gradient*. The normal pressure is <5 mm Hg. Bleeding from portal hypertension is not seen until the portal-hepatic vein gradient is >12 mm Hg.

Primary Prevention

Most often, brisk or massive portal hypertensive bleeding is due to ruptured esophageal or gastric varices. More recently, a diffuse mucosal abnormality termed *portal hypertensive gastropathy* has been described as a frequent cause of hemorrhage. The mortality for first variceal bleeds is approximately 20% for Child A and ≥60% for Child C patients. Because of the often disastrous outcome from variceal hemorrhage, therapy administered to the cirrhotic patient with large varices that have never bled has been studied extensively. Currently, two classes of agents appear effective in preventing the first hemorrhage: noncardioselective β-blockers, especially propranolol, nadolol, and timolol; and long-acting nitrates. β-Blockers have been studied extensively and are reasonably well tolerated and moderately effective in reducing episodes of first hemorrhage. Isosorbide mononitrate appears to be as effective in preventing first variceal hemorrhage. One report, however, found a higher incidence of (nonbleeding) deaths in patients older than 50 years receiving isosorbide mononitrate compared with those who received propranolol. The significance of this possible heightened death rate is uncertain. Endoscopic band ligation is an effective alternative to β-blocker therapy for primary prevention.

Management of Acute Hemorrhage

A patient with acutely bleeding varices represents a medical emergency and should be admitted to the hospital and monitored closely. At the same time that fluid resuscitation is being carried out, a control of bleeding is attempted by simultaneously initiating pharmacotherapy (Table 51.14) and organizing an upper intestinal endoscopy for a direct endoscopic attack on the bleeding source. Octreotide is easier to use than vasopressin and is virtually devoid of significant hemodynamic side effects. It is more effective than vasopressin and is the pharmacologic agent of first choice.

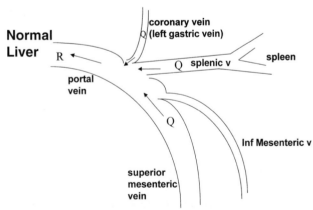

Figure 51.5 Pressure in the normal liver. (Q, volume of blood flow; R, resistance.)

TABLE 51.14

PHARMACOLOGIC STRATEGIES TO CONTROL ACUTE VARICEAL HEMORRHAGE

Option	Agent	Adjunctive Therapy	Concomitant Endoscopic Control
A	Octreotide, 50 μg IV bolus then 50 μg/hr IV	No	Yes
B	Vasopressin, 20 IU in 100 mL D5W over 20 min; then 0.1 IU to 0.4 IU/min	No	Yes
C	Per option B, except infusion rates up to 0.8 IU/min allowed	NTG infusion 40 μg/min and increase by 40 μg/min every 15 min if systolic blood pressure >100 mm Hg. Maximum infusion 400 μg/min or NTG transdermal patch (10 mg over 24 hr) or NTG 0.6 mg SL every 30 min over 6 hr	Yes

D5W, dextrose 5% in water; IV, intravenous; NTG, nitroglycerin; SL, sublingual.

When vasopressin is used, the dosage is limited by the occurrence of significant ischemia of other organs, such as the heart, gut, or kidneys. Bradyarrhythmias may occur. The concomitant use of nitroglycerin (usually as a patch or sublingually) has allowed higher doses of vasopressin. Approximately 60% to 75% of bleeding variceal episodes can be controlled by using these agents.

The use of balloons attached to tubes (Sengstaken Blakemore, Minnesota, or Linton) is also effective. Studies suggest that 85% to 90% of initial control of bleeding varices occurs. A high incidence of early rebleeding occurs once the balloons are deflated or removed, so additional therapy must be planned for most of these patients. Balloon tamponade in our unit is reserved for those in whom pharmacologic therapy (octreotide, vasopressin) has failed to control bleeding.

Endoscopic therapy has been used frequently for the control of the acute bleeding episode. A series of sessions directed at the elimination of esophageal varices is required. Endoscopic sclerotherapy or band ligation is appropriate for the control of bleeding from esophageal varices but not for bleeding from either gastric varices or portal hypertensive gastropathy. Studies indicate that elastic banding of esophageal varices may be more efficient than injection techniques; fewer sessions are needed, and less bleeding occurs.

Where emergency endoscopic services are readily available, the endoscopic control of variceal bleeding is most often used. Adjunctive pharmacotherapy is administered as soon as major variceal hemorrhage is suspected, in preparation for endoscopic control. Octreotide is often given as an intravenous bolus of 50 μg, followed by an infusion of 50 μg per hour. The infusion is continued for up to 5 days. One study has suggested that prolonging treatment with octreotide for 15 days (100 μg subcutaneously three times daily), combined with either β-blocker therapy or

endoscopic sclerotherapy, significantly reduces rebleeding rates during the first 42 days after the index bleed. Rebleeding rates at 6 weeks were lowest (18%) in those who received 15 days of octreotide plus sclerotherapy and highest (82%) in those who received placebo and sclerotherapy.

In the few studies comparing the effectiveness and complication rates of endoscopic and pharmacologic treatment, the results support either approach. A meta-analysis of such studies suggested equivalent efficacy in controlling bleeding and a lower incidence of side effects using drug therapy compared with endoscopic sclerotherapy. Rebleeding rates after the cessation of infusion therapy appear higher, however, than that after sclerotherapy, and the cost may be higher as well. Thus, the debate continues. The importance of this issue to the clinician rests in the observation that both forms of treatment are acceptable and that lack of availability of endoscopic services need not be considered evidence of less than state-of-the-art care. In most centers, these treatment options are both available, and most experts recommend initiating pharmacotherapy and endoscopic therapy simultaneously.

Secondary Prevention

After acute bleeding is controlled, attention moves to a long-term strategy to prevent additional bleeds (secondary prevention). The most frequent therapy has been a series of endoscopic sessions to obliterate varices.

The endoscopic treatment of esophageal varices with band ligation appears superior to injection sclerotherapy. Rebleeding rates are lower, varices are obliterated in fewer sessions, and mortality may also be less. The optimal strategy to prevent bleeding recurrence appears to be with pharmacotherapy plus repetitive band ligation sessions. Nadolol in addition to ligation reduced recurrent hemorrhage from 47% to 21% over 21 months. One report suggests that nadolol combined with isosorbide mononitrate

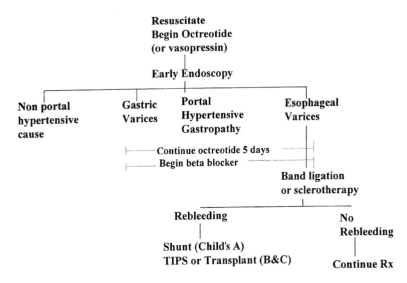

Figure 51.7 Algorithm for management of bleeding cirrhotics. (TIPS, transjugular intrahepatic portosystemic shunt.) (Reproduced with permission from the American College of Gastroenterology. Available at: http://www.acg.gi.org/physicianforum/pated/var_alg2.html.)

is at least as effective at reducing rebleeding as endoscopic ligation.

If bleeding becomes recalcitrant, consideration is given to salvage therapy. Shunt surgery, either central or distal, is considered if the patient is a good surgical risk (Child-Pugh A or B+). A radiologically placed TIPS is used in poorer risk patients or as salvage therapy for the acutely bleeding patient not responsive to other therapy. TIPS was first introduced as a temporizing measure, as a bridge to liver transplantation.

This procedure is performed by invasive radiologists. By puncturing the jugular vein and traversing the superior and inferior vena cava, the hepatic vein is cannulated. A needle is passed through the cannula, and the hepatic vein is punctured. A communication is established between the hepatic vein and the (hypertensive) portal vein. With the fistulous tract established, portal pressure falls. To keep the fistula open, a stent is placed across the track. Preliminary data suggest that bleeding may be controlled in as many as 90% of patients and ascites in 70%. This procedure should be considered in cases in which endoscopic therapy is ineffective. Three prospective studies comparing TIPS with endoscopic sclerotherapy have been reported. In two of these studies, TIPS was more effective in reducing subsequent hemorrhage. In one study only, the mortality for those receiving TIPS was higher. In two of three stud-

ies, the incidence of worsened portosystemic encephalopathy was higher in those treated using TIPS. Until the literature becomes clearer, most will rely first on endoscopic (or pharmacologic) treatment to prevent recurrent hemorrhage, reserving TIPS for patients who fail to respond to or are unlikely to comply with an endoscopic or pharmacologic program. A useful algorithm for portal hypertensive bleeding is shown in **Figure 51.7**. Current first- and second-line treatment for primary prevention, acute hemorrhage, and secondary prevention is indicated in **Table 51.15**.

Hepatic Encephalopathy

Hepatic encephalopathy is chronic liver disease caused by those toxins present in the splanchnic circulation (absorbed from the gastrointestinal tract) being shunted around the liver into the systemic circulation, where they gain access to the central nervous system and exert their deleterious effect. Ammonia, fatty acids, mercaptans, aromatic amino acids, γ-aminobutyric acid (GABA), and endogenous benzodiazepines are all candidate neurotoxins. The central nervous system of cirrhotic patients is much more sensitive to hypnotics, sedatives, and narcotics, all of which may precipitate coma in these patients. The artificial creation of shunts (either surgical or through TIPS) may precipitate hepatic encephalopathy. In acute liver failure,

TABLE 51.15		
VARICEAL HEMORRHAGE MANAGEMENT		
	First Choice	**Second Choice**
Primary prevention	β-blocker[a] $\pm$ IMN	Band ligation
Active bleed	Octreotide/SMN + band ligation	Vasopressin, TIPS, or balloon tamponade
Secondary prevention	Band ligation +β-blocker + IMN	TIPS or shunt

IMN, isosorbide mononitrate; SMN, somatostatin; TIPS, transjugular intrahepatic portosystemic shunt.
[a]β-blocker = noncardioselective (e.g., nadolol, propranolol, timolol).

TABLE 51.16
GRADING OF HEPATIC ENCEPHALOPATHY

Stage	Clinical	Neurologic	Electroencephalography
0	Subtle personality changes (apparent only to family or sophisticated neuropsychiatric testing)	Alert; no asterixis	Normal
1	Definite personality changes; alteration of sleep pattern	Asterixis present	Delta waves present
2	Sleepy; abnormal behavior	Asterixis present	Delta waves present
3	Somnolent but arousable	Asterixis present	Delta waves present
4	Comatose (may respond to painful stimuli)	Asterixis absent	Delta waves present

other mechanisms are operative as well, including the loss of liver function and cerebral edema. Encephalopathy is graded according to severity (Table 51.16).

The treatment of hepatic encephalopathy in cirrhotic patients depends, in part, on the severity. Dietary protein restriction is used in all stages and may be all that is necessary in stage 0 through II encephalopathy. Pharmacotherapy includes lactulose, neomycin, and metronidazole. The use of flumazenil is discussed later in this section. Lactulose has been shown to improve the results of psychometric testing in stage 0 encephalopathy, but the clinical use may be less apparent. We do not routinely use lactulose for very early stage encephalopathy.

Blood in the gut lumen from gastrointestinal bleeding is particularly neurotoxic in cirrhotic patients. Bowel cleansing and reduction or elimination of dietary protein are treatment mainstays. Neomycin, both orally and as enemas, decreases the gut flora that produce many of the toxins. Lactulose acts both as a cathartic and as an ammonia trap (lactulose is fermented, producing acids that favor the equilibrium of $NH_3+ H^+ NH_4$). Ammonium is not absorbed across the gut membrane. Newer data suggest that the mechanism of action of lactulose is multifaceted. Probable actions include (a) a direct effect on ammonia production related to changes in bacterial selection; (b) changes in bacterial protein synthesis and degradation; and (c) a decrease in the 3- to 6-carbon short-chain fatty acids, with a corresponding increase in the nontoxic short chain acetate. Because of reports that endogenous benzodiazepines may play a role in hepatic encephalopathy, the use of a specific benzodiazepine antagonist, such as flumazenil, seems logical. Only a minority of patients with grade III and IV coma appear to achieve a clinical response to flumazenil. This agent should be considered a second-line agent for hepatic encephalopathy. Careful attention to drugs that might provoke encephalopathy is important.

Similar to the rational that lead to the establishment of neomycin for the treatment of hepatic encephalopathy (reduction in bacterial concentration in the bowel), other antiobiotics have been used for the treatment of hepatic encephalopathy including metronidazole (Flagyl) and rifaximin (Xifaxan).

LIVER DISEASE IN PREGNANCY

The pregnant woman with liver disease requires special consideration and knowledge of some liver conditions unique to pregnancy. Liver disease in pregnancy is uncommon but often is serious. Some key data about liver diseases associated with pregnancy are presented in Table 51.17.

TABLE 51.17
LIVER SYNDROMES SEEN IN PREGNANCY

Disease	Trimester	Signs/Symptoms	Outcome	Recurrence
Acute fatty liver of pregnancy	3	Malaise, nausea, vomiting, abdominal pain, jaundice, portosystemic encephalopathy may occur	Mortality 10%–25% for mother and infant; treatment, immediate delivery	Rare
HELLP syndrome	3	*Hemolysis, elevated liver enzymes, low platelets*	Mortality for mother 5%; for infant 10%–60%	Rare
Intrahepatic cholestasis	3	Pruritus, increased ALT/AST, bilirubin seldom exceeds 5 mg %	Benign course; treat symptomatically	Common
Hepatic rupture	3	Toxemia usually present; sudden abdominal catastrophe	Mortality >50% for mother and fetus	Rare

ALT, alanine transaminase; AST, aspartate transaminase.

Acute fatty liver of pregnancy most often presents dramatically with signs and symptoms of acute liver failure between weeks 30 and 38 of gestation. Vomiting, jaundice, and encephalopathy are frequent. Laboratory tests reveal hyperbilirubinemia (usually <15 mg/dL) and moderately elevated ALT and AST values (usually <1,000). The alkaline phosphatase may be modestly elevated, and evidence of liver synthetic failure as measured by prolonged pro times is frequent; ammonia levels may rise. Leukocytosis is prominent. Because of the rarity of the condition and the frequency with which it may be mimicked by other liver disorders such as viral hepatitis, a liver biopsy is recommended. Histologic findings of preserved liver architecture, foamy cytoplasm, and microvesicular fat are diagnostic. Therapy should not be delayed. Prompt delivery of the infant is the treatment. In the event liver failure advances despite delivery, liver transplantation may be required.

*H*emolysis, *e*levated *l*iver enzymes, *l*ow *p*latelets (HELLP syndrome) is part of the spectrum of preeclampsia-eclampsia. Most patients, therefore, have arterial hypertension and frequently other features, such as edema, excessive weight gain, and sometimes renal abnormalities. Nausea, vomiting, and upper abdominal pain are frequent in HELLP. Laboratory values in HELLP include features of microangiopathic hemolytic anemia, elevated bilirubin and lactic dehydrogenase levels, and platelet counts <100,000. Transaminases usually are only slightly elevated. The complications of HELLP are many, including organ damage as a consequence of microangiopathy and progression of eclampsia. Particularly feared complications include hepatic hematomas and hepatic rupture, which is a surgical emergency. Treatment is directed toward reducing blood pressure, correcting the coagulopathy, and assessing for liver hemorrhage. For mature fetuses over 35 weeks of gestation, immediate delivery is recommended.

Intrahepatic cholestasis of pregnancy poses little risk to the mother but is associated with excessive fetal death either in utero or because of prematurity. The disorder most often presents in the third trimester as pruritus, but occasionally it may be seen much earlier in pregnancy. In fewer than 10% of patients, jaundice is seen. Abnormal laboratory tests include AST and ALT elevations in addition to a slight elevation of bilirubin levels. Tests usually associated with cholestasis (e.g., GGTP, alkaline phosphatase, 5′ nucleotidase) are not more elevated in this disorder than in normal pregnancies. The serum bile acid levels, however, are markedly elevated and serve as a useful marker for this complication. Treatment consists of antihistamines to relieve pruritus. Other agents of possible benefit in this disorder are ursodiol, 10-day pulse therapy using dexamethasone, and possibly *S*-adenosyl-L-methionine.

ACUTE LIVER FAILURE

Acute liver failure is a syndrome characterized by the rapid onset of severe liver dysfunction in a patient who has no prior history of liver disease. Jaundice, coagulopathy, and encephalopathy are the major clinical manifestations. Acute liver failure occurs because of either massive or submassive hepatic necrosis. In the former, the disease runs its course within 8 weeks of onset; in the latter, up to 26 weeks may elapse. An improvement in mortality has accompanied an improved understanding of the nature of complications for some but not all causes of acute liver failure. With intensive supportive measures, survival rates for established acute liver failure range from 10% to 25% for most causes. Liver transplantation improves survival rates to 50% to 85%. Early transfer to a center with expertise in the management of this syndrome, particularly in a center that offers liver transplantation, is necessary for optimal salvage.

Common causes for acute liver failure are severe viral hepatitis (A, B [sometimes complicated by delta virus], or C), drug intoxication (especially acetaminophen taken in a suicide attempt), and occasionally mushroom poisoning (usually *Amanita* sp.). Table 51.18 indicates the etiology of acute liver failure in one North American liver unit. Other possible causes include ischemia, acute Budd-Chiari, Wilson disease, and fatty liver of pregnancy. Some drugs that may precipitate acute liver failure are noted in Table 51.19.

The basis for acetaminophen liver injury is particularly well understood. Ninety percent or more of the drug is metabolized to form nontoxic glucuronide or sulfate conjugates, which are excreted in bile. A small percentage of acetaminophen metabolism occurs by means of an alternative pathway that uses cytochrome P450 IIE. Drug metabolized through this pathway produces a toxic metabolite, *N*-acetyl-*p*-benzoquinoneimine, which is rapidly transformed to form mercapturic acid metabolites of acetaminophen, a reaction that requires glutathione. When normal pharmacologic doses of acetaminophen are consumed, glutathione stores are adequate and

TABLE 51.18

DIAGNOSIS OF ACUTE LIVER FAILURE IN 61 PATIENTS

Diagnosis	Percent (%)	Survival Rate (%)
Non-A, non-B hepatitis	28	24
Acetaminophen	25	67
Hepatitis B	16	10
Drug reaction	10	17
Ischemic hepatitis	8	40
Delta hepatitis	5	67
Wilson disease	3	0
Hepatitis A	2	0
Reye syndrome	2	0
Amanita mushroom	2	0

Reproduced with permission from Donaldson BW, Gopinath R, Wanless IR, et al. The role of transjugular biopsy in fulminant liver failure: relationship to other prognostic indicators. *Hepatology* 1993;18:1370–1376.

TABLE 51.19

DRUGS THAT MAY CAUSE ACUTE LIVER FAILURE

Common	Infrequent	Rare	Synergistic Toxicity
Acetaminophen overdose	Isoniazid	Carbamazepine	Alcohol/Acetaminophen
	Valproate	Ofloxacin	Trimethoprim-sulfamethoxazole
	Halothane	Ketoconazole	Rifampin/Isoniazid
	Phenytoin	Lisinopril	Acetaminophen/Isoniazid
	Propylthiouracil	Labetalol	
	Amiodarone	Etoposide (VP-16)	
	Disulfiram	Imipramine	
	Dapsone	Interferon-α flutamide	

Reproduced with permission from Lee WM. Acute liver failure. *N Engl J Med* 1993;329:1862–1870.

N-acetyl-p-benzoquinoneimine does not accumulate. However, glutathione can be depleted easily by large amounts of acetaminophen. N-acetyl-p-benzoquinoneimine accumulates and causes cell death by covalently binding to intracellular proteins. Chronic alcoholism and certain medications increase cytochrome P450 enzyme levels and so make acetaminophen toxic at a daily dose much lower than those usually considered toxic.

Early recognition of the patient with acetaminophen overdose leads to treatment that may prevent liver injury. N-acetylcysteine administered within 10 hours of ingestion is highly effective in preventing hepatic necrosis. More recent evidence suggests that although later administration may not prevent hepatic necrosis, better outcome ensues when N-acetylcysteine is given up to 36 hours after ingestion. Acetaminophen blood levels may assist in the management of such cases by defining patients particularly at risk for hepatic necrosis. Blood levels <200 mg/L 4 hours after ingestion (or 100 mg/L after 8 hours or 50 mg/L at 12 hours) are unlikely to be associated with hepatic damage and may not require specific protective treatment. Nomograms relating plasma acetaminophen levels to the risk of hepatic damage are available. Despite remarkable hepatic dysfunction caused by massive doses of acetaminophen, recovery is the rule. In one large liver failure referral center, only 110 (20%) of 548 patients transferred with signs of severe hepatic impairment from acetaminophen died, and 44 (8%) received liver transplants.

Selected Management Issues in Acute Liver Failure

Problems posed by established acute liver failure include:

- Sepsis
- Coagulopathy
- Renal failure
- Encephalopathy
- Acute cerebral edema
- Metabolic disorders

Sepsis is likely to develop, in part because the acute liver failure patient is immunocompromised. A report of selective gut decontamination in a group of patients with acute liver failure suggests that the incidence of enterobacterial infections can be nearly eliminated. Forty-seven percent of patients developed infection with enterobacteria (*E. coli*, *Klebsiella* sp., *Proteus* sp., *Enterobacter* sp., *Serratia* sp.) before the introduction of selective gut decontamination, whereas only 3% developed such infections when given selective decontamination. Norfloxacin 400 mg every 24 hours with nystatin 1,000,000 U every 6 hours was the regimen most often used. The incidence of other gram-negative and gram-positive infections was not decreased. The effect on mortality was hard to compare directly because patients treated before selective decontamination was used also were treated in an era when transplantation was never used.

In patients who survive for more than a few days, invasive fungal infections (typically *Candida* or *Aspergillus*) may occur in up to one-third. These infections are difficult to diagnose antemortem. Common sources include indwelling vascular catheters and pulmonary reservoirs. A patient who appears to improve but then relapses may have developed invasive fungal infection. Those with renal insufficiency particularly are at high risk. An unexplained temperature elevation (or one that persists after all identified bacterial infections are being treated appropriately), especially if the white blood cell count is elevated, should raise the index of suspicion for a fungal coinfection. Our approach in all patients with acute liver failure is to administer norfloxacin and nystatin (Mycostatin) to achieve selective gut decontamination, even in the absence of established infection. Frequent chest radiographs and culture for bacteria and fungi are done. The threshold to begin broad-spectrum antibiotics is quite low. In a patient who does not respond, a further search for fungal infection is considered on a case-by-case basis.

The patient with acute liver failure has some degree of hepatic encephalopathy. The differential diagnosis of neurologic deterioration in a liver failure patient includes cerebral edema, hypoglycemia, infection, and intracerebral bleeding. Encephalopathy in acute liver failure has, at least in part, a different basis from that occurring in the cirrhotic patient, and neither lactulose nor neomycin improves encephalopathy from acute liver failure. More recent studies indicate an association between the level of ammonia in experimental acute liver failure and decreases in brain function, suggesting that ammonia is of key importance in the encephalopathy that develops after both acute and chronic liver injury.

Acute cerebral edema frequently produces tonsillar herniation and death through brainstem compression. The pathophysiology of cerebral edema is poorly understood. A combination of cytotoxic and vasogenic mechanisms are probably responsible for impaired neuronal Na^+/K^+ adenosine triphosphatase activity, a disrupted blood-brain barrier, and the accumulation of osmotically active amino acids in the brain cells. The frequency of cerebral edema occurring in fulminant hepatic failure may be as high as 85%.

Recognition of significant cerebral edema is difficult on clinical grounds. Headache, projectile vomiting, bradycardia, and papilledema usually are absent. Other noninvasive measures, such as CT scanning, are relatively insensitive in identifying this rapidly progressive complication. In one center in which the routine placement of an epidural pressure transducer was placed in 15 patients with fulminant hepatic failure, elevated intracranial pressure (>15 mm Hg) was identified in 11 (73%). Routine CT scans showed evidence of effacement or flattening of cortical sulci, a reduction in size, a narrowing or obliteration of the cerebral ventricles or cisterns, or the presence of generalized decreased attenuation of the hemispheres in only 27% of cases in which increased intracranial pressure had been identified by pressure measurement.

Measures useful in lowering the intracranial pressure include elevation of the head of the bed by 30 degrees, hyperventilation of the intubated patient to a PCO_2 of 30 mm Hg, mannitol administration, and barbiturate-induced coma. If mannitol is required, it is given in a bolus of 0.5 to 1.0 g/kg to keep the serum osmolality in the range of 310 to 320 mOsm/L. Mannitol cannot be used in oliguric patients who do not exhibit a diuretic response to mannitol. Barbiturate coma lowers intracranial pressure by causing cerebral vasoconstriction and by decreasing both cerebral oxygen demand and neuronal metabolic activity. Corticosteroids, such as dexamethasone, are uniformly unhelpful in preventing or treating the cerebral edema seen in acute liver failure.

The identification of early indicators of prognosis in acute liver failure is essential. Late-occurring clinical or laboratory features are not helpful in planning therapy or deciding on liver transplantation. More helpful indicators are those easily monitored aspects of a case at the outset (Table 51.20). The etiology of the acute liver failure is the most powerful in predicting outcome. Those whose acute liver failure is due to hepatitis A, for example, have a 45% survival rate. Acetaminophen-induced liver failure, hepatitis B, and idiosyncratic drug reactions have a survival rate of 34%, 23%, and 14%, respectively. The worst prognosis is from non-A, non-B–induced acute liver failure; a meager 9% survive. Age is also an important determinant of survival, especially for acute liver failure caused by factors other than acetaminophen. Patients under the age of 10 years or older than 40 years are particularly likely to do poorly.

The grade of encephalopathy on admission plays a role in the early prediction of outcome, although the relationship is complicated and apparently paradoxical. For example, in liver failure not caused by acetaminophen, survival was lowest (12%) in those admitted with grade 0 to II coma compared with those with grade III through IV coma (20% survival). Finally, the duration of jaundice before encephalopathy plays a prognostic role. When this interval is ≤7 days, the survival rate is 34%, but when it is >7 days, this rate is only 7%. For acetaminophen-induced acute liver failure, an initial arterial blood pH <7.30 also was associated with a poorer outcome. Key points in the management of acute liver failure are summarized in Table 51.21. Survival

---

TABLE 51.20

FEATURES ASSOCIATED WITH POOR PROGNOSIS IN ACUTE LIVER FAILURE

Acetaminophen	Other Causes
pH <7.30	Pro time INR >6.5
or	or
(a) Pro time INR >6.5 and	Any three of the following:
(b) Creatinine >3.4 mg/dL and	(a) Age <10 or >40 yr
(c) Portosystemic encephalopathy grade III or IV	(b) Etiology non-A, non-B, halothane, drug reaction
	(c) Jaundice preceded portosystemic encephalopathy >7 day
	(d) Pro time INR >3.5
	(e) Bilirubin >17.6 mg/dL

INR, international normalized ratio; pro time, prothrombin time.
Reproduced with permission from O'Grady JG, Alexander GJM, Haylar KM, et al. Early indicators of prognosis in fulminant hepatic failure. *Gastroenterology* 1989;97:439–445.

TABLE 51.21

MANAGEMENT OF THE ACUTE LIVER FAILURE PATIENT

- Transfer to intensive care unit if stage III or IV coma develops
- Obtain emergent computed tomographic scan of the head
- Stat neurosurgery consult for evaluation and placement of intracranial pressure monitor
- Treat cerebral edema aggressively
- Elective endotracheal intubation in stage III coma to protect airway
- Frequent surveillance cultures
- Selective gut decontamination protocol; norfloxacin, mycostatin, and oral antibiotic paste while intubated
- Low threshold to empirical use of antibiotics if infection suspected
- Dialysis support either for fluid removal or hemodialysis
- Swan-Ganz catheter placement for hemodynamic monitoring and resuscitation
- Gastrointestinal bleeding prophylaxis with histamine blocker ± sucralfate

rates for emergency liver transplantation for acute liver failure range from 50% to 85%. For patients with conditions other than acetaminophen-induced hepatic necrosis, no variable at the time of admission other than cause (Wilson disease did best; idiosyncratic drug reaction did worst) predicted survival after transplantation. Considering changing variables during hospitalization, serum creatinine is the only factor that emerges from stepwise logistic regression analysis as predicting outcome.

PRIMARY LIVER CANCER (HEPATOMA AND CHOLANGIOCARCINOMA)

Hepatoma

Substantial variation occurs in the geographic and racial incidence of hepatocellular carcinoma (hepatoma). Etiology varies in high- and low-incidence regions. In high-incidence regions (Africa, south of the Sahara; Taiwan; Southeast China; and other parts of the Far East), the age-adjusted incidence is >20 per 100,000 per year. In North America, hepatoma is much less common, between 3 and 5 cases per 100,000 per year. In high-incidence areas, the age of onset is young in Africa but much older (sixth decade of life) in the Far East. In low-incidence areas, older onset is the rule. Men are affected more commonly than women (4:1 to 8:1 in high-incidence areas, but only 2.5:1 in low-incidence areas). Malignant hepatic tumors produce one or more of the following:

- Upper abdominal discomfort or pain
- Palpable or visible mass
- Cachexia
- Intractable ascites

Because many malignant tumors occur in the setting of advanced cirrhosis, confusion with the effects of cirrhosis may lead to diagnostic delay. It is not infrequent that hepatoma is diagnosed only at necropsy in a patient who has had a rapid downhill course attributed to decompensated cirrhosis.

Strong epidemiologic evidence incriminates environmental factors in the pathogenesis of hepatoma, especially hepatitis B and C infection, aflatoxins, and cirrhosis. At least 80% of cases of hepatoma worldwide are associated with evidence of persistent hepatitis B infection. HBV carriers run a higher risk of developing this cancer. This association is particularly relevant in regions of high tumor incidence, but it is also found in the United States. Patients without evidence of current infection usually have evidence of remote infection. The presence of hepatitis B as measured by HBV DNA has been shown in hepatomas from persons without HBsAg positivity. Hepatitis B infection precedes the development of hepatoma by many years (often many decades). Evidence from Japan indicates that hepatitis C may be more powerfully associated with hepatoma formation. In a group of 251 patients with chronic hepatitis B or C followed up prospectively with ultrasound and α-fetoprotein, more than twice as high a percentage (10.4% vs. 3.9%) of hepatitis C patients developed hepatoma over a period of 11 years.

Aflatoxins are metabolites of the ubiquitous fungus *Aspergillus flavus*. Aflatoxin B1 is a potent hepatic carcinogen. The contamination of foodstuffs, particularly stored nuts and grain, has been demonstrated in many tropical and subtropical areas where hepatoma is prominent. The urinary excretion of aflatoxin has been demonstrated in high-incidence regions in China. Aflatoxins, either alone or together with hepatitis B infection, almost certainly contribute to the hepatoma incidence in high-incidence areas but not to hepatoma as seen in the United States.

Cirrhosis stands out as a risk factor in the United States, and alcohol abuse is the most common cause. It seems likely that alcohol per se is not a cause of hepatoma, but it causes the cirrhosis that sets the stage for hepatoma risk. In some U.S. studies, nearly all cases of hepatoma were related to alcoholic cirrhosis. Evidence suggests that even in patients with alcoholic liver disease, hepatitis B or C plays a role, at least as a cocarcinogen. Experts predict a sharp upsurge in hepatoma in the United States as persons who acquired hepatitis C during young adulthood continue to age.

Hemochromatosis, A1AT deficiency, and PBC also carry a heightened hepatoma risk. Miscellaneous causes of hepatoma include sex-steroid ingestion, particularly androgenic steroids, which is of increasing concern among young athletes, some of whom take androgenic steroids to increase muscle mass and athletic performance.

Radiologic investigations play a major role in the diagnosis of hepatoma. Isotopic scans show lesions ≥3 cm. CT scans can detect lesions of approximately 1 to 2 cm. Ultrasonography can distinguish similarly small lesions. CT, particularly dynamic scanning, can detect and define hepatomas with an improved degree of precision (2-cm lesions), and MRI is also helpful.

α-Fetoprotein is a fetal protein whose synthesis is repressed after birth. It is positive in many persons with hepatoma. This test has been used in screening, and when it is unusually high (e.g., >200 ng/mL) may confer reasonable certainty on the nature of a focal liver lesion even without biopsy.

Symptomatic hepatoma carries a grave prognosis. Small asymptomatic lesions may remain so for several years; once symptoms develop, however, life expectancy is only a few months.

A range of treatment options, while not all curative, are now available for patients with hepatocellular carcinoma. Chemotherapy has added little to the quantity or quality of life for those with hepatoma. Treatment options for hepatomas remain few. Percutaneous injection of ethanol for small (<2 cm) solitary hepatomas seems to be as effective as surgical resection. This may be done safely even when the neoplasm is located on the surface of the liver. Intratumor alcohol injections may extend life expectancy when the lesions are small. Chemotherapy has limited success. Doxorubicin (Adriamycin) is the single agent with the most activity against hepatomas, but it increases life expectancy little. Combination chemotherapy has been disappointing. Recombinant interferon (50 million U three times weekly) showed a weak activity (median survival 14.0 weeks compared with 7.5 weeks for untreated patients) in Chinese patients. Liver transplantation is appropriate only for small asymptomatic hepatomas and for the rare fibrolamellar variant.

Cholangiocarcinoma

Cholangiocarcinomas derive from bile duct epithelium and may be distal (near or at the terminus of the common bile duct in the duodenum), middle, or proximal (within the liver parenchyma). When the tumor occurs at the bifurcation of the right and left hepatic duct systems, this tumor is referred to as a *Klatskin tumor*. In the United States, cholangiocarcinoma is seen more frequently than hepatoma. The pathogenesis of cholangiocarcinoma is not clear. Sclerosing cholangitis, with which cholangiocarcinoma may be confused, is said to predispose to bile duct cancer. Cholangiocarcinoma is not associated with cirrhosis, hepatitis B, or exposure to mycotoxins.

The disease usually occurs in patients older than the age of 60 years and is rare before age 40 years. Men are more commonly affected. Patients present most often with signs or symptoms or laboratory abnormalities suggesting complete or partial biliary tract obstruction. The disease is highly suspected after a cholangiogram (endoscopic retrograde cholangiopancreatography or transhepatic cholangiogram) shows the lesion. As noted, cases of diffuse cholangiocarcinoma may be hard to distinguish from sclerosing cholangitis radiologically. Indeed, cancer

may develop in sclerosing cholangitis. Brush cytologic material may be obtained during the diagnostic study. Positive results may be seen in as many as 60% of patients after up to three brushings. The high false-negative rate, however, is disappointing.

Treatment is usually palliative. Surgical removal is not usually possible except for a few lesions located in the distal biliary tree. Cholangiocarcinoma that obstructs high in the biliary tree (e.g., at the bifurcation) may be difficult for the surgeon to bypass, although the surgical placement of stents across the lesion may be possible. Either radiologic or endoscopically placed stents usually are favored for these lesions. For lesions in the common bile duct, both surgery and endoscopically placed stents are technically possible and have a high success rate.

LIVER TRANSPLANTATION

A substantial growth has occurred over the past two decades in the number of patients officially listed for liver transplantation. The growth in liver transplant operations has been much slower. It is estimated that nearly 25,000 patients will be waiting for only 5,300 donor organs. Patients selected for liver transplantation usually have common problems related to end-stage cirrhosis (or to fulminant liver failure). Twenty-nine percent of patients seen in Cleveland's Hepatology Clinic have hepatitis C, and 4% have hepatitis B. Of the hepatomas cases seen, most are associated with either HCV or HBV infection. In some centers, hepatitis C is the leading disease causing the end-stage liver disease that requires transplantation. Some have predicted that a wave of end-stage liver disease resulting from hepatitis C will emerge over the next decade, as the epidemic of high-risk behavior that created a high prevalence of hepatitis C endures long enough for the natural history of HCV infection to play out. Current selection criteria for liver transplantation candidacy are broad, and contraindications are few and diminishing each year. In general, patients are selected for liver transplantation candidacy if one or more of the following apply: (a) end-stage liver disease with a life expectancy of less than a year; (b) quality of life judged sufficiently poor that the risks appear justified; or (c) a liver-based metabolic disease with lethal implications. Those sentinel events in the evolution of cirrhosis that indicate a high likelihood of mortality without transplantation include:

- Child-Pugh score ≥7
- Appearance of ascites
- SBP
- Hepatic hydrothorax
- Hepatorenal syndrome

Portal hypertensive bleeding also carries with it a risk of increased mortality, but in the otherwise well-compensated cirrhotic (Child-Pugh <8), this problem is dealt with best by using measures other than liver transplantation. Age per se is usually not considered a contraindication to liver transplantation, although the chances of a disqualifying coexistent disease goes up with age. Acute liver failure patients are suitable for liver transplantation. It is often logistically difficult, however, to obtain a suitable donor organ in the short "window of opportunity" available in such patients. A consensus conference determination of reasonable minimal criteria for liver transplantation is available.

Liver allocation policies of the United Network for Organ Sharing currently determine minimal eligibility requirements for liver transplantation. An elaborate liver allocation system is currently in place to attempt, insofar as possible, to make the process of allocation of scarce resources as equitable as possible. Until recently, priority of transplantation was based on the severity of liver failure (determined by the Child-Pugh-Turcott score) and the length of time a patient had been on the waiting list. This system of organ allocation was widly criticized for a number of reasons, including the presence of subjective factors such as encephalopathy and ascites leading to inequitable liver allocation. A new allocation system (the MELD system [*M*odel for *E*ndstage *L*iver *D*isease]) was introduced in 2002 and has become the basis for organ allocation for liver transplantation in the United States. The MELD system is a mathematical score driven from three simple laboratory values (serum bilirubin, serum creatinine, and the international normalized ratio [INR]). It has been demonstrated that the MELD score is a good predictor of 3-month and 1-year survival and is applicable to most liver diseases. Exceptions include those with hepatocelluar carcinoma or with hepatopulmonary syndrome despite good hepatic function; the MELD score may falsely predict good survival in these situations. In these special groups of patients, the MELD score is typically adjusted to allow for more timely transplantations. Independent of the MELD score, patients with fulminant liver failure will receive the highest priority for liver transplantation (status 1).

Alcoholic liver disease is no longer considered a contraindication to liver transplantation, particularly in those in whom sufficient personal or family support resources are available to make resumption of alcohol intake less likely. Patients with cholangiocarcinoma do poorly and are not candidates for liver transplantation in most centers. Liver transplantation is the therapy of choice for patients with small hepatocelluar carcinoma. The Milan criteria are most often used to identify patients with hepatocellular carcinomas that would most benefit from liver transplantation. The Milan criteria include patients with a single lesion <5 cm in size or those with up to three lesions each <3 cm in size.

Patients with hepatitis B frequently have disease recurrence in the transplanted organ, sometimes with disastrous consequences. Interferon given after liver transplantation does not appear to prevent recurrence and may provoke increased rates of rejection. More recent evidence suggests that hepatitis B recurrence may be delayed, and possibly prevented, by the regular posttransplantation administration of hyperimmune B globulin to sustain serum anti-HBs titers at a protective level. The use of nucleoside analogs has been discussed herein (viral hepatitis B); these agents also are being explored as tools to reduce the incidence and impact of post–liver transplant hepatitis B recurrence.

A certain aura of inevitability persists about the recurrence of hepatitis C after transplantation. This infection is usually better tolerated than recurrent hepatitis B. Serious hepatic infections are sometimes seen, and fibrosing cholestatic hepatitis has been described. Despite reinfection, many centers report 1- and 3-year survival rates, similar to those for other conditions for which transplantation is done. One concern is the possibility that the time horizon has been too short. Evidence suggests a much higher rate of fibrosis, with some estimates that cirrhosis may develop, on average, within 7 years after transplantation. No strategy has been shown to be of unequivocal value in moderating the outcome of recurrent hepatitis C, although several small pilot studies suggested the combination of pegylated interferon and ribavirin is helpful in eradicating hepatitis C in a small proportion of patients after liver transplantation.

Transplantation for hemochromatosis is associated with a higher than expected mortality and a high incidence of cardiac problems, infection, and immunologic problems, including susceptibility to infection, immunoblastic lymphoma, and cancers. Whether or not iron accumulates in the transplanted liver remains controversial.

Living Related Donors

In many parts of the world, the use of cadaveric organs for transplantation is not possible because of religious or cultural taboos. A viable liver transplantation program can still be affected through the use of living related donors. It has long been recognized in animals and humans that major hepatic resection is well tolerated. In the donor, the remaining liver regenerates; thus, within 2 months, total liver volume is approximately what it had been before resection. Liver segments transplanted into the recipient undergo similar regeneration.

Donor selection must proceed with care. Attention to medical and ethical aspects is mandatory. Many programs specify that the donor be between 20 and 45 years of age and in excellent health, without evidence of liver disease, and ABO compatible with the potential recipient. Liver mass must be estimated, most often with CT scan or MRI. The graft-mass/recipient body weight ratio should be ≥1%. The donor liver must be free of significant steatosis.

The donor operation consists of a left or right partial hepatectomy. A left hemihepatectomy is technically easier and often results in a liver mass of 300 to 500 g. This may be sufficient for a small recipient. More often, a right hemihepatectomy is required, which yields 800 to 900 g of liver.

The results of adult living related donor liver transplantation are comparable with cadaveric transplants. Rare donor deaths have been reported.

REVIEW EXERCISES

QUESTIONS

1. Which of the following approaches has shown to improve liver enzymes and liver histology for nonalcoholic steatohepatitis?
a) Weight loss
b) Control of elevated triglycerides
c) Avoidance of alcohol
d) Control of elevated blood sugar
e) The use of insulin-sensitizing agents

Answer and Discussion

The answer is a. Weight loss in obese patients, the control of elevated triglycerides and diabetes, and the avoidance of alcohol are recommended. Of several treatment strategies tested in clinical trials, weight loss (at least 5%–10% of total body weight) seems to be the most effective. Weight loss in obese patients with steatohepatitis has shown to be associated with normalization of liver enzymes and improved hepatic histology. Newer studies are targeting insulin resistance as a potential underlying mechanism of fatty liver. Clinical trials assessing the use of insulin-sensitizing agents developed for patients with type 2 diabetes mellitus are currently under way.

2. Which of the following identifies a group of patients at substantial risk of dying from alcoholic hepatitis?
a) Child-Pugh score
b) Discriminant function
c) MELD score
d) Milan criteria
e) Ranson criteria

Answer and Discussion

The answer is b. Several studies suggest that steroids improve survival for patients with severe alcoholic hepatitis without gastrointestinal bleeding. The definition of severity requires an evaluation of the bilirubin level and the pro time. The so-called *discriminant function value* identifies a group of patients at substantial risk of dying from alcoholic hepatitis.

Discriminant function:
    4.6 (pro time − control [in seconds]) + (serum bilirubin [mg/dL]) = 32

When severely ill patients with a discriminant function score of ≥32 (without gastrointestinal hemorrhage) are given 40 mg of prednisone daily for 28 days, survival is nearly twice as likely.

3. According to the CDC, in the absence of an outbreak (single case exposure), which of the following contacts should receive hepatitis A postexposure prophylaxis with immune globulin?
a) Household contacts under 12 months of age
b) Office coworkers
c) Sexual contacts 18 to 40 years of age
d) Elementary school contacts
e) All of the above

Answer and Discussion

The answer is a. Immune globulin provides protection against hepatitis A. Formerly, preexposure prophylaxis was recommended for those who travel internationally to endemic regions, but currently such persons are advised to receive active immunization. Postexposure prophylaxis with immune globulin is recommended for (a) household and sexual contacts under the age of 12 months or over the age of 40 years (for those between 12 months and 40 years, hepatitis A vaccine is preferred); (b) in day care centers (if children in diapers attend) but not to elementary or secondary school contacts unless an outbreak (more than a single case) has been identified; (c) within institutions to contacts only; and (d) in hospitals only if an outbreak occurs. Immune globulin is not recommended for coworkers in offices or factories. Restaurant-exposed persons also may get immune globulin unless the contact was more than 2 weeks previous, in which case no vaccine is recommended. Postexposure prophylaxis is not needed for persons who have been immunized.

4. Which of the following is *not* an extrahepatic manifestion of hepatitis C?
a) Glomerulonephritis
b) PCT
c) Cryoglobulinemia
d) Type 2 diabetes
e) Cardiomyopathy

Answer and Discussion

The answer is e. Cardiomyopathy is not an extrahepatic manifestation of hepatitis C. All other choices can be seen along with the addition of lymphoproliferative disorders and leukocytoclastic vasculitis.

5. Which of the following is associated with a low SAAG (<1.1)?
a) Wilson disease
b) Autoimmune hepatitis
c) Ovarian cancer
d) Budd-Chiari syndrome
e) Nonischemic cardiomyopathy

Answer and Discussion

The answer is c. Cirrhotic ascites is similar to serum, except it contains less protein. The SAAG is usually >1.1. This ratio is calculated by subtracting the albumin concentration of ascites from that of serum (albumin ser minus albumin asc). Cardiac ascites will have a similarly high gradient. The SAAG has been established as a clinical valuable test with high specificity to differentiate ascites due to portal hypertension (cirrhosis, Budd-Chiari syndrome, or right heart failure) from other causes of ascites. Low gradients (<1.1) suggest a noncirrhotic (and a noncardiac) cause for ascites, such as malignancy or infection.

SUGGESTED READINGS

Blackard JT, Shata MT, Shire NJ, et al. Acute hepatitis C virus infection: a chronic problem. *Hepatology* 2008;47(1):321–331.

Lin S-M, Sheen I-E, Chien R-N, et al. Long-term beneficial effects of interferon therapy in patients with chronic hepatitis B infection. *Hepatology* 1999;29:971–975.

Lindor K. Ursodeoxycholic acid for the treatment of primary biliary cirrhosis. *N Engl J Med* 2007;357(15):1524–1529.

Lindsay KL, Trep C, Heintges T, et al. Randomized double blind trial comparing pegylated interferon α 2b to interferon α 2b as initial treatment for chronic hepatitis C. *Hepatology* 2001;34: 395–403.

Lo GH, Lai KH, Cheng JS, et al. Endoscopic variceal ligation plus nadolol and sucralfate compared with ligation alone for prevention of variceal re-bleeding. A prospective, randomized trial. *Hepatology* 2000;32:461–465.

Lok AS. Navigating the maze of hepatitis B treatments. *Gastroenterology* 2007;132(4):1586–1594.

Mukherjee S. Sorrell MF. Controversies in liver transplantation for hepatitis C. *Gastroenterology* 2008;134(6):1777–1788.

Polson J, Lee WM; American Association for the Study of Liver Disease. AASLD position paper: the management of acute liver failure. *Hepatology* 2005;41(5):1179–1197.

Starkel P. Genetic factors predicting response to interferon treatment for viral hepatitis C. *Gut* 2008;57(4):440–442.

Villanueva C, Minina J, Ortiz J, et al. Endoscopic ligation compared with combined treatment with nadolol and isosorbide mononitrate to prevent recurrent variceal hemorrhage. *N Engl J Med* 2001;345:647–655.

Wakim-Fleming J, Zein NN. The liver in pregnancy: disease vs benign changes. *Cleve Clin J Med* 2005;72(8):713–721.

Zeuzem S, Feinman V, Rasenack J, et al. Peginterferon α 2a in patients with chronic hepatitis C. *N Engl J Med* 2000;343:1666–1672.

Chapter 52

Pancreatic Diseases

Mansour A. Parsi

POINTS TO REMEMBER:

- The death rate for severe acute pancreatitis can reach 25%.
- The most common causes of acute pancreatitis are alcohol and gallstones.
- Patients with severe pancreatitis require monitoring in an intensive care unit.
- The treatment of chronic pancreatitis is mainly symptomatic.
- The risk factors for developing pancreatic carcinoma include advancing age, cigarette smoking, chronic pancreatitis, and hereditary pancreatitis.

The most common disorders of the exocrine pancreas are acute pancreatitis, chronic pancreatitis, and pancreatic cancer. Since a basic knowledge of the anatomy and physiology of the pancreas is required to better understand the presenting symptoms and sequelae of these disorders, this chapter begins with a short discussion on anatomy and physiology of the pancreas followed by a discussion on each of these conditions.

ANATOMY

The pancreas is a retroperitoneal organ with close proximity to the gastric outlet and the duodenum (Fig. 52.1). This close proximity predisposes these structures to

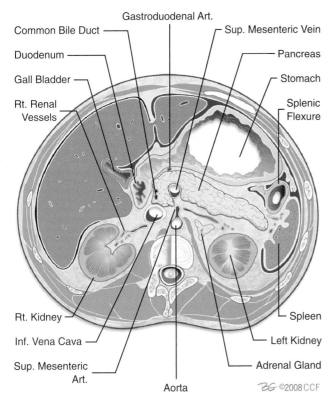

Figure 52.1 Cross-sectional anatomy of the abdomen at the level of the pancreas demonstrating the relationship between the pancreas and surrounding structures.

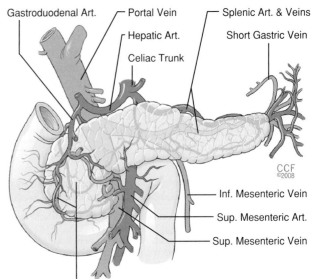

Figure 52.2 Vascular supply of the pancreas.

external compression and obstruction by different processes involving the pancreas, such as acute pancreatitis, large pancreatic cysts, and pancreatic cancer. The distal part of the common bile duct passes through the head of the pancreas and can be externally compressed by inflammation or tumor in the pancreatic head. External compression of the bile duct at this site may lead to elevated liver associated enzymes and/or obstructive jaundice. Jaundice is therefore a common presenting symptom in patients with pancreatic head cancer and can be seen in up to 10% of the patients with acute pancreatitis. Some vital blood vessels such as inferior vena cava, aorta, portal vein, superior mesenteric artery and vein, and the celiac axis are near the pancreas. The close relationship of these vessels to the pancreas is of vital surgical importance. In determining the resectability of a pancreatic lesion, a key step is assessment of involvement of these vessels.

The pancreas has a rich blood supply from branches of the celiac axis and superior mesenteric artery (Fig. 52.2). Due to this dual blood supply, isolated ischemia of the pancreas is exceedingly rare. Blood from the pancreas ultimately drains into the portal vein, which is formed by the junction of the superior mesenteric vein and the splenic vein. The splenic vein runs along the body of the pancreas (Fig. 52.2). Diseases such as pancreatitis and pancreatic cancer can invade the vein, leading to its thrombosis and vascular engorgement of the spleen. The engorgement of

the spleen leads to shunting of the blood through the venous pathways in the upper stomach and development of gastric varices.

PHYSIOLOGY

The functional unit of the pancreas is the pancreatic acinus, composed of acinar and ductal cells. Acinar cells have a rich and highly specialized intracellular matrix for the synthesis, storage, and secretion of large amounts of proteins, mainly as digestive enzymes. The ductal cells primarily secrete water and electrolytes.

The three primary phases of postprandial pancreatic secretion include the cephalic phase, gastric phase, and intestinal phase. The cephalic phase is stimulated by the thought, sight, taste, or smell of food via vagal cholinergic innervation. The gastric phase occurs in response to gastric distention, which also is mediated by vagal cholinergic reflexes. The intestinal phase, which is the major phase of postprandial pancreatic secretion, is regulated primarily by the release of secretin and cholecystokinin (CCK). Secretin released into the blood from the duodenum is responsible for bicarbonate and water secretion from pancreatic ductal cells, while CCK released into the circulation is primarily responsible for digestive enzyme secretion from acinar cells.

Direct pancreatic function tests, which have been developed for diagnosis of chronic pancreatitis, take advantage of this physiology. During these tests, the pancreas is stimulated with either secretin or CCK, and the content of the duodenal secretions are aspirated and analyzed for bicarbonate and digestive enzyme (lipase) concentrations, respectively. The concentration of bicarbonate in the duodenal aspirate reflects the secretory capacity of the pancreatic ductal cells, while the concentration of lipase in the duodenal aspirate reflects the secretory capacity of the pancreatic acinar cells.

ACUTE PANCREATITIS

Epidemiology

Acute pancreatitis is one of the most common disorders of the pancreas. It has been estimated that there are 210,000 admissions for acute pancreatitis each year in the United States. Pancreatitis has many causes, an obscure pathogenesis, and few effective treatments. Most cases are mild (80%), but as many as 20% can be severe. In contrast to mild acute pancreatitis, which has a mortality rate <1%, the death rate for severe acute pancreatitis is much higher and can reach 25% in those with infected pancreatic necrosis.

Pathophysiology

The pathophysiology of acute pancreatitis has been extensively studied in animal models. Although various etiologies produce distinct inciting events, the final common pathway seems to be premature activation of digestive enzymes within the pancreatic acinar cells. Normally, pancreatic enzymes become activated after their release into the duodenum. Activation of pancreatic enzymes within the pancreas (before their release into the duodenum) will lead to pancreatic tissue injury and acute pancreatitis. A systemic inflammatory cascade involving chemokines and cytokines usually follows and can lead to further local and systemic inflammatory responses.

Etiology

Determining the underlying etiology for acute pancreatitis is important, because only by treating the underlying condition can repeated attacks be prevented.

The most common causes of acute pancreatitis are alcohol and gallstones, which combined are responsible for 80% of the cases of acute pancreatitis. Approximately 10% of the cases are idiopathic. The remaining 10% are due to multiple other factors such as autoimmune pancreatitis, microlithiasis, metabolic derangements, infectious agents, and drug-induced pancreatitis (Table 56.1). Although drug-induced pancreatitis is not common, it needs to be considered in every patient, especially in those patients with unexplained recurrent disease. A list of some drugs that have been associated with acute pancreatitis is presented in Table 56.2.

Clinical Presentation

Almost all patients with acute pancreatitis present with abdominal pain. The typical pain is constant, severe, located in the mid-epigastrium or right upper quadrant, and radiates to the back. Some patients express relief of pain when sitting or leaning forward. In the majority of patients, the abdominal pain is accompanied by nausea and vomiting, which may occur without an ileus or gastric outlet obstruction. Unlike patients with ulcer disease, vomiting does not relieve the pain. Patients may have reduced bowel sounds secondary to ileus. Jaundice may be evident in the presence of gallstones or compression of the common bile duct by an edematous pancreatic head. Low-grade fever is reported in 60% of patients. High-grade fever may indicate presence of cholangitis or necrosis of the pancreatic parenchyma. Tachycardia and hypotension are ominous signs and may be due to intravascular volume depletion, increased vacular permeability, vasodilatation, or hemorrhage.

Laboratory features may include a transient mild hypoglycemia, hypocalcemia, hyperbilirubinemia, and mild elevations in the serum alanine transaminase and alkaline phosphatase levels. Patients with a bilirubin level >2.5 times the normal value and a serum alanine transaminase twice the normal value are likely to have gallstone pancreatitis.

TABLE 52.1

ETIOLOGY OF ACUTE PANCREATITIS

Common Etiologic Factors (90%)	Less Common Etiologic Factors (10%)
Gallstones (45%)	Autoimmune
Alcohol (35%)	Drug induced
Idiopathic (10%)	Hereditary
	Iatrogenic (post ERCP, FNA)
	Infectious (mumps, coxsackie, HIV)
	Metabolic (hypertriglyceridemia, hypercalcemia)
	Neoplastic
	Structural (pancreas divisum)
	Traumatic

ERCP, endoscopic retrograde cholangiopancreatography; FNA, fine-needle aspiration.

TABLE 52.2

SOME OF THE DRUGS ASSOCIATED WITH ACUTE PANCREATITIS

ACE inhibitors	6-Mercaptopurine
5-ASA compounds	Pentamidine
Azathioprine	Sulfasalazine
Didanosine	Sulfonamides
Furosemide	Thiazides
NSAIDs	Valproate

ACE, angiotensin-converting enzyme; NSAIDs, nonsteroidal anti-inflammatory drugs.

Diagnosis

Based on the most recent guidelines by the American College of Gastroenterology, a diagnosis of acute pancreatitis requires two of the following three features: (a) abdominal pain characteristic of acute pancreatitis, (b) serum amylase and/or lipase ≥3 times the upper limit of normal, and (c) characteristic findings of acute pancreatitis on computed tomography (CT) scan. This definition allows for the possibility that an amylase and/or lipase might be <3 times the upper limit of normal in acute pancreatitis. In a patient with abdominal pain characteristic of acute pancreatitis and serum enzyme levels <3 times the upper limit of normal, a CT scan must be performed to confirm a diagnosis of acute pancreatitis. In addition, this definition allows for the possibility that the presence of abdominal pain cannot be assessed in some patients with severely altered mental status due to acute or chronic illness.

In general, both amylase and lipase are elevated during the course of acute pancreatitis. Although measurement of amylase is more widely used, serum lipase may be preferable because it remains normal in some nonpancreatic conditions that increase serum amylase, including macroamylasemia, parotitis, and some carcinomas. Both serum amylase and lipase may be elevated in patients with renal insufficiency due to decreased clearance. At a creatinine clearance between 13 and 39 mL per minute, amylase is elevated in somewhat more than half of patients and lipase is only elevated in approximately one-fourth of patients, suggesting an additional advantage for lipase. Once the diagnosis of acute pancreatitis is established, measuring either amylase or lipase on a daily basis has little value in gauging clinical progress or prognosis.

Assessment of Severity

Prognosis in acute pancreatitis depends on the severity of the disease. Mortality in mild forms is rare, while up to 20% of patients with severe acute pancreatitis succumb. Therefore, it is of great importance to predict severity of acute pancreatitis early in the course of the disease, allowing triage to the intensive care unit, more intensive monitoring for signs of multiorgan failure, and more vigorous fluid resuscitation and correction of electrolyte abnormalities.

The severity of acute pancreatitis can be assessed by various methods, including bedside assessment, the use of scoring systems, serum markers, and imaging studies. Unfortunately, none has been shown to be ideal.

Bedside Assessment

Evaluation of cardiovascular and respiratory factors such as hypotension, tachycardia, tachypnea, and hypoxemia has high specificity but low sensitivity (misses a lot of severe

TABLE 52.3

RANSON PROGNOSTIC CRITERIA FOR DETERMINING SEVERITY OF ACUTE PANCREATITIS

At Admission	During Initial 48 Hours
Age >55 yr	Hematocrit decrease >10%
Leukocyte count >16,000 cells/mm^3	Serum urea nitrogen increase >5 mg/dL
Plasma glucose >200 mg/dL	Serum Ca^{2+} <8 mg/dL
Serum lactate dehydrogenase >350 U/L	PAO$_2$ <60 mm Hg
Serum aspartate transaminase >250 U/L	Base deficit >4 mEq/L
	Fluid sequestration >6 L

cases). At the time of admission, clinical judgment should take into account clinical risk factors such as advanced age, comorbid conditions, and obesity (body mass index >30), all of which have been associated with increased mortality.

Scoring Systems

Several multifactorial scoring systems have been developed, with the Ranson criteria and the APACHE II score (Acute Physiology and Chronic Health Evaluation) being the most well known. The Ranson score does not have a high degree of sensitiviy and specificity for the prediction of severe pancreatitis. Still, due to its simplicity, it is commonly used (Table 56.3). Patients with three or more Ranson criteria have traditionally been considered to have severe pancreatitis. Although more reliable, the APACHE II score is complex and cumbersome to calculate. Patients with an APACHE II score ≥8 are considered to have severe pancreatitis.

Laboratory Tests

In severe pancreatitis, there is considerable extravasation of intravascular fluids leading to decreased intravascular volume and increased hematocrit. Hematocrit ≥44 at admission and failure of the admission hematocrit to decrease after 24 hours of hospitalization has been associated with necrotizing pancreatitis and thus has been shown to be a predictor of severe pancreatitis. Recent guidelines by the American College of Gastroenterology recommend obtaining a serum hematocrit at admission, 12 hours after admission, and 24 hours after admission to help gauge the adequacy of fluid resuscitation.

Data from several studies have demonstrated usefulness of C-reactive protein (CRP) measurements in distinguishing mild from severe acute pancreatitis. CRP levels >150 mg/L have been associated with the presence of pancreatic necrosis. Peak levels of CRP are achieved at 36 to 72 hours after the onset of acute pancreatitis. This test is therefore not helpful at admission in assessing severity. CRP levels

>150 mg/L after 48 hours of disease onset, however, may discriminate patients with severe disease.

The degree of elevation in the serum amylase and lipase levels has no prognostic value for determining the severity of pancreatitis.

Imaging Studies

Contrast-enhanced CT, which is indicated in patients with severe pancreatitis, helps to determine whether necrotizing pancreatitis is present. Uniform enhancement on the scan implies an intact microcirculation and is suggestive of mild pancreatitis. Areas of nonenhancement indicate a disruption in pancreatic microcirculation, which is strongly suggestive of pancreatic necrosis and severe pancreatitis.

Since it takes 2 to 3 days for the pancreatic necrosis to develop, a contrast-enhanced CT is rarely required during the first 2 days after the onset of acute pancreatitis.

Treatment

The treatment of mild acute pancreatitis is supportive, using intravenous fluids and analgesia. Fluid resuscitation is particularly important in severe pancreatitis due to considerable extravasation of intravascular fluid into third spaces. Patients with severe pancreatitis are at increased risk of pancreatic necrosis. Approximately one-third of patients with necrotizing pancreatitis develop infected necrosis. Usually, offending organisms are those of intestinal flora, with *Escherichia Coli* being the most common. CT-guided percutaneous fine-needle aspiration (FNA) of necrotic areas in the pancreas with Gram stain and culture is recommended when infected necrosis is suspected. If infection is confirmed, surgical debridement should be strongly considered. Alternative less-invasive approaches, such as endoscopic debridement, may be used in selected cases. Patients with severe pancreatitis require monitoring in an intensive care unit.

Routine use of prophylactic antibiotics in patients with mild pancreatitis or sterile pancreatic necrosis should be discouraged. In patients with pancreatic necrosis who appear septic with leukocytosis, fever, or chills, antibiotic therapy is appropriate during the workup for identification of the underlying cause. Antibacterial agents with good pancreatic tissue penetration are preferred; these include imipenem and ciprofloxacin.

Patients with severe pancreatitis can have systemic complications such as renal failure, acute respiratory distress syndrome, gastrointestinal bleeding, or multiorgan failure. Pancreatic pseudocysts occur in approximately 20% of patients with acute pancreatitis and should be drained only if they cause symptoms.

Patients with gallstone pancreatitis who are deteriorating clinically or have evidence of biliary sepsis should undergo emergent endoscopic retrograde cholangiopancreatography (ERCP) for the removal of impacted gallstones.

CHRONIC PANCREATITIS

Epidemiology

The annual incidence of chronic pancreatitis has been estimated in several studies and ranges from 3 to 10 cases per 100,000 population. In most studies, alcohol abuse accounts for more than two-thirds of all cases of chronic pancreatitis.

Pathophysiology

Multiple hypotheses have been suggested as the main pathophysiological mechanism for development of chronic pancreatitis. Current opinion, however, favors the so-called necrosis-fibrosis hypothesis, in which chronic pancreatitis begins as an acute process and progresses to chronic irreversible damage as a result of repeated acute attacks.

Etiology

In Western countries, the most common cause of chronic pancreatitis is alcohol abuse, which accounts for 70% of cases. Approximately 20% of cases are idiopathic. The remaining miscellaneous causes include prolonged metabolic disturbances (i.e., hypercalcemia, hypertriglyceridemia), cystic fibrosis, hereditary pancreatitis, autoimmune disease, tropical pancreatitis, and recurrent acute pancreatitis due to pancreas divisum.

Clinical Presentation

The two most common clinical presentations of patients with chronic pancreatitis are abdominal pain and weight loss. The mechanism for abdominal pain is controversial, but it may involve inflammation of the pancreas, increased pressure in pancreatic ducts and parenchyma, inflammation in pancreatic nerves and perineural tissue, and pancreatic ischemia. Weight loss initially results from a decreased caloric intake because of fear of precipitating abdominal pain. Later, as the pancreatitis advances, pancreatic insufficiency develops, manifested as malabsorption or diabetes mellitus (DM). In most cases, exocrine pancreatic insufficiency occurs a few years before the development of endocrine insufficiency.

Diagnosis

The diagnosis of chronic pancreatitis is suggested by the history and is confirmed through laboratory tests and imaging studies. Chronic pancreatitis leads to alterations of normal pancreatic structure and function. Diagnostic tests for chronic pancreatitis can therefore be grouped into those tests that detect structural derangements of normal pancreatic architecture and those that detect abnormalities of pancreatic acinar or duct cell function. The structure of the main pancreatic duct and its primary side branches can be assessed by imaging studies such as ultrasound, CT, magnetic resonance cholangiopancreatography (MRCP), or ERCP. Ductal or parenchymal calcifications, characteristic beading of the main pancreatic duct, and ectatic side branches are diagnostic of chronic pancreatitis.

Pancreatic function can be assessed by stimulating the gland with either secretin or CCK with subsequent measurement of electrolyte or enzyme output from the pancreas.

Treatment

The treatment of chronic pancreatitis is mainly symptomatic and directed toward the cardinal features of pain and exocrine and endocrine insufficiency. Patients with chronic pancreatitis should be encouraged to avoid alcohol and smoking. Abstinence from alcohol is important, since functional decline is slower in abstainers. Abstainers also have a better response rate to pain therapy compared with those who continue to drink alcohol.

Abdominal pain in chronic pancreatitis significantly affects the quality of life. Pain management is therefore the cornerstone of therapy in patients with chronic pancreatitis. Patients with increased intraductal pressure may benefit from endoscopic or surgical decompression of the pancreatic duct. Pancreatic enzyme supplementation, in addition to decreasing steatorrhea and improving malabsorption, may lead to relief of pain in a subset of patients. A proton pump inhibitor may be needed to decrease gastric acidity if pancreatic enzyme supplementation is not effective in decreasing steatorrhea. It is also important to rule out other causes of steatorrhea such as celiac disease, Crohn disease, and bacterial overgrowth in such patients.

Treatment of diabetes in patients with chronic pancreatitis is similar to patients with type 1 diabetes. Due to the coexisting deficiency of glucagon, patients with chronic pancreatitis have an increased risk of hypoglycemic events, and effort should be made to prevent such events.

Complications

Complications of chronic pancreatitis include pancreatic pseudocysts, ductal disruption causing pancreatic ascites, and splenic vein thrombosis. Pancreatic pseudocysts occur in approximately 25% of patients. Most pseudocysts resolve in time. Pseudocysts that cause symptoms may need to be drained. The drainage can be done endoscopically, surgically, or radiologically.

Patients with pancreatic ascites require ERCP or MRCP to identify the site of duct disruption. ERCP has the additional advantage of offering therapy in the form of stenting of the pancreatic duct to prevent leakage and allow healing of the disrupted duct. Surgery may become necessary if

endoscopic therapy is not possible or successful. Splenic vein thrombosis occurs in approximately 4% of patients. These patients are predisposed to gastrointestinal bleeding from gastric varices.

PANCREATIC ADENOCARCINOMA

Epidemiology

Pancreatic ductal adenocarcinoma is the fourth leading cause of cancer death in the United States and has the lowest survival rate for any solid cancer. Based on numbers from the American Cancer Society, approximately 32,000 Americans are diagnosed with pancreatic cancer every year. Due to a very high case fatality rate, the total number of deaths from this disease is virtually identical to the number of new cases. Most cancers of the pancreas are adenocarcinomas, with approximately 95% occurring in the exocrine rather than the endocrine pancreas. Over 60% of pancreatic cancers occur in the head of the gland.

Etiology and Risk Factors

The risk factors for developing pancreatic carcinoma include advancing age, cigarette smoking, chronic pancreatitis, and hereditary pancreatitis. DM and obesity may be potential risk factors, but a definite link has not been established. Physical activity and a high intake of fruits and vegetables possibly reduce the risk. Patients with chronic pancreatitis have a relative risk for pancreatic cancer that increases over time. Certain inherited cancer syndromes such as Peutz-Jeghers syndrome or hereditary breast cancer syndromes (BRCA 1 and 2) are also associated with an increased risk of pancreatic cancer.

Clinical Presentation

The clinical presentation of pancreatic adenocarcinoma is pain, jaundice, weight loss, or new-onset DM. As well, patients may have superficial thrombophlebitis, gastrointestinal bleeding, or psychiatric disturbances.

Diagnosis

The diagnosis of pancreatic cancer is typically made radiographically and histologically. The differential diagnosis usually includes chronic pancreatitis, pancreatic endocrine tumors, autoimmune pancreatitis, and lymphoma. Thin-sliced pancreatic CT is the imaging modality of choice for detection of pancreatic cancer. If CT is indeterminate or negative and the clinical suspicion remains high, endoscopic ultrasound may provide further information and also may be used for FNA of the tumor for tissue diagnosis. ERCP as a diagnostic tool for pancreatic cancer has a sensitivity and specificity of 90% to 95%.

Treatment and Prognosis

Surgery offers the only chance for cure; however, only 10% of patients have resectable tumors. The surgery of choice, a Whipple procedure in patients with carcinoma at the head of the pancreas, carries a mortality of approximately 2%. Palliative procedures, such as gastrojejunostomy and endoscopic stenting procedures, are undertaken in patients with metastatic disease. Many attempts at radiation therapy and chemotherapy have met with poor results and have produced no statistically significant beneficial effect on patient survival. Pancreatic ductal carcinoma has a 5-year survival rate of only 1%.

REVIEW EXERCISES

QUESTIONS

1. A 75-year-old man who had open cholecystectomy due to cholecystitis more that 20 years ago underwent ERCP for treatment of choledocholithiasis. Unfortunately, he has developed post-ERCP pancreatitis and has been admitted to your hospital for pain control, intravenous fluid therapy, and observation. On the fourth hospital day, he develops fever (39°C) with a rising white blood cell count. Blood and urine cultures have been obtained. What is the most appropriate imaging study?
a) Ultrasound of the right upper quadrant and the pancreas
b) Contrast-enhanced CT of the abdomen
c) HIDA scan to assess for bile leak
d) Chest CT with intravenous contrast

Answer and Discussion
The answer is b. This man has symptoms suggesting complicated acute pancreatitis. A contrast-enhanced CT is indicated to determine the presence of pancreatic necrosis. The presence of necrosis on CT requires prompt evaluation for infection. FNA with Gram stain has been shown to be most effective at determining the presence or absence of microorganisms.

2. A 35-year-old obese woman who has been hospitalized for acute pancreatitis for a week starts spiking temperatures and becomes hypotensive. Two days before this acute episode, she underwent a contrast-enhanced CT due to continued severe abdominal pain. The CT revealed an area of nonenhancement in the pancreatic body. After adequate resuscitation in the intensive care unit and stabilization of the patient, what is the appropriate next step in the management of this patient?
a) FNA of the pancreatic necrosis
b) Angiography
c) MRI
d) Total parenteral nutrition

Answer and Discussion
The answer is a. The CT scan done 2 days prior to the acute episode had already shown the presence of pancreatic necrosis. The development of fever and hypotension should raise suspicion for infected pancreatic necrosis. FNA of the necrotic material is the best way to detect infection.

3. Gram stain of the FNA of the necrotic pancreatic tissue in the patient above showed gram-negative bacilli. What is the best course of action?
a) Peritoneal lavage
b) Surgical consultation
c) Percutaneous drainage
d) An infectious disease consult

Answer and Discussion
The answer is b. Infected pancreatic necrosis is best managed by surgical debridement.

4. A 21-year-old woman has had recurrent abdominal pain since 3 years of age. She gives a history of similar symptoms in an uncle who died of pancreatic cancer at age 45 years. Plain x-ray films of the abdomen show extensive calcification in the upper abdomen. What is the most likely diagnosis for this patient?
a) Celiac sprue
b) Zollinger-Ellison syndrome
c) Hereditary pancreatitis
d) Gastric carcinoma

Answer and Discussion
The answer is c. This woman has the classic presentation of hereditary pancreatitis: acute bouts of abdominal pain starting in childhood with the eventual development of chronic pancreatitis. Her family history is positive for pancreatitis. Patients with hereditary pancreatitis have a fivefold greater risk for pancreatic cancer than the risk in the average population.

5. A 65-year-old man seeks your advice due to pressure from his wife who thought his color has changed to "yellow" for the past 3 weeks. He does not have any history of liver or bile duct disease. He denies abdominal pain, fever, or chills and says that other than mild fatigue, he feels fine. He does not take any medication on a regular basis. On physical examination, he has scleral icterus, appears jaundiced, and has a palpable but nontender gallbladder. Laboratory evaluation shows the following: total bilirubin, 8.9 mg/dL (reference range, 0–1.5); alkaline phosphatase, 382 U/L (reference range, 40–150), aspartate transaminase, 66 U/L (reference range, 7–40); alanine transaminase, 92 U/L (reference range, 5–50); amylase 23 U/L (reference range, 0–137); normal electrolytes; kidney function; and complete blood count. A right upper quadrant ultrasound shows a dilated intrahepatic biliary tree and distended gallbladder. What is the most likely diagnosis?

a) Acute cholecystitis
b) Chronic pancreatitis
c) Choledocholithiasis
d) Pancreatic cancer

Answer and Discussion

The answer is d. This man has painless jaundice, which along with a palpable, nontender gallbladder (Courvoisier sign) and his age (over 50 years old) is strongly suggestive of pancreatic cancer. Acute cholecystitis, chronic pancreatitis, and choledocholithiasis are usually associated with abdominal pain. Although

chronic pancreatitis and choledocholithiasis can very rarely present this way, pancreatic cancer is more likely.

SUGGESTED READINGS

Banks PA, Freeman ML. The practice parameters committee of the American College of Gastroenterology. Practice guidelines in acute pancreatitis. *Am J Gastroenterol* 2006;101:2379–2400.

Cameron JL, ed. *American Cancer Society Atlas of Clinical Oncology: Pancreatic Cancer.* Hamilton, Ontario: BC Decker, 2001.

Swaroop VS, Chari ST, Clain JE. Severe acute pancreatitis. *JAMA* 2004;291:2865–2868.

Witt H, Apte MV, KeiM V, et al. Chronic pancreatitis: challenges and advances in pathogenesis, genetics, diagnosis, and therapy. *Gastroenterology* 2007;132:1557–1573.

Chapter 53

Esophageal Diseases

Tyler Stevens   Joel E. Richter

POINTS TO REMEMBER:

- Manometry is the definitive test for diagnosing esophageal motility disorders.

- Esophagogastroduodenoscopy (EGD) is the preferred method for identifying reflux esophagitis, infectious esophagitis, and neoplasms.

- In most patients with classic symptoms of heartburn or regurgitation, the history is sufficiently typical to permit a trial of therapy without diagnostic tests.

- Early endoscopy should also be considered in patients with "alarm symptoms" such as weight loss, dysphagia, or anemia.

- Squamous cell carcinoma remains the most common malignant tumor of the esophagus.

The esophagus is tubular organ connecting the oropharynx with the stomach. The pleasures of eating and maintaining adequate nutrition require a normal, healthy esophagus. The esophagus has three major functions:

- To transport ingested material from the oropharynx to the stomach
- To prevent the regurgitation of food and gastric contents from the stomach into the esophagus
- To vent ingested air to reduce abdominal bloating

ANATOMY AND PHYSIOLOGY

The esophagus can be divided into three functional regions:

- Upper esophageal sphincter (UES)
- Esophageal body
- Lower esophageal sphincter (LES)

Upper Esophageal Sphincter

The UES consists of striated muscle, which is formed primarily by the horizontal fibers of the cricopharyngeus muscle at the level of vertebrae C5-C6. Similar to the striated muscles of the oropharynx and upper portion of the esophagus, the UES is innervated and receives motor input directly from the brainstem (i.e., nucleus ambiguus) to the motor endplates in the muscles. The UES is tonically closed, and it opens momentarily in response to a swallow (i.e., the first function). The UES also forms a secondary barrier that prevents the aspiration of gastroesophageal contents (i.e., the second function).

Esophageal Body

The esophageal body consists of an empty tube lined by squamous mucosa, composed of a submucosal layer and two layers of muscles (i.e., the inner circular and outer longitudinal muscles). No serosa overlies the muscle layers. The upper portion of the esophagus primarily is striated muscle, whereas the lower two-thirds predominately is smooth muscle.

The nerve network for the esophageal body lies between the muscle layers. The Meissner (submucosal) plexus is between the muscularis mucosae and the circular muscle layer; the Auerback (myenteric) plexus is between the circular and longitudinal muscle layers. Similar to the LES, innervation of the smooth muscles portion of the esophageal body occurs primarily via the vagus nerve, from neurons arising in the dorsal motor nucleus of the brainstem and from nerve endings in the myenteric plexus.

At rest, the esophageal body is quiet, without motor activity. Normal esophageal motor activity is characterized by the orderly progression (peristalsis) of a contraction along the esophagus in coordination with the relaxation and contraction of the UES and LES. Figure 53.1 represents the pressure sequence of a normal, primary peristaltic wave, as measured with esophageal manometry. The single pressure complex that begins in the pharynx progressively opens the UES and moves sequentially down the esophageal body through an opened LES. The food bolus is pushed ahead by this peristaltic wave through the opened LES and into the stomach. These activities are initiated by the voluntary act of swallowing. Perpetuation through the distal esophagus, however, is controlled by the enteric nervous system.

Lower Esophageal Sphincter

The LES is a high-pressure zone of smooth muscle straddling the diaphragm. It is composed of smooth muscle of the distal esophagus and striated muscle of the crural diaphragm, and it is the major component of the antireflux barrier. At rest, the LES is tonically contracted, which thus prevents the reflux of gastric contents. On swallowing, the LES relaxes and stays relaxed until the peristaltic wave

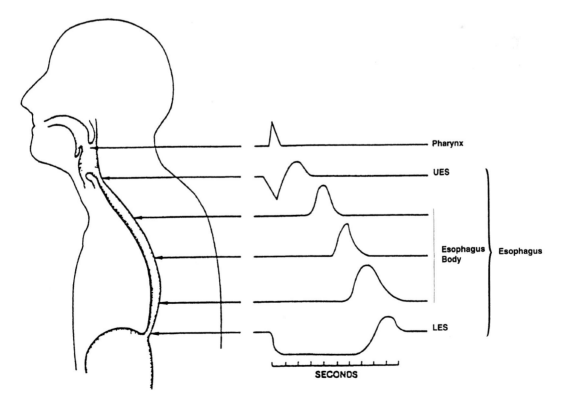

Figure 53.1 Pressure sequences in swallowing. (LES, lower esophageal sphincter; UES, upper esophageal sphincter.)

reaches the end of the esophagus and produces sphincter closure. LES relaxation is vagally mediated via preganglionic cholinergic nerves and postganglionic, noncholinergic, nonadrenergic nerves. Candidates for inhibitory neurotransmitters include vasoactive intestinal polypeptide and nitric oxide.

Tonic contractions of the LES predominantly result from intrinsic muscle activity. LES pressure fluctuates greatly over time, even from minute to minute. Much of this fluctuation results from various extraesophageal factors that modulate LES pressure:

- Food ingested during meals (proteins increase and fats decrease LES pressure)
- Cigarette smoking (decreases LES pressure)
- Gastric distention (decreases LES pressure)

Gastric distention is a critical trigger for transient LES relaxation, which is important in venting ingested gases. In response to transient increases in intra-abdominal pressure, LES pressure increases to a greater degree than the increases occurring in the abdomen below, which thus prevents gastroesophageal reflux (GER). In addition, many hormones and peptides affect LES pressure. Those that increase LES pressure include:

- Gastrin
- Motilin
- Substance P
- Pancreatic polypeptide

Those that decrease LES pressure include:

- Secretin
- Cholecystokinin

- Glucagon
- Vasoactive intestinal polypeptide

DIAGNOSTIC PROCEDURES

A thorough patient history and physical examination are critical in evaluating patients with esophageal disorders. These often identify the appropriate diagnosis and direct further testing (Fig. 53.2).

Imaging Techniques

The barium esophagram is the single most important test for the diagnosis of structural and motor abnormalities of the esophagus. A proper examination should include videotaping of the oropharyngeal and esophageal portions of swallowing, as well as full-column and air-contrast views of the distended esophagus, to identify mucosal irregularities, masses, and regions of luminal narrowing. A solid bolus, such as a marshmallow or tablet, should be administered to any patient with solid food dysphagia in whom a liquid study has been nondiagnostic. Esophageal peristalsis can be assessed in the prone position, with the patient taking five to ten single swallows of barium; this technique approximates esophageal manometry. To identify GER, the cause and extent of barium reflux should be evaluated by rolling the patient from side to side, having the patient cough, and performing the Valsalva maneuver and the water-siphon test.

Solid food scintigraphy, with the patient upright, best approximates normal food ingestion and bolus transport.

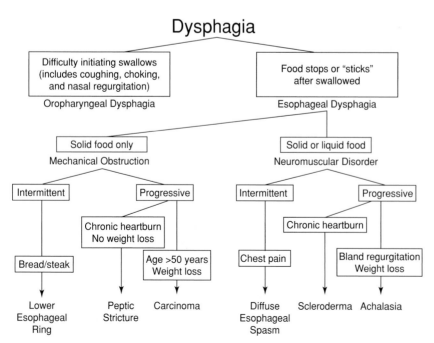

Figure 53.2 Diagnostic approach for patients with dysphagia.

This is an excellent technique for measuring the completeness of LES relaxation and esophageal emptying, and it is especially helpful in patients with achalasia.

Endoscopic ultrasonography, a new imaging technique, is useful in diagnosing and staging both benign and malignant esophageal neoplasms. It is superior to computed tomography in evaluating the depth of tumor infiltration and assessing regional lymph node metastases.

Esophageal Motility Studies

Manometry is the definitive test for diagnosing esophageal motility disorders because it allows an accurate measurement of sphincter pressures and esophageal pressure waves and more completely evaluates abnormalities of esophageal peristalsis. The test is performed by placing a small catheter into the esophagus and measuring changes in intraluminal pressure simultaneously at multiple sites. Normal values for a broad range of ages have been developed with the use of commercially available equipment.

Esophageal manometry does have limitations, however. It accurately records esophageal pressures, but it does not reliably evaluate other important aspects of esophageal function, including completeness of sphincter relaxation, bolus movement, and esophageal emptying. These can best be evaluated with video-imaging techniques or esophageal impedance testing.

Endoscopy and Mucosal Biopsy

Upper endoscopy using biopsy and brush cytology is the best method for identifying mucosal abnormalities of the esophagus. The procedure usually is performed on an outpatient basis with conscious sedation. A small, flexible endoscope, passed orally, permits a thorough evaluation of the esophagus, stomach, and duodenum. EGD is the preferred method for identifying reflux esophagitis, infectious esophagitis, and neoplasms. Mucosal biopsy is most helpful in identifying Barrett esophagus, mild esophagitis, neoplasms, and infectious causes of esophagitis.

Ambulatory Esophageal pH Monitoring

Prolonged ambulatory monitoring of the esophagus for as long as 24 hours is the most reliable means of diagnosing GER. The pH probe is placed transnasally 5 cm above the LES. GER is defined as a decrease in esophageal pH <4. Data are collected in a lightweight box worn on a waist belt, and the information is analyzed by computer. The Bravo pH capsule is a more recent advance in pH monitoring that avoids the need for a nasal tube. It is a tiny device that is attached to the esophageal mucosa at the time of upper endoscopy. pH data is transmitted to the belt pack during a 48-hour period. pH monitoring is usually performed on an outpatient basis, which allows physiological activities to be monitored in the supine and upright po-

sitions, during wakefulness and sleep, during fasting, and after eating. Recording units have an event marker that can be triggered when symptoms occur. This technique allows the accurate quantitation of acid reflux and permits a correlation between acid reflux and subjective symptoms such as chest pain, cough, heartburn, and wheezing. New technology called *pH-impedance* allows us to measure nonacid reflux, which may be helpful with patients having persistent symptoms on proton pump inhibitors (PPI). This technique measures fluid flow independent of pH using a transnasal catheter system and belt pack.

COMMON ESOPHAGEAL DISEASES

Gastroesophageal Reflux Disease

Gastroesophageal reflux disease (GERD)—with heartburn as its major symptom—is the most common disorder of the esophagus, the major indication for antacid consumption, and probably the most prevalent condition originating from the gastrointestinal tract. According to a recent Gallup survey, 44% of adults in the United States experience heartburn at least once every month, and 10% complain of weekly symptoms. More than 40% take antacids for their heartburn, but only 25% discuss this complaint with a physician. Pregnant women have the highest prevalence of heartburn, with at least 25% having daily symptoms, usually in the third trimester.

GERD is defined as the sequelae, both clinical and histopathological, of the chronic movement of gastroduodenal contents into the esophagus. GERD, however, represents a spectrum of disease; for example, it occurs without adverse consequences in many healthy individuals. Episodes of "physiological" reflux typically are postprandial, short lived, and asymptomatic and almost never occur at night. Pathological reflux leads to inflammatory changes and mucosal injury (i.e., reflux esophagitis) and usually is accompanied by symptoms.

Pathophysiology

The pathophysiology of GERD reflects a complex interplay of multiple factors (Fig. 53.3). The common denominator for acid reflux is a creation of a common cavity, representing an equilibration of intragastric and intraesophageal pressures. The LES is the major barrier against GER, with a secondary barrier formed by the crural diaphragm during inspiration, but measurement of a single LES pressure is not very discriminatory. In fact, recent studies determined that transient LES relaxation, occurring with either normal or low LES pressures, is the major mechanism promoting the free reflux of gastric contents. Transient relaxation accounts for nearly all episodes of GER in normal subjects and 65% of episodes in patients with GERD. Other patients experience GER because of very low baseline LES pressures, with either transient increases in intra-abdominal pressure

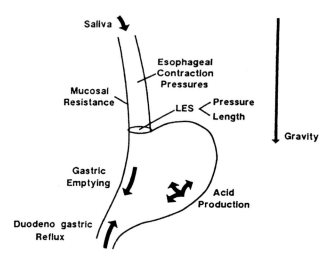

Figure 53.3 Pathogenesis of gastroesophageal reflux disease. (LES, lower esophageal sphincter.)

(i.e., stress reflux) or spontaneous reflux across an atonic sphincter.

Esophageal acid clearance normally occurs as a two-step process:

■ Swallow-induced, peristaltic esophageal contractions rapidly clear fluid volume from the esophagus.
■ The small amount of residual acid is neutralized by saliva, which has a pH of 6.4 to 7.8.

A dysfunction of esophageal clearance mechanisms contributes to esophagitis, particularly in patients with severe motility disorders (e.g., scleroderma) or sicca complex.

Both the nature and volume of gastric contents are important. The primary role of acid is indisputable, but its mechanism of mucosal damage involves the action of co-existing pepsin more than direct damage from acid alone. In animal models, bile salts and pancreatic enzymes can produce esophagitis, but their importance in human disease is unknown. Acid hypersecretory states (e.g., Zollinger-Ellison syndrome) may be associated with a high prevalence of esophagitis. Delayed gastric emptying promotes GER but is an important factor in only 10% to 15% of patients with GERD.

The same degree of acid exposure may lead to variable degrees of mucosal damage, which probably relates to individual variations in esophageal mucosal resistance. Factors contributing to mucosal resistance include:

■ Mucus
■ Bicarbonate ions secreted by submucosal glands
■ Stratified squamous cells and their tight junctions
■ Mucosal blood flow

The relationship between a sliding hiatal hernia and the development of GERD remains controversial. Most patients with esophagitis have a sliding hiatal hernia, but many patients with hiatal hernias do not have GERD. Recent evidence suggests that a large, nonreducible hernia may inter-

fere with normal esophageal clearance by acting as a fluid trap, thus promoting acid reflux during swallow-induced LES relaxations, particularly in the supine position.

Clinical Presentation

The symptoms of GERD include:

■ Heartburn
■ Associated symptoms
■ Dysphagia
■ Odynophagia
■ Regurgitation
■ Water brash
■ Belching

Patients describe their heartburn as a retrosternal burning pain that may also be noted in the epigastrium, neck, throat, and occasionally the back. Frequently, it occurs postprandially and is exacerbated by lying down or bending over. In patients with heartburn, dysphagia is suggestive of a peptic stricture. Other alternative diagnoses include severe inflammation without stricture, peristaltic dysfunction, and an esophageal cancer arising in a Barrett esophagus. Odynophagia usually represents ulcerative esophagitis. The effortless regurgitation of acidic fluid, especially postprandially and at night, is highly suggestive of GERD. Water brash is the sudden appearance in the mouth of a slightly sour or salty fluid from the salivary glands in response to intraesophageal acid exposure.

GERD may present with extraesophageal symptoms, including:

■ Chest pain
■ Respiratory complaints
■ Ear, nose, and throat problems

In these patients, the clinical symptoms of heartburn or regurgitation may be mild or even absent. Recent studies indicate that GERD may be the major cause of noncardiac chest pain in as many as 50% of patients. Chronic cough, recurrent aspiration pneumonia, and pulmonary fibrosis may relate to GERD, and some studies suggest a close association between asthma and GERD, with up to 80% of patients with asthma having evidence of excessive acid reflux on pH testing. Hoarseness, sore throat, halitosis, dental erosions, vocal cord granuloma, and even laryngeal cancer may be caused by the intermittent aspiration of gastric contents.

Diagnosis

In most patients with classic symptoms of heartburn or regurgitation, the history is sufficiently typical to permit a trial of therapy without diagnostic tests. The following situations should lead to early investigation:

■ Esophageal symptoms that do not respond to medical therapy
■ Dysphagia and atypical presentations of suspected GERD

- Possible complications of GERD
- Consideration of antireflux surgery

Tests for GERD evaluate different variables in the disease spectrum; these variables include:

- Potential for reflux
- Hiatal hernia
- Esophageal damage
- Abnormal reflux
- Acid sensitivity

Specific tests include:

- Barium esophagography
- Endoscopy
- Mucosal biopsy
- Manometry
- Acid-perfusion Bernstein test
- 24-hour pH with symptom correlation

There is no single best selection of tests. These tests must be applied selectively, based on the information desired.

All patients with persistent symptoms of GER or with frequent relapses after histamine H_2-receptor antagonist or PPI therapy should have endoscopy to identify possible esophagitis or other complications of GERD. Patients with esophagitis and complications should undergo biopsy to exclude associated malignancies and Barrett esophagus. One must remember, however, that most patients with GERD have no evidence of esophagitis at endoscopy. Early endoscopy should also be considered in patients with "alarm symptoms" such as weight loss, dysphagia, or anemia. EGD may also be considered to screen for Barrett esophagus in patients with chronic reflux symptoms.

Barium esophagography should be the first diagnostic procedure in most patients with dysphagia. Optimally administered, double-contrast barium esophagography detects erosive and ulcerative esophagitis in approximately 90% of patients. The radiologic detection of mild (i.e.,

nonerosive) esophagitis, however, is unreliable. Barium esophagography is also the preferred method for identifying hiatal hernia, and it is good for identifying GER fluoroscopically, particularly when provocative maneuvers are done.

Prolonged esophageal pH monitoring is helpful in patients with atypical presentations or difficult treatment problems, and it has essentially replaced the acid-perfusion Bernstein test. The most common indications for pH monitoring include:

- Noncardiac chest pain
- Suspected pulmonary or ear, nose, and throat presentations of GERD
- Intractable reflux symptoms associated with a negative workup

In addition, prolonged pH monitoring should be conducted before antireflux surgery if there is any question about the diagnosis. A pH evaluation is the single best test for diagnosing GERD, with a sensitivity of 85% and a specificity >95%.

Manometry of LES pressure is not considered to be a sensitive diagnostic test, because fewer than 25% to 50% of patients with GERD have a low resting LES pressure (<10 mm Hg). Manometry is reserved for patients in whom another diagnosis (e.g., achalasia) is suspected, and it is mandatory before antireflux surgery to ensure adequate esophageal pump function.

Treatment

The rationale for GERD therapy depends on a careful definition of specific aims (Table 53.1). In patients without esophagitis, the goal is simply to relieve the acid-related symptoms; in patients with esophagitis, the ultimate goal also is to heal esophagitis while preventing further complications such as strictures and Barrett metaplasia. However, these goals are set against a complex background. GERD is a

TABLE 53.1

GENERAL APPROACH TO THE TREATMENT OF GASTROESOPHAGEAL REFLUX DISEASE

	Symptoms Without Esophagitis	Mild Esophagitis	Severe Esophagitis or Intractable Symptoms
Acute	Lifestyle changes Medications p.r.n. H_2-receptor antagonists Antacids Alginic acid Prokinetics	Lifestyle changes Daily to scheduled medications H_2-receptor antagonists	Lifestyle changes Daily to scheduled medications PPIs
Maintenance	Medications p.r.n. as above	H_2-receptor antagonists	PPIs Antireflux surgery

PPIs, proton pump inhibitors; p.r.n., as needed.

TABLE 53.2

LIFESTYLE MODIFICATIONS FOR PATIENTS WITH GASTROESOPHAGEAL REFLUX DISEASE

Decrease Lower Esophageal Pressure	Improve Acid Clearance	Avoid Direct Esophageal Irritants	Decrease Gastric Distention

Avoid certain foods:
  Fats
  Chocolate
  Coffee
  Carminatives
Avoid certain medications:
  Theophylline
  Progesterone
  Antidepressants
  Nitrates
  Calcium channel blockers
	Elevate head of bed
	Maintain upright position after meals
		Avoid citrus, spicy, or tomato-based products
		Avoid medications causing pill-induced esophagitis
			Avoid large meals
			Take evening meals several hours before retiring; lose weight

chronic condition, and patients with esophagitis generally experience relapse when medical therapy is stopped.

Lifestyle Modification

Lifestyle changes are the cornerstone of effective antireflux treatment in all patients; these are summarized in Table 53.2.

Antacids and Alginic Acid

Antacids and alginic acid are useful for treating mild, infrequent reflux symptoms, especially those brought on by lifestyle indiscretions. However, they are not effective in healing esophagitis. Antacids work primarily by neutralizing acid, albeit for relatively short periods. Therefore, patients need to take these agents frequently, usually 20 to 30 minutes after meals and at bedtime. Aluminium hydroxide antacids that contain alginic acid form a highly viscous solution that floats on the surface of the gastric pool and acts as a mechanical barrier. Recent studies confirm that alginic acid tablets (Gaviscon) effectively prevent acid reflux in the upright position.

Prokinetic Drugs

Bethanechol and metoclopramide (Reglan) are prokinetic drugs that effectively relieve symptoms of heartburn, but their efficacy in treating esophagitis is equivocal. Bethanechol 25 mg or metoclopramide 10 mg is taken 30 minutes before meals and at bedtime. Side effects are common in both young and elderly patients.

H_2-Receptor Antagonists

The use of H_2-receptor antagonists achieved the first real breakthrough in the treatment of GERD, and it continues to be the backbone of therapy for mild reflux esophagitis. Despite advertising to the contrary, all H_2-receptor antagonists (i.e., cimetidine, ranitidine, famotidine, and nizatidine), when properly dosed, are equally effective at improving symptoms of reflux and healing mild to moderate GERD.

These agents are usually given once or preferably twice daily. Recent data on patterns of acid exposure show that most acid reflux occurs during the early evening hours after dinner and that it decreases markedly during the sleeping hours. Therefore, it may be preferable to take an H_2-receptor antagonist 30 minutes after the evening meal rather than at bedtime. Heartburn can be significantly decreased by H_2-receptor antagonists and esophagitis healed in approximately 60% of patients after up to 12 weeks of treatment. Healing rates differ in individual trials, however, depending primarily on the degree of esophagitis before therapy. Mild esophagitis heals in 75% to 90% of patients, whereas moderate to severe esophagitis heals in only 40% to 50% of patients. Studies also suggest that H_2-receptor antagonists are effective in preventing a relapse of GERD in patients with reflux symptoms and mild esophagitis. The H_2-receptor antagonists are available over the counter at lower doses. Their efficacy is similar to that of antacids, although the duration of symptom relief may be longer. The over-the-counter preparations are best used for prophylaxis before refluxogenic activities (i.e., large meals, exercise, etc.).

Proton Pump Inhibitors

Omeprazole (Prilosec), lansoprazole (Prevacid), rabeprazole (Aciphex), and pantoprazole (Protonix) are potent, long-acting inhibitors of both basal and stimulated acid secretion. They act by selective, noncompetitive inhibition of the H^+/K^+ adenosine triphosphatase pump on parietal cells. PPIs completely abolish reflux symptoms in most patients with severe GERD, usually within 1 to 2 weeks; complete healing of esophagitis occurs after 8 weeks in 80% of patients. PPIs are superior to H_2-receptor antagonists, but efficacy is similar across the class of drugs. The newest PPI, however, esomeprazole magnesium trihydrate (Nexium), is a purified form of omeprazole. A recent meta-analysis of 10 trials found a 5% relative increase in healing at 8 weeks with esomeprazole compared with other agents (number needed to treat [NNT] = 25). Symptom relief was 8% superior with esomeprazole than other PPIs. Although statistically significant, the clinical significance of the relative benefit observed for esomeprazole is questionable. However, this PPI may have its best efficacy in those with severe esophagitis where the NNT is 8.

Side effects are minimal with short-term use, but the long-term safety of these drugs is not yet established past 15 years of continuous use. PPIs cause profound hypoacidity that stimulates gastrin release, which in turn promotes the proliferation of enterochromaffinlike cells in the gastric fundus. In the rat model, the prolonged use of omeprazole causes gastric carcinoids; however, such carcinoids have not been reported to date in humans treated for uncomplicated reflux or ulcer disease. The U.S. Food and Drug Administration recently has approved over-the-counter omeprazole (Prilosec) for 2-week use for frequent heartburn. If symptoms persist, then a physician should be seen. This class of drugs is most effective in patients with severe reflux symptoms and severe esophagitis as well as in maintenance therapy to prevent relapse of esophagitis.

Antireflux Surgery

Antireflux surgery, performed either by open or laparoscopic techniques, attempts to maintain a segment of the tubular esophagus below the diaphragm and usually includes wrapping the stomach around the distal esophagus to produce increased LES pressure. Long-term relief of symptoms has occurred in approximately 80% of patients followed for up to 20 years. The preservation of esophageal function, as confirmed with esophageal testing before surgery, is critical for successful antireflux surgery, as is performance of the operation by a skillful surgeon. Indications for antireflux surgery include:

- Severe GERD in younger patients who would otherwise require lifelong medical therapy
- Recurrent, difficult-to-dilate strictures
- Nonhealing ulcers
- Severe bleeding from esophagitis
- Aspiration symptoms from related GERD

Complications of Gastroesophageal Reflux Disease

Peptic Strictures

Peptic strictures represent the end stage of ongoing reflux, mucosal damage, healing, and secondary fibrosis. Patients with strictures present with slowly progressive dysphagia for solids, usually without much weight loss. Radiographically, peptic strictures are commonly found in the lower esophagus and are characterized by smooth-walled, tapered, circumferential narrowings. In all patients, the benign nature of the stricture must be confirmed through endoscopy and biopsy.

Therapy for peptic strictures consists of a careful review of dietary and medication habits, aggressive antireflux therapy, and bougienage. Patients should chew their food well, take fluids liberally, and avoid potentially damaging pills, such as aspirin, nonsteroidal anti-inflammatory drugs (NSAIDs), and potassium chloride. Aggressive acid suppression, particularly with PPIs, may reduce the need for subsequent dilations. Dilating (i.e., stretching) the narrowed distal esophagus with blunt bougies passed either freely or over a guide wire can markedly relieve symptoms of dysphagia.

Barrett Esophagus

Barrett esophagus secondary to severe esophagitis produces a unique reparative process in which the original squamous epithelial lining is replaced by metaplastic columnar epithelium. The prevalence of Barrett esophagus varies depending on the population being studied. Patients with symptomatic GERD have a prevalence rate of 5% to 12%, whereas those with esophagitis, scleroderma, or peptic strictures may have higher rates (11%–44%). The diagnosis is best made with endoscopy and confirmed with biopsy. Barrett epithelium may comprise three types of mucosa, but only the specialized columnar epithelium has malignant potential.

Therapy is no different from that of any other form of esophagitis. The major concerns are the increased prevalence and incidence of esophageal adenocarcinoma. The prevalence rate is estimated at 10%, which is 30- to 40-fold greater than in the general population. The incidence rates are quite variable, however, ranging from 1 in 46 to 1 in 441 patient-years of follow-up. As with colonic adenomas, over time, the columnar lining of the esophagus may evolve through increasing degrees of dysplasia to cancer. For this reason, endoscopic surveillance is recommended in patients with Barrett esophagus to detect high-grade dysplasia (HGD) or early cancer so that curative endoscopic or surgical resection can be performed.

Endoscopic mucosal resection (EMR) involves a variety of techniques to remove focal or nodular areas of dysplasia through the endoscope. Multifocal dysplasia is not easily amenable to EMR. In good surgical candidates, the standard treatment for multifocal HGD is esophagectomy. However, a number of new and less invasive techniques have been explored in recent years. Photodynamic therapy (PDT) involves the intravenous administration of a phototoxic agent (e.g., porfimir sodium, 5-ALA) followed by light treatment through an optical probe passed through the endoscope. A recent multicenter study demonstrated a higher rate of resolution of HGD with PDT compared with medical treatment alone at 5 years (77% vs. 39%, $p < 0.0001$). Problems with PDT include esophageal stricture formation and the necessity to avoid light for up to 30 days following the procedure. There is also a concern of "buried Barrett"—that is, intestinal glands and dypslastic change developing under regenerated epithelium. The circumferential ablation of dypslastic or even nondysplastic Barrett epithelium has been performed using radio frequency ablation (RFA) delivered through a balloon probe inflated in the lower esophagus. Initial studies suggest that RFA is effective and may have a lower rate of strictures and "buried" Barrett metaplasia.

OTHER INFLAMMATORY DISORDERS OF THE ESOPHAGUS

Other disorders of the esophagus are usually acute in onset and characterized clinically by odynophagia and dysphagia. An algorithm for evaluating patients with odynophagia is shown in Figure 53.4.

Eosinophilic Esophagitis

In the past decade, studies have shown an increasing prevalence of children and adults with GERD-like symptoms and esophageal eosinophilia. Eosinophilic esophagitis (EE) is a chronic condition that is more common in males than females and may coincide with atopic conditions and food allergies. In adults, the most common clinical manifestations of EE are medically refractory GERD symptoms, dysphagia, and food bolus impactions. Endoscopy often reveals esophageal narrowing, multiple fixed rings, and longitudinal furrowing. Histologic examination reveals a characteristic increase in esosinophils (<15 eosinophils per high-powered field) in the lamina propria. Treatment for EE currently consists of topical or systemic corticosteroids to relieve the eosinophilic inflammation. PPIs may be helpful

in a subset of EE patients. Esophageal dilation is an ancillary treatment for patients with strictures and dysphagia. However, dilation should be performed carefully due to a higher risk of mucosal tears in these patients.

Infectious Esophagitis

Infections of the esophagus are rare in the general population. When present, however, they should prompt a search for an underlying immune abnormality. Esophageal infection is seen primarily in three groups of immunocompromised patients:

- Patients infected with the HIV
- Patients with cancer and granulocytopenia after chemotherapy
- Organ transplantation patients receiving immunosuppressive therapy

Other predisposing conditions include:

- Malignancy
- Alcoholism
- Diabetes mellitus
- Therapy with corticosteroids or other immunosuppressive agents

The most common causes of infectious esophagitis are:

- *Candida* sp.
- Herpes simplex virus
- Cytomegalovirus

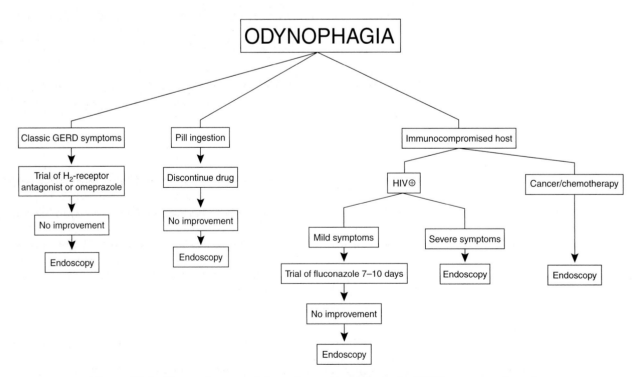

Figure 53.4 Diagnostic approach for patients with odynophagia. (GERD, gastroesophageal reflux disease; HIV, human immunodeficiency virus–positive.) (Adapted with permission from Wilcox CM, Karowe NW. Esophageal infection: etiology, diagnosis, and management. *Gastroenterologist* 1994;2:188–206.)

Candidal esophagitis is most commonly seen in patients who are infected with HIV or have granulocytopenic cancer. Viral esophagitis predominates in patients who have received bone marrow transplants. Both candidal and viral esophagitis are encountered after solid organ transplantation. Other less common causes of infectious esophagitis include:

- *Histoplasma* organisms
- *Mycobacterium tuberculosis*
- *Mycobacterium avium-intracellulare complex*
- *Cryptosporidium* sp.
- *Pneumocystis carinii*
- Epstein-Barr virus
- HIV
- Gram-negative and gram-positive bacteria

Mixed infections are present in approximately 30% of patients, and esophageal infections should be suspected in immunocompromised patients presenting with odynophagia, dysphagia, or chest pain. Oral thrush is commonly sought, but its presence does not preclude infections with organisms besides *Candida*. In addition, its absence does not preclude *Candida*. Double-contrast barium esophagography has neither high sensitivity nor specificity for infectious esophagitis. Endoscopy with brush cytology, biopsy, and culture is the best initial diagnostic test.

Candidiasis is recognized by discrete, 3- to 5-mm, raised yellowish plaques or confluent cheesy exudates. The diagnosis is most easily established by brushing the plaques, smearing the material on a clear glass slide, allowing it to dry, and then applying 10% potassium hydroxide. The specimen is examined for the typical branched hyphae and budding yeast. Fungal cultures and the histologic examination of biopsy specimens are also helpful. The treatment of candidal esophagitis is determined by the severity of the infection and the nature of the underlying immune defect (Table 53.3).

Herpetic esophagitis is characterized by clear vesicles early in its course. Because these vesicles are short lived, however, the usual finding is discrete, small, superficial ulcers with a punched-out appearance and raised yellow edges. The intervening mucosa often appears normal. Brushings and biopsy specimens show cytologic changes that may be suggestive of herpetic infection (i.e., Cowdry type A inclusions).

Cytomegalovirus esophagitis appears as an extensive area of mucosal injury with inflammatory exudate and ulcerations. The ulcers are very deep, progress in size, and occasionally perforate. Biopsy specimens, brush cytologic examination, or viral culture may show evidence of cytomegalovirus. Esophageal ulcerations have been described in patients who undergo HIV seroconversion. These patients present with a syndrome characterized by fever, myalgia, maculopapular rash, and odynophagia. Endoscopy shows multiple discrete esophageal ulcerations, and the electron microscopy of tissue shows retroviral organisms, which thus indicates HIV as the direct cause.

Pill-Induced Esophagitis

More than 50% of cases of pill-induced esophagitis result from tetracycline hydrochloride or tetracycline derivatives, particularly doxycycline. Other commonly prescribed medications causing esophageal injury include:

- Slow-release potassium chloride
- Iron sulfate
- Quinidine sulfate
- Alendronate sodium (i.e., Fosamax)
- NSAIDs

A common factor among these patients is a history of improper pill ingestions. In nearly 50% of reported cases, patients took little or no fluid while swallowing their pills or took their pills just before bedtime. Patients

TABLE 53.3

TREATMENT FOR COMMON ESOPHAGEAL INFECTIONS

Infection	Treatment
Candida	
Minimal compromise (i.e., diabetes, steroids)	Nystatin, 1–3 million U QID; or clotrimazole, 100 mg TID
Acquired immunodeficiency syndrome	Ketoconazole, 200–400 mg daily; or fluconazole, 100 mg daily TS
Failure of above	Amphotericin B, 0.3–56.4 mg/kg/day
Herpes simplex virus	
Immunocompetent patient	Supportive care
	Analgesics
	Topical anesthetics
Immunocompromised patient	
Mild cases	Acyclovir, 200–400 mg PO 5 times daily TS
More severe cases	Acyclovir, 15 mg/kg/day IV
Cytomegalovirus	Ganciclovir, 5 mg/kg IV every 12 hr; or foscarnet, 60 mg/kg/day IV every 8 hr
HIV	Prednisone, 40 mg daily

Modified with permission from Wilcox CM, Karowe NW. Esophageal infection: etiology, diagnosis, and management. *Gastroenterologist* 1994;2:188–206.

with pill-induced esophageal injury generally complain of odynophagia and retrosternal burning; only a minority report that pills get stuck in the chest. Endoscopy, which is the first investigative study, usually reveals discrete ulcers at the aortic arch or distal esophagus.

Pill-induced esophagitis improves after withdrawal of the offending medication. Symptomatic resolution and endoscopic healing are usually evident after 3 days to 6 weeks. In addition to drug discontinuation, other therapies include palliation of odynophagia with viscous lidocaine, prevention of acid reflux, and assurance of adequate nutrition. Rarely, strictures requiring dilation develop. To prevent further pill-induced esophageal injuries, patients should be encouraged to ingest all pills with 8 ounces of water while standing or sitting upright, and they should be discouraged from taking pills just before bedtime.

ESOPHAGEAL MOTILITY DISORDERS

Functional disturbances of the esophagus may result from either neurologic or muscular disorders and may involve the striated muscle, smooth muscle, or both muscle segments. The most common motility abnormalities involve the distal smooth muscle.

Achalasia

Achalasia is characterized by a double defect in esophageal function. The LES does not relax appropriately and thus offers resistance to the flow of liquids and solids from the esophagus into the stomach. In addition, peristaltic muscle movement is lost in the lower two-thirds (i.e., smooth muscle portion) of the esophagus. Achalasia usually develops between 25 and 60 years of age, and men and women are affected equally. The cause is unknown, but the two most popular theories suggest that achalasia is secondary to an infection or a degenerative disease of neurons. In South America, infection with the protozoan *Trypanosoma cruzi* produces ganglion damage and an achalasialike syndrome with megaesophagus, but this is seen rarely in the United States.

Pathophysiology
Abnormalities in both muscle and nerves can be detected in patients with achalasia, but a neural lesion is thought to be of primary importance. Three major neuroanatomic changes are described:

- Loss of ganglion cell within the Auerbach plexus
- Degeneration of the vagus nerve
- Qualitative and quantitative changes in the dorsal motor nucleus of the vagus

Selective damage occurs to inhibitory neurons, with marked reduction in the levels of vasoactive intestinal polypeptide and nitric oxide receptors, which can account for the observed motility disturbances. Further evidence of denervation is the exaggerated contractions in the LES and esophageal body that are observed when these patients are given methacholine; this response indicates denervation hypersensitivity.

Clinical Presentation
Nearly all patients with achalasia have dysphagia for solids, and most also have dysphagia for liquids. The onset is gradual, and most patients have symptoms for an average of 2 years before the diagnosis is made. Postural changes such as throwing the shoulders back, lifting the neck, and performing a rapid Valsalva maneuver help improve esophageal emptying. Fullness in the chest and regurgitation of undigested, nonacidic food are also seen in many patients. Undigested food may be regurgitated postprandially or at night, with the regurgitation causing choking, cough, and aspiration pneumonia. Chest pain occurs in some patients and is more common in younger patients with earlier disease. Surprisingly, heartburn sometimes is described, presumably because of the fermentation of intraesophageal contents. Weight loss is very common and usually increases with disease duration.

Diagnosis
In a patient with suspected achalasia, the first diagnostic test is a barium esophagram. Early in the course of disease, the esophagus may appear normal in diameter but has a loss of normal peristalsis. As the disease progresses, the esophagus becomes more dilated and tortuous, with retained food and presence of air-fluid levels. The distal esophagus is characterized by a smooth, symmetric, tapering, bird-beak appearance. Clues to the diagnosis may also be found on chest radiographs, including

- Widened mediastinum
- Thoracic air-fluid level
- Absence of the gastric air bubble

The diagnosis of achalasia is confirmed through esophageal manometry (Table 53.4). Characteristic manometric features include:

- Absence of peristalsis in the distal smooth muscle esophagus
- Incomplete or abnormal LES relaxation
- Elevated LES pressure
- Elevated intraesophageal pressure relative to gastric pressure

All patients with achalasia should undergo upper gastrointestinal endoscopy to differentiate primary achalasia from pseudoachalasia, which is usually secondary to an adenocarcinoma.

Treatment
The goal of therapy in patients with achalasia is to diminish the high residual LES pressure after swallowing. If esophageal emptying is improved, esophageal stasis and its consequences are reduced. Peristalsis rarely returns, but

TABLE 53.4

MANOMETRIC CHARACTERISTICS OF ESOPHAGEAL MOTILITY DISORDERS

		Spastic Motor Disorder			
	Achalasia	Diffuse Esophageal Spasm	Nutcracker	Hypertensive Lower Esophageal Sphincter	Scleroderma
Striated muscle/ UES	Normal	Normal	Normal	Normal	Normal
Smooth muscle	Aperistalsis	Intermittent peristalsis Simultaneous, repetitive High amplitude Long duration Spontaneous	Normal peristalsis High amplitude	Normal peristalsis	Low-amplitude peristalsis or aperistalsis
LES	Abnormal relaxation High pressure	Occasional LES dysfunction	Normal	High pressure Normal relaxation	Low or no pressure

LES, lower esophageal sphincter; UES, upper esophageal sphincter.

patients feel as if swallowing is nearly normal. Three treatments are available:

- Pharmacologic therapy
- Pneumatic dilation
- Surgical myotomy

Pharmacologic Therapy

Smooth muscle relaxants, including sublingual isosorbide dinitrate, or a calcium antagonist, such as nifedipine, can be used prophylactically with meals or as necessary for pain or dysphagia. These medications provide variable relief of symptoms, but their effectiveness tends to decrease with time. Botulinum toxin injection into the LES during endoscopy has been shown to improve symptoms for 3 months to 1 year. It may be the preferred treatment in the elderly or in subjects with severe comorbid illnesses who are not good candidates for more definitive treatments.

Pneumatic Dilation

Pneumatic dilation involves placing a balloon across the LES and then inflating it to a pressure adequate to tear the muscle fibers of the sphincter. Good to excellent results occur in 50% to 90% of patients. Women and older patients do especially well with pneumatic dilation. The procedure can be performed on an outpatient basis, recovery is rapid, and discomfort is short lived. However, approximately 30% of patients may require subsequent dilations, and perforation is a major complication, reported in approximately 2.5% of patients and usually requiring surgical repair.

Surgical Myotomy

Heller myotomy involves incising the circular muscle of the LES and the more distal esophagus down to the mucosa and allowing the muscle to protrude through the incision. Myotomy produces good to excellent results in 60% to 90% of

patients, and the operative mortality rate is low. Younger subjects and men are the best candidates for surgical myotomy. To prevent postoperative GER, many surgeons now add a loose antireflux operation to the myotomy. Laparoscopic and thoracoscopic techniques for esophageal myotomy have replaced the open procedure, which in the past usually was done through the left chest and had a longer hospitalization and recovery period.

Spastic Motility Disorders

Spastic manometric patterns differ from those of achalasia by the following characteristics:

- Normal peristalsis intermittently interrupted by simultaneous contractions
- High-amplitude or long-duration waves
- Dysfunction of the LES

Confusion has arisen, however, concerning whether these manometric abnormalities represent separate, distinct entities or variations of diffuse esophageal spasm (Table 53.4). The similarities among these disorders in presentation, natural history, and treatment suggest that these syndromes frequently overlap and that they should be designated as spastic motility disorders of the esophagus.

Pathophysiology

The cause and pathogenesis of spastic motility disorders is unknown, and no specific, characteristic pathological lesion is present. These abnormalities commonly are associated with other medical conditions, particularly GER. Central nervous system processing could produce some of these manometric abnormalities. Psychologically stressful interviews, loud noises, or difficult mental tasks can produce simultaneous waves and increase contraction amplitudes in the distal esophagus of both normal persons and patients with spastic motility disorders. These patients also appear to have both a motor and sensory component to their spastic disorder. Acid instillation may stimulate sensitive neural receptors, thus producing esophageal pain at low distention volumes without the accompaniment of noticeable motor changes.

Clinical Presentation

Spastic disorders of the esophagus generally develop during middle age and occur more commonly in women. Dysphagia and chest pain are the cardinal symptoms; most patients present with both. Dysphagia for liquids and solids is present in 30% to 60% of patients. However, the symptom is intermittent and varies daily from mild to very severe, although usually it is not progressive or severe enough to interfere with eating or produce weight loss. Intermittent anterior chest pain, sometimes mimicking that of angina pectoris, is reported by most patients. Episodes of pain last from minutes to hours and may require narcotics or nitroglycerin, which further confuses the distinction between esophageal and cardiac pain. Many patients also have symptoms compatible with that of irritable bowel syndrome, and accompanying urinary and sexual dysfunction may be present in women.

Diagnosis

Spastic motility disorders are best defined using esophageal manometry. A patient's chief symptom is an important factor in identifying the prevalence and type of motility disorder. In patients with diffuse esophageal spasm, the barium esophagram may reveal severe, lumen-obliterating tertiary contractions that trap barium and delay transit and thereby produce a to-and-fro movement of the bolus. Other spastic motility disorders frequently yield a normal barium esophagram. Endoscopy may be done, but its major role is to identify possible structural lesions or rule out reflux esophagitis. Provocative tests, such as the edrophonium chloride and balloon distention tests, may be able to provoke chest pain. Ambulatory 24-hour pH monitoring is useful to identify associated GERD, which is present in 20% to 50% of these patients.

Treatment

Many patients respond favorably to confident reassurance that their chest pain has an esophageal origin and is not coming from the heart. GER should be identified and aggressively treated; otherwise, no single drug has a proved efficacy in the treatment of spastic esophageal motility disorders. Smooth muscle relaxants, such as long-acting nitrates, calcium channel blockers, and anticholinergics, may decrease high-amplitude contractions, but they do not relieve chest pain consistently. Antidepressant medications may reduce the amount of discomfort experienced (as well as the patient's reaction to pain), but the esophageal motility abnormality does not change. Botulinum toxin injections into the lower esophagus may help chest pain and dysphagia. Passive dilation of the esophagus has no value; yet, pneumatic dilation helps some patients with diffuse esophageal spasm or hypertensive LES who complain of severe dysphagia and have documented delays in esophageal emptying. In rare cases, a long surgical myotomy may help the patient. Aggressive interventions must be used cautiously, however, because symptoms may not be relieved.

SCLERODERMA

Esophageal involvement is seen in 70% to 80% of patients with scleroderma, and more than 90% have associated Raynaud phenomenon. Esophageal involvement is seen in patients with either progressive systemic sclerosis or CREST syndrome (*c*alcinosis, *R*aynaud phenomenon, *e*sophageal involvement, *s*clerodactyly, and *t*elangiectasia). The pathophysiology involves an abnormality in muscle excitation and responsiveness resulting from muscle atrophy and decreased cholinergic excitation.

The classic manometric features of advanced scleroderma include (Table 53.4):

- Low LES pressure
- Peristaltic dysfunction of the smooth muscle portion of the esophagus, characterized by low-amplitude contractions or aperistalsis
- Preserved function of the striated esophagus and oropharynx

Because of these manometric abnormalities, patients may have dysphagia and severe GERD. Surprisingly, dysphagia for solids and liquids is reported by fewer than 50% of patients with scleroderma. More severe dysphagia is suggestive of esophagitis, often with an associated stricture. Esophagitis is present in most patients.

The treatment of scleroderma centers around GER and its complications. Patients should chew their food well and drink plenty of fluids. GERD should be identified and aggressively treated using H_2-receptor antagonists or PPIs. Strictures respond to frequent dilations. In severe cases, antireflux surgery may be warranted.

ESOPHAGEAL TUMORS

More than 90% of esophageal tumors are malignant. Squamous cell carcinoma, which is primarily a disease of black men, remains the most common malignant tumor of the esophagus. Associated risk factors are the excessive use of tobacco and alcohol. Conversely, adenocarcinoma, seen mainly in white men, is a recognized complication of Barrett esophagus resulting from chronic GER. Recently, a striking five- to sixfold increase has occurred in the incidence of adenocarcinoma of the esophagus, which has changed the ratio of squamous cell carcinoma cases to adenocarcinoma cases from 90% to 10% to 60% to 40%.

Other types of malignant tumors of the esophagus are rare and include lymphoma and melanoma. Common benign tumors of the esophagus include:

- Leiomyoma
- Lipoma
- Granular cell tumor
- Squamous cell papilloma
- Esophageal cyst

MISCELLANEOUS ESOPHAGEAL DISORDERS

Esophageal Diverticula

An esophageal diverticulum is an outpouching of one or more layers of the esophageal wall. It occurs in three main areas:

- Immediately above the UES (i.e., Zenker diverticulum)
- Near the midpoint of the esophagus (i.e., traction diverticulum)
- Immediately about the LES (i.e., epiphrenic diverticulum)

Zenker diverticulum occurs in older patients who complain of cervical dysphagia, gurgling in the throat, halitosis, regurgitation of foul food, and sometimes a neck mass. It was originally believed to relate to discoordination of UES relaxation, but recent studies show that the sphincter opens incompletely because of reduced muscle compliance. To compensate for this decreased cross-sectional area, the hypopharyngeal bolus pressure increases, which leads to dysphagia and diverticulum formation. Traction diverticula usually are asymptomatic. They are believed to occur secondary either to external inflammatory processes (e.g., tuberculosis) or to a localized segmental motility disorder. Epiphrenic diverticula are invariably associated with esophageal motility disorders, especially achalasia.

Diverticula are best diagnosed with barium esophagography; endoscopy is rarely required. The treatment of symptomatic diverticula requires surgery.

Esophageal Tears and Perforations

Esophageal tears and perforations can result from the following:

- Prolonged and violent vomiting after a meal or alcoholic binge
- Instrumentation of the esophagus
- Ingestion of foods containing bones or sharp foreign objects

A mucosal tear at the gastroesophageal junction is known as a Mallory-Weiss tear. It can be asymptomatic or associated with significant upper gastrointestinal bleeding. In contrast, spontaneous esophageal rupture (i.e., Boerhaave syndrome) is a rare, life-threatening condition characterized by a full-thickness tear of the esophageal wall. Patients with Boerhaave syndrome present with:

- Severe substernal epigastric pain
- Dysphagia
- Odynophagia
- Dyspepsia

Findings include hypotension, fever, tachycardia, and subcutaneous emphysema. Radiographs frequently reveal pleural effusion, parenchymal infiltrates, pneumothorax, pneumomediastinum, and mediastinal widening.

The diagnosis is confirmed with a barium esophagram obtained with the use of a water-soluble contrast agent (e.g., meglumine diatrizoate). On confirmation, a nasogastric tube should be placed to provide continuous suction, and the patient should be given broad-spectrum antibiotics. Small, self-contained leaks can be treated successfully with conservative management, but larger tears require immediate surgery.

Rings and Webs

The lower esophageal (Schatzki) ring, located at the squamocolumnar junction, is the most common source of intermittent dysphagia for solids. Rings are usually found in patients older than 50 years and rarely in those younger than 30 years. The origin of the lower esophageal ring is unknown, but recent studies suggest that it is a complication of GERD. The diagnosis is made with the following:

- Barium swallow examination in the prone position
- Valsalva maneuver
- Having the patient swallow a marshmallow or tablet to bring out the ring

Treatment includes:

- Simple reassurance with guidance for adjustment of eating habits
- Dilation of the ring with a blunt bougie
- Therapy for associated GERD

Webs are membranous narrowings covered entirely by squamous mucosa. They may occur anywhere along the esophagus but are found primarily in the upper 2 to 4 cm. Some webs are congenital; others are associated with iron deficiency anemia (i.e., Paterson-Kelly or Plummer-Vinson syndrome). Most webs are asymptomatic and are discovered as incidental radiologic findings. Symptomatic patients are usually women reporting dysphagia for solids rather than liquids. The diagnosis is made using the lateral view of the barium esophagram. Treatment with bougienage often is successful.

REVIEW EXERCISES

QUESTIONS

1. A patient reports intermittent dysphagia for solid foods only, especially for bread and meat. What is the most likely etiology?
a) Lower esophageal (Schatzki) ring
b) Esophageal cancer
c) Zenker diverticulum
d) Achalasia

Answer and Discussion

The answer is a. A lower esophageal ring presents classically with dysphagia for solids and no weight loss. With esophageal cancer, progressive dysphagia and weight loss is present. Achalasia presents with dysphagia for solids and liquids and regurgitation of nonacidic, undigested food and saliva. Zenker diverticulum is marked by cervical dysplasia, bland regurgitation, and halitosis.

2. Achalasia is usually *not* characterized by which of the following symptoms?
a) Dysphagia for solids and liquids
b) Dysphagia for solids only
c) Bland regurgitation
d) Heartburn

Answer and Discussion

The answer is b. Dysphagia for solids suggests an anatomic (i.e., structural) rather than a functional (i.e., motility) disorder.

3. Which pill is most commonly associated with esophagitis?
a) An NSAID
b) Quinidine
c) Doxycycline
d) Slow-release potassium

Answer and Discussion

The answer is c. All these medications are associated with pill-induced esophagitis. However, the most frequent culprit is doxycycline, as it is a widely used antibiotic. Classically, young adults taking doxycycline for acne present with dysphagia and odynophagia because they take their medication either with a minimal amount of water or immediately before bedtime.

4. Which of the following has been associated with GERD?
a) Noncardiac chest pain
b) Asthma
c) Dental erosion
d) Laryngeal cancer
e) All of the above

Answer and Discussion

The answer is e. More than 50% of patients with noncardiac chest pain have GERD. Extraesophageal presentations of GERD include damage to the lungs (i.e., asthma) and oropharynx (e.g., hoarseness, vocal cord granulomas, dental erosions, laryngeal cancer) secondary to high acid reflux.

5. Which of the following is not true about Barrett esophagus?
a) It results from long-standing acid.
b) The diagnosis is made by endoscopy.
c) The prevalence rate of developing adenocarcinoma is approximately 10%.
d) Endoscopic surveillance is recommended for healthy patients with Barrett esophagus.

Answer and Discussion

The answer is b. The diagnosis of achalasia is *suspected* by endoscopy and confirmed by biopsies showing the presence of specialized columnar mucosa with goblet cells.

SUGGESTED READINGS

Baehr PH, McDonald GB. Esophageal infections: risks factors, presentation, diagnosis and treatment. *Gastroenterology* 1994;106:509–532.

Baron TH, Richter JE. The use of esophageal function tests. *Adv Intern Med* 1993;38:3661–3686.

Biot WJ, Devesa SS, Kneller RW, et al. Rising incidence of adenocarcinoma of the esophagus and gastric cardia. *JAMA* 1991;265:1287–1289.

Clouse RE. Spastic disorders of the esophagus. *Gastroenterologist* 1997;5:112–127.

DeVault KR, Castell DO. Updated guidelines for the diagnosis and treatment of gastroesophageal reflux disease. *Am J Gastroenterol* 1999;94:1434–1442.

Gralnek IM, Dulai GS, Fennerty B, et al. Esomeprazole versus other proton pump inhibitors in erosive esophagitis: a meta-analysis of randomized clinical trials. *Clin Gastroenterol Hep* 2006;4:1452–1458.

Hirano I, Richter JE. ACG practice guidelines: Esophageal reflux testing. *Am J Gastroenterol* 2007;102:668–685.

Lagergren J, Bergstrom R, Lindgren A, et al. Symptomatic gastroesophageal reflux as a risk factor for esophageal adenocarcinoma. *N Engl J Med* 1999;340:825–831.

Marks RD, Richter JE. Peptic strictures of the esophagus. *Am J Gastroenterol* 1993;88:1160–1173.

Overholt BF, Wang KK, Burdick S, et al. Five-year efficacy and safety of photodynamic therapy with Photofrin in Barrrett's high-grade dysplasia. *Gastrointest Endosc* 2007;66:460–468.

Richter JE. Ear, nose and throat and respiratory manifestations of esophageal reflux disease: an increasing conundrum. *Eur J Gastroenterol Hepatol* 2004;16:837–845.

Richter JE. Modern management of achalasia. *Curr Treat Options Gastroenterol* 2005;8:275–283.

Spechler SJ, Goyal RK. The columnar-lined esophagus, intestinal metaplasia and Norman Barrett. *Gastroenterology* 1996;110:614–621.

Spechler SJ, Lee E, Ahnen D, et al. Long-term outcome of medical and surgical therapies of GERD. Follow-up of a randomized controlled trial. *JAMA* 2001;285:2331–2338.

Vigneri S, Termini R, Leandro G, et al. A comparison of five maintenance therapies for reflux esophagitis. *N Engl J Med* 1995;333:1106–1110.

Chapter 54

Peptic Ulcer Disease

Bennie R. Upchurch

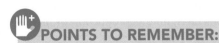

POINTS TO REMEMBER:

- *Helicobacter pylori* is on the decline in the Western world but remains the most common cause of ulcer disease.

- Nonsteroidal anti-inflammatory drugs (NSAIDs) are the second most common cause of ulcer disease, but the cyclooxygenase (COX)-2–selective inhibitors cause much less gastrointestinal toxicity.

- *H. pylori* serology testing has been replaced by breath testing and fecal antigen testing.

- *H. pylori* test and treat strategies are still appropriate in dyspeptic patients under the age of 45 to 50 years without alarm symptoms.

- Proton pump inhibitors (PPI) are the most effective agents for healing ulcers and with available intravenous options have essentially replaced other agents.

- PPI prophylaxis in NSAID users should be reserved for high-risk patients.

EPIDEMIOLOGY

Peptic ulcer disease (gastric ulcer and duodenal ulcer) is a common clinical problem, affecting approximately 4.5 million Americans annually. The lifetime prevalence of peptic ulcer disease is approximately 5% to 10%, but its incidence has been decreasing over the past three to four decades. The prevalence has shifted from a male predominance to similar incidences in men and women. The most important risk factors are infection with *H. pylori* and ingestion of NSAIDs. Factors that clearly are not associated with the development of ulcers include personality, occupation, alcohol consumption, diet, and emotional stress. The prevalence of duodenal ulcer increases with age and is likely related to the increased prevalence of *H. pylori* infection in older age groups, coupled with increased use of NSAIDs. However, with recognition of these factors and trends in current therapy, *H. pylori*–negative, NSAID-negative ulcer disease has become more common in recent years. Race does not seem to play a role, but socioeconomic and geographic factors as they relate to higher prevalences of *H. pylori* infection show a higher prevalence of peptic ulcer disease in some groups. Physician office visits and hospitalizations for peptic ulcer disease have decreased in the last few decades; however, the disease still represents a major financial burden on our health care system by accounting for roughly 10% of medical costs for gastrointestinal illnesses. The mortality rate has decreased modestly in the last few decades and is approximately 1 death per 100,000 cases, with a hospitalization rate of approximately 30 patients per 100,000 cases. Genetic factors may play a role in both duodenal and gastric ulcers. Hypersecretory states, such as Zollinger-Ellison syndrome, antral G-cell hyperplasia, systemic mastocytosis, retained antrum syndrome, and basophilic leukemias are rare causes of peptic ulcer disease.

GASTRODUODENAL PATHOPHYSIOLOGY

The formation of ulcers requires acid and peptic activity in gastric secretions. Acid secretion occurs in the parietal cells located in the oxyntic glands of the fundus and body of the stomach. These cells may be stimulated to secrete acid by three different pathways. The *neurocrine pathway* involves the vagal release of acetylcholine; the *paracrine pathway* is mediated by the release of histamine from mast cells and enterochromaffinlike cells in the stomach; and the *endocrine pathway* is mediated by the release of gastrin from antral G cells. Each of these transmitters has a specific receptor located on the basolateral surface of the parietal cell. The stimulation of these receptors leads to activation of intracellular second-messenger systems: Gastrin and acetylcholine promote the accumulation of intracellular calcium, whereas histamine causes a stimulatory G protein to activate adenylate cyclase, which in turn generates cyclic adenosine monophosphate (cAMP). These intracellular messengers then activate protein kinases, which activate the proton pump—the H^+/K^+ adenosine triphosphatase enzyme, located at the apical surface of the parietal cell—to secrete hydrogen ions in exchange for potassium ions. Prostaglandins and somatostatin inhibit parietal cell function by binding to receptors that act through inhibitory G proteins to inhibit adenylate cyclase. Somatostatin also inhibits gastrin release. Acid is necessary to convert pepsinogen, which is secreted from gastric chief cells, into pepsin, which is a proteolytic enzyme that is inactive at a pH >4. Parietal cells also secrete intrinsic factor, a glycoprotein important in vitamin B_{12} absorption.

Under normal circumstances, gastroduodenal surface epithelial cells resist injury by several protective mechanisms. First, these cells secrete mucins, phospholipids, and bicarbonate to create a pH gradient in the mucous layer between the acidic gastric lumen and the cell surface. Second, the surface cells resist back diffusion of acid by intrinsic mechanisms of cellular integrity. Finally, prostaglandins enhance mucosal protection by increasing mucous secretion, increasing bicarbonate production, maintaining mucosal blood flow, and enhancing the resistance of epithelial cells to injury.

PATHOGENESIS OF PEPTIC ULCER DISEASE

Peptic ulcer disease is the end result of an imbalance between aggressive and defensive factors in the gastroduodenal mucosa. *H. pylori*, NSAIDs, and acid-secretory abnormalities are the major factors that disrupt this equilibrium. Although acid peptic injury is necessary for ulcers to form, acid secretion is normal in almost all patients with gastric ulcers and is increased in approximately one-third of patients with duodenal ulcers. Zollinger-Ellison syndrome accounts for 0.1% of patients who present with peptic ulcer disease. Gastric ulcers tend to occur in areas of non–acid producing cells, such as the antrum, or in areas of atrophic gastritis. A defect in bicarbonate production, and, hence, acid neutralization in the duodenal bulb, also is seen in patients with duodenal ulcer disease. This abnormality resolves with eradication of *H. pylori*, if it is present.

Helicobacter pylori

H. pylori is a gram-negative, curved, flagellated rod found only in gastric epithelium or in gastric metaplastic epithelium. *H. pylori* infection causes chronic active gastritis in all infected patients and used to be found in the overwhelming majority of patients with duodenal and gastric ulcers. Recent data suggest, however, that *H. pylori* infection rates for duodenal ulcer patients in the United States are approximately 73%—far lower than previous estimates of 95%. Furthermore, only a minority of patients infected with *H. pylori*, approximately 15% to 20%, develop peptic ulcer disease. A clear age-related prevalence of *H. pylori* infection is seen in healthy subjects, increasing from 10% in those younger than age 30 years to 60% in subjects older than 60 years in the Western world. The majority are infected early in life, although the mode of transmission remains unknown. *H. pylori* colonization in the United States is more common in minorities, immigrants, and the elderly. The prevalence of *H. pylori* infection in the West is declining and is likely to continue to do so. In contrast, infection is far more common in the developing world, where more than 80% of the population is infected by age 20 years. Infection with *H. pylori* typically is lifelong unless treated.

H. pylori is a noninvasive organism that colonizes the mucous layer overlying gastric epithelium. Factors important in the organism's ability to colonize the stomach include its flagellae, which facilitate locomotion; its ability to adhere to the mucous layer; and its production of urease. Urease increases juxtamucosal pH, which creates a more hospitable microclimate than that of the acidic stomach. Colonization causes acute and chronic inflammation, with the accumulation of neutrophils, plasma cells, T cells, and macrophages accompanied by varying degrees of epithelial cell injury, all of which resolves after treatment.

The ultimate clinical outcome of infection depends on a complex interplay between virulence factors of the organism, the host response, environmental factors, and age at the time of infection. It is now clear that many different strains of *H. pylori* exist, each with different virulence factors. Two such virulence factors are the *vacA* and *cagA* genes, both of which are more common in patients with peptic ulcer disease.

Acute infection results in short-lived acid hyposecretion which then resolves despite the persistence of the organism. Chronic infection increases the basal gastrin, the gastrin response to a meal, basal acid output, and gastrin-stimulated acid output. The regulation of antral G cells may be altered by abnormalities in the ability of adjacent somatostatin-producing D cells to shut down gastrin release. All these abnormalities resolve after eradication of the organism. Gastric ulcers may develop in the setting of intense gastritis associated with infection by certain strains of *H. pylori*. The development of duodenal ulcers is more complex and probably involves enhanced gastric acid secretion caused by the dysregulation of somatostatin and gastrin: Gastrin release is increased, whereas the inhibitory influence of somatostatin is diminished. This results in gastric metaplasia in the duodenum, with subsequent *H. pylori* colonization. Duodenal bicarbonate production is also inhibited by *H. pylori* infection. Atrophic gastritis is another end result of infection that may increase the risk of gastric cancer. Finally, the mucosal lymphocytic response to *H. pylori* infection may lead to a monoclonal B-cell proliferation in mucosa-associated lymphoid tissue (MALT) lymphoma.

Nonsteroidal Anti-Inflammatory Drugs

NSAIDs are among the most widely used classes of drugs in the world. A clear relationship exists between the ingestion of NSAIDs and injury to the gastrointestinal tract. Two types of mucosal injury are caused by NSAIDs. The first form develops after acute ingestion and involves direct topical injury to mucosal cells. The acute ingestion of aspirin enhances mucosal permeability by lowering the mucosal potential difference and enhancing the back diffusion of hydrogen ions. Hyperemia, subepithelial hemorrhage, and superficial erosions are seen endoscopically, although these lesions are typically asymptomatic. Microscopically, a "reactive" pattern of injury is characterized by little or no increase in inflammatory cells. With longer-term NSAID use, these lesions disappear and frank ulceration may develop. Chronic NSAID ingestion inhibits COX, which results in the inhibition of gastroduodenal mucosal prostaglandin synthesis, and, hence, a decrease in mucous and bicarbonate production, mucosal blood flow, epithelial proliferation, and mucosal resistance to injury. Two COX isoenzymes are involved in prostaglandin synthesis. COX-1 is expressed constitutively and is necessary for gastric cytoprotective functions, whereas COX-2 is induced only at sites of tissue inflammation. New NSAIDs that selectively inhibit COX-2 have far less gastrointestinal toxicity.

The use of NSAIDs clearly predisposes patients to ulcers, both duodenal and gastric, as well as to complications of ulcer disease, including hemorrhage, perforation, and obstruction. The risk for gastric ulcers is somewhat greater than that for duodenal ulcers. Endoscopically apparent ulceration occurs in approximately 40% of long-term NSAID users, the majority of whom are asymptomatic. In fact, only approximately 15% of NSAID users have clinical manifestations of ulcer disease, and serious complications are encountered in approximately 2% each year. NSAID-induced ulceration occurs with all nonselective NSAIDs, including low-dose aspirin, although certain compounds, such as salsalate (Disalcid), nabumetone (Relafen), and etodolac (Lodine), may be associated with a decreased risk of ulceration. The administration of COX-2–selective agents, such as celecoxib (Celebrex), results in lower rates of endoscopic ulcers, symptomatic ulcers, and complications such as bleeding, perforation, or obstruction than do conventional nonselective NSAIDs. In fact, the ulcer risk with these agents is no greater than with placebo. Risk factors for NSAID-induced ulceration and complications are shown in Table 54.1. In addition, underlying cardiovascular and cerebrovascular disease may be a risk factor for bleeding peptic ulcer disease as well. Mixed findings have emerged regarding susceptibility to ulcer formation in those taking NSAIDS who are also *H. pylori* positive. A recent meta-analysis has suggested that peptic ulcer disease is significantly more common in NSAID takers who are *H. pylori* positive, thus indicating a possible synergy of both types of damage to the gastroduodenal mucosa.

Helicobacter pylori–*negative Peptic Ulcer Disease*
H. pylori infection is on the decline in the Western world. Because of this decline, the entity of *H. pylori*–negative

TABLE 54.1

RISK FACTORS FOR DEVELOPMENT OF NONSTEROIDAL ANTI-INFLAMMATORY DRUG–INDUCED ULCERS AND COMPLICATIONS

Age >60 yr
Prior peptic ulcer disease or ulcer bleed
High dosage or use of more than one NSAID
Concurrent use of an NSAID and corticosteroids
Concurrent use of a NSAID and anticoagulants
Serious systemic disorder

NSAID, nonsteroidal anti-inflammatory drug.

peptic ulcer disease is becoming more common. In patients with peptic ulcer disease and negative test results for *H. pylori* infection, a number of different diagnoses must be considered (Table 54.2). Many of these patients are acetylsalicylic acid (ASA) or NSAID users who often use over-the-counter medications. Some have a false-negative test result for *H. pylori* because of concurrent PPI use. Others may have Zollinger-Ellison syndrome. In rare cases, Crohn disease may present as gastroduodenal ulceration. This can be diagnosed by the finding of granulomas on biopsy or evidence of Crohn disease in the small bowel.

If all the previously mentioned entities are excluded, then individuals are said to have idiopathic peptic ulcer disease. This entity is characterized by elevated serum gastrin levels, increased gastric acid output, and abnormally rapid gastroduodenal emptying. The treatment of this entity may be more difficult than the treatment of routine peptic ulcer disease.

CLINICAL PRESENTATION

Dyspepsia, the classic symptom of peptic ulcer disease, is defined as a pain centered in the upper abdomen or

TABLE 54.2

ETIOLOGY OF PEPTIC ULCER DISEASE

Helicobacter pylori positive
H. pylori negative
False-negative *H. pylori* test result
Serologic testing in low-prevalence region
Recent use of antibiotics or bismuth
Concurrent use of PPIs with urea breath test or urease test
Atrophic gastritis
NSAID use
Zollinger-Ellison syndrome
Crohn disease
Idiopathic peptic ulcer disease

NSAID, nonsteroidal anti-inflammatory drug; PPIs, proton pump inhibitors.

TABLE 54.3

DIFFERENTIAL DIAGNOSIS OF DYSPEPSIA

Condition	Frequency (%)
Peptic ulcer disease	15–25
GERD	5–15
Functional dyspepsia	60
Gastric cancer	<2

GERD, gastroesophageal reflux disease.

TABLE 54.4

DIAGNOSTIC APPROACHES FOR PATIENTS WITH DYSPEPSIA

Immediate endoscopy *mandatory*
    Alarm signs
    Weight loss
    Anorexia
    Nausea or vomiting
    Evidence of bleeding (anemia, melena)
    Age >45–50 yr with new-onset dyspepsia
    Gastric ulcer or lesion suspicious for cancer on barium
      radiographs
Immediate endoscopy *optional*
    Young patients
    Short duration of symptoms
    Absence of alarm signs
    NSAID use
    Noninvasive *Helicobacter pylori* testing in patients without
      alarm signs
    Positive test results, antimicrobial treatment
    Negative test results, antisecretory treatment

NSAID, nonsteroidal anti-inflammatory drug.

discomfort characterized by fullness, bloating, distention, or nausea. Symptoms may be chronic, recurrent, or of new onset. Dyspepsia is a common clinical problem that may be seen in 25% to 40% of adults. Only 15% to 25% of patients with dyspepsia are found to have a gastric or duodenal ulcer. Up to 60% of patients have no definite diagnosis and are classified as having functional dyspepsia, a condition most likely related to an abnormal perception of events in the stomach caused by afferent visceral hypersensitivity. Other causes of dyspepsia include gastroesophageal reflux disease (GERD) and gastric cancer (Table 54.3). Ulcers may also be asymptomatic, especially in patients ingesting NSAIDs. Patients may present with complications of ulcer disease; hemorrhage may develop in 20%, perforation in 5%, and gastric outlet obstruction in 2%.

DIAGNOSIS OF DYSPEPSIA

General Approaches

Several possible diagnostic approaches are possible in the patient with dyspepsia: (a) instituting a short trial of empiric antisecretory therapy, (b) performing immediate endoscopy, and (c) conducting noninvasive testing for *H. pylori* infection followed by antibiotic treatment of patients with positive test results.

Immediate endoscopic evaluation without a trial of empiric therapy is indicated for individuals with obvious systemic symptoms, such as weight loss, bleeding, nausea, and vomiting, as well as for individuals older than 45 to 50 years with new-onset dyspepsia in whom gastric neoplasia is a consideration (Table 54.4). If a gastric ulcer is found at endoscopy, multiple biopsies and brush cytologic examination are required to exclude a malignancy. Endoscopy is also indicated in patients who fail to respond to empiric therapy. Barium radiography has no role in the evaluation of dyspepsia due to its poor sensitivity and specificity.

Initial noninvasive testing for *H. pylori* followed by antimicrobial therapy in patients with positive test results is a reasonable approach for patients under the age of 45 years with uncomplicated dyspepsia. The rationale for this is that ulcer disease (if present) will heal, and future ulcer diathesis is eliminated. A decision to empirically treat patients with

dyspepsia with antibiotics for presumed *H. pylori* infection without proof of infection is not supported by any model to date, however, and should never be done. The indiscriminate use of antimicrobial therapy also may be associated with illnesses related to alteration of normal human flora; increased resistance of *H. pylori* and other bacteria that are not a target of therapy; and a host of adverse effects, such as *Clostridium difficile* colitis.

Empiric antisecretory therapy with omeprazole is more effective than placebo for the treatment of symptoms of nonulcer dyspepsia, despite an appreciable response to placebo. As the risk of *H. pylori*–induced ulcer disease declines, and because most cases of dyspepsia are not ulcer-related, the test-and-treat approach for *H. pylori* infection likely will become less successful. As the proportion of *H. pylori*–negative ulcers rises, a modest cost advantage may be seen in the use of empiric antisecretory therapy over the test-and-treat approach for *H. pylori* in patients with uninvestigated dyspepsia. Recent data have emerged suggesting that PPIs may predispose to adverse effects such as *C. difficile* colitis, aspiration pneumonia, and hip fractures in certain populations; thus, the benefits of empiric antisecretory treatment must be balanced against the risk in dyspeptic patients.

Diagnostic Tests for *Helicobacter pylori*

H. pylori testing is essential in patients with peptic ulcer disease. A negative test result will focus the subsequent diagnostic evaluation on other causes of peptic ulcer disease, such as NSAID consumption or gastrinoma. An initial negative test result in patients with newly diagnosed peptic ulcer disease should be confirmed by a second test, however,

TABLE 54.5

DIAGNOSTIC TESTS FOR *HELICOBACTER PYLORI*

Nonendoscopic
    Antibody tests (no longer recommended)
        Qualitative (serum or whole blood)
        Quantitative (ELISA)
    Urease tests
        Carbon 13 urea breath test
        Carbon 14 urea breath test
        Carbon 13 urea blood test
    Fecal antigen test
Endoscopic
    Rapid urease test
    Histologic examination
    Culture

ELISA, enzyme-linked immunosorbent assay.

given the importance of diagnosing *H. pylori* infection. Furthermore, a negative test result precludes the use of antimicrobial therapy. Diagnostic tests for the detection of *H. pylori* infection are subdivided into nonendoscopic and endoscopic techniques (Table 54.5). The decline in the prevalence of *H. pylori* in the Western world has resulted in a paradigm shift in testing strategies for *H. pylori* infection. Enzyme-linked immunosorbent assay (ELISA) serologic tests, formerly the cornerstone of *H. pylori* testing, are no longer recommended because of the poor performance characteristics of these tests: sensitivity of 85% and specificity of 79%. The sensitivity (71%) and specificity (88%) of office-based blood and serologic testing is also suboptimal, which makes these tests contraindicated as well. Furthermore, serologic test results may remain positive for up to 3 years after bacterial eradication, which limits the role of such testing in the documentation of eradication. Currently, the only role for serologic testing is in populations with a high background prevalence (>60%).

In the breath test using urea labeled with carbon 13 or carbon 14, *H. pylori* urease splits off labeled carbon dioxide, which may be detected in the breath of the patient. The urea breath tests are more accurate than serologic tests and are now the noninvasive test of choice for diagnosing *H. pylori* infection and documenting successful *H. pylori* eradication after antibiotic therapy. Patients should not receive PPIs for at least 14 days before the administration of breath tests in order to avoid false-negative results.

The stool antigen test is a noninvasive, inexpensive alternative to the urea breath test. In this test, an enzymatic immunoassay detects the presence of *H. pylori* in stool specimens. This technique has excellent sensitivity (93%) and specificity (94%) for the initial diagnosis of *H. pylori* infection. The sensitivity of the test is decreased by the recent use of antibiotics, bismuth, or PPIs. Stool antigen testing can be performed 7 days after the completion of treatment to identify those patients in whom the eradication of *H. pylori* is unsuccessful. Stool antigen testing 7 or more days after the completion of eradication therapy has identified patients with persistent infection in about 95% of cases. A negative stool test 7 days after treatment correctly has identified clearance in 90% of cases. The advantages include the ability for prompt testing after treatment and earlier retreatment for *H. pylori* positivity, especially in those who are at risk for ulcer rebleeding.

If endoscopy is performed, the diagnosis is made by the rapid urease test or histologic examination. In the rapid urease test, mucosal biopsies are directly inoculated into a urea-containing medium with a pH-sensitive indicator that changes color when ammonia is metabolized from urea by the urease of the organism. Recent treatment with antibiotics or PPIs decreases the yield of both these biopsy tests.

Posttreatment testing is mandatory in patients with complicated peptic ulcer disease (i.e., bleeding, perforation, or obstruction), MALT lymphoma, or after resection of early gastric cancer. It also should be performed in all patients with newly diagnosed ulcer disease and in patients concerned about persistent infection. (Because antibiotic treatment suppresses the organism even if it is not eradicated, testing to confirm cure should only be done 4 weeks after the completion of therapy, with the exception of fecal antigen testing.)

TREATMENT OF PEPTIC ULCER DISEASE

Initial Treatment

A number of treatment options are available for the healing of peptic ulcers. Antacids are highly effective agents for healing ulcers and controlling symptoms. From a practical perspective, however, the inconvenient dosing frequency and adverse effects of therapy limit the use of antacids to symptom control only. Antacids neutralize acid that is already secreted. This increases intragastric pH, which also inactivates pepsin. The greatest buffering capacity is achieved when antacids are given 1 hour after eating.

Histamine H_2-receptor antagonists currently have a limited role in the treatment of ulcer disease with the more widespread use of the PPIs. Acid secretion is decreased by the competitive and selective inhibition of the histamine H_2-receptor of the parietal cell. Four different histamine H_2-receptor antagonists are available: cimetidine, ranitidine, famotidine, and nizatidine. All these compounds act by the same mechanism, but all have different relative potencies for inhibiting gastric acid secretion. As a consequence of gastric acid secretion inhibition, gastric pH rises and pepsin activity decreases. This class of drugs is uniformly safe and well tolerated, although the risk of adverse effects is slightly increased with cimetidine because it binds to cytochrome P450 and hence drug interactions are increased. Histamine H_2-receptor antagonists heal 90% to 95% of duodenal ulcers and 88% of gastric ulcers in 8 weeks.

TABLE 54.6

ANTISECRETORY THERAPY FOR PEPTIC ULCER DISEASE

Agent	Duodenal Ulcer		Gastric Ulcer	
	Dose (Milligrams)	Duration (Weeks)	Dose (Milligrams)	Duration (Weeks)
PPI				
Omeprazole	20	4	40	8
Lansoprazole	15	4	30	8
Rabeprazole	20	4	20	8
Pantoprazole	40	4	40	8
Esomeprazole	20	4	40	8

PPI, proton pump inhibitor.

PPIs bind irreversibly to the H^+/K^+-adenosine triphosphatase enzyme of the gastric parietal cell. This blocks the final step of gastric acid secretion in response to any type of stimulation and results in the long-lasting inhibition of gastric acid secretion. For gastric secretory activity to be restored, new enzyme must be resynthesized, which normally takes 2 to 5 days. The PPIs are all remarkably well tolerated. Adverse effects are uncommon and are typically no more common than those experienced with placebo. PPIs achieve duodenal ulcer healing rates at 4 weeks (90%–100%) that typically are seen at 8 weeks with H_2-receptor antagonists. In addition to accelerating duodenal ulcer healing, PPIs typically relieve symptoms more rapidly than histamine H_2-receptor antagonists. In contrast to the dramatic acceleration of duodenal ulcer healing using PPIs, gastric ulcer healing is essentially comparable to that achieved with histamine H_2-receptor antagonists at 8 weeks. The dosing and duration of therapy of the PPIs for peptic ulcer disease is shown in Table 54.6.

Sucralfate is a complex salt of sucrose sulfate and aluminum hydroxide that is as effective as H_2-receptor antagonists in the treatment of duodenal ulcer disease. The evidence for efficacy in gastric ulcer disease is less compelling. With the widespread availability of PPIs for treating peptic ulcer disease, however, this drug rarely is used.

Treatment of *Helicobacter pylori* Infection

The eradication of *H. pylori* accelerates the rate of duodenal and gastric ulcer healing to a point at which it approximates the rate obtained with omeprazole at 4 weeks. The eradication of *H. pylori* essentially cures both duodenal and gastric ulcers and should be attempted in all patients with current or past documented peptic ulcer disease and evidence of infection.

The treatment of *H. pylori* infection is confusing, requires multiple drugs, and remains suboptimal. Despite the in vitro sensitivity of the organism to a variety of antibiotics, the in vivo activity of these same drugs against *H. pylori* is disappointing. For this reason, eradication of the organism

is difficult. Combinations of two antibiotics plus a PPI are used to maximize the chance of eradication. The reported efficacy of these regimens has been approximately 90%. More recent data suggest that the efficacy of these regimens is as low as 70% to 85%, in part due to drug resistance. In over 30 trials involving over 3,900 patients, it has been shown that eradication therapy is superior to ulcer-healing drugs when treating duodenal ulcers in patients who are *H. pylori* positive. No significant differences between the two different treatment regimens were identified in *H. pylori*–positive gastric ulcer patients. Current treatment regimens for *H. pylori* infection are shown in Table 54.7. A reasonable approach is to use either a metronidazole- or clarithromycin-based triple-drug regimen as first-line therapy. Should that fail, then second-line therapy uses the antimicrobial not used or bismuth quadruple therapy.

Factors such as duration of therapy, compliance, and antibiotic resistance, especially to metronidazole and clarithromycin, influence treatment efficacy. Compliance is essential for treatment success. A recent meta-analysis has shown that 1-week and 2-week triple-drug regimens for

TABLE 54.7

PREFERRED THERAPIES FOR *HELICOBACTER PYLORI* INFECTION

Twice-daily PPI[a]
    PPI plus two of the following three agents:
        Amoxicillin, 1 g
        Clarithromycin, 500 mg
        Metronidazole, 500 mg
Quadruple therapy
    PPI twice daily
    Tetracycline, 500 mg QID
    Metronidazole, 500 mg TID
    Bismuth subsalicylate or subcitrate QID

PPI, proton pump inhibitor.
[a]Esomeprazole may be given as 40 mg once daily with any regimen.
Modified from Graham DY. Therapy of *Helicobacter pylori*: current status and issues. *Gastroenterology* 2000;118:S2–S8.

H. pylori eradication are similar in terms of efficacy, safety, and patient compliance. Accordingly, the recent international tendency toward 7- to 10-day regimens over 14-day regimens may improve costs and compliance with therapy, at the expense of minimal reduction in efficacy. In the United States, resistance to metronidazole occurs in approximately 35% of cases and to clarithromycin in 11%. The problem of antibiotic resistance is increasing and in the future may require antimicrobial sensitivity testing before therapy. Given the resistance problems with both metronidazole and clarithromycin, it is recommended that use of these two agents together in the initial treatment of *H. pylori* infection should be avoided. Quinolones have been increasingly used in triple-drug regimens when resistance to traditional agents is a factor. Bismuth quadruple therapy for a 7- to 14-day regimen is another first-line treatment option; however, recent data suggest that a regimen of a PPI, levofloxacin, and amoxicillin is more effective and better tolerated than bismuth quadruple therapy.

Helicobacter pylori and Functional Dyspepsia: Treatment Implications

The role of *H. pylori* in functional dyspepsia has been the subject of intense study. Trials assessing the treatment of *H. pylori* infection in patients with functional dyspepsia indicate that 20% to 25% of these patients experience symptom resolution with effective antibiotic therapy. A recent meta-analysis of randomized, controlled trials of therapy for *H. pylori* in these patients, however, has provided little, if any, support for the use of *H. pylori* eradication therapy in patients with functional dyspepsia. This disorder more likely relates to an abnormal perception of events in the gut resulting from abnormal visceral afferent hypersensitivity.

Interactions Between Nonsteroidal Anti-Inflammatory Drugs and *Helicobacter pylori*: Treatment Implications

The frequency of *H. pylori* infection and NSAID ingestion both increase with age. Some data suggest that *H. pylori* increases, has no effect on, and decreases the risk of bleeding in patients taking NSAIDs, including aspirin. In a landmark study by Chan et al., patients with a history of peptic ulcer disease bleeding who were infected with *H. pylori* and taking aspirin or other NSAIDs were randomly assigned to receive *H. pylori* eradication therapy or treatment with omeprazole 20 mg daily for 6 months. The investigators found that among patients taking low-dose aspirin for cardiac prophylaxis, eradication therapy was equivalent to omeprazole treatment for the prevention of recurrent bleeding, whereas omeprazole therapy was superior to eradication therapy among patients taking other NSAIDs. Therefore, patients with a prior history of peptic ulcer disease or its complications should be tested for *H. pylori* and treated, if necessary, before NSAID therapy is commenced.

TABLE 54.8
STRATEGY FOR PROPHYLAXIS OF NONSTEROIDAL ANTI-INFLAMMATORY DRUG–INDUCED ULCERS

Discontinue NSAIDs
If NSAIDs are necessary, use lowest dose possible
Consider prophylactic therapy for populations at risk:
    Age >60 yr
    Prior peptic ulcer disease
    Prior peptic ulcer bleeding
    Concurrent use of corticosteroids
    Concurrent use of anticoagulants
    High NSAID dosage or use of multiple NSAIDs
If prophylaxis is indicated:
    Omeprazole, 20 mg QD
    Misoprostol, 200 μg TID to QID
    Famotidine, 40 mg BID

NSAIDs, nonsteroidal anti-inflammatory drugs.

Treatment and Prophylaxis of Ulceration Induced by Nonsteroidal Anti-Inflammatory Drugs

For patients who develop ulcers while ingesting NSAIDs, therapy should be stopped, if possible, and the patient placed on conventional doses of H_2-receptor antagonists or PPIs. *H. pylori* infection should be sought and treated if present. For patients who need continued NSAID therapy, the dosage should be reduced as much as possible. Small ulcers ($\leq$5 mm) in the stomach or duodenum will heal with coadministration of histamine H_2-receptor antagonists, whereas larger ulcers require the coadministration of a PPI for healing (Table 54.8).

Given the fact that prophylactic medications are expensive and NSAID use is common, ulcer prophylaxis should be considered only in high-risk individuals. These include (a) those older than 60 years, (b) those with a prior history of peptic ulcer disease or ulcer bleed, (c) those concurrently taking anticoagulants or corticosteroids, and (d) those taking high dosages of NSAIDs. It is important to remember that even low-dose aspirin used for cardiac prophylaxis is a risk factor for bleeding from peptic ulcer disease. There are two options for ulcer prevention: (a) the coadministration of agents that protect the gastroduodenal mucosa or (b) the use of COX-2–selective agents.

Misoprostol is a prostaglandin E1 analog that is effective for the prophylaxis of NSAID-induced ulcers in patients. It decreases the incidence of serious gastrointestinal complications such as bleeding, perforation, and gastric outlet obstruction. It acts by prostaglandin-dependent pathways to decrease gastric acid secretion and enhance mucosal defenses. However, adverse effects with misoprostol are common—especially diarrhea and abdominal cramps—which limit its use. A fixed combination of the NSAID diclofenac sodium and misoprostol (Arthrotec) is also available. Use of this compound results in lower rates of ulcer formation than with placebo.

Several studies suggest that PPIs at standard doses are more effective than either histamine H_2-receptor antagonists or misoprostol for the prevention of NSAID-induced ulcers. Furthermore, PPIs are typically better tolerated than misoprostol. High-dose famotidine 40 mg two times a day is more effective than placebo in preventing both duodenal and gastric ulcers in patients receiving long-term NSAID therapy. Yet, the cost of such a regimen is considerably higher than that of once-a-day omeprazole. The conventional dosages of famotidine and the other histamine H_2-receptor antagonists are effective only for the prophylaxis of duodenal ulcers, not for the prophylaxis of gastric ulcers.

The use of COX-2 agents is a reasonable treatment strategy to consider for high-risk patients instead of coadministration of a PPI or misoprostol. Celecoxib is as effective as diclofenac plus omeprazole in preventing recurrent bleeding in *H. pylori*–negative rheumatoid and osteoarthritis patients who initially have presented with ulcer bleeding while taking NSAIDs. However, low-risk patients may do just as well using nonselective NSAIDs without prophylaxis.

HELICOBACTER PYLORI AND GASTRIC NEOPLASIA

Infection with *H. pylori* is an important risk factor for the development of distal gastric cancer, which is the second leading cause of death from cancer worldwide. Some 40% to 60% of tumors of the gastric body or antrum are associated with *H. pylori* infection. The incidence of gastric cancer in the United States is decreasing, however, and it is estimated that only 1% of infected Americans ever develop cancer. Mass screening for *H. pylori* in middle-aged U.S. adults is not indicated at present.

H. pylori infection also is associated with gastric MALT lymphoma, which is a low-grade, B-cell subtype of non-Hodgkin lymphoma of the stomach. Clinical presentation is nonspecific and is related to the size and location of the tumor(s) in the stomach. Diagnosis is based on the characteristic histologic appearance of destructive lymphoepithelial lesions. Endoscopic ultrasonography is useful in predicting a response to therapy; an excellent response is seen if the tumor is limited to the mucosa or submucosa. The eradication of *H. pylori* may cure up to 70% of individuals with MALT-type lymphoma, especially those with superficial disease.

Maintenance Therapy

Maintenance therapy for ulcer disease with a long-term low dose (i.e., half strength) of any H_2-blocker is an obsolete concept. Before the role of *H. pylori* in peptic ulcer disease was determined, the ulcer relapse rate was reduced to between 10% and 30% at 1 year using this strategy. Today, maintenance therapy is indicated only for a small subset of patients with chronic peptic ulcer disease. Patients

with *H. pylori*–positive peptic ulcer disease should be placed on maintenance therapy if eradication is unsuccessful. Patients with *H. pylori*–negative peptic ulcer disease should be placed on maintenance therapy if they have three or more relapses each year or a history of ulcer complications, such as bleeding or perforation, and multiple other medical problems.

COMPLICATIONS OF PEPTIC ULCER DISEASE

Bleeding Peptic Ulcers

Of those patients with peptic ulcer disease, 15% to 20% develop bleeding, and bleeding ulcer is the most common cause of upper gastrointestinal bleeding. Although bleeding ceases spontaneously in 80% of cases, the mortality of bleeding ulcers is approximately 10%. The major risk factor for bleeding ulcers is consumption of NSAIDs. Patients with bleeding ulcers present with hematemesis, melena, or hematochezia, often without antecedent pain. Clinical predictors for an adverse outcome are shown in Table 54.9.

All patients with upper gastrointestinal bleeding should undergo early upper endoscopy, which allows for both therapeutic intervention and determination of the presence of predictors for rebleeding. Rebleeding rates without endoscopic treatment are approximately 3% for clean-based ulcers, 7% for ulcers with flat spots, 12% to 33% for adherent clots, 50% for nonbleeding visible vessels, and 90% for active arterial spurting from an ulcer. Patients with large ulcers > 1 to 2 cm also have higher rebleeding rates and mortality. Endoscopic therapy using techniques such as bipolar or thermal coagulation combined with the injection with epinephrine decreases subsequent rebleeding and clearly improves the outcome in patients with bleeding ulcers by also decreasing mortality, length of hospital stay, number of blood transfusions required, and the need for emergency surgery. Because most rebleeding occurs within 3 days of initial presentation, patients with active bleeding or stigmata of hemorrhage, such as pigmented spots in an ulcer crater or clot, can typically be discharged within 3 days if they are stable (Table 54.10). Given the excellent prognosis

---

TABLE 54.9

CLINICAL PREDICTORS OF AN ADVERSE OUTCOME IN BLEEDING PEPTIC ULCERS

Hemodynamic instability at presentation
Hematemesis
Hematochezia
Age >60 yr
Ongoing transfusion requirements >6 U for a single bleed
Severe comorbid medical or surgical illnesses
Inpatient hemorrhage
Rebleeding from same lesion while hospitalized

Adapted from Jensen DM. Endoscopic diagnosis and treatment of bleeding peptic ulcers. *Clin Perspect Gastroenterol* 1999;2(2):73–84.

TABLE 54.10

IMPLICATIONS OF STIGMATA OF RECENT HEMORRHAGE ON TREATMENT OF BLEEDING PEPTIC ULCERS

Endoscopic Finding	Endoscopic Therapy	Management
Clean base	No	Regular diet Discharge within 24 hr
Flat spot	No	Regular diet Discharge within 24 hr
Oozing without stigmata	Yes	PPI intravenously, then orally[a] Regular diet Observation for 24–48 hr after treatment
Adherent clot	Yes	PPI intravenously, then orally[a] Regular diet Observation for 48 hr after treatment
Visible vessel	Yes	PPI intravenously, then orally[a] Regular diet Observation for 48 hr after treatment
Active arterial bleeding	Yes	PPI intravenously, then orally[a] Liquid diet Observation for 72 hr after treatment

PPI, proton pump inhibitor.
[a]Intravenous PPI should be the equivalent of omeprazole, 80-mg bolus, followed by continuous infusion of 8 mg/hr. Oral PPI therapy should be the equivalent of omeprazole, 40 mg BID for 3 days, followed by standard-dose PPI or H2-receptor antagonist therapy for ulcer healing.
Adapted from Jensen DM. Endoscopic diagnosis and treatment of bleeding peptic ulcers. *Clin Perspect Gastroenterol* 1999;2(2):73–84.

for patients with clean-based ulcers, discharge within 24 hours of presentation also is reasonable.

Acid-suppression therapy using PPIs decreases rebleeding after the endoscopic treatment of bleeding peptic ulcers. The rationale for aggressive acid suppression is multifactorial: (a) blood clots are unstable at a low pH, and (b) pepsin, which requires a pH <4, can lyse blood clots. At a pH level of 6, platelet aggregation and pepsin inactivation are optimized. In a landmark study, Lau et al. found that intravenous omeprazole (80 mg bolus followed by 8 mg per hour) given for 72 hours was more effective than placebo administration in decreasing rebleeding after endoscopic therapy in patients with actively bleeding ulcers or nonbleeding visible vessels. Both parenteral omeprazole and pantoprazole are now available in the United States. Recent studies suggest that infusion of high-dose omeprazole before endoscopy has accelerated the resolution of signs of bleeding in ulcers and has reduced the need for endoscopic therapy. This method for treating bleeding ulcers also has been shown to be cost-effective when compared with placebo. Previous studies of high-dose oral omeprazole (40 mg two times a day) have shown similar benefit. The standard of care for patients with bleeding peptic ulcers has become treatment with high-dose PPI therapy (the equivalent of omeprazole 40 mg two times a day) as soon as oral medications are permitted or with parenteral PPI therapy for 3 days, followed by conventional-dose PPI therapy for ulcer healing.

Approximately 20% of patients rebleed after initial endoscopic therapy, especially if ulcers are large and deep.

Endoscopic retreatment is effective in approximately 75% of patients; it clearly reduces the need for surgery without increasing the risk of death in these patients and should be offered before alternative modalities are considered. Those in whom retreatment is unsuccessful are candidates for surgical intervention. Alternatively, if they are deemed too high a surgical risk, they may be candidates for angiographic treatment using either intra-arterial vasopressin or embolization techniques.

Patients with bleeding peptic ulcers who are infected with *H. pylori* have a marked decrease in rebleeding after *H. pylori* eradication, whereas failure to cure the infection results in a rebleeding rate of approximately 33% at 1 year. Therefore, all patients with bleeding peptic ulcers should have their *H. pylori* status determined. Eradication therapy should be provided to infected patients and confirmation of eradication performed. Failure to cure *H. pylori* infection mandates long-term, even indefinite, maintenance therapy with antisecretory therapy.

Treatment of Nonhealing Ulcers

Approximately 10% of ulcers fail to heal after standard acid-suppression therapy (i.e., 8 weeks of histamine H_2-receptor antagonists or 4 weeks of PPIs for duodenal ulcers; 12 weeks of H_2-receptor antagonists or 8 weeks of PPIs for gastric ulcers). Persistence of symptoms and macroscopically apparent ulceration are not necessarily correlated.

Factors to be considered when ulcers fail to heal are noncompliance, cigarette smoking, NSAID ingestion, acid hypersecretion, Zollinger-Ellison syndrome, idiopathic acid hypersecretion, cancer (gastric ulcers), and *H. pylori* infection. Each of these issues should be addressed before additional therapy is instituted. Infection with *H. pylori* and the surreptitious use of NSAIDs have emerged as the two leading causes of refractory peptic ulcers. A determination of salicylate levels and platelet aggregation studies may be useful in these patients.

Omeprazole at a dose of 40 mg or other PPIs administered at comparable doses heal almost all peptic ulcer disease refractory to conventional dosages of therapy. The eradication of *H. pylori*, if present, should be attempted in these patients.

Gastric Outlet Obstruction

Gastric outlet obstruction typically is due to either pyloric channel or duodenal ulceration and may be seen in the setting of acute ulceration in which edema, spasm, or inflammation causes gastric outlet obstruction or as a sequela of chronic ulceration with scarring and fibrosis. Patients present with symptoms of early satiety, bloating, nausea, vomiting, and weight loss. Endoscopy is the diagnostic test of choice for gastric outlet obstruction; it should be performed only after adequate gastric decompression and lavage of retained gastric contents. Malignancy accounts for approximately 50% of cases of gastric outlet obstruction and should be excluded with adequate biopsy and cytology samples. Malignancy should be suspected especially in patients older than 55 years with no history of peptic ulcer disease. The treatment of gastric outlet obstruction is aimed at correcting any underlying electrolyte abnormalities resulting from persistent vomiting in conjunction with nasogastric decompression for 3 to 5 days. During that time, a histamine H_2-receptor antagonist or PPI should be administered parenterally as well. Adequacy of response may be assessed empirically with a trial of refeeding. In those patients who respond, the underlying cause of ulcer disease (*H. pylori* infection, NSAID use, or both) should be treated appropriately in conjunction with continued antisecretory therapy. For patients who fail to respond, treatment options include endoscopic balloon dilation or surgery.

Perforation

Peptic ulcer perforation occurs when an ulcer penetrates the full thickness of the stomach or duodenum. This then leads to peritonitis, which if untreated results in sepsis and death. Perforation can occur with either duodenal or gastric ulcers but is a far less common complication than bleeding. Patients present with the sudden onset of severe abdominal pain beginning in the epigastrium and radiating throughout the entire abdomen. Physical examination demonstrates peritoneal findings, including abdominal pain, rebound tenderness, and boardlike rigidity. The clinical suspicion of perforation may be confirmed in most but not all cases by demonstrating pneumoperitoneum with either an upright chest radiograph or upright and supine abdominal radiographs. In less clear-cut cases, computed tomography (CT) or an upper gastrointestinal study using water-soluble contrast may be helpful. Perforation requires surgical intervention. A perforated duodenal ulcer typically is repaired with an omental patch, whereas a perforated gastric ulcer requires either an omental patch or resection.

SURGICAL MANAGEMENT OF PEPTIC ULCER DISEASE

Surgery for peptic ulcer disease has become unusual as an elective procedure but is the mainstay of management for life-threatening or serious complications of ulcer disease not adequately controlled by medical therapy. While previously relied on for recurrent or refractory ulcer disease despite medical therapy, better understanding and management of *H. pylori* has further diminished the role of surgery in these patients. Still, the importance of the availability of experienced surgeons to offer surgical options to those who suffer complications such as nonhealing ulcers, bleeding not amenable or refractory to endoscopic management, perforation, or obstruction should not be underestimated. Exclusion of malignancy remains as an indication for elective surgery in nonhealing ulcers, particularly in those older than 45 to 50 years of age with presumed idiopathic ulceration.

The choice of surgery varies by indication and surgeon preference, but unlike medical management, which has focused less on antisecretory therapies in the last decade, surgical approaches still focus on acid suppression by sectioning the vagus nerve or by partial gastrectomy. Three different types of vagotomy are performed: truncal, selective, and highly selective. This affects gastric motility adversely, and some form of gastric emptying procedure, either pyloroplasty or gastroenterostomy, must be performed. Postoperative complications occur in as many as 20% to 30% of patients and are more commonly related to vagotomy than resection. These can include dumping, postvagotomy diarrhea, anemia, malabsorption, and alkaline reflux gastritis. Most individuals will adapt to these disturbances in digestive function, but 5% may suffer lifetime sequelae and 1% may be permanently debilitated. There is a twofold increase in the risk of adenocarcinoma at the anastomosis or of the gastric remnant 20 years after partial gastrectomy.

Zollinger-Ellison Syndrome

Zollinger-Ellison syndrome is characterized by a marked hypersecretion of acid due to high circulating levels of gastrin caused by the presence of a gastrin-secreting tumor. It accounts for <1% of cases of peptic ulcer disease.

Zollinger-Ellison syndrome should be suspected in patients with recurrent peptic ulcer disease in the absence of *H. pylori* infection or NSAID consumption. Up to 50% of patients may have diarrhea, whereas others also may have symptoms of gastroesophageal reflux and its complications. The diagnosis of Zollinger-Ellison syndrome is made when a high fasting gastrin concentration >1,000 pg/mL is present in the setting of gastric acid hypersecretion (>15 mEq per hour if no gastric surgery and >5 mEq per hour if prior gastric surgery). However, gastrinomas are a relatively uncommon cause of hypergastrinemia. The most common causes of hypergastrinemia are *H. pylori* infection and hypochlorhydria related either to decreased intraluminal acid in the setting of atrophic gastritis or to antisecretory therapy. Other causes of hypergastrinemia include retained gastric antrum (after ulcer surgery), idiopathic G-cell hyperfunction, chronic gastric outlet obstruction, and chronic renal failure. Therefore, acid hypersecretion, as documented by gastric acid analysis, is necessary for the diagnosis of Zollinger-Ellison syndrome.

Surgical therapy is the preferred management of sporadic Zollinger-Ellison syndrome. The tumors are often found in the "gastrinoma triangle" demarcated by the common bile duct, the junction of the second and third portions of the duodenum, and the body of the pancreas, but these tumors also have been found in the heart, bile duct, liver, ovary, kidney, and mesentery. PPIs are the agents of choice to control acid secretion in these patients. Omeprazole or lansoprazole should be commenced at an initial dosage of 60 mg daily, and the dosage should then be titrated to a basal acid output <10 mEq per hour at 24 hours after the last dose of the drug. If >120 mg of a PPI is required, then the dose should be split to twice-daily administration. Long-term therapy with PPIs uniformly results in the continued inhibition of acid secretion, good symptom control, complete healing of any mucosal lesions, and lack of adverse effects. The treatment of Zollinger-Ellison syndrome using PPIs does not result in further elevation of gastrin levels.

STRESS-RELATED MUCOSAL DAMAGE

Stress-related mucosal damage develops in most critically ill patients, and overt upper gastrointestinal bleeding may occur in as many as 15% of untreated patients. Stress-related mucosal injury is caused by mucosal ischemia, which impairs mucosal resistance to acid back-diffusion and the presence of acid. Hyperemia of the mucosa evolves into erosions and then to frank ulceration in the stomach and duodenum. Critical illnesses associated with a risk of stress-related mucosal injury include:

- Burns
- Trauma
- Central nervous system injury
- Prolonged hypotension
- Sepsis
- Respiratory failure
- Hepatic failure
- Multiorgan failure

The mortality rate of patients who progress to bleeding is increased; however, the incidence of major bleeding in critically ill patients has decreased recently. The reason for this is uncertain and cannot necessarily be attributed to the widespread use of prophylactic therapy.

Several prophylactic treatment strategies are effective in preventing upper gastrointestinal bleeding in critically ill patients. Meta-analysis suggests that prophylaxis using antiulcer regimens reduces overt and clinically important gastrointestinal bleeding in critically ill patients. The administration of antacids every 2 hours neutralizes gastric acid but has the disadvantages of inconvenience and increased nursing time and produces diarrhea. The use of sucralfate requires the placement of a nasogastric tube, and a dosage of 1 g every 4 hours was once thought to decrease the risk of late-onset nosocomial pneumonia. Recent data, however, suggest that no difference exists in the rate of ventilator-associated pneumonia with this agent and with H_2-receptor antagonists. H_2-receptor antagonists, given either as a continuous infusion or by bolus injection every 12 hours (in the case of more potent agents such as famotidine), are safe and convenient and should be titrated to produce an intragastric pH >4 to minimize the activity of pepsin. Studies suggest that the administration of H_2-receptor antagonists results in a significantly lower rate of clinically important bleeding than the administration of sucralfate. The role of parenteral PPI use in this setting is currently an active area of study.

Should all patients in the intensive care unit (ICU) receive prophylaxis, especially in this era of cost constraints? The answer is no. A large multicenter Canadian study involving 2,252 medical and surgical ICU patients identified coagulopathy and respiratory failure requiring mechanical ventilation for 48 hours or longer as the only risk factors for clinically significant bleeding in the ICU. Only 1.5% of all patients had clinically significant bleeding in this large study. Therefore, patients with coagulopathy or mechanical ventilation should continue to receive prophylaxis. Other patients who should receive targeted prophylaxis include those with central nervous system trauma, burns, organ transplantation, or a history of peptic ulcer disease with or without bleeding. Admission to the ICU does not automatically warrant prophylaxis for stress gastropathy.

REVIEW EXERCISES

QUESTIONS

1. A 65-year-old woman presents to the office with a complaint of a gnawing epigastric pain. She denies bleeding but has a hemoglobin of 10.9. Her most significant risk factor for ulcer disease is

a) Use of a nonselective NSAID

b) Age

c) Presence of *H. pylori* infection

d) Use of a COX-2 inhibitor

e) Cardiac prophylactic-dose aspirin

Answer and Discussion

The answer is c. *H. pylori* is the most common cause for ulcer disease—especially duodenal ulcer (70%–75%). NSAIDs are causative in approximately 25% of ulcer disease. Ulcers increase with age because these two risk factors increase with age. Cardiac prophylactic doses of aspirin are a risk factor but have a low incidence of ulcer disease (1%). COX-2–selective inhibitors (0.5%) have the same ulcer risk as placebo.

2. A 39-year-old man presents with epigastric fullness and discomfort, which worsens following meals. There is nausea without vomiting. He is a smoker. There is no prior ulcer disease. The single best diagnostic approach would be

a) An initial 8-week trial of a PPI

b) Immediate upper endoscopy

c) Breath testing for *H. pylori* and providing treatment if results are positive

d) Empiric antimicrobial treatment of *H. pylori*

e) Performing a gastric-emptying study

Answer and Discussion

The answer is c. The most appropriate approach in uncomplicated dyspepsia in this young patient would be *H. pylori* breath testing. This test-and-treat method is warranted as a cost-effective approach for a young patient with new-onset dyspepsia, as breath testing is noninvasive. A short course of a PPI is a reasonable strategy, but a full 8-week course would not be warranted. No justification ever exists for treating anyone for *H. pylori* without proof of infection.

Patients younger than 45 to 50 years of age with new-onset dyspepsia without alarm symptoms such as hematemesis, melena, anemia, nausea, vomiting, and weight loss do not warrant immediate upper endoscopy, and the incidence of gastric cancer is low. This patient's symptoms could be related to gastroparesis. However, a gastric-emptying study would not be the best initial diagnostic study.

3. A 34-year-old woman was found to have a duodenal ulcer and *H. pylori* on upper endoscopy with biopsies and was treated with combination lansoprazole, amoxicillin, and clarithromycin (Prevpac) for 10 days. She completed therapy a few days ago but has persistent epigastric discomfort. She is concerned that her ulcer is still there.

Which of the following is most likely accurate?

a) Her *H. pylori* has not been fully eradicated.

b) Her dyspeptic symptoms might persist despite eradication.

c) An immediate *H. pylori* breath test could be repeated to facilitate rescue therapy, if positive.

d) Quadruple therapy with a bismuth and tetracycline combination should be initiated to increase the likelihood of clearance.

e) Performing fecal antigen testing for *H. pylori* in 3 to 4 weeks followed by antibiotic therapy if test results are positive is an excellent way of promptly evaluating and treating treatment failures.

Answer and Discussion

The answer is b. Dyspeptic symptoms frequently may persist long after the course of *H. pylori* eradication therapy. Symptoms, therefore, cannot help to determine if eradication has been achieved. Breath testing would not be accurate this soon after eradication therapy due to the decreased sensitivity from the use of antibiotics and a PPI. Although confirmation of eradication by all testing is most reliable 4 weeks after treatment, fecal antigen testing has the advantage of being a more prompt test to determine treatment failure and can be used as soon as 7 days after the completion of therapy. Quadruple therapy is appropriate as a first-, second-, or even a third-line option. However, in this recently treated patient, it should be initiated only when it has been determined that eradication was unsuccessful.

4. A 41-year-old patient is seen in the emergency room with hematemesis. He smokes, uses NSAIDs on occasion, and has a history of a prior bleeding ulcer. He is otherwise healthy on no medications. The patient is tachycardic and orthostatic on exam. His systolic blood pressure is 90. Hemoglobin is 8.9 g. Gastroenterology consultation has been requested.

Which is the most accurate statement?

a) He should be medically stabilized and then undergo immediate endoscopy.

b) He should be started on an intravenous PPI and monitored for signs of persistent bleeding. Endoscopy should be performed if symptoms persist or worsen.

c) If initial endoscopy fails to stop his bleeding, surgical intervention is needed.

d) Intravenous PPI therapy and eradication of *H. pylori* may be more helpful in this patient than endoscopic management.

Answer and Discussion

The answer is a. This is an unstable patient with risk factors for adverse outcomes with ulcer disease. Medical stabilization is most appropriate, then endoscopy. Intravenous PPI therapy and *H. pylori* eradication are beneficial but not as helpful in this acute bleed as is prompt endoscopic intervention. Rebleeding after initial endoscopic management occurs in 20% to 25% of cases. Repeat endoscopy is very successful, and combined with the use of intravenous PPIs, surgery is needed significantly less often. In addition, interventional radiology procedures in many centers have essentially replaced surgery for intractable gastrointestinal bleeding.

Chapter 55

Colorectal Carcinoma

Carol A. Burke

POINTS TO REMEMBER:

- Sessile separated polyps are a new pathway to colorectal cancer.

- Colon cancer develops in all familial adenomatous polyposis patients by 40 years of age if prophylactic colectomy is not performed.

- New colorectal cancer screening guidelines incorporate CT colonography and stool DNA as options for testing.

- Adjuvant therapy for patients with stage III colon cancer improve overall and disease free survival.

- Folate supplementation is not associated with a reduced risk of recurrent colorectal adenoma.

Colorectal cancer is the second most common cancer and cause of cancer deaths in the United States. As shown in Table 55.1, both men and women face a lifetime risk of 1 in 18 for the development of invasive colorectal cancer. Each year, approximately 154,000 new cases of colorectal cancer are diagnosed and 52,000 deaths occur.[1] The survival benefit from early detection of colorectal carcinoma through the fecal occult blood test (FOBT) and sigmoidoscopy has been proven; however, less than 50% of eligible Americans have undergone screening. More than 45% of patients diagnosed with colorectal cancer present with stage III and stage IV disease, which carry a 5-year survival rate of 50% and 7%, respectively.

ETIOLOGY

In nearly all cases, colorectal carcinoma arises from an adenomatous polyp. Only 2% of adenomas progress to cancer, however. Observational studies suggest that the adenoma-to-carcinoma sequence takes approximately 10 years.[2] The indirect evidence supporting the adenoma-to-carcinoma sequence includes the following:

- Anatomical distribution and patient demographics are similar for both adenoma and colorectal cancer.

- Risk of dysplasia or cancer increases with increasing polyp size and villous architecture, and, in most cases, cancer is associated with the presence of adenomatous polyps.

- Progressive genetic alterations have been found as adenomas progress to cancer.

- Colonoscopic polypectomy has been associated with a diminished incidence of cancer.

RISK FACTORS

Colorectal carcinogenesis results from complex interactions between genetic susceptibility and environmental factors. Epidemiologic studies implicate dietary variables (e.g., high fat, particularly from red meat; excess alcohol ingestion; low fiber) as cofactors in the development of polyps and colorectal cancer. Other environmental risk factors include obesity and smoking. The risk of adenomatous polyps and cancer is low prior to age 40 years, but it increases with age to peak in the seventh and eighth decades of life. A sex or race predilection does not appear to exist, except among African Americans, who have higher colorectal cancer incidence and mortality rates. Approximately 70% of newly diagnosed colorectal cancers arise in patients without known risk factors. In approximately 30% of patients with colorectal cancer, risk factors have been identified (Table 55.2).

A personal history of adenomatous polyps or colorectal cancer increases the risk for metachronous colorectal cancer. First-degree relatives of patients with colorectal cancer have a two- to threefold increased risk for colorectal cancer and adenomatous polyps.[3,4] Recent work has proven that the first-degree family members of patients with adenomatous polyps also have an increased risk of colorectal cancer, particularly when the adenoma is diagnosed prior to age 60 years.[5,6]

Patients with the highest risk of colorectal cancer are those who have germline abnormalities in critical genes that control critical cellular function, as in the hereditary colorectal cancer syndromes. *Familial adenomatous polyposis*

TABLE 55.1

PERCENTAGE OF U.S. POPULATION DIAGNOSED WITH INVASIVE COLORECTAL CANCER

	Birth–39 Years	40–49 Years	50–59 Years	60–69 Years	≥70 Years
Men	0.08	0.92	1.60	4.78	5.65
Women	0.07	0.72	1.12	4.30	5.23

Adapted from Jemal A, Siegel R, Ward E, et al. Cancer statistics, 2008. *CA Cancer J Clin* 2008;58:71–96.

(FAP) is an autosomal dominant disease with nearly 100% penetrance. Germline mutations of the tumor-suppressor gene *APC*, on the long arm of chromosome 5, are detected in up to 90% of FAP patients. *APC* mutations result in the development of hundreds to thousands of colonic adenomas by the second decade of life. Colon cancer develops in all FAP patients by 40 years of age if prophylactic colectomy is not performed. Upper gastrointestinal adenomas are common in this population, and periampullary cancer is the second leading cause of cancer deaths in this group. *Gardner syndrome* is a phenotypic variant of FAP. In addition to colonic polyposis, Gardner syndrome may manifest with benign soft tissue tumors, osteomas, supernumerary teeth, desmoid tumors, and congenital hypertrophy of the retinal pigment epithelium.

Recent studies have identified another genetic cause for multiple colonic adenomas. *MYH*, on chromosome 19, is a base-excision-repair gene. Biallelic germline mutations in *MYH* have been found to be present in 7.5% of individuals with FAP and no detectable *APC* mutation.[7] It also results in a recessive pattern of inheritance to multiple colorectal adenomas and probably an increased risk of colorectal cancer. Biallelic *MYH* mutations are found in 3.9% of individuals with multiple (3–100) lifetime adenomas and in 29% of those with 15 to 100 adenomas.

Hereditary nonpolyposis colon cancer (HNPCC) is an autosomal dominant disease with nearly complete penetrance. Colon cancer occurs in up to 80% of those affected, usually at a young age, and is often right sided. Mutations in at least four genes, called *mismatch repair genes*, result in carcinogenesis in HNPCC. Alterations in the mismatch repair genes prevent the adequate repair of DNA. Germline muta-

tions in one of four mismatch repair genes can be identified in 50% of patients with HNPCC. The diagnosis of HNPCC is made in families that satisfy the Amsterdam criteria:

■ Three or more relatives with colorectal cancer, with one being a first-degree relative of the other two
■ At least two successive generations affected
■ One cancer diagnosed before age 50 years

HNPCC families may have extracolonic cancers, which include other gastrointestinal tumors and urologic and gynecologic malignancies. The risk of endometrial carcinoma has been reported to be as high as 60% in women in HNPCC kindreds.[8] Therefore, aggressive gynecologic screening for endometrial cancer is recommended.

The chronic inflammatory colitides, *ulcerative colitis* and *Crohn's disease*, are associated with a high risk of colorectal cancer. The proximal extent of colonic involvement and the duration of disease (not activity) stratify the level of risk. Risk is highest in patients with pancolitis and negligible in patients with proctitis. After a decade of disease, the cancer risk increases yearly by 1% to 2%.

PATHOGENESIS

Colorectal tumorigenesis results from multiple acquired genetic alterations within tumor tissue. These alterations, in turn, promote malignant transformation (i.e., the development of oncogenes) or loss in the inhibition of cellular proliferation (i.e., the development of tumor-suppressor genes).[9] Mutations in DNA repair (i.e., mismatch repair) genes are implicated in carcinogenesis in patients with HNPCC and in approximately 20% of patients with sporadic colorectal cancer (Table 55.3).

CLINICAL PRESENTATION

Colon polyps and early colon cancer are asymptomatic until they are advanced. Gastrointestinal blood loss is the most common sign and may include a positive FOBT result, iron-deficiency anemia, or hematochezia. When tumors are advanced, unexplained anorexia, weight loss, or symptoms from obstruction or local invasion, such as a change in bowel habits, abdominal pain, or obstruction may occur.

TABLE 55.2

RISK FACTORS FOR COLORECTAL CANCER

Personal history of adenomas or colorectal cancer
First-degree relative younger than 60 years with adenoma or colorectal cancer, or two first-degree relatives of any age with colorectal cancer
Inherited colorectal cancer syndromes
    Hereditary nonpolyposis colorectal cancer
    Familial adenomatous polyposis
Ulcerative colitis and Crohn's disease

TABLE 55.3

GENETIC ALTERATIONS IN COLORECTAL TUMORIGENESIS

Oncogenes	Tumor-Suppressor Genes	Mismatch Repair Genes	Base Excision Genes
12p (k-ras)	5q (APC)	2p (MSH2)	19 (MYH)
	17p (p53)	3p (MLH1)	
	18q (DCC)	2 (PMS1)	
		7 (PMS2)	

DIAGNOSIS

The diagnosis of colorectal polyps and cancer is made most often during a colonic evaluation performed for gastrointestinal symptoms, screening, or surveillance.

Pathology

Polyp is an inexact term that indicates a protuberance of tissue into the colonic lumen. A variety of polyps can be found in the colon. The most common polyp that can become an adenocarcinoma is an adenomatous polyp (Table 55.4). Adenomas account for approximately two of every three colonic polyps. Both the size and the degree of villous features are predictive of the risk of malignancy within the polyp.

Hyperplastic polyps which are serrated lesions are the second most common type of polyp, accounting for 10% to 30% of colonic polyps. Small, hyperplastic polyps, which are most often found in the rectosigmoid, have no clinical significance. Large (greater than 9 mm) hyperplastic polyps and a newly characterized morphologic variant of the hyperplastic polyp called a sessile serrated polyp (SSP) also known as the sessile serrated adenoma (SSA) are believed to be the earliest precursors in the pathway for approximately 20% of colorectal cancers.[10] These lesions are often located in the proximal colon and are distinct from the precancerous, serrated adenoma.

Screening

Various methods are available for colorectal cancer screening, and the cost effectiveness of these modalities has been

TABLE 55.4

CLASSIFICATION OF COLORECTAL POLYPS

Neoplastic	Nonneoplastic
Adenomatous	Hyperplastic
Tubular	Hamartomatous
Tubulovillous	Lymphoid aggregate
Villous	Inflammatory
Serrated adenoma	
Sessile serrated polyp with dysplasia	

established.[11] Any positive finding detected by any of the screening tests warrants colonoscopy.

Fecal Occult Blood Test

The FOBT is the most widely studied screening method. Compliance rates are low, however, possibly because of both the need to follow a special diet (i.e., meatfree, high-residue diet without vegetables having peroxidase activity, such as turnips and horseradish) for at least 24 hours before specimen collection and the need to obtain three separate stool specimens collected at least 1 day apart. A positive finding on one or more samples on an FOBT is a positive test result.

The mortality from colorectal cancer has been shown to be reduced up to 16% in randomized and controlled trials of screening with guaiac FOBT. More sensitive, guaiac based FOBT or immunochemical FOBT (iFOBT) is recommended to replace the less sensitive guaiac based FOBT.[12,13] iFOBT utilizes antibodies to human globin to detect bleeding from colorectal neoplasia. No dietary restrictions are needed. Since globin does not survive passage through the upper GI tract, the test is specific for colorectal bleeding. The accurary of a one times iFOBT has been shown to be greater for cancer and advanced adenoma than the less sensitive guaiac based method.

Sigmoidoscopy

Sigmoidoscopic screening allows a portion of the colorectal mucosa to be visualized directly and a diagnostic biopsy to be *performed* at the time of examination. Both the sensitivity and the specificity are high for the detection of polyps and cancer in the segment of the bowel examined. Unfortunately, however, nearly 40% of polyps and cancers are beyond the limits of detection of the longest (i.e., 60-cm) flexible sigmoidoscope. The detection of adenomas on flexible sigmoidoscopy is considered a positive test result and warrants colonoscopy with polypectomy.

Opinions vary regarding the need for colonoscopy for patients in whom a single tubular adenoma ≥ 1 cm is found on flexible sigmoidoscopy; however, the prevalence of proximal neoplasms in such patients may be substantial enough (7%–9%) to warrant screening colonoscopy.[14]

The results of several case-control studies show a reduction in deaths from colorectal cancer in patients who undergo predominantly rigid sigmoidoscopic examinations. The reported reduction in mortality varies from between 59% and 80%. The most well-known study reviewed the use of sigmoidoscopic screening in 261 patients who died from cancer of the distal colon or rectum, comparing these patients with 868 controls.[15] Screening reduced the rectosigmoid cancer mortality rate by 60%, and the protective effect of sigmoidoscopy was noted to last for up to 10 years. This reduction in mortality may have resulted from earlier detection of cancer and removal of premalignant polyps.

Stool DNA

A variety of mutations are known to be present in colorectal neoplasms. Exfoliated cells carrying mutations from the neoplasm can be shed into the fecal stream and be detected in human stool. One large, multi-center, colorectal cancer screening trial found the accuracy of a multi-target DNA stool assay to detect colorectal cancer to be 52%.[16]

Barium Enema Testing

Double-contrast barium enema testing has the advantage of imaging the entire colon. Recent evidence, however, suggests that it is inaccurate for the detection of polyps and early cancers, and suboptimal for colorectal cancer screening or surveillance. In a prospective study comparing the use of double-contrast barium enema examination and colonoscopy, the miss rate of barium enema testing for polyps >1 cm was 52%.[17]

CT Colonography (CTC)

CTC makes use of computer tomographic images to visualize colorectal polyps. Individuals must undergo bowel preparation and gaseous distension of the colon. A multi-center trial of 2531 patients determined the sensitivity and specificity of CTC versus colonoscopy for the detection of polyps 10 mm and larger in size to be 90% and 86% respectively.[18] Unfortunately the sensitivity for the detection of smaller polyps.

Colonoscopy

Colonoscopy is the only technique with both diagnostic and therapeutic applications. It is considered the gold standard for the detection of colonic neoplasms, and it can be completed in more than 95% of examinations. No published studies have investigated the effectiveness of colonoscopic screening in the prevention of colorectal cancer. In one cohort study of 1,418 patients who underwent colonoscopy and polypectomy, a lower-than-expected incidence of colorectal cancer was observed.[19]

Recommendations

Guidelines for colorectal cancer screening were updated in 2008.[12,13] Recommendations for average-risk patients, for whom screening begins at age 50 years, include the following options:

- Annual high sensitivity FOBT or
- Colonoscopy every 10 years or
- Flexible sigmoidoscopy every 5 years or
- CTC or double-contrast barium enema every 5 years or
- Stool DNA testing, interval uncertain

Patients with a greater-than-average risk of colorectal cancer should undergo colonoscopic surveillance individualized according to the risk of cancer, which involves the following factors.

TABLE 55.5

SURVEILLANCE INTERVAL FOR INDIVIDUALS WITH COLORECTAL NEOPLASIA

Adenoma Characteristics	Surveillance Interval
1–2, <1 cm, tubular adenomas	5–10 years
≥ 3, or ≥1 cm, or *advanced* adenoma (villous component, high-grade dysplasia)	3 years
Curative colon cancer resection	Within 1 year after resection, repeat in 3 years; if normal, repeat in 5 years

Adapted from Levin B, Lieberman DA, McFarland B, et al. Screening and surveillance for the early detection of colorectal cancer and adenomatous polyps, 2008: A joint guideline from the American Cancer Society, the U.S. Multi-Society Task Force on Colorectal Cancer and the American College of Radiology. *CA Cancer J Clin* 2008;58:130–160.

Surveillance

History of Adenomatous Polyps.   Once adenomatous polyps are removed, the next colonoscopy should occur in 3 or 5 to 10 years, depending on the family history, and the size, number, and pathology of the polyps[20,21] (Table 55.5).

Patients who have "advanced" (identified by being >1 cm, or with histology containing villous features or severe dysplasia) or multiple adenomas (≥3) should have their first follow-up colonoscopy in 3 years. Patients who have one or two small, <1 cm, tubular adenomas should have their first follow-up colonoscopy at 5 to 10 years. The surveillance interval is individualized for individuals with large (i.e., >2 cm) sessile polyps, unusually numerous adenomas, adenomas removed piecemeal, or adenomas with malignancy and favorable prognostic features; this period may be as short as 3 to 6 months.

If the first follow-up colonoscopy is normal, or only 1 or 2 small (<1 cm) tubular adenomas are found, the next colonoscopy can be in 5 to 10 years, depending on the aforementioned risk factors.

History of Colorectal Cancer.   In patients who undergo curative surgical intervention for colorectal cancer and have a normal preoperative colonoscopy, the subsequent surveillance examination should occur within 1 year and, if results are negative at that time, 3 years, and, if normal, every 5 years thereafter.

Familial Adenomatous Polyposis.   Patients with FAP should receive genetic counseling and be offered genetic testing. Beginning at puberty, gene carriers or those with indeterminate status should undergo yearly flexible sigmoidoscopy or colonoscopy.

Hereditary Nonpolyposis Colon Cancer. Patients with HNPCC should receive genetic counseling and be offered genetic testing. Colonoscopy should be performed every 1 to 2 years beginning at age 25 (or at an age 10 years younger than the age at which cancer occurred in the relative who developed colon cancer at the youngest age). After age 40 years, surveillance examinations should be conducted yearly. Annual transvaginal ultrasonography and endometrial biopsy should be considered in women older than 25 years.

Ulcerative or Crohn's Colitis. Generally, colonoscopy with biopsies for dysplasia is performed every 1 to 2 years after 8 years of pancolitic disease. Patients with disease involving the left colon should begin surveillance after 12 to 15 years of disease.

Family History of Colon Cancer or Adenomatous Polyps. In an individual with two first-degree relatives who developed colon cancer at any age, or with a first-degree relative diagnosed with adenomatous polyps or colorectal cancer prior to age 60 years, a colonoscopy every 5 years beginning at age 40 (or at an age 10 years younger than the age at which the relative developed cancer) is appropriate. Individuals with one first-degree relative or two second-degree relatives older than age 60 years with colorectal neoplasia should undergo colonoscopy every 10 years, beginning at age 40.

TREATMENT

The curability and chance of recurrence of colorectal cancer, and survival after it, are determined on the basis of the disease stage. For most early-stage tumors (i.e., stages I and II; Table 55.6), surgery alone is curative. For more advanced disease, surgery and adjuvant chemotherapy are recommended to prevent recurrence and prolong survival.

Adjuvant Treatment

Studies over the past 10 years have proven the benefit of adjuvant therapy in decreasing cancer recurrence and prolonging survival in subgroups of patients with colon cancer.[22] Adjuvant chemotherapy with 5-fluorouracil (5-FU)–based therapy, modulated by folinic acid and combined with oxaliplatin, has now become an accepted standard of care for patients with stage III colon cancer. Patients with stage II disease should be encouraged to participate in ongoing trials because adjuvant therapy has no proven survival benefit for these patients.[23] The combination of postoperative radiation and 5-FU significantly reduces the rates of recurrence, cancer-related deaths, and overall mortality in patients with stage II or stage III rectal cancer, compared with radiation therapy alone.[24]

TABLE 55.6

COMPARISON OF DUKES' AND TNM STAGING SYSTEMS

| Stage | TNM System | | | 5-Year Survival (%) |
	Tumor	Node	Metastases	
I	T1 or T2	N0	M0	90
II	T3 or T4	N0	M0	75
III	Any T	N1–N3	M0	35–60
IV	Any T	Any N	M1	<10
Primary tumor (T)				
Tis	Carcinoma in situ			
T1	Tumor invades submucosa			
T2	Tumor invades muscularis propria			
T3	Tumor invades through muscularis propria			
T4	Tumor invades serosa, nodes, and adjacent organs			
Metastases (M)				
M0	No distant metastases			
M1	Distant metastases			
Regional nodes (N)				
N0	Negative nodes			
N1	1–3 Positive nodes			
N2	>3 Positive nodes			
N3	Positive nodes on vascular trunk			

TNM = tumor-node-metastasis.

Hepatic Metastases

The prognosis for patients with hepatic metastases is poor, with virtually no survivors at 3 years. A multi-institutional study reviewing hepatic resection as treatment for colorectal cancer metastases found a 5-year survival rate of 33% and a diseasefree survival rate of 21%.[25] Favorable prognostic factors included a resection margin >1 cm and two or fewer metastases <8 cm.

PREVENTION

Chemoprevention is one of the most exciting potential preventive measures against colorectal neoplasia cancer. In epidemiologic studies, the high consumption of folate, fruits, and vegetables is associated, albeit inconsistently, with a lower risk of colorectal neoplasia. Recently, the analyses from two large studies determined that the intake of high dietary fiber is not associated with a reduced risk of colorectal cancer.[26,27] In addition, a double-blind, placebo-controlled, randomized trial of 1 mg of folate per day in 1,021 men and women found no reduction in colorectal adenoma recurrence in those taking folate.[28]

Nonsteroidal anti-inflammatory drugs (NSAIDs), particularly aspirin, substantially reduce the risk of colorectal cancer by anywhere from 4% to 60%. In two large, prospective double-blind studies, regular aspirin use in dosages similar to those taken for cardioprotection was associated with decreased risk of recurrent colorectal adenomas.[29,30] The cyclooxygenase 2–selective NSAID, celecoxib has been shown to promote the regression of adenomas in patients with FAP.[31] The U.S. Food and Drug Administration (FDA) approved the use of celecoxib 400 mg BID to regress colorectal adenomas, as an adjunct to endoscopic polypectomy, in patients with FAP. Although not FDA approved, there is strong data from large randomized, placebo-controlled trials that both celecoxib[32,33] and rofecoxib[34] are effective for reducing recurrent adenomas in subjects who have undergone polypectomy. Unfortunately, the risk of cardiovascular and thrombotic events is increased with the use of these agents, and thus, they are not recommended for chemoprevention in individuals with sporadic adenomas. A randomized, double-blind, placebo-controlled study detected a significant decrease in the recurrence of adenomas in patients taking 1,200 mg of calcium daily.[35]

CONCLUSION

Colorectal cancer is one of the leading causes of cancer and death from carcinoma in the United States. Increasing awareness regarding the preventable nature of this disease, along with the widespread use of screening, should favorably affect the incidence of colorectal cancer. Colorectal cancer screening and polyp removal can save lives, and the most exciting area of future research is the primary prevention of adenomas and colorectal cancer through chemoprevention.

REVIEW EXERCISES

QUESTIONS

For the cases in questions 1 through 4, choose the appropriate recommendation from the lettered list (each may be used more than once):

1. A single 3-mm rectal adenoma is found on flexible sigmoidoscopy in a 32-year-old woman.
2. A 62-year-old man with an 18-year history of pancolitis just underwent colonoscopy.
3. A 54-year-old woman has a lifelong history of irritable bowel syndrome.
4. A 68-year-old African American man recently underwent removal of an 8-mm villous adenoma.
a) Colonoscopy and polypectomy
b) Yearly fecal occult blood test and flexible sigmoidoscopy every 5 years
c) Colonoscopy at age 40 years
d) Colonoscopy in 5 years
e) Colonoscopy in 3 years
f) Colonoscopy in 1 year

Answers and Discussions

1. The answer is a. Until further studies are performed, all patients with an adenoma detected by flexible sigmoidoscopy should undergo a full colonoscopy to detect synchronous, more proximal neoplasms, as well as polypectomy of all detected polyps.
2. The answer is f. All patients with ulcerative pancolitis who have had the diagnosis for more than 8 years are at increased risk of colorectal dysplasia and cancer. Yearly colonoscopy with four-quadrant biopsy every 10 cm to detect dysplasia is indicated.
3. The answer is b. Patients with irritable bowel syndrome and no risk factors are at average risk for colorectal cancer. Although colonoscopy is the preferred screening strategy, the best answer here is annual fecal occult blood test and flexible sigmoidoscopy every 5 years, which is an appropriate screening method for patients at average risk.
4. The answer is d. The postpolypectomy surveillance interval is 5 years in patients with less than three tubular adenomas <1 cm detected on colonoscopy. New data have shown that those individuals are not at high risk of having numerous, large, or advanced adenomas on their subsequent colonoscopy.

5. A 71-year-old white man underwent complete colonoscopy with removal of two polyps. One was a 7-mm tubulovillous adenoma with severe dysplasia, the other was a 3-mm tubular adenoma. What is the best recommendation in this case?
a) Repeat colonoscopy in 3 to 6 months.
b) Repeat colonoscopy in 1 year.
c) Repeat colonoscopy in 3 years.
d) Repeat colonoscopy in 5 years.

Answer and Discussion

The answer is e. The individuals at higher risk of having recurrent neoplasia on the first postpolypectomy examination are those who had more than two large (>1 cm) or histologically advanced (villous features or severe dysplasia) adenomas. This group of individuals is recommended to have their follow-up colonoscopy in 3 years.

For questions 6 through 10, indicate whether the statement about colorectal cancer and polyps is true or false.

6. A 70-year-old man who underwent curative resection of stage I colon cancer found on a surveillance colonoscopy can wait 1 year until the next examination.
a) True
b) False

Answer and Discussion

The answer is a. A 1-year surveillance interval is recommended after colorectal cancer surgery with curative intent. If the 1-year exam is normal, the next exam is in 3 years and, if negative, every 5 years thereafter.

7. A 53-year-old woman with breast cancer is at increased risk of colorectal cancer and should undergo colonoscopy every 5 years.
a) True
b) False

Answer and Discussion

The answer is b. A personal history of breast cancer is not associated with an increased risk of colorectal carcinoma. Factors that increase the risk of colorectal cancer include a personal or family history of colorectal neoplasia, the inherited colon cancer syndromes, and the chronic colitides, such as ulcerative and Crohn's colitis.

8. A 34-year-old man who has a 52-year-old brother with colon cancer, a sister with endometrial cancer, and a father who died of colon cancer at age 58 years should undergo colonoscopy at age 50 years.
a) True
b) False

Answer and Discussion

The answer is b. This patient's family history should suggest hereditary nonpolyposis colon cancer to the clinician. Although the Amsterdam criteria are not met, the strong family history (in two first-degree relatives) of early-onset colorectal cancer (occurring prior to age 60 years) necessitates colonoscopic surveillance beginning at age 40 years, or 10 years earlier than the age at which cancer was diagnosed in the relative in whom cancer occurred at the youngest age.

9. All patients with a T3 N1 M0 colon cancer should be offered adjuvant leucovorin and 5-fluorouracil-based chemotherapy.
a) True
b) False

Answer and Discussion

The answer is a. The clinician should be familiar with the tumor-node-metastasis cancer staging systems. Adjuvant therapy is recommended only for patients with nodal disease (stage III) colorectal cancer. No benefit was seen in earlier-stage disease.

10. A patient with familial adenomatous polyposis has a 50% chance of transmitting the disease to his or her children.
a) True
b) False

Answer and Discussion

The answer is a. As in all dominantly inherited diseases, such as familial adenomatous polyposis and hereditary nonpolyposis colon cancer, 50% of the offspring are at risk of inheriting the mutation.

11. A 62-year-old woman arrives in your office with recent-onset abdominal pain and a change in bowel habit. She has no family history of cancer and is otherwise in good health. Physical examination reveals some tenderness in the suprapubic area but is otherwise normal. Fecal occult blood test reveals one of six smears to be positive. Which of the following options is most appropriate?
a) Repeat the fecal occult blood test.
b) Schedule a colonoscopy.
c) Order a flexible sigmoidoscopy and, if results are negative, do no further evaluation.
d) Reassure the patient that she has symptoms of irritable bowel syndrome and treat with fiber.

Answer and Discussion

The answer is b. Any patient with symptoms of colorectal cancer should have a complete colonic evaluation. A positive fecal occult blood test result includes a positive finding in any of six sample windows; retesting should not be performed.

12. A 42-year-old father with familial adenomatous polyposis (FAP) has two children, ages 12 and 14 years. He is interested in knowing if his children have FAP. No *APC* mutation was found on his genetic testing, however. What would be the appropriate management of this family?
a) Recommend flexible sigmoidoscopy when the children begin to show symptoms of colonic disease.
b) Offer *MYH* testing to the father
c) Advise the father that he cannot pass FAP on to his children because he has no detectable *APC* mutation.

Answer and Discussion

The answer is b. It is not appropriate to wait for colonic symptoms in individuals "at risk" of FAP. Surveillance should begin at the time of puberty, and colectomy should be performed before bleeding, pain, or cancer develops. About 10% of individuals with FAP are *APC* negative but still have a 50% chance of passing an FAP disease–causing mutation on to their children. It has recently been discovered that biallelic germline mutations in *MYH* account for up to 7.5% of *APC*-negative FAP patients. *MYH* testing should be offered to any patient with multiple adenomas or those with classic FAP who are *APC* negative.

REFERENCES

1. Jemal A, Siegel R, Ward E, et al. Cancer statistics, 2007. *CA Cancer J Clin* 2008;58:71–96.
2. Morson BC. The evolution of colorectal carcinomas. *Clin Radiol* 1984;35:425–431.
3. St. John DJ, McDermott F, Hopper J, et al. Cancer risk in relatives of patients with common colorectal cancer. *Ann Intern Med* 1993;118:785–790.

4. Bazzoli F, Fossi S, Sottili S, et al. The risk of adenomatous polyps in asymptomatic first-degree relatives of persons with colon cancer. *Gastroenterology* 1995;109:783–788.

5. Winawer S, Zauber A, Gerdes H, et al. Risk of colorectal cancer in the families of patients with adenomatous polyps. *N Engl J Med* 1996;334:82–97.

6. Ahsan H, Neugut A, Garbowski G, et al. Family history of colorectal adenomatous polyps and increased risk for colorectal cancer. *Ann Intern Med* 1998;128:900–905.

7. Sieber O, Lipton L, Crabtree M, et al. Multiple colorectal adenomas, classic adenomatous polyposis, and germ-line mutations in *MYH. N Engl J Med* 2003;348:791–798.

8. Brown GJ, St. John DJ, Macrae FA, et al. Cancer risk in young women at risk of hereditary nonpolyposis colorectal cancer: implications for gynecologic surveillance. *Gynecol Oncol* 2001;80:346–349.

9. Vogelstein B, Fearon E, Hamilton S, et al. Genetic alterations during colorectal-tumor development. *N Engl J Med* 1988;319:525–532.

10. East J, Saunders B, Jass J. Sporadic and syndromic hyperplastic polyps and serrated adenomas of the colon: classification, molecular genetics, natural history and clinical management. *Gastroenterol Cl N Amer* 2008;37:25–46.

11. Lieberman DA. Cost-effectiveness model for colon cancer screening. *Gastroenterology* 1995;109:1781–1790.

12. US Preventive Services Task Force. Screening for Colorectal cancer: U.S. Preventive Services Task Force Recommendation Statement. *Annals Int Med* 2008;149:627–637.

13. Levin B, Lieberman D, McFarland B, et al. Screening and surveillance for the early detection of colorectal cancer and adenomatous polyps, 2008: A joint guideline from the American Cancer Society, the U.S. Multi-Society Task Force on Colorectal Cancer and the American College of Radiology. *CA Cancer J Clin* 2008;58:130–160.

14. Lieberman D, Weiss D, Bond J, et al. Use of colonoscopy to screen asymptomatic adults for colorectal cancer. *N Engl J Med* 2000;343:162–168.

15. Selby JV, Friedman GD, Quesenberry CO, et al. Case-control study of screening sigmoidoscopy and mortality from colorectal cancer. *N Engl J Med* 1992;326:653–657.

16. Imperiale TF, Ransohoff DF, Itzkowitz SH, et al. Fecal DNA versus fecal occult blood for colorectal cancer screening in an average risk population. *N Engl J Med* 2004;351:2704–2714.

17. Winawer SJ, Stewart ET, Zauber AG, et al. A comparison of colonoscopy and double-contrast barium enema for surveillance after polypectomy. *N Engl J Med* 2000;342(24):1766–1772.

18. Johnson CD, Chen MH, Toledano AY, et al. Accuracy of CT colonography for detecton of large adenomas and cancers. *N Engl J Med* 2008;359:1207–1217.

19. Winawer S, Fletcher R, Rex D, et al. Colorectal cancer screening and surveillance: clinical guidelines and rationale—update based on new evidence. *Gastroenterology* 2003;124(2):544–560.

20. Winawer SJ, Zauber AG, Fletcher RH, et al. Guidelines for colonoscopy surveillance after polypectomy: a consensus update by the US Multi-Society Task Force on Colorectal Cancer and the American Cancer Society. *Gastroenterology* 2006;130:1872–1885.

21. Rex DK, Kahi CJ, Levin B, et al. Guidelines for colonoscopy surveillance after cancer resection: a consensus update by the American Cancer Society and the US Multi-Society Task Force on Colorectal Cancer. *Gastroenterology* 2006;130:1865–1871.

22. de Gramont A, Tournigand C, Andre T, et al. Adjuvant therapy for stage II and III colorectal cancer. *Semin Oncol* 2007;34(2 Suppl 1):S37–S40.

23. Moertel CG, Fleming TR, Macdonald JS. Intergroup study of fluorouracil plus levamisole as adjuvant therapy for stage II/Dukes' stage B2 colon cancer. *J Clin Oncol* 1995;13:2935–2943.

24. Krook J, Moertel C, Gunderson L, et al. Effective surgical adjuvant therapy for high-risk rectal carcinoma. *N Engl J Med* 1991;324:709–715.

25. Hughes KS, Simon R, Songhorabodi S, et al. Resection of the liver for colorectal carcinoma metastasis: a multi-institutional study of indications for resection. *Surgery* 1986;100:278–284.

26. Michels KB, Fuchs CS, Giovannucci E, et al. Fiber intake and incidence of colorectal cancer among 76,947 women and 47,279 men. *Cancer Epidemiol Biomarkers Prev* 2005;14(4):842–849.

27. Park Y, Hunter DJ, Spiegelman D, et al. Dietary fiber intake and risk of colorectal cancer: a pooled analysis of prospective cohort studies. *JAMA* 2005;294(22):2849–2857.

28. Cole B, Baron J, Sandler R, et al. Folic acid for the prevention of colorectal adenomas: a randomized clinical trial. *JAMA* 2007;297(21):2351–2359.

29. Baron JA, Cole BF, Sandler RS, et al. A randomized trial of aspirin to prevent colorectal adenomas. *N Engl J Med* 2003;348:891–899.

30. Sandler R, Halabi S, Baron J, et al. A randomized trial of aspirin to prevent colorectal adenomas in patients with previous colorectal cancer. *N Engl J Med* 2003;348:883–890.

31. Steinbach G, Lynch PM, Phillips RK, et al. The effect of celecoxib, a cyclooxygenase-2 inhibitor, in familial adenomatous polyposis. *N Engl J Med* 2000;342:1946–1952.

32. Arber N, Eagle CJ, Spicak J, et al. Celecoxib for the prevention of colorectal adenomatous polyps. *N Engl J Med* 2006;355:885–895.

33. Bertagnolli M, Eagle CJ, Zauber AG, et al. Celecoxib for the prevention of sporadic colorectal adenomas. *N Engl J Med* 2006;355(9):873–884.

34. Baron JA, Sandler RS, Bresalier RS, et al. A randomized trial of rofecoxib for the chemoprevention of colorectal adenomas. *Gastroenterology* 2006;131(6):1674–1682.

35. Baron JA, Beach M, Mandel JS, et al. Calcium supplements for the prevention of colorectal adenomas. *N Engl J Med* 1999;340:101–107.

SUGGESTED READINGS

East J, Saunders B, Jass J. Sporadic and syndromic hyperplastic polyps and serrated adenomas of the colon: classification, molecular genetics, natural history and clinical management. *Gastroenterol Cl N Amer* 2008;37:25–46.

Johnson CD, Chen MH, Toledano AY, et al. Accuracy of CT colonography for detecton of large adenomas and cancers. *N Engl J Med* 2008;359:1207–1217.

Levin B, Lieberman D, McFarland B, et al. Screening and surveillance for the early detection of colorectal cancer and adenomatous polyps, 2008: A joint guideline from the American Cancer Society, the U.S. Multi-Society Task Force on Colorectal Cancer and the American College of Radiology. *CA Cancer J Clin* 2008;58:130–160.

US Preventive Services Task Force. Screening for Colorectal Cancer: U.S. Preventive Services Task Force Recommendation Statement. *Annals Int Med* 2008;149:627–637.

Chapter 56

Inflammatory Bowel Disease

Aaron Brzezinski

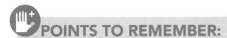

POINTS TO REMEMBER:

- The first susceptibility gene for Crohn's disease has been mapped to chromosome 16 and is referred to as *IBD1*.

- A larger-than-expected number of patients with Crohn's disease are cigarette smokers.

- Patients with ulcerative colitis (UC) have an increased risk of colorectal cancer.

- About 50% to 60% of patients with inflammatory bowel disease (IBD) have extraintestinal manifestations.

- Corticosteroids are indicated in patients with moderate or severely active UC or Crohn's disease, and in patients who fail to respond to 5-aminosalicylic acid or antibiotics.

- Biological agents that block tumor necrosis factor-α are indicated in IBD patients who have refractory disease.

The term *inflammatory bowel disease* (IBD) applies commonly to two diseases of the gastrointestinal system, namely, Crohn's disease and UC. These are chronic diseases of unknown etiology, and their hallmark is a dysregulation of the immune system leading to uncontrolled inflammation primarily in the gastrointestinal system. However, it is important to realize that IBD is a systemic disorder and that patients frequently have extraintestinal manifestations. A greater understanding of the immunologic abnormalities has resulted in more effective treatments; however, the treatments are systemic and have the potential for significant complications. The goals of treatment are aimed at controlling symptoms, limiting morbidity, improving quality of life, and decreasing mortality. Since the characterization of the first Crohn's disease susceptibility gene, the *NOD2/CARD15* mutation on chromosome 16, there have

been numerous genomewide association studies that have led to the recognition of several more genes, such as the interleukin (IL)-23 receptor, that are strongly associated with Crohn's disease. It is hoped that with a better understanding of the function of these mutated genes, there will be better predictors of disease behavior and more effective targeted treatments.

EPIDEMIOLOGY

Over the past 50 years, the incidence of IBD has increased exponentially in industrialized countries. In the United States, Dr. Loftus et al. recently reported the change in incidence of UC and Crohn's disease between 1940 and 2000 in Olmstead County, Minnesota. The incidence of UC increased from 3.1/100,000 in the decade 1940-1949 to 8.8/100,000 in the decade 1990–2000. The annual incidence rates for UC were higher for males than for females (9.8/100,000 vs. 6.5/100,000). The incidence of Crohn's disease also increased from 2.3/100,000 in the decade 1940–1949 to 7.9/100,000 in the decade 1990–2000; however, the annual incidence rates for males and females were similar in Crohn's disease. In 2004, in North America, the estimated incidence rates for UC were between 2.2 and 14.3 cases per 100,000 person years, and between 3.1 and 14.6 cases per 100,000 person years for Crohn's disease.

Kappelman et al. analyzed the information from a large insurance claims database in the United States. For this type of analysis, the identification of cases depends on the criteria used to define a case. When stringent criteria are used, fewer patients are captured, but the data are cleaner; with less stringent criteria, there is a risk of including some cases without the disease. Following a stringent case definition, Kappelman et al. estimated that the prevalence of Crohn's disease in adults was 201 cases per 100,000 persons and 43 per 100,000 in children. The prevalence of UC in adults was 238 cases per 100,000 persons and in children

28 per 100,000. Extrapolating these prevalence estimates to the U.S. population, it was calculated that about 1 million Americans had IBD in 2005. However, if a less stringent case definition had been used by the authors, then a greater number of cases of both Crohn's disease and UC would have been identified, and the overall prevalence of IBD would have increased by 51% for children and by 59% for adults. If this last estimate is used, then there would have been approximately 1.5 million persons with IBD in the United States in 2005.

In patients with Crohn's disease ages 20 to 40 years, there is a female preponderance of 1.3:1. However, in recent reports in the pediatric literature, the ratio is being reversed with a higher number of newly diagnosed Crohn's disease in males than females. There is a bimodal distribution at presentation, with the larger peak occurring between ages 15 and 25 years and a second, lower peak after the sixth decade of life.

ETIOLOGY

The cause of IBD remains elusive; however, it is clear that there are genetic abnormalities and abnormal host–microbial interactions that result in a harmful immune response that leads to intestinal damage. The gastrointestinal tract serves numerous complex functions, including digestion and absorption of nutrients, fluid, and electrolytes, and it also has a pivotal function in immune regulation. The luminal milieu is very complex, and the number of immune cells in the gastrointestinal tract is one of the largest in the human body. IBD is believed to occur when there are genetic abnormalities that result in an inadequate immune response to intestinal microbes. Some of the early information that supports a genetic link in IBD came from twin studies. The concordance for IBD is greater in monozygotic than in dizygotic twins, and greater for Crohn's disease than for UC. The concordance for Crohn's disease in monozygotic twins is 20% to 50% and in dizygotic twins 0% to 7%, and for UC, it is 14% to 19% in monozygotic twins and 0% to 5% in dizygotic twins. Given that the concordance rate is not 100% in monozygotic twins, it is clear that a genetic abnormality is not sufficient to cause the disease, and there must be other factors, possibly environmental or endogenous, that determine the development of the disease.

The first susceptibility gene for Crohn's disease has been the *NOD2/CARD15*, which was mapped to chromosome 16, and it is referred to as *IBD1*. The most compelling evidence for a genetic role of this gene in Crohn's disease comes from the description of three mutations within the *NOD2* gene that is involved in apoptosis and antigen recognition, and the association of genotype-phenotype associations in some patient populations with abnormalities in this gene. In some ethnic groups, Crohn's disease patients with this mutation have primarily strictures in the terminal ileum. With improvement in molecular biology techniques

that have facilitated genetic mapping, numerous genetic mutations have been identified. However, the significance of these mutations in the pathogenesis of IBD remains to be determined.

Abnormalities in the relation between intestinal microbes and the immune system are one of the hallmarks in IBD. These abnormal responses could be related to an abnormal intestinal bacterial milieu, to host abnormalities, or to both. Some of the abnormal immune responses are related to an abnormal bacterial population that causes either a decreased production of protective intestinal byproducts such as short chain fatty acids or an increased production of harmful by-products. Some of the abnormalities related to the host are an increased intestinal wall permeability that allows bacteria or bacterial products to enter the portal circulation.

PATHOGENESIS

As discussed previously, the cause of IBD remains unknown. A genetic predisposition for the disease exists, and there are still unknown environmental factors that trigger the disease. Whereas in 75% to 90% of patients no family history of IBD is present, 10% to 25% have a first-degree relative with the disease. IBD inheritance does not follow a Mendelian pattern, and the lifetime risk of IBD among first-degree relatives of patients is 3 to 20 times higher than in the rest of the population, namely, 9% for offspring and siblings, and 3.5% for parents. Patients with a positive family history of IBD present at a younger age. The concordance rate for Crohn's disease in family members is greater than for UC.

The bacterial population in the gastrointestinal tract varies according to the anatomical location; in the proximal gastrointestinal tract most of the bacteria are aerobes and in the distal gastrointestinal tract, most of the bacteria are anaerobes.

There is also a gradient in the number of microbes in the gastrointestinal tract with the lowest number in the stomach, where the load is 0 to 10^2 and composed predominantly by *Lactobacillus*, *Candida*, *Streptococcus*, and *Peptostreptococcus*; to the distal ileum, where the microbial load is 10^7 to 10^8 and the predominant bacteria are *Clostridium*, *Streptococcus*, *Bacteroides*, *Actinomycinae*, and *Corynebacteria*; to the colon, where the microbial load is 10^{11} to 10^{12} and the predominant bacteria include *Bacteroides*, *Clostridium*, *Bifidobacterium*, and *Enterobacteriaceae*. The total microbial load of the intestine is estimated to be 10^{13} to 10^{14} micro-organisms, and 30% of the stool weight is composed of dead bacteria.

Bacteria in the lumen trigger a series of responses by epithelial cells, macrophages, dendritic cells, T lymphocytes, and B cells. This homeostasis depends on the activation and downregulation of the immune response. A detailed review of the regulation of the immune response is beyond the scope of this chapter, but it is important to mention some of the determinants of such response that include bacterial recognition by toll-like receptors and intracellular NOD-like receptors, production and inactivation of different pathways and proteins such as nuclear factor-B, interferon, interleukins, defensins, prostaglandins, etc. The gastrointestinal system is in a constant state of controlled inflammation because it is continuously exposed to luminal antigens. Therefore, it seems logical that a luminal antigen or antigens can trigger an abnormal inflammatory response. These antigens may be dietary, infectious, or environmental. It is possible that the trigger antigen or antigens are bacterial products such as bacterial wall components, or related to a dysbiosis of the normal intestinal microflora. Even though no unique bacterial abnormality has been identified in IBD, it is clear that bacteria play a major role in the pathogenesis of IBD. This is supported by animal models of IBD, where the disease is not manifested as long as the animal is in a germfree environment.

Whatever the trigger or triggers may be, the mucosal activation of macrophages leads to increased release of proinflammatory cytokines (i.e., IL-1, tumor necrosis factor [TNF]-α, IL-6, IL-8), which in turn results in cell destruction through different mechanisms (including clonal expansion of natural killer cells and cytotoxic T cells); B-cell proliferation (with increased production of mucosal IgG); and increased production of thromboxane A2, leukotriene B, and platelet-activating factor (i.e., proinflammatory mediators that amplify the inflammatory response by recruiting and activating neutrophils).

RISK FACTORS

All populations are at risk, but there are some groups that have a higher risk of developing IBD. Until recently, the incidence of IBD in the United States was greater in Caucasians than in any other ethnic group; however, in a recent report from a large insurance database, the incidence in Americans of African descent and Americans of European descent was similar, and the incidence in Asian and Hispanic descents was lower. The population at greater risk for IBD is Ashkenazi Jews living in Europe and in the United States. In this group, there is a two- to fourfold higher risk for UC and a six- to eightfold higher risk for Crohn's disease compared to the general population living in the same areas. Interestingly, Ashkenazi Jews in Israel have a lower risk of IBD than those in Europe or the United States. This supports the role of environmental factors in the development of IBD. The role of environmental factors is also supported by a rise in the incidence of IBD in ethnic populations that have migrated. In British Columbia, Canada, there has been a sharp rise in the frequency of pediatric IBD in children of Asian ancestry. An interesting association also exists between cigarette smoking and IBD. A larger-than-expected number of patients with Crohn's disease are

cigarette smokers, whereas a lower-than-expected number of patients with UC are cigarette smokers.

Ulcerative Colitis

Clinical Features

The clinical presentation of UC depends primarily on the extent and the severity of the disease. The clinical presentation is also influenced by the age of the patient. The presentation of UC in children is usually with severe and extensive disease, whereas adults usually have milder disease limited to the left colon. In 30% of adults, the disease is limited to the rectum only, and in 60%, it is distal to the splenic flexure. Patients with UC usually present with nonbloody diarrhea that progresses to bloody diarrhea. If the disease involves only the rectum, patients have fecal urgency, tenesmus, and frequent passage of bloody mucus per rectum, but rarely have systemic symptoms. Patients with disease to the splenic flexure have nonbloody diarrhea that becomes bloody over days to weeks. These patients can also have mild systemic symptoms such as malaise and mild abdominal pain, but they are rarely febrile or have weight loss. Patients with more extensive disease are more likely to have severe or fulminant presentations. Less than 15% of patients have a severe or fulminant attack on presentation, but a significant number of these patients undergo colectomy within 1 year of presentation. The mortality rate from the initial attack is <0.5%, but if the patient has severe disease with perforation, the mortality rate is 50%. Massive hemorrhage is rare in UC patients occurring in more than 3% of patients. These patients frequently need urgent colectomy.

Diagnosis

The diagnosis of UC relies on the clinical picture, stool testing, endoscopic appearance, histologic findings, and occasional serologic tests. To provide optimal medical treatment and establish the prognosis, it is important to determine the extent of disease. Histology is the most sensitive way of establishing the extent of the disease, and unless there is a contraindication, a colonoscopy with biopsies is indicated in all patients in whom UC is suspected. In patients with severe or fulminant disease, a limited examination is sufficient. At the time of proctosigmoidoscopy, aspirates of luminal contents can be done for microbiology testing, and biopsies can be obtained for histologic evaluation and stains for cytomegalovirus (CMV). Furthermore, the endoscopic appearance helps guide therapeutic decisions. If there are deep longitudinal ulcers, then the response rate to medical treatment is poor, and early surgery is the best treatment. The response to medical treatment is based on symptoms, physical examination, and laboratory; it is not necessary to repeat a colonoscopy to assess the response to medical treatment.

Stool Tests

Stool studies to exclude bacterial and parasitic infections are indicated at the time of initial presentation. The most common infectious agents that mimic IBD include *Salmonella* species, *Shigella* species, *Campylobacter* species, *Clostridium difficile*, *Yersinia* species, and *Escherichia coli* O157:H7. In populations at risk for infections with *Entamoeba histolytica*, *Strongyloides*, *Mycobacterium avium* complex, or viral infections such as CMV, it is important to do specific tests to exclude the presence of an infection. Treatment with corticosteroids or other immunosuppressive medications in these patients leads to severe complications. Whenever a patient has a "flare-up" or does not respond to medical treatment, it is important to do tests to exclude *C. difficile* infection.

Endoscopy

Rectal involvement is almost universal in untreated patients with UC. The earliest endoscopic findings in patients with UC are blunting of the blood vessel pattern, decreased light reflection, and hyperemia. In patients with more severe inflammation, the mucosa becomes granular and friable, and, finally, with severe disease, the mucosa is ulcerated, and there are frequently mucosal exudates and blood in the intestinal lumen. The mucosa is diffusely involved in a continuous fashion. With long-standing disease, the rectum loses compliance, and the colon becomes tubular in appearance. Inflammatory polyps are frequently seen when the mucosal inflammation subsides. A sharp demarcation between diseased and healthy mucosa may also be seen (Fig. 56.1).

Radiology

The main role of radiologic tests in patients with UC is to exclude complications associated with severe or fulminant

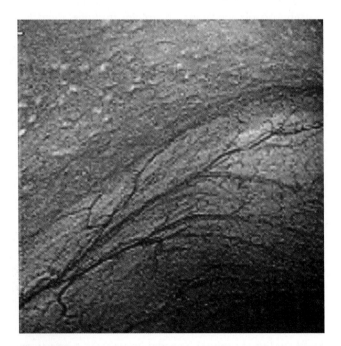

Figure 56.1 Line of demarcation in ulcerative colitis. (See Color Fig. 56.1.)

disease. Such complications include intestinal perforation, colonic dilatation, or pneumatosis coli. Patients taking immunosuppressive medications have a delayed symptomatic presentation when these complications occur, and a plain film of the abdomen is sufficient to exclude such complications. In patients with long-standing UC, the rectal compliance and the haustral folds are lost, and the colon is shortened and narrow ("stem pipe colon"). Pseudopolyps and strictures are visualized in double-contrast enema testing and in CT enterography. If a stricture or a perforation is suspected, patients should undergo a water-soluble contrast enema rather than a barium enema. If a stricture is present, the barium dehydrates and solidifies; if a perforation is present, the barium induces an inflammatory response, it is difficult to remove, and future radiologic tests will be obscured by the remaining barium in the abdominal cavity. When a stricture is found, it is important to exclude malignancy.

Histology

The inflammatory changes in UC are primarily confined to the mucosa. The main findings are cryptitis with crypt abscesses and goblet cell depletion, and an increased number of neutrophils, lymphocytes, plasma cells, and macrophages. In patients with chronic disease, architectural distortion occurs, with crypt atrophy and shortened glands that lose their normal "test tube array" appearance.

Severity

Truelove and Witts proposed a classification of severity based on symptoms and laboratory tests (Table 56.1). This classification is useful to determine severity and establish optimal treatment. Since the initial validation of this index, few modifications have been made, and this includes the addition of endoscopic criteria. There are numerous indices to determine disease severity, but the main use of these indices is in the standardization of clinical trials. A skilled clinician can determine the disease severity by history and physical examination, and with the use of appropriate laboratory and radiologic studies. An ambulatory patient seen in the office that does not have significant systemic symptoms such as fever, abdominal pain, weight loss, and signs or symptoms of dehydration has mild disease. A patient with weight loss, who is complaining of abdominal pain and nocturnal bowel movements, and who is tachycardic and/or febrile has severe disease.

Prognosis

Most patients with UC have intermittent attacks, with remissions lasting from a few weeks to many years. At presentation, 5% to 10% have a severe attack that requires urgent colectomy, and 10% to 15% of patients have chronic active disease. The course and prognosis are largely determined by the extent of the disease. In 50% to 70% of patients presenting with proctitis, the disease remains confined to the rectum; in the other patients, the disease extends

TABLE 56.1

SEVERITY CRITERIA FOR ULCERATIVE COLITIS, MODIFIED

	Mild	Severe	Fulminant
Stool frequency	<4/day	>6/day	>10/day or no bowel movements
Blood in stool	Small amounts	Macroscopic with all bowel movements	Continuous
Temperature	No fever	>37.8°C on 2 of 4 days	>37.8°C
Heart rate	Normal	>90	>90
Hemoglobin	Normal	<75% of normal (12 g/dL)	Transfusion requiring
Erythrocyte sedimentation rate	<30 mm/hr	>30 mm/hr	>30 mm/hr
Radiography	Normal	Thumbprinting	Edematous, dilated
Clinical signs	Normal or mild tenderness	Abdominal tenderness	Abdominal distention, absent bowel sounds, tenderness

Moderate: between mild and severe.
Modified with permission from Truelove SC, Witts LJ. Cortisone in ulcerative colitis. *BMJ* 1955;1:1041–1048.

proximally. With every "flare-up," there is about 60% risk of progression of the disease. The rate of colectomy in the first year in patients with severe diseases is as high as 30%. The risk that colectomy will eventually be required is greater in patients with pancolitis than in patients with limited disease. After the first year, the colectomy rate is 1% per year.

Patients with UC have an increased risk of colorectal cancer. The risk depends on the duration and extent of disease, compliance with medical treatment and surveillance colonoscopy, comorbid conditions such as primary sclerosing cholangitis, and family history. The risk of colorectal cancer increases after 7 years of presentation in patients with pancolitis, and it has been estimated to increase by 0.5% to 1% per year after 15 or 20 years. In patients with left-sided UC, the risk of colorectal cancer is also increased, but this risk begins after 10 to 15 years of presentation. Patients with proctitis have no increased risk of colon cancer compared to the general population and do not require surveillance.

In UC patients, dysplasia can be detected prior to the development of cancer. For this reason, patients who have pancolitis for more than 7 years are advised to undergo surveillance colonoscopies with biopsies. There are different recommendations in regard to the frequency of colonoscopy and biopsies in these patients. Four-quadrant biopsies are obtained at 10-cm intervals, and extra biopsies are taken from suspicious areas, such as strictures or masses. If no dysplasia is found in the biopsies, then the colonoscopy is repeated at 1- to 3-year intervals. The finding of dysplasia should be confirmed by a second expert pathologist. If high-grade dysplasia is found, colectomy is recommended. There is no agreement on whether to recommend colectomy for patients with low-grade dysplasia. If colectomy is not done, then patients should be closely followed up with colonoscopies and biopsies every 3 to 6 months until there is no dysplasia (in which case patients return to yearly surveillance), or if there is progression to high-grade dysplasia, then colectomy is indicated. Because of sampling error, however, dysplasia may be missed using

this approach. The author views dysplasia—whether low or high grade—as premalignant and advises colectomy.

Crohn's Disease

Crohn's disease is a heterogeneous disease that has different clinical presentations, which are determined by the site of involvement and the type of disease (inflammatory, stricturing, or fistulizing). In Crohn's disease, any segment of the gastrointestinal tract can be involved, but the most common distribution is ileocolic disease that is seen in 50% of patients, small bowel involvement alone occurs in 30%, and colonic involvement alone in 20% of the patients. Esophageal and gastroduodenal involvement occurs in 0.5% to 4.0% of patients. Most patients with gastroduodenal involvement also have evidence of Crohn's disease in other segments of the gastrointestinal tract. Clinically, Crohn's disease can be inflammatory, stenotic, fistulizing, or mixed. The signs, symptoms, and treatment depend on the site of involvement and disease behavior.

Clinical Presentation

Patients with ileocolitis usually present with nonbloody diarrhea, crampy abdominal pain (usually worse after meals), weight loss, and low-grade fever, and may also have an inflammatory mass. The onset of symptoms is usually subacute, but it can be acute and confused with appendicitis. On examination, patients are pale, bowel sounds can be decreased, and tenderness to palpation is present in the right lower quadrant of the abdomen, where a palpable mass may be present. More than 90% of patients with ileocecal disease eventually require surgery. The most common indications for surgery are fistulae, abscess, or obstruction.

Crohn's disease of the small intestine was seen more commonly in the terminal ileum. This has changed, and there are more patients that have jejunal Crohn's or extensive disease in the jejunum and ileum. Patients with extensive disease present with diarrhea, abdominal pain suggestive of incomplete small bowel obstruction, and weight loss. Patients with jejunal involvement have abdominal pain, malabsorption, and steatorrhea.

Patients with Crohn's disease of the colon usually have inflammatory disease and present with diarrhea, abdominal pain, and weight loss. Obstruction may occur because of strictures and/or fistulae. When patients need surgery, differentiating Crohn's colitis from UC is of primary importance. In 10% to 15% of patients, however, a specific diagnosis cannot be established; such patients are classified as having "indeterminate colitis." Approximately 50% of patients with Crohn's colitis require surgery, and the most common indications are perianal disease and obstruction. Perianal disease occurs in 30% of patients with Crohn's disease, and approximately 10% of female patients with Crohn's colitis develop rectovaginal fistulas.

Gastroduodenal Crohn's disease may be difficult to distinguish from peptic ulcer disease and nonsteroidal anti-inflammatory drugs (NSAIDs) gastropathy. These patients usually present with nausea, vomiting, and abdominal pain that improves with use of antacids. Gastric outlet obstruction occurs in approximately 30% of patients in this group and is the most common indication for surgery. Patients may develop gastrocolic fistulae, and these usually originate from the colon rather than the stomach. Patients with gastrocolic fistulae frequently have diarrhea, malabsorption, weight loss, and feculent emesis, and may see undigested food in the stool. Rectal and perianal disease can occur without colonic involvement and, at times, before evidence of Crohn's disease is present elsewhere in the gastrointestinal tract. Not infrequently, the symptoms from perianal disease are the most disturbing to patients and are difficult to treat.

Patients with extensive Crohn's disease of the colon have an increased risk of colorectal cancer similar to patients with UC. There are no established guidelines for surveillance in these patients, and it is adequate to follow guidelines similar to those for patients with UC.

Diagnosis

The diagnosis of Crohn's disease is based on clinical, laboratory, radiologic, endoscopic, and histologic criteria. The clinical presentation (described previously) depends on the site of involvement and disease behavior. Physical examination may be normal or may reveal pallor, muscle wasting, palpable right lower quadrant mass, or evidence of perianal disease, such as skin tags, fissures, or fistulae.

Laboratory Testing

Laboratory tests reflect the chronic nature of the disease, and are important to rule out conditions that either mimic or complicate Crohn's disease, such as infections or parasitic enteritis or colitis. Patients are frequently anemic and have leukocytosis, thrombocytosis, and an elevated erythrocyte sedimentation rate or C-reactive protein (CRP). The role of serologic tests in the diagnosis of Crohn's disease is a subject of debate, and a diagnosis of Crohn's

disease cannot be reliably established based only on a positive serology.

Radiology

Contrast studies play a major role in the diagnosis of small bowel and gastroduodenal Crohn's disease. In gastroduodenal Crohn's disease, antral narrowing and duodenal strictures occur. The small intestine is well visualized using a small bowel series; in fact, a dedicated small bowel series provides better mucosal detail than an upper gastrointestinal series with small bowel follow-through. Small bowel enema testing is indicated in very few patients. The findings on radiographs include mucosal ulceration, loop separation, strictures, fistulas, and cobblestoning. The new imaging modalities such as CT enterography and MR enterography are superior to small bowel series in demonstrating intestinal abnormalities. These modalities also delineate the perineum, and help in the diagnosis of complications such as abscesses and fistulae.

Endoscopy

Endoscopic procedures such as colonoscopy and esophagogastroduodenoscopy (EGD) are frequently done to visualize and sample the mucosa (Fig. 56.2). On endoscopy, there are skip lesions, these are areas of abnormal mucosa with intervening normal mucosa. Patients with Crohn's disease may have rectal sparing, and multiple ulcers of different sizes, shapes, and depths can be seen. Aphthoid ulcers are frequently seen in Crohn's disease, but similar lesions can also be seen as a result of the use of some laxatives prior to colonoscopy. Aphthoid ulcers are 3 to 5 mm in size and have a red halo surrounding a white center. The mucosa

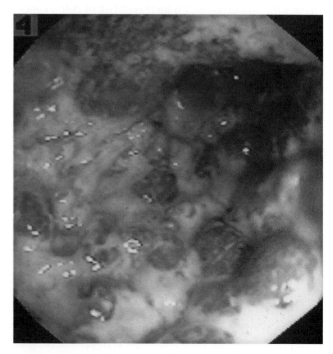

Figure 56.2   Severe Crohn's disease. (See Color Fig. 56.2.)

can have a "cobblestoned" appearance on endoscopy and in contrast x-rays. Fistulae can be seen, but imaging studies are a better diagnostic modality. A video capsule endoscopy may show subtle lesions in the small intestine in areas that are not accessible by endoscopy; however, some of the lesions can be caused by the use of medications such as NSAIDs, ischemia, or radiation.

Differential Features of Ulcerative Colitis and Crohn's Disease

Distinguishing UC from Crohn's disease can be difficult, especially in patients with fulminant colitis or in patients who have only colonic disease (Table 56.2). Histopathological examination can be useful in making this distinction. The histologic findings seen in Crohn's disease, but not in UC, are noncaseating granulomas, skip lesions, and transmural involvement. A number of serologic tests have been described in patients with IBD, and the value of these tests may be in prognosticating disease behavior rather than in the diagnosis of the disease. Perinuclear antineutrophil cytoplasmic antibodies (pANCAs) are more commonly seen in UC; when positive, these are associated with refractory disease and a higher incidence of pouchitis after surgery. When pANCAs are seen in Crohn's disease, they are associated with left-sided colonic disease that endoscopic ally cannot be differentiated from UC, and better response to treatment. Anti–*Saccharomyces cerevisiae* antibodies (ASCAs) are more commonly seen in Crohn's disease. Patients with Crohn's disease that are ASCA+/pANCA −

have more aggressive disease with strictures and fistula. Other antibodies that have been described are OmpC IgA antibody directed against the outer membrane protein C of *E. coli*, and anti-CBir1 that is a flagellinlike antigen associated with the presence of IBD. The principal differential diagnoses for IBD are infectious enteritis or colitis, ischemia, radiation enteritis, lymphoma, Behçet disease, endometriosis, diverticulitis, and enteropathy or colopathy induced by NSAIDs. A careful history, physical examination, and laboratory tests are critical to exclude conditions that mimic IBD.

Extraintestinal Manifestations

About 50% to 60% of patients with IBD have extraintestinal manifestations (EIMs), and about 25% have more than 1 EIM. Today, more than 100 EIMs have been described. Some parallel the disease activity, whereas others follow course independent of disease activity. EIMs occur more frequently in patients with colonic disease. The EIMs that parallel disease activity include:

- Peripheral arthritis
- Erythema nodosum
- Pyoderma gangrenosum
- Keratoconjunctivitis
- Episcleritis
- Hypercoagulability (if related to thrombocytosis and acute-phase reactants, not if it is related to primary abnormalities in the coagulation system such as protein S, C deficiency, or factor V Leiden mutations)

TABLE 56.2

DIFFERENTIAL FEATURES OF ULCERATIVE COLITIS AND CROHN'S DISEASE

Clinical Features	Ulcerative Colitis	Crohn's Disease
Rectal bleeding	Usual	Sometimes
Abdominal mass	Absent	Often
Perianal disease	Extremely rare	30%
Upper gastrointestinal symptoms	Unrelated	Frequent
Malnutrition	Rare, mild	Frequent, moderate to severe
Endoscopic and radiologic		
Rectal involvement	Present	Variable
Continuous disease	Always	Rare
Discrete linear ulcers	Rare	Frequent
Aphthoid ulcers	Absent	Common
Cobblestoning	Absent	Common
Skip areas	Absent	Common
Small bowel disease	Absent[a]	Common
Fistulas	Absent	Common
Pathology		
Aphthous ulcers	Absent	Common
Noncaseating granulomas	Absent	10%–30%
Crypt abscess	Common	Frequent
Transmural involvement	Absent	Present
Microscopic skip lesions	Absent	Frequent

[a] Except in backwash ileitis.

Extraintestinal manifestations that run a course independent of disease activity include:

- Ankylosing spondylitis, which more commonly occurs in patients with UC who are HLA-B27 positive
- Sacroiliitis
- Primary sclerosing cholangitis
- Uveitis

Arthritis

The arthritis of IBD is nonerosive, mono- or pauciarticular, asymmetric, and migratory. No synovial destruction is present, and large joints are more commonly affected than small joints. Peripheral arthritis is more common in female patients and correlates with disease activity. Axial arthritis (ankylosing spondylitis) is associated with the presence of HLA-B27 and does not correlate with disease activity.

Skin and Eye Disorders

Erythema nodosum occurs in approximately 3% of patients with IBD. It is characterized by the presence of tender subcutaneous nodules that generally occur along the shins. The area affected is erythematous and exquisitely sensitive to touch.

Pyoderma gangrenosum is characterized by the presence of an ulcerating lesion that becomes purulent and necrotic, and, when it heals, leaves a scar. Commonly found at sites of minimal trauma, these lesions occur both in UC and Crohn's disease. Treatment frequently involves immunosuppressive therapy.

The ocular manifestations of IBD include iritis, keratoconjunctivitis, episcleritis, and uveitis. Patients with uveitis are usually HLA-B27+. The symptoms of uveitis are blurred vision, photophobia, and a painful eye. Some ocular manifestations are medical emergencies, and patients should be evaluated promptly by an ophthalmologist.

Liver Disease

Cholestatic liver disease is the most common manifestation of hepatic involvement in patients with IBD. It occurs in 5% of patients, and it does not parallel disease activity. PSC occurs in 1% to 5% of patients with UC and rarely in patients with Crohn's colitis. The course of PSC is independent of disease activity; PSC can appear either before the diagnosis of UC or be present years after colectomy for UC. In most patients, early diagnosis depends on the detection of biochemical abnormalities, such as an elevated alkaline phosphatase level. The levels of alkaline phosphatase can fluctuate and can even return to normal in patients with established PSC. During the late stages of disease, PSC can be complicated by cholangiocarcinoma.

Treatment of Inflammatory Bowel Disease

The goals of medical treatment in IBD are to improve symptoms, decrease complications, decrease the need for surgical intervention, improve nutrition, and improve the pa-

tient's quality of life. Treatment can be divided into two phases: therapy for the acute attack (induction of remission), and maintenance of remission.

Pharmacologic Treatment

Medications used to treat patients with IBD include:

- 5-Aminosalicylic acid (5-ASA)
- Antibiotics
- Corticosteroids
- Immunosuppressive medications
- Biological medications

5-Aminosalicylic Acid

The 5-ASA drugs (Table 56.3) are anti-inflammatory agents that act at the mucosal level and decrease inflammation, possibly by inhibiting the formation of both prostaglandin and leukotriene metabolites. These medications are used for induction and maintenance of remission in patients with mild to moderately active UC. The effectiveness of 5-ASA in the treatment of Crohn's disease is minimal. In a recent meta-analysis by Hanauer et al., it was determined that even though there is a numerical improvement in the disease activity index compared to placebo, the clinical significance of the administration of 5-ASA 4 g/day was smaller than that needed to establish clinical efficacy.

The therapeutic effect of 5-ASA is topical, not systemic. For the medication to be effective, it must be delivered to the site of disease. 5-ASA is rapidly absorbed in the proximal small bowel, acetylated by the liver, and excreted in the urine. To prevent proximal absorption and allow the 5-ASA to exert its anti-inflammatory effect at the site of inflammation, different delivery methods are available, including the following:

- Creating a larger molecule by binding it to a carrier or another 5-ASA via an azo-bond
- Coating 5-ASA with a pH-sensitive resin
- Using delayed-release preparations

Other 5-ASA preparations currently used are in the form of suppositories and enemas. Suppositories effectively induce remission in patients with ulcerative proctitis; the recommended dosage is 1 g/day for 4 to 6 weeks. Enemas effectively induce remission in patients with proctosigmoiditis; the recommended dosage is 4 g in 60 mL of liquid at bedtime for 4 to 6 weeks. Both suppositories and enemas can maintain remission in patients with ulcerative proctitis or proctosigmoiditis. Topical 5-ASA is more effective than corticosteroids in inducing remission in patients with distal disease.

Azo-Bond Compounds

Sulfasalazine is a 5-ASA molecule bound to sulfapyridine by an azo-bond. It was the first 5-ASA preparation found to be effective in the treatment of IBD. Sulfapyridine serves as a carrier and has no therapeutic effect. The azo-bond

TABLE 56.3

Formulation	U.S. Food and Drug Administration Indication	Common Use and Dose
Azo-compounds		
Sulfasalazine Tablet: 500 mg Azulfidine: 500 mg Tablet, delayed release: 500 mg Azulfidine EN-tabs Tablet, enteric coated: 500 mg Sulfazine EC	Induction and maintenance of remission in mild to moderately active ulcerative colitis Dosing: 2–4 g/day for induction of remission, 1–2 g/day for maintenance	Induction of remission in mild to moderately active ulcerative colitis: 2–6 g/day Maintenance of remission: 2–4 g/day +Folic acid 1 mg/day in all patients Minimal clinical efficacy in Crohn's disease
Olsalazine Capsule: Dipentum: 250 mg	Maintenance of remission of ulcerative colitis in patients intolerant of sulfasalazine 500 mg PO BID with food	Induction and maintenance of remission in mild to moderately active ulcerative colitis in patients allergic to or intolerant of sulfasalazine 500 mg daily PO BID with meals
Balsalazide disodium capsule: Colazal: 750 mg (contains sodium ~86 mg/capsule)	Mild to moderately active ulcerative colitis 2.25 g (three 750-mg capsules) three times/day for 8–12 weeks	Induction and maintenance of remission in mild to moderately ulcerative colitis 2.25 g (three 750-mg capsules) three times/day
pH-sensitive preparations		
Mesalamine, polymer-coated Asacol: 400 mg	Induction of remission in mild to moderately active ulcerative colitis—800 mg three times/day for 6 weeks Maintenance of remission—1.6 g/day in divided doses	Induction and maintenance of remission in mild to moderately active ulcerative colitis: 2.4–4.8 g/day
Multi-Matrix System tablets Lialda 1.2 g	Induction of remission in patients with active ulcerative colitis—2.4–4.8 g once daily for up to 8 weeks	Induction and maintenance of remission in ulcerative colitis: 2.4–4.8 g once daily with food
Delayed-release preparations		
Controlled-release mesalamine, ethylcellulose-coated capsule Pentasa: 250 mg, 500 mg	Induction and maintenance of remission in patients with ulcerative colitis—1 g four times/day	Induction and maintenance of remission in patients with ulcerative colitis—1 g four times/day Minimal effect in Crohn's ileocolitis

is split by an azo-reductase that is produced by colonic bacteria. A therapeutic effect from sulfasalazine is seen in 60% to 80% of patients with mild or moderate UC. The therapeutic dosage is 4 to 6 g daily, divided in four doses. To improve tolerance, the drug is started at a low dose (e.g., 500 mg three or four times a day) and gradually increased. Thirty percent of patients are either allergic to or intolerant of sulfapyridine and require discontinuation of sulfasalazine therapy. The most common side effects include headache, nausea, anorexia, oligospermia, and dyspepsia; less common side effects include skin rash, pruritus, urticaria, and hemolytic anemia. Rarely, patients can develop life-threatening reactions, such as agranulocytosis or anaphylactic reactions. Because sulfapyridine decreases folic acid absorption by competitive inhibition, patients receiving sulfasalazine should take supplemental folic acid (0.4–1.0 mg/day). Sulfasalazine is especially useful in patients with enteropathic arthritis, given that this is usually responsive to this agent and not to 5-ASA alone. Intolerance and allergy to sulfasalazine is usually related to the sulfapyridine rather than to the 5-ASA; therefore, a 5-ASA

compound that does not contain sulfapyridine can be used in these patients. Olsalazine sodium (Dipentum) is a 5-ASA that is bound by an azo-bond to another molecule of 5-ASA. It is safe for patients who are allergic to sulfa. Unfortunately, as many as 17% of patients taking olsalazine develop a secretory diarrhea; this side effect can be minimized by taking the olsalazine with meals.

pH-Sensitive Preparations

There are two pH-sensitive preparations, Asacol and Lialda, available in the United States. Asacol is 5-ASA coated with a methacrylic acid copolymer B (called Eudragit-S) that dissolves at pH 7.0 (i.e., the pH in the distal ileum and the colon). The recommended dose in patients with mild or moderately active UC is 2.4 g/24 hours divided in three or four doses. Tolerance is good, and some patients that do not respond to low dose may respond to a higher dose (i.e., 4.8–6.0 g/24 hours). Asacol is usually well tolerated, but some patients can have diarrhea, headache, or hair loss.

The other pH-sensitive preparation is Lialda; this is a high-strength formulation that has 1.2 g of 5-ASA and uses a Multi-Matrix System technology designed to release 5-ASA throughout the colon. This patented delivery system uses hydrophilic and lipophilic matrices enclosed within a gastroresistant, pH-dependent coating to facilitate prolonged exposure of the colonic mucosa to 5-ASA. One of the advantages of this medication is that it is taken once a day with food, and because it is a high-strength formulation, patients take fewer tablets. Noncompliance is a big problem in IBD patients; it has been reported that as many as 60% of patients stop the medication when they are in clinical remission. Two of the factors commonly cited by patients are the number of tablets and having to take multiple doses per day.

Delayed-Release Preparations

The only delayed-release preparation currently available is Pentasa, which is an ethylcellulose-coated mesalamine preparation that releases 5-ASA throughout the small intestine and the colon. Pentasa is approved by the U.S. Food and Drug Administration (FDA) for use in patients with UC. The effectiveness of this medication in induction of remission in Crohn's disease patients has been contradictory, and in a recent meta-analysis, it was concluded that even though there is a numeric improvement in the disease activity index, its therapeutic effect is unclear. Based on the current information available, it is difficult to recommend the use of Pentasa for the treatment of patients with active Crohn's disease.

Antibiotics

Primary treatment with antibiotics is indicated only in patients with Crohn's disease. Controlled data are available for metronidazole and ciprofloxacin. Metronidazole is effective in patients with Crohn's colitis or perianal disease. The most common side effects leading to discontinuation of metronidazole are gastrointestinal intolerance and peripheral neuropathy. Long-term metronidazole use during pregnancy is contraindicated because of the risk of cleft palate; in addition, all patients should be warned of its potential interaction with alcohol (Antabuse). Patients intolerant to metronidazole can take ciprofloxacin with similar results. In controlled studies, ciprofloxacin was as effective as mesalamine in inducing remission, and the benefit of such intervention lasted 6 to 9 months. Combination treatment using metronidazole and ciprofloxacin is very effective. Other antibiotics, such as clarithromycin, trimethoprim-sulfamethoxazole, or tetracycline, can be tried in patients intolerant of or allergic to metronidazole and ciprofloxacin. Antibiotics may also improve symptoms by treating small intestinal bacterial overgrowth.

Corticosteroids

Corticosteroids play a significant role in the medical treatment of IBD. Corticosteroids are indicated in patients with moderate or severely active UC or Crohn's disease and in patients who fail to respond to 5-ASA or antibiotics. Because of side effects, physicians do not like to prescribe them, and patients do not like to take them. Corticosteroids should not be used for maintenance of remission, not only because of side effects, but also because they do not alter the natural history of the disease. The recommended dose of oral prednisolone or prednisone for adults is 40 to 60 mg/day; in pediatric patients, the dose is 1 mg/kg/day. Once remission is achieved, the dose of corticosteroids is decreased slowly (i.e., 5 mg every 5–7 days). An initial response occurs in 60% to 80% of patients; however, at least 20% do not improve, and another 20% become steroid dependent. With subsequent use, the response to corticosteroids decreases. If there is no significant improvement after 5 to 7 days of starting oral corticosteroids, patients should be admitted to the hospital and treated with either intravenous steroids or other medications.

Patients with more severe attacks are best treated in the hospital with intravenous corticosteroids. Hydrocortisone and methylprednisolone are equally effective. The usual dose of hydrocortisone is 300 mg/24 hours. If the patient fails to respond in 5 to 7 days, surgery or other medical treatments should be considered.

Budesonide is a very potent anti-inflammatory steroid that has a high first-pass rate metabolism in the liver. Because of this, systemic side effects are usually less pronounced, but this does not mean that their use is entirely free of risks. Even in the absence of side effects, with long-term use there is adrenal axis suppression and risk of osteoporosis. Budesonide is available in a formulation that releases the drug in the distal ileum, and at 9 mg/day, its effectiveness in inducing remission is similar to that of prednisone. However, symptomatic improvement occurs later compared to prednisone, this is likely related to fewer side effects such as improved energy and appetite that occur with prednisone. In a maintenance trial, budesonide at 6 mg/day was not more effective than placebo in maintaining remission.

Steroid enemas are useful in patients with ulcerative proctosigmoiditis, and budesonide is as effective as conventional corticosteroids and has fewer short- and long-term side effects. Neither a corticosteroid enema nor budesonide is as effective as topical 5-ASA for patients with limited distal disease. Furthermore, budesonide enemas are not available for clinical use in the United States.

Corticosteroids have significant short- and long-term toxicity. Some of the side effects include osteoporosis, moon face, buffalo hump, striae, posterior subcapsular cataracts, aseptic necrosis of bones, glaucoma, immunosuppression, hyperglycemia, acne, mood swings, insomnia, weight gain, and adrenal insufficiency. Arrest of growth occurs in children, but this can be lessened by administering corticosteroids on alternate days. Patients should be informed of the potential risks of corticosteroids and should wear an alert bracelet. Patients should also be warned of the severe risks of sudden discontinuation of cortico-steroids to prevent adrenal crisis.

Biological Agents

Biological agents that block TNF-α are indicated in IBD patients who have refractory disease. Patients with IBD have elevated levels of TNF-α in the colon, blood, and feces. Because TNF-α is a proinflammatory cytokine, it seems logical that blocking its action would have beneficial effects in these patients. Infliximab is a chimeric monoclonal TNF-α antibody that was approved by the FDA in August 1998 for use in adult patients with Crohn's disease. The initial approval was for the "Treatment of moderately to severely active Crohn's disease for the reduction of the signs and symptoms in patients who have an inadequate response to conventional therapies; and treatment of patients with fistulizing Crohn's disease for the reduction in the number of draining enterocutaneous fistula(s)." The approval was based on two clinical trials, one reported by Targan et al. and the other by Rutgeerts et al. Based on the results of the clinical trials, infliximab 5 mg/kg was used as a single dose in patients with active Crohn's disease. For patients with fistula, the dose was 5 mg/kg at 0, 2, and 6 weeks. Because infliximab was used on an episodic basis, a significant proportion of patients developed anti-infliximab antibodies, resulting in infusion reactions and loss of response. Two subsequent clinical trials, "A Crohn's Disease Clinical Trial Evaluating Infliximab in a New Long-Term Treatment Regimen" ACCENT I and ACCENT II demonstrated the effectiveness of infliximab in maintenance of remission when infliximab was administered every 8 weeks. Based on these trials, the FDA approved the use of infliximab in 2003 "for maintenance of remission in patients with inflammatory or fistulizing disease."

Infliximab was initially approved for use only in adults. In 2006, based on the results from the REACH trial, the FDA approved the use of infliximab in children "with moderately to severely active Crohn's disease, who have had an inadequate response to conventional therapy." The REACH trial was a randomized, multicenter, open-label study designed to evaluate the safety and efficacy of infliximab in pediatric patients with moderate to severe Crohn's disease. One hundred and twelve patients were enrolled; all received the usual induction regimen with infliximab, 5 mg/kg at 0, 2, and 6 weeks. The response rate to this regimen was 88% at week 10. Patients with a response were then randomized to receive infliximab every 8 weeks ($n = 52$) or every 12 weeks ($n = 51$) through week 46. At 54 weeks, the clinical response was maintained in 63% of the patients receiving infliximab every 8 weeks, and 56% maintained clinical. In the group receiving infliximab every 12 weeks, the response rate and remission rates were significantly lower. Importantly, by week 54, 75% of the children receiving infliximab every 8 weeks were able to discontinue steroids. In this study, the response to infliximab was superior to the response rates

seen in adults. This has brought up the notion that using infliximab earlier in the course of the disease may improve long-term outcomes.

The initial studies on the use of infliximab were in patients with Crohn's disease. Between March 2002 and March 2005, there were two multicenter clinical trials on the use of infliximab in patients with active UC. These clinical trials are known as "Active Ulcerative Colitis Trial" ACT 1 and ACT 2. ACT 1 had 62 sites and a total of 364 patients, and ACT 2 had 55 sites and 364 patients were entered in the trial. The subjects in these trials were patients with moderately to severely active UC despite treatment with corticosteroids with or without azathioprine or 6-mercaptopurine. The design was straightforward; patients were randomly assigned to receive either placebo, infliximab 5 mg/kg, or infliximab 10 mg/kg in a 1:1:1 ratio at weeks 0, 2, and 6, and then every 8 weeks through week 46 in ACT 1 and week 22 in ACT 2. In ACT 1, 84/121 (69.4%) of patients receiving infliximab 5 mg/kg and 75/122 (61.5%) of patients receiving 10 mg/kg had a clinical response compared to 45/121 (37.2%) in the placebo group ($p < 0.001$). In ACT 2, 78/121 (64.5%) of patients in the infliximab 5 mg/kg, 83/120 (69.2%) in the infliximab 10 mg/kg, and 36/123 (29.3%) in the placebo group had a response ($P < 0.001$). In this study, the steroid-sparing effect of infliximab in UC patients was shown. Based on this information, in 2006, the FDA approved the use of infliximab for "reducing signs and symptoms, achieving clinical remission and mucosal healing, and eliminating corticosteroid use in patients with moderately to severely active UC who have had an inadequate response to conventional therapy, and for maintaining clinical remission and mucosal healing in patients with moderately to severely active ulcerative colitis (UC), who have had an inadequate response to conventional therapy."

Infusion Reactions

Mild infusion reactions occur in 5% to 13% of patients, but severe infusion reactions requiring discontinuation of the infusion occur in ≤1% of patients. These reactions can be immediate and occur while the medication is being infused, within 2 hours of finishing the infusion, or delayed, occurring 3 to 12 days after the infusion. The most common immediate infusion reactions include fever, chills, headache, chest tightness, shortness of breath, tachycardia, hypo- or hypertension, and rash. These infusion reactions are not true allergic type 1 IgE-mediated reactions; mild reactions usually respond to slowing or stopping the infusion, and the administration of the medication can be completed in most patients. When the reaction is more severe, the symptoms usually respond to the administration of an antipyretic, an antihistamine, and IV steroids. In severe cases, the administration of epinephrine and hospitalization for observation are required; however, in most patients, the infusion can be completed, and the patient is discharged home. It is likely that the infusion reactions are anaphylactoid reactions to the murine component of the medication and not true anaphylactic reactions.

Delayed Reactions

Delayed reactions occur 3 to 12 days after the administration of infliximab. A long hiatus between infusions is a risk factor for such reactions. These reactions result from the activation of circulating antibody-antigen complexes; however, there is no change in levels of serum complement, so these are better termed "serum sickness–like" reactions. Delayed infusion reactions have been reported in as many as 25% of patients that receive infliximab 2 to 4 years after the last dose, and in 60% of patients, such reactions are severe.

Adalimumab

It is known that patients receiving infliximab can develop anti-infliximab antibodies. The patients at higher risk of developing these antibodies are those that receive episodic treatment, with rates reported between 30% and 60%. The most significant determinant for the formation of anti-infliximab antibodies is episodic treatment with long intervals of time between infusions. Patients on a maintenance regimen have a lower frequency of anti-infliximab antibodies with rates between 7% and 10%. Anti-infliximab antibodies are important because patients with high titers have a higher frequency of infusion reactions and/or loss of response. When patients lose response to infliximab, the dose needs to be increased or the frequency of infusions shortened to improve response. This increases the cost of care and decreases patient's quality of life, and eventually side effects or lack of response lead to discontinuation of infliximab. Anti-infliximab antibodies are directed against the murine region of the molecule.

Adalimumab is a recombinant humanized monoclonal IgG1 TNF-α antibody that has only human peptide sequences. The mechanism of action is similar to infliximab; it binds TNF-α with high affinity and neutralizes its activity by blocking the interaction between this cytokine and the cell surface receptors.

Adalimumab was approved by the FDA in February 2007 for "reducing signs and symptoms and inducing and maintaining clinical remission in adult patients with moderately to severely active Crohn's disease who have had an inadequate response to conventional therapy and/or have lost response or become intolerant to infliximab." The main clinical trials on the use of adalimumab in the treatment of Crohn's disease are CLASSIC I and II (CLinical assessment of Adalimumab Safety and efficacy Studied as an Induction therapy in Crohn's), GAIN (Gauging Adalimumab efficacy in Infliximab Nonresponders), and CHARM (Crohn's trial of the fully Human antibody Adalimumab for Remission Maintenance.)

Based on the results of the clinical trials, it was determined that the optimal dose regimen is to administer adalimumab 160 mg subcutaneously at time 0, 80 mg at week 2, and then 40 mg every other week, with the possibility of increasing the frequency of administration to once per week. With this regimen, the response rate at 4 weeks in patients' naïve to infliximab is 50% to 60%, and the remission rate is ~36%. Approximately 80% of the patients that enter into remission with the loading regimen will maintain long-term remission if they continue to receive adalimumab 40 mg SC every other week or weekly. From the patients that improve but do not achieve remission, 46% will be in remission after 1 year if they continue a regimen of adalimumab 40 mg SC every other week or weekly.

An important group of patients that can benefit from adalimumab are those with a previous response to infliximab and that have to discontinue its use either because of infusion reactions or loss of response. Based on the GAIN study, with a loading regimen of adalimumab 160 mg SC followed 2 weeks later by 80 mg, 21% achieve remission at week 4, and 52% will have improvement in symptoms. It is possible that with scheduled administration of adalimumab 40 mg SC every other week or weekly, some of these patients will continue to improve.

The CLASSIC I trial, was a randomized, double-blind, placebo-controlled, dose-ranging trial to evaluate the efficacy of adalimumab in induction of remission in patients with Crohn's disease naïve to treatment with anti–TNF-α antibodies. The highest remission rate, 36%, was seen in patients that received adalimumab 160 mg SC at time 0 and 80 mg 2 weeks later. The response rate in that group was 50% to 59%. Patients that were in remission at week 4 of CLASSIC I were eligible for enrollment in the CLASSIC II study. The objective of CLASSIC II was to evaluate long-term efficacy and safety of adalimumab maintenance therapy. The design of the study is complex, and only some of the results are presented here. There were 55 patients in remission at time of enrollment. In the group that received adalimumab 40 mg every other week, the remission at week 56 was maintained in 79% (15/19). In the group that received adalimumab 40 mg weekly, 83% (15/18) were in remission, and in the placebo group, 44% (8/18) were in remission. The patients that were not in remission at time of enrollment received adalimumab 40 mg every other week, with the possibility of dose escalation to 40 mg/week. At 56 weeks, the remission rate in this group was 46%.

The GAIN trial was a study where patients with Crohn's disease that had either lost response or developed infusion reactions to infliximab were randomized to receive either adalimumab 160 mg SC at 0 weeks and 80 mg 2 weeks later or placebo at 0 and 2 weeks. A total of 325 patients were enrolled, and 301 patients completed the trial. Twenty-one percent (34 of 159) of patients in the adalimumab group versus 7% (12 of 166) of those in the placebo group achieved remission at week 4 (P <0.001). Improvement was observed at week 4 in 52% (82 of 159) of patients in the adalimumab group versus 34% (56 of 166) of patients in the placebo group ($P = 0.001$).

The CHARM study is a very large phase 3, randomized, double-blind, placebo-controlled, 56-week study conducted in patients with moderate to severe CD regardless of previous TNF-α antibody use. A total of 854 patients were enrolled and received open-label adalimumab 80 mg SC followed by a 40-mg dose at week 2. Response was evaluated at week 4, and 778 patients were randomized to receive placebo ($n = 261$), adalimumab 40 mg every other week ($n = 260$), or adalimumab 40 mg weekly ($n = 257$). The response rate to the induction regimen was 58%. Patients were evaluated at weeks 26 and 56. The response rate in the patients receiving adalimumab every other week at weeks 26 and 56 was 40% and 36%, respectively; in the group receiving adalimumab 40 mg weekly the response at week 26 was 47%, and at week 56, it was 41%; and in the placebo group, the responses were 17% at week 26 and 12% at week 56.

Certolizumab

Certolizumab pegol is a humanized Fab' fragment of an anti–TNF-α monoclonal antibody with a high affinity for TNF-α linked to polyethylene glycol; it is currently approved in Switzerland for the treatment of patients with Crohn's disease, but is not FDA approved for use in the United States. Unlike other monoclonal antibodies such as infliximab and adalimumab, it does not contain an Fc portion and, therefore, does not induce in vitro complement activation, antibody-dependent cellular cytotoxicity, or apoptosis. Two recent trials, PRECISE 1 and PRECISE 2 (Pegylated Antibody Fragment Evaluation in Crohn's Disease: Safety and Efficacy) were published in 2007.

Both studies enrolled adult patients with moderate to severely active Crohn's disease. In PRECISE 1, patients were randomized to an induction regimen with either certolizumab 400 mg or placebo at 0, 2, and 4 weeks and then every 4 weeks for a 26-week treatment phase. The response rates in the entire group at week 6 were 35% in the certolizumab group and 27% in the placebo group ($P = 0.02$). At weeks 6 and 26, the rates of remission in the two groups did not differ significantly ($P = 0.17$). When patients were stratified according to CRP, the response rate at week 6 in patients with baseline CRP > 10 mg/L was 37% in the patients receiving certolizumab and 26% in the placebo group ($P = 0.04$).

In PRECISE 2, 668 patients received an induction regimen with certolizumab 400 mg at 0, 2, and 4 weeks. The response rate at week 6 was 64% (428/668), and the remission rate was 43% (289/668). Response was maintained through week 26 in 62% of patients with a baseline CRP level of ≥ 10 mg/L who were receiving certolizumab and in 34% of those receiving placebo ($P < 0.001$). There was a marked difference in response rates between both clinical trials. It is possible that the difference was related to how patients report symptoms when they know that they are participating in a placebo-controlled trial.

The use of infliximab is likely the most significant event in the medical treatment of IBD in the past 40 years. It is clear that the use of anti–TNF-α antibody improves the course of the disease. Treatment with infliximab and adalimumab has resulted in fewer hospitalizations and surgeries, discontinuation of corticosteroid use, and improved quality of life, and despite its cost, its use is cost effective. However, it is important to remember that the use of these medications is not without risks. There are numerous complications that have been reported, and it is important to review the package inserts to become familiar with these.

The most common complication is the formation of antibodies against the medication, these antibodies are medication specific. In patients with Crohn's disease receiving infliximab, the frequency of anti-infliximab antibodies is ~9%; in patients receiving adalimumab, the frequency of antiadalimumab antibodies is ~5%; and in patients receiving certolizumab, the frequency of anticertolizumab antibodies is ~8%. The other complications are related to TNF-α blockade; they are "class side effects." When patients have such complications, it is not appropriate to try a different TNF-α antibody. Infections are one of the most common and significant complications related to the use of these medications. Infections can be either secondary to reactivation of "latent organisms" or opportunistic infections, particularly those in which the infection is controlled by macrophages. Some of the most significant infections that have been reported include tuberculosis, aspergillosis, histoplasmosis, bacterial infections such *Listeria monocytogenes*, and viral infections such as CMV. Other complications that have been reported are lymphoma, demyelination either in the central or peripheral nervous system, liver toxicity, drug-induced systemic lupus erythematosus, and worsening of congestive heart failure. A recent cluster of young patients with hepatosplenic lymphoma was reported. Hepatosplenic lymphoma is a rare and highly fatal form of T-cell lymphoma. So far, all the cases have occurred in children and young adults, and all of the patients were receiving either azathioprine or 6-mercaptopurine and infliximab. This type of lymphoma has also been reported in immunosuppressed patients. Until this report, it was common practice to use the combination of infliximab and azathioprine or 6-mercaptopurine; currently, it is recommended to use anti–TNF-α monotherapy. There are many infrequent complications that have been reported. A mild-to-moderate increase in liver enzymes has been seen in patients treated with infliximab. Severe hepatic disease has been observed in <0.08/1,000 patients, and a causal relationship with infliximab has not been established.

Infliximab may worsen congestive heart failure and should not be used in patients with heart failure NY class 3 or 4. Infliximab and other agents that inhibit TNF-α have been associated in rare cases with optic neuritis, peripheral neuropathy, seizures, and new onset or exacerbation of clinical symptoms and/or radiographic evidence of central nervous system demyelinating disorders, including multiple sclerosis. Infliximab therapy is frequently associated with autoimmunity with the formation of antinuclear antibodies (ANAs) and antibodies to double-stranded DNA. Drug-induced lupus reactions without end-organ damage occur rarely. ANAs are associated with female sex and with the occurrence of papulosquamous or butterfly rash. The development of ANAs is no reason to discontinue therapy with infliximab.

Immunosuppressive Drugs

The main indications for the use of immunosuppressive drugs in patients with IBD are refractory disease, steroid-dependent disease, and unhealed fistulas. Substantial patient experience exists with 6-mercaptopurine (6-MP) and azathioprine, an S-substituted form of 6-MP. There is also experience with the use of methotrexate and cyclosporine. The exact mechanism by which immunosuppressive drugs reduce symptoms in patients with IBD is unclear, but improvement may result from blocking lymphocyte proliferation and activation, as well as through an effect on humoral responsiveness.

The therapeutic benefit of 6-MP and azathioprine is slow in onset. Response is seen 2 to 3 months after initiation of the drug, and therapeutic benefits have been observed even as late as 12 months after the initiation of treatment. These medications allow a reduction or discontinuation of steroid therapy in 60% to 80% of patients who are steroid dependent, improve symptoms in approximately 70% of patients with refractory disease, and promote fistula healing in approximately 60% of patients. In patients with UC, benefit is observed in ∼50% of patients. Given that surgery is seen as "curative" in UC, the role of these medications in treating these patients is less clear. The main side effects of 6-MP and azathioprine are pancreatitis (3%), allergic-type reactions (2%), bone marrow suppression (2%), and a small increased risk of lymphoma. There are two metabolites of these medications that are useful for the management of patients that do not respond to treatment. 6-Thioguanine (6-TG) is associated with clinical response and bone marrow toxicity, and 6-methylmercaptopurine (6-MMP) is associated with liver toxicity. The relative accumulation of these metabolites depends on genetic polymorphism of the enzymes that participate in the metabolism of these drugs.

There is controversy on how high is the risk of lymphoma in patients receiving either 6-MP or azathioprine. However, it is clear that the benefit outweighs the risks. Current practice is to start either of these medications early in the course of the disease. A randomized trial involving a pediatric population compared treatment with prednisone alone to treatment with prednisone plus 6-MP in children with new-onset Crohn's disease. The addition of 6-MP significantly decreased the number of exacerbations and need to use prednisone over the 18-month duration of

the trial. When using these medications, it is important to monitor complete blood count (CBC) with differential and liver tests. There are various schedules that can be followed; this author orders a CBC/differential once a week × 4, then every 2 weeks × 4, then once per month for 1 year, and then every 3 months. Liver tests are done at 4 weeks and then every 3 months. Depending on response and blood results, the dose of the medication is increased or decreased.

Cyclosporine is a potent immunosuppressant that is frequently used to prevent rejection in patients undergoing organ transplantation. Cyclosporine does not maintain remission in patients with IBD, and main indication is in patients with severe UC who do not respond to intravenous corticosteroids and want to avoid surgery. Because of significant side effects, this medication should be used only by experienced physicians, and preferably in tertiary care centers. The most common side effects include nephrotoxicity, seizures, paresthesia, hypertrichosis, hypertension, and infections.

FK-506 is an oral medication with a similar mode of action to cyclosporine and a better safety profile. In a study from Japan, Ogata et al. tested the efficacy and safety of FK-506 in patients with refractory UC. The study was a double-blind placebo-controlled trial with 60 patients. Patients were randomized to receive KF-506 orally with two different blood level targets, high trough (HT) or low trough (LT), or placebo. The response at 2 weeks in the HT was 68.4%, in 38.1% and in the placebo 10.0%. Remission at 2 weeks was seen in 20.0% in the HT group, 10.5% in the LT groups compared with 5.9% in the placebo group at week. In a 10-week open-label extension trial, the response in the placebo group significantly increased with therapy from 10.0% to 57.9%.

Methotrexate has been shown to be effective in the treatment of patients with Crohn's disease. Feagan et al. reported the results of a double-blind, placebo-controlled trial in patients with chronic active Crohn's disease refractory to prednisone. The remission rate in the patients receiving methotrexate 25 mg once per week by intramuscular injection for 16 weeks was 40%. Furthermore, the dose of prednisone in patients on methotrexate at the end of 16 weeks was also lower. To determine whether methotrexate was effective for maintenance of remission, patients that were in remission after 16 to 24 weeks of treatment with methotrexate 25 mg given intramuscularly once weekly were randomly assigned to receive either methotrexate at a dose of 15 mg intramuscularly once weekly or placebo for 40 weeks. The remission rate at week 40 was 65% in the treatment group, as compared with 39% in the placebo group. Because methotrexate is a folic acid antagonist, patients on methotrexate should take folic acid 1 mg daily. The most serious toxicities of methotrexate are hypersensitivity pneumonitis, teratogenicity, hepatotoxicity, and bone marrow suppression. Patients should be strongly advised against drinking alcohol, and women with childbearing potential should practice adequate contraception. The risk of hepatotoxicity is greater in patients who are obese and in those who consume alcohol.

Alternative Treatments

Fish oil is an inhibitor of the activity of leukotriene and other proinflammatory cytokines. It has successfully been used as primary therapy or adjuvant treatment with corticosteroids in patients with UC and Crohn's disease. The main limitations to its use are that, with consumption of the recommended daily dose of 1 to 1.5 g of omega 3 fatty acids per day, patients experience dyspeptic symptoms and develop a fishy odor.

Transdermal nicotine has been used in patients with refractory UC. It is more effective in ex-smokers. The dosage is 15 to 24 mg/24 hours. Patients who have never smoked cigarettes have poor tolerance and response to this agent. Transdermal nicotine is not effective in maintaining remission.

Surgery

Between one-third and one-half of patients with IBD require surgery. Patients with UC and extensive Crohn's colitis require surgery because of failure to respond to medical treatment, hemorrhage, toxic dilatation, perforation, strictures causing obstruction, and dysplasia or cancer. The type of surgery performed in patients with Crohn's disease differs from that used in patients with UC. Depending on the indication, patients with Crohn's disease may undergo a segmental resection, strictureplasty, or both. Patients with UC should undergo total colectomy, regardless of the extent of the disease. When a pelvic pouch from the terminal ileum and an anal anastomosis is done, patients do not need a permanent ileostomy. A total colectomy with an ileal pouch-anal anastomosis is not curative. Patients experience complications such as inflammation of the mucosa of the pouch (pouchitis) that in most patients is acute, but in some patients is a chronic disease. During surgery, a short segment of colonic mucosa is left in the anal canal, and this can become inflamed and bleed (cuffitis). There is also decreased fertility in women and a small risk of impotence in men.

Symptomatic recurrence is frequent in patients with Crohn's disease. Approximately 50% of the patients require additional surgery within 5 to 10 years of the previous surgery. On endoscopy and biopsies, the recurrence rate is near 100% at 1 year. Postoperative recurrence can be delayed, and the need for steroid use or surgery can be decreased with the use of medications such as 6-MP/azathioprine. It is likely that infliximab will have a similar effect, but the clinical trial to answer this question has not been completed. Whether to start medications postoperatively to delay disease recurrence cannot be recommended to all patients. However, all patients with Crohn's disease should quit cigarette smoking, and none should take NSAIDs.

Systemic Complications

Systemic complications are more common in patients with Crohn's disease than in patients with UC. The most common systemic complications are weight loss, malabsorption, kidney stones, gallstones, thrombotic and embolic events, sepsis, and amyloidosis. Many of the systemic complications in patients with Crohn's disease relate to the involvement of the small intestine and depend on the extent of disease. Weight loss is common, and the most common cause for this is decreased oral intake, either because of anorexia or because of postprandial symptoms. Malabsorption results from extensive mucosal involvement, which leads to decreased absorptive surface area or to a protein-losing enteropathy. Gastrocolic or enterocolic fistula can result in malabsorption because the small intestine is bypassed. Other causes of malabsorption include bile salt depletion causing steatorrhea and small intestinal bacterial overgrowth.

Gallstones and kidney stones are complications that relate primarily to alterations of small bowel physiology. Gallstones are related to a decreased absorption of bile salts, kidney stones occur because of an increased absorption of oxalate and dehydration. Vitamin B_{12} is selectively absorbed in the distal 100 cm of the terminal ileum. When the terminal ileum is diseased or removed surgically, patients develop vitamin B_{12} malabsorption. In such patients, the optimal route for supplementation is parenteral. Likewise, hydroxy bile acids are absorbed in the distal 100 cm of the terminal ileum. Thus, when <100 cm of the terminal ileum are diseased or surgically removed, the malabsorbed hydroxy bile acids enter the colon and cause a secretory diarrhea. This form of diarrhea is called "choleretic diarrhea" and usually responds to bile salt sequestrants such as cholestyramine. Conversely, when more than 100 cm of terminal ileum is surgically removed, the bile salt pool is depleted, and patients develop steatorrhea and malabsorption. When there is depletion of bile salts, there is also malabsorption of lipid-soluble vitamins and calcium. These patients are treated with a reduced-fat diet, empiric use of pancreatic enzymes, and medium-chain triglycerides orally.

Another complication that leads to malabsorption in patients with Crohn's disease is small bowel bacterial overgrowth. Bacterial overgrowth results from strictures, fistulas, or surgery.

Colorectal cancer and sepsis are the leading causes of mortality in patients with Crohn's disease. Hypercoagulability, which leads to thrombotic and embolic phenomena in patients with IBD, is the third leading cause of disease-related mortality in patients with IBD. Thromboembolism occurs in 1% to 6% of IBD patients, and 25% of these patients die during the first event. Some of the conditions that lead to thromboembolic events in these patients include activated protein C resistance (related to a mutation in factor V Leiden) and hyperhomocysteinemia. These disorders occur with greater frequency in patients with IBD than in the general population. Other abnormalities that contribute to the hypercoagulable state in these patients are a decreased antithrombin III level, thrombocytosis, leukocytosis, and abnormal fibrinolysis. Amyloidosis, particularly renal, was a frequent complication, but it is rarely seen now. Other rare extraintestinal complications of IBD include pancreatitis, immune-mediated neutropenia, and immune-mediated thrombocytopenia.

REVIEW EXERCISES

QUESTIONS

A 30-year-old white woman presents to your office because of diarrhea and tender nodules on her legs. Three years before this episode, she was on vacation in Mexico and developed bloody diarrhea on return home. She was treated with ciprofloxacin, 750 mg two times a day for 7 days, and the diarrhea resolved. A year later, she had a similar episode of diarrhea that was diagnosed as irritable bowel syndrome. She discontinued cigarette smoking after an episode of shortness of breath and sharp chest pain that lasted 1 week 2 months earlier. Four weeks before consultation, she developed four red "lumps" on her legs that were extremely painful to touch. She was started on ibuprofen and 2 weeks later developed bloody diarrhea. Her symptoms are predefecational cramps that are followed by small, loose bowel movements and, at times, bloody mucus. On two occasions, she has had nocturnal bowel movements.

She has no systemic symptoms. Her past medical history is unremarkable. She takes ibuprofen for menstrual cramps and is on birth control pills.

On examination, she is in no distress. She has a heart rate of 84 beats/minute, respiratory rate of 16 breaths/minute, and a temperature of 37.6°C.

Examination of the abdomen reveals normal bowel sounds; the abdomen is soft but tender to palpation in the left lower quadrant. Rectal examination reveals soft stool with bloody mucus. On the shins, she has four quarter-size brown nodules.

1. Which is the most likely diagnosis?
a) Irritable bowel syndrome
b) Infectious diarrhea
c) Ulcerative colitis
d) Crohn's disease
e) Collagenous colitis

Answer and Discussion

The answer is c. The patient has new-onset ulcerative colitis, which is mild.

2. Which is the best diagnostic test to confirm your impression?
a) Complete blood cell count/differential
b) Stool test for *Clostridium difficile*
c) Flexible sigmoidoscopy with biopsies
d) Air-contrast barium enema
e) Small bowel series

Answer and Discussion

The answer is c. Her symptoms are suggestive of distal ulcerative colitis, and this can be confirmed by sigmoidoscopy and biopsy.

3. Once you confirmed the diagnosis, you recommend
a) Admission to hospital
b) Metronidazole (Flagyl) 500 mg orally three times a day for 1 week
c) Fiber and an anticholinergic agent
d) Prednisone 40 mg orally once a day
e) 5-ASA enemas at bedtime

Answer and Discussion

The answer is e. The best initial treatment is a topical 5-ASA product.

4. Over the next 3 months, the patient's symptoms worsen despite your initial therapy. Which of the following do you recommend now?
a) Ciprofloxacin 750 mg BID
b) Prednisone 60 mg/day
c) Infliximab infusions 5 mg/kg at 0, 2, and 6 weeks
d) 6-Mercaptopurine daily
e) Surgery

Answer and Discussion

The answer is b. Corticosteroids play a significant role in the medical treatment of irritable bowel syndrome. Corticosteroids are indicated in patients with moderate or severely active ulcerative colitis (UC) and in patients who fail to respond to 5-ASA or antibiotics. Immunosuppressive and biological agents are indicated in steroid refractory or dependent patients. Patients with UC require surgery because of failure to respond to medical treatment, hemorrhage, toxic dilatation, perforation, strictures causing obstruction, and dysplasia or cancer.

5. A 34-year-old patient with a 12-year history of ulcerative colitis comes with her husband for advice regarding the use of medications in pregnancy. She developed bloody diarrhea when she was 22 years old. The initial presentation was severe and was treated with prednisone. She was able to wean off prednisone and has remained on sulfasalazine since then. She has mild flare-ups every year during spring. These are controlled by increasing the dose of sulfasalazine from 2 g/day that she takes for maintenance of remission to 4 g/day. She is otherwise healthy and takes a multivitamin "when I remember." What is your recommendation to the patient regarding the use of sulfasalazine in pregnancy?
a) Sulfasalazine should not be used during pregnancy because of the risk of kernicterus; therefore, discontinue and start another 5-ASA.

b) Discontinue sulfasalazine and do not institute treatment unless there is an exacerbation.

c) Continue sulfasalazine at the present dose.

d) Add folic acid 1 mg orally once a day.

e) Discontinue sulfasalazine postpartum to decrease the risk of kernicterus and start another 5-ASA medication.

Answer and Discussion

The answer is d. All 5-ASA compounds are safe during pregnancy and lactation. The treatment with 5-ASA should be continued during pregnancy to decrease the risk of a flare-up with potentially disastrous consequences. Sulfasalazine contains sulfapyridine, and all sulfas have the potential for inducing kernicterus. However, this is only a theoretical concern; sulfasalazine has been available since the early 1940s, and there are no reports of kernicterus in association with sulfasalazine. The patient should take folic acid at a minimum dose of 1 mg/day. Sulfasalazine interferes with folic acid absorption, and folic acid decreases the risk of spina bifida.

SUGGESTED READINGS

Baert F, Noman M, Vermeire S, et al. Influence of immunogenicity on the long-term efficacy of infliximab in Crohn's disease. *N Engl J Med* 2003;348(7):601–609.

Brzezinski A. Medical treatment of Crohn's disease. *Clin Colon Rectal Surg* 2001;14:167–173.

Cho J. The *Nod2* gene in Crohn's disease: implications for future research into the genetics and immunology of Crohn's disease. *Inflamm Bowel Dis* 2001;7(3):271–275.

Colombel JF, Sandborn WJ, Rutgeerts P, et al. Adalimumab for maintenance of clinical response and remission in patients with Crohn's disease: the CHARM trial. *Gastroenterology* 2007;132(1):52–65.

Hanauer SB, Feagan BG, Lichtenstein GR, et al. Maintenance infliximab for Crohn's disease: the ACCENT I randomised trial. *Lancet* 2002;359:1541.

Hanauer SB, Sandborn WJ, Rutgeerts P, et al. Human anti-tumor necrosis factor monoclonal antibody (adalimumab) in Crohn's disease: the CLASSIC-I trial. *Gastroenterology* 2006;130:323–333.

Hanauer SB, Stromberg U. Oral Pentasa in the treatment of active Crohn's disease: a meta-analysis of double-blind, placebo-controlled trials. *Clin Gastroenterol Hepatol* 2004;2:379.

Högenauer C, Wenzl HH, Hinterleitner TA, et al. Effect of oral tacrolimus (FK 506) on steroid-refractory moderate/severe ulcerative colitis. *Aliment Pharmacol Ther* 2003;18(4):415–423.

Jess T, Riis L, Vind I, et al. Changes in clinical characteristics, course, and prognosis of inflammatory bowel disease during the last 5 decades: a population-based study from Copenhagen, Denmark. *Inflamm Bowel Dis* 2007;13(4):481–489.

Kappelman MD, Rifas-Shiman SL, Kleinman K. The prevalence and geographical distribution of Crohn's disease and ulcerative colitis in the United States. *Clin Gastroenterol Hepatol* 2007;1424–1429.

Loftus CG, Loftus EV Jr, Scott Harmsen WS, et al. Update on the incidence and prevalence of Crohn's disease and ulcerative colitis in Olmsted County, Minnesota, 1940–2000. *Inflamm Bowel Dis* 2007;13(3):254–261.

Mackey AC, Green L, Liang LC, et al. Hepatosplenic T cell lymphoma associated with infliximab use in young patients treated for inflammatory bowel disease. *J Pediatr Gastroenterol Nutr* 2007;44:265–267.

Ogata H, Matsui T, Nakamura M, et al. A randomised dose finding study of oral tacrolimus (FK506) therapy in refractory ulcerative colitis. *Gut* 2006;55:1255–1262.

Papadakis KA, Shaye OA, Vasiliauskas EA, et al. Safety and efficacy of adalimumab (D2E7) in Crohn's disease patients with an attenuated response to infliximab. *Am J Gastroenterol* 2005;100:75–79.

Sandborn WJ, Feagan BG, Stoinov S, et al. Certolizumab pegol for the treatment of Crohn's disease. *N Engl J Med* 2007;357:228–238.

Sandborn WJ, Rutgeerts P, Enns R, et al. Adalimumab induction therapy for Crohn disease previously treated with infliximab: a randomized trial. *Ann Intern Med* 2007;146:829–838.

Sands BE, Anderson FH, Bernstein CN, et al. Infliximab maintenance therapy for fistulizing Crohn's disease. *N Engl J Med* 2004;350:876.

Schreiber S, Khaliq-Kareemi M, Lawrance IC, et al. Maintenance therapy with certolizumab pegol for Crohn's disease. *N Engl J Med* 2007;357:239.

Chapter 57

Diarrhea and Malabsorption

Edy E. Soffer   *John A. Dumot*

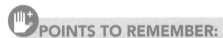POINTS TO REMEMBER:

- Osmotic diarrhea tends to stop during fasting and is associated with an osmotic gap.
- Dysmotility-induced diarrhea is generally a diagnosis of exclusion.
- Foodborne illness with *Escherichia coli* is the most common cause of traveler's diarrhea.
- Diarrhea is almost universally present in malabsorption.
- Conditions that impair gastrointestinal motility can result in bacterial overgrowth.
- In lymphocytic or collagenous colitis, the endoscopic and radiologic appearance of the colon is normal.

DIARRHEA

Diarrhea is best defined by increased stool weight, essentially as the result of increased water content. For most individuals eating a Western-type diet, diarrhea implies a 24-hour stool output in excess of 200 g. A more practical definition is abnormal looseness of the stools, which is usually associated with increased stool weight and frequency of bowel movements.

Approximately 8 to 9 L of fluid enter the intestine daily; 1 to 2 L represent food and liquid intake, and the rest is from endogenous sources such as salivary, gastric, pancreatic, biliary, and intestinal secretions. After small bowel absorption, only 1 to 2 L are presented to the colon; most of it is absorbed as it passes through the colon, leaving a stool output of up to 100 to 200 g daily.

Mechanisms of Diarrhea

Water is absorbed passively in the gut, dependent on osmotic gradient. Consequently, diarrhea is due to an excess of osmotically active substances in the stool, which results in the decreased absorption of nutrients and electrolytes or excess secretion of any combination of electrolytes, water, or nutrients. The intestinal motility and mucosal integrity also play a key role in stool formation. Four mechanisms should be considered in the evaluation of patients with diarrhea: osmotic, secretory, altered motility, and exudative.

Osmotic Diarrhea

Osmotic diarrhea results from the presence of a poorly absorbable solute that causes excessive water output. The presence of the poorly absorbable solute exerts an osmotic pressure effect across the intestinal mucosa. Because the diarrhea is caused by the solute, it tends to stop during fasting and is associated with an osmotic gap. In addition, a stool "osmotic gap" occurs. Normally, stool osmolality can be accounted for by normal concentrations of stool electrolytes. A reasonable estimate of the stool osmolality can be made by adding the serum concentration of sodium and potassium, and by multiplying by 2 for the associated anions. If a nonabsorbable solute is present in the fecal fluid, the concentrations of stool electrolytes are lower. Therefore, adding stool sodium and potassium concentrations and multiplying by 2 (for their associated anions) will result in a stool osmolality value that is lower than the serum osmolality. Because of technical problems associated with measuring total fecal osmolality, one can use the electrolyte estimate method and compare it to the expected serum osmolality, which should be 290 mOsm.

For example, in using stool electrolyte concentrations to estimate the stool osmolality, if stool sodium [Na^+] is 100 mmol and stool potassium [K^+] is 5 mmol, then the expected stool osmolality would be

$$(100 + 5) \times 2 = 210\,\mathrm{mOsm}$$

In a study in which diarrhea was induced in normal volunteers using different agents, it was observed that in secretory diarrhea, the osmotic gap was always <50 mOsm, whereas in all forms of osmotic diarrhea, the gap was always considerably >50 mOsm.

To calculate the osmotic gap, consider that estimated serum osmolality is usually 290 mOsm. Thus,

$$290 \text{ mOsm} - \text{calculated stool osmolality} = \text{gap}$$

Using the previous example,

$$290 - 210 = 80 \text{ mOsm}$$

The 80 mOsm is greater than the expected 50 mOsm. Thus, unaccounted osmotically agents or unabsorbable solutes account for the "gap." Also, fecal fluid with a pH level of <5.6 helps distinguish diarrhea due to malabsorption of sugars such as lactulose.

The causes of osmotic diarrhea include:

- Disaccharidase deficiency, such as lactose intolerance
- Malabsorption of osmotically active nutrients, especially in maldigestion due to pancreatic insufficiency
- Poorly absorbed sugars, such as lactulose, sorbitol, and mannitol, found in laxatives and artificial sweeteners
- Laxatives or antacids containing magnesium, sodium citrate, and sodium phosphate
- Antacids containing magnesium

Secretory Diarrhea

In secretory diarrhea, an abnormal ion transport occurs across intestinal epithelial cells as the result of the active secretion of ions. In this case, no osmotic gap occurs, and because the diarrhea is not related to the intestinal content, it typically will not cease with fasting. The most striking example of secretory diarrhea is bacterial toxin–associated diarrhea, as occurs in cholera.

The causes of secretory diarrhea include:

- Infections, such as *Vibrio cholerae*
- Mucosal inflammation, such as celiac sprue or collagenous colitis
- Stimulants, such as phenolphthalein, senna, docusate sodium, bile, and fatty acids
- Hormonal causes, such as tumors producing vasoactive intestinal peptide, gastrin, calcitonin, carcinoid tumor, and hyperthyroidism

Altered Motility

Motility disturbances of the gastrointestinal (GI) tract can result in decreased absorption. Any anatomical disruption, such as gastrectomy, vagotomy, or intestinal resection, could produce diarrhea. Proving motility as the sole cause of diarrhea is very difficult, however. Dysmotility-induced diarrhea is generally a diagnosis of exclusion. A consequence of reduced intestinal motility may be bacterial overgrowth, which would aggravate the diarrhea and cause fat malabsorption.

The causes of diarrhea due to altered motility include:

- Irritable bowel syndrome
- Postsurgical (vagotomy, cholecystectomy, gastrectomy, and intestinal resection), fistulas, diabetic neuropathy
- Hyperthyroidism

Exudative Diarrhea

Extensive injury of the small bowel or colon mucosa may result in fluid and protein loss into the intestinal lumen and ensuing diarrhea. Exudation is rarely the only mechanism accounting for the diarrhea.

The causes of exudative diarrhea include inflammatory bowel disease (IBD) and invasive bacterial infections (*Shigella, Salmonella*).

It is important to keep in mind that more than one mechanism may contribute to the patient's symptoms. For example, in infectious and inflammatory conditions, both malabsorption (leading to osmotic diarrhea) and active secretion may coexist.

Evaluation of Diarrhea

History and Physical Examination

Conducting a careful interview can provide valuable clues that will aid in choosing the most appropriate and cost-effective investigations. Of particular usefulness is the duration of diarrhea. Acute diarrhea is usually infectious in origin and, for the most part, resolves without intervention. Chronic diarrhea, defined as lasting more than 4 weeks, is unlikely to be infectious. The presence of blood is also a useful clue, suggesting infections by invasive organisms, inflammation, ischemia, or neoplasm. Large-volume diarrhea suggests small bowel or proximal colonic disease, whereas small, frequent stools associated with urgency suggest left colon or rectal disease. All current and recent medications should be reviewed, specifically new medications, antibiotics, antacids, and alcohol abuse. Nutritional supplements should be reviewed, including the intake of "sugarfree" foods (containing nonabsorbed carbohydrates); fat substitutes; milk products or shellfish; or the heavy intake of fruits, fruit juices, or caffeine. The social history should include travel; source of drinking water (treated city water or well water); and the consumption of raw milk, exposure to farm animals that may spread *Salmonella* or *Brucella*, and sexual orientation. Familial occurrence of celiac disease, IBD, or multiple endocrine neoplasia syndromes should also be checked.

Physical examination in acute diarrhea is helpful in determining the severity of disease and hydration status. In chronic diarrhea, findings such as oral ulcers and pyoderma gangrenosum suggest IBD; dermatitis herpetiformis is associated with celiac disease, and lymphadenopathy with lymphoma.

Further evaluation by laboratory tests and the appropriate selection of tests depend to a great extent on the duration

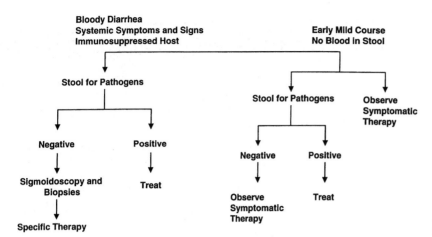

Figure 57.1 Algorithm for the evaluation of acute diarrhea.

and severity of diarrhea and the presence of blood, overt or occult, in the stool.

Acute Diarrhea

Acute diarrhea is defined as lasting less than 4 weeks; it is commonly caused by infectious organisms or toxins. It is usually self-limited and, in the absence of blood in the stool, remains mostly undiagnosed. If a patient is seen early in the course of illness and has no systemic symptoms or blood in the stool, and if diarrhea is mild, then observation and follow-up are most appropriate. Otherwise, and particularly in the presence of blood, stool should be sent for evaluation for infectious organisms and treatment instituted when appropriate. If organisms are not identified, sigmoidoscopy should be performed and biopsies obtained. Further investigations will depend on the results of sigmoidoscopy (e.g., if IBD is suspected), severity of diarrhea, immune status of the host, and presence of systemic toxicity.

Traveler's diarrhea is the most common affliction of a highly mobile population. Foodborne illness with *Escherichia coli* is the most common cause of traveler's diarrhea. Watery diarrhea 5 to 15 days after arrival, with a range 3 to 31 days, is common. *E. coli* is the leading cause and responsible for more cases than all other infectious agents combined. *Campylobacter* infections are responsible for more than *Shigella* and *Salmonella* combined. Other infectious agents include *Vibrio parahaemolyticus*, rotavirus, Norwalk virus, adenovirus, coxsackievirus, *Clostridium difficile*, *Clostridium perfringens*, *Bacillus cereus*, *Staphylococcus aureus*, *Entamoeba histolytica*, and *Vibrio cholerae*. Other organisms make up the remaining cases.

Treatment includes the replacement of fluid loss and the administration of loperamide or diphenoxylate (which should be discontinued after 2 days, or immediately in the presence of blood, mucus, or fever). Bismuth subsalicylate 30 mL eight times a day can shorten the course of traveler's diarrhea and may also be used for prevention at 2.4 g/day. Short-course broad-spectrum antibiotics using fluoroquinolone or trimethoprim/sulfamethoxazole plus loperamide have been the standard for severe cases, but data remain unconvincing, and theoretical risks do exist for selecting out invasive or resistant organisms. Rifaximin (Xifaxan) 200 mg three times a day for 3 days has recently been approved for traveler's diarrhea. Its use is indicated in patients 12 years or older for diarrhea caused by noninvasive strains of *E. coli*.

A general algorithm for the evaluation of acute diarrhea is shown in Figure 57.1.

Chronic Diarrhea

Clinicians have many tests at their disposal for evaluating a patient with chronic diarrhea, and proper judgment should be used in the choice of the most appropriate tests. The duration of diarrhea, evidence of systemic involvement, nutritional deficiencies, and previous investigations should guide the evaluation. Unlike acute diarrhea, chronic diarrhea of infectious etiology is uncommon. Immune-compromised hosts are more susceptible to *C. difficile*, *Cryptosporidium*, *Cyclospora*, *Giardia*, *Aeromonas*, *Amoebae*, *Plesiomonas*, *Campylobacter*, and *Tropheryma whipplei*.

Weight loss and evidence of nutritional deficiencies suggest malabsorption caused by small bowel or pancreatic pathology, the latter implicated by a history of excessive alcohol intake or abdominal pain. Chronic bloody diarrhea suggests IBD, particularly ulcerative colitis. Chronic diarrhea with no evidence of nutritional or metabolic deficiency suggests lactose intolerance; irritable bowel syndrome, particularly when associated with abdominal pain; microscopic colitis; fecal incontinence; or surreptitious laxative abuse. Colon cancer should always be excluded. In the absence of nutritional deficiencies, large-volume diarrhea with features of a secretory process usually prompts a search for hormone-producing tumors, but these are rarely found. A general algorithm for the approach to chronic diarrhea is illustrated in Figure 57.2.

Treatment

When possible, therapy is directed toward the underlying etiology. When no specific therapy is available or no cause

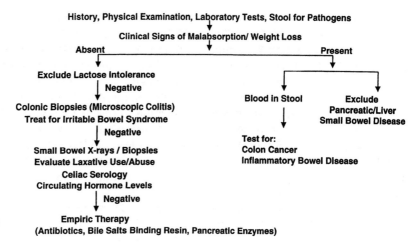

Figure 57.2 Algorithm for the approach to chronic diarrhea.

is found, it is appropriate to give empiric therapy (e.g., an antibiotic for possible bacterial overgrowth or giardiasis, cholestyramine for bile acid malabsorption) or nonspecific therapy with constipating agents, such as loperamide (Imodium); diphenoxylate/atropine sulfate (Lomotil); or, in more severe cases, codeine, paregoric, or a trial of long-acting somatostatin analog.

MALABSORPTION

The main purpose of the GI tract is to digest and absorb major nutrients (fat, carbohydrates, and protein), essential micronutrients (vitamins and trace elements), water, and electrolytes. Digestion involves both the mechanical and biochemical breakdown of food. Mechanical breakdown is achieved by mastication and gastric trituration, and its biochemical counterpart by a complex enzymatic process that depends on gastric, pancreatic, and biliary secretions; this process is completed by enzymes located at the brush border of enterocytes. The final products are then absorbed through the intestinal brush border. The controlled release of food from the stomach, its normal progression through the intestine, and adequate intestinal surface area are important factors. The term *malabsorption* is used in reference to all aspects of the impaired assimilation of nutrients.

Most food components can be absorbed throughout the length of the small intestine, whereas some can be absorbed only at specific segments (e.g., vitamin B_{12} and bile acids in the terminal ileum). The primary absorptive function of the colon is the salvage of water and electrolytes. Malabsorption results from abnormal digestion, abnormal absorption, or both. The digestive process starts in the stomach, with acid and pepsin, and continues in the upper small bowel, with bile and pancreatic enzymes such as lipase, amylase, and trypsin. As a result, fats are broken down to fatty acids and monoglycerides, proteins to amino acids and peptides, and carbohydrates into monosaccharides and disaccharides. Further breakdown of these nutrients takes place at the brush border of the intestinal

mucosal cells by disaccharidases and oligopeptidases, with final absorption across the large surface area of the small intestine. The products of absorption reach the circulation either through the mesenteric vasculature or through lymphatics.

Of all the nutrients ingested, lipids require the most complex digestive process before being absorbed. Lipolysis starts in the stomach and is completed in the jejunum by pancreatic lipase. This results in the formation of free fatty acids and glycerol. Bile salts manufactured in the liver are necessary to facilitate absorption through micellar formation. Bile salts are then reabsorbed in the terminal ileum to be used over and over again (enterohepatic circulation). Therefore, fat malabsorption can occur because of gastrectomy, pancreatic insufficiency, advanced liver disease, biliary obstruction, or surgically absent or markedly diseased ileum. Bile salt action also can be impaired by deconjugation, which occurs in the presence of bacterial overgrowth.

The causes of malabsorption include:

- Defect in intraluminal phase: pancreatic insufficiency, bile salt deficiency, bacterial overgrowth
- Mucosal defect: disaccharidase deficiency, celiac sprue, Whipple's disease, Crohn's disease, abetalipoproteinemia
- Infections: giardiasis, tropical sprue
- Lymphatic obstruction: intestinal lymphangiectasia, lymphoma
- Surgical resection or extensive mucosal disease: gastrectomy, Crohn's disease, ileal resection, lymphoma
- Drugs: neomycin, laxatives, cholestyramine

Clinical Presentation

The symptoms of malabsorption are multiple. Diarrhea is almost universally present in malabsorption. Stools are often described as bulky and sticky. Floating stools do not necessarily indicate malabsorption. Abdominal pain is mild unless an inflammatory etiology (IBD) or pancreatic disease is present. Weight loss can be mild or advanced, depending on the severity of malabsorption. Malabsorption may lead to multiple manifestations due to various nutritional deficiencies, such as anemia due to iron, vitamin B_{12}, or folic acid deficiency; hypocalcemia; and a bleeding tendency due to vitamin K deficiency, among others.

The past history can provide important clues. A surgical history should be taken, with particular attention to the exact site and extent of any organ resection. A history of alcohol or previous attacks of abdominal pain may lead to the diagnosis of chronic pancreatitis. A drug history must be taken, along with a travel history and inquiry about sexual practices.

Laboratory Testing

When malabsorption is suspected, blood tests usually include a measurement of albumin, carotene, cholesterol, calcium, and folic acid levels, and a measure of prothrombin time. These data are helpful in assessing the severity of malabsorption, but do not aid in the differential diagnosis. Many other tests are available in diagnosing malabsorption; the more clinically useful tests are discussed in the following sections.

Fecal Fat Analysis

The simplest way to detect stool fat is to perform a Sudan stain on a stool smear. This test has limited sensitivity because of the stain's affinity for dietary triglyceride and its lipolytic products only, but it has the advantage of simplicity and low cost. A more sensitive test for steatorrhea is the quantitative measurement of fat in the stool. Stool is collected for 3 consecutive days and analyzed for fat content while the patient is eating a diet containing 80 to 100 g of fat daily. Normal fat excretion should not exceed 6 g daily. The test is cumbersome and does not identify the cause of fat malabsorption, but it yields an accurate quantification of stool fat excretion.

Tests of Pancreatic Exocrine Function

Intubation studies of the duodenum near the ampulla of Vater provide the best index of pancreatic function. After stimulation of the pancreas, duodenal contents are aspirated and analyzed for bicarbonate and enzyme output. These tests are invasive and time consuming, however, and are therefore not suitable for screening. Pancreatic calcifications seen on abdominal radiographs or CT indicate the presence of chronic pancreatitis in late stages, but are usually not present early on. Abnormal ductal anatomy can be demonstrated by endoscopic retrograde cholangiopancreatography (ERCP), but this test is invasive and has dangerous side effects. MRI and endoscopic ultrasound (EUS) technology have replaced ERCP for diagnostic purposes. EUS can be combined with pancreatic function testing with the secretagogues cholecystokinin for lipase output concentration or secretin for bicarbonate output concentration.

Small Intestine Biopsy

Small intestine mucosal biopsy is a key diagnostic test in diseases that affect the cellular phase of absorption. In some diseases, the histologic features are diagnostic, whereas in others the findings are suggestive. Endoscopic biopsies from the duodenum and jejunum have replaced biopsies obtained by specially designed per-oral capsules. Several biopsy samples should be taken from the distal duodenum to increase the diagnostic yield. The use of small bowel biopsy specimens in malabsorption is categorized in Table 57.1.

D-Xylose Absorption Test

D-Xylose is a five-carbon monosaccharide that, when given in a large dose, can cross the intestinal mucosa largely by passive diffusion. The test is performed by having a patient ingest 25 g of D-xylose; urine is collected for the next 5 hours. Healthy individuals excrete more than 4.5 g of D-xylose in 5 hours. The test reflects the permeability and surface area of the mucosa and serves as an indicator of mucosal integrity. False-positive abnormally low results may occur in the presence of poor renal function, large amounts of edema, or ascites. Abnormal results may also be seen in the presence of bacterial overgrowth, but these may normalize after treatment with antibiotics. Many institutions have abandoned this test, and it remains only of historical importance.

Radiographic Studies

Barium studies of the small bowel in malabsorption are usually nonspecific. They are helpful in the presence of distinct anatomical changes, however, such as small bowel diverticulosis, lymphoma, Crohn's disease, strictures, and enteric fistulas.

Schilling Test

The absorption of vitamin B_{12} requires several steps. First, it binds to salivary R protein. In the duodenum, pancreatic

TABLE 57.1	
SMALL BOWEL BIOPSY IN DIAGNOSING MALABSORPTION	
Often Diagnostic	**Abnormal But Not Diagnostic**
Whipple's disease	Celiac sprue
Amyloidosis	Systemic sclerosis
Eosinophilic enteritis	Radiation enteritis
Lymphangiectasia	Bacterial overgrowth syndrome
Primary intestinal lymphoma	Tropical sprue
Giardiasis	Crohn's disease
Abetalipoproteinemia	
Agammaglobulinemia	
Mastocytosis	

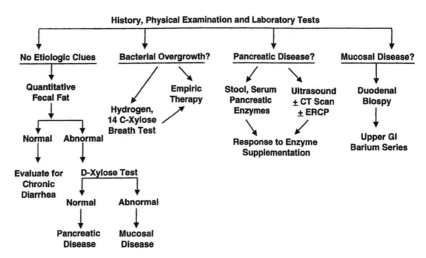

Figure 57.3 Evaluation of a patient with suspected malabsorption. CT = computed tomography; ERCP = endoscopic retrograde cholangiopancreatography; GI = gastrointestinal. (Adapted from Riley SA, Marsh MN. Maldigestion and malabsorption. In: Feldman M, Sleisenger MH, Scharschmidt BF, et al., eds. *Sleisenger & Fordtran's Gastrointestinal and Liver Disease: Pathophysiology, Diagnosis, Management*, 6th ed. Philadelphia: WB Saunders, 1998;1501–1522.)

proteases hydrolyze the R protein, allowing the vitamin to bind with the intrinsic factor secreted by gastric parietal cells. The vitamin B_{12}–intrinsic factor complex is then absorbed by specific receptors found on enterocytes in the distal ileum. Consequently, the malabsorption of vitamin B_{12} can occur because of a lack of intrinsic factor (pernicious anemia or gastric resection), pancreatic insufficiency, bacterial overgrowth, or ileal resection or disease. The Schilling test helps identify the cause of vitamin B_{12} deficiency. The test consists of several phases:

- Phase 1: After 1 mg of vitamin B_{12} is injected to saturate the hepatic storage, the patient ingests radiolabeled vitamin, and urine is collected for measurement of radioactivity.
- Phase 2: If malabsorption is diagnosed, the test is repeated while the patient is given oral vitamin B_{12} and intrinsic factor. If malabsorption is corrected, pernicious anemia is diagnosed.
- Phase 3: If malabsorption is still present, and the test remains abnormal despite treatment with antibiotics, an ileal disease is diagnosed.

Breath Tests

Breath tests rely on the principle that the bacterial degradation of luminal compounds releases gases that can be measured in the breath. In disaccharidase deficiency, the oral ingestion of specific carbohydrates (e.g., lactose) will result in colonic fermentation due to malabsorption in the small bowel, with increased hydrogen in the breath. In the presence of bacterial overgrowth, orally ingested glucose will be fermented in the small bowel, instead of being absorbed, thus resulting in increased breath hydrogen. The measurement of radioactive carbon in the breath (^{14}C) has been used in tests devised to measure malabsorption of fat and bile acids, as well as for bacterial overgrowth (^{14}C-xylose). The radioactive tests are cumbersome, and their use in clinical practice is limited.

Approach to Suspected Malabsorption

Because of the large number of available diagnostic tests, a rational use of these tests is necessary when a patient with suspected malabsorption is being evaluated (Fig. 57.3). The best screening test for steatorrhea is the 72-hour fecal fat analysis. The test is cumbersome and difficult to obtain in practice, and many physicians rely on the qualitative fecal fat as the initial investigation. Alternatively, test selection may depend on the clinical presentation. The presence of cholestatic hepatobiliary disease is usually quite obvious clinically. When weight loss, nutritional deficiencies, and diarrhea are present, a qualitative stool analysis should be done to establish the presence of steatorrhea.

The absence of a history of excessive alcohol intake, previous episodes of pancreatitis, or abdominal pain makes the presence of chronic pancreatitis unlikely. A urinary D-xylose test or a small bowel biopsy then may be performed to determine whether mucosal disease is present. If these tests are normal, then enzyme tests can be done, along with abdominal radiography, to look for pancreatic disease. If tests are nonrevealing, or the D-xylose test is abnormal in the presence of a normal mucosal biopsy, a hydrogen breath test can be done and small bowel films obtained to test for bacterial overgrowth. When abdominal pain suggestive of a pancreatic origin is present, magnetic resonance cholangiopancreatography, EUS, or CT of the pancreas may be performed first to exclude chronic pancreatitis or pancreatic cancer.

When diarrhea is associated with cramps and flatulence with minimal or no weight loss and no nutritional deficiencies, the possibility of carbohydrate malabsorption, particularly lactose intolerance, should be entertained.

Treatment

The treatment of malabsorption depends on the underlying condition. It consists of dietary manipulations in celiac sprue, antibiotic therapy in bacterial overgrowth, enzyme supplementation in pancreatic insufficiency, surgery for small bowel obstruction, or parenteral nutrition when treatment options have failed to maintain an adequate nutritional status. Empiric treatment using pancreatic enzyme supplementation or an antibiotic for suspected bacterial overgrowth or giardiasis is occasionally given when the etiology remains unclear.

CELIAC SPRUE

Celiac sprue, also known as *nontropical sprue* or *gluten-sensitive enteropathy*, is characterized by intestinal mucosal injury resulting from an immunologic intolerance to gluten in genetically predisposed individuals. The prevalence of the disease among relatives of patients with celiac sprue is approximately 10%. Celiac sprue is strongly associated with human leukocyte antigen class II molecules, in particular HLA-DQ2 and HLA-DQ8. The disease is induced by exposure to the storage proteins found in grain plants, such as wheat (which contains gliadin), barley, rye, and oats, and their products. The exposure initiates a cellular immune response that results in mucosal damage, particularly in the proximal intestine. Recent investigations suggest that an enzyme, tissue transglutaminase, may be the autoantigen of celiac sprue.

Clinical Presentation

Celiac disease may present with the classic constellation of symptoms and signs of a malabsorption syndrome. Conversely, the presentation may be atypical, with nonspecific GI symptoms such as bloating, chronic diarrhea without steatorrhea, flatulence, lactose intolerance, or deficiency of a single micronutrient, such as iron-deficiency anemia. Up to 50% of celiac patients do not have diarrhea. Non-GI complaints, such as depression, fatigue, and arthralgia, and manifestations such as osteoporosis or osteomalacia, may predominate. Several diseases are associated with a higher incidence of celiac disease; these include dermatitis herpetiformis, type I diabetes mellitus, autoimmune thyroid disease, and selective immunoglobulin A deficiency.

Diagnosis

Although celiac disease is part of the differential diagnosis of every malabsorption syndrome, a high index of suspicion should be kept in mind for patients with atypical presentations. Intestinal biopsy is the most valuable test in establishing the diagnosis of celiac sprue. A spectrum of pathological changes occur, ranging from normal villous architecture with an increase in mucosal lymphocytes and plasma cells (infiltrative lesion) to partial or total villous atrophy. Although abnormal findings on intestinal biopsy are nonspecific, they are highly suggestive, particularly because most other conditions that can mimic celiac disease, such as Crohn's disease, lymphoma, tropical sprue, graft-versus-host disease, or immune deficiency, may be distinguished on clinical grounds. A clinical response to a gluten-free diet in the presence of an abnormal biopsy should establish the diagnosis and preclude the need, in adults, to document healing by repeat biopsies. Serologic blood tests are helpful for screening patients and the asymptomatic relatives of celiac sprue patients. The panel used in our lab includes a total immunoglobulin A (IgA) level, endomysial IgA, gliadin IgG and IgA, and transglutaminase IgA levels. In patients with low total IgA levels, normal antibody levels are unreliable; these patients should undergo small bowel biopsy. The proper management of patients with serologic evidence of celiac disease and normal biopsies is unknown, but a clinical response to a glutenfree diet should raise the possibility of the biopsies being a false-negative result.

Treatment

A strict, lifelong adherence to a glutenfree diet is the only treatment for celiac disease. Specific nutritional supplementation should be provided to correct deficiencies, particularly of iron, vitamins, and calcium. Clinical response may be seen within a few weeks. Patients should be followed to ensure adequate response and proper adherence to diet. Long-term prognosis is excellent for patients who adhere to a glutenfree diet, although a slight increase in the incidence of malignancies may be present, particularly lymphoma.

BACTERIAL OVERGROWTH SYNDROME

The proximal small bowel normally contains only a small number of bacteria, less than a thousand per milliliter of fluid, with no anaerobic *Bacteroides* organisms and few coliforms. An overgrowth of bacteria can result in diarrhea and malabsorption through several mechanisms:

- Deconjugation of bile salts leading to impaired micelle formation and fat malabsorption
- Patchy injury to enterocytes on the intestinal mucosal surface
- Direct use of nutrients, such as uptake of vitamin B_{12}, by gram-negative organisms
- Secretion of water and electrolytes, secondary to byproducts of bacterial metabolism, such as hydroxylated bile acids and organic acids

Associated Conditions

The most important factor in maintaining the relative sterility of the upper gut is a normal motor function, with other factors being gastric acid and intestinal immunoglobulins. Consequently, conditions that impair GI motility can result in bacterial overgrowth. GI stasis may be caused by a motility disorder (scleroderma, intestinal pseudo-obstruction, diabetes) or anatomical impairment (blind loops, obstruction, and diverticulosis). Achlorhydria, pancreatic insufficiency, and immunodeficiency syndromes are also associated with bacterial overgrowth.

Diagnosis

The direct culture of a jejunal aspirate is the most definitive diagnostic test, but it is invasive and uncomfortable. The ^{14}C-xylose breath test is the most appropriate test, whereas the glucose breath hydrogen test is the simplest, although not as sensitive or specific. An empiric therapeutic trial of an antibiotic is an acceptable alternative.

Treatment

When appropriate, specific therapy should be provided, such as surgery for intestinal obstruction. More commonly, patients are treated with an antibiotic effective against aerobic and anaerobic enteric organisms. Tetracycline, trimethoprim/sulfamethoxazole, and metronidazole, in combination with a cephalosporin, are suitable agents. A single course of therapy for 7 to 10 days may be therapeutic for months. In other patients, intermittent therapy (1 week out of every 4) or even continuous therapy for 1 or 2 months may be needed.

LYMPHOCYTIC OR COLLAGENOUS COLITIS

This is a relatively common disease or spectrum of diseases, which is characterized by chronic diarrhea and mucosal abnormalities consisting of infiltration of the lamina propria and epithelium with lymphocytes, increased subepithelial collagen plate (in collagenous colitis), or both. In lymphocytic or collagenous colitis, the endoscopic and radiologic appearance of the colon is normal. The mean age at presentation is in the sixth decade, with a female predominance. An association with autoimmune disorders and celiac sprue has been noted. Typically, patients exhibit no biochemical deficiencies, and the diagnosis can be made only through random biopsies from the colon.

Sulfasalazine, mesalamine, budesonide, and systemic steroids have clinical benefit, but large controlled trials are lacking. In a recent study involving a small number of patients, high-dose bismuth subsalicylate resolved diarrhea and colitis in most patients. Symptomatic therapy using antidiarrheal agents may be the only treatment necessary in some patients.

DIARRHEA IN AIDS

In up to two-thirds of patients with AIDS, diarrhea develops during the course of their disease. An increasing array of infectious and noninfectious etiologies is recognized as causing diarrhea in this population. These include pathogens found in immunocompetent hosts, those related to sexually transmitted organisms, and organisms associated with the immunocompromised host, as well as noninfectious causes. Stool analysis is the most productive investigation, followed by colonoscopy. Upper endoscopy may be done if the workup for small bowel pathogens is negative.

The causes of diarrhea in patients with AIDS include

- Organisms affecting immunocompetent hosts: *Salmonella, Shigella, C. difficile, Giardia lamblia, Entamoeba histolytica*
- Sexually transmitted pathogens: *Neisseria gonorrhoeae, Chlamydia trachomatis, Treponema pallidum*
- Organisms affecting immunocompromised hosts: *Mycobacterium avium*-intracellulare, cytomegalovirus, *Cryptosporidium*, microsporidia
- Malignancy: Kaposi's sarcoma, non-Hodgkin's lymphoma
- AIDS enteropathy

REVIEW EXERCISES

QUESTIONS

1. A 68-year-old woman reports diarrhea and occasional fecal incontinence. She is otherwise healthy; her appetite is good, and her weight stable. Which of the following helps you decide whether her diarrhea is significant?
a) Passage of liquid stools
b) Frequent passage of stools
c) Presence of large bowel movements
d) 24-Hour stool weight >250 g
e) History of fecal incontinence

Answer and Discussion

The answer is e. The history of fecal incontinence should always be considered significant and evaluated. In a patient with fecal incontinence who is otherwise healthy, the involuntary loss of stool can be perceived as diarrhea. Although liquid stools are usually associated with increased weight, stool weight remains the only objective way of assessing the degree of diarrhea (thus, answer d is also considered an acceptable answer, but not the best answer).

2. Which of the following features can help distinguish osmotic from secretory diarrhea?
a) Secretory diarrhea decreases or disappears with fasting.
b) There is usually no osmotic gap in secretory diarrhea.
c) Osmotic diarrhea is often accompanied by bleeding.
d) Stool weight is higher in osmotic diarrhea due to the nonabsorbable solutes.

Answer and Discussion

The answer is b. Because secretory diarrhea is associated either with the active secretion of electrolytes and water or impaired absorption, no increase in osmotic gap occurs in this condition. Secretory diarrhea is usually not affected by food intake. Osmotic diarrhea is not accompanied by bleeding. Stool volumes may be high in either osmotic or secretory diarrhea. The nonabsorbable solutes in osmotic diarrhea do not cause the stool weight to rise.

3. A 42-year-old man presents with a 2-year history of diarrhea and weight loss. No bleeding is present. He admits to heavy alcohol intake in the past but has been without alcohol for several years. His diabetes is well controlled with insulin. He underwent cholecystectomy 6 years ago. Laboratory tests are normal, except for mild anemia, and radiographs of the small bowel are reported as normal. Which should be the next test?
a) Endoscopic retrograde cholangiopancreatography
b) Small bowel biopsy
c) 72-Hour stool collection for volume and fat
d) Glucose hydrogen breath test
e) Colonoscopy with biopsy

Answer and Discussion

The answer is c. This man has several potential reasons for diarrhea: (a) alcohol intake, which raises the possibility of pancreatic insufficiency; (b) diabetes, which can lead to bacterial overgrowth or autonomic impairment (diabetic diarrhea); and (c) cholecystectomy. Given the weight loss (suggestive of malabsorption), a 72-hour collection would be helpful in determining whether steatorrhea is present; this result would be highly suggestive of pancreatic insufficiency or possibly bacterial overgrowth. Although endoscopic retrograde cholangiopancreatography and invasive tests can provide evidence of chronic pancreatitis, they do not necessarily indicate the presence of pancreatic insufficiency. A colonoscopy would be reasonable in this man, but it would not help determine the presence of steatorrhea, which is likely in this patient.

4. A 59-year-old African American woman presents with a 6-year history of diarrhea and occasional abdominal pain. Laboratory and stool tests are normal. With which of the following would you proceed?
a) Upper gastrointestinal endoscopy and biopsy
b) Treatment with an anticholinergic
c) Colonoscopy and random biopsies
d) Hydrogen breath test or lactosefree diet for lactose intolerance

Answer and Discussion

The answer is d. Given the history of chronic diarrhea with no evidence of laboratory abnormalities or any suggestion of systemic abnormalities, lactose intolerance is likely, particularly in an African American person. The test is simple and noninvasive, and response to a lactosefree diet will confirm the diagnosis with no need for further testing.

5. A 55-year-old woman with diarrhea is found to have lymphocytic colitis. She has iron-deficiency anemia, and the diarrhea is difficult to control. With which would you proceed?
a) Iron supplementation
b) Antigliadin antibody
c) Small bowel radiograph
d) 72-Hour stool collection for fat
e) Upper endoscopy and small bowel biopsy

Answer and Discussion

The answer is e. Lymphocytic colitis is usually not associated with anemia. Because the diarrhea is difficult to control and the patient also has iron-deficiency anemia, the possibility of celiac disease should be kept in mind. An upper gastrointestinal (GI) endoscopy and small bowel biopsy to exclude celiac, as well as other upper GI sources for anemia, would be the most appropriate way to proceed.

SUGGESTED READINGS

Dieterich W, Ehnis T, Bauer M, et al. Identification of tissue transglutaminase as the autoantigen of celiac disease. *Nat Med* 1997; 3:797–801.

Eherer AJ, Fordtran JS. Fecal osmotic gap and pH in experimental diarrhea of various causes. *Gastroenterology* 1992;103:545–551.

Fine KD, Lee EL. Efficacy of open-label bismuth subsalicylate for the treatment of microscopic colitis. *Gastroenterology* 1998;114:29–36.

Fine KD, Schiller LR. AGA technical review on the evaluation and management of chronic diarrhea. *Gastroenterology* 1999;116:1464–1486.

Goggins M, Kelleher D. Celiac disease and other nutrient-related injuries to the gastrointestinal tract. *Am J Gastroenterol* 1994; 89(Suppl):S2–S17.

Grohmann GS, Glass RI, Pereira HG, et al. Enteric viruses and diarrhea in HIV-infected patients. *N Engl J Med* 1993;329:14–20.

Kotler DP, Orenstein JM. Chronic diarrhea and malabsorption associated with enteropathogenic bacterial infection in a patient with AIDS. *Ann Intern Med* 1993;119:127–128.

Matteoni C, Wang N, Goldblum J, et al. Celiac disease is highly prevalent in lymphocytic colitis. *J Clin Gastroenterol* 2001;32:225–227.

Phillips S, Donaldson L, Geisler K, et al. Stool composition in factitial diarrhea: a 6-year experience with stool analysis. *Ann Intern Med* 1995;123:97–100.

Saslow SB, Camilleri M. Diabetic diarrhea. *Semin Gastrointest Dis* 1995;6:187–193.

Shamir R. Advances in celiac disease. *Gastroenterol Clin North Am* 2003;32:931–947.

Trier JS. Diagnosis of celiac sprue. *Gastroenterology* 1998;115:211–216.

Wilcox CM, Schwartz DA, Cotsonis G, et al. Chronic unexplained diarrhea in human immunodeficiency virus infection: determination of the best diagnostic approach. *Gastroenterology* 1996;110:30–37.

Chapter 58

Coronary Artery Disease

Sarinya Puwanant   Richard Grimm

 POINTS TO REMEMBER:

- In patients with coronary stenosis, the flow of blood is preserved at rest until the lumen diameter is reduced by 90% to 95%, at which time rest pain occurs.

- The gold standard of coronary artery disease (CAD) is stenosis >50% diameter (some centers use >70%) at coronary angiography.

- In patients with high or low probability of disease, the usefulness of noninvasive testing for diagnostic purposes is limited.

- Cardiac imaging is currently performed by (a) anatomical imaging, including multislice computed tomography (MSCT) and magnetic resonance imaging (MRI), which directly visualize the coronary arteries; or (b) functional imaging, including single photon emission computed tomography (SPECT), echocardiography, positron emission tomography (PET), or MRI, which evaluate the physiological consequences of CAD.

- No single test is optimal for the diagnosis of significant CAD in the population as a whole, but the two major determinants of appropriate testing modality are the interpretability of the stress ECG and the ability of the patient to exercise maximally.

- Stress imaging typically is used in patients with non-diagnostic ST segments. This includes patients with the following conditions:

  Complete left bundle-branch block
  Left ventricular hypertrophy with strain
  Digitalis therapy
  Resting ST-segment changes (ST depression >1 mm)
  Wolff-Parkinson-White syndrome

- Dobutamine stress MRI with a standard dobutamine-atropine stress protocol increases sensitivity from 74% to 86% and specificity from 70% to 86% compared with dobutamine stress echocardiography in detecting CAD ≥50% coronary luminal stenosis.

- Given consistently high negative predictive value based on currently available data and technology, multislice computed tomographic angiography (MSCTA) is a useful noninvasive tool for excluding obstructive CAD rather than predicting who has obstructive disease and needs further an invasive cardiac catheterization.

The diagnostic approach to the evaluation of patients with CAD is in the midst of a significant overhaul. Although exercise stress testing has traditionally been the method of choice in determining functional severity of coronary stenosis and prognosis and coronary angiography has been the method of choice to identify CAD, several other methods are vying for credibility as testing methods most adept at identifying and characterizing plaque burden and vulnerable plaque and, hence, prognosis. These include electron beam tomography (EBT); MRI; intravascular ultrasound (IVUS); serum markers of inflammation (i.e., C-reactive protein); and, most notably, MSCT. Due to the relatively preliminary nature of these data as well as the lack of adequate outcome information at the present time, it would be premature to include a definitive discussion of these methods with this review. The more conventional approach will therefore be discussed with the recognition that exercise stress testing will likely be paired with one of several diagnostic modalities to identify CAD in a more thorough and comprehensive evaluation of such patients.

WHAT IS "SIGNIFICANT" CORONARY ARTERY DISEASE?

In patients with coronary stenosis, the flow of blood is preserved at rest until the lumen diameter is reduced by 90% to 95%, at which time rest pain occurs. Patients with milder lesions develop ischemia during stress, when despite dilation of the distal coronary vasculature, coronary flow becomes restricted by the stenosis. This usually occurs with stenosis >50% and almost always with lesions >70% of the artery diameter. In the 50% range, flow reduction is modulated by collateral flow, location and length of stenosis, relation to bends and bifurcations, and other variables. Thus, the gold standard of CAD is stenosis >50% diameter (some centers use >70%) at coronary angiography.

There certainly are a number of problems with this criterion, including poor correlation between severity of stenosis and reduction of flow and interobserver variability in subjective interpretation. Nonetheless, a reference standard is needed, and this is the best that is currently available.

STATISTICAL APPROACH TO ASSESSING STRESS TESTS

No noninvasive test used for the diagnosis of CAD is perfect. The aim of testing is to inform the ordering physician about the likelihood of disease being present as well as its severity and prognosis.

The accuracy of the diagnostic noninvasive test is defined in relation to a gold standard—the coronary angiogram. Several statistic values are used to measure the ability of noninvasive tests to predict the presence of significant coronary stenosis (Table 58.1). Sensitivity and specificity are the most widely used because they depend less on disease prevalence than the other variables.

Applying the Bayes theorem, the posttest probability of disease depends not only on the accuracy of the test but also on the pretest probability of CAD (Table 58.2).

The pretest probability is dependent on age, gender, and symptom status (Table 58.3). Accordingly, the elderly

---

TABLE 58.1

STATISTICAL TERMS OF DIAGNOSTIC TEST ACCURACY

Sensitivity: True positives/All patients with CAD
Specificity: True negatives/All patients without CAD
PV of positive test: True positives/All positive tests
PV of negative test: True negatives/All negative tests
Accuracy: All correct results/All patients

CAD, coronary artery disease; PV, positive value.

TABLE 58.2

BAYES THEOREM

$$\text{Posttest probability} = \frac{\text{Pretest probability} \times \text{Sensitivity}}{\text{Pretest probability} \times \text{Sensitivity} + [(1\text{-Pretest probability}) \times (1\text{-Specificity})]}$$

---

male with typical anginal chest pain has the highest pretest probability, whereas the young female with nonanginal chest pain has the least pretest probability. Additionally, a history of prior myocardial infarction and electrocardiographic Q wave dramatically increases the pretest probability. The relationship between accuracy, pretest probability, and posttest probability is summarized in Figure 58.1, which shows that patients with a very low (<10%) (*Patient 3*) or very high (>90%) (*Patient 1*) pretest probability of disease will remain in these categories regardless of test results and accuracy. Thus, in patients with high or low probability of disease, the usefulness of noninvasive testing for diagnostic purposes is limited. This is the reason why noninvasive testing should be performed in individuals with intermediate pretest probability (*Patient 2*).

The ordering physician should determine the pretest probability in each patient prior to referral for noninvasive testing. These tests may, however, provide useful prognostic data (e.g., exercise capacity, site and extent of ischemia, severity of left ventricular dysfunction), which may influence treatment. The following sections assume that appropriate decisions about investigation are made on clinical grounds, even though in clinical practice, these "rules" often are broken. Low pretest probability will refer to that <10%, intermediate pretest probability will refer to that between 10% and 90%, and high pretest probability will refer to that >90%.

DIAGNOSTIC TESTS

There is a bewildering number of combinations of stress ECG and/or imaging techniques for the detection of CAD (Table 58.4). Cardiac imaging is currently performed by (a) anatomical imaging, including MSCT and MRI, which directly visualize the coronary arteries; or (b) functional imaging, including SPECT, echocardiography, PET, or MRI, which evaluate the physiological consequences of CAD.

No single test is optimal for the diagnosis of significant CAD in the population as a whole, but the two major determinants of appropriate testing modality are the interpretability of the stress ECG and the ability of the patient to exercise maximally. Patients who can exercise maximally should do so, because exercise testing provides useful functional and prognostic information independent of

TABLE 58.3

PRETEST PROBABILITY BY AGE, GENDER, AND SYMPTOM

Age (Years)	Nonanginal Chest Pain		Atypical Angina		Typical Angina	
	Men	Women	Men	Women	Men	Women
30–39	4	2	34	12	76	26
40–49	13	3	51	22	87	55
50–59	20	7	65	31	93	73
60–69	27	14	72	51	94	86

whether ischemia is detected. If the ECG is nondiagnostic (discussed later), an imaging test should be performed, and this should be planned for all patients who undergo pharmacologic stress because of an inability to exercise. The latter groups (nondiagnostic ECGs) now constitute the majority of tests performed in most tertiary centers (Fig. 58.2).

EXERCISE ELECTROCARDIOGRAPHY

Who Should Undergo Exercise Electrocardiography?

Patients should undergo exercise ECG if they can exercise maximally and have an interpretable ST segment. In contrast to the expense of imaging tests (which can exceed $1,000), exercise ECG is "low-tech" and relatively inexpensive. It is difficult to obtain current, specific cost and charge data at most institutions, but the multiples between different tests change little. Table 58.5 lists these multiples for costs, reimbursements, and charges involved with the common diagnostic methodologies.

Despite the potential cost savings of a given methodology, its effectiveness must be considered as well. Exclusive use of standard exercise ECG would have clear disadvantages in relation to accuracy. Only about one-third of patients exercise maximally and have an interpretable stress ECG, and among these patients, equivocal results (e.g., borderline ST-segment changes without angina) may necessitate the performance of a stress-imaging test.

Indications for exercise ECG tests in addition to those used for the diagnosis of CAD are:

- Diagnostic evaluation of chest pain
- Physiological significance of known CAD
- Prognosis of CAD (especially after myocardial infarction)
- Evaluation of therapy (e.g., drug, percutaneous transluminal coronary angioplasty, coronary artery bypass graft)
- Screening for CAD in "at-risk" individuals
- Evaluation of arrhythmias, pacing, and chronotropic competence
- Heart failure (especially evaluation of treatment)
- Estimation of functional capacity
- Follow-up of patients with congenital and valvular diseases

Provided that the contraindications are observed, exercise ECG testing is quite safe, with a recorded serious-event rate of 1:1,000 or lower. Contraindications are:

- Acute myocardial infarction (within 2 days)
- High-risk unstable angina
- Uncontrolled cardiac arrhythmias causing symptoms or hemodynamic compromise
- Symptomatic severe aortic stenosis
- Uncontrolled symptomatic heart failure
- Acute pulmonary embolism or pulmonary infarction
- Acute myocarditis or pericarditis
- Acute aortic dissection

Lesser degrees of these problems, especially after treatment, may benefit from exercise testing. Relative contraindications include:

- Left main coronary stenosis
- Moderate stenotic valvular heart disease
- Electrolyte abnormalities
- Severe arterial hypertension
- Tachy- or bradyarrhythmias
- Hypertrophic obstructive cardiomyopathy and other forms of outflow tract obstruction

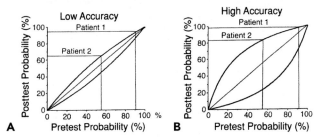

Figure 58.1 Relation of pretest and posttest probability with tests of low accuracy **(A)** and high accuracy **(B)**.

TABLE 58.4

DIAGNOSTIC TEST MODALITIES FOR DETECTION OF CORONARY ARTERY DISEASE

1. ECG Testing
   Exercise ECG test (treadmill, bicycle)
2. Cardiac Imaging
   2.1. Functional Imaging

Stress imaging and perfusion study	Exercise	**Stress Modalities** Pharmacological Agent	Pacer, Cold
	■ Treadmill	■ Dobutamine	
	■ Bicycle	■ Dipyridamole-Adenosine	
	Commonly used examples		
a) Stress echocardiography	Exercise stress echocardiography	Dobutamine stress echocardiography	
b) Stress nuclear test			Uncommon
■ SPECT	Exercise SPECT	Dipyridamole/Adenosine SPECT	
■ Thallium-201			
■ Tc-MIBI			
■ Other technecium-99m			
■ PET	Exercise PET	Dipyridamole/Adenosine PET	
c) Stress cardiac MRI		Dobutamine/Adenosine stress cardiac MRI	
■ Stress-induced wall motion abnormality			
■ Perfusion imaging			

   2.2. Anatomical Imaging
   Direct visualization of coronary arteries
   a) Multislice coronary CT scan
   b) Coronary MRA

CT, computed tomography; ECG, electrocardiogram; MRA, magnetic resonance angiography; MRI, magnetic resonance imaging; PET, positron emission tomography; SPECT, single photon emission computed tomography.

■ Mental or physical impairment leading to the inability to exercise adequately
■ High-degree atrioventricular block

Performing Exercise Electrocardiography

A test is identified as being "positive" by a horizontal or downsloping ST-segment depression >0.1 mV (Fig. 58.3). Upsloping ST depression is accepted if it occurs 0.08 seconds after the J point, but this is less specific than the other changes. Unless it occurs in leads with Q waves, ST-segment elevation is a reliable sign of transmural ischemia. The area of ST depression detected during exercise stress test poorly correlates with localization of wall motion abnormalities and ischemia distribution, whereas the area of ST elevation correlates well with ischemia distribution localization. The presence of angina, exercise capacity, hypotensive response, and dysrhythmia during testing also provide adjunctive poor prognostic information. These data have been combined into various global exercise scores, but these scores have not been widely accepted.

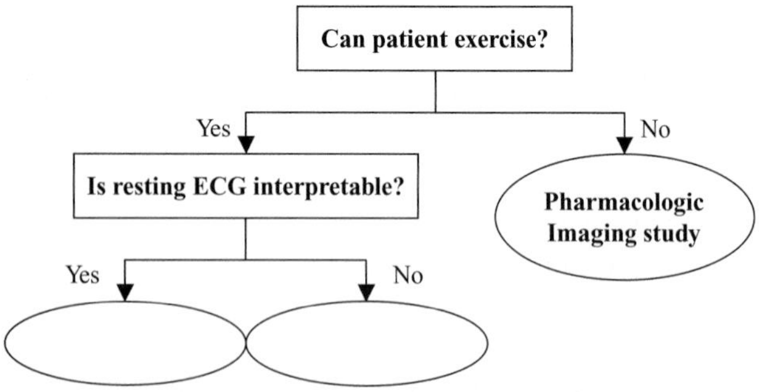

Accuracy of Exercise Electrocardiography

Results of studies having minimal referral bias have shown that both the sensitivity and specificity of standard exercise

Figure 58.2 Schematic algorithm for selection of diagnostic tests.

TABLE 58.5

COSTS, REIMBURSEMENTS, AND CHARGES FOR COMMON DIAGNOSTIC METHODOLOGIES AS A MULTIPLE OF THE COST FOR AN EXERCISE STRESS ELECTROCARDIOGRAM

	Charges	Reimbursement (Medicare)	Cost
Exercise ECG	2.5	0.4	1.0
Exercise [201]Tl	13.3	3.2	5.1
Exercise echocardiography	7.7	1.6	1.4
Coronary angiography	31.8	9.1	13.4

ECG, electrocardiogram; ^{201}Tl, thallium-201.

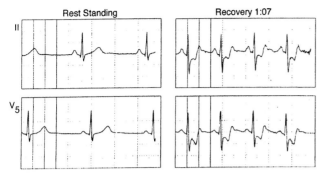

Figure 58.3 Exercise-induced ST-segment depression consistent with myocardial ischemia.

ECG is in the mid-70% range (Table 58.6). The accuracy is somewhat lower in female subjects, but the reasons for this are not well understood.

Selection of exercise ECG testing must be made with the knowledge that this technique is less accurate than are stress-imaging approaches. Equivocal results such as a negative test response in a high-probability patient may occur, thus causing a stress-imaging test or angiography to be performed to clarify the matter.

STRESS-IMAGING TECHNIQUES

Who Should Undergo Stress Imaging?

Stress imaging typically is used in patients with nondiagnostic ST segments. This includes patients with the following conditions:

- Complete left bundle-branch block
- Left ventricular hypertrophy with strain
- Digitalis therapy
- Resting ST-segment changes (ST depression >1 mm)
- Wolff-Parkinson-White syndrome
- Electrically paced ventricular rhythm

Stress imaging also is used in patients who require pharmacologic stress because of their inability to exercise maximally, such as those with the following conditions:

- Peripheral vascular disease
- Orthopedic problems (e.g., back, legs)
- Chronic respiratory disease
- Cerebrovascular disease
- Medications, poor motivation
- Poor physical capacity

To these, one also might add patients with normal resting ST segments in whom exercise ECG may be unreliable, such as women and patients with left ventricular hypertrophy.

Performing Stress Imaging

Stress Echocardiography
Stress echocardiography involves comparison of regional function, including new regional wall motion abnormality, a global ejection fraction, and an end-systolic volume, at rest as well as both during and after stress (by either exercise or dobutamine) to identify myocardial ischemia. Usually, this process is facilitated by a side-by-side display of digitized images in a cine-loop format. Its accuracy, however, depends on the ability of the observer to identify often subtle changes in regional function. The clinical interpretation of all stress-imaging approaches involves some degree of subjectivity, but a trained observer is especially important during stress echocardiography.

Stress Nuclear Perfusion Study
The basic principle of nuclear imaging involves in detection of tracer emissions, which are indicators of myocardial blood flow and/or myocardial metabolism, by a scanning camera. Standard nuclear methodologies comprise stress ventriculography and myocardial perfusion imaging. The commonly used pharmacologic agents with stress nuclear perfusion study are two vasodilators—dipyridamole and adenosine—which cause an increase in coronary blood flow. Dobutamine, instead, is reserved for patients who are contraindicated to dipyridamole and adenosine.

Single Photon Emission Computed Tomography
The most widely used perfusion imaging technique is SPECT in association with either treadmill or pharmacologic (dipyridamole or adenosine) stress. Tracers labeled with thallium-201 (^{201}Tl) or technecium-99m (^{99m}Tc) (methoxyisobutylisonitrile [MIBI]) are primarily used to assess both myocardial perfusion and viability. Thallium is innately unfavorable for imaging because of its low-energy photon emission, which leads to tissue attenuation and scatter; unfavorable radiation dosimetry, which also contributes to low photon counts; and long half-life, which precludes a true resting scan and leads to ambiguity regarding the presence of infarction and ischemia. These constraints are not shared by ^{99m}Tc, however, which has been attached

TABLE 58.6		
EXERCISE ELECTROCARDIOGRAPHY: SENSITIVITY AND SPECIFICITY		
	Sensitivity (n [%])	Specificity (n [%])
Sketch (1980)	40/59 (68)	39/48 (81)
Melin (1981)	73/99 (74)	43/61 (70)
Patterson (1982)	27/50 (54)	35/46 (76)
Weintraub (1984)	73/101 (72)	37/46 (80)
Hung (1985)	99/117 (85)	34/54 (63)
Combined male patients	312/426 (73)	188/255 (74)
Hung (1986)	20/28 (71)	38/64 (59)
Melin (1985)	27/44 (61)	72/91 (79)
Combined female patients	47/72 (65)	110/155 (71)

to various isonitriles, the most widespread of which is MIBI. The benefits of MIBI include a better image quality; a small increment of accuracy, particularly in the posterior territories of the heart, which are the most poorly visualized areas at ^{201}Tl imaging; ability to perform ventriculography simultaneously with perfusion measurements; imaging for exclusion of false-positive perfusion defects resulting from soft tissue attenuation; and absence of redistribution, thus allowing injection of this tracer at one time and imaging at a later time, which is useful in the emergency room or during acute intervention.

Recent work has combined the benefits of [201]Tl (i.e., assessment of viability, lesser expense) with those of MIBI (i.e., absence of washout, high-quality images), thus producing a dual-isotope approach that enhances the performance speed of nuclear scintigraphic studies. The benefits of using MIBI in this approach, however, are obtained at a significant increase in cost.

Positron Emission Tomography

PET is a sophisticated imaging technique that may be used to examine myocardial perfusion using the tracers ^{13}N-ammonia, ^{15}O-water, or [82]Rb. This technology provides accurate measurements of myocardial perfusion, glucose metabolism, and fatty acid metabolism, but further development of PET for diagnostic purposes has been inhibited by its cost. Whether the expense of PET is justified on the basis of better prognostic assessment or prevention of a substantial number of unnecessary catheterizations remains unresolved.

Stress Cardiac Magnetic Resonance Imaging

The basic principle of cardiac MRI is based on a release of energy of the hydrogen atom in the electromagnetic radiation form that is detected and processed to the image. The static and cine cardiac images can be obtained by using ECG or respiratory-gated image technique.

Perfusion Imaging

Gadolinium is a primary contrast agent used as a perfusion agent. Since the gadolinium intensity parallels with coronary blood flow, the functional significance of obstructive coronary lesion and/or the presence of ischemia can be detected by an area of delay or absence of gadolinium perfusion into the myocardium during stress testing using vasodilators (dipyridamole or adenosine). Furthermore, not only ischemia but also myocardial scar and viability can be assessed by cardiac MRI technique.

Stress-induced Wall Motion Abnormality

Similar to stress echocardiography, wall thickening, ejection fraction, end systolic volume, and wall motion abnormality at rest and during stress testing using dobutamine can be accurately assessed by cine cardiac MRI. Cardiac MRI has superior spatial resolution compared with that found in echocardiography. Additionally, the image quality is not limited in a patient with a poor acoustic window.

Although cardiac MRI is a promising cardiac imaging technique, it is limited in patients with atrial fibrillation or arrhythmia and a pacemaker or defibrillator. Furthermore, its expensive cost, a requirement of skilled equipment-operated personnel, and portable capability make it somewhat less attractive compared with echocardiography in particular clinical settings.

Accuracy of Stress Imaging

Tomographic myocardial perfusion imaging (i.e., SPECT) offers a greater sensitivity for CAD than planar approaches, but this may occur at the cost of lower specificity (Table 58.7). To an extent, this may reflect referral bias. Perfusion scintigraphy has a particularly low specificity in subgroups of patients with left ventricular hypertrophy and left bundle-branch block. Thus, whereas perfusion scintigraphy has the benefit of much experience with its use, recent concerns have focused on its cost as well as on its

TABLE 58.7

EXERCISE THALLIUM SPECT DIAGNOSIS OF CORONARY ARTERY DISEASE: SENSITIVITY AND SPECIFICITY

	Sensitivity (%)			
	Overall	No Myocardial Infarction	Specificity (%)	Myocardial Infarction (in Coronary Artery Disease) (%)
Tamaki (n = 104)	96	96	91	39
DePasquale (n = 210)	95	92	74	26
Iskandrian (n = 461)	82	78	60	18
Maddahi (n = 183)	95	90	56	47
Mahmarian and Verani (1991) (n = 360)	87	79	87	33
Van Train (n = 262)	94	90	43	40
Total	90	85	70	31

SPECT, single photon emission computed tomography.

TABLE 58.8

ACCURACY OF POSITRON EMISSION TOMOGRAPHY FOR DETECTION OF CORONARY ARTERY DISEASE

	Tracer	Myocardial Infarction (%)	Sensitivity (n [%])	Specificity (n [%])
Schelbert (1982)	^{13}N	?	31/32 (97)	13/13 (100)[a]
Yonekura (1987)	^{13}N	43	37/38 (97)	13/14 (93)[a]
Tamaki (1988)	^{13}N	74	47/48 (98)	3/3 (100)[a]
Go (1990)	^{82}Rb	47	142/152 (93)	39/50 (78)
Stewart (1991)	^{82}Rb	42	50/60 (83)	19/21 (90)

[a]Including normal volunteers.
^{13}N, nitrogen-13; ^{82}Rb, rubidium-82

false-positive rate. It remains an excellent choice, however, in patients with previous infarction and at centers without a major commitment to high-quality stress echocardiography.

The accuracy of PET for the diagnosis of CAD is >90%, although many of the studies have been small and have included an unacceptable number of patients with previous myocardial infarction (Table 58.8). Comparisons of cardiac PET with SPECT have shown a benefit to PET in terms of accuracy, which mirrors the underlying benefits of PET regarding accurate localization of tracer, ability to obtain high counts (and, therefore, excellent image quality), and capacity to perform attenuation correction. Clinically, these benefits include a better ability to resolve moderate (i.e., 50%–70% diameter) coronary stenosis, reduction of false-positive results because of soft tissue attenuation artifacts, and ability to accurately diagnose CAD involving the posterior parts of the heart (reflecting the benefits of attenuation correction, reduction of scatter, and higher counts). Both the cost and availability of PET, however, mandate a selective and sparing use of this technology. For diagnostic purposes, its high specificity is attractive in patients with a lower probability of CAD, and its high diagnostic accuracy is attractive in patients for whom angiography is inappropriate. It also may be useful for studying patients who otherwise are difficult to image (e.g., obese patients). Nonetheless, the major value of PET relates to evaluating the physiological significance of known coronary lesions as well as investigating issues of myocardial viability.

The sensitivity and specificity of exercise echocardiography for identification of CAD are approximately 85% each (Table 58.9). As with other noninvasive tests, however, these values vary among studies relative to the mix of patients, and particularly relative to the prevalence of multivessel disease and previous infarction, which augment the recorded sensitivity of all stress-imaging tests. Two particular problems for stress echocardiography are identification of multivessel disease in patients without previous infarction and detection of ischemia in the setting of resting wall motion abnormalities. Currently, stress echocardiography

has the disadvantage of involving subjective interpretation. However, it has advantages in relation to cost, safety, and patient convenience. In addition, it may be the test of choice for patients with left ventricular hypertrophy and, possibly, those with left bundle-branch block.

A recent meta-analysis has shown that the stress-induced wall motion abnormalities using MRI demonstrated a sensitivity of 83% and specificity of 86% in detecting ≥50% diameter stenosis using conventional invasive coronary angiography as a gold standard. Perfusion imaging demonstrated a corresponding sensitivity of 91% and specificity of 81% on a per-patient analysis.

Notably, the ECG component of either dipyridamole or dobutamine stress is insensitive for the identification of myocardial ischemia. Consequently, if either dipyridamole or dobutamine is selected as a stressor in these patients, a stress-imaging technique should be performed as well.

COMPARATIVE STUDIES

The sensitivity of stress imaging exceeds that of exercise ECG. This result can be readily anticipated from the "ischemic cascade" (Fig. 58.4).

TABLE 58.9

DIGITAL EXERCISE ECHOCARDIOGRAPHY: SENSITIVITY AND SPECIFICITY

	Sensitivity (n [%])	Specificity (n [%])
Armstrong (1987)	40/51 (78)	19/22 (86)
Ryan (1988)	31/40 (78)	24/24 (100)
Crouse (1991)	170/175 (97)	34/53 (64)
Marwick (1992)	96/114 (84)	31/36 (86)
Quinones (1992)	64/86 (74)	21/26 (81)
Hecht (1993)	127/137 (93)	37/46 (80)
Ryan (1993)	192/211 (91)	76/98 (78)
Combined	720/814 (88)	242/305 (79)

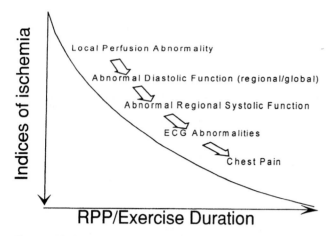

Figure 58.4 The "ischemic cascade," during which less sensitive tests become positive at higher workloads. (RPP, rate-pressure product.)

The overall accuracy of stress echocardiography is comparable to that of nuclear scintigraphy. Scintigraphy has a slightly higher sensitivity, however, and echocardiography has a higher specificity. The strengths of stress echocardiography are its speed, cost, accuracy in patients with left ventricular hypertrophy or left bundle-branch block, and acquisition of data about resting left ventricular function, valves, and pericardium. Scintigraphy is more sensitive for single-vessel disease, better for recognizing multivessel disease, and may be better for distinguishing ischemia and infarction. It also is more quantitative, although both techniques require both technical and interpretive expertise. Adenosine SPECT perfusion imaging is the test of choice in patients with conduction abnormalities (i.e., left bundle-branch block) requiring a functional study.

Dobutamine stress MRI with a standard dobutamine-atropine stress protocol increases sensitivity from 74% to 86% and specificity from 70% to 86% compared with dobutamine stress echocardiography in detecting CAD ≥50% coronary luminal stenosis. In patients who are not contraindicated in performing MRI, stress and perfusion cardiac MRI study is an attractive imaging modality used as either an initial diagnostic test or an alternative stress-imaging study, particularly in the individual who has a potentially poor acoustic window for echocardiography and contraindication for nuclear stress test. Furthermore, cardiac MRI can be considered as a "one-stop-shop" for ischemia (by stress MRI or MRI perfusion study), myocardial viability and scar (by contrast enhancement), ventricular performance, and coronary anatomy (by coronary magnetic resonance angiography [MRA]) evaluation.

The decision between echocardiography, nuclear testing, or cardiac MRI is made predominantly on the basis of local expertise and availability. This is particularly true for stress echocardiography, which undoubtedly is the most technically demanding of the techniques.

EVALUATION OF PATIENTS UNABLE TO EXERCISE

As discussed, pharmacologic stress ECG (without imaging) is not a good option in patients who are unable to exercise. Because myocardial perfusion scintigraphy essentially depends on the evaluation of differences in regional hyperemia, coronary vasodilators (e.g., dipyridamole, adenosine) are the optimal pharmacologic stressors for this test. For echocardiography, dobutamine is a better stressor than coronary vasodilators, which rarely cause ischemia in a functional sense.

Exercise and pharmacologic stress-imaging tests have comparable accuracy. The additional data provided by exercise, however—including correlation of stress with daily life, exercise capacity, and ST-segment and rhythm evaluation—all favor the use of exercise whenever a patient can exercise maximally.

CARDIAC IMAGING FOR DIRECT VISUALIZATION OF THE CORONARY ARTERIES

Contrast-enhanced noninvasive coronary angiography, including MSCT and coronary MRA, is an emerging noninvasive imaging tool allowing direct visualization of the coronary arteries after administration of contrast agents (iodinated contrast for CT and gadolinium for cardiac MRI). Those can provide not only qualitatively and quantitatively evaluated obstructive CAD but also nonobstructive atherosclerotic plaque (calcified, soft, or noncalcified plaque) information (Figure 58.5). The latter, as well as noninvasive strategy, cause those imaging modalities to be more attractive compared with conventional invasive coronary angiogram or "luminogram."

Who Should Undergo Imaging for Direct Visualization of the Coronary Arteries?

Although there are no universally accepted indications or guidelines for contrast-enhanced MSCT and coronary MRA due to insufficient available data, the ACCF/ACR/SCCT/SCMR/ASNC/NASCI/SCAI/SIR recommend that MSCT is appropriate in patients with chest pain syndrome or acute chest pain with intermediate pretest probability, patients with chest pain syndrome with uninterpretable or equivocal stress test, evaluation of suspected coronary anomalies, and evaluation of coronary arteries in patients with new-onset heart failure. In the near future, the usefulness of plaque information, as well as improved spatial and temporal resolution technology, will likely allow MSCT to play a major role in aggressive primary prevention, intensify medical therapy, and screen for the need of invasive coronary angiography in patients with atherosclerotic risk factor(s). Risk of radiation and contrast exposure should be

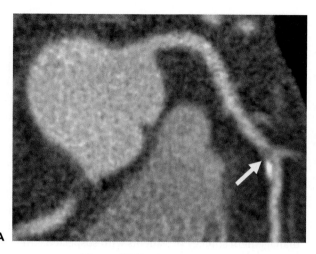
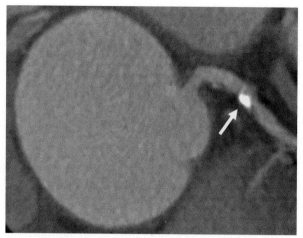

Figure 58.5 Coronary arterial plaque visualized by multislice computed tomography. (**A,** mixed soft plaque at the proximal LAD coronary artery; **B,** calcified plaque at the proximal LAD.)

considered before ordering the test. Patients with renal insufficiency, obesity (body mass index >40 kg/m^2), arrhythmia (including atrial fibrillation and high-grade atrioventricular block), tachycardia, coronary calcium score >600, inability to hold the breath, or claustrophobia should not undergo an MSCT scan.

Generally, MSCT can provide superior spatial resolution of coronary artery stenoses as well as plaque morphology compared with that found in coronary MRA. MRA is usually performed as a hybrid or subsequent test complement to functional cardiac MRI study (perfusion or viability). MRI is, however, limited in patients with a pacemaker, defibrillator or cardiac resynchronization therapy, arrhythmia, claustrophobia, inability to hold the breath, and renal insufficiency.

Since not all obstructive coronary lesions are flow-limiting or ischemia-producing lesions, a functional study (such as stress-imaging or perfusion-imaging study) in addition to the anatomical information is required to provide clinical significance (or ischemic burden data) of such anatomically obstructive coronary lesions prior to consideration for cardiac catheterization.

Performing Imaging for Direct Visualization of the Coronary Arteries

Cardiac Computed Tomography

Contrast-enhanced Multislice Computed Tomographic Angiography

The advanced technology of MSCTA allows high-quality imaging of the beating heart and its vessels with a high spatial resolution and an improved temporal resolution. Cardiac image acquisitions are obtained in multiple cardiac phases during a single breath-hold (<10 seconds). A bolus of contrast (approximately 100 mL) with a relatively high iodine concentration (400 mg iodine/mL) is required to assess obstructive CAD and plaque information. Both 16- and

64-slice MSCTA scanners provides adequate visualization of the coronary arteries and plaque information, although the 64-slice scanner reduces the breath-hold requirement by allowing faster acquisition of all slices. Compared with conventional coronary angiography (luminography), the radiation exposure for MSCTA is generally higher (8–21 vs. 2–10 mSv); however, image acquisition with prospective ECG-gating technique can reduce the radiation exposure.

Coronary Calcium Imaging

CAC can be quantitatively evaluated in the scale of the calcium score by both electron beam computed tomography (EBCT) scan and MSCT scan techniques. For obligatory CAC detection, a contrast administration is not required. Furthermore, the radiation exposure for the calcium score obtained with MSCT is small (2–4 mSv). The considerable amount of CAC or a high CAC score (>600) can cause overestimation of the severity of coronary obstruction, so-called "blooming artifact"; thus, the CAC screening prior to MSCT scanning can minimize the likelihood of an MSCT that cannot be interpreted.

Coronary Magnetic Resonance Angiography

Acquisition of coronary MRA can be obtained with either breath-hold or respiratory-gated techniques. Gradient-echo technique has been used for coronary MRA that detects coronary blood flow. The major advantages of coronary MRA over contrast-enhanced MSCTA are MRA is free of radiation exposure and provides better temporal resolution.

Accuracy of Coronary Artery Imaging

Multislice Coronary Computed Tomographic Angiography

Published data pertaining to the accuracy of MSCTA has been based on patients with known or suspected CAD. On a per-segment analysis, the average sensitivity and specificity for detecting at least one coronary artery with >50% luminal stenosis are 83% (30%–99%) and 92% (64%–98%), respectively. The corresponding average positive and negative predictive values are 67% (14%–91%) and 97% (83%–99%), respectively. Given the consistently high negative predictive value based on currently available data and technology, MSCTA is a useful noninvasive tool for excluding obstructive CAD rather than predicting who has obstructive disease and needs further an invasive cardiac catheterization.

Coronary Calcium Score

The CAC is a marker of atherosclerosis, but it does not necessarily indicate the presence of obstructive CAD. Furthermore, the absence of CAC does not exclude noncalcified coronary plaque. Since the accuracy of the CAC in terms of diagnosis of obstructive CAD is modest, it is not recommended to establish the presence of CAD.

Coronary Magnetic Resonance Angiography

A recent meta-analysis evaluating the accuracy of coronary MRA as compared with conventional invasive coronary angiography in patients with known or suspected CAD has shown that the average sensitivity and specificity for detecting coronary artery are 73% (75% for vessel-level analysis and 88% for subject-level analysis) and 86% (85% for vessel-level analysis and 56% for subject-level analysis), respectively. This implies that MRA is a reasonable noninvasive tool for exclusion of significant CAD in patients referred for diagnostic invasive coronary angiography; however, the available published data is not sufficient to use coronary MRA as a screening tool, especially in patients with a low pretest probability of CAD.

PROGNOSIS

In clinical practice, diagnosis rarely is separate from prognostic assessment. In addition, further investigations rarely are determined by the prediction of CAD alone but on the basis of an assessment of the severity and, hence, the implications of the diagnosis in each individual.

The outcome of patients with CAD is determined by their left ventricular function, amount of jeopardized myocardium, exercise capacity, and noncardiac factors such as age and diabetes. As functional testing provides most of these data, it is not surprising that its predictive power exceeds that of coronary angiography, which supplies anatomic data. At exercise testing, exercise capacity, hypotension, and dysrhythmias predict outcome at exercise testing more so than ST-segment changes. At imaging, the extent of ischemic or all abnormal myocardium is the strongest predictor of outcome. The future of coronary plaque characterization and burden as assessed by MSCTA and its prognostic value in predicting cardiovascular outcomes is expected to exceed current methodologies.

CONCLUSIONS

Recent advances in stress testing have enhanced our ability to identify CAD by noninvasive means. Over the last decade, SPECT, stress echocardiography, and PET have become accepted clinical tools, and some initial data point toward their specific utility in individual situations. Recently, a rapid revolution of advanced tomographic imaging technology has permitted cardiac MRI and MSCT to become attractive imaging modalities in evaluation of significant and presignificant CAD. Nonetheless, the standard exercise ECG stress test remains the backbone of functional testing for CAD. Indeed, the challenge of the next few years will be to incorporate these new techniques into a cost-effective management strategy of patients with suspected CAD.

REVIEW EXERCISES

QUESTIONS

1. A 56-year-old woman with arthritis has atypical pain but a normal ECG. The best diagnostic option is
a) Stress (exercise or dobutamine) ECG
b) Coronary angiography
c) Exercise echocardiography
d) Dipyridamole-thallium imaging
e) None of the above

Answer and Discussion

The answer is d. This is a 56-year-old woman who is described as having arthritis. Therefore, exercise stress will likely result in the patient being unable to exercise maximally or even at all. Because the patient is a female with atypical pain, she would be considered to have an intermediate pretest probability and therefore would be a good candidate for a stress-imaging study. Proceeding directly to coronary angiography with such a relatively low pretest probability would potentially subject the patient to an unnecessary invasive test.

2. A 28-year-old woman presents with left-sided pain at rest and exercise. The best diagnostic option is
a) Exercise ECG
b) Coronary angiography
c) Exercise echocardiography
d) Exercise thallium imaging
e) None of the above

Answer and Discussion

The answer is e. This patient has a very low pretest probability for having CAD (approximately 4%) due to her age, gender, and the atypical nature of the pain. Because of this low pretest probability, the accuracy of a given test will not significantly affect the posttest probability of disease. It is only in those patients with an intermediate pretest likelihood of disease where the accuracy of the test will have a significant effect on posttest probability. Therefore, none of the choices provides the best diagnostic option, as that likely includes consideration of another etiology for the pain other than cardiac.

3. A 68-year-old man presents with central retrosternal pain at exercise. The best diagnostic option is
a) Exercise ECG
b) Coronary angiography
c) Exercise echocardiography
d) Exercise thallium imaging
e) None of the above

Answer and Discussion
The answer is b. This patient would have a high pretest probability of disease; therefore, coronary angiography would provide information on the site, the severity, and extent of the disease. Although an exercise electrocardiographic study as well as an imaging study with echocardiography or thallium perfusion imaging would be useful in risk stratifying such a patient, the definitive diagnosis in detecting disease in this patient population with such a high pretest probability would be coronary angiography.

4. A 48-year-old man with hypertensive left ventricular hypertrophy complains of atypical chest pain. The best diagnostic option is
a) Exercise ECG
b) Coronary angiography
c) Exercise echocardiography
d) Dipyridamole-thallium imaging
e) None of the above

Answer and Discussion
The answer is c. An exercise ECG stress test is likely to be nondiagnostic in patients with left ventricular hypertrophy. Because of the resting secondary ST-T wave repolarization changes characteristic of left ventricular hypertrophy, a false-positive result is likely and may therefore inappropriately lead to further testing. A coronary angiogram would lead to undue risk from an invasive procedure, particularly in a 48-year- old man with atypical pain. A dipyridamole-thallium study is also limited by the potential of falsely positive perfusion defects that likely are secondary to subendocardial ischemia due to abnormal coronary flow reserve seen in hypertrophied hearts despite the presence of normal epicardial vessels. Exercise echocardiography has been demonstrated to be more specific in this patient population, as the basis for this test is an assessment of left ventricular function rather than perfusion, which can be affected by abnormalities in coronary flow reserve.

5. Problems may occur with exercise thallium imaging, except in patients with
a) Left bundle-branch block
b) Left ventricular hypertrophy
c) Female sex
d) Obesity, posterior circulation disease
e) Left anterior descending (LAD) CAD.

Answer and Discussion
The answer is e. Abnormalities may be seen on thallium SPECT imaging in patients with left bundle-branch block secondary to abnormalities in septal conduction. Additionally, patients with left ventricular hypertrophy may also manifest false-positive findings on thallium SPECT imaging that likely are related to coronary flow reserve–related abnormalities, which are characteristic of this patient population. Attenuation defects may be seen in the female population as a result of breast tissue, which may manifest as falsely positive defects particularly in the LAD territory. Nuclear perfusion imaging, specifically thallium SPECT imaging, may be limited in obese patients with potentially false-positive abnormalities arising in the segments served by the posterior circulation and related to the relatively low-energy emissions typical of the ^{201}Tl radioisotope and its relative inability to penetrate large masses of soft tissue. Therefore, the best answer in this case is LAD disease, as this is a patient population that can be identified with a high degree of sensitivity using nuclear SPECT perfusion imaging.

6. A 52-year-old woman has an ECG that cannot be interpreted as well as atypical pain. The least expensive option for further imaging is
a) Exercise thallium
b) Coronary angiography
c) Exercise echocardiography
d) Dipyridamole PET
e) None of the above

Answer and Discussion
The answer is c. Although highly accurate for the diagnosis of CAD, both exercise thallium and dipyridamole PET imaging are relatively expensive and would not qualify as the least expensive option. In addition to being very expensive, a coronary angiogram would subject the patient to an undue relative risk, especially given the relatively low pretest probability of disease (approximately 30%). An exercise echocardiogram would provide the advantage of both a highly accurate diagnostic imaging study as well as a cost benefit of roughly only one and one-half times the cost of an exercise ECG examination.

7. A 52-year-old man needs a femoropopliteal bypass. What would you recommend first for risk stratification?
a) Exercise ECG
b) Coronary angiography
c) Dobutamine echocardiography

d) Dipyridamole-thallium imaging
e) Clinical evaluation

Answer and Discussion

The answer is e. The question specifically requests a recommendation for an initial assessment of risk stratification in this 52-year-old man requiring femoropopliteal bypass surgery. The initial risk stratification should therefore include a clinical examination that initially is directed at determining the presence of angina pectoris—age over 70 years, history of prior heart failure, history of prior myocardial infarction, or the presence of diabetes mellitus. Only when one or more of the above risk factors can be identified should one proceed to a stress-imaging examination. If none of the above risk factors is identified, this patient would have a very low perioperative risk of a cardiac event of approximately 3%, based on the data of Eagle et al.

8. The following probably constitute significant CAD, except
a) Proximal LAD stenosis of 80%
b) LAD stenosis of 60% with angina
c) Right coronary artery stenosis of 50%
d) Left circumflex coronary artery stenosis of 50% with positive exercise ECG

Answer and Discussion

The answer is c. Significant CAD is typically considered to be present with lesions >50% or 70% of the artery diameter. Coronary stenoses in the 50% range may or may not be functionally significant in terms of a reduction in coronary flow, as flow reduction is modulated by collateral vessels, location, and length of stenoses and related to bends and bifurcations as well as other variables. Coronary artery stenoses >90% have been demonstrated to restrict flow at rest without the provocation of stress. Therefore, in this question, a proximal LAD stenosis of 80% almost certainly is considered significant disease, and an LAD stenosis of 60% in the presence of typical angina pectoris also quite likely represents significant flow-limiting coronary disease. Finally, a left circumflex coronary stenosis of 50% with the presence of positive exercise ECG changes is likely to represent significant CAD, yet a right coronary stenosis of 50% in the absence of a functional test that is positive for ischemia or the presence of concomitant symptoms may or may not represent the presence of significant stenosis.

9. Which of the following patients has the greatest probability of CAD?
a) A 48-year-old woman with atypical chest pain
b) A 25-year-old man with typical angina
c) A 45-year-old man with atypical chest pain
d) A 70-year-old man with atypical chest pain

Answer and Discussion

The answer is d. Based on the Diamond and Forester estimate of pretest probability of disease, which is based on age, gender, and symptoms of chest pain, a 70-year-old man with atypical chest pain is likely to have a pretest probability of disease approximating 70%. Of note, the 25-year-old man with typical angina also would have a significant but slightly lower pretest probability of disease. A 45-year-old man with atypical chest pain would have a pretest probability of approximately 46%, whereas a woman of similar age with atypical symptoms would have a dramatically lower pretest probability of disease, estimated to be approximately 13% and reflecting the delayed onset of disease among the female population, which likely is related to the protective effect of estrogen.

10. In what proportion of patients is an exercise ECG adequate for the diagnosis of CAD?
a) Most (approximately 80%).
b) The majority (approximately 60%).
c) The minority (approximately 40%).
d) Few (approximately 10%).

Answer and Discussion

The answer is c. Exercise stress ECG testing is of benefit and useful in a patient who is able to maximally exercise and has a normal resting ECG. Studies have demonstrated that a significant proportion of subjects presenting for an evaluation of coronary disease are either unable to exercise (or cannot exercise maximally) or have ECGs that cannot be interpreted at rest. For this reason, the minority of patients meet both criteria—namely, they have a normal resting ECG and are able to maximally exercise.

11. What is the accuracy of exercise ECG for the diagnosis of CAD?
a) Sensitivity 85%, specificity 85%
b) Sensitivity 85%, specificity 65%
c) Sensitivity 75%, specificity 75%
d) Sensitivity 75%, specificity 95%

Answer and Discussion

The answer is c. More recent investigations that have evaluated the accuracy of exercise electrocardiography have done so in a more sound manner by attempting to limit selection bias and have demonstrated sensitivities and specificities in the 75% range. The sensitivity and specificity of the test in the female population is somewhat lower, at 65% and 71%, respectively.

12. In a patient with intermediate pretest CAD probability, which of the following tests is least sensitive?
a) Stress echocardiography
b) Exercise thallium SPECT

c) Exercise ECG

d) Exercise nuclear ventriculography

Answer and Discussion

The answer is c. Reported sensitivities of stress echocardiography, exercise thallium SPECT imaging, and exercise nuclear ventriculography are approximately 85%, 90%, and 80%, respectively. Reported sensitivities of approximately 75% for exercise ECG make this the least sensitive test of those listed.

13. In a middle-aged woman with atypical pain, which of the following tests is most accurate?

a) Exercise ECG

b) Exercise thallium SPECT

c) PET

d) Exercise nuclear ventriculography

Answer and Discussion

The answer is c. In this middle-aged woman with atypical chest pain, an exercise ECG test is subject to a false-positive result, as ST-T wave abnormalities are relatively common in the female population for reasons that are as yet not well understood. Exercise thallium SPECT imaging, although a more sensitive test, is limited by its reported specificity in large part related to breast attenuation, obesity, and artifacts in the posterior circulation. Exercise nuclear ventriculography is a relatively poorly sensitive study for the detection of CAD. PET imaging, on the other hand, is both highly sensitive as well as highly specific and is particularly good in the female population, as attenuation artifacts are largely eliminated primarily related to the high-energy radioisotopes that are utilized for this imaging procedure.

14. In a patient with left ventricular hypertropy and atypical pain, which of the following tests is most accurate?

a) Exercise ECG

b) Exercise thallium SPECT

c) PET

d) Exercise echocardiography

Answer and Discussion

The answer is d. In this patient with left ventricular hypertrophy and atypical chest pain, the least accurate test would be exercise ECG testing due to the presence of uninterpretable secondary ST-segment repolarization abnormalities commonly seen on the baseline ECG in patients with left ventricular hypertrophy. Of note, recent data would suggest that even in patients without resting electrocardiographic abnormalities but with evidence for left ventricular hypertrophy, the propensity for false-positive stress ECG abnormalities is

significant. It is suspected that abnormalities in coronary flow reserve with resultant subendocardial ischemia in the absence of epicardial vessel disease is responsible for these false-positive perfusion abnormalities noted on nuclear perfusion imaging whether this is thallium SPECT imaging or myocardial PET imaging.

SUGGESTED READINGS

Berman DS, Kiat HS, van Train KF, et al. Myocardial perfusion imaging with technetium-99m-sestamibi: comparative analysis of available imaging protocols. *J Nucl Med* 1994;35:681–688.

Danias PG, Roussakis A, Ioannidis JP. Diagnostic performance of coronary magnetic resonance angiography as compared against conventional X-ray angiography: a meta-analysis. *J Am Coll Cardiol* 2004;44:1867–1876.

Detrano R, Froelicher VF. Exercise testing: uses and limitations considering recent studies. *Prog Cardiovasc Dis* 1988;31:173–204.

Diamond GA, Forrester JS. Analysis of probability as an aid in the clinical diagnosis of coronary artery disease. *N Engl J Med* 1979;300:1350–1358.

Fletcher GF, Balady G, Froelicher VF, et al. AHA Medical/Scientific Statement. Exercise standards. A statement for healthcare professionals from the AHA. *Circulation* 1995;91:580–615.

Gibbons RJ, Balady GJ, Bricker JT, et al; American College of Cardiology/American Heart Association Task Force on Practice Guidelines. ACC/AHA 2002 guideline update for exercise testing: summary article. *Circulation* 2002;106(14):1883–1892.

Hendel RC, Patel MR, Kramer CM, et al. ACCF/ACR/SCCT/ SCMR/ASNC/NASCI/SCAI/SIR 2006 appropriateness criteria for cardiac computed tomography and cardiac magnetic resonance imaging: a report of the American College of Cardiology Foundation Quality Strategic Directions Committee Appropriateness Criteria Working Group, American College of Radiology, Society of Cardiovascular Computed Tomography, Society for Cardiovascular Magnetic Resonance, American Society of Nuclear Cardiology, North American Society for Cardiac Imaging, Society for Cardiovascular Angiography and Interventions, and Society of Interventional Radiology. *J Am Coll Cardiol* 2006;48:1475–1497.

Kahn JK, McGhie I, Akers MS, et al. Quantitative rotational tomography with ^{201}Tl and ^{99m}Tc-methoxyisobutylisonitrile. A direct comparison in normal individuals and patients with coronary artery disease. *Circulation* 1989;79:1282–1290.

Mahmarian JJ, Verani MS. Exercise thallium-201 perfusion scintigraphy in the assessment of coronary artery disease. *Am J Cardiol* 1991;67:2D–11D.

Marwick T, Willemart B, D'Hondt AM, et al. Selection of the optimal nonexercise stress for the evaluation of ischemic regional myocardial dysfunction and malperfusion: comparison of dobutamine and adenosine using echocardiography and Tc-99m MIBI single photon emission computed tomography. *Circulation* 1993;87:345–354.

Nagel E, Lehmkuhl HB, Bocksch W, et al. Noninvasive diagnosis of ischemia-induced wall motion abnormalities with the use of high-dose dobutamine stress MRI: comparison with dobutamine stress echocardiography. *Circulation* 1999;99:763–770.

Picano E, Lattanzi F, Orlandini A, et al. Stress echocardiography and the human factor: the importance of being expert. *J Am Coll Cardiol* 1991;17:666–669.

Pryor DB, Shaw L, McCants CB, et al. Value of the history and physical in identifying patients at increased risk for CAD. *Ann Intern Med* 1993;118:81–90.

Chapter 59

Clinical Electrocardiography

Curtis M. Rimmerman

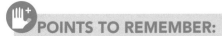
POINTS TO REMEMBER:

- The initial interpretive step for each ECG is to identify atrial activity and determine the cardiac rhythm.

- A varying PR interval supports the possibilities of atrioventricular dissociation of differing types of heart block, both requiring further detailed analysis.

- If >120 msec, a careful assessment of the QRS complex morphology is important, as complete left or right bundle-branch block may exist. Complete left bundle-branch block represents a QRS complex duration >120 msec, the absence of a Q wave (septal depolarization) in leads I and V_{5-6}, an upright QRS complex in leads I and V_{5-6}, and ST segment depression and T-wave inversion in leads I and V_{5-6}.

- To successfully interpret ECGs, a deliberate, consistent, and reproducible approach is essential. Through experience and repetition, the interpreter will demonstrate improved interpretive abilities and confidence, rendering greater diagnostic accuracy.

THE RECOMMENDED APPROACH TO ECG INTERPRETATION

To assure accurate and consistent ECG interpretation, a systematic approach is required. ECG interpretation is not an exercise in pattern recognition. Instead, it requires an interpreter with an inquisitive mind who strives to understand why the ECG demonstrates a specific morphology. This requires a thorough understanding of the cardiac conduction sequence, cardiac anatomy, and cardiac physiology.

Similar cardiac pathology is manifest differently on the surface ECG depending on the ECG lead undergoing analysis. For instance, precordial lead V_1 predominantly overlies the right ventricle. Right ventricular cardiac electrical events are often best seen in this lead. Conversely, precordial lead

V_6 overlies the left ventricle and predictably best represents left ventricular cardiac electrical events. Knowledge of ECG anatomical correlates helps to plan an interpretation strategy, reducing the likelihood of overlooking an important finding. Additionally, oftentimes the ECG serves as the first indicator of occult cardiac pathology. Interpretation is most rewarding when the interpreter deduces a disease state and alerts the clinician to the findings. With experience, certain ECG findings are identified simultaneously, together representing a unifying cardiac diagnosis. A recommended systematic approach to ECG interpretation is outlined below.

CARDIAC RHYTHM DETERMINATION

The initial interpretive step for each ECG is to identify atrial activity and determine the cardiac rhythm. If P waves are present, it is important to precisely measure the P-wave to P-wave interval. This determines the atrial depolarization rate. After identifying the dominant P-wave morphology, the P-wave frontal plane axis is ascertained. A normal P-wave frontal plane axis reflects a sinus node origin, demonstrating a positive P-wave vector in leads I, II, III, and aVF. An abnormal P-wave axis supports an ectopic, non–sinus node P-wave origin. Possible atrial rhythms including the following:

1. *Normal sinus rhythm:* A regular atrial depolarization rate of sinus node origin between 60 and 100 per minute demonstrating a positive P-wave vector in leads I, II, III, and aVF.
2. *Sinus bradycardia:* A regular atrial depolarization rate of sinus node origin <60 per minute demonstrating a positive P-wave vector in leads I, II, III, and aVF.
3. *Sinus tachycardia:* A regular atrial depolarization rate of sinus node origin >100 per minute demonstrating a positive P-wave vector in leads I, II, III, and aVF.
4. *Sinus arrhythmia:* A normal P-wave morphology and frontal plane axis of sinus node origin with an atrial

depolarization rate between 60 and 100 per minute demonstrating a P-wave to P-wave cycle length variation >160 msec.

5. *Atrial fibrillation:* A rapid, irregular, and disorganized atrial depolarization rate of 400 to 700 per minute without discrete P waves. Atrial activation is represented by fibrillatory waves. In the absence of atrioventricular block, the ventricular response is irregularly irregular. The fibrillatory waves can vary in amplitude between patients, generating a subclassification of atrial fibrillation as either coarse or fine.

6. *Atrial flutter:* A rapid, regular atrial depolarization rate of 250 to 350 per minute, felt most commonly to represent an trial re-entrant circuit. The atrial waves are termed "F waves" and demonstrate a "saw-toothed" appearance, best seen in leads V_1, II, III, and aVF. The ventricular rate is either regular or irregular depending on the atrioventricular conduction ratio.

7. *Atrial tachycardia:* A regular automatic tachycardia from a single ectopic atrial focus demonstrating a P wave possessing an abnormal frontal plane axis. The typical atrial rate is between 180 and 240 per minute. The ventricular rate is either regular or irregular depending on the atrioventricular conduction ratio.

8. *Wandering atrial pacemaker:* The atrial depolarization rate is between 60 and 100 per minute. The P-wave to P-wave interval varies, reflecting the different foci of atrial activation. To satisfy this diagnosis, more than three atrial foci and P-wave morphologies are present on a single 12-lead ECG.

9. *Multifocal atrial tachycardia:* A tachycardic heart rhythm with an atrial depolarization rate >100 per minute with a P wave preceding each QRS complex. On a single 12-lead ECG, P waves of at least three different morphologies are necessary to satisfy the diagnostic criteria. The PR intervals vary, and the ventricular response is irregularly irregular given the unpredictable timing of atrial depolarization. Nonconducted atrial complexes during the absolute ventricular refractoriness are often present.

10. *Ectopic atrial rhythm:* A regular atrial depolarization rate of nonsinus node origin between 60 and 100 per minute. The P-wave frontal plane axis is abnormal, reflecting the nonsinus node single atrial focus origin.

11. *Ectopic atrial bradycardia:* A regular atrial depolarization rate of nonsinus node origin <60 per minute. The P-wave frontal plane axis is abnormal, reflecting the nonsinus node single atrial focus origin.

12. *Sinus node re-entrant rhythm:* A re-entrant circuit involving the sinus node and perisinus nodal tissues. The P-wave morphology and frontal plane axis are normal given the sinus node origin. Atrial depolarization is regular at a rate between 60 and 100 per minute. This dysrhythmia is characterized by abrupt onset and termination.

13. *Sinus node re-entrant tachycardia:* A re-entrant circuit involving the sinus node and perisinus nodal tissues. The P-wave morphology and frontal plane axis are normal given the sinus node origin. Atrial depolarization is regular at a rate >100 per minute. This dysrhythmia is characterized by abrupt onset and termination.

14. *Atrioventricular nodal re-entrant tachycardia:* This dysrhythmia is dependent on the presence of two separate atrioventricular nodal pathways with slowed conduction in one pathway and unidirectional conduction block in the other pathway. Electrocardiographic criteria include a ventricular rate between 140 and 220 per minute and a regular rhythm with abrupt onset and termination. Dysrhythmia onset is often initiated by a premature atrial complex. Inverted P waves may occur prior to the QRS complex, within the QRS complex, or after the QRS complex within the ST segment. The QRS complex may be conducted normally or aberrantly.

15. *Supraventricular tachycardia:* A global term encompassing regular tachycardia dysrhythmias originating within the atria or the atrioventricular junction. This term is best utilized in the presence of a regular narrow complex tachycardia, where identifiable atrial activity is not readily identified and the exact determination of the supraventricular rhythm disturbance is not possible from the 12-lead ECG.

When ECG evidence for atrial depolarization is absent, it is important to identify a subsidiary pacemaker origin such as the atrioventricular junction. Several different types of atrioventricular junctional rhythms exist, including the following:

1. *Junctional rhythm:* This dysrhythmia may occur in the setting of digitalis intoxication with suppression of sinus node activity and sinus exit block. A subsidiary pacemaker such as the atrioventricular junction assumes the primary pacemaker role at a regular rate of approximately 60 per minute.

2. *Junctional bradycardia:* This dysrhythmia originates within the atrioventricular node and represents a regular heart rhythm generated from a subsidiary pacemaker at a rate <60 per minute. Retrograde P waves representing atrial activation may be present and can occur before, within, or after the QRS complexes.

3. *Junctional tachycardia:* The ventricular rate is regular and typically between 120 and 200 per minute. The atrioventricular junction serves as the primary cardiac pacemaker. Retrograde P waves may precede, be superimposed, or follow the QRS complexes depending on the level of junctional tachycardia origin.

4. *Accelerated junctional rhythm:* The rhythm is regular with a rate between 60 and 100 per minute. The atrioventricular junction serves as the cardiac pacemaker. Retrograde P waves may precede, be superimposed, or follow the QRS complexes depending on the level of junctional rhythm origin.

5. *Junctional escape rhythm:* This dysrhythmia commonly occurs in the setting of digitalis intoxication with suppression of sinus node activity and sinus exit block. With depression of the sinus node, a subsidiary pacemaker such as the atrioventricular junction assumes the primary pacemaker role at a rate between 40 and 60 per minute.

Each ECG should also be assessed for the presence of an independent ventricular rhythm. Possible ventricular rhythm disturbances include the following:

1. *Ventricular tachycardia:* A sustained cardiac rhythm of ventricular origin occurring at a regular rate of 140 to 240 per minute. Common features include a widened QRS complex, frontal plane QRS complex left axis deviation, precordial lead QRS complex concordance, atrioventricular dissociation, capture complexes, and fusion complexes.

2. *Polymorphic ventricular tachycardia (torsades de pointes):* A paroxysmal form of ventricular tachycardia with a nonconstant R-to-R interval, a ventricular rate of approximately 225 to 250 per minute, QRS complexes of alternating polarity, prolongation of the QT interval at arrhythmia onset, and a changing QRS complex amplitude often resembling a sine wave pattern.

3. *Ventricular fibrillation:* A terminal cardiac rhythm with chaotic ventricular activity without organized ventricular depolarization.

4. *Ventricular parasystole:* An independent ventricular rhythm with regular discharge and ventricular depolarization. This is characterized by varying coupling intervals, a constant R-to-R interectopic complex interval, and the presence of fusion complexes when the parasystolic focus discharges simultaneously with native ventricular depolarization.

5. *Idioventricular rhythm:* A regular rhythm at a ventricular rate <60 per minute. Widened QRS complexes are present, with the ventricular complexes commonly dissociated from the atrial activity. This rhythm disturbance is often seen in abnormalities of advanced atrioventricular conduction, where the ventricle serves as a subsidiary pacemaker and escape rhythm.

6. *Accelerated idioventricular rhythm:* A regular rhythm at a ventricular rate of 60 to 100 per minute. Widened QRS complexes are present with the ventricular complexes commonly dissociated from the atrial activity. This rhythm disturbance is often seen in abnormalities of advanced atrioventricular conduction, where the ventricle serves as a subsidiary pacemaker and escape rhythm.

ELECTROCARDIOGRAM INTERVALS

PR interval: Early identification and accurate determination of the PR interval is important. A constant PR interval of normal duration (120–220 msec) reflects normal intra-atrial conduction, atrioventricular nodal conduction, and atrioventricular association. A varying PR interval supports the possibilities of atrioventricular dissociation of differing types of heart block, both requiring further detailed analysis. A shortened PR interval may reflect facile intra-atrial and atrioventricular conduction or ventricular preexcitation. A prolonged PR interval reflects delayed intra-atrial and/or atrioventricular conduction.

R-to-R interval: A precise measurement of the R-wave to R-wave interval determines the ventricular rate of depolarization. In the presence of normal atrioventricular conduction, the ventricular rate will equal the atrial rate. If an atrioventricular conduction abnormality exists, a determination of the atrioventricular conduction ratio (number of P waves for each QRS complex) is performed. In the presence of atrioventricular dissociation or complete heart block, two independent cardiac rhythms exist originating from separate cardiac foci, each necessitating interpretation. Important forms of atrioventricular conduction abnormalities include the following:

1. *Second-degree Mobitz type I Wenckebach atrioventricular block:* This implies atrioventricular conduction block within the atrioventricular node superior to the bundle of His. Progressive PR-interval prolongation transpires with a P wave and a nonconducted QRS complex representing conduction cycle termination. Grouped QRS complexes are a common finding. Varying atrioventricular conduction ratios are often present. A common atrioventricular conduction ratio is 4:3.

2. *Second-degree Mobitz type II atrioventricular block:* This conduction disturbance occurs at the level of the atrioventricular node below the bundle of His. This patient subgroup requires pacemaker placement unless this conduction disturbance is readily reversible. A common atrioventricular conduction ratio is 2:1. This dysrhythmia is characterized by lack of progressive PR-interval prolongation and an abrupt nonconducted QRS complex. This patient subgroup has a high propensity to progress to more advanced forms of atrioventricular block.

3. *Advanced atrioventricular block:* This is also known as high-grade atrioventricular block and is present when the atrioventricular conduction ratio is 3:1 or greater in the presence of a nontachycardic atrial rhythm. Unless readily reversible, permanent pacemaker placement is warranted.

4. *Complete heart block:* In complete or third-degree heart block, atrioventricular conduction is absent. Instead, the atrial and ventricular rhythms are independent. The ventricular rhythm is regular and reflects an escape rhythm between 20 and 60 per

minute. The QRS complexes may be of normal duration, indicating the presence of an atrioventricular junctional escape rhythm, or prolonged in the presence of a ventricular escape rhythm.

5. *Variable atrioventricular conduction:* This is most commonly manifest during atrial flutter and atrial tachycardia at an atrial rate >130 per minute. At elevated atrial rates, physiological conduction block occurs at the level of the atrioventricular node variably and unpredictably. The atrioventricular node serves as a "gatekeeper" to prevent accelerated and potentially unstable elevated ventricular rates.

QRS complex interval: The QRS complex duration is best measured in the limb leads from R-wave onset (Q-wave onset, if present) to S-wave offset. A normal QRS complex interval is <100 msec. If >100 msec but <120 msec, the QRS complex conduction delay is best classified as nonspecific. If the QRS complex duration is >120 msec but without a specific ascribable morphology, it is still best classified as nonspecific intraventricular conduction delay. If >120 msec, a careful assessment of the QRS complex morphology is important, as complete left or right bundle-branch block may exist. Complete left bundle-branch block represents a QRS complex duration >120 msec, the absence of a Q wave (septal depolarization) in leads I and V_{5-6}, an upright QRS complex in leads I and V_{5-6}, and ST segment depression and T-wave inversion in leads I and V_{5-6}. Complete right bundle-branch block represents a QRS complex duration >120 msec, widened terminally slowed S waves in leads I and V_{5-6}, a widened RSR′ QRS complex morphology in leads V_{1-2}, and ST segment depression and T-wave inversion in leads V_{1-2}.

QT interval: Unlike the other cardiac intervals, the QT interval demonstrates heart rate interdependence. The QT interval duration is inversely proportional to the R-to-R cycle length. The QTc interval represents the QT interval divided by the square root of the R-to-R interval. This adjusts the QT interval for the heart rate and standardizes this measurement. This is a cumbersome manual measurement and calculation for each ECG. At present, ECG machines provide a comprehensive printout of all cardiac intervals, including the QTc interval. These values serve as a useful reference but are not without limitation and potential error. The interpreter is encouraged to verify the accuracy of the computer-generated intervals for each tracing. For the QT interval, a fairly accurate shortened approach involves visually assessing this interval in limb lead II. If the QT interval is <50% of the R-wave to R-wave interval, prolongation is not likely present. If the QT interval is >50% of the R-wave to R-wave interval, this usually reflects prolongation that is best confirmed with a manual measurement

by the interpreter. Causes of a prolonged QT interval include the following:

1. Idiopathic long QT interval syndrome
2. Central nervous system event
3. Hypocalcemia
4. Cardiac antiarrhythmic medication
5. Psychotropic medicine
6. Hypothyroidism

The presence of a shortened QT interval, which may represent an underlying electrolyte disturbance, is best done by careful interval assessment and visual inspection. It often is first suggested by a truncated ST segment. This is an easily overlooked ECG finding that reinforces the need for a consistent and diligent interpretation approach. Causes of QT interval shortening include the following:

1. Digitalis administration
2. Hypercalcemia

QRS COMPLEX FRONTAL PLANE AXIS

The QRS complex frontal plane axis is next assessed for each ECG. The QRS complex vector is carefully assessed in each limb lead. An isoelectric vector is concluded if the area of possibility (R wave) is equal to the area of negativity (Q wave plus S wave).

A simplified approach is as follows:

1. Assess the QRS complex vector in leads I and aVF. If both are negative, the QRS complex frontal plane axis is between zero and positive 90 degrees and therefore normal.
2. If the QRS complex vector is positive in lead I and negative in lead aVF, assess the QRS complex vector in lead II. If the lead QRS complex vector is positive, the QRS complex frontal plane axis is between zero and negative 30 degrees, best classified as QRS complex frontal plane left axis deviation.
3. If the QRS complex vector is positive in lead I and negative in leads aVF and II, the QRS complex frontal plane axis is greater than negative 30 degrees, reflecting left anterior hemiblock.
4. If the QRS complex vector is negative in lead I and positive in leads III and aVF, QRS complex right axis deviation is present.

ELECTROCARDIOGRAM MORPHOLOGIES

Once the cardiac rate, rhythm, intervals, and QRS complex frontal plane axis are assessed, it is appropriate to proceed with identification of specific ECG morphologic findings. The approach of addressing the P wave first, the QRS complex second, and the ST-T waves last is both systematic and logical.

P wave: Besides P-wave identification and P-wave frontal plane axis determination, specific P-wave morphologies suggest underlying conduction and structural cardiac pathology. The P-wave morphology is best assessed in leads V_1 and II. Important findings in these leads include left atrial abnormality and right atrial abnormality. The ECG findings of left atrial abnormality include a prominent terminally negative or biphasic P wave in lead V^1. This reflects delayed left depolarization manifest as a terminally negative P-wave vector with left atrial depolarization transpiring opposite lead V^1. In lead II, the P-wave duration is prolonged to >110 msec with a bifid positive vector. The second or terminal component of this positive P-wave vector represents delayed left atrial depolarization. The ECG finding of right atrial abnormality demonstrates a P-wave amplitude of ≥ 2.5 mm in lead II. Given the anterior P-wave vector in the presence of right atrial abnormality, a tall P wave of ≥ 1.5 mm is often seen in lead V_1. It is not possible to discern from the surface ECG if an atrial abnormality represents chamber enlargement and/or delayed conduction. The less specific term, abnormality, therefore is most appropriate.

QRS complex: Evaluation of the QRS complex morphology is an important individual step. It is best to proceed with an initial careful evaluation for the presence or absence of Q waves. Q waves of diagnostic duration in most circumstances represent an underlying myocardial infarction. In the inferior and lateral leads, Q waves of ≥ 40 msec duration represent a myocardial infarction. In leads V_{2-4}, a Q wave of diagnostic duration is ≥ 25 msec. In the presence of a myocardial infarction, Q waves are most commonly grouped into ECG "regions," reflecting a specific coronary artery distribution. When a Q wave is identified, it is helpful to evaluate contiguous leads integrating a working knowledge of coronary artery anatomy. For instance, in the presence of an inferior myocardial infarction, careful evaluation for the presence of a posterior, lateral, and right ventricular myocardial infarction is prudent. Alternatively, when an anterior myocardial infarction is noted, lateral and apical involvement may be seen.

Q waves can also demonstrate a pseudoinfarction pattern and thus not reflect a true myocardial infarction. This is most commonly seen in the presence of the Wolff-Parkinson-White syndrome. The pseudoinfarction Q waves instead reflect ventricular pre-excitation. The delta wave possesses a negative vector, indicating ventricular conduction opposite the ECG led. This is most often seen in the inferior, lateral, and high lateral leads. *A prominent R wave in lead V_1 in isolation should be interpreted with caution.* It is unusual to diagnose an isolated true posterior myocardial infarction. Other causes such as ventricular pre-excitation,

counterclockwise cardiac rotation, right ventricular hypertrophy, and right ventricular conduction delay should be carefully considered. QRS complex frontal plane right axis deviation and left posterior fascicular block are other causes of a pseudoinfarction pattern. In these examples, the pseudoinfarction Q waves are located inferiorly.

ST segment: The ST segment is the segment between the terminal aspect of the QRS complex (also known as the J point) and T-wave onset. As part of a complete ECG interpretation, each ST segment is assessed for deviation from the ECG baseline. The isoelectric comparative segment on the ECG is the TP segment. This is the segment between the terminal aspect of the T-wave and P-wave onset. Most often, ST segment deviation is best termed *nonspecific*, as the exact cause is not discernible from the ECG alone, instead requiring a complete clinical history and medication record.

Causes of ST segment elevation include the following:

1. *Acute myocardial injury:* Convex upward (coved) ST segment elevation confined to at least two contiguous ECG leads.
2. *Pericarditis:* Diffuse concave upward ST segment elevation not confined to contiguous ECG leads.
3. *Left ventricular aneurysm:* Most commonly, right precordial lead convex upward (coved) ST segment elevation overlying the infarct zone persisting for months to years.

Causes of ST segment depression include the following:

1. *Myocardial ischemia:* Most commonly, exercise-induced ST segment depression as seen during stress testing. ST segment depression often reflects coronary artery disease and myocardial ischemia. Horizontal and/or downsloping ST segment depression demonstrates greater specificity.
2. *Non–Q-wave myocardial infarction:* Horizontal and/or downsloping ST segment depression with supporting clinical and laboratory markers of acute myocardial injury.
3. *Cardiomyopathy:* Abnormal ST segments, including ST segment depression, are often present in both dilated and hypertrophic cardiomyopathic forms.
4. *Ventricular hypertrophy:* Downsloping ST segment depression is commonly present in both left and right ventricular hypertrophy.
5. *Supraventricular tachyarrhythmias:* Paroxysmal ST segment depression is frequently present at high heart rates during supraventricular tachycardic rhythms. These findings may persist after arrhythmia cessation. They may or may not represent coexistent myocardial ischemia; oftentimes, further corroborative testing is necessary.

T wave: The T wave begins at the terminal aspect of the ST segment and ends at the onset of the TP segment.

Precise identification of the exact beginning and end of the T wave is often difficult. T-wave abnormalities are seen in many clinical conditions and are not a specific finding. T-wave abnormalities are found in the following circumstances:

1. Cardiomyopathies
2. Ventricular hypertrophy
3. Electrolyte disturbances
4. Valvular heart disease
5. Coronary artery disease
6. Central nervous system event
7. Wolff-Parkinson-White syndrome
8. Pericarditis
9. Medication administration
10. Hyperventilation
11. Positional change

U wave: The U wave is variably present on the ECG. When seen, it begins at the terminal aspect of the T wave and ends within the TP segment. Often, T-wave and U-wave fusion is present; therefore, it is not possible to separately measure the T-wave and U-wave duration. Both positive and negative U waves may exit. The U wave generally does not exceed 25% of the T-wave amplitude and is best seen in leads V_{2-3}.

Causes of a positive U wave include the following:

1. Bradycardia
2. Central nervous system disease

3. Cardiac antiarrhythmic medication
4. Electrolyte disturbances
   a. Hypokalemia
   b. Hypomagnesemia

Causes of negative U waves include the following:

1. Left ventricular hypertrophy
2. Coronary artery disease

CONCLUSION

To successfully interpret ECGs, a deliberate, consistent, and reproducible approach is essential. Through experience and repetition, the interpreter will demonstrate improved interpretive abilities and confidence, rendering greater diagnostic accuracy. The once complex and intimidating ECG will now represent a routine tracing, which is readily interpreted. The former student will assume the role of knowledgeable educator.

ELECTROCARDIOGRAM FIGURE 59.1

Clinical History

A 56-year-old man who underwent a cardiac transplant procedure 6 weeks prior to this ECG secondary to an

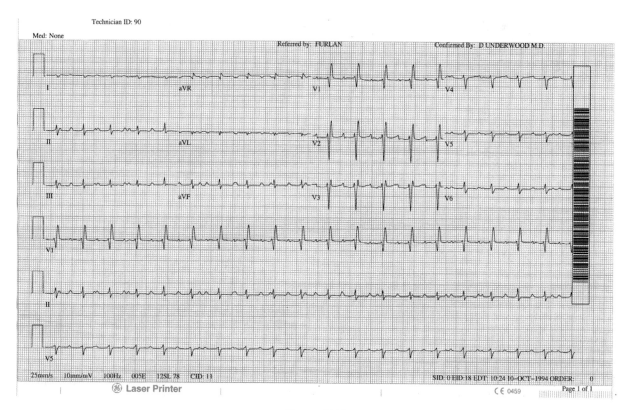

Figure 59.1

idiopathic nonischemic dilated cardiomyopathy and recurrent ventricular tachycardia. His medications at the time of this ECG included digoxin, furosemide, lisinopril, potassium, and aspirin.

Interpretation and Comments

The cardiac rhythm is sinus tachycardia, as the P waves demonstrate a normal axis with a constant P:P interval preceding each QRS complex at a regular rate >100 per minute. A second set of P waves is noted at a constant P:P interval at a slightly longer P:P interval compared with the conducted P waves. This represents the native atrium in this cardiac transplant patient, which is still depolarizing via the native sinus node. The donor P wave immediately preceding each QRS complex demonstrates first-degree atrioventricular block. Diffuse nonspecific ST-T changes are present. QRS complex frontal plane right axis deviation is present, as the QRS complex vector is negative in lead I and positive in leads II, III, and aVF. Low-voltage QRS complexes are seen in the limb leads, as each complex is <5 mm in amplitude. A rsR′ QRS complex morphology is present in lead V_1 with an overall normal QRS complex duration supporting incomplete right bundle-branch block.

The presence of dual-functioning atria in a recent cardiac transplant patient is a common finding. The native atria gradually extinguish themselves, and the donor atria become the dominant atrial pacemaker. The presence of incomplete right bundle-branch block in a post cardiac transplant patient is also a common finding.

ELECTROCARDIOGRAM FIGURE 59.2

Clinical History

A 70-year-old woman who presents for a general physical examination. She has a history of coronary artery obstructive disease and is status post myocardial infarction of unknown location 4 years prior to this ECG. Other comorbid conditions include extensive past tobacco use, hypertension, and gastroesophageal reflux disease. Her medications at the time of this ECG included potassium, thyroxine, triamterene-hydrochlorothiazide, and naprosyn.

Interpretation and Comments

Normal sinus rhythm is present. As demonstrated on this tracing, second-degree Mobitz type I Wenckebach atrioventricular block is most readily identified by the grouped QRS complexes. A group of six QRS complexes exist in the center of the tracing. This represents a 7:6 Wenckebach conduction cycle. Note the prolonged PR interval at Wenckebach cycle onset, progressive PR interval prolongation and a nonconducted QRS complex. The third QRS complex occurs after a pause. This represents a junctional escape complex.

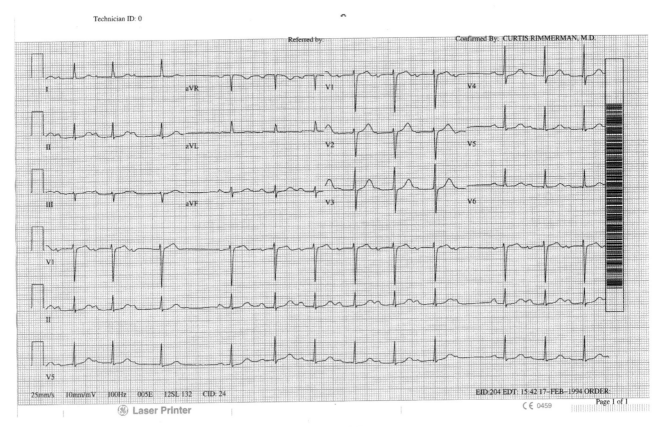

Technician ID: 0

Referred by: Confirmed By: CURTIS RIMMERMAN, M.D.

25mm/s   10mm/mV   100Hz   005E   12SL 132   CID: 24   EID:204 EDT: 15:42 17–FEB–1994 ORDER:

Page 1 of 1

CE 0459

⑯ Laser Printer

Figure 59.2

Second-degree Mobitz type I Wenckebach atrioventricular block supports atrioventricular block at a level above the bundle of His and confers a more favorable prognosis. The greatest percentage of PR interval prolongation in a typical Wenckebach cycle occurs with the second PR interval.

ELECTROCARDIOGRAM FIGURE 59.3

Clinical History

A 41-year-old man with myelodysplastic syndrome and insulin-requiring diabetes mellitus admitted for a bone marrow transplantation. His serum potassium at the time of this ECG was 3.4 meq/L.

Interpretation and Comments

This ECG emphasizes the necessary methodical approach to interpretation. This demonstrates normal sinus rhythm. When assessing the intervals, it is most notable for a prolonged QT interval. This is best assessed in the limb leads. This assessment needs to be adjusted for heart rate as the QT interval becomes longer with a slower heart rate. A reliable method of assessing the QT interval is to look, for example, in lead I. If the QT interval is >50% of the R:R interval, it likely is prolonged. This is the case for this tracing. Associated nonspecific ST-T changes are best seen in

the precordial and high lateral leads. In lead V_4 there is a terminal positivity to the T wave, which represents an upright U wave. Therefore, this apparent prolongation of the QT interval is more accurately described in this instance as a prolonged QT-U interval. This reflects hypokalemia.

This ECG demonstrates the common findings seen in hypokalemia. Prolongation of the QT interval, prominent U waves and T-wave flattening are evident.

ELECTROCARDIOGRAM FIGURE 59.4

Clinical History

A 39-year-old woman unrestrained passenger who suffered an aortic transection distal to the left subclavian artery from a motor vehicle accident. This ECG was taken postoperatively, shortly after thoracic aorta repair.

Interpretation and Comments

The heart rate and cardiac rhythm are both normal. This represents normal sinus rhythm. This ECG is most notable for diffuse ST segment elevation not confined to a particular coronary artery territory, which is most consistent with acute pericarditis. Lead aVR is helpful, as there is elevation of the atrial repolarization segment. This segment is termed

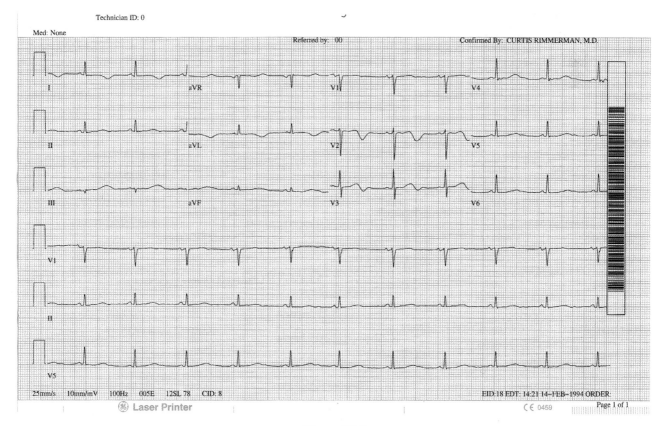

Figure 59.3

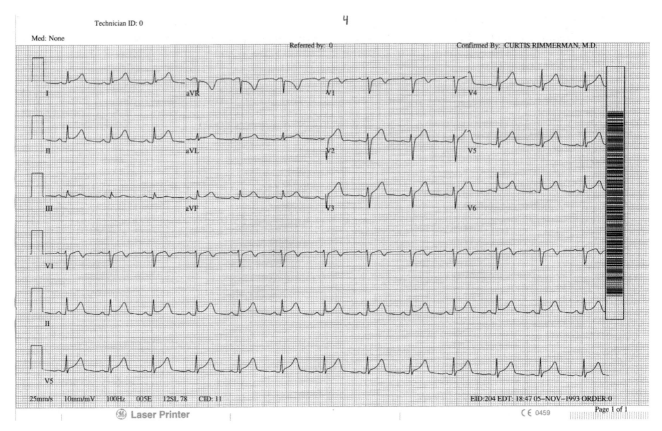

Figure 59.4

the *PR segment* and is located between the terminal aspect of the P-wave and QRS complex onset.

When the PR segment is elevated in lead aVR, this serves as a specific sign for pericarditis. This may be the only ECG finding supporting pericarditis and remains an important marker to identify.

ELECTROCARDIOGRAM FIGURE 59.5

Clinical History

A 59-year-old man with coronary artery disease status post remote percutaneous transluminal coronary angioplasty of the right coronary artery who re-presents with chest discomfort. A myocardial infarction was excluded by cardiac enzymes, and a subsequent stress test was normal. The patient was felt to be suffering from noncardiac musculoskeletal chest discomfort.

Interpretation and Comments

The cardiac rhythm demonstrates a regular bradycardia with retrograde P waves after each QRS complex. The P waves are negative in the inferior leads, as the initial wave of depolarization is traveling superiorly, which is opposite the normal direction of conduction. The QRS complex is of normal duration. This represents junctional brady-

cardia. The causes of this could be many, including sinus node disease, medication administration, increased vagal tone, atrial conduction system disease, myocardial ischemia, and valvular heart disease. Prominent positive U waves are present in leads V_{2-4}.

In this instance, the R:R interval is constant with absent atrial activity prior to each QRS complex. Depending on the relative retrograde versus antegrade conduction rates, a retrograde P wave may occur before, within, or after the QRS complex. In this example, antegrade conduction from the atrioventricular junction to the ventricle is faster than retrograde conduction from the atrioventricular junction to the atrium and therefore explains the P wave occupying the proximal ST segment after the QRS complex.

ELECTROCARDIOGRAM FIGURE 59.6

Clinical History

A 46-year-old man with a myocardial infarction 2 years before this ECG who presented to the emergency room with a 6-hour history of acute severe substernal chest discomfort. The patient underwent emergent cardiac catheterization and percutaneous transluminal coronary angioplasty of a severe proximal left anterior descending coronary artery stenosis.

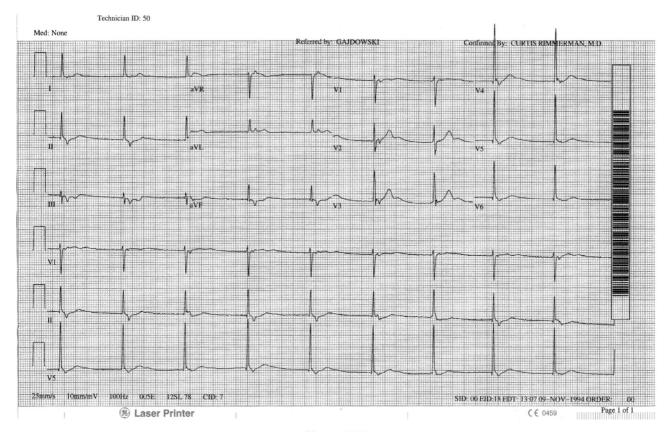

Figure 59.5

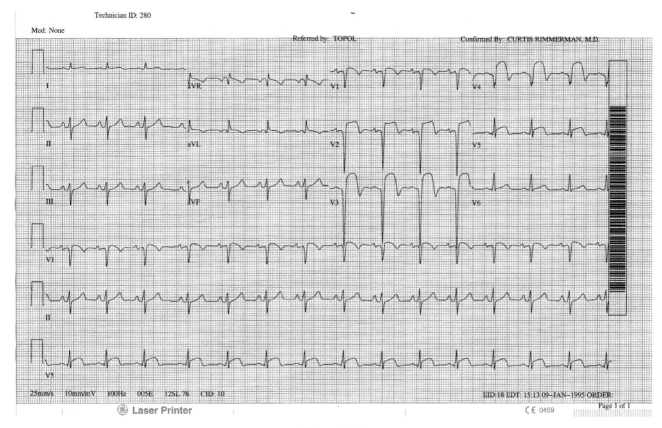

Figure 59.6

Interpretation and Comments

The cardiac rhythm is regular with a normal P-wave axis denoting normal sinus rhythm. A leftward QRS complex frontal plane axis is present in the setting of a normal QRS complex duration, fulfilling the criteria for left anterior hemiblock. Most striking on this ECG is the maximal 7-mm ST segment elevation noted in leads V_{2-5}, I, and aVL with Q-wave formation indicating an extensive anterolateral myocardial infarction–acute. There is an ongoing acute myocardial injury pattern with terminal T-wave inversion representing an involving acute infarction.

This ECG is an example of an evolving extensive anterolateral myocardial infarction. There is concomitant injury and infarction occurring, as prominent Q waves are present with ST segment elevation. Presumably, the left anterior descending obstruction is proximal to the first septal perforated branch, as ST segment elevation is present in lead V_1.

ELECTROCARDIOGRAM FIGURE 59.7

Clinical History

A 56-year-old man with severe left ventricular systolic dysfunction in the setting of normal coronary arteries who is awaiting cardiac transplantation. His medications include thyroxine, furosemide, hydralazine, isosorbide dinitrate, captopril, and amiodarone.

Interpretation and Comments

The cardiac rhythm is regular and rate <60 per minute, reflecting sinus bradycardia. PR interval prolongation is best seen in leads I and II, which is consistent with first-degree atrioventricular block. The QRS complex is significantly widened with a complete left bundle-branch block morphology. The widened QRS complex represents delayed conduction within the left ventricle.

The ECG finding of complete left bundle-branch block is pathological and often reflects significant underlying cardiac pathology. In this instance, it reflects advanced left ventricular systolic dysfunction, which is a common finding in the presence of complete left bundle-branch block. Conduction to the ventricles is blocked via the left bundle branch. Ventricular depolarization is slowed and transpires transseptally via the right bundle branch.

ELECTROCARDIOGRAM FIGURE 59.8

Clinical History

A 61-year-old man with coronary artery disease and ischemic left ventricular systolic dysfunction who presents urgently to the hospital with an acute chest discomfort syndrome. His medications include potassium, isosorbide mononitrate, furosemide, glyburide, lisinopril, and warfarin.

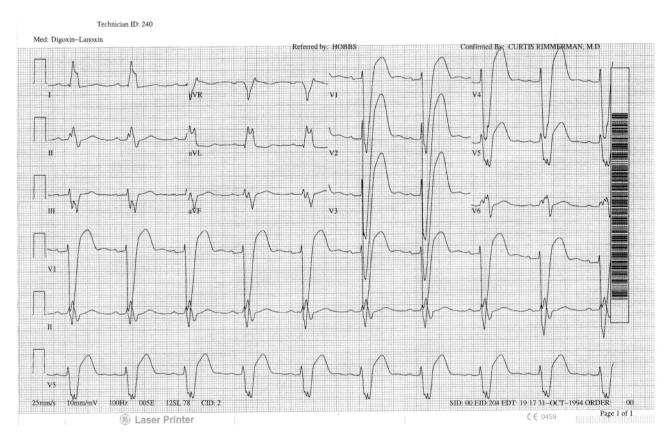

Figure 59.7

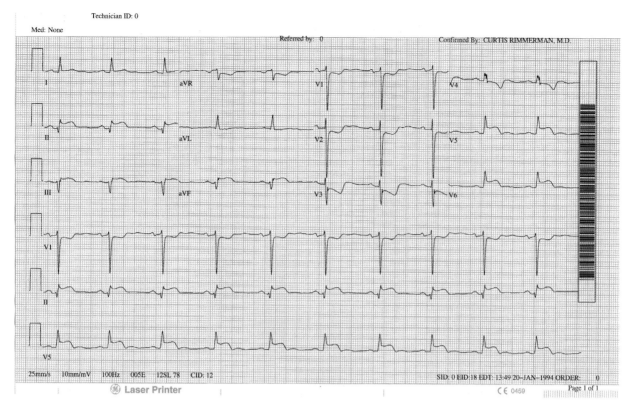

25mm/s   10mm/mV   100Hz   005E   12SL 78   CID: 12   SID: 0 EID: 18 EDT: 13:49 20–JAN–1994 ORDER: 0

Laser Printer   C E 0459   Page 1 of 1

Figure 59.8

Interpretation and Comments

P waves occur at regular intervals at a rate slightly >60 per minute, indicating normal sinus rhythm. Two millimeters of ST segment elevation is noted in leads II, III, and aVF, and 3 mm of ST segment elevation is noted in leads V_{5-6}, suggesting an inferolateral myocardial infarction–acute and acute myocardial injury. Downsloping ST segment depression is noted in leads V_{1-4}. These are reciprocal changes and may represent transpiring posterior myocardial injury. Follow-up ECGs would be helpful to look for "growth" of the R wave in the anterior precordium, suggesting a posterior myocardial infarction. Left atrial abnormality is present, as reflected by a broaden P wave in lead wave II and a terminally negative P wave in lead V_1.

Unlike a myocardial infarction, an acute injury pattern implies a lack of Q-wave formation and greater potential reversibility to the ongoing process. When an acute inferior injury pattern is present, it is important to assess for both posterior and lateral involvement, as demonstrated on this ECG. The lateral ST segment elevation suggests a larger myocardial injury pattern with greater myocardial territory involvement portending a worse prognosis.

ELECTROCARDIOGRAM FIGURE 59.9

Clinical History

A 45-year-old man who presented to an outside emergency room with a one-half hour history of acute chest discomfort radiating to both shoulders and hands. The patient underwent urgent cardiac catheterization that demonstrated a 100% proximal right coronary artery occlusion with superimposed thrombosis. The patient underwent successful percutaneous transluminal coronary angioplasty. Cardiac enzymes were positive for acute myocardial injury.

Interpretation and Comments

The cardiac rhythm is normal sinus rhythm. The most prominent finding on this ECG is the upwardly coved 3-mm ST segment elevation in lead V_1. This lead overlies the right ventricle and is consistent with a right ventricular myocardial infarction–acute. A more subtle finding is the <1-mm ST segment elevation and small Q-wave formation in leads III and aVF. This represents an inferior myocardial infarction–acute, less notable than the concomitant right ventricular myocardial infarction–acute. The right coronary artery occlusion is anatomically proximal to the right ventricular marginal branch of the right coronary artery. Right ventricular leads would be helpful to confirm this finding but almost certainly should demonstrate the acute right ventricular myocardial infarction.

On this tracing, the prominent ST segment elevation in leads V_{1-2} representing acute right ventricular myocardial injury clues the interpreter to the subtle ST segment elevation in leads III and aVF. It is unusual for an acute right ventricular myocardial infarction to be so prominent

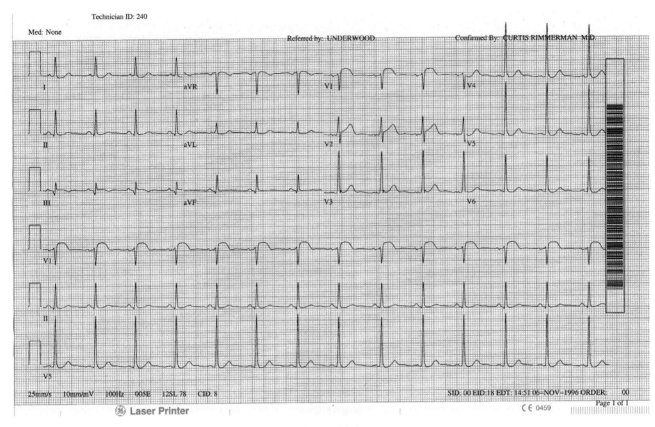

Figure 59.9

electrocardiographically in the absence of significant inferior ST segment elevation.

ELECTROCARDIOGRAM FIGURE 59.10

Clinical History

A 72-year-old woman who presented to the hospital after 3 hours of severe epigastric pressure with associated vomiting, nausea, and profuse diaphoresis. Serial cardiac enzymes documented acute myocardial injury. Medications at the time of this ECG included fentanyl, glyburide, ranitidine, lisinopril, intravenous heparin, and intravenous nitroglycerin.

Interpretation and Comments

A P wave precedes each QRS complex. This represents normal sinus rhythm, as the atrial rate is approximately 70 per minute. Inferior ST segment elevation with terminal T-wave inversion is seen. This represents an inferior myocardial infarction–acute and acute myocardial injury with reciprocal ST segment depression in leads I and aVL. Lateral ST segment depression is seen. Approximately 1 mm of ST segment elevation is present in lead V_1. In the setting of an acute inferior myocardial infarction, this represents a concomitant right ventricular myocardial infarction–acute. Further verification of this finding could be obtained by

obtaining a right-sided precordial tracing. A prominent baseline artifact is also demonstrated, making assessment of the P-wave morphology difficult.

In the presence of acute inferior myocardial injury, it is important to assess leads V_{1-2} for both ST segment elevation and R-wave prominence, which may reflect right ventricular myocardial injury or a posterior myocardial infarction, respectively. In the presence of acute right ventricular myocardial injury, this suggests a proximal right coronary artery occlusion prior to the origin of the right ventricular marginal branch. An inferior myocardial infarction with right ventricular myocardial involvement portends a worse prognosis with greater potential complications and more extensive myocardial injury.

ELECTROCARDIOGRAM FIGURE 59.11

Clinical History

A 79-year-old woman who 5 days prior to this ECG experienced acute-onset chest discomfort and an ECG consistent with an acute inferior myocardial infarction. Following her myocardial infarction convalescence, a cardiac catheterization demonstrated severe three-vessel coronary artery disease. This ECG was obtained prior to anticipated coronary artery bypass graft surgery. Left ventriculography at the time of her cardiac catheterization demonstrated proximal and mid inferior wall akinesis. Her medications

Technician: 10

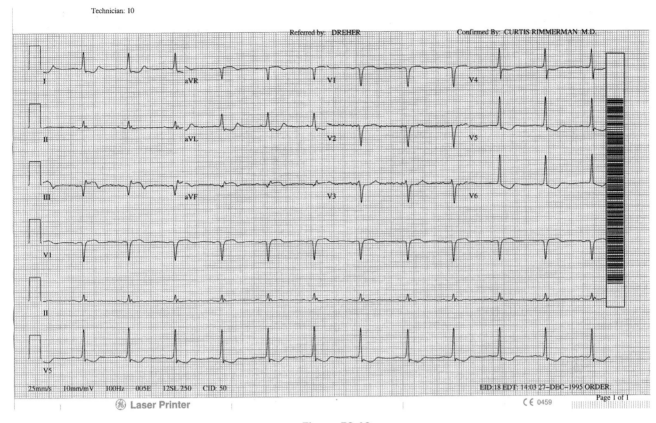

Figure 59.10

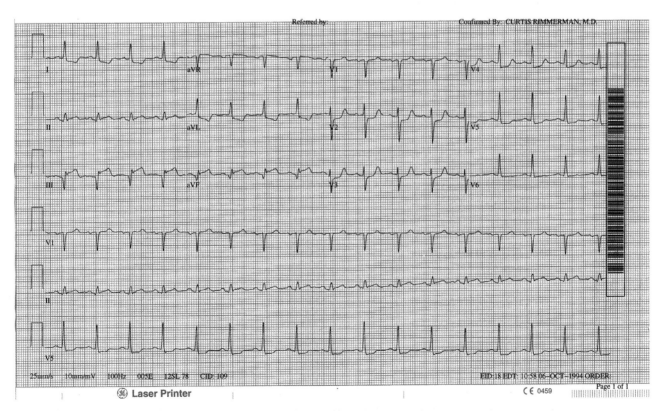

Figure 59.11

included metoprolol, intravenous heparin, intravenous nitroglycerin, and temazepam.

Interpretation and Comments

This ECG demonstrates a P wave with a normal axis preceding each QRS complex at a regular rate >100 per minute. This represents sinus tachycardia. Q-wave formation and ST segment elevation are noted in the inferior leads, reflecting an inferior myocardial infarction–acute. Reciprocal ST segment depression is present in leads V_{2-5}, I, and aVL, which may reflect a more extensive myocardial infarction. The ST segment in lead V_1 is isoelectric; therefore, no ECG evidence of acute right ventricular myocardial injury is present.

This ECG suggests inferior acute myocardial injury. However, by history, this patient suffered a myocardial infarction 5 days prior to this ECG. This ECG represents an acute infarction that is slow to evolve and resolve, raising the possibility of ongoing myocardial injury versus the interval development of an inferior wall ventricular aneurysm.

ELECTROCARDIOGRAM FIGURE 59.12

Clinical History

A 43-year-old man admitted in urgent hospital transfer after a 1-day history of acute chest discomfort. The patient was taken urgently to the cardiac catheterization laboratory,

where a 90% mid left anterior descending coronary artery stenosis involving a second diagonal branch was present. The patient underwent successful angioplasty and stent deployment.

Interpretation and Comments

The cardiac rhythm is normal sinus rhythm at an atrial rate of 60 per minute with a positive QRS complex vector in lead I and negative QRS complex vectors in leads II, III, and aVF, fulfilling the criteria for left interior hemiblock. Marked J-point elevation, ST segment elevation, and ST segment straightening are seen in leads V_{2-6}, I, and aVL. This represents the very early onset of acute myocardial injury over an extensive anterolateral distribution. This is an anterolateral myocardial infarction–acute. The patient is best served with urgent myocardial revascularization.

Obtaining an ECG at such an early juncture of acute myocardial injury is unusual and generally is obtained in a hospitalized setting. Most often, when patients present to an outside physician, the ECG will have evolved beyond the hyperacute findings demonstrated on this tracing.

ELECTROCARDIOGRAM FIGURE 59.13

Clinical History

A 65-year-old man referred for coronary artery bypass graft surgery in the setting of pulmonary edema and advanced

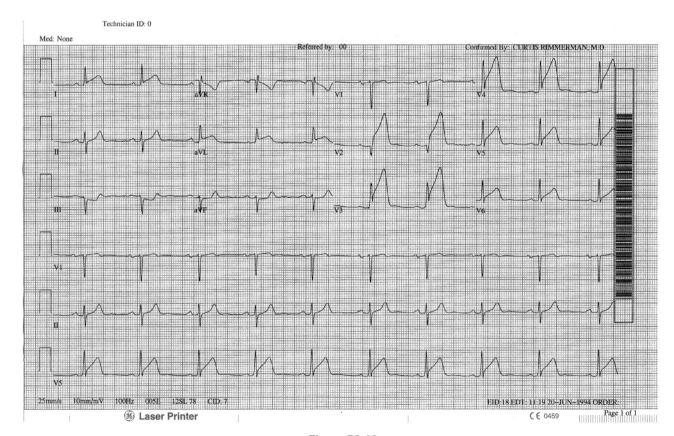

Figure 59.12

Technician ID: 10

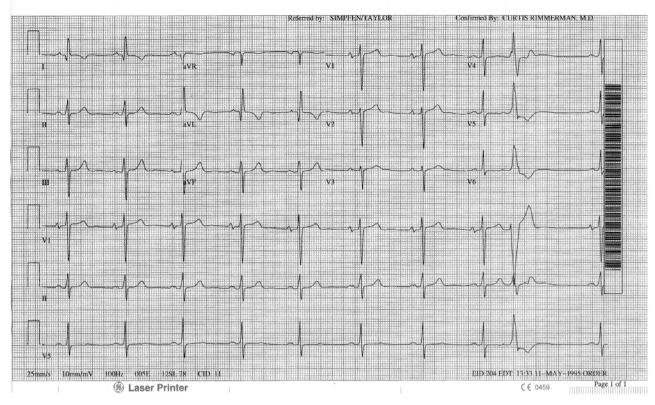

Figure 59.13

coronary artery disease. A recent cardiac catheterization demonstrated moderately severe left ventricular systolic dysfunction and anterolateral akinesis. The most advanced coronary artery obstruction was in the diagonal branch of the left anterior descending coronary artery. Medications at the time of this ECG included atenolol, aspirin, simvastatin, and isosorbide mononitrate. Comorbidities included hypertension and long-term tobacco use.

Interpretation and Comments

Sinus bradycardia is present, as the P waves are regular at a rate slightly <60 per minute. A prominent bifid P wave in lead II and a terminally negative P wave in lead V_1 are both consistent with left atrial abnormality. Toward the right hand portion of the ECG, a premature ventricular complex is present, widened, and different in morphology than the native QRS complex. Most important, Q waves of diagnostic width are present in leads I and aVL, reflective of a high lateral myocardial infarction–age indeterminate. There are associated ST-T changes in leads V_{4-6} but no Q waves. This infarction is limited to the high lateral leads and is best termed a high lateral myocardial infarction–age indeterminate.

This infarction most likely represents the left circumflex coronary artery distribution but may also represent a ramus intermedius branch or a diagonal branch of the left anterior descending coronary artery. The high lateral leads

demonstrate significant coronary artery territory overlap. The exact delineation of the coronary artery representing this ECG region is most confidently concluded at the time of cardiac catheterization.

ELECTROCARDIOGRAM FIGURE 59.14

Clinical History

A 59-year-old woman who suffered a bradycardic cardiac arrest in the setting of an acute subarachnoid hemorrhage. The patient eventually recovered and was discharged from the hospital. During her hospitalization, an echocardiogram demonstrated normal left ventricular function and no evidence of a prior myocardial infarction.

Interpretation and Comments

This ECG is one typically seen in patients acutely admitted to a neurosurgical intensive care unit with a catastrophic central nervous system event such as a subarachnoid hemorrhage. Sinus slowing, generally in the form of sinus bradycardia, exists. Nonspecific ST-T changes are present with deep T-wave inversion in the high lateral leads. There is a markedly prolonged QT interval in all leads.

Another consideration would be diffuse myocardial ischemia. This would be best determined at the bedside by performing a detailed history and physical examination

Technician: 10

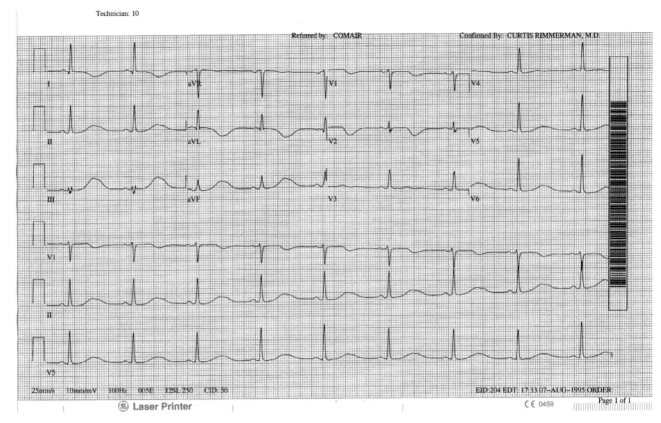

Figure 59.14

and obtaining serial serum cardiac enzymes. Note the normal appearance of both the PR and QRS complex intervals, as cerebrovascular events predominantly demonstrate abnormal ventricular repolarization.

ELECTROCARDIOGRAM FIGURE 59.15

Clinical History

A 65-year-old man with a nonischemic dilated cardiomyopathy and moderately severe left ventricular systolic dysfunction who returns for cardiology follow-up in the setting of nonsustained ventricular tachycardia. His medications included mexiletine, aspirin, enalapril, and atenolol. A prior cardiac catheterization demonstrated mild coronary artery disease.

Interpretation and Comments

The fourth QRS complex is preceded by an upright P wave and normal PR interval. This represents normal sinus rhythm. Frequent premature ventricular complexes are noted throughout the ECG. This represents nonsustained ventricular tachycardia, as three premature ventricular complexes occur in succession. A terminally negative P wave in lead V_1 suggests left atrial abnormality. A Q wave is present in leads II, III, and aVF without associated ST-T changes. It appears to be 30 msec in duration. This is not of sufficient

duration to confidently diagnose a prior inferior myocardial infarction.

In this instance, it is best to suggest the possibility of an inferior myocardial infarction of indeterminate age but not conclusively diagnose it. Further clinical correlation would be necessary. This demonstrates a limitation of the ECG found in daily practice in an attempt to accurately diagnose the presence or absence of an inferior myocardial infarction. The presence of frequent premature ventricular complexes may portend a worse prognosis.

ELECTROCARDIOGRAM FIGURE 59.16

Clinical History

A 42-year-old man who is self-referred for evaluation of heart palpitations. His medications included ibuprofen and ranitidine.

Interpretation and Comments

This ECG demonstrates normal sinus rhythm with a shortened PR interval and a slurred QRS upstroke indicative of ventricular pre-excitation and the Wolff-Parkinson-White syndrome. The third and eighth QRS complexes are preceded by a premature P wave. These are premature atrial complexes.

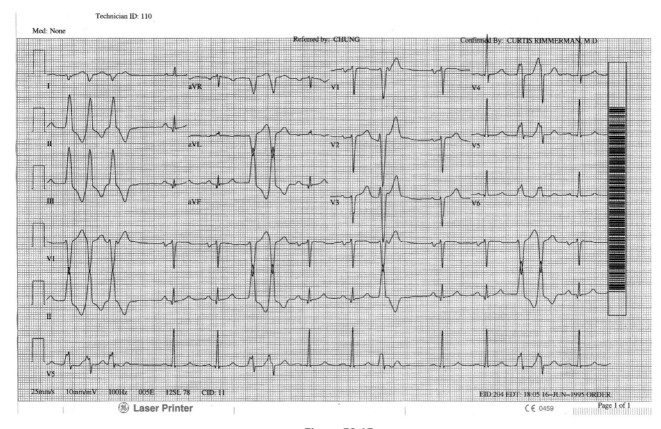

Figure 59.15

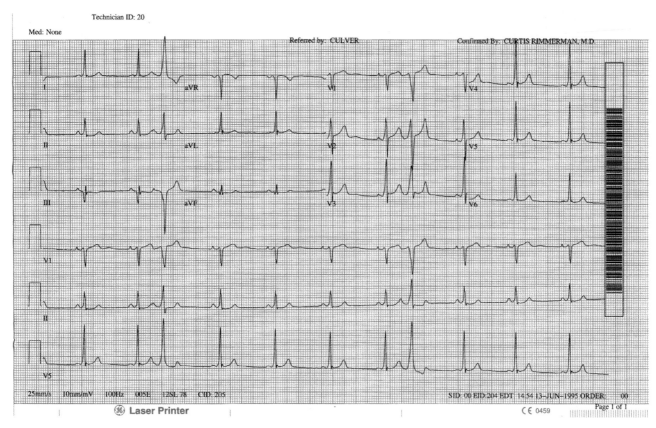

Figure 59.16

Note that the QRS complexes associated with the premature atrial complexes demonstrate a greater degree of ventricular pre-excitation. This is an expected finding, as the accessory pathway, unlike the atrioventricular node, demonstrates facile conduction at this shorter cycle length and is able to conduct preferentially without block. This demonstrates the facility of conduction within the accessory pathway and why arrhythmias such as atrial fibrillation are clinically dangerous, as the accessory pathway can conduct at very high heart rates and generate hemodynamically unstable cardiac rhythms.

ELECTROCARDIOGRAM FIGURE 59.17

Clinical History

A 72-year-old woman with recent onset angina pectoris accepted in hospital transfer for planned coronary artery bypass graft surgery. Her medications included glucotrol, thyroxine, omeprazole, lisinopril, and furosemide. Cardiac risk factors include non–insulin-requiring diabetes mellitus and hypertension.

Interpretation and Comments

This ECG demonstrates atrial fibrillation without identifiable P-wave activity in the setting of an irregularly irregular ventricular response. Acceleration-dependent complete right bundle-branch block is present. With QRS complex

cycle length slowing, as seen between the 10th and 11th QRS complexes, the complete right bundle-branch block transitions to an incomplete right bundle-branch block. This suggests the presence of an acceleration-dependent complete right bundle-branch block. Broad Q waves are seen in the inferior leads, reflecting an inferior myocardial infarction–age indeterminant.

Oftentimes, the electrocardiographer can work backward from an ECG and deduce a significant portion of the clinical history. It is likely that this patient suffered an inferior myocardial infarction in the past and subsequently developed atrial fibrillation and acceleration-dependent complete right bundle-branch block on an ischemic basis.

ELECTROCARDIOGRAM FIGURE 59.18

Clinical History

A 42-year-old man with end-stage liver disease secondary to chronic hepatitis C infection who presents to the hospital with an altered mental status, acute renal failure, and a serum potassium level of 8.2 meq/L.

Interpretation and Comments

Normal sinus rhythm is present, as the P waves are upright in the limb leads and precede each QRS complex with a constant PR interval. The PR interval is prolonged at approximately 240 msec, supporting first-degree atrioventricular

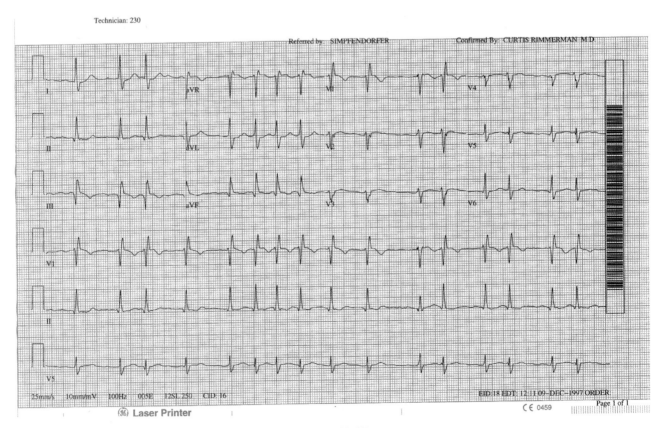

Figure 59.17

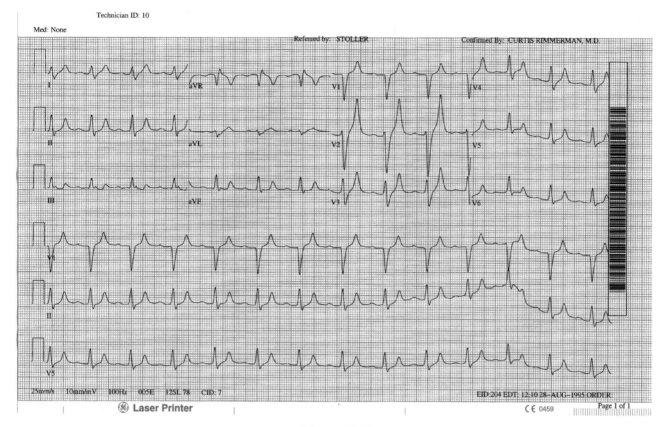

Technician ID: 10

Med: None

Referred by: STOLLER   Confirmed By: CURTIS RIMMERMAN, M.D.

25mm/s   10mm/mV   100Hz   005E   12SL 78   CID: 7   EID 204 EDT: 12:10 28–AUG–1995 ORDER:

Laser Printer   CE 0459   Page 1 of 1

Figure 59.18

block. The QRS complex is widened to a nonspecific degree, and the T waves are narrow based and peaked in all leads. This combination of findings, including first-degree atrioventricular block, a nonspecific intraventricular conduction delay, and peaked T waves, all suggest advanced hyperkalemia.

It is important to identify abnormalities suggesting hyperkalemia, as the ECG may represent the first clinical clue. If the potassium level continues to rise, further QRS widening will ensue, progressing to eventual asystole.

ELECTROCARDIOGRAM FIGURE 59.19

Clinical History

A 35-year-old woman with a history of mitral valve endocarditis status post St. Jude mitral valve replacement who presents for elective hip replacement. Her medications included warfarin, lisinopril, and meperidine.

Interpretation and Comments

Normal sinus rhythm is present. The 4th P wave is premature and does not conduct to the ventricle. This represents a nonconducted premature atrial complex. This is repeated on the right-hand portion of this tracing. The 5th and 10th QRS complexes are conducted with complete right bundle-

branch block aberrancy. These are premature atrial complexes, as the QRS complex is preceded by P wave seen as a positive deflection in lead V_1 within the terminal aspect of the T wave. This is otherwise a normal ECG.

Compared to the nonconducted premature atrial complexes, the conducted premature atrial complexes with complete right bundle-branch block aberrancy have a longer preceding RP internal. At this slightly longer RP interval, the right bundle branch remains refractory. The left bundle branch is able to conduct normally, resulting in ventricular depolarization.

ELECTROCARDIOGRAM FIGURE 59.20

Clinical History

An 87-year-old man with a history of gastritis and benign prostatic hypertrophy admitted to the hospital with acute-onset abdominal pain. The patient subsequently underwent an exploratory laparotomy for a small bowel obstruction. His past medical history is notable for a myocardial infarction 26 years prior to this ECG.

Interpretation and Comments

Prominent baseline artifact, particularly on the left-hand side of this ECG, is present. This represents the best obtainable tracing for this patient. Despite the artifact,

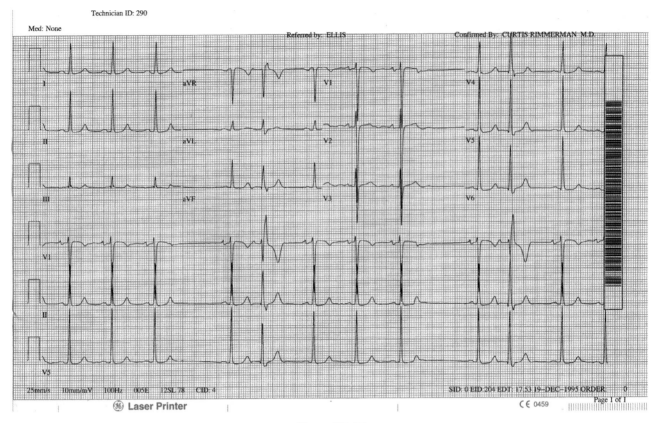

Figure 59.19

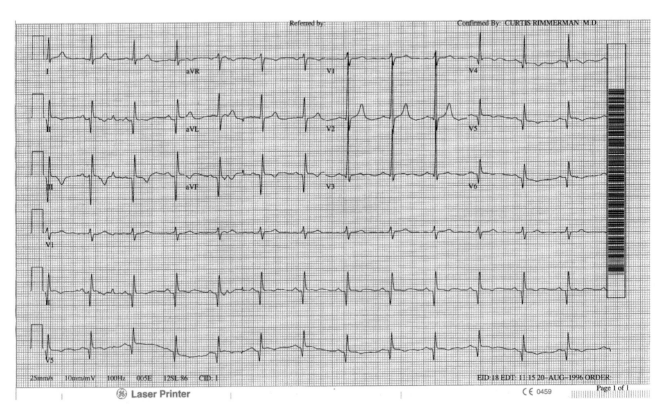

Figure 59.20

pathological findings are seen. The cardiac rhythm is normal sinus rhythm. Deep and wide Q waves are present inferiorly and laterally with prominent R waves in leads V_{1-2}. These findings together support the presence of an inferolateral myocardial infarction–age indeterminate.

Baseline artifact can interfere with ECG interpretation. Focusing on the most readily interpretable lead and working "backward" to those leads with greater artifact is a helpful approach. In lead II, a possible P wave exists between the second and third QRS complexes. This is not repeated throughout the tracing and does not interfere with the P:P cycle length. This is artifactual in origin.

ELECTROCARDIOGRAM FIGURE 59.21

Clinical History

A 47-year-old woman with dialysis requiring renal failure secondary to long-standing hypertension who presented to the hospital with recent-onset shortness of breath. At the time of this ECG, her serum calcium was 7.2 mg/dL, and her serum potassium was 6.4 meq/L.

Interpretation and Comments

This ECG was obtained at half standardization. Therefore, each complex is one-half the voltage of a standard ECG. The atrial rate is 60 per minute, regular, and of normal

axis. This represents normal sinus rhythm. The QRS complexes are also normal. A prolonged QT interval is present, and the ST segment is straightened, as seen in patients with hypocalcemia. Peaked T waves, particularly noted in leads V_{4-6}, are narrow based and symmetric, denoting hyperkalemia.

This combination of findings is commonly seen in a chronic renal failure patient, reflecting both hypocalcemia and hyperkalemia. The ECG may serve as the initial clinical clue for the presence of these electrolyte abnormalities. The patient also demonstrates QRS complex voltage consistent with left ventricular hypertrophy. This is not diagnosed on this ECG given the absence of secondary ST-T changes, also known as a left ventricular strain pattern. Diagnosing left ventricular hypertrophy solely on the basis of increased QRS complex voltage suffers from reduced specificity.

ELECTROCARDIOGRAM FIGURE 59.22

Clinical History

A 51-year-old man with rheumatic heart disease status post aortic and mitral valve reparative surgery who re-presents with anemia and laboratory studies consistent with hemolysis. A repeat echocardiogram demonstrated severe aortic and mitral insufficiency, and the patient was referred for repeat cardiac surgery.

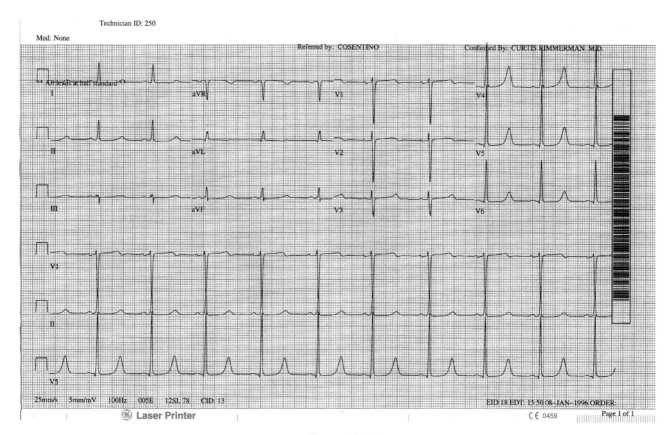

Figure 59.21

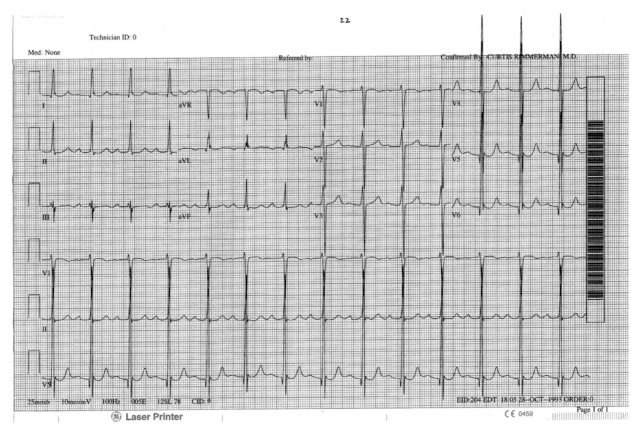

Figure 59.22

Interpretation and Comments

P waves precede each QRS complex with a constant PR interval. The P waves are of normal axis, representing normal sinus rhythm at a rate of approximately 85 per minute. The PR interval is prolonged at 280 msec. This represents first-degree atrioventricular block. The QRS complex voltage is prominent in the precordial leads, satisfying the criteria for left ventricular hypertrophy. Subtle nonspecific ST-T changes are also seen, possibly secondary to left ventricular hypertrophy.

This ECG demonstrates the diastolic or volume overload pattern of left ventricular hypertrophy. Narrow deep Q waves are present in leads V_{5-6}, consistent with the patient's history of aortic and mitral insufficiency. In a pressure overload or systolic pattern of left ventricular hypertrophy, the narrow and deep Q waves typically are absent.

ELECTROCARDIOGRAM FIGURE 59.23

Clinical History

A 65-year-old man admitted to the hospital for evaluation of acute renal failure in the setting of Wegener granulomatosis. His past medical history includes paroxysmal atrial fibrillation and hypertension. His medications include prednisone, omeprazole, cyclophosphamide, verapamil, and bumetanide.

Interpretation and Comments

No discernible atrial activity is seen on this ECG. This represents atrial fibrillation. The ventricular response is irregularly irregular at a rate of approximately 100 per minute. Elevation of the atrial repolarization segment in lead aVR is present. This suggests pericarditis. Nonspecific ST-T changes are also noted throughout the tracing.

In the presence of ST segment elevation, it is important to differentiate acute myocardial injury from pericarditis, as each clinical entity has distinct treatment plans. In the case of pericarditis, it most commonly demonstrates widespread ST segment elevation and elevation of the PR or atrial repolarization segment in lead aVR. Unlike in acute myocardial injury, reciprocal ST segment depression is not commonly seen in the setting of pericarditis. The absence of reciprocal ST segment depression and the PR segment elevation favors the diagnosis of pericarditis.

ELECTROCARDIOGRAM FIGURE 59.24

Clinical History

A 19-year-old man with end-stage renal disease of unknown etiology requiring dialysis who presented to the hospital with symptoms of shortness of breath and chest

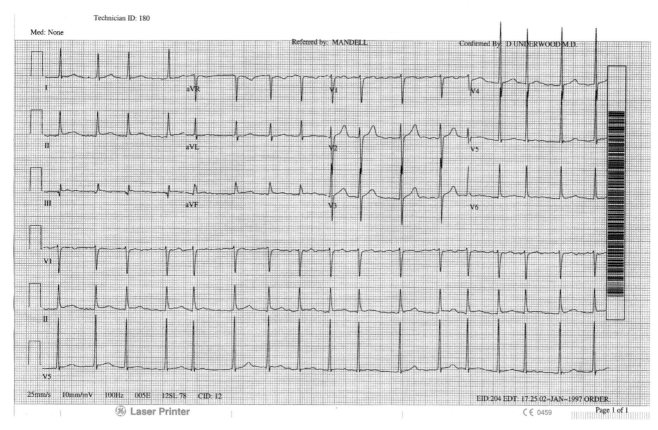

Figure 59.23

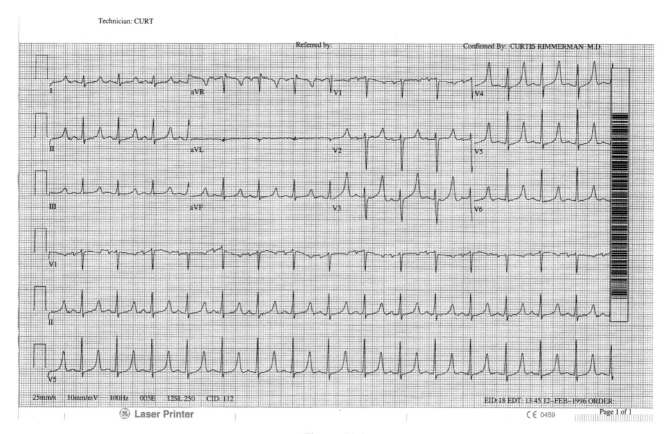

Figure 59.24

x-ray confirmation of pulmonary edema. His serum potassium at the time of admission was 6.8 meq/L. His serum calcium was 6.0 mg/dL.

Interpretation and Comments

The baseline artifact on this ECG makes the interpretation of the atrial rhythm initially difficult. Lead II supports the presence of P waves prior to each QRS complex with a normal PR interval at a rate of approximately 95 per minute. This represents normal sinus rhythm. In lead II, it is important not to confuse the P wave that immediately precedes the QRS complex with the peaked T wave that is more prominent and precedes the P wave. Assessing the cardiac intervals, a prolonged QT interval is present. The ST segment is straightened, and the T waves are symmetric, narrow based, and peaked.

This combination of ECG findings suggests both hypocalcemia and hyperkalemia, as is often seen in patients with chronic renal disease. The finding of hypocalcemia on an ECG is supported by a prolonged QT interval that is greater than one-half of the R:R limb lead interval. It is also supported by the ST segment straightening best seen in this instance in lead V2. When suspecting hyperkalemia on an ECG, not only is the absolute T-wave amplitude important, but equally valuable is the finding of both narrowed-based and symmetric T waves resembling a high pitched tent.

ELECTROCARDIOGRAM FIGURE 59.25

Clinical History

A 28-year-old man status post orthotopic liver transplantation secondary to chronic hepatitis B infection contracted 10 years prior to this ECG who re-presents to the hospital with epigastric pain, nausea, and hematemesis. His medications at the time of this ECG included cyclosporine, prednisone, and omeprazole. His admission serum chemistries were notable for a serum potassium level of 2.3 meq/L.

Interpretation and Comments

The cardiac rhythm is normal sinus rhythm. Inspection of the cardiac intervals demonstrates a markedly prolonged QT interval in all leads. Lead V2 demonstrates a second upright deflection immediately following the T wave. This represents prominent positive U waves. The QT interval prolongation is more accurately termed *QT-U interval prolongation*. Electrolyte disturbances such as hypokalemia and concomitant medications are important diagnostic considerations.

It is important to have an organized approach to ECG interpretation. This includes assessment of the cardiac intervals for each tracing. In this instance, the ECG may serve as the initial indicator of a life-threatening serum electrolyte abnormality.

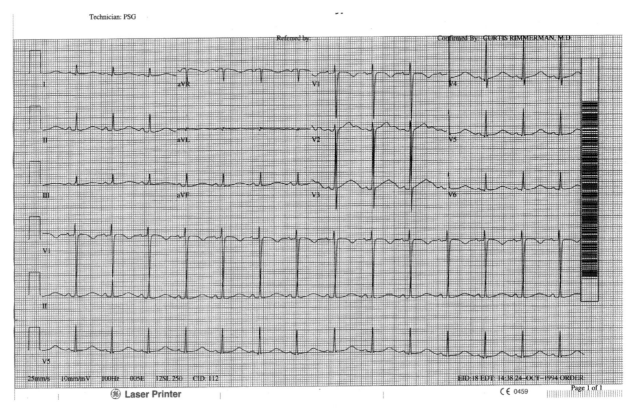

Figure 59.25

ELECTROCARDIOGRAM FIGURE 59.26

Clinical History

A 52-year-old man with recently diagnosed multiple myeloma and a serum calcium level of 13.1 mg/dL.

Interpretation and Comments

This ECG demonstrates normal sinus rhythm. The QRS complexes are normal both in duration and morphology. The only identifiable abnormality is a short QT interval with a truncated ST segment. This is abnormal and represents an ECG marker of hypercalcemia.

This ECG emphasizes the need to carefully assess the ECG intervals on each tracing. The routine ECG may be the only clinical marker of underlying serum electrolyte disturbances. It is important to readily identify these abnormalities, as prompt clinical treatment frequently is warranted.

ELECTROCARDIOGRAM FIGURE 59.27

Clinical History

A 74-year-old man with hypertrophic obstructive cardiomyopathy who is being seen in follow-up in the psychiatric department for chronic depression. His cardiac medications included verapamil and atenolol.

Interpretation and Comments

The atrial rhythm is regular at a rate <60 per minute with a normal P-wave axis. This satisfies the ECG criteria for sinus bradycardia. This ECG is obtained at half standardization. Despite this, prominent QRS complex voltage is seen in the precordial leads and inferiorly. A tall R wave is present in leads V_{1-2}. This suggests the presence of both left ventricular hypertrophy with secondary ST-T changes and right ventricular hypertrophy. This is an example of biventricular hypertrophy with secondary ST-T changes. Prominent Q waves are seen in this patient with hypertrophic obstructive cardiomyopathy, reflecting septal depolarization.

In this diagnostic setting, prominent septal Q waves are frequently present, as seen on this ECG. It is important to distinguish Q waves secondary to septal depolarization from the possibility of an underlying age-indeterminant myocardial infarction. Oftentimes, this is not possible and requires further adjunctive testing.

ELECTROCARDIOGRAM FIGURE 59.28

Clinical History

A 42-year-old woman with primary pulmonary hypertension and severe right ventricular systolic dysfunction admitted for further evaluation and treatment of worsening right-sided congestive heart failure. Her medications

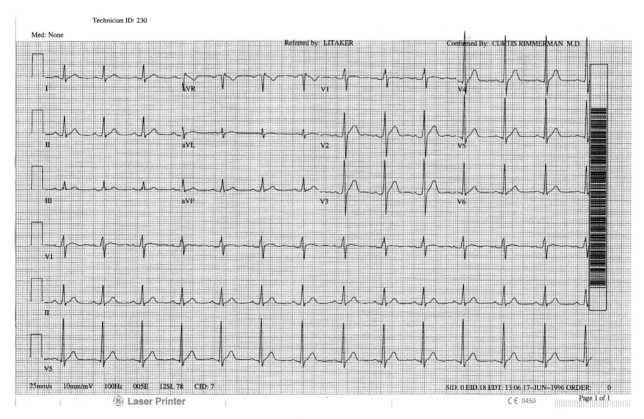

Figure 59.26

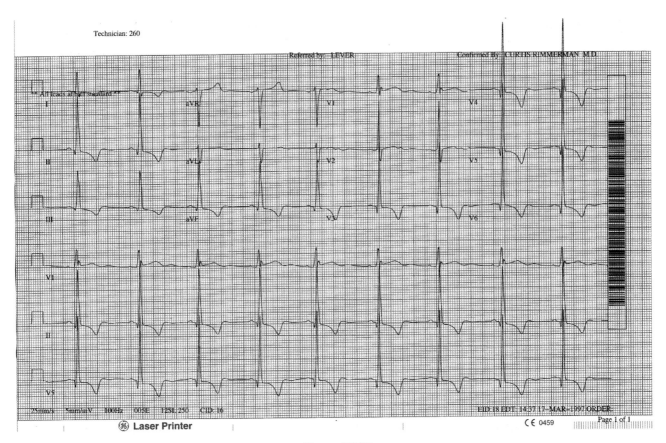

Figure 59.27

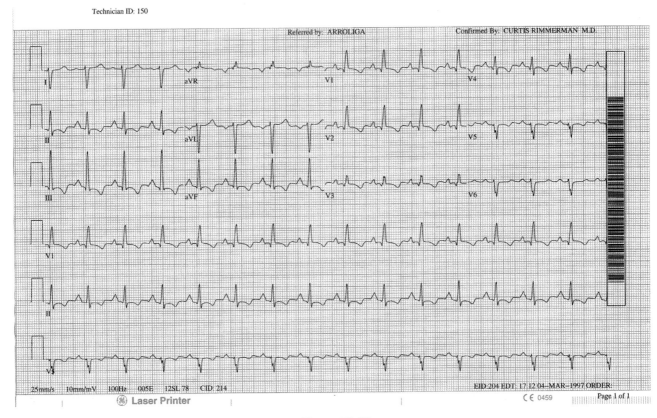

Figure 59.28

included warfarin, nifedipine, furosemide, potassium, and inhaled bronchodilators.

Interpretation and Comments

The cardiac rhythm is normal sinus rhythm. The P wave in lead II is both broadened and heightened at 3 mm. This supports right atrial abnormality. The QRS complex frontal plane axis demonstrates right axis deviation, as the QRS complex vector is negative in lead I and positive in leads II, III, and aVF. A small Q wave and prominent R wave with a normal QRS complex duration is seen in leads V_{1-2}, reflecting right ventricular hypertrophy with secondary ST-T changes. Note the poor R-wave progression throughout the precordium given the right ventricular hypertrophy and resultant counterclockwise cardiac rotation.

This ECG demonstrates the common features of right ventricular pressure overload, including right atrial abnormality, right axis deviation, and right ventricular hypertrophy with secondary ST-T changes.

ELECTROCARDIOGRAM FIGURE 59.29

Clinical History

A 53-year-old woman who was seen in the emergency room with an acute upper gastrointestinal distress syndrome. She

has a long-standing history of tobacco use. Her medications included Ranitidine. A serum potassium level was not checked at the time of this ECG.

Interpretation and Comments

The cardiac rhythm is normal sinus rhythm as each P wave is upright in leads I, II, and III and precedes each QRS complex with a constant PR interval. The QRS complexes are also normal as are the cardiac intervals. The T waves appear narrow-based and peaked suggesting hyperkalemia. Negative U waves are present in leads V_{3-6}. These occur at the terminal portion of the T wave.

Negative U waves most commonly occur in the presence of left ventricular hypertrophy and/or myocardial ischemia. The possibility of underlying coronary artery disease and myocardial ischemia warrants further evaluation. The peaked T waves should prompt a serum electrolyte investigation.

ELECTROCARDIOGRAM FIGURE 59.30

Clinical History

An 82-year-old woman who presents to the hospital with acute-onset severe shortness of breath. Her past medical history includes hypertension and gout. Her admission

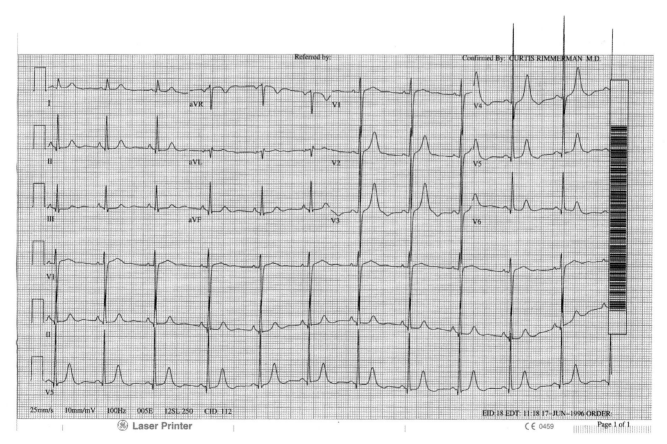

Figure 59.29

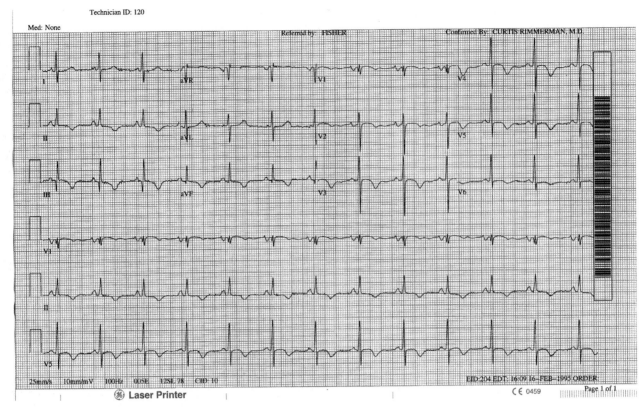

Technician ID: 120

Med: None

Referred by: FISHER   Confirmed By: CURTIS RIMMERMAN, M.D.

25mm/s   10mm/mV   100Hz   00SE   12SL 78   CID: 10   EID:204 EDT: 16:09 16-FEB-1995 ORDER:

Laser Printer   CE 0459   Page 1 of 1

Figure 59.30

blood gas demonstrates advanced hypoxemia, and a V/Q scan has been interpreted as high probability for a pulmonary embolism.

Interpretation and Comments

This ECG demonstrates normal sinus rhythm, as the P-wave vector in leads I, II, and III is upright with a constant PR interval. Left atrial abnormality is suggested by a terminally negative P wave in lead V_1. Diffuse nonspecific ST-T changes are noted of uncertain origin. No other abnormalities are seen on this tracing.

Given the history of acute pulmonary embolism, in retrospect, subtle but present ST segment elevation is noted in leads V_{1-2}. This may represent acute right ventricular myocardial injury secondary to the pulmonary embolism and presumed acute-onset pulmonary hypertension. A prominent S wave is present in lead I, a Q wave in lead III, and T-wave inversion in lead III. This is the so-called S1-Q3-T3 pattern described in the setting of an acute pulmonary embolism.

ELECTROCARDIOGRAM FIGURE 59.31

Clinical History

A 44-year-old woman with a several hour history of "rapid heart beating" and mild shortness of breath. Her past medical history includes hypertension. Her medications include lisinopril. The patient received intravenous adeno-

sine, which promptly converted this dysrhythmia to normal sinus rhythm.

Interpretation and Comments

On this tracing, no readily identifiable sinus P waves are seen. A regular narrow complex supraventricular tachycardia at a rate of approximately 160 per minute is identified. Lead I demonstrates a small deflection at the terminal portion of the QRS complex occupying the proximal portion of the ST segment. This is also seen in lead V_1, where an apparent terminal r' QRS complex pattern reflects atrial activity. This represents retrograde P waves. Diffuse nonspecific ST-T changes are seen. These may be related to the tachycardia. It would be prudent to repeat the tracing during an arrhythmiafree interval to document ST-T wave change resolution.

Given the short PR interval, this dysrhythmia most likely represents typical atrioventricular nodal re-entrant tachycardia, where antegrade conduction occurs via the slow atrioventricular nodal pathway and retrograde conduction occurs via the fast atrioventricular nodal pathway. If this arrhythmia is recurrent and disabling, this patient would be appropriately considered for radio frequency ablation.

ELECTROCARDIOGRAM FIGURE 59.32

Clinical History

A 77-year-old woman who was accepted in hospital transfer after suffering an acute inferior myocardial infarction

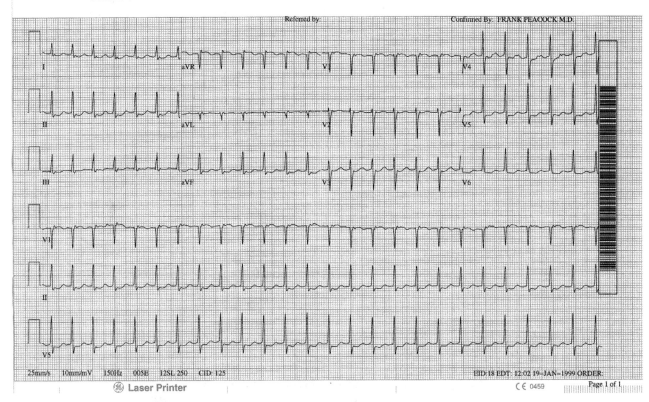

Figure 59.31

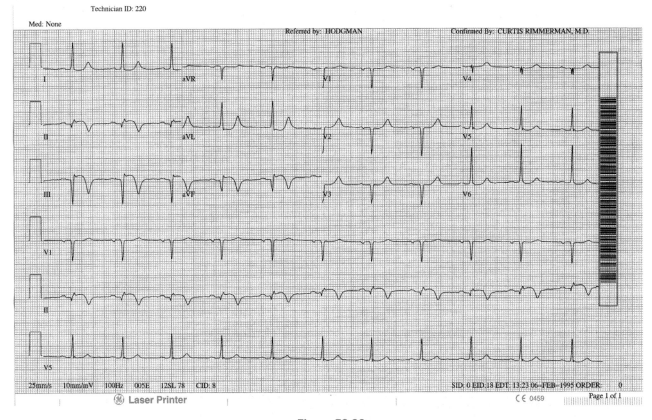

Figure 59.32

10 days prior to this ECG. Comorbidities include hypertension and a prior cerebral aneurysm repair. Her medications include nifedipine, triamterene-hydrochlorothiazide, and aspirin.

Interpretation and Comments

Normal sinus rhythm is present, as the P-wave axis is normal. The atrial rate is regular at approximately 70 per minute. ST segment elevation with prominent Q-wave formation is seen in the inferior leads. Terminal T-wave inversion is present. This represents an inferior myocardial infarction–acute and acute myocardial injury. Q waves are present in leads V_{2-4} without associated ST segment elevation. This represents an anterior myocardial infarction–age indeterminate. The ST segment depression in leads I and aVL reflects reciprocal changes from the acute inferior myocardial infarction.

This ECG is atypical, as the myocardial infarction of 10 days duration demonstrates persistent ST segment elevation. This could represent several possibilities, including ongoing myocardial ischemia and repetitive myocardial injury and/or the interval development of a ventricular aneurysm. Careful clinical evaluation of this patient would be warranted.

ELECTROCARDIOGRAM FIGURE 59.33

Clinical History

A 58-year-old woman who is being evaluated preoperatively prior to a bilateral mastectomy for cancer of the breast. Her cardiac history includes a normal cardiac catheterization prompted by a chest discomfort syndrome 2 years before this ECG. There is no clinical history of palpitations, presyncope, or prior myocardial infarction.

Interpretation and Comments

Normal sinus rhythm and a short PR interval are both present. A slurred upstroke to the QRS complex is noted, particularly in the chest leads, consistent with ventricular pre-excitation. The fifth QRS complex represents a premature ventricular complex. An apparent inferoposterior myocardial infarction is present, and clinical correlation would be necessary. This most likely instead represents a pseudoinfarction pattern in the setting of the Wolff-Parkinson-White syndrome.

Careful inspection of the cardiac intervals is an important step for ECG interpretation. A shortened PR interval is often the first clue to the presence of an accessory pathway. Once a shortened PR interval is seen, it is important to look for evidence of ventricular pre-excitation in the form of a delta wave. A pseudo-infarction pattern is most often

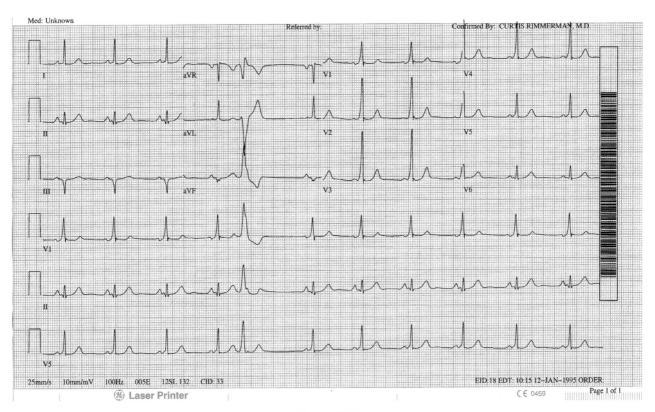

Figure 59.33

located inferiorly and/or laterally depending on accessory pathway location. If a prior myocardial infarction is suspected, a cardiac imaging study may be indicated.

ELECTROCARDIOGRAM FIGURE 59.34

Clinical History

A 56-year-old man with rheumatoid arthritis who is seen in the outpatient department for a follow-up evaluation. He has no cardiac history and is on no cardiac medications.

Interpretation and Comments

This ECG demonstrates sinus bradycardia, as the atrial rate is approximately 50 per minute with a normal P-wave axis. The third P wave is premature with a normally conducted QRS complex representing a premature atrial complex. The fifth P wave is also a premature atrial complex and is followed by a prolonged PR interval and a QRS complex with a complete left bundle-branch block aberrancy. In contrast to the prior premature atrial complex, this occurs with a shorter RP interval, greater intra-atrial and atrioventricular nodal delay, and subsequent ventricular aberration. The last premature atrial complex is an interpolated premature atrial complex, as it does not reset the sinus node. It also demonstrates aberrant conduction, but its shorter QRS

complex duration does not satisfy the criteria for complete left bundle-branch block. Diffuse nonspecific ST-T changes are also seen.

Premature atrial complexes with complete left bundle branch aberrancy are less common compared to complete right bundle-branch block aberrancy, as the refractory period of the left bundle branch is shorter. The premature atrial complexes conduct with a prolonged PR interval given the short preceding RP interval and the reciprocal relationship between the preceding RP interval and subsequent PR interval. This is an example of concealed conduction.

ELECTROCARDIOGRAM FIGURE 59.35

Clinical History

A 26-year-old man with severe rheumatic aortic insufficiency seen in preoperative cardiac evaluation prior to anticipated aortic valve replacement. A recent echocardiogram demonstrated severe aortic insufficiency, a dilated left ventricle with mildly reduced left ventricular systolic function, and left ventricular hypertrophy.

Interpretation and Comments

This ECG is obtained at half standardization. The cardiac rhythm is normal sinus rhythm. The P wave is prolonged in lead II and terminally negative to a slight degree in lead

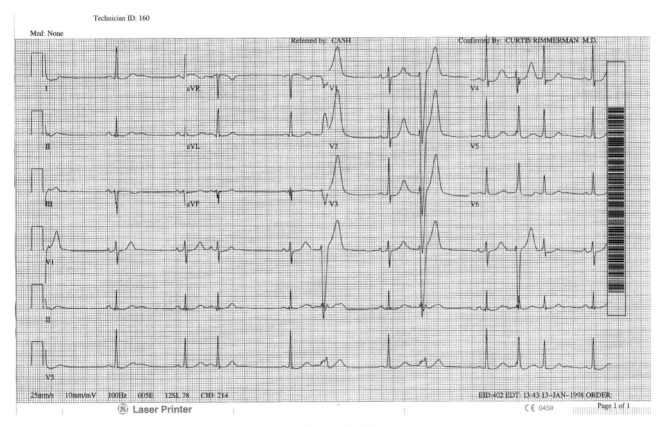

Figure 59.34

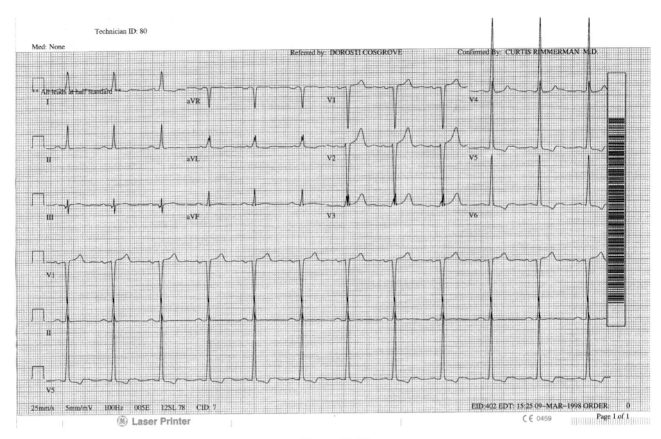

Technician ID: 80

Med: None

Referred by: DOROSTI COSGROVE   Confirmed By: CURTIS RIMMERMAN M.D.

** All leads at half standard **

I   aVR   V1   V4

II   aVL   V2   V5

III   aVF   V3   V6

V1

II

V5

25mm/s   5mm/mV   100Hz   005E   12SL 78   CID: 7   EID:402 EDT: 15:25 09-MAR-1998 ORDER: 0

℗ Laser Printer   CE 0459   Page 1 of 1

Figure 59.35

V_1, supporting left atrial abnormality. Prominent precordial QRS complex voltage is present with secondary ST-T changes indicative of a strain pattern, satisfying the ECG criteria for left ventricular hypertrophy with secondary ST-T changes. In leads V_{5-6}, after the termination of the T wave and prior to the onset of the P wave, an additional small negative deflection is seen, representing a negative U wave. This further supports the diagnosis of left ventricular hypertrophy.

The presence of a negative U wave suggests one of two etiologic possibilities: left ventricular hypertrophy and coronary artery disease. In this circumstance, given the patient's young age and known severe aortic insufficiency, left ventricular hypertrophy is the most likely possibility.

ELECTROCARDIOGRAM FIGURE 59.36

Clinical History

A 72-year-old woman with a history of insulin-requiring diabetes mellitus who is accepted in hospital transfer with the suspected diagnosis of status epilepticus. The patient was diagnosed with metabolic encephalopathy. Her neurologic status failed to improve, and she subsequently expired.

Interpretation and Comments

The cardiac rhythm is an ectopic atrial rhythm, as P waves occur at regular intervals with a negative P-wave vector evi-

dent in the inferior leads. A prolonged QT interval, nonspecific ST-T changes, and deep T wave inversion are present.

These ECG findings are consistent with the patient's clinical history of a recent central nervous system event and increased intracranial pressure. The differential diagnosis of these findings includes a central nervous system event, electrolyte abnormalities, and diffuse myocardial ischemia.

ELECTROCARDIOGRAM FIGURE 59.37

Clinical History

A 22-year-old woman who presents for evaluation of dysplastic nevi. She has known dextrocardia and is not taking any medications.

Interpretation and Comments

This tracing demonstrates an abnormal P-wave axis with a negative P-wave vector in leads I and aVL. The differential diagnosis of this finding is misplaced limb leads versus dextrocardia. A prominent R wave is seen in lead V_1 with R-wave regression, as one proceeds from leads V_{2-6}. This finding in combination with the negative P-wave vector in the high lateral leads confirms the presence of dextrocardia. This ECG otherwise demonstrates normal sinus rhythm with premature atrial complexes in a pattern of atrial bigeminy.

Recognizing the presence of dextrocardia is important, as normal ECGs can be interpreted as significantly

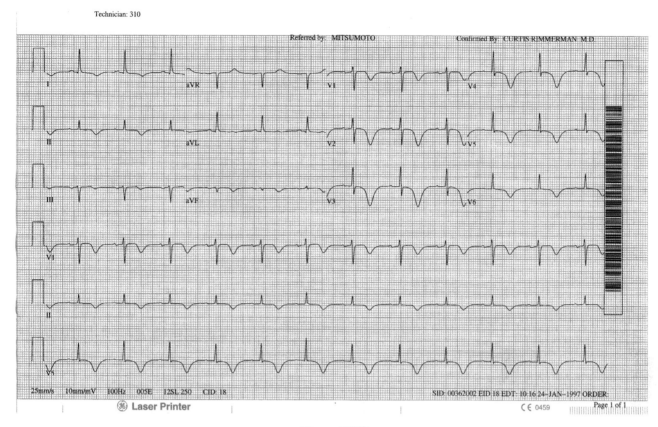

Figure 59.36

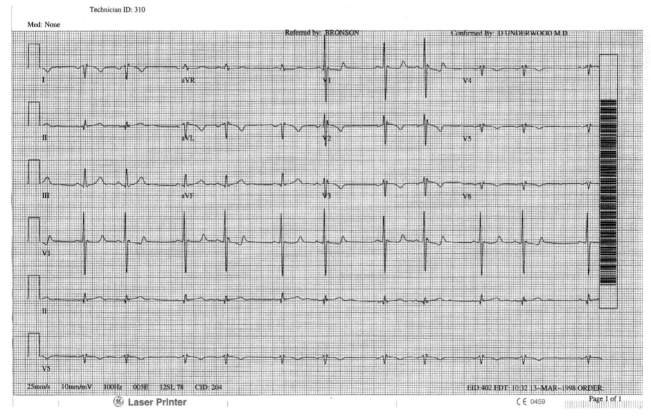

Figure 59.37

abnormal. On first glance, the frontal plane QRS complex axis appears deviated extremely rightward, possibly even suggesting a high lateral myocardial infarction. The important diagnostic clue present on this ECG is the negative P-wave vector in leads I and aVL. This finding, together with R-wave regression seen in leads V_{2-6}, confirms the presence of dextrocardia.

ELECTROCARDIOGRAM FIGURE 59.38

Clinical History

A 48-year-old man with severe mitral stenosis referred for mitral valve reparative surgery. He is not taking any medications. A recent echocardiogram confirmed the presence of severe mitral stenosis, a dilated right ventricle with moderately severe systolic dysfunction, moderately severe tricuspid insufficiency, and severe pulmonary hypertension.

Interpretation and Comments

This ECG demonstrates normal sinus rhythm, as the P-wave axis is normal and the atrial rate is slightly <100 per minute. In lead II, the P wave is 120 msec wide and demonstrates an amplitude of 3 mm, satisfying the criteria for right atrial abnormality. In lead V_1, a deep terminally negative P wave is present, supporting left atrial abnormality. The QRS complex frontal plane axis demonstrates right axis deviation, as the QRS complex vector is negative in lead I and positive in leads II, III, and aVF. A minuscule R wave is seen in lead V_1 followed by a small Q wave and a large R' deflection. This, in the setting of right atrial abnormality, QRS complex right axis deviation and a normal QRS complex duration supports the presence of right ventricular hypertrophy with secondary ST-T changes.

This tracing demonstrates the common ECG features of advanced mitral stenosis. These include left atrial abnormality, right atrial abnormality, QRS complex right axis deviation, and right ventricular hypertrophy with secondary ST-T changes.

ELECTROCARDIOGRAM FIGURE 59.39

Clinical History

A 22-year-old woman admitted to the hospital for evaluation and treatment of schizophrenia. She is not taking any medications.

Interpretation and Comments

This is a normal ECG. The cardiac rhythm is normal sinus rhythm, as the P-wave axis in leads I, II, and III is normal and the atrial rate is approximately 70 per minute. T-wave

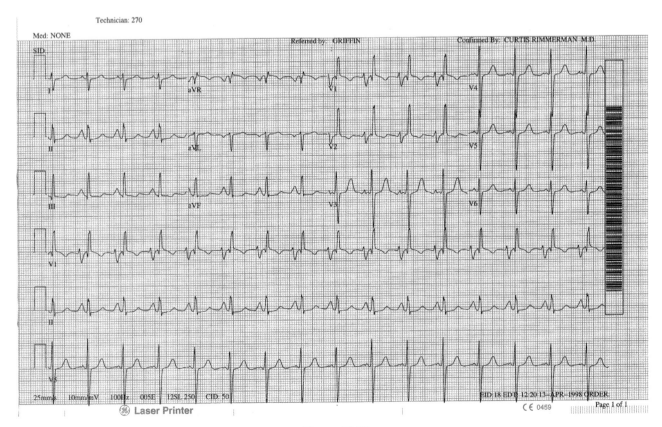

Figure 59.38

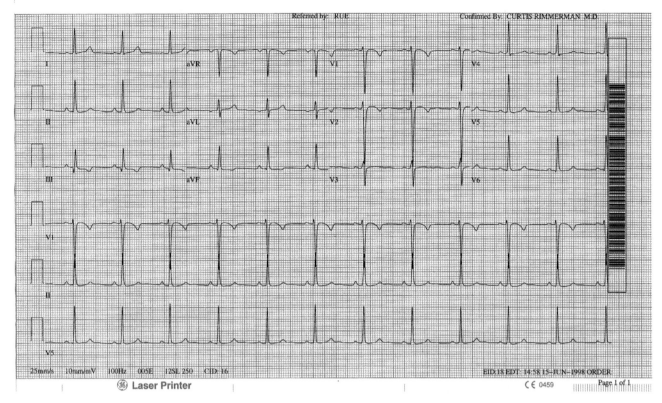

Technician: 220

Figure 59.39

inversion is present in leads V_{1-2}. In a younger patient, this is a normal finding and reflects a persistent juvenile T-wave pattern.

It is important to recognize normal variants when interpreting ECGs. The persistent juvenile T-wave pattern is a normal variant and should not be confused with underlying cardiac pathology such as myocardial ischemia or cardiomyopathy.

ELECTROCARDIOGRAM FIGURE 59.40

Clinical History

A 65-year-old man resting comfortably on a left ventricular assist device with severe left ventricular systolic dysfunction awaiting cardiac transplantation. He has severe ischemic left ventricular systolic dysfunction. The patient underwent successful cardiac transplantation.

Interpretation and Comments

This ECG demonstrates a wide QRS complex tachycardia at a cycle length of 250 msec corresponding to a ventricular rate of approximately 240 per minute. A monophasic QRS complex is seen in lead V_1, and the QRS complex is significantly widened with frontal plane QRS complex left axis

deviation. These findings together support the presence of ventricular tachycardia. No capture complexes, fusion complexes, or identifiable atrial activities are seen.

The regular-appearing QRS complexes with a "sawtooth" pattern resemble flutter waves. This is often called *ventricular flutter*, which is a more descriptive term.

ELECTROCARDIOGRAM FIGURE 59.41

Clinical History

A 65-year-old man with advanced coronary artery disease and resultant severe left ventricular systolic dysfunction who is awaiting cardiac transplantation. This ECG was obtained while the patient was fully conscious and dependent on a left ventricular assist device. The patient underwent successful cardiac transplantation surgery.

Interpretation and Comments

The ECG baseline is chaotic, without discernible organized atrial or ventricular activity. This represents ventricular fibrillation and is a terminal heart rhythm.

This is a rare opportunity to obtain a recording of ventricular fibrillation on a 12-lead ECG. There is a complete absence of organized cardiac electrical activity.

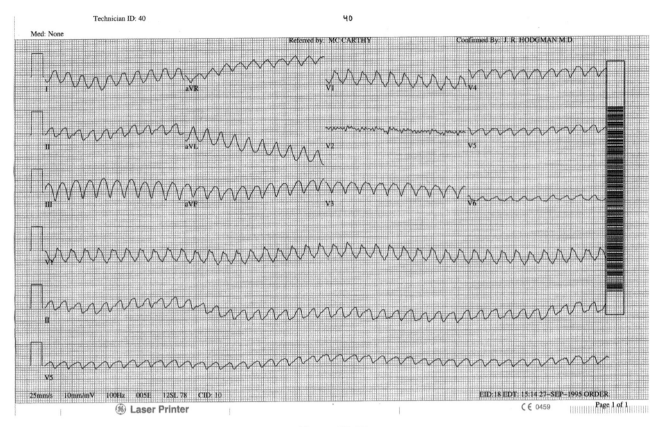

Figure 59.40

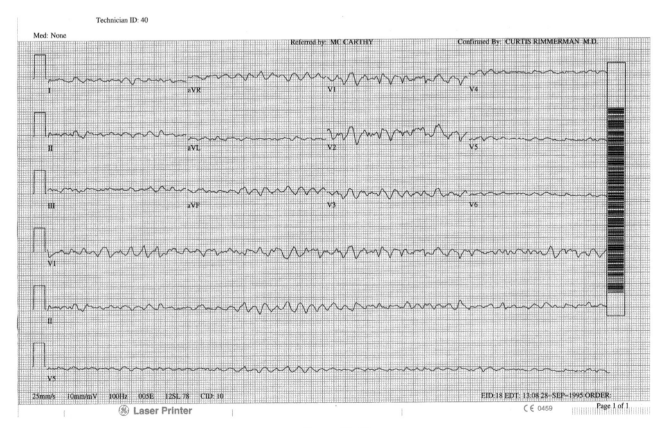

Figure 59.41

ELECTROCARDIOGRAM FIGURE 59.42

Clinical History

A 19-year-old man seen preoperatively prior to intended ostium secundum atrial septal defect repair. A recent echocardiogram demonstrated a moderate-sized ostium secundum atrial septal defect with left-to-right shunt flow, a dilated right ventricle with normal right ventricular systolic function, and moderate pulmonary hypertension.

Interpretation and Comments

The cardiac rhythm is normal sinus rhythm, as a P wave of normal axis precedes each QRS complex. The QRS complex frontal plane axis demonstrates right axis deviation, as the QRS complex vector is negative in lead I and positive in leads II, III, and aVF. A rsR' QRS complex morphology is noted in lead V_1. This represents an unusual pattern of right ventricular conduction delay and in the setting of QRS complex right axis deviation raises the possibility of an atrial septal defect.

The right ventricular conduction delay as seen in lead V_1 is characteristic of an atrial septal defect. Unlike an ostium primum atrial septal defect where the QRS complex frontal plane axis is deviated leftward, in the setting of an ostium secundum atrial septal defect, the QRS complex vector is normal or deviated rightward. In this circumstance, the rightward deviation of the QRS complex vector is secondary to the volume overload of the right ventricle given the left-to-right interatrial shunt.

ELECTROCARDIOGRAM FIGURE 59.43

Clinical History

A 67-year-old woman with coronary artery disease who underwent multivessel coronary artery bypass graft surgery 1 year prior to this ECG. She now presents for evaluation of a recent syncopal episode.

Interpretation and Comments

When QRS complexes of differing morphology appear on a surface ECG, it is important to identify the native QRS complex from an aberrantly conducted or ectopic QRS complex. The last five QRS complexes represent the native QRS complex in the setting of normal sinus rhythm and nonspecific ST-T changes. The initial portion of the ECG illustrates an example of acceleration-dependent complete left bundle-branch block. The third and ninth P waves are premature, representing premature atrial complexes. After the latter premature atrial complex, the subsequent

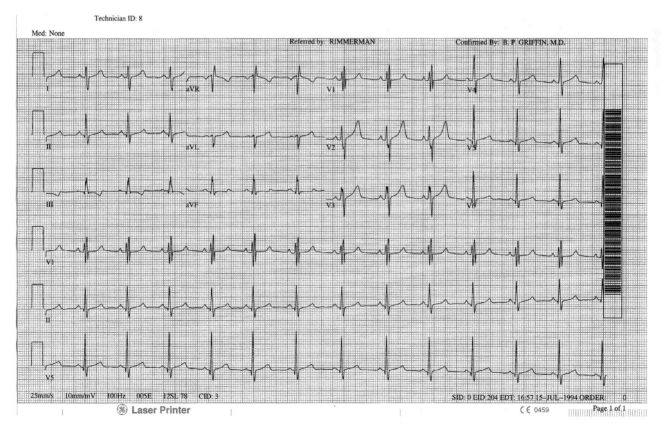

Figure 59.42

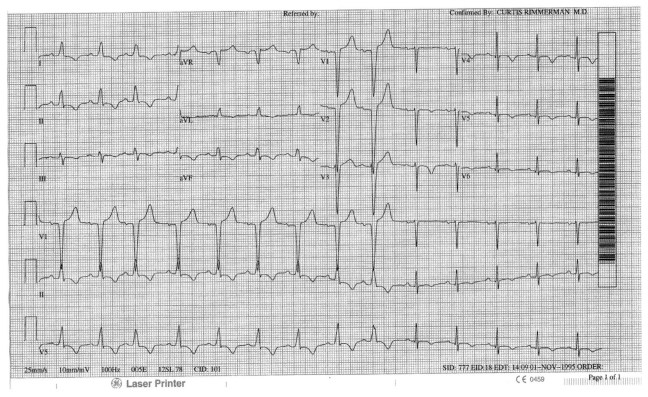

Figure 59.43

R:R cycle is slightly prolonged, allowing for recovery of the left bundle branch and normalization of QRS complex conduction. This permits a more accurate assessment of the native ST segments and T waves, which are masked by the complete left bundle-branch block. This may in fact reflect underlying myopathic and/or coronary artery disease that is otherwise not seen secondary to the complete left bundle-branch block.

In this instance, a premature atrial complex allows for recovery of the left bundle-branch block and normalized conduction. In the absence of this premature atrial complex, complete left bundle-branch block would be manifest for the entirety of the ECG, and the interpretation of ST-T changes would not be possible. Acceleration-dependent complete left bundle-branch block is not a normal finding and in this instance reflects this patient's underlying coronary artery disease.

ELECTROCARDIOGRAM FIGURE 59.44

Clinical History

A 77-year-old man with moderate left ventricular systolic dysfunction status post two coronary artery bypass grafting procedures admitted to the hospital with recurrent congestive heart failure and newly discovered atrial flutter.

Interpretation and Comments

Atrial flutter is readily identifiable in leads II, III, aVF, and V$_1$. The ventricular response demonstrates variable atrioventricular conduction ranging from a 2:1 to 4:1 conduction ratio. Q waves are present in leads II, III, and aVF, consistent with an inferior myocardial infarction–age indeterminant. Nonspecific ST-T changes are seen anterolaterally and are likely related to the suspected underlying ischemic heart disease.

Atrial arrhythmias are frequent in patients who have ischemic heart disease and particularly in those patients who have suffered a myocardial infarction. In the setting of reduced left ventricular systolic function, atrial arrhythmias are commonly the inciting factor for congestive heart failure development.

ELECTROCARDIOGRAM FIGURE 59.45

Clinical History

A 66-year-old man with a long-standing history of atrial dysrhythmias who is status post aortic valve replacement for endocarditis. He returns for an outpatient cardiology follow-up evaluation. Complete heart block ensued, necessitating permanent pacemaker placement.

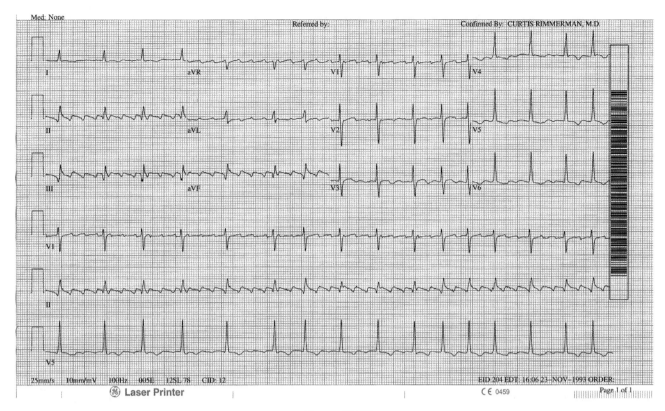

Figure 59.44

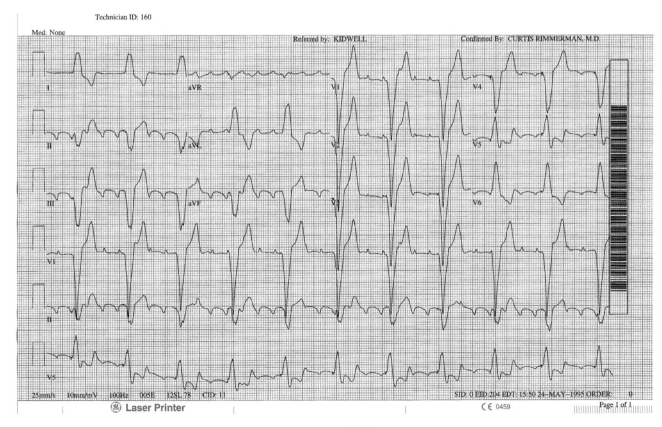

Figure 59.45

Interpretation and Comments

Regular atrial activity with a negative vector is seen in the inferior leads. Atrial activity is also readily seen in leads V_{1-2}. This either represents slow atrial flutter or an ectopic atrial tachycardia. Widened regular QRS complexes occur at regular intervals not related to atrial activity. These have a complete left bundle-branch block configuration. Careful inspection at the beginning of each QRS complex demonstrates a small, sharp deflection, indicating an electronic ventricular pacemaker. This is best seen in lead V_4. This ECG therefore demonstrates atrial flutter, complete heart block, and a ventricular pacemaker.

When a complete left bundle-branch block QRS complex morphology is present, it is important to look for ventricular pacemaker deflections. Frequently, pacemaker deflections are diminutive and potentially overlooked, as demonstrated on this tracing.

ELECTROCARDIOGRAM FIGURE 59.46

Clinical History

A 77-year-old woman who is seen in cardiology follow-up as an outpatient. She has a known history of hypertrophic obstructive cardiomyopathy, as diagnosed by both heart catheterization and transthoracic echocardiogram. At the time of her heart catheterization approximately 15 years prior to this ECG, the patient had a measurable left ventricular outflow tract gradient of 50 mm Hg.

Interpretation and Comments

Sinus bradycardia is present, as the atrial rate is slightly <60 per minute with a normal P-wave axis. Prominent QRS complex voltage is seen with T-wave inversion. These findings together suggest voltage criteria for left ventricular hypertrophy with secondary ST-T changes. The symmetric T-wave inversion is atypical for a strain pattern, as seen in left ventricular hypertrophy. A concomitant process such as ischemic heart disease, electrolyte disturbance, or an atypical form of hypertrophic cardiomyopathy merits consideration. A biphasic terminally negative P wave is seen in lead V_1, denoting left atrial abnormality. Also note, as indicated on the far left-hand portion of the ECG, that this tracing is performed at half standardization. The voltage is twice that recorded. The tracing is performed at half standardization to permit the QRS complexes to appear within the interpretive portion of the ECG.

The symmetric T-wave inversion in the setting of prominent QRS complex voltage is suggestive of Yamaguchi disease. This is an atypical form of hypertrophic obstructive cardiomyopathy that primarily involves the cardiac apex.

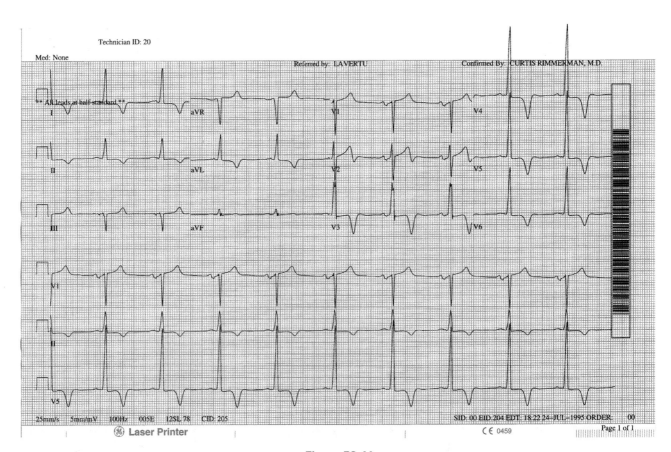

Figure 59.46

ELECTROCARDIOGRAM FIGURE 59.47

Clinical History

A 67-year-old man admitted acutely to the hospital for evaluation and treatment of new-onset atrial fibrillation. His past medical history includes emphysema, long-standing tobacco and alcohol use, and an abdominal aortic aneurysm repair. Medications at the time of this ECG included inhalers and lisinopril.

Interpretation and Comments

No identifiable atrial activity is seen with a ventricular rate >100 per minute. QRS complexes occur in an irregularly irregular pattern both consistent with atrial fibrillation and a rapid ventricular response. Left anterior hemiblock is seen, as the QRS complex vector is positive in lead I and negative in leads II, III, and aVF. Diffuse nonspecific ST-T changes are also present. On the right-hand portion of the ECG, best seen in the lead V_1 rhythm strip, a QRS complex is conducted with complete right bundle-branch block aberrancy. This follows a long–short R:R interval and is an example of Ashman phenomenon.

The presence of Ashman phenomenon is common in the setting of atrial fibrillation with a rapid ventricular response. The refractory period of the right bundle branch is directly proportional to the preceding R:R cycle length.

When the preceding R:R cycle is relatively prolonged and followed by a short R:R cycle, right bundle-branch block aberration and the Ashman phenomenon commonly are present. This reflects normal physiology and is not pathological.

ELECTROCARDIOGRAM FIGURE 59.48

Clinical History

A 69-year-old woman with coronary artery disease status post percutaneous transluminal coronary angioplasty of her right coronary artery 3 years prior to this ECG who presents in follow-up to the outpatient cardiology clinic. Comorbidities include diffuse peripheral vascular disease, hypertension, and hypercholesterolemia. Medications at the time of this ECG included aspirin, lisinopril, thyroxine, diltiazem, and atenolol.

Interpretation and Comments

The right-hand portion of this ECG demonstrates normal sinus rhythm, as each QRS complex is preceded by a P wave of normal axis with a constant PR interval. Immediately preceding the last three QRS complexes is an irregularly irregular ventricular response in the setting of no identifiable atrial activity. This represents an episode of paroxysmal atrial fibrillation with a rapid ventricular response.

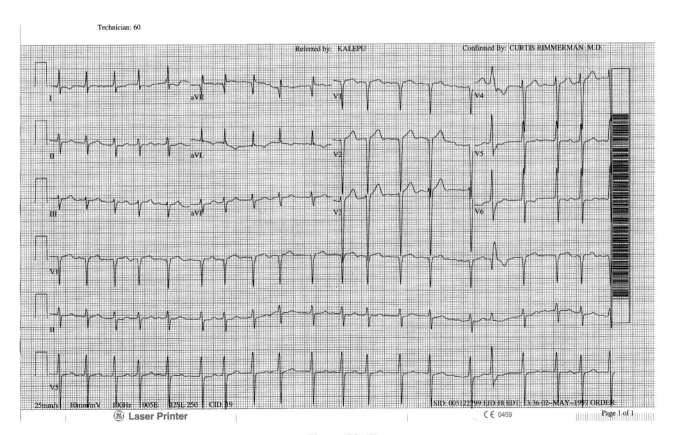

Figure 59.47

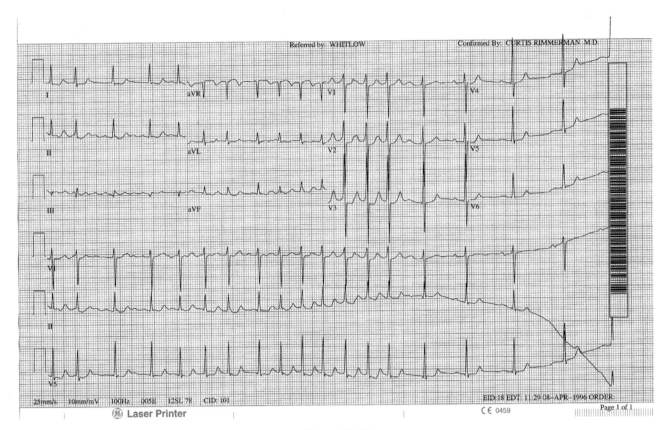

Figure 59.48

Nonspecific ST-T changes and a wandering baseline artifact are also seen.

This is a timely ECG that happens to demonstrate a self-terminating paroxysm of atrial fibrillation with resumption of normal sinus rhythm. This is an unusual and fortuitous finding on the surface ECG. Oftentimes, patients will note palpitations for which Holter monitor recordings are required to document paroxysmal dysrhythmias as depicted on this ECG. The atrial fibrillation conducts with a rapid ventricular rate. This ECG demonstrates a clinical finding that may result in medication adjustments such as the addition of digoxin and warfarin.

ELECTROCARDIOGRAM FIGURE 59.49

Clinical History

A 77-year-old woman with a history of paroxysmal atrial fibrillation who returns for routine cardiac assessment and pacemaker interrogation. Her medications included amiodarone, digoxin, and furosemide.

Interpretation and Comments

Atrial and ventricular pacing deflections occur at regular intervals throughout the ECG. This represents an atrioven-

tricular pacemaker. There are apparent pauses on the ECG. These pauses are preceded by a ventricular pacemaker deflection without a subsequent QRS complex, representing pacemaker capture failure.

This represents ventricular pacemaker capture failure. This is an abnormal finding that requires further clinical evaluation and interrogation of both the pacemaker generator, pacemaker lead placement, and pacemaker lead stability.

ELECTROCARDIOGRAM FIGURE 59.50

Clinical History

A 46-year-old woman with severe hypertension status post cadaveric renal transplantation one year prior to this ECG referred to the cardiology clinic for evaluation of recent onset palpitations and a suspected slow heart rate. A cardiac catheterization several months prior to this ECG demonstrated near normal coronary arteries with advanced left ventricular hypertrophy. The patient was on numerous medications at the time of this ECG including diltiazem, clonidine, doxazosin, and immunosuppressive agents for her renal transplant. Her serum potassium was normal.

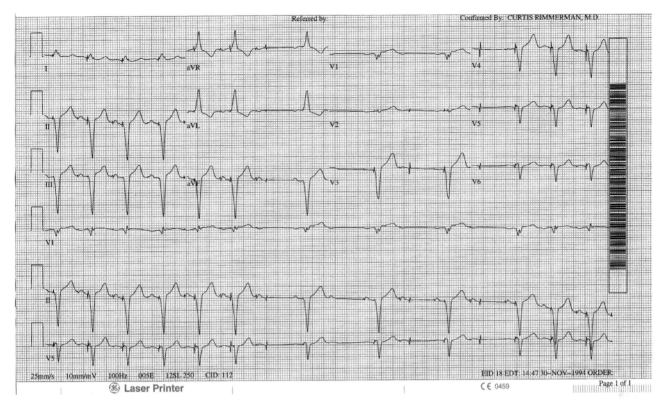

Figure 59.49

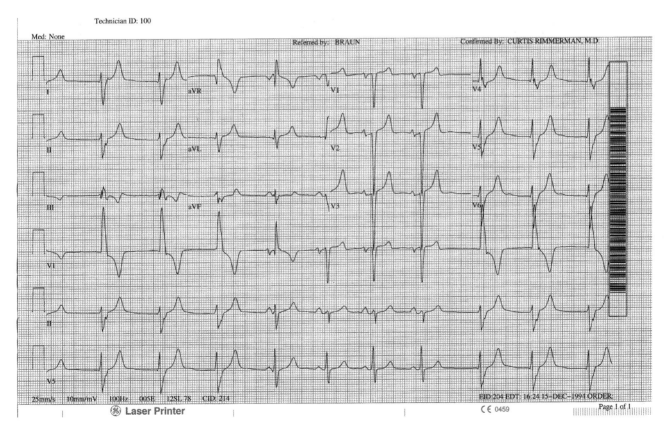

Figure 59.50

Interpretation and Comments

The fifth through seventh QRS complexes are preceded by upright P waves with a constant PR interval. They occur at a regular rate of approximately 75 per minute, representing normal sinus rhythm. The P-wave vector is terminally negative in lead V_1, suggesting left atrial abnormality. Following the seventh QRS complex, a sinus pause ensues and a wide QRS complex rhythm follows. This same rhythm is also seen at the onset of the ECG. This represents a ventricular escape rhythm. The fourth QRS complex is intermediate between the ventricular escape rhythm and the native QRS complex and represents a fusion complex. The ventricular escape rhythm conducts with a far-leftward QRS complex frontal plane axis and a complete right bundle-branch block morphology, reflecting a left posterior fascicular origin. R-wave progression is slow, suggesting the possibility of a septal myocardial infarction of indeterminate age. This would need clinical correlation and adjunctive testing, as a small R wave is still present and identifiable in both leads V_2 and V_3.

Given the presence of the ventricular escape rhythm, the electrocardiographic diagnosis of left ventricular hypertrophy is not possible. Despite this, left ventricular hypertrophy is suspected, as the S waves are deep in leads V_{2-3} and left atrial abnormality is present as well. A repeat ECG in the absence of the ventricular escape rhythm would be helpful to better delineate the QRS complex morphology and QRS complex voltage in leads V_{4-6}.

ELECTROCARDIOGRAM FIGURE 59.51

Clinical History

A 76-year-old man with a remote extensive anterolateral myocardial infarction and subsequent left ventricular aneurysm formation who returns for outpatient evaluation of his implantable cardiac defibrillator. He presently is asymptomatic. The patient has a past history of drug-refractory ventricular tachycardia and an abdominal aortic aneurysm repair. His medications at the time of this ECG included aspirin, digoxin, and nadolol.

Interpretation and Comments

The cardiac rhythm is normal sinus rhythm with an atrial rate of approximately 60 per minute in the setting of a normal P-wave axis. Left anterior hemiblock is present, as the QRS complex vector is positive in lead I and negative in leads II, III, and aVF. Q-wave formation is present in leads V_{2-4}, and ST segment elevation is seen in leads V_{2-6}. This suggests an anterolateral myocardial infarction–acute and acute myocardial injury.

Persistent ST segment elevation in the setting of an age-indeterminant myocardial infarction is consistent with a left ventricular aneurysm. When suspected electrocardiographically, clinical correlation is necessary.

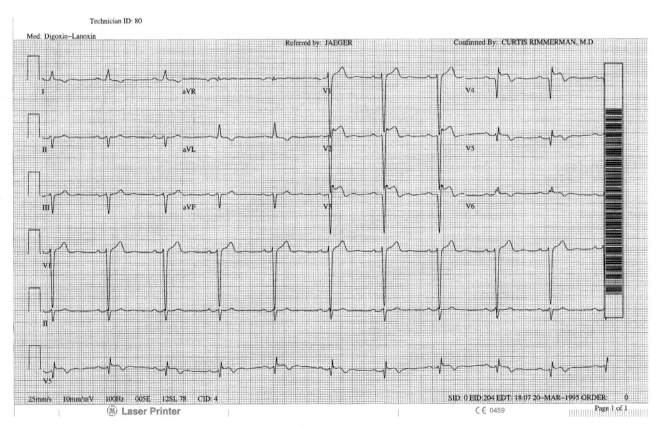

Figure 59.51

ELECTROCARDIOGRAM FIGURE 59.52

Clinical History

A 54-year-old woman who is immediately postoperative bioprosthetic aortic valve replacement secondary to aortic stenosis. Comorbid conditions include hypertension, non–insulin-requiring diabetes mellitus, and dialysis requiring renal insufficiency.

Interpretation and Comments

Successive pacemaker deflections are seen separated by a RP interval of 250 msec. This represents an atrioventricular pacemaker. The ventricular paced QRS complexes alternate in morphology. This is the ECG finding of electrical alternans, as seen in patients with a large pericardial effusion.

This patient was status post recent cardiac surgery and was suffering from a large postoperative pericardial effusion at the time of this ECG. If a pericardial effusion is not suspected clinically, the ECG may be the first clinical clue to its presence and therefore serves an important clinical role.

ELECTROCARDIOGRAM FIGURE 59.53

Clinical History

A 73-year-old man with severe ischemic left ventricular systolic dysfunction who is recently status post a second coro-

nary artery bypass graft operation. Comorbid conditions include hypertension, non–insulin-requiring diabetes mellitus, and chronic atrial fibrillation.

Interpretation and Comments

This patient demonstrates atrial fibrillation, as no discrete atrial activity is seen. The QRS complexes occur at a regular rate of approximately 85 per minute and are normal in duration. This represents an accelerated junctional rhythm and in the setting of atrial fibrillation denotes atrioventricular dissociation. Diffuse nonspecific ST-T changes are also seen.

This patient is recently status post open heart surgery. This is a common clinical setting for accelerated junctional rhythms. This ECG does not imply complete heart block, as the atrioventricular junction represents the dominant pacemaker. Another possibility is digitalis toxicity. This warrants further clinical investigation.

ELECTROCARDIOGRAM FIGURE 59.54

Clinical History

A 34-year-old woman with a history of an atrioventricular canal and ostium primum atrial septal defect status post surgical repair who is readmitted for a cardiac evaluation. She is experiencing paroxysmal atrial dysrhythmias and is not taking any medications.

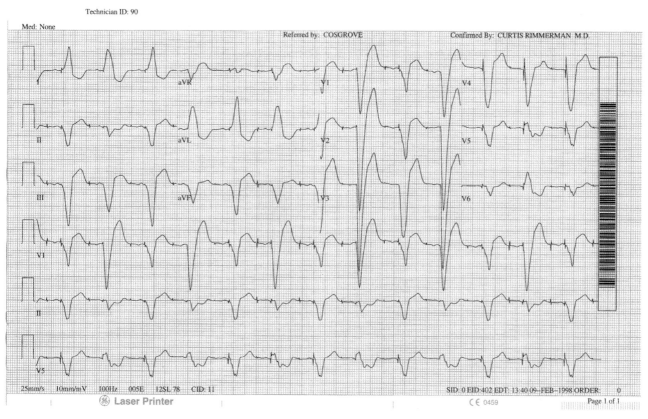

Figure 59.52

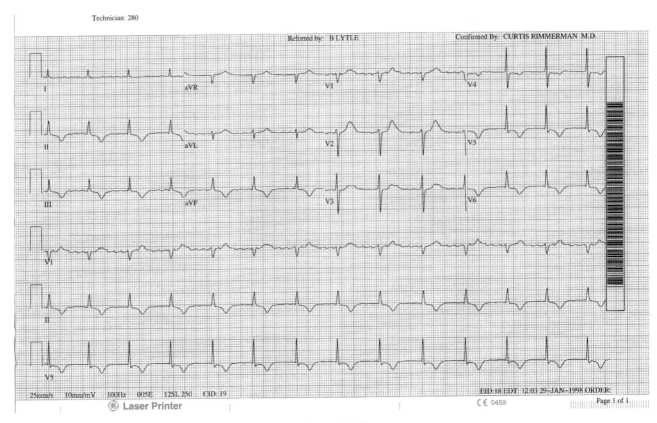

Figure 59.53

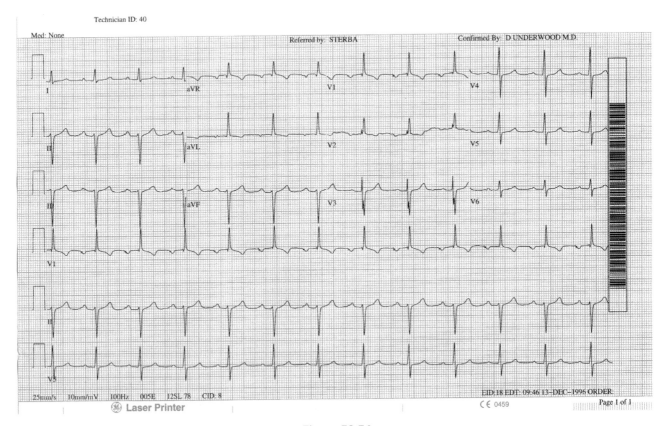

Figure 59.54

Interpretation and Comments

This patient is known to have an ostium primum atrial septal defect. The ECG demonstrates a group of findings consistent with this diagnosis. The atrial rhythm is normal sinus rhythm. The PR interval is prolonged at 240 msec, representing first-degree atrioventricular block. The P wave is terminally negative in lead V_1 and broadened in lead II, suggesting left atrial abnormality. The QRS complex axis is deviated leftward, satisfying the criteria for left axis deviation, as the QRS complex frontal plane vector is positive in lead I and deeply negative in leads II, III, and aVF. An rsR′ QRS complex is seen in lead V_1 with a normal QRS complex duration supporting incomplete right bundle-branch block.

A narrow rsR′ QRS complex morphology in the presence of left axis deviation and left atrial abnormality are a group of findings consistent with the diagnosis of an ostium primum atrial septal defect.

ELECTROCARDIOGRAM FIGURE 59.55

Clinical History

A 38-year-old man who presents with severe dyspnea of 1 week duration. An echocardiogram demonstrated a large pericardial effusion, with evidence supporting cardiac tamponade. The patient underwent urgent surgical pericardial drainage.

Interpretation and Comments

The cardiac rhythm is sinus tachycardia, as the P waves are of normal axis and precede each QRS complex at an atrial rate slightly >100 per minute. The frontal plane QRS complex axis demonstrates right axis deviation, as the QRS complex vector is negative in lead I and positive in leads II, III, and aVF. There are diffuse low-voltage QRS complexes. Nonspecific ST-T changes are seen as well. Alternation of the QRS complex voltage, best seen in rhythm strip lead V_1, is apparent. This alternation occurs with every other QRS complex and is termed *electrical alternans*. Electrical alternans is an ECG marker of a large pericardial effusion.

The ECG findings of diffuse low-voltage QRS complexes and electrical alternans suggest the presence of a significant pericardial effusion and cardiac tamponade. The electrical alternans is secondary to the beat-to-beat variability of cardiac position. This is sometimes referred to as a "swinging heart."

ELECTROCARDIOGRAM FIGURE 59.56

Clinical History

A 22-year-old woman with primary pulmonary hypertension admitted for treatment of worsening right-sided congestive heart failure.

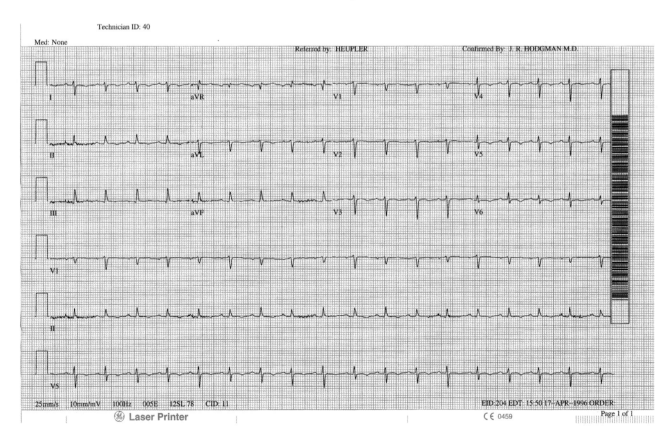

Figure 59.55

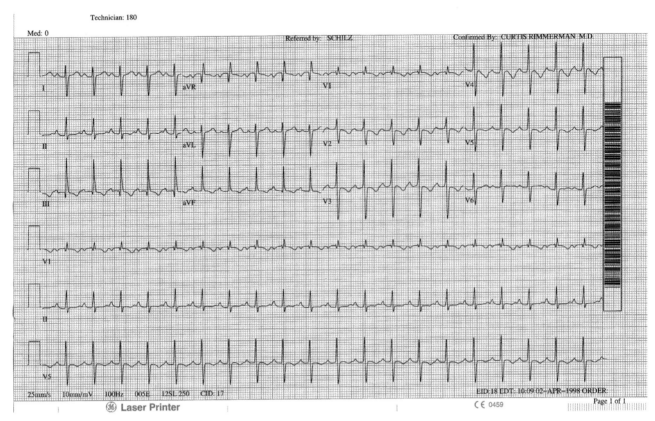

Figure 59.56

Interpretation and Comments

This ECG demonstrates sinus tachycardia, as the P-wave axis is normal in leads I, II, and III and the atrial rate is approximately 125 per minute. Frontal plane QRS complex right axis deviation is present, as the QRS complex vector is negative in lead I and positive in leads II, III, and aVF. An rsr' QRS complex is present in lead V_1, and prominent R waves are seen in leads V_{2-3} with associated ST-T changes. This finding, together with frontal plane QRS complex right axis deviation, supports right ventricular hypertrophy with secondary ST-T changes.

The criteria for right ventricular hypertrophy include frontal plane right axis QRS complex deviation and prominent R waves in leads V_{1-2}. The associated asymmetric ST segment depression in leads V_{1-3} represents a right ventricular strain pattern secondary to the right ventricular hypertrophy.

ELECTROCARDIOGRAM FIGURE 59.57

Clinical History

A 73-year-old man with coronary artery disease who is status post four-vessel coronary artery bypass graft surgery 2 years prior to this ECG. He now returns for an outpa-

tient cardiology follow-up evaluation. He has a history of a prior inferior myocardial infarction. Comorbidities include non–insulin-requiring diabetes mellitus. His medications include aspirin and vitamin E.

Interpretation and Comments

P waves occur at regular intervals, with a normal P-wave axis at an atrial rate of approximately 90 per minute representing normal sinus rhythm. A bifid P wave is seen in lead II with marked terminal P-wave negativity in lead V_1, supporting left atrial abnormality. QRS complexes occur at regular intervals at a rate slightly >60 per minute. In lead V_1, the P waves are not associated with the QRS complexes and do not demonstrate constant PR intervals. This supports the presence of complete heart block and an accelerated junctional rhythm given the normal duration QRS complex.

This patient did not have a permanent pacemaker implanted, as the accelerated junctional rhythm occurred at a sufficient heart rate to maintain hemodynamic stability without symptoms of fatigue or cerebral hypoperfusion. While suggested by the medical history, no evidence of an inferior myocardial infarction is seen on this ECG.

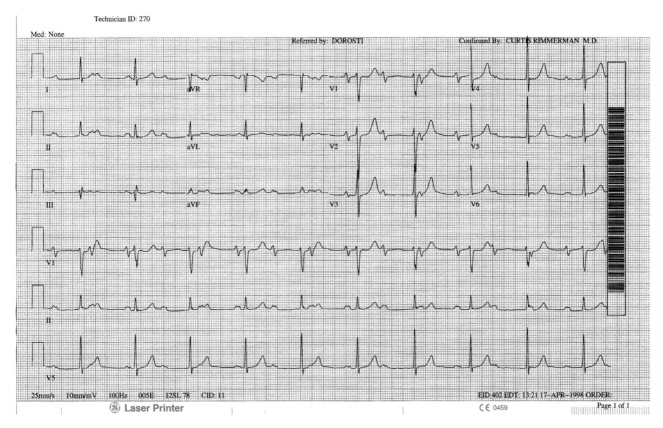

Figure 59.57

ELECTROCARDIOGRAM FIGURE 59.58

Clinical History

A 76-year-old woman with a history of endometrial carcinoma status post resection who is readmitted to the hospital with shortness of breath in the setting of lymphangitic pulmonary metastasis. She has had recurrent pleural effusions. Her past history includes paroxysmal atrial fibrillation. Her medications include aspirin, prednisone, atenolol, and hydrochlorothiazide.

Interpretation and Comments

P waves of differing morphology precede each QRS complex with a varying PR interval duration. There are greater than three P-wave morphologies on this 12-lead ECG with the ventricular rate >100 per minute, satisfying the criteria for multifocal atrial tachycardia. Both the first and last QRS complexes are conducted with incomplete right bundle-branch block aberrancy. Diffuse nonspecific ST-T changes are present.

Multifocal atrial tachycardia is a common dysrhythmia in patients with pulmonary disease. It represents a chaotic atrial rhythm, as multiple atrial foci exist, frequently originating in both atria and discharging without predictability. The best form of treatment for this atrial dysrhythmia is to treat the underlying pulmonary pathology. In this patient population, it oftentimes is difficult to achieve ventricular rate control.

ELECTROCARDIOGRAM FIGURE 59.59

Clinical History

A 71-year-old woman with long-standing hypertension and hypertensive heart disease documented on a recent echocardiogram. The patient was admitted to the hospital at the time of this ECG for antiarrhythmic therapy initiation in the setting of recurrent and drug refractory atrial arrhythmias.

Interpretation and Comments

Normal sinus rhythm is present, as the first P wave is of normal axis and precedes the QRS complex. A bifid P wave is noted in lead II, which reflects left atrial abnormality. The atrial rhythm varies on this ECG. Subsequent to the initial P wave, a series of P waves occur, which represents a paroxysm of ectopic atrial tachycardia. The eighth P wave, which precedes the fifth QRS complex, represents a normal sinus complex. This is followed by a normal sinus complex; subsequently, toward the middle of the tracing, another paroxysm of ectopic atrial tachycardia with second-degree Mobitz type I Wenckebach atrioventricular block ensues.

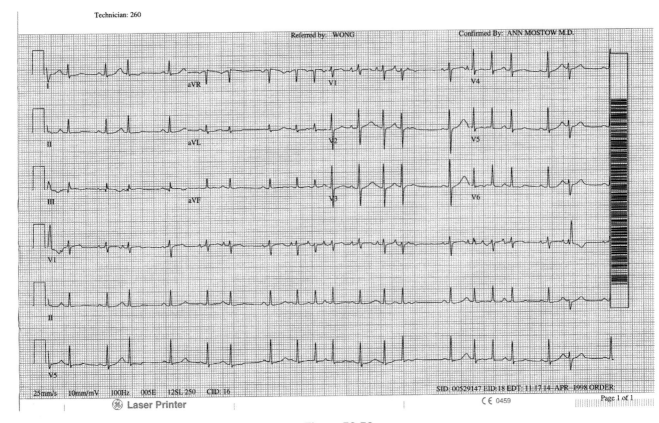

Figure 59.58

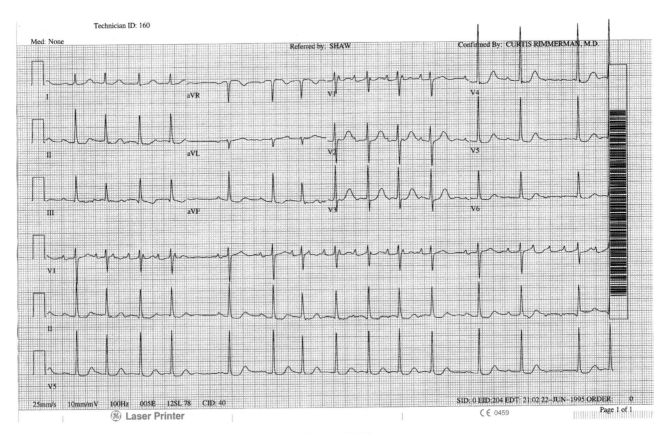

Figure 59.59

Toward the right-hand portion of the ECG, the paroxysmal ectopic atrial tachycardia recurs with variable atrioventricular conduction. Nonspecific ST-T changes are also seen.

In the presence of ectopic atrial tachycardia with variable atrioventricular block, consideration should be given to digitalis intoxication. Other potential etiologies include hypertensive heart disease and mitral valve disease.

ELECTROCARDIOGRAM FIGURE 59.60

Clinical History

A 76-year-old woman with dialysis requiring renal failure who is recently postoperative exploratory laparotomy for an ischemic bowel. The patient became septic, hypotensive, and hyperkalemic. This ECG represents her terminal heart rhythm prior to expiring.

Interpretation and Comments

Sinus tachycardia is present. The PR interval is prolonged, representing first-degree atrioventricular block. The QRS complex is markedly prolonged, evidenced by a nonspecific intraventricular conduction delay. This patient suffers from extreme hyperkalemia, likely in the 7.5 to 8.0 meq/L range. This represents a preterminal ECG in this patient with acute renal failure and sepsis refractory to treatment.

In extreme forms of hyperkalemia, ventricular arrhythmias are common, as is profound widening and prolongation of all ECG intervals. The ST segment elevation in lead V_{2-3} has been termed a dialyzable current of injury.

ELECTROCARDIOGRAM FIGURE 59.61

Clinical History

A 65-year-old woman status post recent mitral valve and tricuspid valve repair in the setting of severe coronary artery obstructive disease and prior coronary artery bypass graft surgery.

Interpretation and Comments

The fourth, fifth, and sixth QRS complexes occur at regular intervals without identifiable preceding atrial activity. This represents a junctional escape rhythm, as the QRS complex is of normal duration. There are associated nonspecific ST-T changes. Preceding the third QRS complex is a P wave with a normal axis. This represents a sinus capture complex. This is followed by a period of sinus arrest and a junctional escape complex that initiates the junctional escape rhythm.

This patient is status post recent cardiac surgery. The epicardial pacemaker was turned off for this ECG and restarted toward the end of the recording. In the setting of valvular

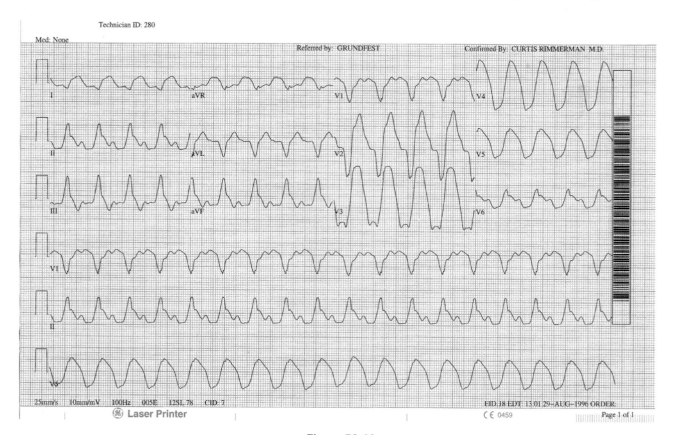

Figure 59.60

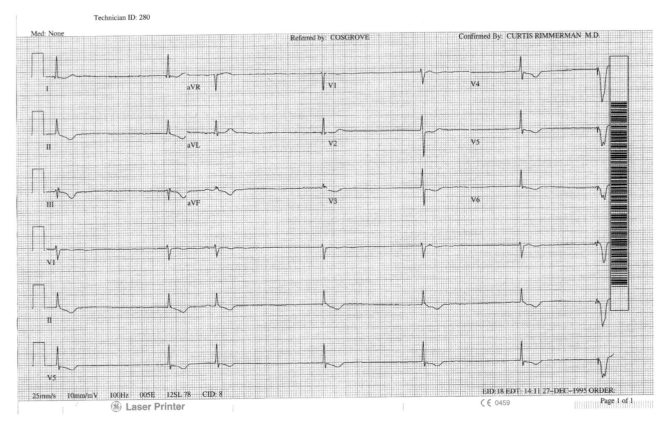

Technician ID: 280

Med: None
Referred by: COSGROVE   Confirmed By: CURTIS RIMMERMAN M.D.

Figure 59.61

heart surgery, depression of the native conduction system is a common finding in the immediate postoperative period.

ELECTROCARDIOGRAM FIGURE 59.62

Clinical History

A 76-year-old man with recent syncope admitted for evaluation. He has a history of a remote inferior myocardial infarction.

Interpretation and Comments

The atrial rhythm is best discerned in the lead V_1 rhythm strip. P waves occur at regular intervals, with a normal P-wave axis denoting normal sinus rhythm. The second QRS complex is preceded by a P wave. The fourth QRS complex is also preceded by a P wave, with both PR intervals of equal duration. This suggests the presence of intact atrioventricular conduction. The P wave following the second QRS complex fails to conduct to the ventricle and instead is followed by a ventricular paced complex. This is an example of second-degree Mobitz type II atrioventricular block. The P wave demonstrates a terminally negative vector in lead V_1 consistent with left atrial abnormality. The P wave is also bifid in lead II. The QRS complex morpho-

logy demonstrates a rSR' pattern in lead V_1 consistent with complete right bundle-branch block. In the nonventricular paced QRS complexes in leads II, III, and aVF, prominent Q waves are seen, indicating an inferior myocardial infarction–age indeterminant.

This patient demonstrates advanced atrioventricular block given the second-degree Mobitz type II atrioventricular block and complete right bundle-branch block. A ventricular pacemaker appropriately was implanted.

ELECTROCARDIOGRAM FIGURE 59.63

Clinical History

A 51-year-old woman with metastatic breast carcinoma who is undergoing a bone marrow transplantation. Her serum potassium level at the time of this ECG was 2.9 mmol/L.

Interpretation and Comments

The extreme left-hand portion of this ECG demonstrates upright P waves in leads I, II, and III, suggesting normal sinus rhythm. A prolonged QT interval is present with nonspecific ST-T changes. The first QRS complex is reflective of normal sinus rhythm and a native QRS complex. This is followed by a premature ventricular complex, and a

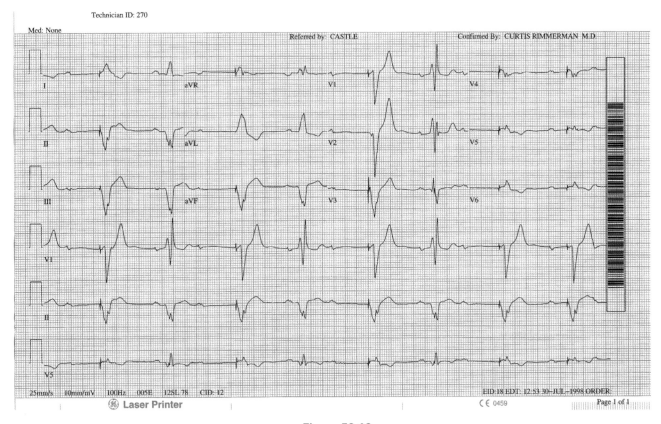

Figure 59.62

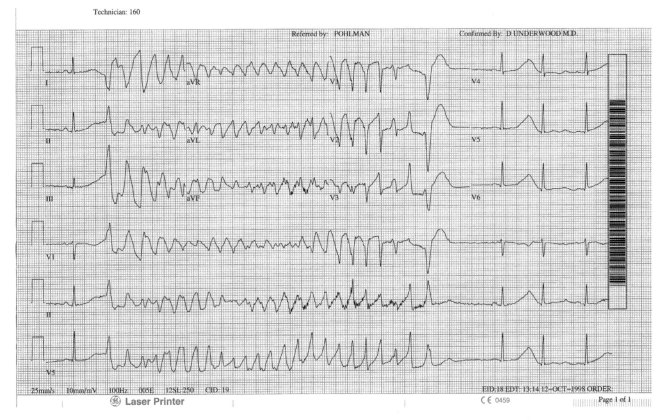

Figure 59.63

disorganized wide QRS complex tachycardia ensues. The wide QRS complex tachycardia has a changing or rotating axis consistent with torsades de pointes. A fine baseline artifact is present.

Torsades de pointes is a potentially fatal ventricular arrhythmia, in this instance triggered by extreme hypokalemia. It also can be seen in the presence of antiarrhythmic therapy initiation. It is characterized as a wide QRS complex ventricular tachycardia with a varying QRS complex axis, as depicted on this ECG. Prompt correction of any underlying metabolic disturbance and withdrawal of potentially contributing medications is essential.

ELECTROCARDIOGRAM FIGURE 59.64

Clinical History

A 68-year-old man with biopsy-proven amyloidosis who is being seen in the congestive heart failure clinic. On echocardiography, the patient has severe left ventricular systolic

dysfunction. He currently suffers from intractable congestive heart failure.

Interpretation and Comments

P waves occur at regular intervals and appear of normal axis with a positive P-wave vector in leads II, III, and aVF at a rate slightly >100 per minute, which is consistent with sinus tachycardia. In lead V_1, the P wave demonstrates terminal negativity consistent with left atrial abnormality. The limb lead QRS complex voltage is diminutive, consistent with low-voltage QRS complexes. Q waves are present in leads V_{1-2}, with a diminutive R wave in lead V_3. This is suggestive but not diagnostic of a septal myocardial infarction of indeterminate age. Lateral nonspecific ST-T changes are also seen in leads V_{5-6}.

This ECG demonstrates common findings seen in advanced cardiac amyloidosis. These findings include low-voltage QRS complexes and a pseudoinfarction pattern present in leads V_{1-3}. An echocardiogram did not support the regional finding of a septal myocardial infarction.

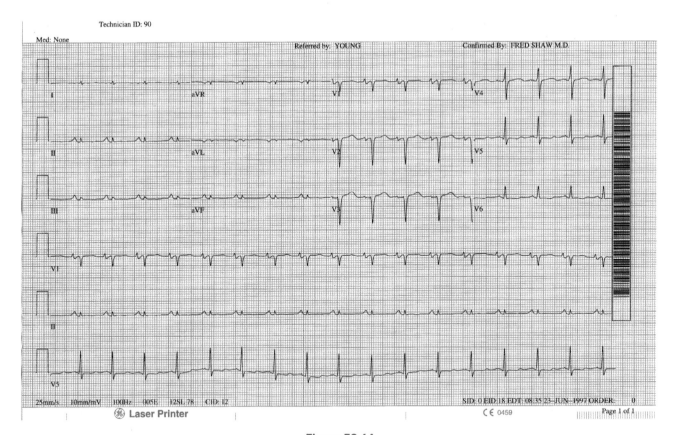

Figure 59.64

Chapter 60

Valvular Heart Disease

Carmel Halley   Brian P. Griffin

POINTS TO REMEMBER:

- Valvular heart disease may cause problems when the valve becomes stenotic; when it is regurgitant; or, as frequently occurs, a combined stenotic and regurgitant lesion is present.

- Stenotic lesions produce problems by reducing cardiac output, particularly during stress, and by increasing the pressure in the chambers proximal to the valve.

- Conversely, regurgitant lesions cause problems by increasing the volume load on the ventricles.

- Echocardiography is the most important test currently used for the diagnosis of valvular heart disease.

- Planimetry using two-dimensional echocardiography can directly measure the area of the valve opening in mitral stenosis.

- The qualitative and quantitative assessment of regurgitant lesion severity is done by using the flow disturbance associated with the regurgitation on color flow mapping.

- The general principles for treating patients with valvular heart disease are as follows:
  1. Assess the severity of symptoms.
  2. Determine the nature of the valvular lesion and its severity.
  3. Assess the effects of the lesion on ventricular function.
  4. Assess for other cardiac (or other) pathologies.

- There have been recent major changes to the American Heart Association (AHA) guidelines for endocarditis prophylaxis.

- The new AHA guidelines recommend that prophylaxis should be used only in patients with underlying cardiac conditions associated with the highest adverse outcome from infective endocarditis. These conditions include prosthetic heart valves, previous infective endocarditis, certain classes of congenital heart disease, and in valvulopathy occurring post cardiac transplantation.

Valvular heart disease remains an important cause of cardiac morbidity, despite a decline in the incidence of rheumatic valvular disease in the developed world. Congenital valvular anomalies (e.g., bicuspid aortic valve, which is seen in approximately 2% of the population) and myxomatous degeneration of valvular tissue (e.g., mitral valve prolapse) are the most common conditions encountered today.

Valvular heart disease may cause problems when the valve becomes stenotic; when it is regurgitant; or, as frequently occurs, a combined stenotic and regurgitant lesion is present. Multiple valves often are affected either by the primary disease process (e.g., rheumatic fever) or secondarily affected by the pressure or volume effects of another valve lesion. For instance, tricuspid regurgitation commonly is associated with mitral disease because mitral disease increases pulmonary pressures, thus causing the right ventricle to dilate. Right ventricular dilatation causes the tricuspid valve ring or annulus to dilate and, thus, causes the valve to leak.

Stenotic lesions produce problems by reducing cardiac output, particularly during stress, and by increasing the pressure in the chambers proximal to the valve. The heart chambers respond to increased pressure first by hypertrophying and then by dilating. Conversely, regurgitant lesions cause problems by increasing the volume load on the ventricles. For instance, in mitral and aortic regurgitation, the left ventricle dilates to maintain a normal cardiac output. Eventually, with more severe degrees of regurgitation, ventricular dilatation fails to compensate for the regurgitation, and cardiac output falls.

CLINICAL PRESENTATION

Many patients with valvular heart disease are asymptomatic for years. The onset of symptoms often is insidious, and

779

patients often unwittingly decrease their activities to reduce their symptoms. An acute onset of symptoms may signal valvular disruption (e.g., acute myocardial infarction with papillary muscle rupture or after endocarditis), an acute volume load (e.g., as in pregnancy), or the onset of a tachyarrhythmia (e.g., atrial fibrillation). Symptoms include dyspnea, chest discomfort, syncope, palpitations, embolization, and fatigue.

- Dyspnea is the most common symptom in valvular heart disease. It usually results from high pulmonary venous pressures, which increase the transudation of fluid into the alveoli and result in diminished gas exchange. It is seen relatively early in mitral stenosis and later in the course of aortic and mitral regurgitation as well as the course of aortic stenosis. It is important to determine the limitations caused by the dyspnea, because therapeutic interventions usually are based on the severity of symptoms rather than on the severity of the disease process itself.
- Chest discomfort may be anginal because of oxygen supply and demand mismatch (e.g., aortic or mitral stenosis) or nonanginal (e.g., mitral valve prolapse).
- Syncope usually results from an inability to increase cardiac output during peripheral vasodilatation (e.g., with exercise). It is seen in conditions that severely limit cardiac output (e.g., aortic stenosis, mitral stenosis with pulmonary hypertension).
- Palpitations result from an arrhythmia (e.g., atrial fibrillation in mitral disease).
- Embolic events may occur when material on abnormal valves (e.g., calcium) embolizes. An important cause of embolization is endocarditis, and another important cause of embolization is thrombus formation in the left atrium accompanying mitral valve disease.
- Fatigue is common in all forms of valvular heart disease, particularly those associated with low cardiac output (e.g., mitral or aortic stenosis).

DIAGNOSIS

Physical Examination

The physical examination is critical to the evaluation of patients with valvular heart disease. It is important to examine thoroughly all aspects of the cardiovascular system. These aspects include the following:

- *Pulse:* The pulse is best palpated at the carotid artery. The rhythm, rate, and character (e.g., slow upstroke in aortic stenosis, collapsing in aortic regurgitation) should be assessed.
- *Venous pressure:* Venous pressure height and wave pattern should be assessed. Valvular disease is characterized by large A waves in pulmonary hypertension and

pulmonary stenosis and large V waves in tricuspid regurgitation.
- *Blood pressure:* A narrow pulse pressure (i.e., difference between systolic and diastolic blood pressure) is present in aortic stenosis; wide pulse pressure with low diastolic pressure is present in aortic regurgitation.
- *Facies:* Cyanotic facies often is marked peripherally in low output disorders; mitral facies (i.e., purplish red cheeks) is noted in mitral stenosis.

Heart Examination

Palpation

The patient should be palpated for cardiomegaly and the position of the apex beat as well as for the following:

- *Thrills:* Thrills occur with significant valvular lesions and result from turbulent blood flow at the site of the valve lesion. They can be systolic or diastolic in timing, and they are most common with aortic stenosis, ventricular septal defect, and pulmonic stenosis. Diastolic thrills are less common, but they occur with mitral stenosis and aortic regurgitation.
- *Character of apex beat:* Tapping is less sustained than normal in mitral stenosis and is more sustained than normal or heaving in left ventricular hypertrophy.
- *Right ventricular heave:* Right ventricular heave is felt along the left sternal border in right ventricular hypertrophy.
- *Other sounds:* The second heart sound often is palpable in pulmonary hypertension, and S_3 and S_4 may be palpable as well.

Auscultation

The patient should be auscultated for the following:

- *First heart sound:* The first heart sound is loud in mitral and tricuspid stenosis and soft in mitral regurgitation. Later, with calcification of a stenosed mitral valve, the first heart sound again becomes softer.
- *Second heart sound:* The second heart sound has a loud pulmonary component in pulmonary hypertension and a soft aortic component in severe aortic stenosis.
- *Third heart sound:* The third heart sound is a low-pitched, filling sound best heard with the bell of a stethoscope. It is common during severe mitral regurgitation and left ventricular dilatation and may be physiological in young people.
- *Fourth heart sound:* The fourth heart sound is the atrial filling sound. It is heard during conditions with left ventricular hypertrophy (e.g., aortic stenosis).
- *Opening snap:* The opening snap is heard at the lower left sternal border during mitral stenosis. The opening snap follows S_2. The shorter the time interval between S_2 and the opening snap, the more severe the mitral stenosis.

- *Ejection sounds:* Early systolic sounds at the base of the heart are heard in congenitally abnormal but mobile valves (e.g., bicuspid aortic valve).
- *Mid-systolic clicks:* Systolic sounds are heard with myxomatous mitral valve prolapse because of tensing of the redundant leaflets.

Murmurs should be assessed in terms of timing, location, intensity, and provocative maneuvers. Timing involves

- Systolic
- Ejection (peaking in mid-systole), as in aortic stenosis, pulmonic stenosis, hypertrophic cardiomyopathy
- Pansystolic (heard throughout systole, may encompass S_1 and S_2), as in mitral regurgitation, tricuspid regurgitation
- Late systolic, as in mitral valve prolapse, ischemic mitral regurgitation because of papillary muscle dysfunction
- Diastolic
- Early, decrescendo, as in aortic regurgitation, pulmonary regurgitation
- Mid-diastolic, as in mitral stenosis, tricuspid stenosis
- Presystolic (late diastole), as in mitral stenosis in normal sinus rhythm

Location involves

- Apical, as in mitral murmurs; aortic murmur may radiate to the apex
- Base, as in aortic, pulmonary murmurs
- Sternal border, as in tricuspid murmurs, aortic and pulmonary regurgitation
- Radiation, to axilla with mitral, to neck and apex with aortic

Regarding intensity, the severity of the lesion often relates to the loudness of the murmur in systolic murmurs (e.g., aortic stenosis, mitral regurgitation). The severity of diastolic murmurs relates more to the duration of the murmur than to intensity.

Provocative maneuvers include the following:

- *Respiration:* Right-sided lesions are louder with inspiration (i.e., increased flow through the right heart). Left-sided lesions are louder with expiration.
- *Valsalva:* The Valsalva maneuver decreases intracardiac volume and reduces the intensity of most murmurs. Exceptions are the murmurs of hypertrophic cardiomyopathy, which become louder, and of mitral valve prolapse, which become longer and louder. A reduction in intracardiac volume accentuates outflow obstruction in hypertrophic cardiomyopathy and prolapse in mitral valve prolapse syndrome.
- *Position:* With standing, intracardiac volume decreases; therefore, most murmurs decrease in intensity (except those of hypertrophic cardiomyopathy and mitral valve prolapse). Squatting accentuates intracardiac volume. Therefore, most murmurs become louder, but those of

mitral valve prolapse and hypertrophic cardiomyopathy usually decrease.

Studies

Electrocardiography
During electrocardiography, the clinician should look for atrial fibrillation, left or right atrial enlargement, and signs of left ventricular or right ventricular hypertrophy.

Chest Radiography
A chest radiograph is useful in detecting cardiac chamber enlargement, pulmonary venous hypertension, and more overt signs of pulmonary congestion.

Doppler Echocardiography
Echocardiography is the most important test currently used for the diagnosis of valvular heart disease. It can define the specific valves that are affected, type of lesion (i.e., stenosis or regurgitation), and severity of the lesion. Transesophageal echocardiography is especially useful when chest wall images are poor, after a prosthesis has been implanted, and when looking at the left atrium for thrombus.

Severity of Stenosis

Planimetry using two-dimensional echocardiography can directly measure the area of the valve opening in mitral stenosis. This is the most reliable measurement in mitral stenosis, but it often is technically difficult.

Velocity across the valve as measured by Doppler can be converted to a pressure gradient using the Bernoulli equation:

$$\text{Pressure gradient} = 4 \times \text{velocity}^2$$

Thus, for example, if a peak velocity measured across the aortic valve is 4 m/s, then the peak pressure gradient across the valve is 64 mm Hg.

The pressure gradient depends on the flow across the valve. The higher the flow for any given area, the higher the pressure gradient will be (Fig. 60.1). Therefore, pressure gradients should be interpreted with knowledge of the cardiac output and function.

Estimation of Valve Area
The continuity equation usually is applied to the aortic valve. Because of the law of conservation of mass-energy, the flow into the valve is equivalent to that leaving the valve. Flow (F) is the product of the cross-sectional area (A) at a given point and the velocity (v) at that point, or

$$F = Av$$

The velocity (v_p) and cross-sectional area (A_p) below the aortic valve in the left ventricular outflow tract can be

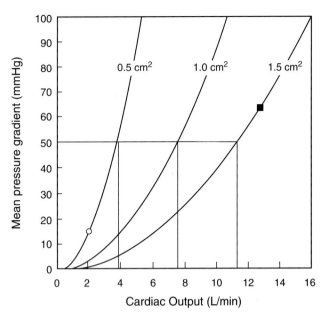

Figure 60.1 Relationship of flow to pressure gradient and valve area. A mean pressure gradient of 50 mm Hg across the aortic valve is possible with a valve area of 0.5 to 1.5 cm², depending on the flow (i.e., cardiac output) through the valve.

measured readily, as can the velocity at the site of maximal narrowing at the aortic valve (v_d), which is the highest velocity recorded (Fig. 60.2). The cross-sectional area at the valve itself (A_d) can be derived as

$$A_d = A_p v_p / v_d$$

Pressure Half-time

In mitral stenosis, the severity of stenosis inversely relates to the time it takes for the initial pressure to decrease to half its original value. The valve area has been empirically derived as

$$220/\text{Pressure half-time}$$

The shorter the pressure half-time, the less severe the stenosis.

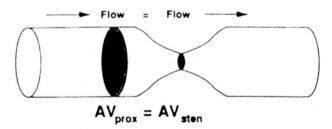

Figure 60.2 Flow is the product of area and velocity at a given point, and the continuity equation uses this to calculate the aortic valve area. Flow in the left ventricular outflow tract below the valve can be calculated from the known velocity (V) and area (A) at this level (AV_{prox}). The stenotic valve area can be derived from the velocity at this point (AV_{sten}) as $\dfrac{A_{prox} V_{prox}}{V_{sten}}$.

Assessment of Regurgitant Lesions

The qualitative and quantitative assessment of regurgitant lesion severity is done by using the flow disturbance associated with the regurgitation on color flow mapping. Quantitative assessment uses the determination of flow across the regurgitant valve and across a normal valve. Regurgitant flow is the total flow through the regurgitant valve minus that through the normal valve. The regurgitant fraction equals the regurgitant volume divided by the total volume flow (i.e., forward plus backward).

Newer methods are becoming available to measure regurgitant flow and the size of the regurgitant orifice directly. These use the flow field that is proximal to the regurgitant orifice (proximal convergence).

Assessment of Effects of Valvular Disease on Ventricular Function

Increasing ventricular size over time in the absence of symptoms is an indication for surgical intervention in patients with mitral and aortic regurgitation. The response of the left ventricle, both in size and function, to exercise stress is increasingly used to assess the effect of valvular regurgitation on contractile function and to help determine optimal timing for surgery.

Cardiac Catheterization

Cardiac catheterization is less critical today because of reliable, noninvasive measures. It still is used, however, when a discrepancy occurs between clinical findings and noninvasive techniques or to confirm noninvasive findings in selected patients. It also is necessary when coronary disease is suspected or must be excluded (e.g., in patients who need surgery).

With cardiac catheterization, the pressure gradients across the valves can be measured directly rather than simply being derived, as they are with Doppler. The effects of maneuvers, such as exercise, also can be used to determine the severity of a lesion. Valve area is derived empirically using the Gorlin equation from the flow (thermodilution or Fick technique) and the pressure gradient across the valve.

Regurgitation usually is assessed semiquantitatively, by the direct injection of dye into the left ventricle to assess mitral regurgitation or into the aorta to assess aortic regurgitation. The opacification of the chamber receiving the regurgitant flow is then determined.

TREATMENT

The general principles for treating patients with valvular heart disease are as follows:

1. Assess severity of symptoms.
2. Determine the nature of the valvular lesion and its severity.

3. Assess the effects of the lesion on ventricular function.
4. Assess for other cardiac (or other) pathologies.

Intervention is indicated in the following situations:

- Limiting symptoms with significant stenosis
- Limiting symptoms with significant regurgitation
- Significant left ventricular dysfunction or progressive left ventricular dilatation attributable to the valve lesion in severe mitral or aortic regurgitation or aortic stenosis (Newer guidelines suggest that mitral valve repair surgery in asymptomatic patients with severe mitral regurgitation and preserved left ventricular size and systolic function is reasonable if the surgery is performed in an experienced surgical center and there is a high [>90%] likelihood of successful repair without residual regurgitation.)

There have been recent major changes to the AHA guidelines for endocarditis prophylaxis. Previously, prophylaxis for endocarditis was indicated whenever blood flow was turbulent at a structurally abnormal valve, and although the benefits of prophylaxis had never been fully established, it was usual clinical practice to err on the side of administration. However, the new guidelines recommend that prophylaxis should only be used in patients with underlying cardiac conditions associated with the highest adverse outcome from infective endocarditis. These conditions include prosthetic heart valves, previous infective endocarditis, certain classes of congenital heart disease, and in valvulopathy occurring post cardiac transplantation.

SPECIFIC VALVE LESIONS

Mitral Stenosis

Mitral stenosis is twice as common in women as in men. It usually is rheumatic in origin, although congenital mitral stenosis also occurs. The valve becomes fibrosed and tends to calcify with time. The reduction in the size of the mitral valve orifice lowers the cardiac output, and it tends to raise left atrial and pulmonary venous and arterial pressures. In patients with severe mitral stenosis, pulmonary hypertension as high as that of the systemic vasculature may occur. Flow across the mitral valve occurs in diastole and is critically dependent on the heart rate; therefore, the reduction of diastolic filling time caused by increased heart rate worsens the symptoms and can cause acute pulmonary edema. Symptomatic deterioration often results from the onset of atrial fibrillation.

The complications of mitral stenosis may include atrial arrhythmia, atrial fibrillation, and thromboembolism. Left atrial enlargement and atrial fibrillation predispose patients to atrial thrombus and thromboembolism. This may occur in as many as 25% of those who are not anticoagulated, and it often occurs silently.

Diagnosis

The symptoms of mitral stenosis are:

- Dyspnea
- Fatigue
- Hemoptysis (from pulmonary venous hypertension)
- Angina; syncope, if there is pulmonary hypertension
- Edema secondary to right heart failure

The signs of mitral stenosis are

- Tapping apex beat from a loud first heart sound if the valve is pliable
- Diastolic thrill in severe stenosis (classically described as like a purring cat)
- Palpable P_2, if there is pulmonary hypertension
- Loud S_1, because the valve remains open at the end of diastole and shuts abruptly with the onset of systole; as the valve calcifies, the S_1 gets softer
- Opening snap indicates a pliable valve and disappears as the valve calcifies. The opening snap often is heard at the left sternal border rather than at the apex and with the diaphragm rather than with the bell of the stethoscope
- Diastolic murmur with presystolic accentuation in sinus rhythm, best heard at apex with the bell of the stethoscope and the patient on his or her left side
- Associated pulmonary hypertension leads to a loud P_2, right ventricular heave, tricuspid regurgitation, and pulmonary insufficiency (i.e., Graham-Steel murmur)
- Occasionally, no murmur is heard if flow through the valve is low (e.g., as with severe pulmonary hypertension)

Signs indicating severe stenosis include a long diastolic murmur, a short duration of the interval between S_2 and the opening snap (thus indicating high atrial pressure even at the end of systole), and a loud P_2.

Differential Diagnosis

The differential diagnosis of diastolic murmur includes tricuspid stenosis, Austin-Flint murmur of aortic regurgitation (i.e., aortic regurgitant jet hits the mitral valve and prevents full diastolic opening), left atrial myxoma, and cor triatriatum. Silent mitral stenosis with pulmonary hypertension simulates primary pulmonary hypertension.

Studies

Electrocardiography shows left atrial enlargement, right atrial enlargement, right axis, and right ventricular hypertrophy. Chest radiography may show left atrial enlargement, prominence of main pulmonary artery Kerley B lines with edema, and pulmonary hemosiderosis. Doppler echocardiography reveals

- The appearance of doming of the mitral valve, which has a restricted opening. The opening may be measured directly by planimetry in the short axis (Fig. 60.3), which

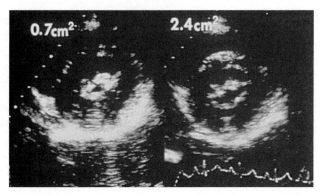

Figure 60.3 Planimetry of the mitral valve by echocardiography. The mitral valve area increases after balloon valvuloplasty **(right)** compared with baseline **(left)**.

usually is the most reliable method for assessing severity of the narrowing.

- A pressure gradient across the valve (normal <5 mm Hg) may be as high as 20 mm Hg in those with severe mitral stenosis. The valve area also is derived empirically from the pressure half-time.
- A decrease in valve area (normal 4–6 cm^2) to <1 cm^2 in patients with critical mitral stenosis.
- A mitral valve score based on thickness, calcification, mobility, and involvement of subvalvular apparatus on transthoracic echocardiography. This score is used to determine the likelihood of success for percutaneous mitral valvuloplasty. The score may vary from 0 to 16. If the score is >8, valvuloplasty will have less chance of success.
- The possible presence of associated lesions such as mitral, aortic, or tricuspid regurgitation.

Stress echocardiography is increasingly used to assess functional capacity and the effects of exercise on valve pressure gradients and pulmonary pressures (as derived from the velocity of tricuspid regurgitation). This is especially useful when patients have severe stenosis but deny symptoms or when the degree of stenosis apparently is mild but the symptoms are more severe than would be anticipated.

Cardiac catheterization is used to determine the presence of accompanying coronary disease, and it also is useful in confirming the severity of mitral disease. Knowledge regarding the effect of exercise on the mitral pressure gradient may be useful when the severity of the lesion is in doubt. Cardiac catheterization is necessary for percutaneous mitral valvuloplasty (Fig. 60.4).

Treatment

Survival rates are lower among patients with mitral stenosis in whom symptoms have appeared. Patients increasingly are treated with balloon valvuloplasty, which at 2 years has results similar to those of open mitral commissurotomy regarding symptoms and valve area. Balloon valvuloplasty is feasible if the valve is pliable and relatively uncalcified (as assessed by the echocardiographic splitability score), if no more than mild mitral regurgitation is present (i.e., mitral regurgitation usually increases one grade with the balloon procedure), if no thrombus is present in the left atrium (i.e., a thrombus could be dislodged by wires during valvuloplasty), and if severe tricuspid regurgitation is absent (i.e., severe tricuspid regurgitation often persists after a balloon procedure).

Asymptomatic patients usually can be treated conservatively. Indications for intervention in patients without symptoms include significant pulmonary hypertension, prophylaxis in those undergoing major surgery during which a large volume shift might be encountered, or women of childbearing age with severe stenosis who wish to start a family.

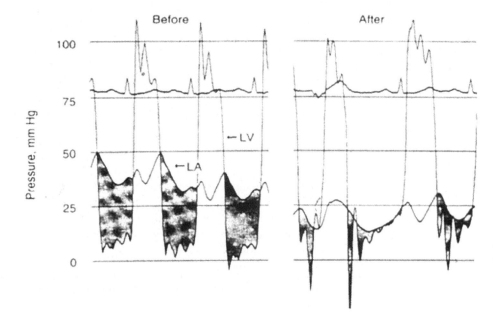

Figure 60.4 The mitral valve gradient is the *shaded* area between the left atrial (*LA*) and left ventricular (*LV*) pressure in diastole. **Left:** The gradient before percutaneous valvuloplasty. **Right:** The reduced gradient after successful balloon valvuloplasty.

With symptomatic patients, intervention with balloon valvuloplasty or surgery may be considered. Valve replacement is indicated in patients with calcified valves or severe mitral regurgitation.

Patients with mitral stenosis must be monitored closely during pregnancy because the volume load and tachycardia may cause severe, symptomatic deterioration even in those with mild mitral stenosis. The risk of heart failure is greatest during the first trimester and at delivery. Careful monitoring and slowing of the heart rate allows most patients with mitral stenosis to carry their pregnancies to term without intervention. In those with severe, symptomatic deterioration, commissurotomy (preferably with a balloon) is indicated.

With medical treatment, the control of heart rate in patients with atrial fibrillation is important. In older patients who are not considered to be good surgical candidates, rate control and diuretics may effectively reduce symptoms. In younger patients, prophylaxis against rheumatic fever usually is required. Patients with chronic atrial fibrillation and mitral stenosis have a high risk for thromboembolism and should receive anticoagulation.

Surgical treatment consists of open commissurotomy, in which the fused mitral valve leaflets are opened under direct vision by the surgeon or by prosthetic valve insertion.

Mitral Regurgitation

Etiology
Primary mitral regurgitation is an abnormality of the valve or apparatus. The causes of primary mitral regurgitation are:

- Rheumatic, more often men than women
- Myxomatous, as in mitral valve prolapse
- Congenital, as in endocardial cushion defects with primum atrial septal defect
- Endocarditis, as in bacterial and marantic infections, Libman-Sacks vegetations in lupus
- Ischemic, as in papillary muscle dysfunction or rupture

Secondary mitral regurgitation results from dilatation of the left ventricle from any cause. This can include ischemia, cardiomyopathy, or aortic valve disease.

Pathophysiology
When volume load occurs on the left atrium and left ventricle, the left ventricle initially responds by pumping more vigorously and emptying more completely. Subsequently, progressive dilatation occurs, with eventual impairment of left ventricular function. This may be permanent despite valve surgery.

Diagnosis
Mitral regurgitation often is asymptomatic for many years. Dyspnea and heart failure are the most common symptoms, and right-sided heart failure with hepatic congestion and cachexia also are seen.

No specific pulse findings are present. The jugular venous pressure often is elevated because of right-sided heart failure.

The murmur generally is holosystolic, louder in expiration, best heard at the apex, and radiates to the axilla. A murmur that radiates to the back indicates a posterior-directed jet (e.g., anterior prolapse of the mitral valve). It often is associated with an S_3 gallop, which is consistent with severe mitral regurgitation and a dilated left ventricle. S_1 usually is soft, and S_2 may be loud in patients with pulmonary hypertension.

Studies
Electrocardiography shows a volume overload pattern and left atrial enlargement. It allows the anatomy of the valve and cause of the leak to be delineated precisely. Such imaging also is useful in determining the severity of the leak, either semiquantitatively by the size and extent of the regurgitant jet on color Doppler or quantitatively as the regurgitant volume. The leak can be quantified by a new color Doppler technique proximal to the hole through which the leaks occur (i.e., regurgitant orifice). The size of the regurgitant orifice also can be estimated; in patients with severe mitral regurgitation, it usually is >0.3 cm^2.

Over time, any change in size of the chambers, particularly the left ventricle, is useful for monitoring the progress of the lesion and determining the need for surgery. The contractile function of the left ventricle is difficult to assess accurately through noninvasive means, because the ventricle is volume loaded and ejects much of its blood back into the lower pressure left atrium. Left ventricular function always appears to be better than it really is when using ejection indices such as ejection fraction. An ejection fraction $<60\%$ should suggest possible contractile dysfunction in this condition. Therefore, in the presence of mitral regurgitation, preserved systolic function is defined as an ejection fraction $>60\%$ and an end-systolic dimension <40 mm.

Increasingly, left ventricular volume measurements are made to determine the appropriate timing of surgery. Our group have used the response of the left ventricle to exercise stress as a means of determining contractile reserve in this condition. A failure of the left ventricle to decrease in size at peak exercise, or of the ejection fraction to increase, is indicative of left ventricular dysfunction, which is often manifest postoperatively.

Chest radiography shows left atrial and left ventricular enlargement as well as congestive changes (Fig. 60.5), and cardiac catheterization can determine the severity of mitral regurgitation (using ventriculography) or the presence of coronary disease. Large V waves in pulmonary wedge tracings also suggest severe mitral regurgitation. A succession of pressure-volume loops, as defined using high-fidelity catheters and by changing the loading conditions, allows myocardial elastance to be measured. This is the best

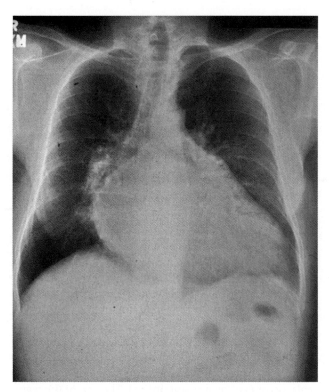

Figure 60.5 Chest radiograph of a patient with chronic mitral regurgitation showing left atrial and left ventricular enlargement.

load-independent measure of true contractile function in this condition. It remains a research tool, however, because it is difficult to measure and requires catheterization as well as intravenous pressors and vasodilators for its measurement.

Treatment

Medical Treatment

No treatment is needed for mild regurgitation, but these patients should undergo serial echocardiography. Afterload reduction usually is not indicated in those with primary mitral regurgitation, because this has not been shown to postpone surgical intervention. If congestive heart failure is present, treatment includes diuretics, digoxin, and afterload reduction. In patients with secondary mitral regurgitation, the primary disease should be treated. Vasodilators or afterload reduction should be used in patients with cardiomyopathy.

Surgical Treatment

Patients with mitral regurgitation eventually develop heart failure. The onset of heart failure is associated with reduced survival rates, as is significant ventricular dysfunction. Mitral regurgitation should be corrected before the signs of left ventricular dysfunction or failure become overt. Indications for surgery, therefore, are severe mitral regurgitation with symptoms of heart failure, dyspnea, evidence of deteriorated left ventricular function, or progressive left ventricu-

lar enlargement. In asymptomatic patients, an end-systolic dimension >40 mm is considered to be an indication for surgery. Because patients with mitral regurgitation should have hyperdynamic function, even a low-normal left ventricular ejection fraction (i.e., <60%) should be considered to be a sign of incipient left ventricular dysfunction, and surgery should be recommended accordingly. With exercise, those patients in whom the left ventricular ejection fraction fails to increase, or the end-systolic volume fails to decrease, likely have contractile dysfunction and should be considered for early surgery (Fig. 60.6). Also, in asymptomatic patients with severe regurgitation and preserved systolic function, mitral valve repair is a reasonable approach if the surgery is performed in a high-volume surgical center and if the likelihood of successful repair is >90%.

Surgical therapy includes mitral valve repair and mitral valve replacement. Mitral valve repair is the surgical intervention of choice. It is successful in selected patients, especially those with myxomatous valves (i.e., prolapse) or mitral regurgitation from ischemia. It is less likely to be feasible, however, in patients with endocarditis or rheumatic disease. Mitral valve repair has a lower mortality than replacement (i.e., <1%) and allows a better preservation of left ventricular systolic function through the conservation of valve-supporting structures. Freedom from reoperation at 20 years has been reported in >90% of patients who have undergone repair for mitral valve prolapse.

Mitral valve replacement is indicated when repair is not feasible, especially in rheumatic or elderly patients with calcified valves. Replacement has both a higher mortality (i.e., <5%) and morbidity than valve repair.

Emerging Treatment: Percutaneous Valve Repair

Percutaneous mitral valve repair involves a catheter-based treatment in which coaptation of the mitral leaflets is achieved by devices deployed at the time of cardiac catheterization. The types of devices under investigation can be classed into two functional approaches: one in which a clip is used to approximate the center of the mitral valve leaflets, thus giving a double orifice valve in an approach that models the surgical Alfieri edge-to-edge repair; and the other in which a flexible ring is deployed and tightened in the coronary sinus so as to reduce the mitral annulus area. The former is more suitable to repair of mitral valve prolapse, while the latter is felt to be more suited toward repair of functional regurgitation. Currently, clinical trials are under way in both types of approach.

Mitral Valve Prolapse

Mitral valve prolapse is a relatively common condition that is associated with myxomatous degeneration of the mitral valve. It occurs in 1% to 2% of the population and is equally prevalent in men and women. An increased amount of acid mucopolysaccharides accumulates in the valve tissue to cause prolapse. Mitral valve prolapse is associated with

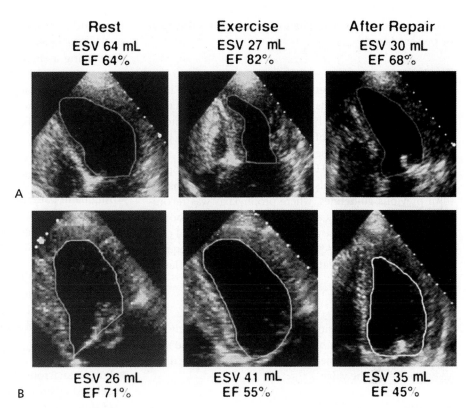

Rest
ESV 64 mL
EF 64%

Exercise
ESV 27 mL
EF 82%

After Repair
ESV 30 mL
EF 68%

A

B

ESV 26 mL
EF 71%

ESV 41 mL
EF 55%

ESV 35 mL
EF 45%

Figure 60.6 Effects of exercise on left ventricular ejection fraction (*LVEF*) and end-systolic volume (*ESV*) in patients A **(top three panels)** and B **(bottom three panels)**, both of whom have severe mitral regurgitation. In patient A, LVEF increases at peak exercise and ESV decreases, thus indicating preserved left ventricular systolic function. The LVEF remains normal after mitral valve repair. In patient B, LVEF declines and ESV increases at peak exercise, thus indicating latent left ventricular dysfunction, which becomes overt once the volume-loading effects that mask it are removed after mitral valve repair.

Marfan's syndrome, but it usually occurs as an isolated entity involving the mitral valve. Occasionally, however, the tricuspid and the aortic valves also are involved. In prolapse, the annulus may be dilated, and elongation of the chordae occurs. The valve leaflets often are redundant, with excess tissue that causes them to prolapse. The degree of abnormality tends to increase with age.

Mitral valve prolapse is associated with a spectrum of abnormality, varying from asymptomatic to severe heart failure resulting from mitral regurgitation. Mitral valve prolapse often is a relatively benign condition, especially in women. In many women, prolapse becomes less prominent with age, which may reflect a relative disproportion between the size of the valve leaflets and the ventricle, which is lessened as the ventricle dilates with increasing age. Men, on the other hand, are more prone to the complications of mitral valve prolapse and are at least twice as likely as women to require surgical intervention for mitral regurgitation. Mitral valve prolapse often is associated with ventricular arrhythmia in the form of ectopy and more rarely with sustained ventricular tachycardia and sudden death.

Diagnosis

Mitral valve prolapse often is asymptomatic at presentation and detected by a mid-systolic click on auscultation. Another presentation is with congestive heart failure from severe mitral regurgitation that results from acute chordal rupture. Patients with prolapse and regurgitation are prone to endocarditis, and they may present as such.

In young women especially, a syndrome of chest pain of nonanginal quality, paresthesia, and arrhythmia (especially ventricular ectopy) is seen. These symptoms have been attributed to autonomic imbalance, but they are as common in matched populations without prolapse as in those with prolapse.

Signs are a mid-systolic click, with or without a systolic apical murmur. The murmur typically occurs after the click in late systole, but in those with more severe prolapse, the murmur may be holosystolic. Clicks may be present even without echocardiographic prolapse. Maneuvers that decrease intracardiac volume accentuate the click and murmur, causing them to begin earlier in systole.

Studies

Electrocardiography commonly shows inferior T-wave inversion. Mitral valve prolapse is a cause of false-positive stress ECGs.

Echocardiography reveals late systolic prolapse of the posterior leaflet on M mode as well as thickening and redundancy of the leaflets and chordae. Prolapse of either or both leaflets (posterior is much more common) can be seen on a two-dimensional echocardiogram. It is important to make the diagnosis with the parasternal or apical long-axis views rather than with the apical views. In apical views, apparent prolapse of the mitral leaflets occurs even in normal patients because the mitral annulus is not a flat plane but is saddle-shaped. Thus, in this view, the mitral leaflets often appear to be displaced superior to the annular plane. Mitral regurgitation of varying severity may be present as well.

Treatment

If severe mitral regurgitation is present, surgery is indicated. Reassuring patients of the relatively benign nature of this condition often is beneficial. Autonomic symptoms and ventricular ectopy often respond to treatment with β-blockade (in small doses).

According to recent AHA guidelines, antibiotic prophylaxis is not indicated. This represents a significant change from previous guidelines, where prophylaxis was recommended for dental work and selected procedures if both a click and a murmur were present, in the presence of a click and echocardiographic evidence of prolapse and regurgitation, or in high-risk features such as thickened leaflets.

Aortic Stenosis

Aortic stenosis is increasingly common. Approximately 2% of the population has a bicuspid aortic valve, and 80% of cases occur in male subjects. Aortic stenosis may occur at, above, or below the valve.

Etiology

The causes of aortic (valvular) stenosis are congenital (bicuspid, occasionally unicuspid), rheumatic, or degenerative (valvular calcification). Bicuspid valves are familial and occur in approximately 10% of first-degree relatives. Degenerative aortic valve disease has been shown to have histologic characteristics similar to that of atherosclerosis. The progression of stenosis is promoted by hyperlipidemia, and lipid-lowering agents may slow the rate of progression. Subaortic (nonvalvular) stenosis occurs because of a congenital membrane that is seen below the aortic valve in the left ventricular outflow tract. Hypertrophic cardiomyopathy is a dynamic obstruction of the left ventricular outflow tract as the left ventricle contracts. Supravalvular aortic stenosis is associated with hypercalcemia.

Pathophysiology

The obstruction of the aortic valve initially leads to increased left ventricular hypertrophy and then to left ventricular dilatation and failure. The normal aortic valve opens from 3 to 4 cm^2. The valve area is >1.5 cm^2 in patients with mild aortic stenosis, 1.0 to 1.5 cm^2 in those with moderate stenosis, and <1 cm^2 in those with severe stenosis. Critical aortic stenosis is present when the valve area is <0.75 cm^2. A normalization of the valve area, as based on the body surface area, often is useful. A valve area <0.5 cm^2/m^2 is considered to be critical stenosis.

The pressure gradient across the valve also is used to indicate the severity of aortic stenosis, but this depends on the flow. In patients with normal heart function and without significant aortic regurgitation, a mean gradient of 50 mm Hg by Doppler or a peak-to-peak gradient of 50 mm

Hg at cardiac catheterization is consistent with severe aortic stenosis. In patients with heart failure, flow may be reduced, thus giving a small gradient across the aortic valve and underestimating the degree of stenosis. Aortic regurgitation increases the flow across the valve and, in turn, the gradient for any degree of stenosis. It generally is best to measure the valve area rather than rely on the pressure gradient alone.

Diagnosis

The symptoms of aortic stenosis are

- Angina in patients without coronary disease because of mismatch between the blood supply and demand, especially of the subendocardium of the hypertrophied heart
- Dyspnea because of increased pulmonary capillary pressure
- Syncope caused by an inability of the heart to increase output with systemic vasodilatation, thus leading to decreased cerebral perfusion; arrhythmia also can cause syncope or sudden death in these patients

The signs of aortic stenosis are:

- Pulse is anacrotic (i.e., pulsus parvus et tardus), with slow delayed upstroke. This is the most reliable physical sign of significant aortic stenosis.
- Pulse usually is best examined at the carotid artery.
- Systolic thrill often is felt in patients with critical aortic stenosis.
- In young people with mobile valves, an ejection click may be heard.
- A harsh ejection systolic murmur over the aortic area, radiating to the neck, usually with a soft S_2 and S_4, is heard. The murmur often radiates to the apex as well.

Studies

Electrocardiography reveals left atrial enlargement and left ventricular hypertrophy. Doppler echocardiography reveals a thickened, abnormal valve, and this study can define the severity of the lesion with the pressure gradient and valve area. Cardiac catheterization is used to assess the valve area and pressure gradient, but it usually is not indicated if Doppler gradients appear to be reliable and the patient is under 40 years of age and does not have angina.

Treatment

Survival rates are lower among patients in whom symptoms have appeared. Once left ventricular dysfunction or congestive heart failure occurs, the 2-year survival rate is low.

Asymptomatic patients with severe aortic stenosis, except for young patients with severe congenital aortic stenosis, have a relatively low risk of death. In studies, patients who died suddenly with aortic stenosis usually had the onset of symptoms before death. In older patients, especially those with calcific aortic stenosis, the asymptomatic interval in severe aortic stenosis usually is relatively short (typically 2–3 years).

Therefore, patients with symptoms of syncope, angina, or dyspnea and severe aortic stenosis should be considered for surgery. No treatment usually is indicated in patients without symptoms, except in those with severe stenosis and resultant left ventricular dysfunction or in those with severe aortic stenosis and pressure gradients >100 mm Hg; these patients may have an increased risk of sudden death. Patients with asymptomatic, severe aortic stenosis must be monitored closely using serial echocardiography at 6-month intervals (at least) and must be alerted to report their symptoms. In older patients with calcific aortic stenosis, elective surgery may be considered, even among those who are asymptomatic, given the high likelihood of its being necessary anyway. The recent American College of Cardiology (ACC)/AHA guidelines suggest that elective surgery for severe aortic stenosis may be considered even in asymptomatic patients if the mortality associated with valve replacement is ≤1% in the institution where surgery is being considered. Asymptomatic patients with severe aortic stenosis should avoid heavy exertion, and young patients with aortic stenosis should refrain from competitive sports.

In young patients with fused commissures, aortic valvotomy provides good palliation for years. Often, this treatment results in significant aortic regurgitation, but it also obviates a prosthesis while growth is still occurring. Prosthetic valve replacement may be either mechanical or bioprosthetic. Biological valves should be avoided in young patients, because early degeneration is common. The mortality typically is from 2% to 3%, although it is lower in young patients.

Homograft implantation using cadaveric human valves have good intermediate-term results but in the long term are not superior to bioprosthetic valves in their durability. This procedure does not require long-term anticoagulation, but reoperation (if required) is difficult, as the entire homograft may become heavily calcified. Aortic valve repair is possible at some centers in selected patients with congenitally bicuspid valves.

The Ross procedure involves the autotransplantation of the native pulmonic valve to the aortic position and a pulmonary homograft to the pulmonary position. This is indicated in adolescent patients, because the autograft grows with the patient and anticoagulation is not required. The procedure, however, is technically complex, and long-term complications include degeneration of the pulmonic homograft and neoaortic root dilation and resultant aortic regurgitation.

Balloon valvuloplasty accomplished with percutaneous dilatation of the aortic valve is feasible in patients with congenital stenosis and even calcific stenosis. Results are better in younger patients. In older patients, it is used as a palliative procedure in those who cannot withstand surgery, and most often as a bridge to surgery. Short-term hemodynamic results are reasonable, and early restenosis (<6 months) is the rule. Survival rates are not affected in those patients who cannot undergo valve replacement. Morbidity and mortality, however, are substantial (i.e., 5%). This procedure is not an alternative to surgery in older patients.

Percutaneous aortic valve replacement either via a retrograde aortic approach or, when this is not possible due to severe peripheral vascular disease, via a transapical approach represents an emerging treatment option for severe aortic stenosis. Small clinical trials have been performed in elderly high–surgical risk patient populations and have demonstrated feasibility of this approach in humans with an improvement in aortic valve area. Futher clinical trials are ongoing in larger numbers comparing this technique with either surgical valve replacement or with balloon valvuloplasty in inoperable patient groups.

Aortic Regurgitation

Etiology

The causes of aortic regurgitation include:

- Congenital anomaly (e.g., bicuspid valve, aortic valve prolapse)
- Rheumatic disease
- Diseases of the aorta, such as aortic root aneurysm because of Marfan's syndrome or aortic dissection involving the ascending aorta; the mechanism of aortic regurgitation usually involves dilatation of the aortic root with poor coaptation of leaflets
- Aortitis caused by connective tissue disease or syphilis
- Endocarditis
- Degeneration (an area of leaflet coaptation becomes friable with aging)

Aortic regurgitation is rarely, if ever, caused by ischemic heart disease.

Pathophysiology

Aortic regurgitation causes volume overload of the left ventricle, which dilates to compensate for the volume load. Left ventricular dilatation is well tolerated for a long time, but eventually it leads to impaired systolic function and heart failure. The pressure gradient between the aorta and left ventricle is greatest at aortic valve closure and decreases progressively throughout diastole, thus giving rise to the decrescendo nature of the aortic regurgitation murmur.

Diagnosis

Aortic regurgitation often is asymptomatic for years. If it is acute, such as in dissection or endocarditis, it may give rise to congestive symptoms that are poorly tolerated. Chest pain of an anginal nature also may be reported.

The signs of aortic regurgitation are:

- High-volume pulse with rapid falloff as blood leaks back into the left ventricle (i.e., collapsing or Corrigan water-hammer pulse). Increased capillary pulsation also is seen (i.e., Quincke pulse) at the nail bed, where alternate flushing and pallor of the skin is seen when light pressure is applied to the nail tip. Other signs of severe aortic regurgitation are pistol-shot femoral artery pulses and the Duroziez sign (i.e., a to-and-fro murmur over the femoral artery when it is lightly compressed with a stethoscope).

- The pulse pressure is widened, with a high systolic and a low diastolic pressure.
- Prominent pulsation of the carotid arteries is seen.
- The apex beat is hyperdynamic, and a diastolic thrill may be felt on occasion.
- The murmur of valvular aortic regurgitation is decrescendo and is heard over the aortic area and along the left sternal border. The murmur is best heard during expiration, with the patient leaning forward. When aortic regurgitation results from aortic root dilatation, the murmur frequently is heard at the right rather than the left sternal border.
- Aortic regurgitation usually is associated with an ejection systolic murmur, even in patients without clinically significant stenosis. The ejection murmur reflects increased flow across the aortic valve.
- S_3 and S_4 may be heard.
- During severe aortic regurgitation, the jet may impinge on the opening of the anterior mitral valve leaflet and cause a mid-diastolic murmur (i.e., Austin-Flint murmur).

Studies

Electrocardiography reveals diastolic volume overload and left ventricular hypertrophy. Doppler echocardiography can quantify and determine the mechanism of the aortic regurgitation. Serial echocardiography is used to follow left ventricular size and function over time. The chest radiography shows cardiomegaly and a prominent aorta.

Cardiac catheterization aortography is used to determine semiquantitatively the severity of aortic regurgitation. It currently is the gold standard for assessing such severity.

Treatment

Acute, severe aortic regurgitation needs urgent surgical treatment. Afterload reduction using sodium nitroprusside can stabilize the patient while he or she is waiting for surgery. Intra-aortic balloon counterpulsation increases the severity of aortic regurgitation by increasing the diastolic pressure in the aorta, and it should not be used to treat this condition.

Chronic aortic regurgitation is well tolerated for many years. Valve surgery is indicated once symptoms occur or left ventricular dysfunction manifests. After left ventricular dysfunction is present for more than 1 year, it may not normalize, even after aortic valve replacement. Sudden death is more likely once left ventricular size is greatly increased; therefore, a careful follow-up of patients with significant regurgitation is required.

Echocardiography is used to follow both the size and function of the left ventricle. Even in asymptomatic patients, surgery should be considered if left ventricular function is impaired (ejection fraction $\leq 50\%$) or if left ventricle end-systolic dimension is >5.5 cm even if ejection fraction is normal, because surgical intervention in patients with large ventricles is associated with poor outcome. Surgery may be considered at smaller end-diastolic and end-systolic dimensions if the left ventricular enlargement is rapidly progressive or left ventricular function is declining or in patients of small stature. In asymptomatic patients with left ventricular dilatation but with normal left ventricular systolic function, afterload reduction with vasodilators may be considered with the aim of prolongation of this compensated phase, although the effectiveness of this approach has been recently challenged. Valve surgical options are similar to those for aortic stenosis, except that aortic valve repair is more likely to be possible in patients with aortic regurgitation as compared with those with aortic stenosis.

Tricuspid Stenosis

Tricuspid stenosis is less common than mitral stenosis. Tricuspid stenosis occurs in 5% to 10% of patients with severe mitral stenosis. Carcinoid is an additional rare cause.

Tricuspid stenosis leads to elevated right atrial pressure. In turn, this leads to peripheral edema, ascites, and low cardiac output.

Diagnosis

Isolated tricuspid stenosis is rare, but it may lead to low cardiac output and peripheral edema. The signs include a jugular pressure with a large A wave if the patient is in normal sinus rhythm. Elevated jugular venous pressure is present as well. Auscultation reveals a diastolic murmur similar to that of mitral stenosis, except that it is best heard during inspiration and over the left sternal margin and xiphoid.

Studies

Electrocardiography shows right atrial enlargement. Doppler echocardiography is used to measure the gradient across the tricuspid valve.

Treatment

Right-sided symptoms should be treated with diuretics first. Balloon valvuloplasty is feasible in suitable candidates, and surgical treatment should be considered in patients undergoing mitral surgery, if the mean tricuspid gradient is >4 or 5 mm Hg. If surgical repair is unsuccessful, prosthetic replacement usually is performed using a tissue valve (because of the increased risk of thrombosis with mechanical prostheses at this position).

Tricuspid Regurgitation

Tricuspid regurgitation may be either primary or secondary. Primary tricuspid regurgitation usually results from rheumatic disease. Other causes include carcinoid, congenital abnormalities (e.g., Ebstein anomaly), right ventricular ischemia or infarction, tricuspid valve prolapse, trauma, or endocarditis.

Secondary tricuspid regurgitation results from conditions that cause pulmonary hypertension, with resultant right ventricle dilatation and dilatation of the tricuspid annulus. Tricuspid regurgitation leads to reduced cardiac output, with peripheral edema as well as hepatic and gastrointestinal congestion.

Diagnosis

Tricuspid regurgitation causes symptoms of low cardiac output (e.g., fatigue) or right-sided failure (e.g., anorexia) from passive congestion of the liver and gastrointestinal tract. The signs include large V waves in the jugular venous pulse. Auscultation reveals a pansystolic murmur, which is heard best during inspiration at the left sternal border and subxiphoid area.

Studies

Electrocardiography reveals right atrial enlargement and right ventricular hypertrophy. Doppler echocardiography can be used to determine both the severity of the regurgitation and its cause.

Treatment

Isolated, severe tricuspid regurgitation may not require any treatment apart from diuretics. Surgical repair or replacement might be considered in patients with congestive symptoms that are refractory to medical treatment. In patients with secondary tricuspid regurgitation, the primary condition should be treated. In those with tricuspid regurgitation secondary to mitral or aortic valve disease, however, tricuspid annuloplasty should be considered at the time of surgery for the primary condition.

Diet Drugs and Valve Disease

Certain anorexigenic drugs, either alone or in combination, have been associated with a valvulopathy. Drugs involved include phentermine, fenfluramine, and dexfenfluramine. The valvulopathy occurs mainly at the mitral and aortic valves and has similarities to rheumatic disease, carcinoid syndrome, and ergot valve disease. The pathophysiology of the valve lesion currently is unknown, although serotonin has been implicated, given the similarity to carcinoid syndrome. The predominant hemodynamic abnormality is regurgitation rather than stenosis. Valvulopathy consists of thickening and restriction of the valve leaflets and supporting structures. A minority of patients taking the drugs develop valvulopathy, although some patients have required surgical repair or replacement of the affected valves. The longer the duration of treatment with these anorexigenic agents, the more likely a valvulopathy will develop. Improvement in the valvulopathy after cessation of the anorexigenic agents has been reported. Patients who have taken anorexigenic drugs should undergo physical examination of the heart, and echocardiography is recommended if any clinical suspicion of valve disease emerges.

REVIEW EXERCISES

QUESTIONS

1. The most common cause of mitral regurgitation in the United States is
a) Rheumatic disease
b) Myxomatous disease (prolapse)
c) Endocarditis
d) Hypertension
e) None of the above

Answer and Discussion

The answer is b. Mitral valve prolapse is the most common cause of mitral regurgitation in the United States.

2. Which of the following is untrue about mitral stenosis?
a) It is more common in men.
b) It is usually rheumatic in origin.
c) It is associated with a diastolic murmur.
d) A presystolic murmur is heard in mitral stenosis in those in sinus rhythm.
e) The duration of the diastolic murmur predicts severity of the stenosis.

Answer and Discussion

The answer is a. Mitral stenosis is more common in women than in men.

3. All of the following are indications for surgery in severe mitral regurgitation, *except*
a) Shortness of breath on exertion
b) Left ventricular ejection fraction of 45%
c) Dilated left ventricle (end-systolic dimension 5 cm)
d) Frequent ventricular ectopy
e) Recurrent atrial fibrillation

Answer and Discussion

The answer is d. Frequent ventricular ectopy is common and does not necessarily improve with surgery. It is not considered an indication for valve surgery in mitral regurgitation.

4. Consider the following hemodynamic data: left atrial pressure, 25 mm Hg; left ventricular pressure, 120/10 mm Hg; aortic pressure, 120/80 mm Hg; and cardiac index, 1.9 L/minute/m². These are most consistent with which valvular lesion?
a) Mitral stenosis
b) Mitral regurgitation
c) Aortic stenosis
d) Aortic regurgitation
e) None of the above

Answer and Discussion
The answer is a. High left atrial pressure with a pressure gradient across the mitral valve in diastole and a low cardiac output diagnose mitral stenosis.

5. Recognized complications of isolated mitral stenosis include all of the following, *except*
a) Atrial fibrillation
b) Pulmonary hypertension
c) Atrial thrombus
d) Right heart failure
e) Left ventricular enlargement

Answer and Discussion
The answer is e. Isolated mitral stenosis does not cause left ventricular enlargement; left ventricle size is normal or small due to reduced inflow to the left ventricle.

6. The following statements concerning surgical correction of mitral regurgitation are correct, *except*
a) Repair is most likely to be possible in rheumatic valves.
b) Repair has a lower complication rate than prosthetic replacement.
c) Left ventricular function declines more after prosthetic replacement than with repair.
d) Surgery is indicated in severe mitral regurgitation with symptomatic deterioration.
e) Men are more likely to require surgical correction of regurgitation than women.

Answer and Discussion
The answer is a. Mitral valve repair is most likely to be successful in mitral valve prolapse and least likely in rheumatic disease and endocarditis.

7. Common symptoms of aortic stenosis include all of the following, *except*
a) Dyspnea
b) Syncope
c) Ankle edema
d) Angina
e) Fatigue

Answer and Discussion
The answer is b. Ankle edema is uncommon in aortic stenosis.

8. The most reliable physical finding in predicting severe aortic stenosis is
a) Loudness of the murmur
b) Absent first heart sound
c) Loud second heart sound
d) Delayed carotid upstroke
e) Left ventricular heave

Answer and Discussion
The answer is d. Delayed carotid upstroke is the most reliable predictor of severe aortic stenosis.

9. Surgical intervention is indicated in severe aortic stenosis for all of the following, *except*
a) Recent exercise-induced syncope
b) Left ventricular ejection fraction of 45% with normal coronary vessels
c) Shortness of breath on walking two blocks
d) Associated significant aortic regurgitation
e) Exertional chest pain usually relieved by rest

Answer and Discussion
The answer is d. Aortic regurgitation does not affect the decision regarding surgery in aortic stenosis. Surgery is indicated for symptoms and left ventricular dysfunction.

10. Consider the following hemodynamic data: left atrial pressure, 15 mm Hg; left ventricular pressure, 220/15 mm Hg; aortic pressure, 100/60 mm Hg; and cardiac index, 1.9 L/minute/m^2. These are most consistent with which valvular lesion?
a) Tricuspid stenosis
b) Mitral stenosis
c) Aortic stenosis
d) Aortic regurgitation
e) Tricuspid regurgitation

Answer and Discussion
The answer is c. Low cardiac output and large pressure gradient between the left ventricle and aorta in systole diagnose aortic stenosis.

11. Indications for surgical treatment in severe aortic regurgitation include the following, *except*
a) Left ventricular ejection fraction of 53%
b) Increasing left ventricular size on sequential echo (left ventricular end-systolic dimension 6 cm)
c) Shortness of breath
d) Aortic root size >6 cm
e) Anginal chest pain

Answer and Discussion
The answer is a. Reduced left ventricular ejection fraction, to <50%, is considered an indication for surgery.

12. A 27-year-old woman has recent onset of shortness of breath going upstairs and a history of palpitations. Physical examination reveals a regular pulse, loud S$_1$, and an apical diastolic murmur. The most likely diagnosis is
a) Aortic stenosis
b) Mitral stenosis
c) Aortic regurgitation
d) Tricuspid stenosis
e) None of the above

Answer and Discussion
The answer is b. Mitral stenosis.

SUGGESTED READINGS

Bonow RO, Carabello BA, Kanu C, et al. ACC/AHA 2006 guidelines for the management of patients with valvular heart disease: a report of the American College of Cardiology/American Heart Association Task Force on Practice Guidelines (writing committee to revise the 1998 Guidelines for the Management of Patients With Valvular Heart Disease): developed in collaboration with the Society of Cardiovascular Anesthesiologists: endorsed by the Society for Cardiovascular Angiography and Interventions and the Society of Thoracic Surgeons. *Circulation* 2006;114(5):e84–e231.

Griffin BP, Rimmerman CM, Topol EJ, eds. Valvular Heart Disease section. In: *The Cleveland Clinic Cardiology Board Review*. Philadelphia: Lippincott Williams & Wilkins, 2006.

Griffin BP, Topol EJ, eds. *Manual of Cardiovascular Medicine*, 2nd ed. Philadelphia: Lippincott Williams & Wilkins, 2004.

Hayek E, Gring CN, Griffin BP. Mitral valve prolapse. *Lancet* 2005; 365:507–518.

Levine HJ, Gaasch WH. Vasoactive drugs in chronic regurgitant lesions of the mitral and aortic valves. *J Am Coll Cardiol* 1996;28:1083.

Wilson W, Taubert KA, Gewitz M, et al. Prevention of infective endocarditis: guidelines from the American Heart Association: a guideline from the American Heart Association Rheumatic Fever, Endocarditis, and Kawasaki Disease Committee, Council on Cardiovascular Disease in the Young, and the Council on Clinical Cardiology, Council on Cardiovascular Surgery and Anesthesia, and the Quality of Care and Outcomes Research Interdisciplinary Working Group. *Circulation* 2007;116(15):1736–1754.

Chapter 61

Arrhythmias

Mina K. Chung

POINTS TO REMEMBER:

- Automaticity is the property of a cell or fiber to initiate a spontaneous impulse without previous stimulation. Spontaneously discharging cardiac cells that initiate spontaneous action potentials during phase 4 diastolic depolarization result in automaticity.

- Unlike automaticity, which does not require previous stimulation to occur, triggered activity is initiated by oscillations in the membrane potential (i.e., afterdepolarizations) that are induced by preceding action potentials.

- The most common mechanism of tachyarrhythmias is reentry.

- In narrow QRS complex tachycardias, the relationship of the QRS complex and P waves can be important in establishing the diagnosis.

- The diagnosis of wide complex tachycardia (WCT) often can be established on the basis of clinical presentation, physical examination, ECG findings, and provocative maneuvers. As a general rule, however, treat as a ventricular tachycardia (VT) when in doubt, particularly in patients with structural heart disease.

- QRS complex morphology can help to distinguish supraventricular tachycardia (SVT) with aberrancy from VT. QRS concordance in leads V_1 through V_6 is predictive of VT but also can be seen in patients with Wolff-Parkinson-White syndrome.

- Age, valvular disease, congestive heart failure, hypertension, and diabetes mellitus are independent risk factors for atrial fibrillation. Other associated conditions include rheumatic heart disease (especially mitral valve disease), nonrheumatic valvular disease, cardiomyopathies, congenital heart disease, pulmonary embolism, thyrotoxicosis, chronic lung disease, sick sinus syndrome, and degenerative conduction system disease, Wolff-Parkinson-White syndrome, pericarditis, neoplastic disease, postoperative states, and normal hearts affected by high adrenergic states, alcohol, stress, drugs (especially sympathomimetics), excessive caffeine, hypoxia, hypokalemia, hypoglycemia, or systemic infection.

Cardiac arrhythmias can be categorized on the basis of mechanisms, rates, and associated risk. When considering rate, tachycardias generally consist of arrhythmias with rates >100 beats per minute. Significant bradycardias generally consist of arrhythmias with rates <60 beats per minute. The appropriate diagnosis and assessment of the risk associated with arrhythmias are important to their treatment.

TACHYARRHYTHMIAS

Mechanisms

The mechanisms underlying cardiac arrhythmias usually are categorized into disorders of impulse formation, impulse conduction, or a combination of both.

Disorders of Impulse Formation

Automaticity

Automaticity is the property of a cell or fiber to initiate a spontaneous impulse without previous stimulation. Spontaneously discharging cardiac cells that initiate spontaneous action potentials during phase 4 diastolic depolarization result in automaticity. Cells that can exhibit spontaneous phase 4 diastolic depolarization are located in the sinus node, atria, atrioventricular junction, and His-Purkinje system. Normal automaticity generally occurs in normal cells with normal membrane resting potentials. It can be suppressed by overdrive pacing but generally resumes after the termination of pacing. The rate at which the sinus node discharges usually is faster than, and suppresses, the discharge rate of other potential latent or subsidiary automatic pacemaker sites. Normal or abnormal automaticity at the sinus node or other ectopic sites, however, can lead to rates that are faster and can gain control of the cardiac rhythm for one or more cycles. This may manifest if the discharge rate of the sinus node slows or that of the latent pacemaker increases. Subsidiary pacemakers can become dominant in the settings of acidosis, ischemia, sympathetic stimulation, and use of certain drugs.

Abnormal Automaticity. Normal myocardial cells maintain membrane resting potentials at approximately −90 mV, and they depolarize only when stimulated. Abnormal automaticity, however, can occur in cells with reduced maximum diastolic potentials, often at membrane potentials of −50 to −60 mV. The partial depolarization and failure to reach or maintain the normal maximum diastolic potential may induce automatic discharge. Examples of tachycardias that likely result from abnormal automaticity include accelerated junctional rhythm (i.e., nonparoxysmal junctional tachycardia), accelerated idioventricular rhythms, certain atrial tachycardias, some VTs in patients without structural heart disease, exercise-induced VT, VT during the first several hours of myocardial infarction (MI), and some VTs in patients with marked electrolyte imbalance.

Triggered Activity

Unlike automaticity, which does not require previous stimulation to occur, triggered activity is initiated by oscillations in the membrane potential (i.e., afterdepolarizations) that are induced by preceding action potentials. Afterdepolarizations that occur before full repolarization is completed are called *early afterdepolarizations* (EAD); those that occur after completion of repolarization, during phase 4, are called *delayed afterdepolarizations* (DAD). If afterdepolarizations reach threshold potential, an action potential can be generated, which potentially can trigger another or repetitive afterdepolarization(s).

Early Afterdepolarizations. Occurring during phase 2 or 3 of the action potential, EADs are thought to be responsible for VTs associated with prolonged repolarization, such as long QT syndromes (acquired or congenital) and torsades de pointes (TdP). Rapid rates and magnesium both suppress EADs as well as these arrhythmias. Experimentally, EADs can be produced by hypoxia and cesium as well as class IA (e.g., quinidine) and III potassium channel blocker (e.g., sotalol) antiarrhythmic agents.

Delayed Afterdepolarizations. Occurring after repolarization during phase 4, DADs have been demonstrated in Purkinje fibers as well as in atrial and ventricular fibers exposed to digitalis. Faster rates may augment DADs and are associated with an increase in intracellular calcium overload. Clinically, DADs have been classically implicated in digitalis toxicity as well as in those tachyarrhythmias associated with catecholamine excess, acidosis, MI, and certain VTs (e.g., catecholaminergic polymorphic ventricular tachycardia [CPVT].

Disorders of Impulse Conduction

Conduction delay or block can produce bradyarrhythmias or tachyarrhythmias. The most common mechanism of tachyarrhythmias is reentry. Classically, reentry requires:

- Alternate or separate pathways of conduction as defined by anatomic barriers (e.g., myocardial scar, atrioventricular node, or an accessory pathway) or functional properties (e.g., no anatomic boundaries but contiguous fibers with different electrophysiological properties, such as local differences in refractoriness, excitability, or anisotropic intercellular resistances)
- An area of unidirectional block in one pathway
- An area of conduction in the alternate pathway that is slow enough for the propagating and returning impulse to meet and excite tissue proximal to the block that has recovered (Fig. 61.1)

Reentry is thought to be the mechanism underlying many recurrent paroxysmal tachycardias, including

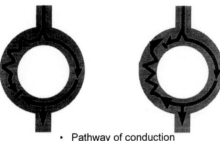

- Pathway of conduction
- Unidirectional block
- Slow conduction

Figure 61.1   Reentry.

atrial flutter, atrioventricular nodal reentry, atrioventricular reentry involving accessory pathways (including Wolff-Parkinson-White syndrome), and most VTs associated with ischemic heart disease and previous MI.

Diagnosis

Patient History and Physical Examination

A key to diagnosing and appropriately treating patients with arrhythmias is the determination of the underlying, predisposing cardiac substrate. Known structural heart disease, particularly in patients with known coronary artery disease or ischemic or nonischemic cardiomyopathies, can greatly influence both treatment and diagnosis. Patients presenting with wide QRS complex tachycardias and previous MI almost always have VT. Triggering agents (e.g., inotropic or QT-prolonging drugs) or events may be important to longer-term treatment and the subsequent prevention of arrhythmias. In addition to hemodynamic status and the evidence of underlying ventricular dysfunction, helpful physical findings include evidence of atrioventricular dissociation (i.e., cannon A waves in the jugular venous pulse) and termination or slowing with vagal maneuvers (e.g., carotid sinus massage, Valsalva maneuver, cough, cold-water immersion) or adenosine.

Differential Diagnosis

Tachyarrhythmias can be classified into wide versus narrow QRS complex and regular versus irregular tachycardia (Table 61.1). An ECG evaluation of tachycardias should begin by assessing the rate, regularity, and QRS complex width. Narrow QRS complex tachycardias, which are defined as tachycardias with a QRS complex width <120 ms, implies ventricular activation over the rapidly conducting His-Purkinje system, which in turn suggests an SVT (a tachycardia requiring atrial or atrioventricular junctional tissue for initiation or maintenance). Irregularity of the ventricular rate during an SVT suggests atrial fibrillation, atrial flutter with variable block, or multifocal atrial tachycardia. A wide QRS complex tachycardia may result from VT or SVT and is discussed later.

TABLE 61.1

DIFFERENTIAL DIAGNOSIS OF TACHYCARDIAS

Regular Rhythm	Irregular Rhythm
Narrow QRS complex	
Atrial tachycardia	Atrial fibrillation
Sinus tachycardia	Atrial flutter, variable AV block
Sinus node reentry	Multifocal atrial tachycardia
Ectopic atrial tachycardia	
Atrial flutter, fixed AV block	
AV nodal reentrant tachycardia	
Orthodromic AV reentry	
Wide QRS complex	
VT	VT
SVT	Atrial fibrillation with
Preexisting BBB	Preexisting BBB
Functional BBB	Functional BBB
Preexcitation	Preexcitation
Antidromic AV reentry	TdP
Bystander accessory pathway	

AV, atrioventricular; BBB, bundle-branch block; SVT, supraventricular tachycardia; TdP, torsades de pointes; VT, ventricular tachycardia.

Narrow QRS Complex Tachycardias

ECG evaluation of narrow QRS complex tachycardias should include assessment of:

- Rate
- Regularity
- QRS complex width
- Atrial activation pattern and relationship to the QRS complex (RP/PR relationship, morphology of the P wave)
- QRS complex morphology
- Effect of bundle-branch block (BBB) aberration (if present)
- Mode of initiation
- Effect of vagal maneuvers and drugs

SVTs may be classified as:

- Sinus node tachycardias
  - Inappropriate sinus tachycardia
  - Sinus node reentry
- Atrial tachycardias
  - Automatic
  - Reentrant
  - Ectopic
- Atrial flutter
- Atrial fibrillation
- Multifocal atrial tachycardia
- Junctional tachycardias
  - Nonparoxysmal
  - Automatic
- Atrioventricular nodal reentry
  - Typical
  - Atypical

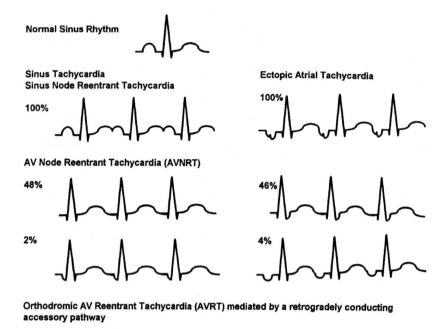

Figure 61.2 Relationships and configurations of QRS and P waves in supraventricular tachycardia. (AV, atrioventricular.) (Adapted from Josephson ME. *Clinical Cardiac Electrophysiology: Techniques and Interpretation*, 2nd ed. Malvern, PA: Lea & Febiger, 1993:269.)

■ Atrioventricular reciprocating tachycardia and other SVTs associated with accessory pathways

In narrow QRS complex tachycardias, the relationship of the QRS complex and P waves can be important in establishing the diagnosis. Figure 61.2 shows the QRS complex and P-wave relationships and configurations commonly seen in patients with various SVTs, and these conditions are discussed further in later sections on specific arrhythmias. In typical atrioventricular nodal reentrant tachycardia (AVNRT), which is characterized by near simultaneous atrial and ventricular activation, the P wave is buried in the QRS complex, and it either is not visible or is detected at the end of the QRS complex (within 80 ms) in 94% of cases. In 2% of cases, the P wave barely precedes the QRS complex and can be diagnostic. Atypical AVNRT occurs in 4% of cases and is characterized by a long RP interval and a short PR interval, with inverted P waves in the inferior (i.e., II, III, aVF) leads. In orthodromic atrioventricular reentrant tachycardia (AVRT) mediated by a retrograde-conducting accessory pathway, the retrograde P wave often can be detected early in the ST segment. Slowly conducting retrograde accessory pathways can have long RP intervals. Atrial tachycardias, sinus tachycardia, and sinoatrial node reentrant tachycardia have long RP and short PR intervals, with the P-wave morphology differing from that of sinus rhythm in ectopic atrial tachycardias but being similar in sinoatrial node reentrant tachycardia or sinus tachycardia. Thus, close examination of the PR and RP intervals can be helpful.

The differential diagnosis of short RP (i.e., RP interval shorter than the PR interval) and long RP (i.e., RP interval longer than the PR interval) SVTs is further illustrated in Figure 61.3. Short RP narrow complex tachycardias most likely result from AVNRT or orthodromic AVRT mediated by a retrograde-conducting accessory pathway; atrial tachycardia is a much less likely cause. Long RP narrow complex tachycardias result from atrial (or sinus) tachycardias, atypical AVNRT, or orthodromic AVRT mediated by a slow-retrograde-conducting accessory pathway.

Wide QRS Complex Tachycardias

WCT has a QRS duration of 120 ms or longer with a ventricular rate of 100 beats per minute or more.

The differential diagnosis of WCT includes:

■ VT
■ SVT
　■ SVT with preexisting BBB or intraventricular conduction defect
　■ SVT with aberrant His-Purkinje system conduction (i.e., functional BBB)
　■ Ashman phenomenon after long–short RR interval
　■ Rate-related, acceleration-dependent BBB
　■ Maintenance of functional BBB by transseptal concealed conduction (i.e., linking)
　■ SVT with antegrade conduction via an accessory pathway
　■ Antidromic SVT with antegrade conduction via an accessory pathway
　■ Atrial fibrillation/flutter/tachycardia with antegrade conduction via an accessory pathway

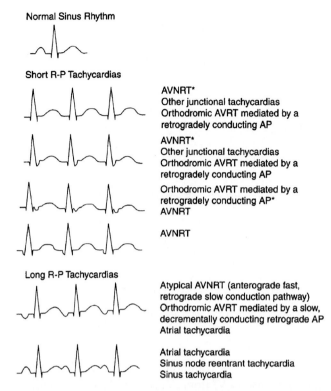

Figure 61.3 Differential diagnosis of supraventricular tachycardias by RP/PR relationships and P-wave configurations. (*, most common; AP, accessory pathway; AVNRT, atrioventricular nodal reentrant tachycardia; AVRT, atrioventricular reentrant tachycardia.) (Adapted from Josephson ME. *Clinical Cardiac Electrophysiology: Techniques and Interpretation*, 2nd ed. Malvern, PA: Lea & Febiger, 1993:270.)

- AVNRT with antegrade conduction down a bystander accessory pathway
- SVT with slowed conduction because of electrolyte or metabolic imbalance or an antiarrhythmic drug

The diagnosis of WCT often can be established on the basis of clinical presentation, physical examination, ECG findings, and provocative maneuvers. As a general rule, however, treat as a VT when in doubt, particularly in patients with structural heart disease.

Clinical Presentation

In multiple studies, VT was the correct diagnosis in more than 80% of patients presenting with WCT. VT is more likely to occur in older patients, but age alone is not a useful marker. In very young patients (<20 years), SVT is a more frequent cause of WCT. VT can occur in younger patients with structurally normal hearts, but this is less common. Hemodynamic instability is a poor discriminating factor, because hemodynamic stability depends on rate, ventricular function, cardiac disease, and concomitant pharmacologic therapy. A history of structural heart disease, particularly of coronary artery disease with previous MI, is important. In patients with a history of MI, 98% of WCTs result from VT; a history of MI and symptoms of tachycardia starting only after the MI strongly favor VT.

Physical Examination. Rate and blood pressure are not useful in determining the cause of WCTs. The finding of atrioventricular dissociation, however, strongly favors VT. This is because approximately two-thirds of patients with VT have atrioventricular dissociation at electrophysiology study, and atrioventricular dissociation is rare in SVT. An asynchronous contraction of the atria and ventricles can cause cannon A waves in the jugular venous pulsation, wide split heart sounds, variable S_1, and variability in blood pressure resulting from changes in stroke volume with atrioventricular dissociation.

Provocative Maneuvers. Vagal maneuvers can depress sinus node automaticity and slow atrioventricular nodal conduction. A gradual slowing of the rate of the WCT suggests sinus tachycardia. A termination of the rhythm suggests reentry involving the atrioventricular node or sinus node (e.g., sinoatrial node reentrant tachycardia, AVNRT, AVRT). Transient atrioventricular block with continuing atrial activation suggests atrial tachycardia, atrial fibrillation, or atrial flutter. VT rarely is affected by vagal maneuvers.

It is important that intravenous verapamil not be used to treat WCT, because hemodynamic collapse and death have been reported, regardless of the cause of the WCT. Adenosine has a much shorter duration of action (i.e., seconds) and is delivered intravenously as a 6- to 12-mg rapid bolus. Like vagal maneuvers, adenosine can terminate supraventricular arrhythmias resulting from reentry involving the atrioventricular or sinus node, or it can allow the demonstration of atrial flutter waves, atrial tachycardia, or atrial fibrillation. Some uncommon forms of VT in structurally normal hearts can be terminated by vagal maneuvers or adenosine.

Electrocardiographic Findings. In patients with preexisting complete BBB, the QRS complex is wide, and a comparison with previous ECGs can be helpful. The QRS complex may be wide in any supraventricular rhythm, however, if functional aberrancy occurs. Patients receiving antiarrhythmic drugs, particularly class IC agents, may develop rate-related aberrancy. Preexcitation via an anterograde-conducting accessory pathway (i.e., Wolff-Parkinson-White syndrome) also causes a wide QRS complex. The ECG should be analyzed with specific attention paid to the atrioventricular relationship, presence of capture or fusion beats, and QRS duration, axis, and morphology.

Fusion beats (Fig. 61.4) occur when conducted supraventricular impulses depolarize the ventricle coincident with ventricular depolarization from the VT circuit. A narrower, usually intermediate-width QRS complex results. Narrow beats during WCT strongly favor the diagnosis of VT, but they are not pathognomonic (e.g., premature ventricular contraction [PVC] during SVT with BBB could also result in a narrower QRS complex).

Capture beats (Fig. 61.4) represent the conduction of a supraventricular impulse to the ventricle and

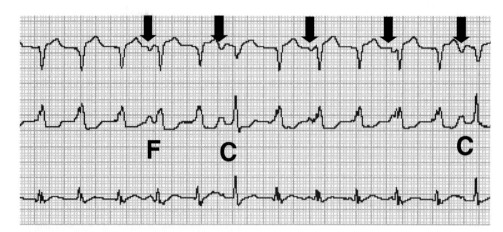

Figure 61.4   Ventricular tachycardia confirmed by the presence of fusion (*F*) and capture (*C*) beats. Atrioventricular dissociation is evident, with *arrows* indicating P waves. Ventricular fusion beats occur with a narrower QRS when the ventricle is activated from two different sites (e.g., supraventricular conduction to the ventricles during VT or premature ventricular complex during SVT with aberrancy). Sinus capture beats during VT are a form of fusion, but the narrow complexes occur with a shorter coupling interval (than the VT interval), denoting a sinus beat has captured the ventricle during VT. This indicates that the rhythm is VT, as a shorter coupling interval during SVT with aberrancy would result in no change in or a wider QRS duration.

depolarization before it is depolarized by the VT circuit. It appears as a narrow complex beat with a shorter coupling interval than the tachycardia interval, which indicates that the WCT is VT. Capture beats virtually exclude SVT with aberrancy, because they occur after a shorter interval with a narrow QRS complex; aberrancy is more likely to occur with wider QRS complexes after shorter rather than longer intervals.

Atrioventricular dissociation (Fig. 61.4) strongly favors the diagnosis of VT, but this feature is not always identifiable on surface ECGs. One-third of VTs may have 1:1 ventriculoatrial (VA) conduction. Even so, variable retrograde VA conduction, or VA Wenckebach conduction, strongly suggests VT. Rare SVTs may exhibit VA dissociation (e.g., automatic junctional tachycardia with retrograde block). The recording of an atrial electrogram through a right atrial or an esophageal electrode may facilitate assessment.

QRS complex morphology can help to distinguish SVT with aberrancy from VT. QRS concordance in leads V_1 through V_6 is predictive of VT but also can be seen in patients with Wolff-Parkinson-White syndrome. Delayed or slowed initial QRS deflection suggests VT. The QRS complex morphology can be classified into a left BBB or a right BBB pattern on the basis of QRS polarity in V_1. Right BBB morphology has a predominantly positive QRS deflection, and left BBB morphology a predominantly negative QRS deflection, in V_1. In right BBB morphology WCT (Fig. 61.5), a monophasic R, qR, RS, or R greater than r′ pattern in V_1 favors VT. In V_6, a QS, QR, or monophasic R pattern also favors VT. In contrast, triphasic complexes in V_1 or V_6 favor SVT. In left BBB morphology WCT (Fig. 61.6), an R in V_1 or V_2 of ≥40 ms, notched downstroke on the S wave in V_1 or V_2, any Q in V_6, or more than 60 ms from the QRS onset to the S nadir in V_1 or V_2 favors VT.

Brugada Criteria. A commonly used four-level algorithm for distinguishing VT from SVT (i.e., the Brugada criteria) is shown in **Figure 61.7**. This algorithm was prospectively validated for more than 500 WCTs with electrophysiological diagnoses. It had a high sensitivity (0.987) and specificity (0.965). Using these criteria, if no RS can be identified in any precordial lead, VT is diagnosed. If an RS complex is present and the RS interval is longer than 100 ms, VT is diagnosed. If the RS interval is shorter than 100 ms, evidence of atrioventricular dissociation indicates VT. If none of the

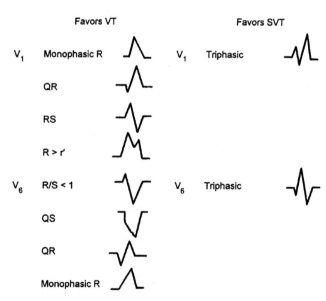

Figure 61.5   Right bundle-branch block morphologic criteria for distinguishing ventricular tachycardia (*VT*) from supraventricular tachycardia (*SVT*). (Adapted from Wellens HJJ, Bar FWHM, Lie KI. The value of the electrocardiogram in the differential diagnosis of a tachycardia with a widened QRS complex. *Am J Med* 1978;64: 27–33.)

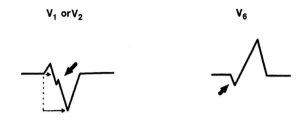

V₁ orV₂   **V₆**

1   R in V₁ or V₂ ≥ 40 ms sec.

2   >60 msec from QRS onset to S nadir in V₁ or V₂.

3   Notched downstroke S wave in V₁ or V₂.

4   Any Q in V₆.

Figure 61.6 Left bundle-branch block morphologic criteria for ventricular tachycardia in leads V₁ and V₆. (Adapted from Kindwall KE, Brown J, Josephson ME. Electrocardiographic criteria for ventricular tachycardia in wide complex left bundle-branch block morphology tachycardias. *Am J Cardiol* 1988;61:1279–1283.)

first three criteria is met, then morphologic criteria for VT are analyzed in leads V₁ or V₂ as well as V₆. If both leads fulfill the criteria for VT, then VT is diagnosed; otherwise, the diagnosis of SVT with aberrancy is made by exclusion of VT.

Other ECG clues include the consistent initiation of WCT by premature atrial contractions, which favors a supraventricular rhythm. The initiation of WCT preceded by constant PP intervals, but a short PR interval (with the QRS complex fused to the P wave) in patients without preexcitation, suggests VT. Grossly irregular RR intervals suggest atrial fibrillation. If a rapid, irregular WCT has beat-to-beat variation in the QRS complex duration,

Wolff-Parkinson-White syndrome should be suspected. A comparison with previous sinus rhythm ECGs is helpful to determine preexisting preexcitation or baseline BBB/intraventricular conduction defect.

A QRS complex duration of longer than 140 ms with WCT of right BBB morphology, or of longer than 160 ms with left BBB morphology, favors the diagnosis of VT. Most SVTs with aberrancy have QRS complex durations of ≤140 ms, but wide QRS complex durations can be seen with preexcitation and marked baseline intraventricular conduction defects. In addition, 15% to 35% of patients with VT also may have QRS complex durations of ≤140 ms.

QRS axis deviation with a right superior axis (i.e., negative in I, aVF) suggests VT. Left superior axis (i.e., left axis deviation; negative in aVF, II; positive in I) in WCT with right BBB morphology suggests VT, but it is not helpful in WCT with left BBB morphology.

Management

For hemodynamically unstable WCT, including pulmonary edema or severe angina, cardioversion should be performed. Sedation should be given before cardioversion if the patient is awake. For hemodynamically stable WCT, a clinical history (including cardiac disease, previous arrhythmias, previous MI, drug use) should be elicited and physical examination performed (including inspection for cannon A waves). A 12-lead ECG and laboratory studies to exclude electrolyte and metabolic abnormalities, ischemia, hypoxia, or drug toxicity should be obtained. If the diagnosis is in doubt, placement of an esophageal lead can be considered. Adenosine, 6 to 12 mg delivered intravenously as a rapid bolus, can be given if there is evidence for SVT. Lidocaine or procainamide can be attempted as well, and

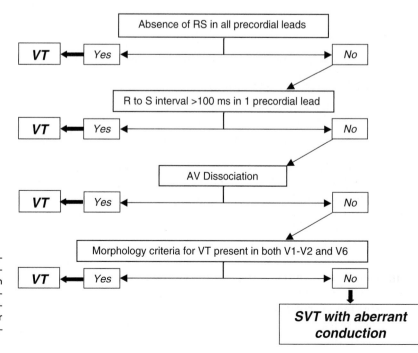

Figure 61.7 Brugada criteria for distinguishing ventricular tachycardia (*VT*) from supraventricular tachycardia (*SVT*) in tachycardia with widened QRS complexes. (Adapted from Brugada P, Brugada J, Mont L, et al. A new approach to the differential diagnosis of a regular tachycardia with a wide QRS complex. *Circulation* 1991;83:1649–1659.)

if the WCT persists, intravenous amiodarone can be considered. Cardioversion under anesthesia or overdrive pace termination can be attempted for persistent WCT. If WCT is incessant, consider the possibility of electrolyte abnormalities, digitalis toxicity, acute severe ischemia, reperfusion arrhythmias, proarrhythmia, or TdP. Consideration also should be given to empiric MgSO$_4$, treatment for acute ischemia or MI, and intravenous amiodarone.

An evaluation after the termination of WCT should include a consideration of electrophysiological testing, if WCT etiology remains indeterminate. Subsequent therapy depends on the diagnosis but can include pharmacologic, ablation, or device therapies.

SPECIFIC SUPRAVENTRICULAR ARRHYTHMIAS

Atrial Premature Depolarizations

Atrial premature depolarizations can be frequent and occasionally symptomatic. Although not associated with significant risk, they can be associated with underlying cardiovascular or pulmonary disease. Treatment generally includes reassurance, avoidance of precipitating factors (e.g., caffeine, sympathomimetic agents), occasionally β-blockers or calcium channel blockers, and rarely class I or III antiarrhythmic drugs or ablation.

Sinus Tachycardia

Sinus tachycardia is defined in an adult as a sinus rate >100 beats per minute. The sinus node is located in the high right atrium and is sensitive to catecholamines and autonomic tone. Therefore, sinus tachycardia may be secondary to many physiological and pathological states. It is a normal response to exertion, anxiety, and a variety of stresses, including fever, hypotension, hypovolemia, hyperthyroidism, congestive heart failure, pulmonary embolism, myocardial ischemia or infarction, inflammation, and drugs such as catecholamines, caffeine, alcohol, or nicotine. Because of the location and automatic properties associated with the sinus node, physiological sinus tachycardia has normal P-wave morphology (i.e., upright in II, III, and aVF) and exhibits gradual rate acceleration and deceleration that varies with changes in the autonomic tone and volume. Treatment should focus on the cause of sinus tachycardia, avoidance of stimulants, fluid replacement in patients with hypovolemia, fever reduction, and, possibly, β-blockers or calcium channel blockers.

Inappropriate Sinus Tachycardia

Inappropriate sinus tachycardia, in which otherwise healthy patients have chronic, nonparoxysmal sinus tachycardia without apparent cause or at an inappropriate rate, may result from increased automaticity, increased sympathetic tone, increased sensitivity to catecholamines, decreased vagal tone, or an automatic atrial focus located near the sinus node. Treatment may require β-adrenergic blockers, calcium channel blockers, digitalis, or sinus node catheter modification or surgical ablation.

Sinus Node Reentry

Sinus node reentry, which only rarely occurs, may be difficult to distinguish from sinus tachycardia. However, the onset typically is sudden and paroxysmal, and it often is precipitated by a premature atrial beat, which is important in establishing the diagnosis. The heart rate can vary from 80 to 200 beats per minute but generally is slower than in other SVTs, with an average rate of 130 to 140 beats per minute. The rate also can fluctuate with the autonomic tone. P-wave morphology demonstrates a high-to-low atrial activation sequence (i.e., upright in II, III, aVF) that is identical to sinus rhythm in morphology. The PR interval relates to the SVT rate, with a long RP interval and a shorter PR interval. Atrioventricular block can occur (e.g., Wenckebach) without affecting the tachycardia. Vagal maneuvers (e.g., carotid sinus massage, Valsalva maneuver) or adenosine can slow and terminate the tachycardia. Drugs, such as β-blockers or calcium channel blockers, as well as class I or III antiarrhythmic agents, also have been used successfully. Surgical or radiofrequency catheter ablation occasionally may be indicated.

Atrial Tachycardias

Tachycardias originating in the atria at sites other than the sinus or atrioventricular node are called *atrial*, or *ectopic atrial*, *tachycardias*. Heart rates generally are regular, ranging from 100 to 250 (generally 150–200) beats per minute, with a P-wave morphology differing from that in sinus rhythm and isoelectric periods between P waves, thus distinguishing it from atrial flutter or atrial fibrillation. A long RP interval (with a shorter PR interval) that is variable in duration usually is present. Atrioventricular conduction block (i.e., spontaneous Wenckebach second-degree atrioventricular block or atrioventricular block induced by carotid sinus massage, other vagal maneuvers, or adenosine) typically does not terminate the tachycardia. A positive or biphasic P wave in aVL suggests a right atrial origin. A positive P wave in V$_1$ suggests a left atrial focus. At physical examination, rapid A waves in the jugular venous pulse may be evident.

Atrial tachycardia can occur paroxysmally in short, nonsustained runs or in longer, sustained runs, and they occasionally may be incessant, potentially leading to a tachycardia-mediated cardiomyopathy. It often is associated with significant structural heart disease, pulmonary disease, hyperthyroidism, or digitalis intoxication. Three mechanisms of atrial tachycardias have been described: abnormal automaticity, reentry, and triggered activity. In general, and depending on the clinical situation, treatment in patients not receiving digitalis may include atrioventricular node–blocking agents (e.g., calcium channel blockers,

β-adrenergic blockers, digitalis); class IA, IC, or III antiarrhythmic agents; or surgical or radiofrequency catheter ablation.

Atrial Tachycardia With Block Resulting from Digitalis Toxicity

In digitalis toxicity, the concomitant impairment of atrioventricular conduction can cause atrial tachycardia with block, and triggered activity (i.e., DAD) is believed to be the mechanism responsible for the atrial tachycardia. This may occur in patients with atrial fibrillation or flutter, but it can be distinguished by isoelectric periods between P waves. Treatment includes cessation of digitalis, administration of potassium (if the potassium level is not already elevated) and, depending on the ventricular rate and presence of other digitalis-toxic arrhythmias, potentially a β-adrenergic blocker, lidocaine, or phenytoin.

Automatic Atrial Tachycardia

Automatic atrial tachycardia generally is characterized by a warm-up phenomenon, in which the heart rate gradually accelerates after initiation. Usually, it can be overdrive suppressed, but not terminated, through pacing. Automatic atrial tachycardia can occur in all age groups and can be seen in association with MI, lung disease, alcohol ingestion, and metabolic abnormalities.

Reentrant Atrial Tachycardia

Reentrant atrial tachycardia can result from anatomic abnormalities, including surgical scars or atriotomy incisions. It can be initiated by premature atrial stimuli that induce conduction delay or block, usually can be terminated through atrial pacing, and not uncommonly is associated with atrial flutter.

Multifocal Atrial Tachycardia

Multifocal atrial tachycardia is characterized by a heart rate >100 beats per minute; multiple (three or more) P-wave morphologies; and variable PP, PR, and RR intervals. The multiple P-wave morphologies result from multiple depolarizing foci in the atria. The irregularly irregular ventricular rate can mimic atrial fibrillation, and a differentiation from "coarse" atrial fibrillation can be made by isoelectric periods between P waves. Multifocal atrial tachycardia predominantly occurs in patients who are elderly or critically ill with advanced chronic pulmonary disease. Other commonly associated conditions include pneumonia, infection or sepsis, postoperative states, lung cancer, pulmonary embolism, cor pulmonale, congestive heart failure, hypertensive heart disease, and other acute cardiac or pulmonary processes. Rarely, digoxin toxicity, hypokalemia, and hypomagnesemia may be associated. Multifocal atrial tachycardia also may progress to atrial fibrillation. In critically ill patients, it is associated with a high hospital mortality. Treatment is directed toward the underlying disease, which often is pulmonary. Antiarrhythmic agents often are ineffective, and β-blockers can be effective but often are contraindicated in patients with severe bronchospastic disease. Verapamil, amiodarone, and potassium, as well as magnesium replacement, have been helpful. The mechanism underlying multifocal atrial tachycardia may be enhanced automaticity or triggered activity.

Atrial Flutter

The incidence of atrial flutter is lower than that of atrial fibrillation, and two general categories of atrial flutter have been described. The typical (i.e., type I) form is caused by macroreentry in the right atrium. Atrial depolarization in this reentrant circuit typically propagates in the counterclockwise direction, craniocaudally down the free wall, through the cavotricuspid isthmus (between the tricuspid valve and inferior vena cava), and caudalcranially up the atrial septum. This pattern of atrial activation inscribes the typical sawtooth flutter waves on the surface ECG (Fig. 61.8) that typically are negative in the inferior leads (i.e., II, III, aVF). Clockwise propagation along the posterior corridor also can occur, producing positive flutter waves in the inferior leads. The atrial rate usually is 250 to 350 beats per minute, but this may be slowed by class IA, IC, and III antiarrhythmic drugs. Type I atrial flutter often can be terminated through atrial pacing. It also can be cured, with a success rate of 75% to 90%, by radiofrequency catheter ablation, in which the application of radiofrequency energy produces a line of conduction block across the cavotricuspid isthmus.

Atypical (i.e., type II) atrial flutter has an atrial rate that usually is 250 to 400 beats per minute and may not be influenced or terminated through atrial pacing. Atrial flutter/tachycardias due to reentrant circuits around areas of atrial scars or prior incisions may have slower rates, depending on the size of the macroreentrant pathway and atrial conduction times. In type II atrial flutter, the right atrial posterior corridor, as described in type I atrial flutter, is generally not a critical component of the reentrant circuit, with other right or left atrial pathways of conduction participating in the arrhythmia.

In untreated patients with type I atrial flutter, the atrial rate usually is 300 beats per minute, with 2:1 atrioventricular conduction and a ventricular rate of 150 beats per minute. Slower rates may occur with treatment (e.g., atrioventricular node–blocking agents) or atrioventricular nodal disease. The ventricular response often occurs with 2:1, 4:1, alternating 2:1/4:1, or variable conduction patterns. Thus, the ventricular rate may be constant or variable and irregular. Occasionally, 1:1 atrioventricular conduction can be seen in patients with preexcitation syndromes (e.g., Wolff-Parkinson-White syndrome), with hyperthyroidism, or in children, and this can be a medical emergency. Slowing of the atrial rate, as occurs with the administration of antiarrhythmic agents, also may result in 1:1 atrioventricular conduction. Vagal maneuvers or adenosine can help

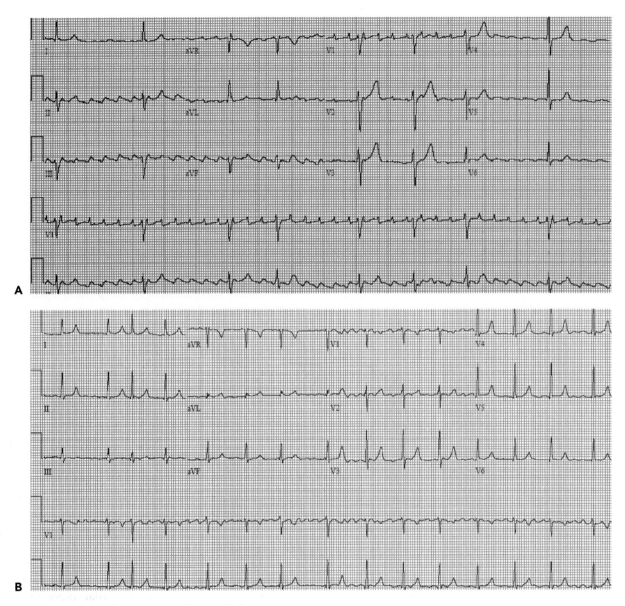

Figure 61.8   Atrial flutter **(A)** and atrial fibrillation **(B)**.

to establish the diagnosis by blocking the ventricular response and enhancing appreciation of the flutter waves. Esophageal or intracardiac atrial electrogram recordings can help in patients for whom the diagnosis remains unclear.

Paroxysmal atrial flutter can occur in patients without structural heart disease, but chronic, persistent atrial flutter most often occurs in patients with underlying heart disease. Conditions associated with atrial flutter include coronary artery disease, rheumatic heart disease, cardiomyopathy, hypertensive heart disease, pulmonary disease with or without cor pulmonale, hyperthyroidism, alcohol ingestion, pericarditis, acute MI, pulmonary embolism, septal defects, congenital heart disease, after surgical repair of congenital defects or valve disease, and other causes of atrial dilatation. In patients treated with class IC antiarrhythmic drugs that can significantly slow conduction, a

recurrence of atrial arrhythmias often occurs in the form of type I atrial flutter and tachycardia because significant slowing of conduction can facilitate reentry along the typical atrial flutter posterior corridor circuit.

The treatment of atrial flutter commonly involves controlling the ventricular response with agents such as verapamil, diltiazem, β-adrenergic blockers, or digoxin. Synchronized direct current (DC) cardioversion is effective and may require only low energies (i.e., 25–100 J). Rapid atrial overdrive pacing may terminate type I atrial flutter. Antiarrhythmic agents (i.e., class IA, IC, III) have been used successfully, but because the facilitation of atrioventricular conduction may occur during the use of class IA agents with vagolytic activity or class I or III agents that slow the atrial rate enough to allow 1:1 conduction, concomitant negative dromotropic (i.e., atrioventricular nodal slowing) agents may be required. The long-term prevention of atrial flutter has been difficult with medical treatment. As noted, however, type I atrial flutter can be cured, with a success rate of 75% to 90%, using radiofrequency catheter ablation. Atypical atrial flutters also may be approached with catheter ablation methods and advanced mapping techniques, although with success rates that are lower than those for type I atrial flutter. Radiofrequency ablation also has been used successfully as adjunctive therapy in patients on antiarrhythmic agents to cure the atrial flutter that can be facilitated by these agents.

Atrial Fibrillation

Atrial fibrillation is the most common sustained tachyarrhythmia. The incidence of atrial fibrillation increases with age. The most common underlying cardiovascular diseases associated with atrial fibrillation are hypertension and ischemic heart disease. Age, valvular disease, congestive heart failure, hypertension, and diabetes mellitus are independent risk factors for atrial fibrillation. Other associated conditions include rheumatic heart disease (especially mitral valve disease), nonrheumatic valvular disease, cardiomyopathies, congenital heart disease, pulmonary embolism, thyrotoxicosis, chronic lung disease, sick sinus syndrome and degenerative conduction system disease, Wolff-Parkinson-White syndrome, pericarditis, neoplastic disease, postoperative states, and normal hearts affected by high adrenergic states, alcohol, stress, drugs (especially sympathomimetics), excessive caffeine, hypoxia, hypokalemia, hypoglycemia, or systemic infection.

During atrial fibrillation, an electrical activation of the atria occurs in rapid, multiple waves of depolarization, with continuously changing, wandering pathways. Intra-atrial activation can be recorded as irregular, rapid depolarizations, often at rates exceeding 300 to 400 beats per minute. On the surface ECG, atrial fibrillation is characterized by an absence of discrete P waves, the presence of irregular fibrillatory waves, or both, as well as an irregularly irregular ventricular response. Complete BBB or aberrancy (e.g., Ashman phenomenon) can mimic VT. On physical examination, the pulse is irregularly irregular, variable stroke volumes may produce pulse deficits, and the jugular venous waveform lacks A waves. Mechanically, this pattern of rapid, disordered atrial activation results in a loss of coordinated atrial contraction. Irregular electrical inputs to the atrioventricular node lead to irregular ventricular rates.

Focally initiating atrial fibrillation is now recognized as a common cause of atrial fibrillation, particularly in lone atrial fibrillation that occurs in the absence of structural heart disease. Focally discharging triggers most frequently arise from the ostia of the pulmonary veins, and catheter or surgical pulmonary vein ostial isolation may achieve long-term cure, even in patients with structural heart disease.

One of the most important clinical consequences of atrial fibrillation is its association with thromboembolic events and stroke. A useful scoring system for assessing

TABLE 61.2

STROKE RISK ACCORDING TO THE CHADS$_2$ INDEX IN THE NATIONAL REGISTRY OF ATRIAL FIBRILLATION PARTICIPANTS WITH NONVALVULAR ATRIAL FIBRILLATION ($n = 1733$) NOT TREATED WITH ANTICOAGULATION

CHADS$_2$ Risk Criteria	Score
Prior stroke or TIA	2
Age >75 yr	1
Hypertension	1
Diabetes mellitus	1
Heart failure	1

CHADS$_2$ Score	Adjusted Stroke Rate, Percent per Year (95% CI)
0	1.9 (1.2–3.0)
1	2.8 (2.0–3.8)
2	4.0 (3.1–5.1)
3	5.9 (4.6–7.3)
4	8.5 (6.3–11.1)
5	12.5 (8.2–17.5)
6	18.2 (10.5–27.4)

CHADS$_2$, cardiac failure, hypertension, age, diabetes, and stroke (doubled); CI, confidence interval; TIA, transient ischemic attack. Adapted from van Walraven WC, Hart RG, Wells GA, et al. A clinical prediction rule to identify patients with atrial fibrillation and a low risk for stroke while taking aspirin. *Arch Intern Med* 2003;163:936–943; and Gage BF, Waterman AD, Shannon W, et al. Validation of clinical classification schemes for predicting stroke: results from the National Registry of Atrial Fibrillation. *JAMA* 2001;285:2864–2870.

thromboembolic risk is the CHADS$_2$ Index (Table 61.2), which helps to identify patients at high and low risk for stroke. Recommended guidelines for antithrombotic therapy are listed in Tables 61.3 and 61.4.

Acute Treatment

The acute treatment of atrial fibrillation that is symptomatic with an increased heart rate should include the consideration of urgent cardioversion if the patient is hemodynamically unstable (e.g., hypotensive) or has evidence of ischemia or pulmonary edema. For moderate to severe symptoms, acute control of the ventricular rate usually can be achieved using intravenous β-adrenergic blockers, verapamil, diltiazem, or digoxin (Table 61.5). Digoxin can be used safely in patients with heart failure, but it has a delayed peak onset of heart rate–lowering effect, a narrow therapeutic window, and is less effective in the rate control of paroxysmal atrial fibrillation or rapid rates during hyperadrenergic states when the vagal tone is low (such as in the intensive care unit) because of increased sympathetic tone. Pharmacologic or electrical cardioversion, the use of antiarrhythmic agents, and anticoagulation should be considered. Pharmacologic conversion can be attempted intravenously, using ibutilide, amiodarone or procainamide, or orally, using class I or III antiarrhythmic agents (Table 61.6). If the duration of atrial fibrillation is more than

TABLE 61.3

AMERICAN COLLEGE OF CARDIOLOGY/AMERICAN HEART ASSOCIATION/EUROPEAN SOCIETY OF CARDIOLOGY GUIDELINES FOR ANTITHROMBOTIC THERAPY FOR PATIENTS WITH ATRIAL FIBRILLATION

Risk Category	Recommended Therapy
No risk factors	Aspirin 81–325 mg daily
One moderate risk factor	Aspirin 81–325 mg daily or warfarin (INR 2.0–3.0, target 2.5)
Any high risk factor or >1 moderate risk factor	Warfarin (INR 2.0–3.0, target 2.5)[a]

Less-validated or Weaker Risk Factors	Moderate Risk Factors	High Risk Factors
Female gender	Age ≥75 yr	Previous stroke, TIA, or embolism
Age 65–74 yr	Hypertension	Mitral stenosis
Coronary artery disease	Heart failure	Prosthetic heart valve[a]
Thyrotoxicosis	LV ejection fraction ≤35%	
	Diabetes mellitus	

INR, international normalized ratio; LV, left ventricular; TIA, transient ischemic attack.
[a]If mechanical valve, target INR >2.5.
Adapted from Fuster V, Ryden LE, Cannom DS, et al. ACC/AHA/ESC 2006 guidelines for the management of patients with atrial fibrillation–executive summary. *Circulation* 2006;114;700–752.

TABLE 61.4

GUIDELINES FOR ELECTRICAL OR PHARMACOLOGIC CARDIOVERSION

Class I Recommendations
1. For AF of ≥48 hr duration, or when AF duration is unknown, anticoagulation (e.g., warfarin INR 2.0–3.0) is recommended for at least 3 wk prior to and 4 wk after cardioversion.
2. For AF >48 hr duration requiring immediate cardioversion because of hemodynamic instability, heparin should be administered concurrently (unless contraindicated) by an initial IV bolus injection followed by a continuous infusion (adjusted to aPTT 1.5–2.0 times the reference control value). Thereafter, oral anticoagulation (INR 2.0–3.0) should be provided for at least 4 wk, as for patients undergoing elective cardioversion. Limited data support subcutaneous administration of low molecular weight heparin in this indication.
3. For AF <48 hr duration associated with hemodynamic instability (angina pectoris, MI, shock, or pulmonary edema), cardioversion should be performed immediately without delay for prior initiation of anticoagulation.

Class IIa Recommendations
1. During the 48 h after onset of AF, the need for anticoagulation before and after cardioversion may be based on the patient's risk of thromboembolism.
2. As an alternative to anticoagulation prior to cardioversion of AF, it is reasonable to perform TEE in search of thrombus in the left atrium or left atrial appendage.
2a. For patients with no identifiable thrombus, cardioversion is reasonable immediately after anticoagulation with unfractionated heparin (e.g., initiated by IV bolus injection and an infusion adjusted to aPTT 1.5–2.0 times the control value until oral anticoagulation has been established with an oral vitamin K antagonist [e.g., warfarin] as evidenced by an INR ≥2.0). Thereafter, continuation of oral anticoagulation (INR 2.0–3.0) is reasonable for at least 4 wk, as for patients undergoing elective cardioversion. Limited data are available to support the subcutaneous administration of a low molecular weight heparin in this indication.
2b. For patients in whom thrombus is identified by TEE, oral anticoagulation (INR 2.0–3.0) is reasonable for at least 3 wk prior to and 4 wk after restoration of sinus rhythm, and a longer period of anticoagulation may be appropriate even after apparently successful cardioversion, because the risk of thromboembolism often remains elevated in such cases.
3. For patients with atrial flutter undergoing cardioversion, anticoagulation can be beneficial according to the recommendations as for patients with AF.

Long-term anticoagulation beyond the fourth week after cardioversion should be considered if other indications for long-term anticoagulation also exist, as listed in Table 61.3.

AF, atrial fibrillation; INR, international normalized ratio; IV, intravenous; MI, myocardial infarction;
TEE, transesophageal echocardiography.
Adapted from Fuster V, Ryden LE, Cannom DS, et al. ACC/AHA/ESC 2006 guidelines for the management of patients with atrial fibrillation—executive summary. *Circulation* 2006;114;700–752.

TABLE 61.5

MEDICAL TREATMENT FOR VENTRICULAR RATE CONTROL IN SUPRAVENTRICULAR ARRHYTHMIAS, INCLUDING ATRIAL FIBRILLATION

Agent	Loading Dose	Maintenance Dose	Side Effects/Toxicity	Comments
Digoxin	0.25–0.50 mg IV, then 0.25 mg IV every 4–6 hr to 1 mg in the first 24 hr	0.125–0.250 mg PO or IV every day	Anorexia, nausea, AV block, ventricular arrhythmias; accumulates in renal failure	Used in congestive heart failure, vagotonic effects on the AV node, delayed onset of action, narrow therapeutic window, less effective in paroxysmal atrial fibrillation or high adrenergic states
β-Adrenergic blockers	—	—		Effective in heart rate control even with exercise, rapid onsets of action
Propranolol	1 mg IV every 2–5 min to 0.1–0.2 mg/kg	10–80 mg PO TID to QID	Bronchospasm, congestive heart failure, decreased blood pressure	—
Metoprolol	5 mg IV every 5 min to 15 mg	25–100 mg PO BID	—	—
Esmolol	500 μg/kg IV over 1 min	50 μg/kg IV for 4 hr, repeat load as needed and increase maintenance to 20–50 μg/kg/min every 5–10 min as needed	—	Esmolol, short acting
Calcium channel blockers	—	—	Decreased blood pressure, congestive heart failure	Rapid onset, can be used safely in chronic obstructive pulmonary disease and diabetes mellitus
Verapamil	2.5–10.0 mg IV over 2 min	5–10 mg IV every 30–60 min or 40–160 mg PO TID	Increased digoxin level	—
Diltiazem	0.25 mg/kg over 2 hr, repeat as needed every 15 min at 0.35 mg/kg	5–15 mg/h IV or 30–90 mg PO QID	—	—
Sotalol	—	80–240 mg PO BID	Bradycardia, congestive heart failure, bronchospasm, decreased blood pressure, increased QT, TdP, proarrhythmia	—
Amiodarone	600–1,600 mg/day, divided	100–400 mg PO daily	Bradycardia, pulmonary, thyroid, liver, skin, gastrointestinal, ophthalmologic	Drug interactions
Adenosine	6–18 mg IV rapid bolus	—	Transient sinus bradycardia, sinus arrest, AV block, flushing, chest discomfort, bronchospasm; may precipitate atrial fibrillation by shortening of atrial refractoriness	Not effective in controlling ventricular rate in atrial fibrillation flutter, but may be useful diagnostically; can terminate reentrant paroxysmal supraventricular achycardias using the AV node

AV, atrioventricular; TdP, torsades de pointes.

TABLE 61.6

CLASS I AND III ANTIARRHYTHMIC AGENTS

Antiarrhythmic Drug	Dose	Side Effects/Comments
Class I Sodium channel blockers		
Class IA		Increased QT, proarrhythmia/TdP, potential increased AV node conduction can be seen with all three
Quinidine	200–400 mg PO TID to BID	Diarrhea, nausea, increased digoxin levels
Procainamide	10–15 mg/kg IV at 50 mg/min or 500–1,000 mg PO every 6 hr sustained release)	Decreased blood pressure, congestive heart failure, drug-induced lupus; metabolite N-acetylprocainamide (class III) can accumulate in renal failure
Disopyramide	100–300 mg PO TID	Anticholinergic effects (e.g., urinary retention, dry eyes/mouth), congestive heart failure
Class IB		
Lidocaine	50–100 mg IV (0.5–1.5 mg/kg) bolus, infusion of 1–4 mg/min, and rebolus in 5–15 min	Reduce dosage in congestive heart failure, elderly, hepatic dysfunction, bradycardia, hypotension, CNS side effects (tremors, seizures, altered mental status)
Mexiletine	150–300 mg PO every 8 hr	Gastrointestinal side effects (nausea, vomiting) common, may be minimized by dosing with meals; CNS effects (tremor, dizziness, nervousness)
Tocainide	400–600 mg PO every 8 hr	Gastrointestinal side effects (nausea, vomiting), CNS less common (dizziness, vertigo, nervousness); rare but potentially life-threatening agranulocytosis and pulmonary fibrosis
Phenytoin	100 mg PO every 8 hr; loading up to 1 g in divided doses; or 20–50 mg/min IV to maximum 1 g	Rarely used as an antiarrhythmic agent outside of digitalis toxicity; CNS side effects common; dermatologic reactions
Class IC		Proarrhythmia
Flecainide	50–200 mg PO BID	Visual disturbance, dizziness, congestive heart failure; avoid in coronary artery disease or left ventricular dysfunction
Propafenone	150–300 mg PO TID	Congestive heart failure, ? avoid in coronary artery disease/left ventricular dysfunction, β-blocker effects can slow metabolizers
Class IA/B/C		
Moricizine	200–300 mg PO TID	Proarrhythmia, dizziness, gastrointestinal/nausea, headache, caution in coronary artery disease/left ventricular dysfunction
Class III Potassium channel blockers		
Sotalol	80–240 mg PO BID	Congestive heart failure, bronchospasm, bradycardia, increased QT, proarrhythmia/TdP; renally excreted
Bretylium	5–10 mg/kg IV bolus; 1–2 mg/min IV infusion	Hypotension; transient increased arrhythmias possible due to initial norepinephrine release; reduce dose in renal failure
Amiodarone	600–1,600 mg/day loading in divided doses PO, 100–400 mg PO daily maintenance; IV available	Pulmonary toxicity, bradycardia, hyperthyroidism or hypothyroidism, hepatic toxicity, gastrointestinal (nausea, constipation), neurologic, dermatologic, and ophthalmologic side effects, drug interactions
Ibutilide	1.0 mg IV over 10 min, may repeat in 10 min	Monitor for QT prolongation, TdP
Dofetilide	125–500 μg PO every 12 hr; initial dose: CrCl (mL/min) >60: 500 μg BID; 40–60: 250 μg BID; 20–40: 125 μg BID.	In-hospital initiation mandated; exclude if CrCl <20 mL/min; monitor for QT prolongation, proarrhythmia/TdP; headache, muscle cramps

AV, atrioventricular; CNS, central nervous system; TdP, torsades de pointes.

48 hours, anticoagulation using warfarin for 3 weeks versus transesophageal echocardiographically guided cardioversion using anticoagulation should be considered (Table 61.4). For shorter durations of atrial fibrillation (i.e., <48 hours), anticoagulation still should be considered if the patient has underlying heart disease or risk factors for thromboembolism. Anticoagulation also should be considered for the pericardioversion period.

Long-term Treatment

The long-term treatment of atrial fibrillation should include evaluation for underlying structural heart disease, risk factors, and, potentially, other precipitating arrhythmias. Anticoagulation using warfarin or aspirin should be considered (Table 61.3). Control of the ventricular rate using β-blockers, calcium channel blockers, or digoxin also may be required (Table 61.5). In addition, restoring and maintaining sinus rhythm through cardioversion, maintenance antiarrhythmic therapy, or both can be considered. The Atrial Fibrillation Follow-up Investigation of Rhythm Management (AFFIRM) study, a large randomized trial of rate- vs. rhythm-control strategies for atrial fibrillation, showed no significant survival benefit for either approach, although a trend toward better survival was observed in the rate control arm. Nevertheless, for first-onset atrial fibrillation, or continued symptoms despite rate control, a rhythm control strategy still may be of some benefit. Available primary antiarrhythmic agents that may effectively maintain sinus rhythm include class IA (i.e., quinidine, procainamide, disopyramide), class IC (i.e., flecainide, propafenone), class IA/B/C (i.e., moricizine), and class III (i.e., sotalol, amiodarone, dofetilide) antiarrhythmic drugs (Table 61.6). Nonpharmacologic approaches include permanent pacemaker implantation for symptomatic bradyarrhythmias or tachycardia-bradycardia syndrome and include the use of mode-switching, dual-chamber devices for paroxysmal atrial fibrillation. Implantable defibrillators with programmable atrial therapies may be useful for some patients but are limited by discomfort from shocks. Strategies with the aim of curing atrial fibrillation include catheter or surgical ablation directed toward achieving electrical isolation of the pulmonary vein ostia. Catheter ablation of atrial fibrillation can be considered for symptomatic patients who have not responded to antiarrhythmic therapy. Radiofrequency energy is applied to the antra of the pulmonary vein ostia in a segmental or circumferential manner to isolate the ostia. Connecting areas between the ostia and fractionated electrical potentials may also be targeted. The maze procedure is a surgical option that was designed to cure atrial fibrillation by dividing the atria into mazelike corridors and blind alleys, which limit the development of reentry by limiting the available path length. Much of the success of this procedure likely has been due to surgically created pulmonary vein isolation. Currently, surgical ablation has the most use as a concomitant procedure during cardiac operations. For patients in whom mainte-

nance of sinus rhythm is poorly maintained and for whom rate control is suboptimal, complete atrioventricular junction ablation with the implantation of a rate-responsive, permanent pacemaker has produced symptomatic benefit, particularly in patients with difficult-to-control ventricular rates. However, atrioventricular junction ablation aims to create complete heart block, which renders the patient pacemaker dependent.

Junctional Tachycardias

Abnormal junctional tachycardias can be divided into nonreentrant and reentrant tachycardias.

Nonparoxysmal Junctional Tachycardia

Nonparoxysmal atrioventricular junctional tachycardia is characterized by gradual onset and termination, and it likely results from accelerated automatic discharge in or near the bundle of His. In this form of accelerated junctional rhythm, atrioventricular junctional tissue may exhibit faster discharge rates or usurp the dominant pacemaker status during sinus slowing. Heart rate generally ranges from 70 to 130 beats per minute, but it can be faster. Nonparoxysmal atrioventricular junctional tachycardia occasionally occurs in patients with underlying heart disease, such as acute MI, myocarditis, after open heart surgery (particularly valve procedures), or with digitalis intoxication. It also can occur in otherwise healthy, asymptomatic individuals. In infants or children, it is associated with a high mortality. Incessant tachycardia may lead to a tachycardia-mediated cardiomyopathy. Treatment generally is supportive and directed toward the underlying disease. Standard treatment for digitalis toxicity may be required. β-adrenergic blockers and class IA, IC, and III antiarrhythmic agents have been used, as has radiofrequency catheter ablation.

Atrioventricular Nodal Reentrant Tachycardia

The most common form of paroxysmal reentrant SVT is AVNRT, which accounts for 60% to 70% of patients with paroxysmal SVT. Reentry occurs within the atrioventricular node and perinodal tissue, and at least two functional pathways of conduction can be demonstrated within the atrioventricular node in patients with AVNRT (Fig. 61.9). Typically, one (fast) pathway conducts rapidly, with a relatively long refractory period. A second (slow) pathway conducts more slowly and usually with a shorter refractory period. During sinus rhythm, conduction generally occurs over the fast pathway. A premature atrial depolarization that blocks conduction in the fast pathway because of the longer refractory period, however, still may conduct over the slow pathway. If conduction through this pathway is slow enough that the fast-pathway refractory period ends and the impulse can travel retrogradely back to the atrium, and anterogradely through the slow pathway, then atrioventricular node reentry can occur. In common, or

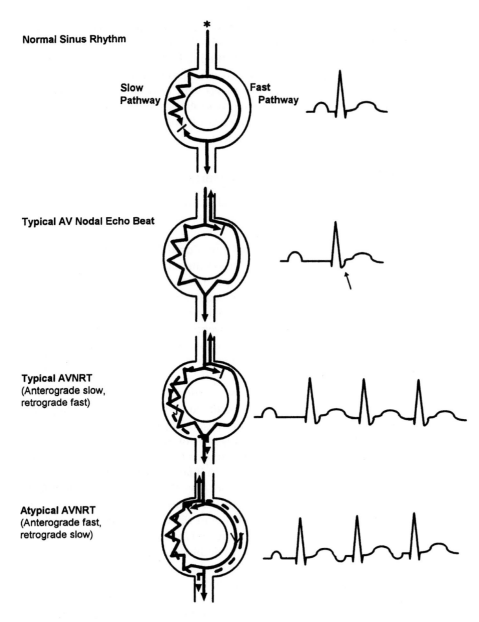

Figure 61.9 Atrioventricular nodal reentrant tachycardia.

typical, AVNRT, anterograde conduction occurs via the slow pathway and retrograde conduction via the fast pathway. Rapid retrograde activation of the atrium via the fast pathway occurs nearly simultaneously with the ventricular activation, and it usually causes the P wave to be simultaneous with, or buried within, the QRS complex. In 5% to 10% of patients with AVNRT, atypical or uncommon AVNRT occurs, in which anterograde conduction takes place via the fast pathway and retrograde conduction via the slow pathway. This causes retrograde P waves that usually are negative in the inferior leads (i.e., II, III, aVF) and are separated from the QRS complex, with an RP interval that is longer than the PR interval (i.e., a mechanism of long RP tachycardia).

Clinically, AVNRT commonly occurs in patients with no structural heart disease, and 70% of patients are women. It may occur at any age, but most patients present during the fourth or fifth decade of life. Symptoms may in-

clude palpitations, lightheadedness, near syncope, weakness, dyspnea, chest pain, rarely syncope, and frequently neck pounding with prominent A waves that can be seen on the jugular pulse, representing atrial contraction against a closed tricuspid valve.

Electrocardiographically, the rate of AVNRT usually is 150 to 200 beats per minute, although rates as high as 250 beats per minute can occur. The initiation of typical AVNRT usually occurs with a premature atrial contraction that is followed by a long PR interval, thus indicating blocked conduction in the fast pathway and conduction down the slow pathway. Because atrial and ventricular activation occur simultaneously during the tachycardia, P waves generally are buried in the QRS complex. A pseudo r′ in V_1 may be seen during typical AVNRT (Fig. 61.10). A longer RP interval indicates retrograde conduction via a slower retrograde pathway.

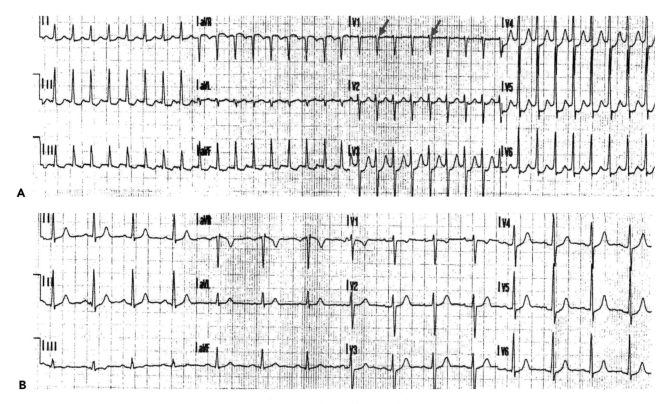

Figure 61.10   **A:** Atrioventricular nodal reentrant tachycardia. The small r' in V$_1$ (*arrows*) is characteristic and represents retrograde atrial activation occurring nearly simultaneously with ventricular activation. **B:** Sinus rhythm after conversion of AVNRT. The r' in V$_1$ is no longer present.

Treatment

Vagal maneuvers (e.g., carotid sinus massage, Valsalva maneuver) may slow or terminate the tachycardia. Adenosine, 6 to 12 mg administered as a rapid intravenous bolus, is the initial drug of choice. Termination of a narrow complex tachycardia by vagal maneuvers or adenosine can be helpful diagnostically by suggesting that the atrioventricular node may be a component of the circuit (in contrast to atrial tachycardias, in which atrioventricular block can be produced with continued tachycardia). β-adrenergic blockers, verapamil, or diltiazem also can be successful. The long-term use of these agents or of class IA, IC, or III antiarrhythmic drugs can be successful, but radiofrequency or cryo catheter ablation of the slow atrioventricular nodal pathway has become the standard therapy for cure of AVNRT, having success rates that can exceed 95% with <1% risk of inducing complete atrioventricular block or the need for a permanent pacemaker.

Supraventricular Tachycardia Mediated by Accessory Pathways

Accessory pathways are bands of excitable conducting tissue that connect the atrium and the ventricle, thus bypassing either all or part of the normal atrioventricular conduction system. Preexcitation syndromes are disorders in which anterograde ventricular or retrograde atrial activation occurs, either in part or totally, through anomalous pathways distinct from the normal conduction system. Anterograde conduction (i.e., from atrium to ventricle) via an accessory pathway during sinus rhythm causes manifest ventricular preexcitation (i.e., Wolff-Parkinson-White syndrome). This results in wide QRS complexes because the accessory pathway inserts into the ventricular myocardium, with activation occurring from myocyte to myocyte rather than via the faster conducting His-Purkinje system. On ECG, a short PR interval and a delta wave (i.e., initial slurring of the QRS complex) usually are seen. Approximately 1 to 3 per 1,000 ECGs show ventricular preexcitation. Accessory pathways that conduct only in the retrograde direction are called *concealed* (i.e., no ventricular preexcitation or delta wave seen on surface ECG), yet these still may participate in SVT. Typical accessory pathways conduct rapidly and nondecrementally. Variant accessory pathways include those with slow, decremental conduction and connections from the atrium to the distal atrioventricular node, the atrium to the His bundle, and the atrium to the right bundle, distal Purkinje network, or apex via a duplicate atrioventricular node/His bundle–like connection (i.e., Mahaim fiber). Congenital abnormalities associated with accessory pathways include Ebstein anomaly, coarctation of the aorta, hypertrophic cardiomyopathy, ventricular septal defects, and transposition of the great arteries.

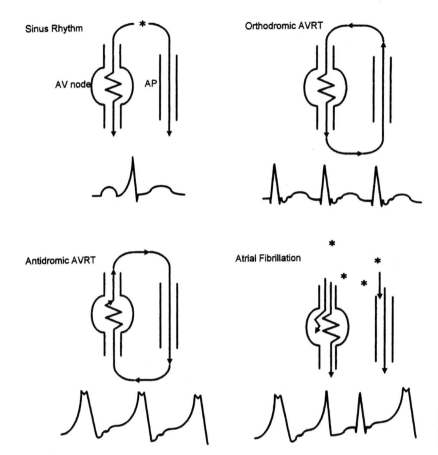

Figure 61.11 Tachycardias associated with accessory pathways. (AVRT, atrioventricular reentrant tachycardia.)

Atrioventricular Reentrant Tachycardia

During AVRT, the accessory pathway, as well as the atria and ventricles, are essential parts of the circuit (Fig. 61.11). In orthodromic AVRT, anterograde conduction occurs via the atrioventricular node and retrograde conduction via the accessory pathway. In antidromic AVRT, anterograde conduction occurs via an accessory pathway and retrograde conduction via the atrioventricular node or a second accessory pathway. Other accessory pathway–associated tachycardias include atrial fibrillation, atrial flutter, atrial tachycardia, or AVNRT, with conduction via a bystander accessory pathway, in which the accessory pathway is not integral to the tachycardia but conducts to the ventricle. Slowly conducting, concealed accessory pathways, which usually are located in the posteroseptal region, can mediate near incessant orthodromic SVT, with retrograde, slow conduction via the accessory pathway (i.e., permanent form of junctional reciprocating tachycardia); these can present as a tachycardia-mediated cardiomyopathy. The most common tachycardias associated with accessory pathways are discussed in the following sections; their treatment is summarized in Table 61.7.

Orthodromic Atrioventricular Reentrant Tachycardia

Orthodromic AVRT is the most common SVT in patients with accessory pathways, occurring in 90% of those who

are symptomatic. Anterograde conduction occurs via the atrioventricular node and His-Purkinje system, inscribing a narrow QRS complex (with no preexcitation) on the surface ECG, unless BBB aberrancy occurs (Fig. 61.12). Because retrograde conduction occurs via the accessory pathway, patients with either manifest or concealed accessory pathways can experience orthodromic AVRT. The rate of the tachycardia usually is 150 to 250 beats per minute, and the tachycardia usually initiates with an atrial or ventricular premature depolarization. Because the atria and ventricles are requisite parts of the circuit, a 1:1 relationship must be present. The demonstration of atrioventricular dissociation or intermittent atrioventricular block during SVT excludes AVRT as a diagnosis. The P wave commonly is visualized in the early part of the ST segment, with a constant RP interval despite the tachycardia rate. Spontaneous or induced BBB during orthodromic AVRT that slows the tachycardia rate indicates the participation of an accessory pathway ipsilateral to the side of the BBB (Fig. 61.13). For example, during orthodromic AVRT using a left free wall accessory pathway as the retrograde limb, the production of block in the left bundle forces ventricular activation to occur via the right bundle, thus requiring conduction through a longer ventricular myocardial path back up to the accessory pathway and slowing the tachycardia cycle length.

Short-term treatment of the two common, regular, narrow complex tachycardias (i.e., orthodromic AVRT and

TABLE 61.7

MANAGEMENT OF PREEXCITATION SYNDROMES

Initial evaluation
  Determine presence or absence of symptoms.
  Characterize symptoms, including frequency and severity.
  Determine previous treatment regimens and effectiveness.
  Document specific arrhythmias present during symptoms.
  Determine presence of concomitant heart disease.
Acute treatment of arrhythmias associated with preexcitation
  syndromes
  Orthodromic SVT
    Vagal maneuvers (e.g., Valsalva, carotid sinus massage)
    Adenosine IV (6–12 mg rapid bolus)
    Verapamil IV (5–10 mg), β-blocker, or diltiazem
    Procainamide IV (1 g over 20–30 min)
    Cardioversion
  Antidromic SVT (retrograde conduction may occur via a second
    AP or the AV node)
    Procainamide IV
    Cardioversion
  Atrial fibrillation (avoid digoxin and verapamil, which may
    accelerate ventricular rate)
    Procainamide IV
    Cardioversion
Long-term treatment of patients with preexcitation syndromes
  Pharmacologic management
    Concealed AP
      Digoxin/verapamil/β-blocker
      Class IC: flecainide/propafenone
      Class IA: disopyramide/quinidine/procainamide
      Class III: sotalol/amiodarone
    Manifest AP
      Class IC: flecainide/propafenone
      Class IA: disopyramide/quinidine/procainamide
      Class III: sotalol/amiodarone
  Indications for nonpharmacologic management
    Life-threatening ventricular rate during atrial
      fibrillation/flutter
    SVT refractory to medical therapy
    Intolerance to medical therapy
    Alternate first-line therapy in patients with symptomatic
      arrhythmias, high-risk occupations, or preference for
      nonpharmacologic treatment
  Nonpharmacologic approaches
    Radiofrequency catheter ablation
    Surgical ablation (rarely required)
Indications for electrophysiology studies
  Delineation of the mechanism of arrhythmias
  Localization/mapping of pathways for ablation
  Assess efficacy of antiarrhythmic agents
  Assessment of the refractory periods of the AP as an indicator
    of the risk of sudden death

AP, accessory pathway; AV, atrioventricular; SVT, supraventricular tachycardia.

precipitate atrial fibrillation with a rapid ventricular response. In patients with very rapid SVT and hemodynamic impairment, DC cardioversion is the initial treatment of choice. Longer-term treatment may include β-blockers; verapamil; diltiazem; digoxin; or class IA, IC, or III antiarrhythmic drugs. Radiofrequency catheter ablation, however, can be curative with high success rates; in many patients, it can be considered as a first-line or early therapeutic option.

Antidromic Atrioventricular Reentrant Tachycardia

Antidromic AVRT is uncommon, occurring in <5% to 10% of patients with Wolff-Parkinson-White syndrome. The anterograde limb of the circuit is an accessory pathway. In 33% to 60% of patients with antidromic AVRT, however, multiple accessory pathways are present, and the retrograde limb may be via either the atrioventricular node or another accessory pathway. Because ventricular activation occurs via an accessory pathway, the QRS complex is wide, bizarre, and preexcited. Mahaim fibers, which are accessory pathways with decremental conduction properties that connect the atrium to the distal right bundle branch or apex via a duplicate atrioventricular node/His bundle–like connection, also can mediate a form of antidromic AVRT with left BBB morphology. In antidromic AVRT, if the atrioventricular node makes up the retrograde limb, then vagal maneuvers or adenosine may terminate the tachycardia, but these measures will not be effective if both limbs are accessory pathways. In the short-term, treatment may require DC cardioversion or procainamide.

Atrial Fibrillation and Wolff-Parkinson-White Syndrome

In patients with manifest accessory pathways having a short refractory period, rapid conduction to the ventricles during atrial fibrillation via the accessory pathway can provoke ventricular fibrillation. The shortest preexcited RR interval during atrial fibrillation gives an indication of the refractory period of the accessory pathway. Short refractory periods (<250 ms) are associated with an increased risk of sudden death. Diagnostically, atrial fibrillation with ventricular preexcitation should be suspected for rapid, irregularly irregular rhythms with varying QRS morphology and widths due to variable degrees of ventricular fusion (Fig. 61.14). Verapamil can increase the ventricular rate during atrial fibrillation; intravenous verapamil may precipitate ventricular fibrillation and should not be given. The treatment of choice is procainamide or DC cardioversion.

SPECIFIC VENTRICULAR ARRHYTHMIAS

VT is defined as three or more consecutive ventricular beats at a rate of 100 beats per minute or more. Nonsustained VT is defined as VT lasting three or more beats under 30 seconds in duration and that does not require intervention for termination. Sustained VT is VT lasting 30 seconds or more

AVNRT) is similar because the atrioventricular node is an integral part of the circuit in the anterograde direction. To terminate the tachycardia, vagal maneuvers or adenosine are the first options of choice, followed by intravenous β-adrenergic blockers, verapamil, or diltiazem. Adenosine can shorten atrial refractory period and occasionally may

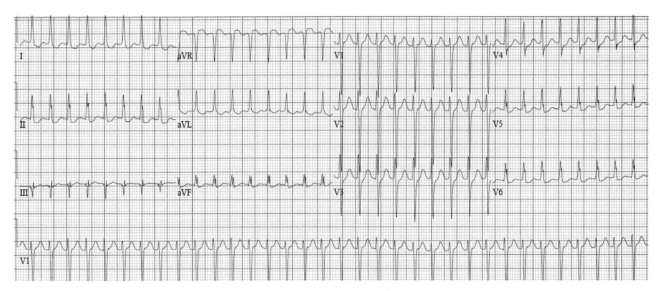

Figure 61.12   ECG of orthodromic atrioventricular reentrant tachycardia. A narrow QRS complex occurs (in the absence of aberration). This confirms anterograde conduction occurring through the atrioventricular node. Thus, this acute SVT can usually be treated successfully with atrioventricular node–blocking maneuvers or drugs (e.g., vagal maneuvers, adenosine, beta-blockers).

or requiring intervention for termination. QRS complex morphology may be either monomorphic (i.e., uniform) or polymorphic (i.e., variable). The usual heart rate of VT ranges from 100 to 280 beats per minute. VT is wide because of the slower rate of conduction through ventricular tissue, compared with that through Purkinje fibers. Hemodynamic stability depends on the rate, underlying cardiac disease, ventricular function, and concomitant pharmacologic treatment. VA dissociation occurs in 60% to 70% of these patients, but it may be evident on surface ECGs only in one-third of patients.

Premature Ventricular Depolarizations

Isolated premature ventricular depolarizations are not associated with significant risk in patients without structural heart disease, but frequent or complex premature ventricular complexes can be markers for a potential increased risk in those with structural heart disease. The treatment of isolated, symptomatic premature complexes generally includes an assessment of risk in the presence of structural heart disease or risk factors, avoidance of precipitating factors (e.g., caffeine, sympathomimetic agents), and reassurance, with the administration of occasional β-blockers or (rarely) other antiarrhythmic agents for persistently symptomatic patients. An electrophysiology study, using mapping and catheter ablation of focally originating premature ventricular complexes or tachycardias, also has been performed for frequent or refractory symptoms.

Sustained Ventricular Tachycardia or Fibrillation: Aborted Sudden Cardiac Death

The patient who survives hemodynamically compromising sustained ventricular arrhythmias or aborted sudden cardiac death in the absence of reversible causes or acute MI faces a high recurrence rate. The implantation of a cardioverter-defibrillator (ICD) is usually indicated. Randomized studies, such as the Antiarrhythmics versus Implantable Defibrillator (AVID) trial, have demonstrated the superiority of ICDs over medical therapies using antiarrhythmic drugs in these high-risk patients.

Ventricular Tachyarrhythmias After Myocardial Infarction

Premature ventricular complexes, nonsustained or sustained VT, ventricular fibrillation, and polymorphic VT can occur during the acute phases of ischemia and infarction.

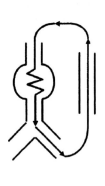
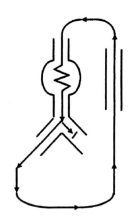

Orthodromic AVRT   Orthodromic AVRT with Ipsilateral BBB

Figure 61.13   Orthodromic atrioventricular reentrant tachycardia with bundle-branch block ipsilateral to the accessory pathway.

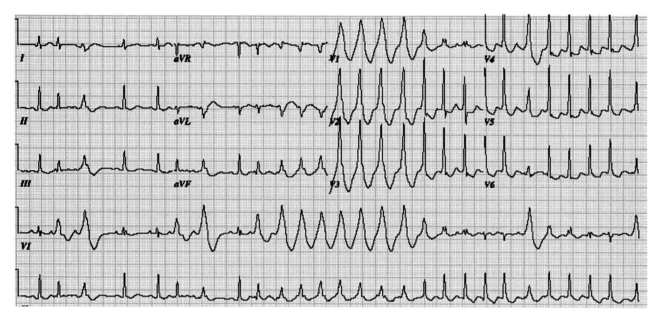

Figure 61.14 Atrial fibrillation with Wolff-Parkinson-White syndrome (ventricular preexcitation). The rhythm is irregular and often rapid. The QRS is variable in morphology and duration due to variable degrees of fusion between conduction through the atrioventricular node and an anterogradely conducting accessory pathway.

Coronary reperfusion has been associated with accelerated idioventricular rhythms and ventricular tachyarrhythmias. Nonsustained or sustained VT, which often results from reentry, can occur late after MI.

Use of lidocaine as prophylaxis for ventricular fibrillation in patients with suspected acute MI has been controversial. Prophylactic lidocaine may produce a small decrease in the incidence of ventricular fibrillation. It has not been shown to improve the mortality, however, and significant side effects can occur. Potential adverse effects include asystole, bradyarrhythmias, neurologic symptoms, seizures, respiratory arrest, nausea, and vomiting. Current data suggest that the routine use of prophylactic lidocaine in patients with suspected acute MI should be avoided when facilities and personnel for prompt resuscitation are available, but when defibrillation is unavailable, prophylactic lidocaine might be beneficial.

The short-term treatment of ventricular arrhythmias after MI depends on the hemodynamic status of the patient and presence of ongoing or recurrent ischemia (as well as other precipitating factors). The long-term prognosis depends on the timing of these arrhythmias in relation to the acute infarction as well as to the degree of ventricular dysfunction. Asymptomatic premature ventricular complexes or nonsustained VTs generally do not require short-term therapy, but they may be associated with an increased mortality when they are frequent or complex, detected late in the course of MI, or associated with left ventricular dysfunction. Accelerated idioventricular rhythms have been associated with coronary reperfusion, but they have not been specific or highly sensitive as predictors of reperfusion and generally do not require specific short-term therapy.

Early VT and sustained fibrillation are associated with an increased in-hospital mortality. Among hospital survivors, however, it may not signify a worsened long-term prognosis. Short-term therapy may require DC countershock, antiarrhythmic therapy, correction of electrolyte and metabolic imbalances, or assessment and treatment of associated recurrent or ongoing ischemia.

Long-term treatment requires assessment of prognostic significance. Frequent or complex ventricular arrhythmias occurring after the acute phase of MI (i.e., the first 48–72 hours) are more frequent in patients with significant myocardial dysfunction. They also are an independent prognostic factor. Empiric suppression of PVCs or nonsustained VT using antiarrhythmic agents, however, with the possible exception of amiodarone, is associated with the potential for an increased mortality. Patients more than 1 month after MI with left ventricular ejection fraction (LVEF) of ≤30% are indicated for ICD implantation based on superior survival seen in the Multicenter Automatic Defibrillator Implantation Trial II (MADIT II). Results of the Sudden Cardiac Death in Heart Failure Trial (SCDHeFT) support ICD implantation in patients with LVEF of ≤35% and New York Heart Association (NYHA) functional class II or greater congestive heart failure. For patients with nonsustained VT and an LVEF <40% after MI, consideration should be given for electrophysiology study with implantation of an ICD if the study induces sustained VT or reproducible ventricular fibrillation. Sustained ventricular arrhythmias after the acute phase of MI are associated with a high rate of recurrence, and ICD implantation usually is indicated. Beta-blockers and angiotensin-converting enzyme inhibitors also have been associated with improved survival rates in many studies and should be routinely advocated in the absence of contraindications.

Ventricular Arrhythmias Associated With Nonischemic Cardiomyopathy

Sustained ventricular arrhythmias, including in sudden cardiac death survivors, are associated with a high rate of recurrence, and ICD implantation usually is indicated. VT or fibrillation associated with nonischemic cardiomyopathy may result from reentry, triggered activity, or increased automaticity.

The presence of nonsustained VT in patients with nonischemic cardiomyopathy has been associated with an increased risk of mortality. The roles of prophylactic ICD implantation and empiric amiodarone in heart failure patients were subjects of large multicenter trials. The Defibrillators in Non-Ischemic Cardiomyopathy Treatment Evaluation (DEFINITE) randomized patients with nonischemic cardiomyopathy and LVEF ≤35% and PVCs or nonsustained VT to single-chamber ICD implantation or standard medical therapy. A reduction in all-cause mortality that did not reach statistical significance ($p = 0.08$) and a significant reduction in sudden death from arrhythmia was reported in the ICD group. SCDHeFT randomized nonischemic and ischemic cardiomyopathy patients with NYHA functional class II or III heart failure symptoms and LVEF ≤35% to ICD implantation, amiodarone, or placebo. No significant survival benefit was reported in the amiodarone group, compared with placebo, but ICD implantation resulted in a significant reduction in mortality. Based on re-

sults of the SCDHeFT trial, ICD implantation is justified for patients with nonischemic or ischemic cardiomyopathy, LVEF ≤35%, and NYHA FC II or greater heart failure symptoms.

A form of macroreentry caused by bundle branch reentry is more common in patients with nonischemic dilated cardiomyopathy and preexisting His-Purkinje system disease, as can be manifested by an intraventricular conduction delay in sinus rhythm, most commonly of the left BBB type. Bundle-branch reentrant VT most commonly presents as a rapid VT of left BBB morphology, although rare right BBB morphologies have been described. This arrhythmia potentially can be cured by selective radiofrequency ablation of one of the bundle branches (most commonly the right), but many of these patients will also meet indications for ICD implantation.

Arrhythmogenic Right Ventricular Dysplasia

Arrhythmogenic right ventricular dysplasia (ARVD) is a form of cardiomyopathy that predominantly involves the right ventricle with hypokinetic and thinned areas that often have fatty infiltration. The disease can present with symptomatic ventricular arrhythmias or sudden death. ARVD can cause ventricular arrhythmias in patients with an apparently normal left ventricle. VTs associated with ARVD generally have left BBB morphology, often multiple in morphology and often precipitated by exercise. The ECG in sinus rhythm may display anterior T-wave abnormalities or an epsilon wave (Fig. 61.15) at the end of the QRS, beginning of the ST segment, most evident in lead V_1

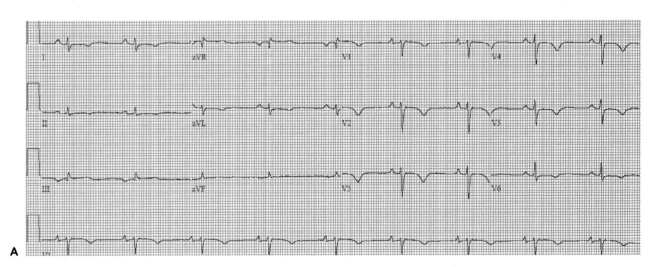

A

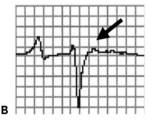

B

Figure 61.15 Arrhythmogenic right ventricular dysplasia: anterior T-wave abnormalities **(A)** and epsilon wave **(B)**.

or V_2. A signal-averaged ECG may show late potentials, and cardiac magnetic resonance imaging or computed tomography may show characteristic abnormalities of the right ventricle. The left ventricle may also be involved. Pharmacologic therapies using antiarrhythmic drugs, surgery, ICD therapy, and radiofrequency ablation have been used as treatments of ventricular arrhythmias in patients with ARVD. ARVD often is familial and has been associated with mutations in desmosomal system genes.

Ventricular Tachycardias in Patients With Structurally Normal Hearts

Syndromes of repetitive, monomorphic, nonsustained, or sustained VT and paroxysmal VTs can present in patients with structurally normal hearts.

Outflow tract VT (arising from the right or left ventricular outflow tract) can present with symptomatic, minimally symptomatic, or asymptomatic frequent, repetitive, or paroxysmal nonsustained or sustained VT, or with frequent symptomatic PVCs. It may be precipitated by stress, exercise, or high catecholamine states. Vagal maneuvers or adenosine may terminate the tachycardia. The PVCs or VT are monomorphic (Fig. 61.16) and characterized by left BBB morphology with an inferior axis (i.e., tall positive QRS in aVF, II, and III). The VT may not be inducible with programmed ventricular extrastimulation (i.e., at electrophysiology study) but may occur during rapid pacing or infusion of isoproterenol. The mechanism may result from triggered activity or increased automaticity. Radiofrequency catheter ablation has been effective in abolishing the right ventricular outflow tract focus. Left ventricular outflow tract or aortic cusp sites have also been targets for ablation. Treatment also may include β-blockers, calcium channel blockers, and type I or III antiarrhythmic agents.

Idiopathic left ventricular or *fascicular tachycardia* may present as a paroxysmal VT and usually can be induced through programmed ventricular extrastimulation, rapid pacing, isoproterenol, or exercise. It is characterized by right BBB morphology, usually with left superior axis (i.e., left-axis deviation; negative in II and aVF) (Fig. 61-17), and it usually arises in the left inferoposterior septum through a mechanism believed to result from fascicular reentry or triggered activity. It may be terminated or suppressed by verapamil or diltiazem, and it has been successfully treated using radiofrequency catheter ablation, usually at sites where the VT is preceded by a fascicular potential.

Torsades de Pointes and Long QT Syndromes

A form of polymorphic VT associated with prolonged QT intervals, TdP is a potentially life-threatening condition that can occur as a complication of several medications or in association with congenital long QT syndromes. The heart rate ranges from 150 to 250 beats per minute, with twisting of the QRS complexes around the baseline (Fig. 61.18). QT prolongation and QTU abnormalities are characteristic but may be present only in beats preceding TdP. TdP

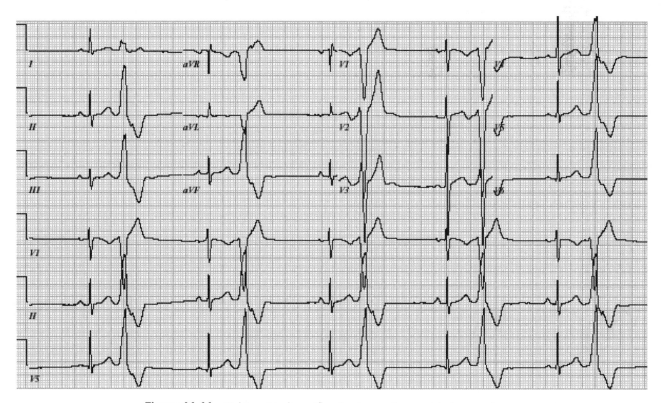

Figure 61.16 Right ventricular outflow tract premature ventricular complexes.

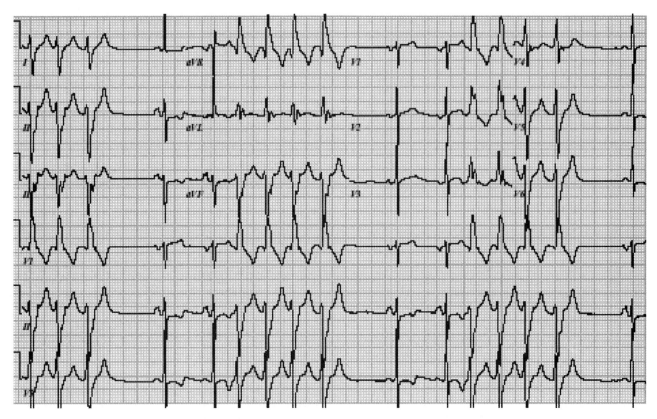

Figure 61.17 Left ventricular fascicular tachycardia.

typically is rate dependent, and sinus bradycardia, bradycardia resulting from atrioventricular block, or abrupt prolongation of the RR interval (e.g., with a pause after a premature complex) can trigger its onset. It usually initiates with "long–short" coupled intervals, which may occur because of a PVC on the previous, long QT–associated T wave. A pause followed by a subsequent sinus or supraventricular beat and another PVC with a short coupling interval then may initiate TdP.

Acquired or congenital forms of long QT syndromes can predispose an individual to TdP. Congenital syndromes include the Romano-Ward syndrome (i.e., autosomal dominant) and Jervell and Lange-Nielsen syndrome (i.e., recessive, associated with deafness). Linkage studies have revealed multiple separate loci (including on chromo-somes 3, 4, 7, 11, and 21) that cause abnormalities in potassium (K^+) or sodium (Na^+) channels. Major long QT syndromes identified thus far with their respective genetic and ion channel defects are summarized in Table 61.8.

So-called acquired long QT syndromes, many of which are associated with drugs that can prolong repolarization, are more commonly encountered, but most are likely associated with similar ion channel abnormalities. Drugs or conditions associated with TdP include:

- Antiarrhythmic drugs that prolong QT interval
    - Quinidine
    - Procainamide (including its metabolite N-acetyl-procainamide)
    - Disopyramide

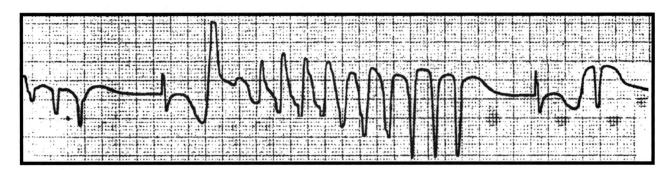

Figure 61.18 Torsades de pointes.

TABLE 61.8

LONG QT SYNDROMES

	Chromosome	Clinical Characteristics	Gene	Ion Current Change	Frequency
LQT1	11	Events during exercise, swimming; broad T wave	KCNQ1	↓ IKs α subunit	55–60%*
LQT2	7	Events during auditory stimuli, startle, emotion; notched or low T wave	KCNH2 (HERG); KCNE2	↓ IKr α subunit	35–40%*
LQT3	3	Events during sleep; bradycardia; long flat ST	SCN5A	↑↑ INa	3–5%*
LQT4	4		ANK2 (Ankyrin)	Unknown	rare
LQT5	21		minK/KCNE1	↓ IKs β subunit	rare
LQT6	21		MiRP1/KCNE2	↓ IKr α subunit	rare
LQT7	17	Andersen's syndrome: intermittent muscle weakness; ventricular ectopy	KCNJ2	↓ IKir2.1	rare
JLN1	11	Deafness; autosomal recessive	KCNQ1	↓ IKs	rare
JLN2	21	Deafness, autosomal recessive	KCNE1	↓ IKs	rare

*Percent of Romano-Ward syndrome (autosomal dominant LQTS).

- Sotalol
- Amiodarone
- Ibutilide
- Dofetilide
- Bepridil
- Tedisamil
- Tricyclic antidepressants
- Phenothiazines
- Nonsedating antihistamines
  - Terfenadine
  - Astemizole
- Antibiotics
  - Erythromycin
  - Pentamidine
  - Trimethoprim-sulfamethoxazole
  - Ampicillin
  - Ketoconazole
  - Itraconazole
  - Spiramycin
- Other QT-prolonging drugs
  - Probucol
  - Ketanserin
  - Cisapride
- Organophosphates
- Electrolyte abnormalities
  - Hypokalemia
  - Hypomagnesemia
  - Hypocalcemia (uncommon)
- Bradyarrhythmias
- Hypothyroidism
- Liquid protein and other diets, anorexia
- Central nervous system abnormalities, particularly affecting sympathetic outflow
  - Subarachnoid hemorrhage
  - Brain stem, cervical cord lesions

Treatment includes the avoidance of offending agents and may require an acceleration of the heart rate, which can be accomplished through either pharmacologic agents (e.g., isoproterenol) or pacing, and intravenous magnesium. Lidocaine, mexiletine, or phenytoin can be tried as well.

Brugada's Syndrome

Brugada's syndrome is a cause of sudden death, often at night. It is a common cause of nocturnal sudden cardiac death in young healthy males in southeast Asia (sudden unexpected nocturnal death syndrome) and may cause some cases of sudden infant death syndrome. Primary ventricular fibrillation (and rarely sustained VT) may occur in up to one-third of patients with Brugada syndrome. The ECG shows right BBB–like morphology with J-point elevation in leads V_1 to V_3 and persistent descending ST elevation in the right precordial leads (Fig. 61-19). These characteristic changes may not be present at all times and may be worsened or unmasked by sodium channel blockers (e.g., flecainide, procainamide, ajmaline). Loss of function mutations in the SCN5A gene, which codes for the α-subunit of the sodium channel (the same gene that causes LQT3 but with loss of function rather than gain of function) have been identified in Brugada's syndrome with autosomal dominant inheritance, although genetic heterogeneity and variable penetrance have been identified. High-risk factors include a history of aborted sudden cardiac death, syncope, prior ventricular arrhythmias, spontaneous ST elevation, and inducible VT/VF (ventricular tachycardia/ventricular fibrillation, although the role of electrophysiological testing is controversial. Lower-risk indicators are asymptomatic patients with a diagnostic ECG only after provocative challenge. There has been no effective drug therapy identified. Amiodarone and β-adrenergic blockers are inadequate. ICD implantation is appropriate for those surviving aborted sudden cardiac death or sustained VT/VF or who have syncope. ICD implantation in asymptomatic patients is controversial.

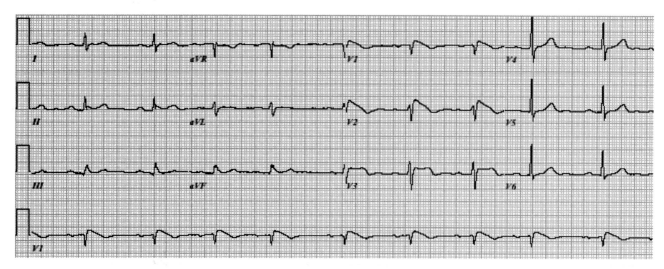

Figure 61.19   ECG in Brugada's syndrome.

Catecholaminergic Polymorphic Ventricular Tachycardia

Polymorphic VT not associated with long QT may be associated with ischemia or electrolyte abnormality, but a syndrome of CPVT has been recognized. Clinical features include syncope, polymorphic VT during exercise or acute emotion, absence of structural heart disease, and a family history of sudden death. The age of onset is usually in childhood, but late onset (in the fourth decade of life) has been reported. CPVT can cause sudden cardiac death and has been postulated to cause some cases of sudden infant death syndrome. An exercise stress test may provoke the arrhythmia, characterized by a fast, bidirectional or polymorphic VT that may self-terminate or degenerate to ventricular fibrillation. Mutations in genes controlling intracellular calcium (e.g., ryanodine release channel [RYR2] or calsequestrin [CASQ2]) have been identified. A form of ARVD (ARVD2) associated with apical morphologic changes and CPVT has been associated with RYR2 mutation; other loci are also postulated. Beta-blockers may be effective, and repeat stress testing may be helpful to assess efficacy. ICDs are indicated for cardiac arrest survivors or sustained VT/VF.

PHARMACOLOGIC THERAPY FOR TACHYARRHYTHMIAS

The most commonly accepted classification of antiarrhythmic drugs is the Vaughan-Williams classification (Harrison modification). All drug classifications possess shortcomings, and specific agents may block more than one ion channel with effects that are characteristic of multiple classes. This scheme, however, has proved useful. Class I antiarrhythmic drugs block Na^+ channels, thereby decreasing action potential upstroke velocity (i.e., phase 0) and slowing conduction. Class I drugs are further divided

into three subdivisions. Class IA agents, which prolong repolarization or action-potential duration, have a moderate effect on conduction slowing and the depression of phase 0. Class IB drugs have little effect on conduction and phase 0 in normal tissue, but they exhibit moderate effects in abnormal tissue. In addition, they show either no effect or a shortening of repolarization–action potential duration. Class IC agents have a marked effect on conduction slowing and phase 0, with mild or no effects on repolarization or action potential duration. Class II contains the β-adrenergic blocking agents, and class III potassium channel–blocking agents prolong repolarization/action potential duration. Class IV contains calcium channel blockers. Commonly used antiarrhythmic agents and their suggested dosages are listed in Tables 61.5 and 61.6.

BRADYARRHYTHMIAS

Sinus Node Dysfunction

Sinus node dysfunction includes a range of abnormalities, including sinus bradyarrhythmias (e.g., sinus pauses, sinus bradycardias, chronotropic incompetence, sinus arrest, sinoatrial exit block), sick sinus syndrome, and tachycardia-bradycardia syndrome (e.g., paroxysmal or persistent atrial tachyarrhythmias with periods of bradyarrhythmia). Other forms of sinus node dysfunction that cause tachycardias (e.g., sinus tachycardia, inappropriate sinus tachycardia, sinus node reentry) were discussed previously.

Sinus Bradycardia

Sinus bradycardia, which generally is defined as sinus rates <60 beats per minute, is common in young, healthy adults (especially in athletes), with normal rates during sleep falling to as low as 35 to 50 beats per minute. It usually is benign, but it can be associated with diseases such as hypothyroidism, vagal stimulation, increased intracranial pressure, MI, and drugs such as β-blockers (including those used for glaucoma), calcium channel blockers, amiodarone, clonidine, lithium, and parasympathomimetics. Treatment often is unnecessary if the patient is asymptomatic. Patients with chronic bradycardia or chronotropic incompetence and symptoms of congestive heart failure or low cardiac output, however, may benefit from permanent pacing.

Sinus Pauses or Sinus Arrest

Sinus pauses or arrest may result from degenerative changes of the sinus node, acute MI, excessive vagal tone or stimuli, digitalis toxicity, sleep apnea, or stroke. Symptomatic or very long pauses may require permanent pacing.

Sinoatrial Exit Block

Sinoatrial exit block results from a block in conduction from the sinus node to the atria. It usually appears as the absence of a P wave, with the sinus pause duration being a multiple of the basic PP interval (i.e., type II). In type I (Wenckebach pattern) sinoatrial exit block, the PP interval shortens before the pause, and the pause is less than two PP intervals. Sinoatrial exit block usually is transient but may be caused by drugs, vagal stimulation, or degenerative disease of the sinus node and atrium. Therapy for symptomatic sinoatrial exit block involves the avoidance of precipitating factors and, potentially, pacing for persistent symptoms.

Sick Sinus Syndrome

Sick sinus syndrome includes a variety of sinus nodal disorders, such as inappropriate sinus bradycardia; sinus pauses, arrest, or sinoatrial exit block; combinations of sinoatrial and atrioventricular conduction abnormalities; and tachycardia-bradycardia syndrome, in which periods of rapid atrial tachyarrhythmias, as well as periods of slow atrial and ventricular rates, occur. Treatment depends on the basic rhythm disturbance. Drug therapy for rapid atrial arrhythmias may aggravate the bradyarrhythmias, and permanent pacing may be required.

Hypersensitive Carotid Sinus Syndrome

Carotid sinus hypersensitivity can produce sinus arrest or atrioventricular block that leads to syncope, and it may be demonstrable with carotid sinus massage. Two types of responses are noted. Through carotid sinus massage, a cardioinhibitory component, with pauses of longer than 3 seconds, or a vasodepressor component, with a decrease in systolic blood pressure, may be provoked. Symptomatic patients may require pacemaker implantation to treat the cardioinhibitory component. Continued symptoms caused by vasodepressor reactions, even after pacemaker implan-

tation, may require further treatment, including support stockings, high-sodium diets, or sodium-retaining drugs.

Atrioventricular Dissociation

Atrioventricular dissociation refers to an independent depolarization of the atria and ventricles. It may be caused by:

- Physiological interference resulting from a slowing of the dominant pacemaker (e.g., sinus node) and the escape of a subsidiary or latent pacemaker (e.g., junctional or ventricular escape)
- Physiological interference resulting from the acceleration of a latent pacemaker that usurps control of the ventricle (e.g., accelerated junctional tachycardia or VT)
- Atrioventricular block preventing the propagation of the atrial impulse from reaching the ventricles, thus allowing a subsidiary pacemaker (e.g., junctional or ventricular escape) to control the ventricles

Note that patients with complete atrioventricular block have atrioventricular dissociation and, generally, a ventricular rate that is slower than the atrial rate. Patients with atrioventricular dissociation, however, may have complete atrioventricular block or dissociation resulting from physiological interference, with the latter typically having an atrial rate that is slower than the ventricular rate.

Atrioventricular Block

Atrioventricular block occurs when the atrial impulse either is not conducted to the ventricle or is conducted with delay at a time when the atrioventricular junction is not refractory. It is classified on the basis of severity into three types: first-, second-, and third-degree atrioventricular block.

In first-degree atrioventricular block, conduction is prolonged (PR interval >200 ms), but all impulses are conducted. The conduction delay may occur in the atrioventricular node, the His-Purkinje system, or both. If the QRS complex is narrow and normal, the atrioventricular delay usually occurs in the atrioventricular node.

In second-degree atrioventricular block, an intermittent block in conduction occurs. In Mobitz type I (i.e., Wenckebach) second-degree atrioventricular block, a progressive prolongation of the PR interval occurs before the block in conduction. In the usual Wenckebach periodicity (Fig. 61.20), the PR interval gradually increases, but with a decreasing increment, thus leading to a gradual shortening of the RR intervals. The longest PR interval usually precedes the block, and the shortest PR interval usually occurs after the block, thereby resulting in the long RR interval of the blocked impulse being shorter than twice the basic PP interval. Variants of this pattern are not uncommon. In Mobitz type II second-degree atrioventricular block, PR intervals before the block are constant, and sudden blocks in P-wave conduction occur (Fig. 61.21). Advanced or high-degree atrioventricular block refers to a block of two or

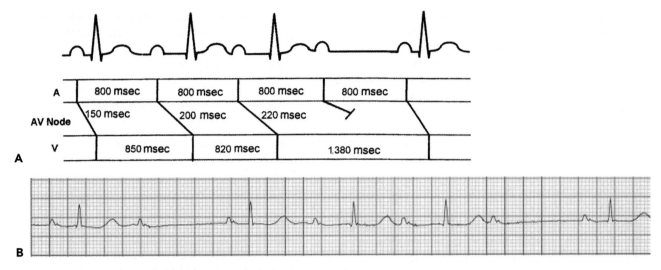

Figure 61.20 Second-degree atrioventricular block Mobitz type I (Wenckebach) periodicity. **A:** Ladder diagram of Wenckebach periodicity. **B:** ECG of 4:3 second-degree atrioventricular block Mobitz type I.

more consecutive impulses. In Mobitz type I block, the level of the block is almost always at the atrioventricular node. Rarely, type I Wenckebach periodicity in the His-Purkinje system may be seen in patients with BBB. In contrast, Mobitz type II block is almost always at the level of the His-Purkinje system and has a higher risk of progressing to complete atrioventricular block.

In third-degree (i.e., complete) atrioventricular block, no impulses are conducted from the atria to the ventricles (Fig. 61.22). The level of the block can occur at the atrioventricular node (usually congenital), His bundle, or in the His-Purkinje system (usually acquired). Escape beats that are junctional at rates of 40 to 60 beats per minute generally occur with congenital complete atrioventricular block. Escape beats that are ventricular in origin often are slow, ranging from 30 to 40 beats per minute.

Indications for Permanent Pacing

Conditions for which permanent pacing is or is not indicated are outlined in Table 61.9, based on a three-part classification of indications:

- *Class I:* Conditions for which evidence and/or general agreement exists that permanent pacemakers should be implanted

- *Class IIa:* Conditions for which pacemakers are reasonable to implant
- *Class IIb:* Conditions for which pacemakers may be considered.
- *Class III:* Conditions for which pacemakers should not be implanted since pacemakers are not helpful and may be harmful

Indications for Temporary Pacing

In general, temporary pacing is indicated for patients with medically refractory, symptomatic bradyarrhythmias without contraindications to pacing. In the absence of acute MI, particularly while awaiting the implantation of a permanent pacemaker (if indicated), temporary pacing can be warranted for patients with medically refractory, symptomatic or hemodynamically compromising sinus node bradyarrhythmias, second- or third-degree atrioventricular block, or third-degree atrioventricular block with a wide QRS complex escape rhythm or a ventricular rate <50 beats per minute.

In the presence of acute MI, temporary pacing is indicated for:

- Third-degree atrioventricular block
- Second-degree atrioventricular block

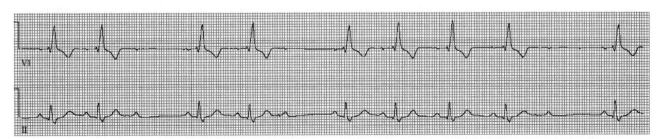

Figure 61.21 Second-degree atrioventricular block, Mobitz type II.

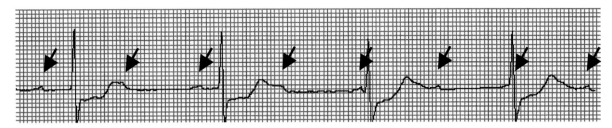

Figure 61.22 Third-degree atrioventricular block with junctional escape beats. P waves are indicated by the *arrows*.

TABLE 61.9

INDICATIONS FOR PERMANENT PACEMAKERS

Disorder	Class of Indication	Indication
SND	I	1. SND with documented symptomatic bradycardia, including as a consequence of necessary long-term drug therapy or frequent sinus pauses producing symptoms 2. Symptomatic chronotropic incompetence
	IIa	1. SND with heart rates <40 beats/min, no clear associations between symptoms and bradycardia 2. Syncope of unexplained origin with clinically significant SND found at electrophysiologic testing
	IIb	1. In minimally symptomatic patients, chronic heart rate <40 beats/min while awake
	III	1. No symptoms 2. Symptoms clearly documented as not associated with slow heart rate 3. Symptomatic bradycardia due to nonessential drug therapy

Acquired AVB	I	1. Advanced 2nd- or 3rd-degree AVB at any anatomic level associated with:
		  a. Bradycardia with symptoms (including heart failure) or ventricular arrhythmias presumed due to AVB
		  b. Arrhythmias and other medical conditions needing drugs that result in symptomatic bradycardia
		  c. Periods of asystole ≥3.0 secs or escape rate <40 bpm, or escape rhythm that is below the AV node, in awake, asymptomatic patients
		  d. In awake, asymptomatic patients with atrial fibrillation and bradycardia with 1 or more pauses of ≥5 secs
		  e. AV junction ablation
		  f. Postoperative AVB not expected to resolve
		  g. Neuromuscular diseases (e.g. myotonic muscular dystrophy, Kearns-Sayre syndrome, Erb's limb-girdle dystrophy, peroneal muscular atrophy) with AVB, with or without symptoms, as progression of AVB may be unpredictable
		2. 2nd degree AVB at any level with symptomatic bradycardia
		3. Asymptomatic persistent 3rd-degree AVB at any anatomic site with average awake ventricular rates of ≥40 bpm if LV dysfunction or cardiomegaly is present or if the site of block is below the AV node

	IIa	1. Persistent 3rd degree AVB with escape rate >40 bpm in asymptomatic adults without cardiomegaly 2. Asymptomatic 2nd-degree AVB at intra- or infra-His levels found at electrophysiology study 3. 1st- or 2nd-degree AVB with symptoms similar to those of pacemaker syndrome 4. Asymptomatic type II 2nd degree AVB with narrow QRS (Type II 2nd degree AVB with wide QRS, including isolated RBBB, is a class I recommendation)
	IIb	1. Neuromuscular diseases with any degree of AVB (including 1st degree), with or without symptoms, as progression of AVB may be unpredictable 2. AVB in the setting of drug use and/or toxicity when block is expected to return even after drug is withdrawn
	III	1. Asymptomatic 1st-degree AVB 2. Asymptomatic 2nd-degree AVB type I at the AV node level 3. AVB expected to resolve and unlikely to recur (e.g., drug toxicity, Lyme disease, transient increases in vagal tone or hypoxia in sleep apnea syndrome in absence of symptoms)

(Continued)

TABLE 61.9

INDICATIONS FOR PERMANENT PACEMAKERS (*Continued*)

Disorder	Class of Indication	Indication
AV block associated with myocardial infarction	I	1. Persistent advanced 2nd-degree AVB with alternating BBB or 3rd-degree AVB with block within or below the His-Purkinje system after ST elevation MI 2. Transient advanced (2nd or 3rd degree) infranodal AVB and associated BBB. If the site of AVB is uncertain, EPS may be necessary. 3. Persistent and symptomatic 2nd- or 3rd-degree AVB
	IIb	Persistent 2nd- or 3rd-degree AVB at the AV node level even without symptoms
	III	1. Transient AVB in the absence of intraventricular conduction defects or in the presence of isolated left anterior fascicular block 2. New BBB or fascicular block without AVB 3. Persistent asymptomatic 1st-degree AVB with BBB or fascicular block
Bifascicular or trifascicular block	I	1. Advanced 2nd degree AVB or intermittent 3rd-degree AVB 2. 2nd-degree type II AVB 3. Alternating BBB
	IIa	1. Syncope not demonstrated to be due to AVB when other likely causes, including ventricular tachycardia, have been excluded 2. HV interval ≥100 ms or nonphysiologic pacing-induced infra-His block found at electrophysiologic study
	IIb	1. Neuromuscular diseases with bifascicular or any fascicular block with or without symptoms
	III	Asymptomatic fascicular block without AV block or fascicular block with associated 1st-degree AV node block
Neurocardiogenic syncope or carotid sinus hypersensitivity	I	Recurrent syncope from spontaneously occurring carotid sinus stimulation and carotid sinus pressure that induces ventricular asystole of >3 secs
	IIa	1. Syncope without clear provocative events and with a hypersensitive cardioinhibitory response of ≥3 secs
	IIb	1. Significantly symptomatic neurocardiogenic syncope associated with bradycardia documented spontaneously or at tilt-table testing
	III	1. Hypersensitive cardioinhibitory response to carotid sinus stimulation that is asymptomatic or with vague symptoms 2. Situational vasovagal syncope in which avoidance behavior is effective and preferred
Obstructive Hypertrophic Cardiomyopathy	IIb	1. Medically refractory, symptomatic hypertrophic obstructive cardiomyopathy with significant resting or provoked LV outflow tract obstruction
	III	1. Asymptomatic or medically controlled patients with hypertrophic obstructive cardiomyopathy or dilated cardiomyopathy 2. Symptomatic patients without LV outflow tract obstruction
CRT in Patients with Severe Systolic Heart Failure	I	1. For LVEF ≤35%, QRS duration ≥0.12 sec and sinus rhythm, CRT with or without an ICD is indicated for treatment of NYHA functional class III or ambulatory class IV heart failure symptoms with optimal recommended medical therapy
	IIa	1. For LVEF ≤35%, QRS duration ≥0.12 sec and AF, CRT with or without an ICD is indicated for treatment of NYHA functional class III or ambulatory class IV heart failure symptoms with optimal recommended medical therapy 2. For LVEF ≤35%, NYHA functional class III or ambulatory class IV heart failure symptoms with optimal recommended medical therapy who have frequent dependence on ventricular pacing
	IIb	1. For LVEF ≤35%, NYHA functional class I or II symptoms with optimal recommended medical therapy and who are undergoing implantation of a permanent pacemaker and/or ICD with anticipated frequent ventricular pacing
	III	1. Asymptomatic patients with reduced LVEF in the absence of other indications for pacing 2. Functional status and life expectancy are limited predominantly by chronic noncardiac conditions
After Cardiac Transplantation	I	1. Persistent inappropriate or symptomatic bradycardia not expected to resolve; and other Class I indications for permanent pacing
	IIb	1. Relative bradycardia is prolonged or recurrent, limiting rehabilitation or discharge after postop recovery 2. Syncope after cardiac transplantation even when bradyarrhythmia has not been documented

SND, sinus node dysfunction; AVB, atrioventricular block; BBB, bundle branch block; LV, left ventricular; LVEF, left ventricular ejection fraction. CRT = cardiac resynchronization therapy. ICD = implantable cardioverter-defibrillator; AF, atrial fibrillation [Modified from Epstein AE, et al. ACC/AHA/HRS 2008 Guidelines for Device-Based Therapy of Cardiac Rhythm Abnormalities: A Report of the American College of Cardiology/American Heart Association Task Force on Practice Guidelines (Writing Committee to Revise the ACC/AHA/NASPE 2002 Guideline Update for Implantation of Cardiac Pacemakers and Antiarrhythmia Devices): Developed in Collaboration with the American Association for Thoracic Surgery and Society of Thoracic Surgeons. *Circulation* 2008;117;e350-e408]

- Mobitz II with anterior MI
- Mobitz II with inferior MI and wide QRS complex or recurrent block with narrow QRS complex
- Mobitz I with marked bradycardia and symptoms
- Atrioventricular block associated with marked bradycardia and symptoms (e.g., hypotension, heart failure, low cardiac output)
- BBB
  - New bifascicular block
  - Alternating BBB
  - New BBB with anterior MI
  - Bilateral BBB of indeterminate age with anterior or indeterminate MI
  - Bilateral BBB with first-degree atrioventricular block

SUGGESTED READINGS

Antiarrhythmics Versus Implantable Defibrillators (AVID) Investigators. A comparison of antiarrhythmic-drug therapy with implantable defibrillators in patients resuscitated from near-fatal ventricular arrhythmias. *N Engl J Med* 1997;337:1576–1583.

Atrial Fibrillation Follow-Up Investigation of Rhythm Management (AFFIRM) Investigators. A comparison of rate control and rhythm control in patients with atrial fibrillation. *N Engl J Med* 2002;347:1825–1833.

Brugada P, Brugada J, Mont L, et al. A new approach to the differential diagnosis of a regular tachycardia with a wide QRS complex. *Circulation* 1991;83:1649–1659.

Epstein AE, et al. ACC/AHA/HR 2008 guidelines for device-based therapy of cardiac rhythm abnormalities. A report of the American College of Cardiology/American Heart Association Task Force on Practice Guidelines. *Circulation* 2008,117:e350–3408.

Fuster V, Ryden LE, Cannom DS, et al. ACC/AHA/ESC 2006 guidelines for the management of patients with atrial fibrillation—executive summary. *Circulation* 2006;114;700–752.

Moss AJ, Zareba W, Hall WJ, et al., Multicenter Automatic Defibrillator Implantation Trial II Investigators. Prophylactic implantation of a defibrillator in patients with myocardial infarction and reduced ejection fraction. *N Engl J Med* 2002;346:877–883.

Chapter 62

Adult Congenital Heart Disease

Yuli Y. Kim   Richard A. Krasuski

 POINTS TO REMEMBER:

- There are two populations of adult congenital patients: those who have been managed and followed throughout their pediatric years, and those who present de novo (previously unrecognized adults who may or may not be symptomatic at the time of diagnosis).

- The congenital diseases commonly encountered in adults are atrial septal defect (ASD), ventricular septal defect (VSD), and patent ductus arteriosus (PDA) (shunt lesions); coarctation of the aorta and pulmonary stenosis (PS) (obstructive lesions); and tetralogy of Fallot (TOF), corrected transposition of the great arteries, and Ebstein anomaly (complex lesions).

- If congenitally bicuspid aortic valve and mitral valve prolapse are excluded, ASD is the most common form of congenital heart disease in adults, constituting approximately 22% to 25% of these patients.

- Because of the reduced life expectancy of patients with uncorrected ASDs, those who have a significant shunt, classically defined as a Qp:Qs shunt fraction >1.5 to 1, symptoms, or evidence of right heart dilation should be offered closure.

- The majority (~70%) of VSDs are located in the membranous septum, approximately 20% in the muscular portion of the trabecular septum (muscular VSD), about 5% in the infundibular septum beneath the pulmonary valve (subpulmonary VSD), and about 5% in the inlet septum near the tricuspid valve (atrioventricular [AV] canal-type VSD).

- Indications for VSD repair include a significant left-to-right shunt (Qp:Qs >1.5), chamber enlargement due to left ventricular volume overload, elevated pulmonary artery resistance, symptoms of conges-

tive heart failure, or significant aortic regurgitation in the case of infundibular VSD.

- Some adults with PDA will develop signs of congestive heart failure from chronic left-to-right shunting.

- If the PDA is amenable, transcatheter closure by an Amplatzer ductal occluder (AGA Medical; Golden Valley, MN) is the treatment of choice for adults, with surgery being reserved for very large PDAs.

- Untreated patients with aortic coarctation have poor survival, with an estimated mortality of 75% by 46 years of age and median age of death being only 31 years.

- Stent implantation for coarctation became a treatment option in the early 1990s and is preferred in adults and adult-size adolescents.

- Tetralogy of Fallot is characterized by pulmonic stenosis, overriding aorta, interventricular communication, and right ventricular hypertrophy with considerable variability in morphology.

With advances in surgical technique and medical therapies, the number of adults with congenital heart disease in the United States is estimated to be over 800,000 (1) and will soon begin to outnumber children with congenital heart disease (2). There are two populations of adult congenital patients: those who have been managed and followed throughout their pediatric years, and those who present de novo (previously unrecognized adults who may or may not be symptomatic at the time of diagnosis). These young, middle-aged, and older adults require a lifetime of follow-up, ideally from specialists. Despite the need for specialized care for this rapidly growing subset of the population, the majority of adults with congenital heart disease are followed primarily by a generalist. Therefore, it is essential that *all* physicians familiarize themselves with the unique clinical presentations of these patients, including the anatomy, physiology, and natural history in order to facilitate proper management and referral.

Congenital disease can be grouped into shunt lesions, obstructive lesions, and complex lesions—cyanotic or acyanotic. The congenital diseases most commonly encountered in adults are ASD, VSD, and PDA (shunt lesions); coarctation of the aorta and PS (obstructive lesions); and TOF, corrected transposition of the great arteries, and Ebstein anomaly (complex lesions).

ATRIAL SEPTAL DEFECT

If congenitally bicuspid aortic valve and mitral valve prolapse are excluded, ASD is the most common form of congenital heart disease in adults, constituting approximately 22% to 25% of these patients (3). There are three major types of ASDs: ostium secundum, ostium primum, and sinus venosus (Fig. 62.1). There is an uncommon type of ASD called a *coronary sinus septal defect*, or "unroofed" coronary sinus type, as well. ASDs account for 7% to 11% of all cardiac defects in general. The female-to-male ratio is approximately 2:1.

Some 65% to 75% of all ASDs are of the ostium secundum type and represent true defects of the atrial septum in the region of the fossa ovalis. Ostium primum defects occur in the inferior-anterior portion of the septum and account for 15% to 20% of ASDs. They fall within the spectrum of AV canal defects and are frequently associated with a cleft anterior mitral valve leaflet and Down syndrome. Sinus venosus defects make up 5% to 10% of ASDs and occur at the junction of the right atrium and the superior

vena cava. They are associated with anomalous pulmonary venous drainage of the right upper pulmonary veins.

In young adults, the dominant shunt is from left to right, because left atrial pressure exceeds right atrial pressure during the majority of the cardiac cycle. Immediately after atrial systole, the right atrial pressure may briefly exceed that of the left, and blood may shunt right to left. The degree of left-to-right shunting depends on the size of the defect as well as the diastolic properties of the ventricles.

Clinical Presentation

The most common symptoms of ASD are dyspnea, palpitations, and exercise intolerance. Late findings include atrial flutter (and less commonly atrial fibrillation) resulting from atrial stretch in response to long-standing left-to-right shunting. Patients can develop right heart failure and occasionally may present with a stroke or transient ischemic attack symptoms due to paradoxical embolization. Pulmonary vascular disease leading to pulmonary hypertension develops in 5% to 10% of patients with untreated ASD (4), although the pathogenesis of this process is not thought to be solely attributable to increased left-to-right flow.

On physical examination, patients usually are acyanotic. There may be a wide, fixed-split S2, which is the hallmark auscultatory feature of ASD. Evidence of increased pulmonary flow can be palpated as a right ventricular lift or a focal thrill in the left second intercostal space, which represents a dilated pulmonary artery. A soft systolic pulmonic outflow murmur can also be heard here. Findings of pulmonary hypertension such as a loud P2 may be present.

Radiographic Features

Depending on the degree of shunting, right heart dilatation may be appreciated on chest x-ray. Enlarged central pulmonary arteries and prominent vascular markings represent increased flow to the lungs. If significant pulmonary hypertension has developed, however, the lung fields may be oligemic.

Electrocardiographic Features

First-degree AV block suggests primum ASD but can be seen in older patients with secundum defects. An incomplete right bundle-branch block or RSR' pattern in V_1 is found in secundum ASD, whereas primum ASD will have a complete right bundle-branch block. Typically, there is right axis deviation in secundum ASD and left axis deviation in primum ASD.

DIAGNOSIS

The diagnosis of ASD is made primarily by echocardiography, and oftentimes transesophageal echocardiography

Types of Atrial Septal Defects

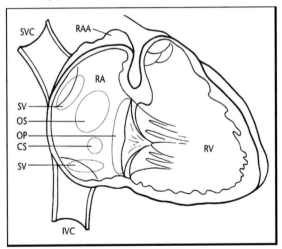

Figure 62.1 Diagrammatic representation of the various forms of atrial septal defects as viewed from the right side. These include ostium secundum (*OS*), ostium primum (*OP*), sinus venosus (*SV*), and coronary sinus (*CS*) type defects. (IVC, inferior vena cava; RA, right atrium; RAA, right atrial appendage; RV, right ventricle; SVC, superior vena cava.)

is required in the adult patient. Cardiac catheterization is not necessary for diagnostic purposes, although a "step-up" in venous saturation at the level of the right atrium can be demonstrated. Cardiac magnetic resonance imaging (MRI) is useful in delineating anatomy and identifying anomalous pulmonary venous connection in cases of sinus venosus defects.

Management

Because of the reduced life expectancy of patients with uncorrected ASDs, those who have a significant shunt, classically defined as a Qp:Qs shunt fraction >1.5 to 1, symptoms, or evidence of right heart dilation should be offered closure. There are certain circumstances in which closure should not be pursued, including advanced pulmonary hypertension (or Eisenmenger's syndrome) and severe left ventricular dysfunction (5). Surgical closure is required for primum and sinus venosus defects, but transcatheter closure is the preferred technique for secundum ASDs, provided the anatomy is suitable. Dual antiplatelet therapy with aspirin and clopidogrel for 4 to 6 months is required after percutaneous closure. Prophylactic antibiotics are not indicated for isolated ASDs except for recent device closure in which case it is recommended for 6 months post procedure (6).

VENTRICULAR SEPTAL DEFECT

VSD is a common anomaly, occurring in approximately 10% of adult patients with congenital heart disease (3)

and is the most common congenital defect in children (Fig. 62.2). They are frequently found in conjunction with other cardiac anomalies, including coarctation of the aorta and PDA. VSDs are also a component of other major congenital diseases, including TOF, persistent truncus arteriosus, and tricuspid atresia. They are classified according to location in either the membranous or muscular septum. Defects in the muscular septum are further categorized according to location in the inlet, trabecular, and infundibular portions. The majority (~70%) of VSDs are located in the membranous septum, ~20% in the muscular portion of the trabecular septum (muscular VSD), about 5% in the infundibular septum beneath the pulmonary valve (subpulmonary VSD), and about 5% in the inlet septum near the tricuspid valve (AV canal–type VSD) (7).

The size of the VSD, ventricular pressure, and pulmonary vascular resistance are determinants of hemodynamic significance. Without pulmonary hypertension or right ventricular outflow tract obstruction, left ventricular pressure is higher than right ventricular pressure, leading to left-to-right shunting. Over time, the pulmonary vascular bed may develop changes in response to increased volume load, resulting in pulmonary hypertension, as described previously with ASD. If the pulmonary hypertension is severe enough, this can create a bidirectional shunt with reversal of flow, leading to right-to-left shunt and cyanosis (Eisenmenger's syndrome).

Some VSDs close spontaneously, and this occurs most often in childhood. The process by which they close varies according to the type of VSD. Small restrictive muscular VSDs can spontaneously close by muscular growth. Perimembranous defects may close by aneurysm formation of

Locations of VSDs

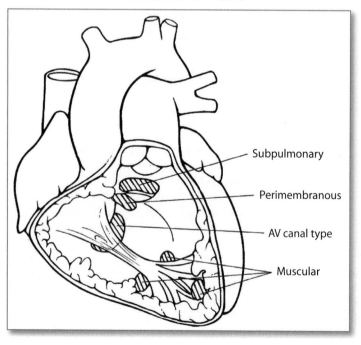

Subpulmonary

Perimembranous

AV canal type

Muscular

Figure 62.2 Diagrammatic representation of four forms of ventricular septal defect as viewed from the right ventricle. The subpulmonary defect has also been referred to as a subaortic or supracrystal defect. The AV canal–type defect has also been referred to as an ostium primum defect.

the tricuspid valve. The right coronary cusp of the aortic valve can prolapse to close over an infundibular VSD (also known as subaortic or supracristal VSD), resulting in aortic insufficiency (8).

Clinical Presentation

The most common symptoms in adult patients with VSDs are dyspnea and exercise intolerance. Symptoms are related to the amount of shunting and the degree of pulmonary hypertension. On physical examination, the classic auscultatory finding is a holosystolic murmur, the intensity of which depends on the velocity of flow. Small defects will cause higher-pitched, loud murmurs and may have an associated thrill. Larger defects are quieter, often without a thrill. The large volume load to the left side of the heart can manifest as a diastolic flow rumble across the mitral valve as well as a laterally displaced apical impulse. In cases of right-to-left shunting or no shunting at all, the murmur often is absent. The second heart sound may be prominent due to pulmonary hypertension. There may be a diastolic murmur of aortic insufficiency in cases of infundibular VSDs.

Radiographic Features

Small VSDs will have no specific radiographic findings, but larger defects will demonstrate cardiomegaly, which is left atrial and left ventricular enlargement due to volume overload from left-to-right shunting. Increased pulmonary vascular markings also are present. In contrast, Eisenmenger's syndrome results in vascular pruning.

Electrocardiographic Features

Similar to radiography, patients with small defects will not manifest any ECG abnormalities. Patients with large VSDs may have evidence of left ventricular hypertrophy and left atrial enlargement. With elevated pulmonary artery pressures, right axis deviation, right ventricular hypertrophy, and right atrial enlargement can be seen.

Diagnosis

Echocardiography is the mainstay of diagnosis of VSD, and oftentimes transesophageal echocardiography may be required. Cardiac catheterization seldom is required for diagnostic purposes alone but may demonstrate a classic "step-up" in venous oxygen saturation at the level of the right ventricle. Cardiac MRI is helpful in delineating anatomy in the setting of complex associated lesions.

Management

The medical management of the adult patient with symptomatic VSD without Eisenmenger's syndrome should focus on relieving volume overload and address suitability

for closure. On the other hand, those with a small VSD can be followed. Recent guidelines from the American Heart Association do not endorse routine antibiotic prophylaxis against infective endocarditis in the setting of an isolated VSD unless there is cyanosis or Eisenmenger's syndrome (6). Indications for closure include a significant left-to-right shunt (Qp:Qs >2.0), chamber enlargement due to left ventricular volume overload, elevated pulmonary artery resistance, symptoms of congestive heart failure, or significant aortic regurgitation in the case of infundibular VSD (8). Eisenmenger's syndrome, however, is a contraindication to closure due to resultant right ventricular failure post closure. Surgery is the primary means of repair, but phase I clinical trials have shown promise for a transcatheter device approach. Currently, this is only available on an investigational or compassionate-use basis in select medical centers.

PATENT DUCTUS ARTERIOSUS

The ductus arteriosus is a fetal structure connecting the proximal descending aorta just distal to the left subclavian artery to the distal main pulmonary artery (Fig. 62.3). A PDA is abnormal if present weeks after birth, as usually it is functionally closed 48 hours after delivery. It is the second most common congenital heart defect in adults, with a prevalence of approximately 1 in 2000 to 1 in 5000 births (9,10). Risk factors for PDA include premature birth, female sex, maternal rubella, and genetic disorders (11).

Patent Ductus Arteriosus

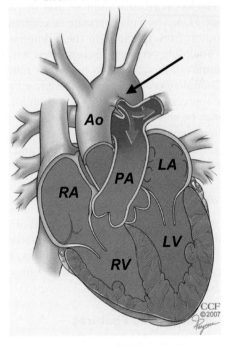

Figure 62.3 Diagrammatic representation of a patent ductus arteriosus (*arrow*). (Ao, aorta; LA, left atrium; LV, left ventricle; PA, pulmonary artery; RA, right atrium; RV, right ventricle.)

Like ASDs and VSDs described earlier, PDA is a shunt lesion that results in left-to-right flow. Likewise, the hemodynamics of the shunt physiology depend on ductal resistance, cardiac output, and systemic and pulmonary resistances—all of which determine the pressure gradient across this shunt (11). Increased pulmonary blood flow will lead to increased preload to the left ventricle, elevating left ventricular end-diastolic and left atrial pressures. And like the other shunt lesions, the long-standing effect of increased flow to the lungs can create pulmonary hypertension and, in its extreme form, Eisenmenger's syndrome. Even if the size of the PDA shunt is small, these patients are at risk for endarteritis with vegetation development usually on the pulmonary arterial side of the ductus.

Clinical Presentation

Adults with PDA may be asymptomatic. Others will develop dyspnea, palpitations, and exercise intolerance. Some adults will develop signs of congestive heart failure from chronic left-to-right shunting. Atrial fibrillation can also result from progressive left atrial hypertension. As is the case for adult congenital heart disease in general, a previously well-tolerated PDA may become manifest in the setting of acquired heart disease such as ischemia, essential hypertension, and valvular disease (11).

The classic auscultatory feature of PDA is the harsh continuous murmur at the left upper sternal border. This murmur involves S2 and is decreased in intensity during diastole. It radiates down the left sternal border and to the back. A large PDA will be a loud "machinery" murmur, whereas a small PDA is a soft, high-frequency, continuous murmur. The left ventricular impulse may be prominent with a large PDA. The pulse pressure is widened due to diastolic runoff from the aorta to the pulmonary artery, leading to bounding peripheral pulses. There may be a diastolic murmur of increased flow across the mitral valve. Again, if Eisenmenger's syndrome is present, a prominent P2 may be appreciated with a right ventricular lift, and the murmur may be soft or inaudible due to minimal shunting. The Eisenmenger patient due to a PDA is cyanotic and may have differential cyanosis with cyanosis and clubbing of the lower extremities only.

Radiographic Features

The chest x-ray may be normal if the amount of shunting is minimal. Cardiomegaly and increased pulmonary vascularity may be appreciated in larger PDA shunts. The main pulmonary artery often is enlarged. The PDA may be calcified in older adults.

Electrocardiographic Features

Again, in the case of a small PDA, the ECG is often normal. Left ventricular hypertrophy and left atrial enlargement may be seen. With Eisenmenger's syndrome, right ventricular hypertrophy and right atrial enlargement may be appreciated.

Diagnosis

Transthoracic echocardiography is the initial diagnostic modality of choice, with transesophageal echocardiography required for cases in which there are inadequate windows. Cardiac catheterization is not utilized in the diagnosis of PDA.

Management

In general, closure of the PDA is recommended for all patients at the time of diagnosis to prevent the risk of endarteritis, left heart failure, and development of pulmonary vascular disease. If the lesion is amenable, transcatheter closure by an Amplatzer ductal occluder is the treatment of choice for adults, with surgery being reserved for very large PDAs. Percutaneous deployment of coil occluders is utilized for small PDAs or residual leaks (12). Transcatheter procedural success is excellent, with >95% closure rates at 6 months and 1 year. Complications are rare and include device embolization, partial obstruction of the pulmonary artery, and pseudoaneurysm (13). Dual antiplatelet therapy is recommended for 4 to 6 months post procedure along with antibiotic prophylaxis for 6 months.

Patients with pulmonary vascular disease or Eisenmenger's syndrome may not be candidates for closure due to the risk of right ventricular decompensation post procedure. These patients may be managed with selective pulmonary vasodilator therapy and considered for closure later if pulmonary vascular resistance improves to an acceptable level (11).

COARCTATION OF THE AORTA

Aortic coarctation usually presents as a discrete narrowing in the thoracic aorta in the region of the ligamentum arteriosum (Fig. 62.4). It accounts for 7% of congenital heart lesions, with a slight male predominance of 1.5 to 1 (14,15). It is a diffuse arteriopathy characterized by cystic medial necrosis, increased collagen deposition, and decreased smooth muscle mass (16,17). Associated lesions include bicuspid aortic valve in 22% to 42% of cases (18), intracranial aneurysms in 10% (19), and less commonly VSDs, Shone's syndrome (serial left-sided obstructive lesions including parachute mitral valve), and Turner's syndrome.

The major physiological consequence of this stenotic lesion is the increased afterload due to obstruction of flow from the left ventricle. This creates significant hypertension in the aorta and branch vessels proximal to the coarctation site. Distal to the coarctation, there is diminished flow and collaterals may form to supplement areas of relative hypoperfusion.

Coarctation of the Aorta

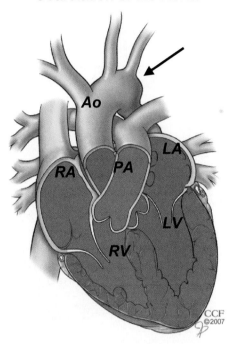

Figure 62.4 Diagrammatic representation of a classical isolated coarctation of the aorta (*arrow*). (LA, left atrium; LV, left ventricle; PA, pulmonary artery; RA, right atrium; RV, right ventricle.)

Untreated patients have poor survival, with an estimated mortality of 75% by 46 years of age and median age of death being only 31 years (20). Causes of death are related to uncontrolled hypertension, congestive heart failure, infective endocarditis, aortic rupture or dissection, and cerebral hemorrhage. Because these patients are at risk for premature coronary and cerebrovascular disease, they should be managed aggressively and early on.

Clinical Presentation

Clinically, most adult patients are asymptomatic but may have minor symptoms such as headaches, epistaxis, dizziness, claudication, and palpitations (7). They present with hypertension—classically, upper extremity hypertension with diminished or delayed femoral pulses. Blood pressure measurements will depend on the location of the coarctation in relation to the left subclavian artery. Therefore, blood pressure should be measured in all four extremities. There may be a soft systolic murmur at the left upper sternal border that radiates to the interscapular area, representing flow across the coarctation itself. A loud A2 can be heard. If there is an associated bicuspid aortic valve, a systolic ejection click may be appreciated as well. The presence of a continuous murmur over the precordium and back indicates the development of collaterals.

Radiographic Features

The classic finding on chest radiography is the "3," or "reverse E" sign, representing a dilated left subclavian artery

above the coarctation and poststenotic aortic dilatation beyond the coarctation. Cardiomegaly from long-standing hypertension may be appreciated. Rib notching is caused by enlarged intercostal artery collaterals. There may be an enlarged ascending aorta, which usually suggests an associated bicuspid aortic valve.

Electrocardiographic Features

Long-standing hypertension can cause left ventricular hypertrophy, which can be appreciated on ECG.

Diagnosis

Echocardiography is a useful initial tool for the evaluation of suspected aortic coarctation. However, cardiac MRI increasingly is being utilized to carefully delineate aortic anatomy to help determine the best reparative approach. In adults, cardiac catheterization may yield better information than echocardiography in determining anatomy and pressure gradients but is not considered a first-line diagnostic tool.

Management

An ophthalmologic examination is warranted to evaluate for hypertensive retinopathy. Medical therapy is limited to antihypertensive medications. For repair, several factors need to be considered, including age, anatomy of coarctation, history of prior repair, and institutional expertise. For native coarctation in infants and children younger than 1 year, surgical repair is the treatment of choice, with the end-to-end anastomosis being the preferred method. Stent implantation became a treatment option in the early 1990s and is preferred in adults and adult-size adolescents. Balloon angioplasty with or without stent implantation is the accepted treatment approach in recurrent coarctation. Safety and efficacy are excellent for transcatheter repair by experienced operators, but long-term outcomes are still accruing for this newer technique. Dual antiplatelet therapy is recommended for 4 to 6 months after stent implantation in addition to infective endocarditis prophylaxis for 6 months.

PULMONARY STENOSIS

PS is the most common form of right-sided obstruction. The lesion can be at the level of the valve (valvar), above the valve (supravalvar), or in the outflow tract (infundibular) (21). The natural history of PS is quite favorable, with survival comparable to that of the general public (22). It may be associated with various genetic disorders, including Noonan, Williams, and Alagille syndromes.

Clinical Presentation

Patients may be asymptomatic. With more severe PS, they may present with dyspnea, fatigue, palpitations, exercise intolerance, or even syncope (21). Right atrial pressure may become elevated, creating a "stretched" and subsequently patent foramen ovale, leading to right-to-left flow and cyanosis.

On inspection, a prominent jugular "a" wave may be appreciated, representing forceful atrial contraction into a noncompliant right ventricle. A right ventricular lift can be palpated when at least moderate to severe PS is present. A systolic ejection click that decreases with inspiration and a crescendo–decrescendo systolic ejection murmur may be auscultated at the left upper sternal border. A right-sided S4 may be heard with severe PS.

Radiographic Features

The chest radiograph typically is normal unless there is evidence of right ventricular failure, in which case right ventricular and right atrial enlargement may be seen. A prominent pulmonary artery representing a dilated main and left pulmonary artery may be appreciated. With severe PS, there may be oligemic lung fields.

Electrocardiographic Features

The ECG may be normal with mild PS; however, with severe PS, there may be evidence of right ventricular hypertrophy, right axis deviation, and right atrial enlargement.

Diagnosis

The diagnosis of PS is made by echocardiography. Cardiac MRI may add additional data regarding branch pulmonary artery stenosis. Cardiac catheterization is not needed to make the diagnosis.

Management

Management requires determining the exact level(s) of obstruction and the severity of the lesion. Mild PS with a peak systolic Doppler gradient of <30 mm Hg can be followed every 2 to 3 years (22). For isolated simple PS, percutaneous balloon valvuloplasty is the procedure of choice. In the presence of symptoms and peak systolic gradient >50 mm Hg and <2+ pulmonic insufficiency (PI), balloon valvuloplasty is a class I indication for repair (23). Procedural results are excellent, with a low restenosis rate if there is no residual gradient (24,25). Surgical repair using commisurotomy is indicated for more complex lesions, and valve replacement may be necessary if there is significant accompanying pulmonary insufficiency.

TETRALOGY OF FALLOT

TOF is the most common cyanotic congenital cardiac defect, with a frequency of 356 per million live births (26). It is characterized by pulmonic stenosis, overriding aorta, interventricular communication, and right ventricular hypertrophy with considerable variability in morphology (27).

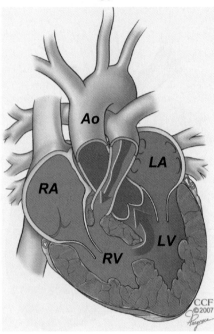

Figure 62.5   Diagrammatic representation of tetralogy of Fallot. The lesions found in the anomaly include pulmonic stenosis (usually subvalvular), a VSD, an overriding aorta, and right ventricular hypertrophy. (LA, left atrium; LV, left ventricle; PA, pulmonary artery; RA, right atrium; RV, right ventricle.)

Associated defects include a right-sided aortic arch in 25%, secundum ASD in 15%, left superior vena cava in 5%, and anomalous coronary arteries in 10% (28).

The clinical presentation of unrepaired patients with TOF depends largely on the amount of right outflow tract obstruction; the amount of aortic override; and, to a lesser degree, systemic vascular resistance. All these factors dictate the amount of right-to-left shunting across the VSD. With severe right ventricular outflow tract obstruction, there is severe hypoxemia, whereas with mild obstruction, there may be left-to-right shunting resulting in a "pink tet."

Adult TOF patients will likely present after primary repair (a classic repair consisting of a VSD patch, a right ventricular outflow tract patch, and infundibular resection) or a repair preceded by a palliative systemic-to-pulmonary artery shunt procedure. The repaired patient will no longer be cyanotic but can present with a host of other problems that require lifelong follow-up, including pulmonic insufficiency, ventricular tachycardia, atrial arrhythmias, right heart failure, and aortic dilatation. They are also at increased risk for sudden cardiac death.

Clinical Presentation

The adult patient with TOF is often asymptomatic. If unrepaired, the patient likely is cyanotic, although severe cyanosis or a history of classic "squatting" (as seen in the pediatric population) is uncommon. If repaired, the patient may present with late symptoms such as dyspnea, exercise intolerance, palpitations, right heart failure, syncope, and even death (21).

On physical examination, patients may be cyanotic or have digital clubbing. Those who have undergone a previous Blalock-Taussig shunt between the subclavian artery to pulmonary artery may have a diminished pulse on that side. The jugular venous pressure is normal unless there is right ventricular dysfunction. There may be a right ventricular lift on palpation. On auscultation, a variable right ventricular outflow murmur may be heard at the left upper sternal border. There is a single S2 (pulmonic component is not audible), and an aortic ejection click may be appreciated due to a dilated overriding aorta. The diastolic murmur of pulmonic insufficiency must be actively sought in the same area and can produce a to-and-fro quality. A holosystolic murmur of the VSD may be appreciated if unrepaired or a high-frequency systolic murmur auscultated if there is a VSD patch leak. There may a systolic murmur of tricuspid regurgitation at the lower left sternal border as well.

Radiographic Features

Findings on chest radiography depend on prior surgical interventions. The presence of a right aortic arch may be determined. The silhouette of a "boot-shaped" heart is caused by the upturning of the apex from right ventricular hypertrophy. Pulmonary vascular markings depend on the amount of relative blood flow and the presence of branch pulmonary artery stenosis. Prior conduits or evidence of right ventricular outflow tract repair may be appreciated.

Electrocardiographic Features

The ECG usually demonstrates sinus rhythm with right ventricular hypertrophy. Most patients who have undergone prior repair will have a right bundle-branch block. Both atrial and ventricular arrhythmias may be present.

Management

For patients who are unrepaired or status post palliative shunt, a relatively well-balanced situation must be present. These patients need to be monitored for progressive right ventricular outflow tract obstruction, right heart failure, cyanosis, paradoxical emboli, and arrhythmias.

In the post repair patient, management is focused on residual lesions, their location, and severity. Cardiac MRI is considered the gold standard in evaluating the right ventricle and assessing the amount of pulmonic insufficiency. It can provide important anatomical information, including branch pulmonary artery stenosis, presence of aortopulmonary collaterals, aortic dilatation, VSD patch leak, recurrent right ventricular outflow tract obstruction, and right ventricular outflow tract aneurysm.

An important sequela post repair is pulmonic insufficiency. Patients need to be followed for resultant right

ventricular enlargement, right ventricular failure, exercise intolerance, arrhythmias, and sudden cardiac death to determine timing for reintervention. Pulmonary valve replacement is the procedure of choice for severe pulmonic insufficiency, when deemed appropriate. A yearly ECG should be obtained, as QRS duration has been found to be predictive of sudden cardiac death (29).

CORRECTED TRANSPOSITION OF THE GREAT ARTERIES

Congenitally corrected transposition of the great arteries (ccTGA) or L-loop transposition is an unusual cardiac malformation, found in <1% of all forms of congenital heart disease (Fig. 62.6). The defining feature of ccTGA is atrioventricular (AV) and ventriculoarterial discordance. Blood flows from the right atrium to a right-sided, morphologic left ventricle through the pulmonary artery to the lungs. Pulmonary venous return to the left atrium goes to a left-sided, morphologic right ventricle, out the aortic valve, and to the aorta. In essence, the systemic ventricle is the morphologic right ventricle, whereas the venous ventricle is the morphologic left ventricle. The natural history of this arrangement is progressive systemic ventricular failure and

Congenitally-corrected Transposition of the Great Arteries

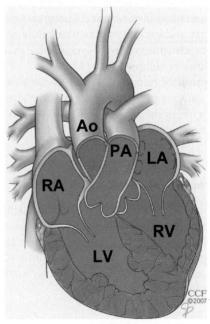

Figure 62.6 Diagrammatic representation of congenitally corrected transposition showing that the right atrium (*RA*) sits above a morphologic left ventricle (*LV*) connected by a morphologic mitral valve. Pulmonary venous return is to a morphologic left atrium (*LA*) that sits above a morphologic tricuspid valve connected to a systemic morphologic right ventricle (*RV*). The aorta (*Ao*) is anterior and to the left of the pulmonary artery. (Ao, aorta; LA, left atrium; LV, left ventricle; PA, pulmonary artery; RA, right atrium; RV, right ventricle.)

systemic AV valvular insufficiency, even in the absence of other anomalies.

ccTGA often is accompanied by other congenital anomalies. Associated lesions include VSD (70%); PS (~40%), which is usually subvalvar; and Ebstein-like abnormalities of the left-sided systemic AV valve in 90% (30). Conduction abnormalities are common, and the development of complete heart block occurs at an incidence of 2% per year (31).

It is important to mention another form of transposition of the great arteries called *complete transposition of the great arteries*, or D-loop transposition. The defining feature of this condition is ventriculoarterial discordance in which the aorta arises from the morphologic right ventricle, and the pulmonary artery arises from the morphologic left ventricle, although AV concordance is maintained. This results in the systemic and pulmonary circulations to run in parallel and is incompatible with life unless there is some type of communication between the two systems (ASD, VSD, or PDA).

Clinical Presentation

Symptoms and clinical presentation depend on the presence and severity of associated lesions, and it is not uncommon for patients to present in adulthood for the first time. Often, patients are asymptomatic, since physiological blood flow preserved. However, with time, patients can present with dyspnea, fatigue, exercise intolerance, or congestive heart failure in the setting of progressive AV valvular insufficiency and systemic ventricular failure. Patients can also present with presyncope or syncope due to conduction abnormalities or complete heart block.

On physical examination, a loud A2 can be appreciated due to an anterior and leftward aorta as the anatomic relationship between the great vessels is altered. There may be a systolic murmur of systemic AV valvular insufficiency as well.

Radiographic Features

The chest radiograph can demonstrate a straight left heart border as a result of the anatomic configuration of the great vessels. Dextrocardia occurs in ~20% of these patients and can be appreciated on x-ray. Sequelae from associated defects such as increased pulmonary vascular markings from a VSD can be seen.

Electrocardiographic Features

The typical ECG shows left axis deviation and Q waves in leads III and aVF as well as septal Q waves over the right precordial leads because septal activation is now occurring from right to left (32). As a result, the ECG can be misinterpreted as an inferior myocardial infarction. Varying degrees of AV block may be seen.

Diagnosis

The diagnosis can be made with echocardiography, and the key feature of AV and ventriculoarterial discordance must be demonstrated. The morphologic right ventricle usually can be identified by its heavier trabeculations and the presence of a moderator band. The tricuspid valve is also displaced more apically than the mitral valve. Cardiac catheterization is not necessary for the diagnosis of ccTGA but can be helpful with regard to the hemodynamic significance of associated anomalies and to evaluate the coronary arteries if surgery is planned.

Management

Because ccTGA likely presents with other associated defects, management depends on the presence of these lesions. Medical therapy for isolated ccTGA involves periodic Holter monitoring for conduction abnormalities. The lifetime prevalence of complete heart block is >30%. The use of agents in the treatment of congestive heart failure for morphologically normal hearts has been extrapolated to this population, such that angiotensin-converting enzyme inhibitors, beta-blockers, and diuretics are routinely used despite the lack of strong data. Yearly imaging with echocardiography and/or cardiac MRI is warranted.

Systemic AV valve repair or replacement may be necessary in adult patients with worsening AV valvular insufficiency. Perioperative mortality is acceptable in experienced centers. Other operative techniques such as the "double-switch" repair (atrial baffle and arterial switch) have generally not been performed in adult patients.

EBSTEIN ANOMALY

Ebstein anomaly of the tricuspid valve represents 0.5% of congenital heart defects. Anatomically, it is characterized by adherence of the septal and posterior leaflets to the underlying myocardium; apical displacement of the annulus; and the classic "atrialization" of the right ventricle, which becomes disproportionately dilated (33) (Fig. 62.7). An associated ASD or patent foramen ovale is found in 80% to 94% of cases (34). Other lesions that can be found with Ebstein anomaly include bicuspid aortic valve, pulmonary atresia, subaortic stenosis, aortic coarctation, mitral valve prolapse, VSD, and PS. As mentioned above, ccTGA can have an associated Ebstein anomaly or an "ebsteinoid" tricuspid valve (which does not fit the classic morphology). Maternal lithium has been linked to Ebstein anomaly, but most cases are sporadic.

The pathophysiology of Ebstein anomaly is right ventricular dysfunction and tricuspid valve regurgitation. The right atrium acts as a passive reservoir for this regurgitant flow and progressively dilates. This not only contributes further to poor forward flow through the right ventricle but enlarges any associated interatrial communication. This

Ebstein Anomaly

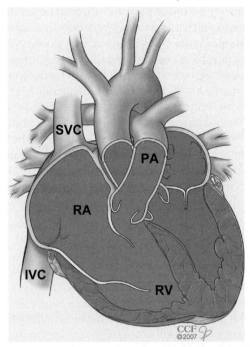

Figure 62.7 Diagrammatic representation of Ebstein anomaly showing the downward displacement and elongated leaflets of the tricuspid valve. (IVC, inferior vena cava; PA, pulmonary artery; RA, right atrium; RV, right ventricle; SVC, superior vena cava.)

results in right-to-left flow and cyanosis. Patients with Ebstein anomaly are at risk for arrhythmias and sudden cardiac death. Therefore, the natural history of this lesion varies from early death to adult survival, depending on the degree of tricuspid valve involvement and the presence and type of arrhythmias.

Clinical Presentation

There is a wide spectrum of presentation. Patients may be diagnosed in infancy with cyanosis and congestive heart failure or present later in life as adolescents or adults with progressive right heart failure, cyanosis, arrhythmias, or even sudden death. Symptoms include decreased exercise tolerance and fatigue. Palpitations can represent the development of tachyarrhythmias. Paradoxical embolization and brain abscess may also result in the presence of an interatrial communication.

The downward displacement of the septal leaflet creates a substrate for accessory pathways. Wolff-Parkinson-White syndrome is found in 10% to 25% of patients with Ebstein anomaly. Supraventricular arrhythmias such as atrial fibrillation or flutter can develop in the setting of a markedly dilated right atrium. This, in the setting of accessory pathway(s), is poorly tolerated and can be lethal.

On physical examination, the jugular venous pressure is normal due to a highly compliant right atrium. There may be cyanosis and digital clubbing. A systolic murmur

of tricuspid insufficiency can be appreciated at the lower left sternal border. A persistent and widely split S2 is typical.

Radiographic Features

The chest radiograph can vary from normal to the classic Ebstein silhouette of a "globe-shaped" heart with a narrow waist. Pulmonary vascularity can vary.

Electrocardiographic Features

The ECG in Ebstein anomaly almost invariably is abnormal. It can demonstrate tall, broad P waves ("Himalayan P waves") from right atrial enlargement and complete or incomplete right bundle-branch block. First-degree AV block is often found.

Diagnosis

Echocardiography is the diagnostic modality of choice for Ebstein anomaly, where the apical displacement of the septal leaflet and tethering of the septal leaflet can be demonstrated with careful interrogation. Other characteristic findings such as atrial enlargement and the presence of an atrialized right ventricle can be shown. Cardiac catheterization largely has been replaced by noninvasive echocardiography and is not necessary for the diagnosis.

Management

Medical management consists of congestive heart failure treatment such as diuretics and digoxin. Infective endocarditis prophylaxis is appropriate. Catheter ablation of accessory pathways or supraventricular arrhythmias should be performed in these patients or at the time of surgical repair. Surgical correction is recommended for those with New York Heart Association functional class III and IV symptoms despite medical therapy. The tricuspid valve may be repaired or may need to be replaced in addition to closure of an interatrial communication.

REVIEW EXERCISES

QUESTIONS

1. A 36-year-old man presents to the emergency room with sudden onset of atrial fibrillation. He is hemodynamically stable but has a systolic murmur at the left upper sternal border radiating to the back, a widely fixed split second heart sound, and a diastolic flow rumble along the right lower sternal border. The most likely diagnosis is

a) VSD
b) ASD
c) PS
d) Aortic stenosis

Answer and Discussion

The answer is b. ASD commonly presents in the adult, and the first symptom may be the sudden onset of atrial flutter or atrial fibrillation. At least 12% to 15% of adult patients have atrial fibrillation preoperatively. Physical findings that demonstrate this as an ASD are the murmur of increased pulmonary blood flow at the left upper sternal border radiating to the back, the pathognomonic finding of a fixed split-second heart sound, and the diastolic flow rumble along the right mid-right lower sternal border (functional tricuspid stenosis), which suggests that this patient has a large left-to-right shunt at atrial level. Adult patients with ASD tend to have large defects that raise the question of whether somewhat smaller defects in childhood actually get stretched and become larger defects in adults with significant left-to-right shunts. ASDs are also more common in women, with a female-to-male ratio of 2 to 3:1.

2. A 22-year-old professional basketball player was noted to have an unusual murmur on her sports physical before the season began. The doctor thought he heard a continuous murmur at the left upper sternal border associated with a slightly widened pulse pressure and brisk to abounding pulses. The most likely diagnosis is
a) VSD
b) ASD
c) Coarctation of the aorta
d) PDA

Answer and Discussion

The answer is d. Many adult patients with patent ductus are asymptomatic, depending on the size of the left-to-right shunt and the size of the ductus. Frequently, the condition is discovered by the unusual quality of a continuous murmur at the left upper sternal border that can sound like an innocent venous hum. Because a patent ductus is an aortopulmonary runoff, however, the pulse pressure frequently is widened, and the pulses are brisk to bounding. Today, most lesions of ductus can be closed in the catheterization laboratory without surgery.

3. A 32-year-old woman is noted to have a systolic blood pressure of 170/100 mm Hg. She has a prominent aortic ejection click and murmurs heard over the ribs on both sides anteriorly and over the back posteriorly. In addition, no pulses are palpable in the lower extremities, and she complains of mild claudication with exertion. The most likely diagnosis is
a) ASD
b) Aortic stenosis
c) Coarctation of the aorta
d) VSD

Answer and Discussion

The answer is c. Adult patients with coarctation almost always present with systolic hypertension, and diastolic hypertension may occasionally be seen as well. A bicuspid aortic valve is noted in a significant proportion of patients with coarctation; therefore, an aortic ejection click may be heard. These patients frequently have collateral murmurs from intercostal arteries heard over the anterior and posterior chest as well as increased collaterals from the thyrocervical trunk. The pulses in the lower extremity may be weak to absent. If the coarctation is severe enough, the individuals may complain of claudication with exercise. The approach to correction in adult patients is usually percutaneous stent placement.

4. A 42-year-old man presents for his first visit to your clinic. He has always been cyanotic, clubbed, and physically restricted. His hematocrit is 68%, with a hemoglobin level of 24 g. He has never undergone surgery, and his oxygen saturation on room air is 62%. Cardiac catheterization demonstrates a large VSD, overriding aorta, and severe calcification of the entire right ventricular outflow tract with small pulmonary arteries bilaterally. The diagnosis in this patient is
a) Double-outlet right ventricle
b) Truncus arteriosus
c) TOF
d) AV canal

Answer and Discussion

The answer is c. TOF is the most common form of cyanotic congenital heart disease in adolescents and adults. The hallmark of tetralogy is severe valvular and subvalvular PS associated with a large VSD. Patients shunt right to left at the ventricular level; therefore, they are cyanotic and clubbed. In addition, cyanotic patients are polycythemic; once their hematocrit is >65%, they are at increased risk for stroke or spontaneous cerebral hemorrhage. The approach to tetralogy is surgical, with relief of the right ventricular outflow tract obstruction and closure of the VSD.

5. A 30-year-old woman presents to your office with the murmur of mitral regurgitation. She has been known to have a complete heart block since childhood and is now somewhat fatigued and short of breath. You notice that on her chest radiograph she has a completely straight left heart border. The most likely diagnosis in this patient is
a) VSD
b) Rheumatic mitral regurgitation
c) Corrected transposition of the great arteries
d) PDA

Answer and Discussion

The answer is c. Patients with congenitally corrected transposition frequently present as adults. Although a morphologic right atrium is connected to a morphologic left ventricle via the mitral valve, the blood flows from that ventricle to the pulmonary artery. It returns then to a morphologic left atrium, which crosses a tricuspid valve into a morphologic right ventricle that pumps blood out the aorta, and the aorta is anterior and to the left. Patients with this condition frequently present in adulthood because the blood is flowing from inverted ventricles but out the appropriate arteries. Patients with corrected transposition, however, are either born with complete heart block or develop heart block at a rate of 2% per year. In addition, they often have VSD and PS. The chest radiograph shows a completely straight left heart border because of the anterior and leftward position of the aorta. Patients also frequently have an Ebstein-like malformation of the left-sided AV valve (tricuspid valve), and that valve is frequently regurgitant.

6. A 28-year-old man has been known to have Wolff-Parkinson-White syndrome with episodes of supraventricular tachycardia. You order a chest radiograph and are surprised at the significant cardiomegaly, with what appears to be marked right atrial enlargement. The patient also has a murmur of tricuspid regurgitation. The most likely diagnosis is
a) ASD
b) VSD
c) Tricuspid stenosis
d) Ebstein anomaly

Answer and Discussion
The answer is d. Ebstein anomaly is the only congenital cardiac defect commonly associated with preexcitation syndromes like Wolff-Parkinson-White. Patients frequently have significant tricuspid regurgitation with a markedly dilated right atrium. Ebstein patients are prone to all rhythm disorders, including both atrial and ventricular arrhythmias, and they have a significant incidence of sudden death.

REFERENCES

1. Warnes CA, Liberthson R, Danielson GK, et al. Task force 1: the changing profile of congenital heart disease in adult life. *J Am Coll Cardiol* 2001;37(5)1170–1175.
2. Marelli AJ, Mackie AS, Ittu RI, et al. Congenital heart disease in the general population: changing prevalence and age distribution. *Circulation* 2007;115(2):163–172.
3. Fuster V, Brandenburg RO, McGoon, et al. Clinical approach and management of congenital heart disease in the adolescent and adult. *Cardiovasc Clin* 1980;10(3):161–197.
4. Steele PM, Fuster V, Cohen M, et al. Isolated atrial septal defect with pulmonary vascular obstructive disease—long-term follow-up and prediction of outcome after surgical correction. *Circulation* 1987;76(5):1037–1042.
5. Webb G, Gatzoulis MA. Atrial septal defects in the adult: recent progress and overview. *Circulation* 2006;114(15):1645–1653.
6. Wilson W, Taubert KA, Gewitz M, et al. Prevention of infective endocarditis: guidelines from the American Heart Association: a guideline from the American Heart Association Rheumatic Fever, Endocarditis, and Kawasaki Disease Committee, Council on Cardiovascular Disease in the Young, and the Council on Clinical Cardiology, Council on Cardiovascular Surgery and Anesthesia, and the Quality of Care and Outcomes Research Interdisciplinary Working Group. *Circulation* 2007;116(15):1736–1754.
7. Wu JC, Child JS. Common congenital heart disorders in adults. *Curr Probl Cardiol* 2004;29(11):641–700.
8. Minette MS, Sahn DJ. Ventricular septal defects. *Circulation* 2006;114(20):2190–2197.
9. Mitchell SC, Korones SB, Berendes HW. Congenital heart disease in 56,109 births. Incidence and natural history. *Circulation* 1971;43(3):323–332.
10. Therrien J, Webb G. Clinical update on adults with congenital heart disease. *Lancet* 2003;362(9392):1305–1313.
11. Schneider DJ, Moore JW. Patent ductus arteriosus. *Circulation* 2006;114(17):1873–1882.
12. Inglessis I, Landzberg MJ. Interventional catheterization in adult congenital heart disease. *Circulation* 2007;115(12):1622–1633.
13. Pass RH, Hijazi Z, Hsu DT, et al. Multicenter USA Amplatzer patent ductus arteriosus occlusion device trial: initial and one-year results. *J Am Coll Cardiol* 2004;44(3):513–519.
14. Keith JD. Prevalence, incidence and epidemiology. In: Keith JD, Rowe RD, Vlad P, eds. *Heart Disease in Infancy and Childhood.* New York: MacMillan, 1978:3–13.
15. Keith JD. Coarctation of the aorta. In: Keith JD, Rowe RD, Vlad P, eds. *Heart Disease in Infancy and Childhood.* New York: MacMillan, 1978:736–757.
16. Isner JM, Donaldson RF, Fulton D, et al. Cystic medial necrosis in coarctation of the aorta: a potential factor contributing to adverse consequences observed after percutaneous balloon angioplasty of coarctation sites. *Circulation* 1987;75(4):689–695.
17. Niwa K, Perloff JK, Bhuta SM, et al. Structural abnormalities of great arterial walls in congenital heart disease: light and electron microscopic analyses. *Circulation* 2001;103(3):393–400.
18. Aboulhosn J, Child JS. Left ventricular outflow obstruction: subaortic stenosis, bicuspid aortic valve, supravalvar aortic stenosis, and coarctation of the aorta. *Circulation* 2006;114(22):2412–2422.
19. Connolly HM, Huston J 3rd, Brown RD Jr, et al. Intracranial aneurysms in patients with coarctation of the aorta: a prospective magnetic resonance angiographic study of 100 patients. *Mayo Clin Proc* 2003;78(12):1491–1499.
20. Campbell M. Natural history of coarctation of the aorta. *Br Heart J* 1970;32(5):633–640.
21. Bashore TM. Adult congenital heart disease: right ventricular outflow tract lesions. *Circulation* 2007;115(14):1933–1947.
22. Hayes CJ, Gersony WM, Driscoll DJ, et al. Second natural history study of congenital heart defects. Results of treatment of patients with pulmonary valvar stenosis. *Circulation* 1993;87(Suppl 2):I28–I37.
23. Bonow RO, Carabello BA, Kanu C, et al. ACC/AHA 2006 guidelines for the management of patients with valvular heart disease: a report of the American College of Cardiology/American Heart Association Task Force on Practice Guidelines (writing committee to revise the 1998 Guidelines for the Management of Patients With Valvular Heart Disease): developed in collaboration with the Society of Cardiovascular Anesthesiologists: endorsed by the Society for Cardiovascular Angiography and Interventions and the Society of Thoracic Surgeons. *Circulation* 2006;114(5):e84–e231.
24. Jarrar M, Betbout F, Farhat BM, et al. Long-term invasive and non-invasive results of percutaneous balloon pulmonary valvuloplasty in children, adolescents, and adults. *Am Heart J* 1999;138(5 Pt 1):950–954.
25. Sadr-Ameli MA, Sheikholeslami F, Firoozi I, et al. Late results of balloon pulmonary valvuloplasty in adults. *Am J Cardiol* 1998;82(3):398–400.
26. Hoffman JI, Kaplan S. The incidence of congenital heart disease. *J Am Coll Cardiol* 2002;39(12):1890–1900.
27. Anderson RH, Weinberg PM. The clinical anatomy of tetralogy of Fallot. *Cardiol Young* 2005;15(Suppl 1):38–47.

28. Dabizzi RP, Teodori G, Barletta GA. Associated coronary and cardiac anomalies in the tetralogy of Fallot. An angiographic study. *Eur Heart J* 1990;(8):692–704.
29. Gatzoulis M, Till J, Somerville J, et al. Mechanoelectrical interaction in tetralogy of Fallot: QRS prolongation relates to right ventricular size and predicts malignant ventricular arrhythmias and sudden death. *Circulation* 1995;92(2):231–237.
30. Warnes CA. Transposition of the great arteries. *Circulation* 2006;114(24):2699–2709.
31. Huhta JC, Maloney JD, Ritter DG, et al. Complete atrioventricular block in patients with atrioventricular discordance. *Circulation* 1983;67(6):1374–1377.
32. Khairy P, Marelli AJ. Clinical use of electrocardiography in adults with congenital heart disease. *Circulation* 2007;116(23):2734–2746.
33. Attenhofer Jost CH, Connolly HM, O'Leary PW, et al. Ebstein's anomaly. *Circulation* 2007;115(2):277–285.
34. Brickner ME, Hillis LD, Lange RA. Congenital heart disease in adults. Second of two parts. *N Engl J Med* 2000;342(5):334–342.

Chapter 63

Acute Coronary Syndromes

Hani Jneid   *Curtis M. Rimmerman*   *A. Michael Lincoff*

POINTS TO REMEMBER:

- Acute coronary syndromes (ACS) represent a spectrum of ischemic heart events that share a common pathophysiology and encompass the following entities: unstable angina; non–ST elevation myocardial infarction (NSTEMI), and ST elevation myocardial infarction (STEMI).

- ACS usually is caused by an unstable atheromatous plaque that fissures or ruptures in an epicardial coronary artery, which results in the formation of a superimposed platelet and fibrin thrombus.

- Unstable plaques associated with ACS are most often lipid-rich, atheromatous lesions with a thin fibrous cap and increased macrophage infiltration, whereas stable plaques causing chronic stable angina generally possess a thick fibrous cap and less lipid core and inflammatory burden.

- The diagnosis of a STEMI can be made on the basis of ECG criteria, including ST segment elevation >1 mm in at least two contiguous leads. Reciprocal ST segment depression is an associated and helpful finding that makes the possibility of acute pericarditis mimicking acute STEMI less likely.

- Serial testing of serum cardiac enzyme levels should be performed routinely in patients with a suspected ACS.

- Troponins T and I are components of the cardiac myocyte contractile apparatus and are highly specific for a cardiac origin. They are also highly sensitive for the detection of myocardial necrosis and are available in rapid assay forms. Troponins begin to rise 3 hours after onset of chest pain and last longer in the circulation (7–14 days) than creatine kinase (CK).

- The mainstay of treatment for acute STEMI is immediate reperfusion therapy based on the observation that myocardial necrosis occurs as a wavefront over 4 to 6 hours after coronary artery occlusion.

- Indications for fibrinolytic therapy in patients with acute myocardial infarction (MI) include ST segment elevation in two or more contiguous leads or new (or presumably new) left bundle-branch block, with ischemic symptoms <12 hours in duration.

- Randomized clinical trials have shown that primary percutaneous coronary intervention (PCI; PCI as the primary means of reperfusion used instead of fibrinolytic therapy) is associated with a lower mortality and reduced rates of intracranial hemorrhage when compared with fibrinolytic therapy.

ACS represent a spectrum of ischemic heart events that share a common pathophysiology and encompass the following entities:

- Unstable angina
- NSTEMI
- STEMI

Some also include sudden cardiac death, defined as an unexpected cardiac death occurring within 1 hour of chest discomfort onset.

EPIDEMIOLOGY

In 2004, the estimated number of hospital discharges with the primary diagnosis of ACS was 840,000. However, this number was a conservative estimate, and when including secondary discharge diagnoses, the corresponding number of inpatient hospital discharges in 2004 is >1.5 million hospitalizations for ACS. Based on the 2007 report on heart disease and stroke statistics by the American Heart Association, the estimated annual incidence of MI (STEMI and NSTEMI) is 565,000 new events and 300,000 recurrent events annually. Approximately 25% of patients with STEMI die, with half of these deaths occurring in the prehospital setting before effective treatment can be given. Invariably, these prehospital deaths are arrhythmogenic in origin. To minimize out-of-hospital mortality, a multidisciplinary approach should be implemented including patient education, rapid patient evaluation and triage, prompt initiation of therapies, and ready access to public external defibrillators for witnessed out-of-hospital ventricular dysrhythmias. In the case of STEMI, successful early infarct-related coronary artery reperfusion reduces both the infarct size and the incidence of subsequent complications, including congestive heart failure, arrhythmia, and death.

PATHOPHYSIOLOGY

An ACS usually is caused by an unstable atheromatous plaque that fissures or ruptures in an epicardial coronary artery, which results in the formation of a superimposed platelet and fibrin thrombus. The unstable plaque and the superimposed thrombus can result in the rapid diminution or interruption of regional myocardial blood flow, which in cases of total or nearly total occlusion can cause acute myocyte ischemia and infarction. While patients presenting with unstable angina and NSTEMI often have subocclusive or intermittently occlusive thromboses, patients with STEMI usually present with an occlusive thrombus and thus require immediate reperfusion therapy.

Unstable plaques associated with ACS are most often lipid-rich, atheromatous lesions with a thin fibrous cap and increased macrophage infiltration, whereas stable plaques causing chronic stable angina generally possess a thick fibrous cap and less lipid core and inflammatory burden.

Most coronary artery unstable plaques leading to ACS were not flow-limiting prior to fissuring or rupture (70% of these plaques have <50% angiographic stenosis). Unstable plaques do not occur in isolation in the coronary arteries of patients with an ACS: Up to 40% of patients with an acute MI in one study had multiple complex plaques with angiographic features of instability (thrombus, ulceration, etc.). This is in line with the accumulating evidence demonstrating the diffuse nature of coronary artery inflammation rather than its focal nature. Sometimes, the terms *vulnerable* or *high-risk plaque* are used interchangeably with the term *unstable plaque*.

CLINICAL PRESENTATION

The classic symptoms of ACS include chest discomfort, pain, or heaviness. Associated symptoms include dyspnea, palpitations, light-headedness, nausea, vomiting, and diaphoresis. Symptoms develop mostly in the central or left chest area, with radiation to the jaw, neck, shoulders, back, and arms but almost never below the waist. The discomfort is usually not highly localized, does not vary with position or inspiration (as does pleuropericarditic pain), and is not reproducible by palpation (as is costochondritis).

Usually, if the duration of unstable angina symptoms extends beyond 20 minutes, a MI documentable by positive cardiac enzymes transpires secondary to irreversible myocyte necrosis. Fleeting chest pain of few seconds duration is usually not related to ischemic heart disease.

Most chest discomfort episodes representing an unstable coronary syndrome occur at rest or with minimal physical activity, although strenuous activity is well known to trigger acute ischemic events, especially among patients who exercise infrequently. Circadian variation in ACS onset is well described, with a peak occurrence in the morning, and is believed to be secondary to an increase in catecholamine release and platelet aggregability.

The differential diagnosis of chest pain encompasses multiple other conditions, some of which can be life threatening (Table 63.1). Aortic dissection and pulmonary embolism are particularly important to consider and

TABLE 63.1

DIFFERENTIAL DIAGNOSIS OF NONISCHEMIC CHEST PAIN

Chest pain from other cardiovascular causes
Pericarditis
Dissection of the aorta
Pulmonary embolism/Infarction
Chest pain from gastrointestinal causes
Esophageal reflux
Esophageal spasm
Esophageal rupture
Gallstone colic
Peptic ulcer disease
Chest pain from other causes
Tietze's syndrome (pain associated with tender swelling of the costochondral joints)
Chest wall pain
Spontaneous pneumothorax
Herpes zoster
Mondor's disease (phlebitis of the veins in the left breast region)

differentiate in a timely manner. Aortic dissection is abrupt in onset, perceived as "ripping" chest, interscapular, or back pain. These qualities distinguish it from chest pain of ischemic origin, in which the discomfort is less severe and intensifies gradually. Patients with an acute aortic dissection often have a history of hypertension (often severe) and manifest pulse deficits and a widened mediastinum on the chest radiograph.

Pulmonary embolism is characterized by pleuritic chest pain that worsens while in a supine position, accompanied by dyspnea, tachycardia, tachypnea, and unexplained hypoxemia. The chest radiograph typically is normal. Frequently, a history of recent prolonged immobility and/or a hypercoagulable state are present, making the clinical and medical history diagnostically important.

Chest pain alleviation using nitroglycerin has little diagnostic utility in patients presenting with chest pain. In one study of 223 patients presenting to the emergency room with chest pain, response to nitroglycerin was equally present among patients with cardiac and noncardiac chest pain. In addition, patients with esophageal spasm are known to exhibit symptomatic relief secondary to smooth muscle relaxation with nitrate therapy.

Angina pectoris usually is a diagnosis made by the medical history. However, the medical history, physical examination, 12-lead ECG, and initial cardiac biomarker tests should all be used to assign patients with chest pain into one of four categories: a noncardiac diagnosis, chronic stable angina, possible ACS, and definite ACS.

DIAGNOSIS

Physical Examination

During an ACS, patients often appear to be restless and are unable to assume a comfortable position. Diaphoresis and skin pallor often are visible, and the pulse is regular and rapid. The blood pressure response varies, including

- Hypertension (in the setting of increased adrenergic stimulation)
- Normal blood pressure
- Hypotension (particularly in patients with large infarction or ischemia)

The jugular venous pulse usually is normal, unless a right ventricular infarct or congestive heart failure occur. Rales may be present on pulmonary examination, reflecting an increase in left ventricular end-diatolic pressure secondary to a large burden of ischemia and/or left-sided infarction. Cardiac examination frequently demonstrates an S_4 gallop, and a dyskinetic cardiac apex may be palpable precordially, particularly during an anterolateral infarction. A new third heart sound usually reflects a more extensive ischemia or infarction. Newly audible systolic murmurs during an ACS may be related to a transient or persistent mitral regurgitation and usually indicate papillary muscle dusfunction or rupture secondary to ischemia or infarction.

Electrocardiography

Diagnostic Findings

If the initial ECG is not diagnostic but the patient remains symptomatic and a high clinical suspicion for ACS exists, serial ECGs at 15- to 30-minute intervals or continuous 12-lead ECG monitoring should be performed.

The diagnosis of STEMI can be made on the basis of ECG criteria, including ST segment elevation >1 mm in at least two contiguous leads. Reciprocal ST segment depression is an associated and helpful finding that makes the possibility of acute pericarditis mimicking acute STEMI less likely. Electrocardiographically, ST segment elevation is thought to represent acute myocardial injury, whereas Q-wave formation is most appropriately labeled as infarction, and Q waves in the setting of ST segment elevation are best labeled as acute infarction. In the absence of ST segment elevation, Q waves represent an MI of indeterminate age. Unlike right bundle-branch block, left bundle-branch block obscures Q waves and interferes with the ability to diagnose Q waves, unless Q waves develop newly in the presence of left bundle-branch block, in which setting they should be considered pathological. Premature ventricular complexes with a complete right bundle-branch morphology and, thus, a left ventricular origin, may manifest Q waves. When present, they can be a useful diagnostic adjunct for the presence of coronary artery disease. Tall and peaked T waves have been noted in the early phases of acute STEMI and are termed *hyperacute T waves*. On the other hand, common ECG findings of unstable angina and NSTEMI include ST segment depression, T-wave inversion, or even nonspecific ECG changes.

A 12-lead ECG may also provide a crude estimate of the infarct size or the "myocardium in jeopardy" during an

ACS. For example, when the ECG demonstrates ST segment elevation in leads V_{2-6}, I, and aV_L, it usually indicates an extensive anterolateral STEMI. Ischemia or infarction involving the left circumflex coronary artery may be apparent in leads V_5, V_6, I, and aV_L. However, it can also be "silent" on a 12-lead ECG, and this is why it is advisable to obtain supplemental ECG leads V_{7-9} when left circumflex occlusion is suspected in the absence of major changes on 12-lead ECG.

Although the ECG is an indispensable adjunct to the patient history and physical examination, it may sometimes provide inconclusive information despite a transpiring ACS presentation. In the Thrombolysis in Myocardial Infarction (TIMI) III trial, with 1,473 patients enrolled having unstable angina or NSTEMI, 9% of patients demonstrated absence of ischemic ECG changes on 12-lead ECG.

ST Segment Elevation and Q Waves

Historically, MI has been classified as transmural and nontransmural, or Q-wave and non–Q-wave MI, based on the presence or absence of Q waves on the ECG along with evidence of elevated cardiac enzymes. However, Q-wave infarction is not always associated with a transmural infarction, and a non–Q-wave infarction is not always a nontransmural infarction. Significant overlap occurs, as shown in histopathological studies. The development of Q waves depends to some extent on the speed and completeness of spontaneous or therapeutic coronary reperfusion. Patients with Q-wave infarcts tend to have larger infarcts and less prominent coronary collaterals, lower ejection fraction, and higher peak cardiac enzyme levels. In-hospital mortality is greater among patients with Q-wave infarction, which is likely attributable to larger infarct size. Postinfarction ischemia, however, is more common in those patients with non–Q-wave infarctions, as is reinfarction.

With the advent of reperfusion therapy for acute STEMI, a more important distinction at presentation (than the presence of Q waves) is based on the presence or absence of ST segment elevation on initial ECG (i.e., STEMI vs. NSTEMI). With STEMI, early coronary angiography typically demonstrates an occlusive thrombus in >80% of patients, compared with only 10% to 20% of patients without ST segment elevation. Fibrinolytic therapy or PCI is recommended for patients with STEMIs (or new bundle-branch block) presenting within 12 hours of onset of symptoms. Thus, the identification of ST segment elevation on the ECG represents a key finding dictating the acute management of these patients.

Laboratory Studies

With the discovery and clinical introduction of the highly sensitive cardiac troponins, clinicians can detect minimal degrees of myocardial necrosis. The diagnosis of an acute MI can be made either histopathologically or inferred by the rise of cardiac markers in the presence of any of the following: ischemic symptoms, ECG evidence of myocardial ischemia or infarction, and/or direct visualization of a fresh coronary thrombus with a disrupted plaque on coronary angiography.

Serial testing of serum cardiac enzyme levels should be performed routinely in patients with a suspected ACS. Successful reperfusion (spontaneous, pharmacologic, or mechanical) results in a higher and earlier peak of enzyme levels secondary to a "washout" phenomenon, which serves as a useful indicator of reperfusion success.

Troponins T and I

Serum marker troponins T and I are components of the cardiac myocyte contractile apparatus and are highly specific for a cardiac origin. They are also highly sensitive for the detection of myocardial necrosis and are available in rapid assay forms. Troponins begin to rise 3 hours after onset of chest pain and last longer in the circulation (7–14 days) than CK. This reduces their value for detection of reinfarction, in which setting CK-MBs become the markers of choice (Fig. 63.1). Troponin levels should also be interpreted with caution in the presence of renal failure. With rapid assay forms available, these biomarkers permit prompt patient triage and help dictate therapy. It is also important to note that patients with elevated troponins and normal CK-MB levels have worse outcomes compared with patients who have ischemic symptoms but no elevation in cardiac markers (i.e., unstable angina patients). This substantiates the adverse prognostic importance of detecting myocardial necrosis (often a surrogate for the presence of thombotic coronary artery disease), irrespective of its extent.

Creatine Kinase

The measurement of the CK-MB isoenzyme level continues to be a useful laboratory test for the diagnosis of acute MI and comes second to troponins in specificity for diagnosing acute MI. Initial elevations are detected 4 hours after acute injury. Levels tend to peak at approximately 24 hours and return to baseline within 48 to 72 hours. Levels should be obtained at initial presentation, 8 to 12 hours, and 16 to 24 hours after the onset of chest discomfort (Fig. 63.1).

Nonspecific Markers

The elevation of levels of white blood cell count, serum myoglobin, lactate dehydrogenase (LDH) and its isoenzymes (mainly LDH1), and aspartate aminotransferase represent nonspecific biochemical markers for the detection of MI. Myoglobin is one of the earliest cardiac markers to rise (1–4 hours) and used to be important in the emergency room setting. Levels of LDH exceed the normal range 24 to 48 hours after the acute event and peak at approximately 78 to 96 hours (Fig. 63.1). Fractionation of total LDH is, however, important because LDH1 is the specific cardiac marker that should be measured. Importantly, total

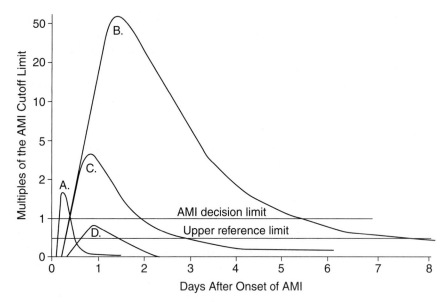

Figure 63.1 Plot of the appearance of cardiac markers in blood versus time after onset of symptoms. *Peak A*, early release of myoglobin or CK-MB isoforms after AMI; *peak B*, cardiac troponin after AMI; *peak C*, CK-MB after AMI; *peak D*, cardiac troponin after unstable angina. Data are plotted on a relative scale, where 1.0 is set at the AMI cutoff concentration. (Reproduced with permission from Wu AH, Apple AS, Gibler WB, et al. National Academy of Clinical Biochemistry Standards of Laboratory Practice: recommendations for the use of cardiac markers in coronary artery diseases. *Clin Chem* 1999;45(7):1104–1121.)

CK (without the MB fraction) and all the aforementioned nonspecific markers should no longer be utilized as primary tests for the detection of myocardial injury.

Although markers of myocardial necrosis are helpful in the diagnosis of MI, other emerging markers have important prognostic value. Myeloperoxidase (a marker of leukocyte activation) and brain natriuretic peptide (BNP; a marker of neurohormonal activation) predict future cardiovascular events in patients presenting to the emergency room with chest pain and in patients with ACS. High-sensitivity C-reactive protein (hs-CRP), a marker of inflammation, stands as an independent prognostic marker for recurrent events after an ACS, including death, MI, and restenosis after PCI.

A multimarker approach (e.g., simultaneous assessment of troponin, CRP, and BNP, and others) to risk stratify non–ST elevation ACS, in particular, may be superior to single biomarker assessment.

TREATMENT

All patients with ACS warrant hospitalization and telemetry monitoring. Those who develop an acute MI, manifest persistent ischemic symptoms, or develop hemodynamic or electrical instability should be observed in the intensive care unit.

Oxygen

The routine administration of oxygen during the initial peiord after an ACS is recommended. Higher-dose mask oxygen or endotracheal intubation may be necessary in patients with severe pulmonary edema or congestive heart failure.

Antiplatelet Therapy

The prompt administration of 160 to 325 mg of aspirin (to be chewed) is indicated for all patients presenting with ACS, and daily use of aspirin should be continued indefinitely thereafter. As more rapid buccal absorption is observed with non–enteric-coated aspirin, it is advisable not to use enteric formulations during acute MI or ischemia. The Second Interventional Study of Infarct Survival (ISIS-2) examined the efficacy of aspirin and demonstrated a reduction of 23% in the 35-day mortality in patients presenting with STEMI (Fig. 63.2). Aspirin reduces the incidence of coronary reocclusion and recurrent myocardial ischemia and infarction. In the absence of acute ischemic symptoms, 81 mg of aspirin daily is as effective for secondary prevention and has less gastroenterologic toxicity than larger doses of aspirin.

Data from the Clopidogrel in Unstable Angina to Prevent Recurrent Ischemic Events (CURE) trial showed a 20% additional reduction in the composite endpoint of cardiovascular death, MI, and stroke in patients with unstable angina and NSTEMI randomized to dual antiplatelet therapy with aspirin and clopidogrel compared with aspirin alone. The benefit was evident as early as 2 hours after the acute event and persisted for the total follow-up period of 12 months. Both the CLARITY-TIMI 28 (Clopidogrel as Adjunctive Reperfusion Therapy) and COMMIT-CCS-2 randomized trials also showed salutary cardiovascular effects of using clopidogrel in addition to aspirin after STEMI. Based on the two aforementioned trials, it is recommended to add clopidogrel to all STEMI patients, irrespective of whether patients receive reperfusion therapy, for at least 14 days (and preferably for a total of a 12-month period). It is thus recommended to use clopidogrel, with a loading dose of 300 mg, in addition to aspirin in all patients presenting with ACS. The use of a loading dose in the elderly

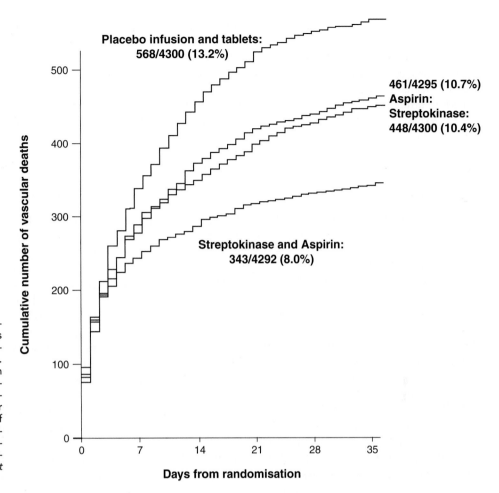

Figure 63.2 Cumulative vascular mortality after STEMI for days 0 to 35 in the Second Interventional Study of Infarct Survival. (Reproduced with permission from ISIS-2 Collaborative Group. Randomised trial of intravenous streptokinase, oral aspirin, both, or neither among 17,187 cases of suspected acute myocardial infarction: ISIS-2. ISIS-2 (Second International Study of Infarct Survival) Collaborative Group. *Lancet* 1988;2(8607):349–360.)

(>75 years of age) receiving a fibrinolytic agent for STEMI has not been studied and therefore is not recommended.

Glycoprotein IIb/IIIa inhibitors effectively block the final common pathway of platelet aggregation and are thus the most potent antiplatelet therapy available. Each platelet contains thousands of glycoprotein IIb/IIIa receptors on its surface; these receptors undergo conformational changes on platelet activation, enabling them to bind fibrinogen dimers and cross-link platelets. Abciximab, a chimeric human-murine monoclonal antibody with a high affinity to the glycoprotein IIb/IIIa receptor and a long physiological half-life (12 hours), is the pharmacologic agent of choice as an adjunct therapy in patients with STEMI or non–ST segment elevation ACS undergoing PCI and for all patients undergoing high-risk PCI. However, patients with STEMI who are treated with fibrinolytic therapy do not benefit from the addition of abciximab. In addition, there is no benefit of adding abciximab to patients presenting with unstable angina and NSTEMI but not undergoing early revascularization. The small molecules, eptifibatide (a synthetic peptide inhibitor) and tirofiban (a nonpeptide mimetic), which are glycoprotein IIb/IIIa inhibitors with shorter half-lives (90–120 minutes), have proven benefits as adjunct therapy before the catheterization and revascularization of patients with unstable angina and NSTEMI and in those patients receiving medical treatments alone.

In patients with a history of gastrointestinal bleeding, medications to minimize the risk of recurrent bleeding (especially proton-pump inhibitors) should be prescribed when using antiplatelet agents.

Anticoagulant Therapy

Anticoagulants should be used in all patients presenting with ACS. The duration and type of agent used vary with the patients' clinical presentation, physicians' preference, and institutional practices.

Unfractionated heparin, an antithrombin, is the traditional anticoagulant used and is advocated to use for 48 hours after ACS onset (given the limited medical evidence available for unfractionated heparin and the risk of heparin-induced thrombocytopenia), unless other indications for anticoagulation exist. Recent studies have demonstrated the salutary benefits of various anticoagulants, such as fondaparinux (a synthetic factor Xa inhibitor), and the low molecular weight heparin (LMWH) drugs reviparin (not available in the United States) and enoxaparin. The latter agents are advocated for extended use beyond the

48-hour period (unlike unfractionated heparin) and preferably for the duration of the index hospitalization (up to 8 days). However, caution should be exercised when using these agents in patients with renal insufficiency (as they are cleared by the renal route) and in other settings. Moreover, fondaparinux should not be used alone during PCI for STEMI or NSTEMI, given the apparent increased risk for catheter-related thrombosis when this agent is used without factor IIa inhibition, but instead should be supplemented with another additional anticoagulant such as unfractionated heparin. LMWH, in particular, offers the advantages of subcutaneous dosing compared with unfractionated heparin as well as reduced protein binding, platelet activation, monitoring requirements, and heparin-induced thrombocytopenia. In trials comparing enoxaparin to unfractionated heparin in the settings of STEMI or non–ST segment elevation ACS, enoxaparin was associated with lower rates of reinfarction but higher risk of bleeding. Bivalirudin, a direct thrombin inhibitor, has also been increasingly used because of its short-half life and low bleeding risk. Bivalirudin has shown to be as effective as the combination of heparin and GPIIb/IIIa inhibitors in reducing ischemic events but safer with respect to bleeding rates among patients with non–ST segment elevation ACS and STEMI.

After the administration of streptokinase for STEMI, unfractionated heparin does not reduce ischemic events and increases hemorrhage rates. Unless indicated for other reasons, unfractionated heparin is thus not recommended in the immediate period after treatment with streptokinase (although reviparin, a LMWH, was shown to reduce ischemic events with streptokinase in the CREATE trial). On the other hand, for the fibrin-specific agents (alteplase, reteplase, and tenecteplase [TNK]), unfractionated heparin has been associated with improved reperfusion rates.

All anticoagulants should be discontinued after PCI in patients with ACS and noncomplicated course.

Reperfusion Therapy

The mainstay of treatment for acute STEMI is immediate reperfusion therapy based on the observation that myocardial necrosis occurs as a wavefront over 4 to 6 hours after coronary artery occlusion. The operative paradigm is that early reperfusion arrests this wavefront, salvages myocardium, preserves left ventricular function, and reduces mortality. Multiple large-scale, placebo-controlled trials have demonstrated that fibrinolytic agents administered during the initial 6 hours after symptom onset reduce short-term (4–5 week) mortality by 25% to 35% in patients with acute STEMI. Primary PCI (usually angioplasty with or without stenting) is a viable alternative to pharmacologic reperfusion, with evidence of greater efficacy than fibrinolytic therapy when performed at expert centers and in a timely manner.

It is important to minimize total ischemic time (time from onset of symptoms of STEMI to initiation of reperfusion therapy). Goals are defined as time from a first-medical-contact-to-balloon within 90 minutes for primary PCI, and fibrinoytic drug delivery within 30 minutes of patients' presentation to the hospital. To improve systems of care for STEMI patients, efforts are under way to expand the use of prehospital 12-lead ECG programs by emergency medical systems.

Fibrinolytic Therapy

Indications for fibrinolytic therapy in patients with acute MI include ST segment elevation in two or more contiguous leads or new (or presumably new) left bundle-branch block, with ischemic symptoms <12 hours in duration. Clinical benefit is noted to be greater with larger (i.e., anterior) infarcts, in diabetic patients, and in patients with previous MI. A clear relationship exists between the magnitude of treatment benefits and time to therapy, with the greatest benefit observed with shorter ischemic time (i.e., door-to-needle time <30 minutes). The value of fibrinolytics 12 to 24 hours after symptom onset is less clear. Patients with ongoing chest discomfort and ST segment elevation are more likely to benefit from PCI. In TIMI IIIB, patients with NSTEMI had higher reinfarction rates with fibrinolytics compared with placebo. Fibrinolytics should therefore not be administered to NSTEMI patients.

Four fibrinolytic agents are currently approved in the United States for the treatment of acute MI. The first of these, streptokinase, is a non–fibrin-specific agent and produces the lowest rate of acute infarct vessel recanalization. Better rates of patency are achieved using the second- and third-generation agents (alteplase, reteplase, and TNK). These latter agents vary with regard to circulating half-life and fibrin specificity. Mortality of patients receiving alteplase, reteplase, and TNK therapy is lower than that with streptokinase. TNK, a mutant of alteplase with higher fibrin specificity, is a newly approved fibrinolytic with similar efficacy to alteplase but offers the advantage of administration in a single and rapid bolus over 5 seconds (compared with reteplase, which is administered as two boluses 30 minutes apart).

The principal limitation of fibrinolytic therapy is bleeding, most notably intracranial hemorrhage. Rates of intracranial hemorrhage after fibrinolysis have been documented in recent trials to range as high as 0.9% and may be higher in clinical practice. Risk factors for intracranial hemorrhage include female gender, advanced age, low body weight, concurrent warfarin therapy, excessive heparinization, and use of fibrinolytic agents other than streptokinase.

Absolute contraindications for fibrinolytic administration reflect predominantly bleeding risk and include:

- Intracranial neoplasm or arteriovenous malformation
- Active internal bleeding (excluding menses)

- Cerebrovascular accident within the prior year or any prior intracranial hemorrhage
- Suspected aortic dissection

Relative contraindications for fibrinolytic administration include:

- Blood pressure >180/110 mm Hg on presentation
- History of cerebrovascular accident more than 1 year prior
- History of chronic, severe hypertension
- Anticoagulant therapy with international normalized ratio >2.0
- Active peptic ulcer
- Pregnancy
- Recent trauma or internal bleeding (within 2–4 weeks)
- Noncompressible vascular puncture within the prior 24 hours
- Cardiopulmonary resuscitation
- Recent major surgery

Mechanical Reperfusion

There essentially are three types of mechanical reperfusion: primary PCI (where PCI is used as the reperfusion modality instead of fibrinolytic therapy), rescue PCI (where PCI is used once fibrinolytic therapy fails), and adjunctive PCI (PCI after successful fibrinolytic therapy—although the benefit of PCI in this setting has generally been difficult to prove).

Overall, randomized clinical trials have shown that primary PCI (PCI as the primary means of reperfusion used instead of fibrinolytic therapy) is associated with a lower mortality and reduced rates of intracranial hemorrhage when compared with fibrinolytic therapy. Whenever feasible in a timely manner (door-to-balloon <90 minutes), primary PCI is preferred to fibrinolytic therapy in patients with STEMI. Primary PCI may also be applied to patients for whom fibrinolysis is relatively or absolutely contraindicated. In the high-risk subset of patients with acute MI presenting with cardiogenic shock, primary PCI is clearly the preferred modality of therapy. Limitations of primary PCI include the requirement for specialized facilities with skilled and experienced personnel.

Pharmacologic reperfusion is not uniformly successful in restoring antegrade flow in the infarct artery. In such situations, prompt coronary angiography with rescue PC should be performed. It is advisable to continuously check the 12-lead ECG for signs of successful reperfusion after administration of fibrinolytic therapy, with 90 minutes after its initiation considered as the best time point for evaluating the need for rescue PCI. If <50% ST segment resolution in the lead showing the greatest degree of ST segment elevation is evident at 90 minutes after fibrinolytic therapy administration, it is likely that this treatment has failed to produce reperfusion and thus rescue PCI should be undertaken. Notably, the presence or absence of is-

chemic discomfort may be unreliable for identifying failed reperfusion.

In patients with cardiogenic shock, severe congestive heart failure, or hemodynamically compromising ventricular arrhythmias, prompt coronary angiography with possible PCI is a useful approach even after initiation of fibrinolytic therapy and regardless of the time elapsed since its initiation. Coronary arteriography may also be considered as part of an invasive strategy for risk assessment after fibrinolytic therapy or for patients not undergoing primary reperfusion.

The open artery hypothesis suggests that late patency of an infarct artery is associated with improved left ventricular function and increased electrical stability. However, the recently published Occluded Artery Trial (OAT) tested routine PCI against medical therapy for total coronary occlusion 3 to 28 days after MI in stabilized patients and found no benefits beyond optimal medical therapy with routine PCI strategy. However, the study included only patients who were clinically stable and excluded those with New York Heart Association class III or IV heart failure, rest angina, renal insufficiency, left main or three-vessel disease, clinical instability as well as those with severe inducible ischemia. Although additional data demonstrated modest benefits from opening occluded arteries late in stable patients, mostly in preventing left ventricular dilation, this remains to be proven in the future.

Finally, although *facilitated percutaneous coronary intervention* (a term used for the strategy of using adjunct pharmacologic therapy preceding primary PCI in the setting of STEMI) has been associated with many advantages (including earlier time to reperfusion, smaller infarct size, improved patient stability, and lower infarct artery thrombus burden), increased bleeding complications and additional cost remain important concerns. Recently, the ASSENT-4 PCI and FINESSE trials demonstrated no cardiovascular benefits and increased complications with the facilitated PCI strategy among patients with STEMI.

Coronary Stenting

Coronary stenting has become the preferred modality of percutaneous revascularization, as compared with coronary balloon angioplasty alone, among patients with acute MI as well as those in more elective settings. Stents prevent elastic recoil in the coronary artery after balloon inflation, attenuate the risk of acute closure, markedly diminish the need for emergent coronary artery bypass graft surgery, and reduce restenosis. However, reactive neointimal hyperplasia and consequent restenosis are important limitations to stent use.

The novel drug-eluting stents, which are coated with biological agents (such as sirolimus, paclitaxel, etc.) to inhibit smooth muscle cell proliferation and neointimal hyperplasia, have markedly reduced clinical restenosis (up to 70% compared with the traditional bare-metal stents). For all

ACS patients who undergo PCI and stenting, aspirin 162 to 325 mg daily should be given for at least 1 month after bare-metal stent implantation, and for 3 and 6 months after sirolimus- and paclitaxel-eluting stent implantation, respectively, and then indefinitely at a dose of 75 to 162 mg daily. It is preferred that all post-PCI patients who receive a drug-eluting stent receive clopidogrel 75 mg daily in addition to aspirin for at least 12 months, especially when utilizing drug-eluting stents to decrease the risk of stent thrombosis.

Beta-blockers

In general, β-blockers should be administered as early as possible after ACS, initially as intravenous medication and then as oral therapy. The COMMIT/CCS-2 trial showed, however, an increase in the risk of cardiogenic shock, which counterbalanced the reduction in reinfarction and ventricular fibrillation with the early use of intravenous β-blockers after STEMI. Thus, intravenous β-blocker therapy is reasonable in the early 24 hours when hypertension is present and the patient is at low risk for developing cardiogenic shock. Patients with sinus tachycardia or atrial fibrillation should have left ventricular function rapidly evaluated before administration of intravenous β-blockers.

Oral β-blocker therapy should be administered within 24 hours of presentation to all ACS patients without a contraindication (e.g., heart failure), irrespective of concomitant performance of PCI. By lowering the heart rate, blood pressure, and consequently myocardial oxygen demand, β-blockers reduce the rates of cardiac rupture and ventricular fibrillation, relieve pain, and reduce infarct size. In patients with left ventricular dysfunction after MI (ejection fraction <40%), the β-blocker carvedilol has been specifically shown to reduce long-term mortality. Patients with heart failure, hypotension (blood pressure <90 mm Hg), bradycardia (heart rate <60), or advanced heart block should be excluded. A common protocol is to initiate intravenous metoprolol in three separate 5-mg boluses 5 minutes apart, subsequently beginning oral metoprolol therapy (50 mg every 6 hours), provided the patient is hemodynamically stable and has no evidence of heart failure or shock.

Neuroendocrine Inhibitors

Early in the course of an acute MI, administration of an angiotensin-converting enzyme (ACE) inhibitor reduces mortality. The greatest benefit occurs in those patients with anterior infarctions and heart failure. Therapy with ACE inhibitors should be started promptly (i.e., within 24 hours of presentation), but immediate intravenous therapy is unnecessary and may be detrimental. ACE inhibitors should be given and continued indefinitely for patients recovering from ACS with heart failure, left ventricular dysfunction

(≤40%), hypertension, or diabetes mellitus, unless contraindicated.

If the patient is intolerant to ACE inhibitors, then it is reasonable to use angiotensin receptor blocker (ARB) therapy, especially in the presence of heart failure or left ventricular dysfunction (≤40%). In addition, aldosterone blockers are recommended for ACS patients without significant renal insufficiency or hyperkalemia who are already receiving therapeutic doses of an ACE (or ARB) inhibitor and a β-blocker, have an ejection ≤40%, and have either diabetes or heart failure.

Nitrate Therapy

Nitrate therapy reduces both right and left ventricular preload, produces peripheral vasodilation, and reduces ventricular afterload, thereby lowering myocardial oxygen requirement and work. In addition, it has also direct vasodilator effects on the coronary arteries. The routine administration of nitrate therapy for ACS patients has not been associated with reduced mortality in randomized trials and may even be detrimental in those patients with right ventricular infarction or intravascular volume depletion. Similarly, long-term nitrate administration to these patients does not improve long-term survival and should thus be used predominantly for symptom relief. Nitroglycerin remains helpful in those patients with persistent ischemia, hypertension, or congestive heart failure during the initial 24 to 48 hours after an ACS. Continued use after 24 to 48 hours is appropriate in the settings of recurrent ischemia and persistent heart failure.

Calcium Channel Blockers

Indications for calcium channel blockers in the setting of acute MI are confined to the clinical settings where ischemia or atrial arrhythmias persist and there is a contraindication to the administration of β-blockers. Calcium channel blockers have not been shown to reduce mortality after acute MI, and in some patient subgroups, these agents may cause myocardial depression or heart failure and even increase mortality.

Analgesia

Ongoing chest discomfort causes increased sympathetic output, and therefore increases the heart rate and blood pressure. This ultimately increases myocardial oxygen consumption. Prompt administration of an intravenous analgesic (e.g., morphine sulfate) is therefore recommended. Morphine sulfate also reduces ventricular preload and helps relieve dyspnea, so it is particularly helpful in acute MI complicated with congestive heart failure. On the other hand, acute right ventricular infarction is a preload-sensitive state, in which setting morphine (and especially nitrates) should be used with extreme caution.

Hydroxymethylglutaryl–Coenzyme A Reductase Inhibitors

The Scandinavian Simvastatin Survival Study (4S) demonstrated a 30% mortality reduction in patients with coronary artery disease randomized to simvastatin compared with placebo and was the earliest secondary prevention trial to demonstrate a survival benefit of hydroxymethylglutaryl–coenzyme A (HMG-CoA) reductase inhibitors. Additional trials using various HMG-CoA reductase inhibitors (or statins) showed benefit in both primary and secondary prevention. A recent meta-analysis by Cannon et al. demonstrated that intensive lipid lowering with high-dose HMG-CoA reductase inhibitors (such as 80 mg of atorvastatin or simvastatin) provides a significant benefit over standard-dose therapy for preventing predominantly nonfatal cardiovascular events. Intensive lipid-lowering showed also less progression in atheroma burden (and possibly mild regression) compared with standard-dose lipid-lowering therapy.

HMG-CoA reductase inhibitors are known to exert their benefits through lipid lowering and perhaps through nonlipid actions (so-called pleiotropic effects), such as anti-inflammatory and antithrombotic effects. New lipid-modifying agents have emerged and are targeting the high-density lipoprotein cholesterol component.

SECONDARY PREVENTION GOALS AND ADDITIONAL RECOMMENDATIONS

Secondary prevention goals for patients with ACS include the complete cessation of tobacco (including no exposure to environmental smoke), achieving blood pressure <140/90 mm Hg (<130/80 in patients with diabetes and chronic kidney disease), achieving a low-density lipoprotein cholesterol substantially <100 mg/dL (and preferably <70 mg/dL in high-risk patients), daily walking for 30 minutes (or a minimum of 5 days per week), achieving a body mass index of 18.5–24.9 kg/m^2 and a waist circumference <40 inches for men and <35 inches for women, and achieving a HbA1c <7% in diabetic patients.

All patients with cardiovascular disease should have an annual influenza vaccination. Hormone replacement therapy (estrogen with or without progestin) should not be initiated in postmenopausal women after ACS for secondary prevention, given their prothrombotic hazards. Antioxidants (such as vitamin E) and folic acid are no longer recommended for secondary prevention of ACS. Cardiac rehabilitation, on the other hand, should be recommended particularly to those with multiple modifiable risk factors and those in whom exercise monitoring is needed. Given the increased risk of cardiovascular events among patients taking cyclooxygenase-2 inhibitors and other nonsteroidal anti-inflammatory drugs, these drugs should be discontinued immediately at the time of ACS.

Physicians should also screen ACS patients for the occurrence of depression and refer and treat them when indicated. Selective serotonin reuptake inhibitors are particularly proven to be safe antidepressant therapies after ACS.

HEMODYNAMIC MONITORING

The placement of a pulmonary artery catheter (also called a *Swan-Ganz catheter*) for continuous hemodynamic measurement of right- and left-sided cardiac pressures are indicated in few selected circumstances. These include severe or progressive congestive heart failure (in which volume and inotrope therapies are difficult to titrate), cardiogenic shock, and suspected mechanical complications of acute infarction (e.g., papillary muscle rupture, ventricular septal defect, pericardial tamponade).

Patients with severe congestive heart failure, cardiogenic shock, or both often require intravenous inotropes as well as ventricular preload- and afterload-reducing agents, best administered and dosed with full knowledge of the cardiac-filling pressures. This allows the differentiation in critically ill patients of inadequate left ventricular volumes and an underfilled left ventricle versus a volume-replete state with extensive left ventricular systolic impairment. The routine uncomplicated acute MI, regardless of its location, is not an indication for the placement of a Swan-Ganz catheter, and multiple randomized studies have failed to show benefit from the routine use of this catheter, even among heart failure patients.

INTRA-AORTIC BALLOON COUNTERPULSATION

Intra-aortic balloon counterpulsation is reserved for critically ill patients. Subgroups in which this therapy is indicated include patients with the following conditions:

- Persistent cardiogenic shock despite pharmacologic therapy as a bridge to coronary revascularization
- Refractory arrhythmias resulting in hemodynamic instability
- Refractory postinfarction angina despite maximal antianginal therapy
- Acute mechanical complications of MI (e.g., ventricular septal defect, papillary muscle rupture)
- High-risk PCI (unprotected left main disease, left ventricular dysfunction, target vessel supplying >40% territory, or severe congestive heart failure)

Contraindications to intra-aortic balloon counterpulsation include aortic dissection, aortic aneurysms, peripheral arterial disease, descending aortic and peripheral vascular grafts, and moderate to severe aortic regurgitation.

COMPLICATIONS OF ACUTE MYOCARDIAL INFARCTION

Arrhythmias

With the widespread use of fibrinolytic therapy and primary PCI, severe arrhythmias are observed less frequently in the presence of an acute MI. Arrhythmias are more common in patients with the following conditions:

- Anterior MI
- Large MI
- MI complicated by congestive heart failure
- Hypotension and hypoperfusion
- Older age
- Postinfarction patients with ongoing myocardial ischemia

Atrial Fibrillation

Atrial fibrillation is the most common sustained arrhythmia, occurring in approximately 10% of patients with acute MI. If hemodynamic compromise develops during an episode of atrial fibrillation, prompt electrical cardioversion is indicated. If the patient is not hemodynamically unstable, the initial cautious use of intravenous β-blockers is useful in slowing the ventricular response and attenuating superimposed ischemia. If atrial fibrillation persists, anti-coagulant therapy (such as unfractionated heparin) should be initiated, and cardioverision or antiarrhythmic therapy should be considered.

Ventricular Arrhythmias

Fatal ventricular arrhythmias commonly occur during an acute MI. It is important to distinguish early ventricular fibrillation, which occurs within the first few hours of infarction, from late ventricular fibrillation, which occurs more than 48 hours after infarction (Fig. 63.3). Early ventricular fibrillation suggests a higher immediate mortality that can reach 20%, but those patients who reach hospital discharge have a prognosis similar to those who did not suffer ventricular fibrillation. In contrast, the out-of-hospital mortality is elevated in those patients experiencing late ventricular fibrillation, because this is often associated with larger infarctions, greater left ventricular systolic dysfunction, and congestive heart failure.

The use of routine in-hospital intravenous lidocaine administration during an acute MI has long been abandoned. Lidocaine reduces the incidence of primary in-hospital ventricular fibrillation but does not exert a favorable effect on mortality. In fact, it may have a negative effect on mortality, which likely is related to increased episodes of bradycardia and asystole. The early administration of intravenous β-blockade followed by oral doses exerts a favorable

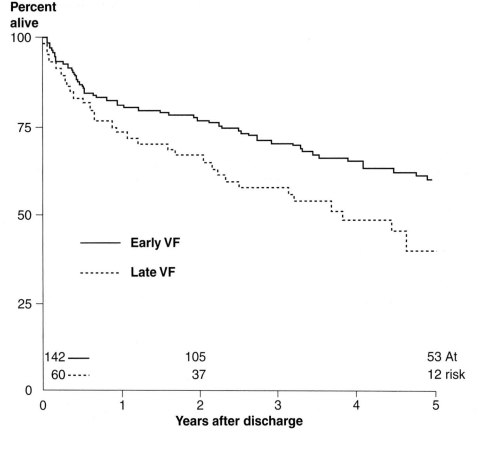

Figure 63.3 Kaplan-Meier survival curves for patients discharged alive after acute myocardial infarction complicated by ventricular fibrillation (*VF*). (VF, ventricular fibrillation.) (Reproduced with permission from Jensen GV, Torp-Pederson C, Kober L, et al. Prognosis of late versus early ventricular fibrillation in acute myocardial infarction. *Am J Cardiol* 1990;66(1):10–15.)

impact on ventricular fibrillation frequency and should be administered routinely to patients with acute infarction devoid of advanced heart block, significant hypotension, or cardiogenic shock. In addition, close monitoring of electrolyte levels, specifically potassium and magnesium levels, is important in arrhythmia prevention. The treatment of ventricular fibrillation requires prompt, unsynchronized electric shock, followed by pharmaceutical therapy, as outlined in the advanced cardiac life support protocol.

Ventricular tachycardia is classified as either nonsustained (<30 seconds) or sustained (>30 seconds). Nonsustained, nonhemodynamically compromising ventricular tachycardia does not require specific treatment other than attenuation of persistent ischemia, normalization of electrolyte levels, and β-blockade. Hemodynamically unstable sustained ventricular tachycardia requires cardioversion with synchronized electric shock. Hemodynamically noncompromising sustained ventricular tachycardia can be treated with cardioversion or pharmacologic agents, including intravenous lidocaine or amiodarone. Drug-refractory sustained ventricular tachycardia in the setting of acute MI is best treated using β-blockade, intravenous amiodarone, balloon pump insertion, and urgent revascularization.

Bradyarrhythmias

Sinus bradycardia is another frequent complication of acute MI, especially in those patients with inferior infarctions and reperfusion of the right coronary artery (the Bezold-Jarisch reflex). Heart block occurs in approximately 10% of patients with acute infarction, and new left or right bundle-branch block also can develop. Patients with heart block or bundle-branch block have greater in-hospital mortality, most likely related to the greater size of their presenting infarction. Atropine is an effective treatment for bradycardia associated with hypotension or ischemia. It is also effective as prompt treatment for ventricular asystole or symptomatic atrioventricular (AV) block.

Temporary pacing is an effective bridge therapy for symptomatic bradycardia and heart block during an acute MI. It can be performed by the transcutaneous or transvenous route. The transcutaneous mode is safer, especially in the setting of fibrinolytic therapy, although this method is uncomfortable and should be reserved for "backup" for patients who do not require ongoing pacing. The transvenous mode is best used in those patients with a high likelihood of proceeding to advanced heart block. Indications for temporary pacing or "backup" pacing include:

- Symptomatic bradycardia unresponsive to drug therapy
- Mobitz type II AV block
- Third-degree heart block
- New bilateral bundle-branch block
- Newly acquired left bundle-branch block

- New right bundle-branch block or left bundle-branch block and first-degree AV block

Relatively few patients with acute infarction require permanent pacemakers. Rhythm disturbances that indicate a need for permanent pacing are persistent second-degree AV block in the His-Purkinje system, complete heart block, and symptomatic AV block.

Mechanical Complications

Acute Mitral Regurgitation

Acute mitral regurgitation, which usually occurs 2 to 7 days after an acute MI, is mostly associated with an inferior MI. It commonly results from a dysfunctional or ruptured posteromedial papillary muscle because of its single blood supply (from the posterior descending coronary artery), as opposed to the anterolateral papillary muscle, which has a dual blood supply (from both the left anterior descending and the left circumflex coronary arteries). Acute mitral regurgitation should be suspected on physical examination when a new holosystolic murmur or acute pulmonary edema develops (although the murmur may not be present with massive regurgitation), and it is best confirmed using two-dimensional echocardiography with color Doppler analysis. It is an indication for prompt surgical repair, with an overall mortality ranging from 40% to 90%.

Ventricular Septal Defect

Similar to acute mitral regurgitation, a ventricular septal defect occurs 3 to 5 days after an acute infarction. A new murmur almost always is audible, occurring in approximately two-thirds of cases in the setting of new ventricular septal defect with an anterior infarction. This defect can also be diagnosed echocardiographically. The mortality without surgery is >90%.

Ventricular Free Wall Rupture

Ventricular free wall rupture occurs approximately 3 to 6 days after an acute infarction and without any clear predilection for infarction location. The mortality approaches 100%. The incidence is thought to be reduced in those patients receiving fibrinolytic therapy and prompt β-blockade at initial presentation by reducing infarct size and left ventricular systolic wall tension.

REVIEW EXERCISES

QUESTIONS

1. Which of the following statements is *incorrect* after acute MI?

a) Even during an acute MI, angiography remains safe to perform.

b) More than 85% of infarct-related arteries are totally occluded during the acute phase of STEMI.

c) The incidence of totally occluded infarct vessels decreases with time after STEMI secondary to spontaneous fibrinolysis.
d) Most patients who die from an acute MI have advanced coronary atherosclerosis involving significant obstruction in at least one coronary artery.
e) None of the above

Answer and Discussion

The answer is e. During an acute MI, angiography remains safe, with primary PCI often considered as the appropriate treatment. Of importance, most infarct-related arteries are occluded during the acute STEMI phase. This is reduced after infarction secondary to spontaneous fibrinolysis. Most patients who die of an acute infarction have advanced coronary atherosclerosis involving a significant coronary obstruction in at least one coronary artery.

2. Which of the following statements concerning risk stratification after an acute MI is false?
a) Women possess an improved postinfarction prognosis compared with that of men.
b) The single most important determinant of both short- and long-term survival is the residual left ventricular systolic function.
c) Silent ischemia, as detected by Holter monitoring, has a similar prognosis to that of symptomatic ischemia after infarction.
d) Diabetes mellitus contributes to an increased postinfarction risk.

Answer and Discussion

The answer is a. Important adverse prognostic predictors after an MI include the extent of left ventricular systolic dysfunction and coexistent morbidity, including diabetes mellitus. Silent ischemia, as detected at Holter monitoring, portends a worse prognosis, as does the female gender.

3. The following items are features of NSTEMI, *except*
a) The residual coronary artery stenosis generally is severe.
b) Prominent collaterals serve the infarct-related artery.
c) A greater likelihood of a previous infarction exists.
d) Recurrent infarction is less likely compared with STEMI patients.

Answer and Discussion

The answer is d. NSTEMI are characterized by the residual, high-grade coronary stenosis, prominent collaterals, and greater likelihood of previous MI. The ejection fraction is lower, but the reinfarction rate is higher compared with that in patients with STEMI.

4. The following statements regarding fibrinolytic therapy are true, *except*

a) An improved mortality has been shown in patients with inferior infarction after fibrinolytic administration.
b) The earlier the fibrinolytic treatment is administered, the greater the impact on survival.
c) Preservation of left ventricular function depends on early fibrinolytic administration.
d) Cardiopulmonary resuscitation is an absolute contraindication for fibrinolytic therapy.

Answer and Discussion

The answer is d. Fibrinolytic therapy is most beneficial within the early phases of an acute MI. Reduced morbidity and mortality is shown for all infarction, including inferior infarction. Enhanced left ventricular systolic function is noted with earlier fibrinolytic administration. Cardiopulmonary resuscitation remains a relative, not an absolute, contraindication to fibrinolytic therapy.

5. Indications for a temporary pacemaker in patients with acute MI include the following, *except*
a) New left anterior fascicular and right bundle-branch block
b) New second-degree Mobitz type I AV block
c) New left bundle-branch block
d) Complete heart block

Answer and Discussion

The answer is b. Indications for temporary pacing during an acute MI include new-onset bifascicular block, second-degree Mobitz type II AV block, and complete heart block. First-degree AV block and Mobitz type I Wenckebach second-degree AV block require careful observation but not temporary pacing.

5. True statements concerning the ECG findings during an acute MI include the following, *except*
a) Sinus tachycardia is frequently present.
b) An accelerated idioventricular rhythm post fibrinolytic therapy warrants urgent electric cardioversion.
c) Atrial dysrhythmias such as atrial fibrillation are commonly observed.
d) The development of complete heart block portends a worse prognosis.

Answer and Discussion

The answer is b. In the presence of an acute MI, increased sympathetic tone often is reflected in the form of sinus tachycardia. Atrial arrythmias frequently are demonstrated in part related to atrial ischemia, increased circulating catecholamines, acutely elevated intracardiac pressures, and cardiac chamber dilatation. Advanced forms of heart block are associated with larger infarction, which portend a worse prognosis. Accelerated idioventricular rhythms frequently manifest after successful reperfusion during the acute myocardial injury phase, rarely require treatment other than careful observation, and represent a noninvasive marker of successful coronary blood flow restoration.

7. In a patient presenting with an acute chest discomfort syndrome and an ECG demonstrating an extensive anterolateral myocardial injury pattern, appropriate treatment measures include the following, *except*

a) The prophylactic placement of an intra-aortic balloon pump to attenuate the degree of myocardial injury given the large MI

b) Intravenous fibrinolytic therapy

c) Intravenous β-blocker administration in the absence of advanced heart failure and hemodynamic compromise

d) An urgent coronary angiography with the goal of performing a PCI and possible coronary stent placement

Answer and Discussion

The answer is a. In the presence of an acute chest discomfort syndrome and an ECG demonstrating acute myocardial injury, the restoration of coronary artery blood flow in the most expedient manner results in reduced morbidity and mortality. This can be achieved by administering intravenous fibrinolytic therapy or proceeding directly with coronary angiography and PCI. β-blockers reduce myocardial oxygen demand, attenuate myocardial ischemia, and limit the size of an infarction. β-blockers should be administered to all acute MI patients in the absence of a hemodynamic contraindication. In the presence of cardiogenic shock, drug-refractory congestive heart failure, and recurrent life-threatening cardiac dysrhythmias believed to be ischemia mediated, the placement of an intra-aortic

balloon pump in the periinfarction period can achieve a positive clinical benefit. The routine use of an intra-aortic balloon pump is not indicated and may subject the patient to excess morbidity secondary to vascular injury, cholesterol and systemic embolization, and infection, all without a tangible benefit. The use of an intra-aortic balloon pump is an individualized decision for each acute MI patient.

SUGGESTED READINGS

Anderson JL, Adams CD, Antman EM, et al. ACC/AHA 2007 guidelines for the management of patients with unstable angina/non ST-elevation myocardial infarction: a report of the American College of Cardiology/American Heart Association Task Force on Practice Guidelines (writing committee to revise the 2002 Guidelines for the Management of Patients With Unstable Angina/Non ST-Elevation Myocardial Infarction). *Circulation* 2007;116(7):e148–e304.

Antman EM, Anbe DT, Armstrong PW, et al. ACC/AHA guidelines for the management of patients with ST-elevation myocardial infarction: a report of the American College of Cardiology/American Heart Association Task Force on Practice Guidelines (committee to revise the 1999 Guidelines for the Management of Patients with Acute Myocardial Infarction). *Circulation* 2004;110(9):e82–e292.

Antman EM, Hand M, Armstrong PW, et al. 2007 focused update of the ACC/AHA 2004 Guidelines for the Management of Patients With ST-Elevation Myocardial Infarction. A report of the American College of Cardiology/American Heart Association Task Force on Practice Guidelines. *Circulation* 2008;117;296–329.

DeWood MA, Spona J, Notske R, et al. Prevalence of total coronary occlusion during the early hours of transmural myocardial infarction. *N Engl J Med* 1980;303:897–902.

ISIS-2 (Second Interventional Study of Infarct Survival) Collaborative Group. Randomized trial of intravenous streptokinase or aspirin, both or neither, among 17,187 cases of suspected acute myocardial infarction: ISIS-2. *Lancet* 1988;2:349–360.

Smith SC, Allen J, Blair SN, et al. AHA/ACC guidelines for secondary prevention for patients with coronary and other atherosclerotic vascular disease: 2006 update: endorsed by the National Heart, Lung, and Blood Institute. *Circulation* 2006;113(19):2363–2372.

Chapter 64

Dyslipidemia

Matthew A. Kaminski   *Leslie Cho*

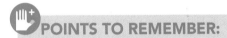**POINTS TO REMEMBER:**

- There is a strong, independent, continuous, and graded relation between total cholesterol (TC) and low-density lipoprotein cholesterol (LDL-C) level and risk for coronary events.

- All adults 20 years of age or older and without a history of coronary artery disease (CAD) or other atherosclerotic disease should have a fasting lipid panel (i.e., TC, LDL-C, high-density lipoprotein cholesterol [HDL-C], and triglycerides [TG]) every 5 years. If a nonfasting lipid panel is obtained and the TC level is 200 mg/dL or the HDL-C is <40 mg/dL, a follow-up fasting lipid panel is recommended.

- The treatment of hyperlipidemia requires two approaches: therapeutic lifestyle changes (TLC) and medications. To achieve target LDL levels, most patients need both approaches simultaneously.

Dyslipidemia is an important correctable risk factor for CAD. There is a strong, independent, continuous, and graded relation between the TC and LDL-C level and the risk for coronary events. This relation has been clearly demonstrated in both men and women and in all adult age groups. More than one-half of U.S. adults have TC levels >200 mg/dL, and of these, one-third have values >240 mg/dL. In general, a 1% increase in LDL-C level leads to a 2% to 3% increase in risk for CAD.[1]

Aggressive lipid-lowering drug treatment of persons at various risk levels reduces CAD morbidity and mortality rates and increases overall survival rate. Although the association between hyperlipidemia and CAD was established two decades ago,[2] the demonstration of a relationship between reduction in serum lipid levels and a reduction in all-cause mortality had to await the development of 3-hydroxy-3-methylglutaryl coenzyme A (HMG-CoA) reductase inhibitors, or "statins." Multiple randomized trials have provided overwhelming evidence of the benefit of statins in both primary and secondary prevention of cardiovascular events.

PRIMARY PREVENTION TRIALS

One of the first major trials of statin efficacy in the primary prevention of coronary events was the West of Scotland Coronary Prevention Study (WOSCOPS).[3] It demonstrated that treatment of men at relatively high risk with profoundly elevated cholesterol levels significantly reduced the risk for heart attack and death from heart disease. The double-blind study randomized 6,600 healthy men with a baseline mean LDL cholesterol level of 193 mg/dL to pravastatin (40 mg per day) or to placebo for an average of 5 years and demonstrated a 31% relative reduction in the incidence of nonfatal myocardial infarction (MI) or CAD death. Recently published data[4] has shown that the statin group continued to experience lower rates of cardiovascular death after 10 years of additional follow-up, even though only one-third continued to take statins during the additional follow-up period.

The Air Force/Texas Coronary Atherosclerosis Prevention Study (AFCAPS/TexCAPS)[5] was published in 1998 and demonstrated benefit among patients with more typical risk profiles, including lower cholesterol values, than those in WOSCOPS. AFCAPS/TexCAPS patients had a baseline mean LDL-C of 150 mg/dL. The study randomized 6,600 patients to lovastatin 20 to 40 mg daily or placebo and demonstrated a 36% relative risk reduction (RRR) for first acute major coronary events in the lovastatin group.

The landmark Heart Protection Study (HPS)[6] was published in 2002. In total, 20,536 subjects were randomized in a 2 × 2 factorial design to daily simvastatin (40 mg) or placebo and to antioxidants or placebo (the antioxidant arm did not show any benefit or harm). The study focused on patients who were deemed at high risk for cardiovascular disease but not thought to merit treatment with statins based on the prevalent clinical practice at that time. Increased risk was defined as presence of or history of CAD, cerebrovascular disease, peripheral arterial disease, diabetes mellitus, or treated hypertension. The baseline mean LDL-C for all patients randomized was 133 mg/dL. Simvastatin therapy was associated with a 13% reduction in all-cause mortality, including an 18% reduction in coronary death rate. The beneficial impact of statin therapy was seen with respect to all cardiovascular end points with significant reductions in risk for nonfatal MI, incidence of first stroke, and coronary and noncornary revascularization. Treating LDL levels <100 mg/dL was also associated with a beneficial reduction in vascular events. The benefit was maintained in patients receiving other cardioprotective medications, such as angiotensin-converting enzyme (ACE) inhibitors, β-blockers, and aspirin. Although not strictly a primary prevention trial, the HPS has provided evidence to support treatment of risk as endorsed by the National Cholesterol Education Program's (NCEP) guidelines.

The Pravastatin in Elderly Individuals at Risk of Vascular Disease (PROSPER) trial,[7] published in 2002, randomized 5,804 patients between the age of 70 and 82 years with a baseline mean LDL-C of 147 mg/dL to placebo or pravastatin. These patients had preexisting coronary, cerebral, or peripheral vascular disease or had a history of smoking, hypertension, or diabetes. The study demonstrated a 15% reduction in the composite of coronary death, nonfatal MI, and stroke over a period of 3 years. The study demonstrated efficacy of primary and secondary prevention in the elderly.

The Antihypertensive and Lipid-Lowering Treatment to Prevent Heart Attack Trial (ALLHAT-LLT),[8] also published in 2002, randomized 10,355 hypertensive patients with one other coronary risk factor and a baseline mean LDL-C of 148 mg/dL to pravastatin 20 to 40 mg per day or usual care. The study did not demonstrate a mortality difference in the two arms after a follow-up period of 4.8 years. This lack of observable difference in outcome might have resulted from the relatively modest LDL reduction (17% with pravastatin vs. 8% in usual care) or the fact that 26% of the patients in the "usual care" group were taking a statin at the end of the trial.

The Anglo-Scandinavian Cardiac Outcomes Trial—Lipid-Lowering Arm (ASCOT-LLA)[9] randomized 10,305 patients with hypertension and at least three other cardiovascular risk factors and a baseline mean LDL-C of 133 mg/dL to atorvastatin 10 mg per day or placebo. The study was stopped prematurely after a median follow-up of 3.3 years by the safety monitoring committee due to a significantly higher incidence of the primary end point (nonfatal MI or fatal coronary heart disease [CHD]) in the placebo group. The study demonstrated an RRR in the primary end point of 36% in the atorvastatin group compared with the placebo group. Further analysis demonstrated that the benefit of statin therapy started after only 1 year of treatment. There was also a significant reduction (RRR of 27%) in the incidence of fatal and nonfatal stroke in the atorvastatin group. This study, like the HPS, provided further evidence of the benefit of statins in patients at high risk for cardiovascular disease without regard for baseline TC or LDL levels.

The Collaborative Atorvastatin Diabetes Study (CARDS)[10] randomized 2,838 diabetic patients with one additional cardiovascular risk factor, no history of cardiovascular disease, and an average baseline LDL-C of only 117 mg/dL to atorvastatin 10 mg per day or placebo. This study was also terminated prematurely due to an excess incidence of the primary end point (a composite of acute coronary events, coronary revascularization, or stroke) in the placebo group after a median follow-up of 3.9 years. Overall, the atorvastatin group had an RRR of 37% for the primary end point and 27% for all-cause mortality. The importance of this trial was in demonstrating the clinical benefit of statin use in diabetic patients regardless of baseline LDL-C level, making a compelling case for statin use in all diabetic patients with at least one additional cardiovascular risk factor. According to NHANES-III data, 82% of diabetic patients in the United States would meet the entry criteria for the CARDS trial.

SECONDARY PREVENTION TRIALS

The Scandinavian Simvastatin Survival Study (4S)[11] was the first secondary prevention trial to demonstrate a clear reduction in total mortality. Simvastatin reduced total mortality among patients with CAD by 30%, largely because of a 42% reduction in deaths from CAD. The 4S treated 4,444 men and women with CAD and mean baseline LDL of 188 mg/dL, with a range of 130 to 266 mg/dL.

The randomized, controlled Cholesterol and Recurrent Events Trial (CARE)[12] was designed to evaluate the effects of treatment with pravastatin on 4,159 persons who had experienced acute MI 3 to 20 months before randomization and had moderately elevated TC levels (mean, 209 mg/dL) and a baseline mean LDL-C of 139 mg/dL. The benefits of pravastatin therapy in preventing recurrent coronary events were similar in the subset analysis of age, sex, ejection fraction, hypertension, diabetes mellitus, and smoking. The RRR was 24% for the primary end point of fatal coronary event or nonfatal MI in the pravastatin group.

The Long-Term Intervention with Pravastatin in Ischemic Disease Study (LIPID)[13] was the first to examine the use of a statin for patients with a history of unstable angina. In total, 9,014 patients with a history of MI or unstable angina with a baseline median LDL-C of 150 mg/dL were randomized to either pravastatin 40 mg daily or placebo. The trial was stopped early due to a 24% reduction in the primary end point of CHD death in the pravastatin group compared with the placebo group. The study also provided new data on noncoronary mortality (i.e., stroke) and on other groups, such as women and patients with diabetes, who previously had been underrepresented in clinical trials. LIPID demonstrated improved CAD outcomes among all subgroups, including those with unstable angina with statin therapy.

The Pravastatin or Atorvastatin Evaluation and Infection Therapy–TIMI 22 (PROVE-IT–TIMI-22)[14] trial was designed to determine whether intensive lipid-lowering therapy in patients with acute coronary syndromes (ACS) reduced major coronary events and mortality more than "standard" lipid lowering. A total of 4,162 patients with a mean LDL-C of 106 mg/dL who had been hospitalized for ACS within the preceeding 10 days were randomized to atorvastatin 80 mg per day or pravastatin 40 mg per day. After 2 years of follow-up, the composite end point of all-cause mortality, MI, unstable angina, coronary revascularization, and stroke was significantly reduced by 16% with atorvastatin compared with pravastatin. High-dose atorvastatin was well tolerated with no cases of rhabdomyolysis. Importantly, the LDL-C attained on atorvastatin 80 mg per day was 33 mg/dL lower than on pravastatin, with a mean of 62 mg/dL. These results suggested that use of intensive lipid-lowering therapy to achieve very low LDL-C levels was of benefit in a group of patients at high risk of recurrent coronary events.

The Treating to New Targets (TNT)[15] trial sought to demonstrate the benefit of intensive lipid-lowering therapy in patients with stable coronary disease. The trial randomized 10,001 patients with clinically evident CHD and baseline mean LDL-C levels <100 mg/dL to atorvastatin 80 mg per day or atorvastatin 10 mg per day. After 4.9 years of follow-up, the group receiving atorvastatin 80 mg per day had a 22% RRR in the primary composite end point of death from CHD, nonfatal MI, resuscitation after cardiac arrest, or fatal or nonfatal stroke compared with the group receiving atorvastatin 10 mg per day. High-dose atorvastatin was remarkably safe, with a 1.2% prevalence in elevation of alanine transaminase/aspartate transaminase (ALT/AST) greater than three times above normal compared with a 0.2% prevalence in the atorvastatin 10 mg group. Rates of myalgias and rhabodmyolysis were similar between the two groups. This study provided very compelling evidence that use of intensive statin therapy to reduce LDL-C to levels <100 mg/dL had marked clinical benefit in patients with stable CHD.

The Incremental Decrease in End Points Through Aggressive Lipid-lowering (IDEAL)[16] trial randomized 8,888 patients with a mean LDL-C of 121 mg/dL and a prior history of acute MI to atorvastatin 80 mg per day or simvastatin 20 mg per day. After 4.8 years of follow-up, there was a nonsignificant difference in the risk of the composite end point of coronary death, acute MI, or cardiac arrest. However, if either stroke or revascularization was added to the primary end point, the results favored the atorvastatin group and the associated hazard ratios were similar to the results of PROVE-IT and TNT. Despite the published negative result of this trial, it provided complementary evidence for the benefit of intensive LDL lowering in patients at high risk of coronary events.

META-ANALYSES

Cholesterol Treatment Trialists' (CTT) Collaborators

The CTT meta-analysis,[17] comprised of 90,056 individuals from 14 randomized trials of statin drugs, demonstrated an impressive 12% reduction in all-cause mortality for each 1 mmol/L (39 mg/dL) reduction in LDL. There was a 19% reduction in coronary mortality and 21% reduction in MI, coronary revascularization, and stroke. Statin use showed benefit within the first year of use but was greater in subsequent years. Statins were also remarkably safe, with no increase in cancer seen and a 5-year excess risk of rhabdomyolysis of 0.1%.

Cannon: Intensive Statin Therapy

The Cannon[18] meta-analysis, comprised of 27,548 patients from four trials, investigated intensive versus standard lipid-lowering therapy and found a significant 16% odds reduction in coronary death or MI in the group that received intensive therapy. There was a nonsignificant trend toward decreased cardiovascular mortality.

MANAGEMENT OF LIPIDS

Despite overwhelming evidence supporting the treatment of dyslipidemia, a large number of patients remain untreated. The NCEP Adult Treatment Panel III (ATP III) has released guidelines for treatment of hyperlipidemia in adults.[19] These guidelines focus on identification of risk of cardiovascular morbidity and appropriate targeting of therapy. The official guidelines were most recently updated in 2004.[20]

RISK STRATIFICATION AND TREATMENT GOALS

All adults 20 years of age or older and without a history of CAD or other atherosclerotic disease should have a fasting lipid panel (i.e., TC, LDL-C, HDL-C, and TG) every 5 years. If a nonfasting lipid panel is obtained and the TC level is 200 mg/dL or the HDL-C is <40 mg/dL, a follow-up fasting lipid panel is recommended (Table 64.1).

The patient's risk of future events is based on presence of known CAD or clinical atherosclerosis in a noncoronary bed, diabetes mellitus (i.e., CAD equivalent), and other risk factors. These include age (men 45 years or older and women 55 years or older) smoking, hypertension (>140/90 mm Hg or use of antihypertensive medication), family history of premature CAD (defined as CAD in first-degree male relatives before age of 55 years and in a first-degree female relative before the age of 65 years), and low HDL-C (<40 mg/dL). A HDL-C ≥60 mg/dL counts as a negative risk factor. Patients are classified into three categories of risk based on these factors.

INITIATION OF THERAPY

The treatment of hyperlipidemia requires two approaches: TLCs and medications. To achieve target LDL levels, most patients need both approaches simultaneously.

TABLE 64.1	
LIPID CLASSIFICATION ACCORDING TO THE NATIONAL CHOLESTEROL EDUCATION PROGRAM III	
Risk Factor	**Goal**
LDL-C	
<100	Optimal
100–129	Near or above optimal
130–159	Borderline high
160–189	High
≥190	Very high
Total cholesterol	
<200	Desirable
200–239	Borderline high
≥240	High
HDL-C	
<40	Low
≥60	High

HDL-C, high-density lipoprotein cholesterol; LDL-C, low-density lipoprotein cholesterol.

CHD risk equivalent: Patients with highest risk of cardiovascular events are those with established CAD or evidence of atherosclerosis in noncoronary beds, diabetics, or patients with presence of multiple risk factors conferring a calculated 10-year risk >20%. These patients are at the highest risk of adverse events and therefore benefit the most from aggressive treatment. NCEP III, whose recommendations were published in 2001, had recommended therapy with a statin and TLCs if LDL-C was ≥130 mg/dL. In patients with LDL-C levels between 100 and 130 mg/dL, it suggested that the clinician use judgment when determining whether to begin treatment with a statin, TLCs, or another agent such as niacin. The 2004 update, however, was more definitive and recommended starting a statin and TLCs for all patients with a CHD risk equivalent with LDL-C levels 100 to 130 mg/dL. This was based on cited evidence from HPS and further supported by CARDS and ASCOT-LLA. In patients who have a baseline LDL-C concentration <100 mg/dL, the 2004 update stopped short of recommending initial use of a statin but acknowledged that there was evidence for statin use in this group regardless of the LDL-C level. It did, however, state that initiation of a statin drug in patients with an initial LDL-C <100 mg/dL who are at "very high risk" for future cardiovascular events, with the goal of lowering the LDL-C to <70 mg/dL, was a "reasonable therapeutic option." The cited evidence included HPS and PROVE-IT–TIMI-22. The publication of TNT provided even more evidence for intensive lipid lowering in all patients with clinically evident CHD. Given the balance of evidence in the most recently published trials and meta-analyses, a reasonable current approach for most clinicians would be to initiate statin therapy in all patients with CHD or a CHD risk equivalent, regardless of baseline LDL-C, with a goal LDL-C ≤70 mg/dL for patients with CHD or at high risk of future cardiovascular events.

Ten-year risk of 10% to 20%: These generally are patients with two or more risk factors for cardiovascular events whose 10-year Framingham risk scores were between 10% and 20%. The target LDL-C for this group is <130 mg/dL. The 2004 ATP III update stated that an LDL-C goal <100 mg/dL is a therapeutic option, and initiation of statin therapy along with TLCs for patients with baseline LDL-C 100 to 130 mg/dL was reasonable. This recommendation was based on evidence from HPS and ASCOT-LLA.

Ten-year risk less than 10% and zero or one risk factor: These patients should be treated with TLC to achieve a target LDL-C level <160 mg/dL. If the LDL-C concentration remains >160 mg/dL after 3 months of TLCs, drug therapy may be considered. Pharmacotherapy is recommended in those with LDL-C levels >190 mg/dL. Factors favoring use of drugs include a 10-year risk close to 10% or the presence of a severe risk factor such as a strong family history of premature CAD, a very low HDL level, poorly controlled hypertension, or heavy smoking.

TYPES OF THERAPY

Therapeutic Lifestyle Changes

TLCs encompass increased physical activity, ideal weight maintenance, and a diet that provides a reduced intake of saturated fat (<7% of total calories) and cholesterol (<200 mg per day). Other TLCs are listed in Table 64.2. Intake of trans-fatty acids should be kept to a minimum. For most patients, it is essential to reduce saturated fat intake over total fat intake; for patients with metabolic syndrome, a fat intake of 30% to 35% may be optimal for reducing lipid and nonlipid risk factors. High-carbohydrate diets may worsen the lipid abnormalities in these patients. Dietary carbohydrates should predominantly be derived from foods rich in complex carbohydrates, such as whole grains, fruits, and vegetables. Daily intake of 5 to 10 g of viscous fiber reduces LDL levels by approximately 5%, and the use of plant stanols and sterols (2–3 g per day) reduces the level by another 6% to 15%. TLCs can achieve an almost 30% reduction in LDL-C in highly motivated individuals and should form the cornerstone of all preventive activity. LDL-C should be measured 6 weeks after initiating TLC diet, and if the goals are not met, intensification of TLCs and use of plant stanols or sterols should be considered. Referral to a dietitian for education and dietary counseling often is invaluable at this stage. If after 3 months of TLCs adequate control is not achieved, drug therapy should be considered.[19]

PHARMACOTHERAPY

Statins

The third report of the NCEP Adult Treatment Panel included HMG-CoA reductase inhibitors, or statins, among

TABLE 64.2

COMPONENTS OF A THERAPEUTIC LIFESTYLE

Component	Recommendation	Approximate LDL Reduction (%)
Diet		
Saturated fat	<7% of total calories	8–10
Dietary cholesterol	<200 mg/day	3–5
Polyunsaturated fat	Up to 10% of total calories	—
Monounsaturated fat	Up to 20% of total calories	—
Total fat	25%–35% of total calories	—
Carbohydrate	50%–60% of total calories	—
Dietary fiber	20–30 g/day	—
Total protein	15% of total calories	—
Therapeutic options for LDL lowering		
Plant stanols/sterols	2 g/day	6–15
Increased viscous soluble fiber	5–10 g/day (consumption of 10–25 g/day may have added benefit)	3–5
Physical activity	Enough moderate activity to expend at least 200 kcal/day	—

LDL, low-density lipoprotein.

the first-line alternatives in the management of hyper-cholesterolemia, given the high efficacy of statins in lowering LDL-C and their demonstrated mortality benefits. The category includes six drugs: lovastatin, simvastatin, pravastatin, fluvastatin, atorvastatin, and rosuvastatin.

When TLCs are inadequate, statins effectively lower TC and LDL-C in patients with mixed hyperlipidemias (i.e., elevated cholesterol and TG levels). Statins are extremely effective in reducing LDL-C in most patients with primary hypercholesterolemia. They decrease TC by 15% to 60% and LDL-C by 20% to 59% and increase HDL-C levels by 5% to 15%. Declines in apo B commensurate with reductions in LDL have been demonstrated. Statins also reduce TG levels by 10% to 25% but have minimal effects on apo AI, apo AII, and lipoprotein (a) (Lp[a]). All statin drugs at the starting dose and within one to two dose titrations are well tolerated, efficacious, and reasonably equivalent with respect to safety profiles.

Statins are remarkably safe drugs with a very low incidence of side effects. They are contraindicated in pregnancy. The most common side effects are mild gastrointestinal disturbances (e.g., nausea, abdominal pain, diarrhea, constipation, flatulence). Headache, fatigue, pruritus, and myalgia are other minor side effects, but none of these complaints usually warrants discontinuation of therapy. Mild, transient elevations in liver enzymes have been reported with all HMG-CoA reductase inhibitors, but it is still unclear if this represents true hepatotoxicity. Marked elevation of transaminases is rare, and statin use in patients with acute or chronic liver disease is one of the few contraindications to therapy. In the HPS, only 0.5% of patients had to stop treatment because of elevated ALT levels. Even when taking the highest dose of atorvastatin (80 mg), patients

in PROVE-IT and TNT had only a 3.3% and 1.1% prevalence, respectively, of transaminase elevation greater than three times above normal. In general, for each doubling of a statin dose, there is a 0.6% increase in risk for elevation of transaminase levels. Current recommendations state that therapy should be discontinued when greater than threefold elevation occurs. Enzyme levels typically return to normal within 2 weeks. Lower doses of the same medication can be reinstituted, or a different statin can be tried.[21]

Monitoring of hepatic aminotransferase levels is recommended for those taking HMG-CoA reductase inhibitors, but the frequency of monitoring has been debated. Current package inserts for all statins recommend obtaining a liver panel prior to initiation of statin therapy, prior to dose titration, and when "clinically indicated." More frequent monitoring is recommended for patients taking the highest dose of a statin. In recent clinical trials, the high-dose statin that appears to have the highest incidence of transaminase elevation is atorvastatin. A panel of hepatologists who examined the potential hepatotoxicity of statins made a recommendation to obtain a liver panel prior to initiating statins as a baseline measurement of hepatic transaminases and bilirubin. If the baseline measurements were within normal limits, the panel recommended follow-up measurement of transaminases only if there was symptomatic or physical evidence of liver disease.[22] An ACC/AHA/NHLBI clinical advisory panel on the safety and use of statins recommends measurement of transaminases at baseline, 12-weeks after starting therapy, and then annually or more frequently if indicated.[23]

Myopathy, a rare but potentially serious side effect of HMG-CoA reductase inhibitors, occurs with muscle pain, stiffness or aching, and elevations in serum creatine kinase

(CK) level to more than ten times the upper limit of normal. Statins should be discontinued immediately if myopathy occurs due to the risk of rhabdomyolysis and associated acute renal failure. Routine monitoring of serum CK levels has not been shown to be of benefit in the absence of suggestive symptoms, however. A panel of muscle experts examining the risk of statin-induced myopathy concluded that measurement of baseline CK levels could be useful, "especially in patients at increased risk for myopathy such as those with renal or hepatic dysfunction or on medications that might affect statin metabolism."[24] The risk of myopathy may be increased in the elderly, in those with a low body mass index, in patients with multisystem disease such as chronic renal failure, in the perioperative period, and in those on multiple medications. In the U.S. Food and Drug Administration's (FDA) Adverse Event Reporting System database up until 2002, the reporting rates per million statin prescriptions was 0.38 cases for myopathy and 1.07 cases of rhabdomyolysis.[24] Death from statin-induced rhabdomyolysis, which is potentially life threatening, is exceedingly rare, with an incidence of 1.5 deaths per 10 million prescriptions. Statin-associated myalgias (muscle symptoms without elevations in serum CK) occur with somewhat higher frequency of about 1.4% to 1.5% in published clinical trials and can appear at any time during statin therapy, even years after initiation of treatment.[25] Muscle symptoms usually resolve with discontinuation of the statin. There is recent evidence that statin inhibition of mitochondrial coenzyme Q10 may be responsible for statin-induced myalgias, and there is anecdotal and evidence from small clinical trials that oral coenzyme Q10 supplementation may decrease symptoms of statin-associated myalgias.[26]

When statins are used in combination with certain pharmaceutical agents, such as erythromycin, gemfibrozil, azole antifungals, cimetidine, methotrexate, or cyclosporine, the risks for CK elevation and myositis increase. These drug combinations should be avoided or used judiciously with interval measurements of CK levels and liver function. Pravastatin and fluvastatin are safer in combination with other drugs, because these two drugs are not metabolized by the cytochrome P450 3A4 microsomal pathways. Verapamil and amiodarone are two commonly used cardiovascular agents that inhibit this pathway, and the concurrent use of simvastatin or lovastatin may therefore predispose to an increased risk of myositis.[23]

Bile Acid Sequestrants

Drugs in this class lower LDL-C by interfering with reabsorption of bile acids in the distal ileum, reducing the amount returned to the liver. They are safe and free of systemic side effects because they are not systemically absorbed; however, gastrointestinal side effects such as constipation are common, and compliance is poor. The average LDL decrease is approximately 20% to 22%, with

a small rise seen in HDL. TG show no change or may rise; thus, they should be avoided in patients with elevated TG. Two small angiographic trials, the NHLBI Type II Interventional Study[27] and the St. Thomas Atherosclerosis Regression Study (STARS),[28] have demonstrated reduced progression of CAD on serial angiograms in men with hypercholesterolemia who were taking cholestyramine. These agents may be of particular benefit in patients with minor elevation in LDL-C, for young patients, for women considering pregnancy, and in combination with a statin in those with very high LDL-C. In a pregnant patient, additional supplementation of iron and folate may be necessary, as resins used over the long term can interfere with their absorption.

Nicotinic Acid

Nicotinic acid (niacin) affects all lipid parameters favorably (i.e., LDL reduction of 5%–25%, TG reduction of 20%–25%, HDL elevation of 15%–30%).[29] It is one of the only agents that reduces Lp(a) significantly (up to 30%). Unfortunately, compliance is poor because of frequent side effects. Flushing and pruritus, gastrointestinal discomfort, glucose intolerance, and hyperuricemia often accompany use of niacin. Hepatotoxicity is rare but is more commonly seen with the sustained-released preparation. It is often heralded by a dramatic reduction in lipid levels or the onset of nausea and vomiting. There are limited data on long-term therapy with this agent. Niacin may be particularly useful for patients who do not have substantial elevations in their LDL-C levels, and low doses may be used to treat diabetic dyslipidemia. High doses should be carefully monitored in diabetics, and the drug should be avoided in those with a history of gout, severe peptic ulcer disease, or active hepatic disease.

Fibrates

Fibrates are effective at lowering TG levels by 20% to 50% and raising HDL by 10% to 35%. The mechanism of action is activation of the nuclear transcription factor PPAR-α with resultant increases in hepatic synthesis of apolipoproteins A-I and A-II (raising HDL) and increase in lipoprotein lipase-mediated lipolysis, thus lowering TG levels. LDL reduction varies with the agent used and may range from 5% to 20% in patients who are not hypertriglyceridemic. Fenofibrate appears to lower LDL more effectively than gemfibrozil. Although a higher mortality rate was seen in the clofibrate arm of the World Health Organization (WHO) clofibrate study,[30] such a finding was not seen in subsequent studies of gemfibrozil or fenofibrate. These agents have been demonstrated to impart a reduction in risk of CAD events and are of use in patients with elevated TGs. The Veterans Affairs High-density Lipoprotein Cholesterol Intervention Trial (VA-HIT)[31] found a reduction in fatal and nonfatal MI with gemfibrozil use in men with CAD who had low HDL levels (mean, 32 mg/dL), but the FIELD trial[32] did not find a significant reduction in the primary end point of CAD death or MI in diabetic patients. Although fibrates are often used in combination with statin therapy to treat mixed dyslipidemia, there are no studies demonstrating reduction in clinical events with this approach. This combination increases the risk of myopathy. For patients with very high TG levels (>1,000 mg/dL), fibrate therapy reduces the risk for pancreatitis.

Cholesterol Absorption Inhibitors

Cholesterol absorption inhibitors, such as ezetimibe, inhibit cholesterol absorption by the enterocyte. It reduces cholesterol absorption from the small bowel by 23% to 50% and reduces serum LDL by an additional 14% to 20% when used in combination with a statin.[33] Reduction in clinical end points or surrogate end points has not been demonstrated for this group of drugs. The ENHANCE study failed to demonstrate any additional benefit of the use of ezetimibe added to statin over statin alone in slowing progression of carotid intimal thickness in a cohort of patients with familial hyperlipidemia. However, a number of large scale studies are in progress seeking to determine the utility of a statin ezetimibe combination on hard cardiovascular end points.

Choice of an Agent and Combination Therapy

The use of statin therapy for treatment of hyperlipidemia should be guided by the expected change in LDL-C levels (Table 64.3). Most statins have a log-linear dose-response pattern, with each doubling of dose associated with a further 7% reduction in LDL-C levels. Adverse effects of statins are also dose dependent and rise with the use of higher doses.

In isolated forms of LDL elevation, the combination of a statin and a bile acid resin exhibits highly complementary mechanism of action. The combination is ideal because of the lack of potentiation of side effects. The sequestrant provides little added toxicity, and the LDL-C lowering needed may not necessitate a full sequestrant dosage. Unfortunately, patient compliance with the combination is poor because of the common side effects of resins. Although the combination may reduce LDL by as much as 70% in some patients, there appears to be a ceiling effect, with no LDL lowering occurring beyond the original level with an increase in dose of either agent.

Combining a statin with niacin is attractive because it can favorably influence all lipid subfractions. The side effects of the combination are increased but not synergistic, and the risk of myopathy may be lower than previously believed. The main serious side effect of the combination is hepatotoxicity, which may be reduced by using extended-release niacin. In small studies using this combination, the risk of hepatotoxicity (i.e., persistent elevation of AST or ALT of more than three times the upper limit of normal) at niacin doses of 2 g per day was about 1%.[34]

The combination of a statin plus fibrate is highly effective at treating mixed hyperlipidemias. Although theoretically appealing, no reduction in clinical events has been demonstrated with this approach. The combination is associated with an increased risk of myopathy. Although earlier work has suggested a higher incidence, later studies suggest that this complication may be seen in approximately 1% of patients with the currently used agents.[35] Because of the marked interference of statin glucuronidation with gemfibrozil and the subsequent elevation of statin concentrations, fenofibrate is the fibrate of choice when fibrates are combined with statins. The combination of a statin plus ezetimibe has been evaluated in small studies and has proved to be highly safe and effective at lowering LDL-C levels. Given the small number of patients treated and short follow-up periods, it is suggested that this combination should be reserved for the patients who fail maximal statin doses or are intolerant of statins.

Therapy of Specific Lipid Disorders

Very high LDL levels usually result from inherited disorders of lipoprotein metabolism and carry a high risk of premature atherosclerosis with attendant morbidity and mortality. Hypothyroidism may be associated with markedly elevated LDL levels and should be ruled out in any patient presenting with elevated LDL level. Most of these patients respond to high-dose statin therapy in addition to dietary restrictions. The addition of a bile acid sequestrant with an additional third agent (i.e., niacin) often is warranted to achieve target levels. Ezetimibe is another agent that may prove useful in this group. Therapy should be begun early, and family members should be screened for hyperlipidemia. Patients with homozygous familial

---

TABLE 64.3

AVERAGE REDUCTION IN LOW-DENSITY LIPOPROTEIN CHOLESTEROL ASSOCIATED WITH THE STARTING DOSE OF STATIN AGENTS

Agent	Average LDL-C Reduction (%)
Lovastatin (20 mg)	24
Pravastatin (20 mg)	24
Simvastatin (20 mg)	35
Fluvastatin (20 mg)	18
Atorvastatin (10 mg)	37
Rosuvastatin (10 mg)	47

LDL-C, low-density lipoprotein cholesterol.

hyperlipidemia are deficient in LDL receptors, and measures that reduce cholesterol absorption (e.g., diet, ileal exclusion, bile acid sequestrants, ezetimibe) or act by LDL receptor upregulation (e.g., statins) are largely ineffective. These patients are treated with LDL apheresis and should be managed in tertiary care centers only.

Elevated TG levels may be caused by many factors, and more than one cause may be active in a given patient. Minor elevations in TG levels (150–299 mg/dL) usually are caused by obesity, sedentary lifestyle, smoking, excess alcohol intake, and high-carbohydrate diets. In other patients, secondary causes such as diabetes, renal failure, Cushing's disease, nephrotic syndrome, or medications (e.g., protease inhibitors, corticosteroids, retinoids, oral estrogens) may be responsible, and genetic causes may be pertinent to others. The therapy for this group of patients involves identification and treatment of secondary cause (if present), change in medications, and lifestyle changes. These patients benefit from total caloric restriction and switching from a very high carbohydrate diet to a more balanced diet. Very high TG levels (≥500 mg/dL) usually result from genetic defects of lipoprotein metabolism; in some patients, there is a combination of factors at play. These patients are at risk for acute pancreatitis (especially with TG levels >1,000 mg/dL), and treatment is directed to prevention of this condition. This is achieved with a combination of dietary measures (using very low fat diets [<15% calories from fat], and substituting medium-chain fatty acids in patients with TG levels >1,000 mg/dL), increasing physical activity, maintaining optimal weight, and initiating fibrates or niacin therapy. Fibrates are especially efficacious in this group. Statins are not especially effective agents for TG reduction and should be considered after the other two agents. Patients with an intermediate rise in TG levels (200–499 mg/dL) are a more heterogenous group with a wide array of underlying pathogenetic mechanisms at play. This pattern often is a result of an intersection of poor lifestyle, secondary causes, and genetic factors. These patients often have other markers of increased atherogenic risk, such as increased small LDL, low HDL, or elevated very low–density lipoprotein (VLDL) remnants. They need to be treated aggressively to bring the LDL level to the target; statins, with their ability to lower non-HDL cholesterol, are the preferred agents. In these patients, after the LDL target has been achieved, the secondary goal is a non–HDL-C level of 30 mg/dL higher than target LDL-C.[19] Non-HDL cholesterol is defined as the difference between the total and HDL cholesterol. Non-HDL cholesterol includes all cholesterol present in lipoprotein particles that are considered atherogenic, including LDL, lipoprotein(a), intermediate-density lipoprotein, and VLDL. High-dose statins often suffice to achieve the LDL-C and non–HDL-C goals, but for most patients, a second agent to lower TGs becomes necessary. The choices are niacin or fibrates in addition to a statin; these combinations carry an increased risk for hepatotoxicity or myopathy, and careful monitoring

therefore is essential. Refractory cases may benefit from fish oil supplements (>3 g per day) which, by reducing VLDL production, can lower the serum TG concentration by as much as 50% or more.[36] However, many currently available over-the-counter fish oil supplements contain <50% active omega-3 fatty acids. The commercial preparation Omacor, which has been available for many years in Europe and is now also available in the United States, contains 90% omega-3 fatty acids. The FDA limited approval for Omacor to the treatment of severe hypertriglyceridemia (≥500 mg/dL) because of concerns that it appears to increase LDL-C levels. Finally, weight loss by obese patients should be encouraged; it is associated with an improvement in the lipid profile and facilitates pharmacologic therapy, if still necessary.

Low HDL cholesterol levels often accompany minor or modest elevations in TG levels. Low HDL has been shown in epidemiologic studies to be an independent risk factor for cardiovascular disease. However, despite a multitude of research on currently available therapies to raise HDL and recent investigation of several newer agents that raise HDL, there has been no conclusive evidence that pharmacologically raising serum HDL-C levels contributes to lower rates of cardiovascular disease. Current guidelines specify that raising HDL should be a teriary goal after LDL and non–HDL-C goals have been reached.[19] In patients who have isolated low HDL levels without any elevation in TG levels, the first goal is to identify and modify lifestyle factors (e.g., high-carbohydrate diet, sedentary lifestyle, obesity, smoking) and medications (e.g., progestational agents, anabolic steroids). The next step encompasses calculation of 10-year risk and treating LDL-C with a statin when appropriate. The AFCAPS/TexCAPS study found a clear benefit for statin therapy in patients with low HDL-C levels.[5] In patients who continue to have low HDL-C levels despite lifestyle modifications and who are at goal for LDL and TGs, niacin therapy is the most reasonable choice to raise HDL-C.

Patients with diabetes are at an increased risk for cardiovascular events and often fare poorly after CAD manifests. Diabetes is associated with an increase in small LDL particles and often is associated with high TG and low HDL levels. Hyperglycemia is an independent risk factor for CAD. Primary prevention is important in this group and was demonstrated to be efficacious in the HPS trial. All diabetic patients, irrespective of LDL-C, should be considered for statin therapy and TLCs. Secondary goals include improved non–HDL-C levels and treatment for elevated TG levels. Blood sugar control and insulin therapy often facilitate the former, but fibrates or low-dose niacin may be necessary in some patients. Diabetes patients also often have coexisting hypertension. Blood pressure control and smoking cessation are essential, because both interventions are highly effective at reducing cardiovascular events in this population.

CONCLUSIONS

There is a clear association between elevated serum LDL-C and the risk of coronary events. Aggressive lowering of LDL-C with lifestyle modifications and pharmacologic therapy, particularly with statins, of persons at various risk levels reduces CAD morbidity and mortality rates and increases overall survival. This is especially true in patients with existing CHD or patients with equivalent CHD risk, such as those with diabetes mellitus.

REVIEW EXERCISES

QUESTIONS

1. A 51-year-old woman with a history of diabetes mellitus, hypertension, and CAD presents with history of statin intolerance. She was on Zocor 20 mg per day after her coronary artery bypass graft in 2000. She did well with Zocor until 3 years ago, when she had some vague muscle aches. Her primary physician drew a CK level, which was 500. She was told to stop Zocor. Her CK normalized, and her vague muscle ache resolved. Her fasting lipid panel was again drawn 3 months later. At that time, her LDL was 180; TRG, 500; and HDL, 27. She was started on Lipitor 40 mg and again after a few months had more vague muscle aches. Again, CK was drawn, and it was elevated at 600. What systemic diseases are known to effect CK levels?
a) Hypothyroidism
b) Acute renal failure
c) Biliary obstruction
d) All of the above
e) None of the above

Answer and Discussion
The answer is d. Hypothyroidism, acute renal failure, and biliary obstruction can increase the statin levels and should be ruled out by history, physical examination, and laboratory testing.

2. What common medications also effect CK levels in patients taking statin therapy?
a) Amiodarone
b) Verapamil
c) Fluconazole
d) Cyclosporine
e) HIV protease inhibitors
f) All of the above

Answer and Discussion
The answer is f. The risk of myopathy is greater in patients receiving concurrent therapy with medications that inhibit CYP3A4. These include macrolide antibiotics, antifungals, HIV protease inhibitors, fibrates, and commonly prescribed cardiac medications.

3. What is the difference between rosuvastatin and pravastatin with the rest of statin medications?
a) Rosuvastatin and pravastatin are not metabolized by CYP3A4 and are hydrophilic. However, there are limited data on muscle toxicity with these agents.
b) Rosuvastatin and pravastatin are metabolized by CYP3A4 and are hydrophobic. There is good data that these agents cause less muscle toxicity.
c) Rosuvastatin and pravastatin are not metabolized by CYP3A4 and are hydrophilic. There is good data that these agents cause less muscle toxicity.
d) Rosuvastatin and pravastatin are metabolized by CYP3A4 and are hydrophobic. However, there are limited data on muscle toxicity with these agents.
e) None of the above

Answer and Discussion
The answer is a. Rosuvastatin and pravastatin are not metabolized by CYP3A4 and are hydrophilic. However, there are limited data on muscle toxicity with these agents. There have been case reports of rhabdomyolysis with rosuvastatin.

4. A 65-year-old man with CAD, hypertension, and hyperlipidemia presents to you for follow-up. He is doing well and denies any pain. He recently underwent angioplasty to his left anterior descending artery with a drug-eluting stent. He is on aspirin 81 mg per day, Norvasc 10 mg per day, and Lipitor 10 mg per day. His fasting lipid shows LDL of 70; TRG, 100; and HDL, 19. What should you do next?
a) Increase his Lipitor dose.
b) Change from Lipitor to Crestor.
c) Add Tricor to his statin.
d) Add niacin to his statin dose.

Answer and Discussion
The answer is d. Add niacin to his statin. Unfortunately, the patient has low HDL. His LDL and TGs are well controlled. Therefore, the best thing for this patient is to increase his HDL with niacin. Further increase in his statin will not adequately raise his HDL.

5. A diet high in trans-fat will cause which kind of lipid abnormalities?
a) High HDL, low LDL
b) High HDL, high LDL
c) Low HDL, low LDL
d) Low HDL, high LDL
e) No significant effect on HDL or LDL but will increase TGs

Answer and Discussion
The answer is d. Low HDL and high LDL. A diet high in trans-fat will also increase TGs.

REFERENCES

1. Chen Z, Peto R, Collins R, et al. Serum cholesterol concentration and coronary heart disease in population with low cholesterol concentrations. *BMJ* 1991;303(6797):276–282.
2. Stamler J, Wentworth D, Neaton JD. Is relationship between serum cholesterol and risk of premature death from coronary heart disease continuous and graded? Findings in 356,222 primary screenees of the Multiple Risk Factor Intervention Trial (MRFIT). *JAMA* 1986;256(20):2823–2828.
3. Shepherd J, Cobbe SM, Ford I, et al. Prevention of coronary heart disease with pravastatin in men with hypercholesterolemia. West of Scotland Coronary Prevention Study Group. *N Engl J Med* 1995;333(20):1301–1307.
4. Ford I, Murray H, Packard CJ, et al. Long-term follow-up of the West of Scotland Coronary Prevention Study. *N Engl J Med* 2007;357(15):1477–1486.
5. Downs JR, Clearfield M, Weis S, et al. Primary prevention of acute coronary events with lovastatin in men and women with average cholesterol levels: results of AFCAPS/TexCAPS. Air Force/Texas Coronary Atherosclerosis Prevention Study. *JAMA* 1998;279(20):1615–1622.
6. Heart Protection Study Collaborative Group. MRC/BHF Heart Protection Study of cholesterol lowering with simvastatin in 20,536 high-risk individuals: a randomised placebo-controlled trial. *Lancet* 2002;360(9326):7–22.
7. Shepherd J, Blauw GJ, Murphy MB, et al. Pravastatin in elderly individuals at risk of vascular disease (PROSPER): a randomised controlled trial. *Lancet* 2002;360(9346):1623–1630.
8. Major outcomes in moderately hypercholesterolemic, hypertensive patients randomized to pravastatin vs usual care: the Antihypertensive and Lipid-Lowering Treatment to Prevent Heart Attack Trial (ALLHAT-LLT). *JAMA* 2002;288(23):2998–3007.
9. Sever PS, Dahlof B, Poulter NR, et al. Prevention of coronary and stroke events with atorvastatin in hypertensive patients who have average or lower-than-average cholesterol concentrations, in the Anglo-Scandinavian Cardiac Outcomes Trial—Lipid-Lowering Arm (ASCOT-LLA): a multicentre randomised controlled trial. *Lancet* 2003;361(9364):1149–1158.
10. Colhoun HM, Betteridge DJ, Durrington PN, et al. Primary prevention of cardiovascular disease with atorvastatin in type 2 diabetes in the Collaborative Atorvastatin Diabetes Study (CARDS): multicentre randomised placebo-controlled trial. *Lancet* 2004;364(9435):685–696.
11. Randomised trial of cholesterol lowering in 4444 patients with coronary heart disease: the Scandinavian Simvastatin Survival Study (4S). *Lancet* 1994;344(8934):1383–1389.
12. Sacks FM, Pfeffer MA, Moye LA, et al. The effect of pravastatin on coronary events after myocardial infarction in patients with average cholesterol levels. Cholesterol and Recurrent Events Trial investigators. *N Engl J Med* 1996;335(14):1001–1009.
13. Prevention of cardiovascular events and death with pravastatin in patients with coronary heart disease and a broad range of initial cholesterol levels. The Long-Term Intervention with Pravastatin in Ischaemic Disease (LIPID) Study Group. *N Engl J Med* 1998;339(19):1349–1357.
14. Cannon CP, Braunwald E, McCabe CH, et al. Intensive versus moderate lipid-lowering with statins after acute coronary syndromes. *N Engl J Med* 2004;350(15):1495–1504.
15. LaRosa JC, Grundy SM, Waters DD, et al. Intensive lipid-lowering with atorvastatin in patients with stable coronary disease. *N Engl J Med* 2005;352(14):1425–1435.
16. Pedersen TR, Faergeman O, Kastelein JJ, et al. High-dose atorvastatin vs usual-dose simvastatin for secondary prevention after myocardial infarction: the IDEAL study: a randomized controlled trial. *JAMA* 2005;294(19):2437–2445.
17. Baigent C, Keech A, Kearney PM, et al. Efficacy and safety of cholesterol-lowering treatment: prospective meta-analysis of data from 90,056 participants in 14 randomised trials of statins. *Lancet* 2005;366(9493):1267–1278.
18. Cannon CP, Steinberg BA, Murphy SA, et al. Meta-analysis of cardiovascular outcomes trials comparing intensive versus moderate statin therapy. *J Am Coll Cardiol* 2006;48(3):438–445.
19. Executive Summary of The Third Report of The National Cholesterol Education Program (NCEP) Expert Panel on Detection, Evaluation, and Treatment of High Blood Cholesterol in Adults (Adult Treatment Panel III). *JAMA* 2001;285(19):2486–2497.
20. Grundy SM, Cleeman JI, Merz CN, et al. Implications of recent clinical trials for the National Cholesterol Education Program Adult Treatment Panel III guidelines. *Circulation* 2004;110(2):227–239.
21. Fletcher GF, Bufalino V, Costa F, et al. Efficacy of drug therapy in the secondary prevention of cardiovascular disease and stroke. *Am J Cardiol* 2007;99(6C):1E–35E.
22. Cohen DE, Anania FA, Chalasani N. An assessment of statin safety by hepatologists. *Am J Cardiol* 2006;97(8A):77C–81C.
23. Pasternak RC, Smith SC Jr, Bairey-Merz CN, et al. ACC/AHA/NHLBI Clinical Advisory on the Use and Safety of Statins. *Stroke* 2002;33(9):2337–2241.
24. Thompson PD, Clarkson PM, Rosenson RS. An assessment of statin safety by muscle experts. *Am J Cardiol* 2006;97(8A):69C–76C.
25. Davidson MH, Robinson JG. Safety of aggressive lipid management. *J Am Coll Cardiol* 2007;49(17):1753–1762.
26. Marcoff L, Thompson PD. The role of coenzyme Q10 in statin-associated myopathy: a systematic review. *J Am Coll Cardiol* 2007;49(23):2231–2237.
27. Brensike JF, Levy RI, Kelsey SF, et al. Effects of therapy with cholestyramine on progression of coronary arteriosclerosis: results of the NHLBI Type II Coronary Intervention Study. *Circulation* 1984;69(2):313–324.
28. Watts GF, Lewis B, Brunt JN, et al. Effects on coronary artery disease of lipid-lowering diet, or diet plus cholestyramine, in the St Thomas' Atherosclerosis Regression Study (STARS). *Lancet* 1992;339(8793):563–569.
29. McKenney J. New perspectives on the use of niacin in the treatment of lipid disorders. *Arch Intern Med* 2004;164(7):697–705.
30. A co-operative trial in the primary prevention of ischaemic heart disease using clofibrate. Report from the Committee of Principal Investigators. *Br Heart J* 1978;40(10):1069–1118.
31. Rubins HB, Robins SJ, Collins D, et al. Gemfibrozil for the secondary prevention of coronary heart disease in men with low levels of high-density lipoprotein cholesterol. Veterans Affairs High-Density Lipoprotein Cholesterol Intervention Trial Study Group. *N Engl J Med* 1999;341(6):410–418.
32. Keech A, Simes RJ, Barter P, et al. Effects of long-term fenofibrate therapy on cardiovascular events in 9795 people with type 2 diabetes mellitus (the FIELD study): randomised controlled trial. *Lancet* 2005;366(9500):1849–1861.
33. Knopp RH, Gitter H, Truitt T, et al. Effects of ezetimibe, a new cholesterol absorption inhibitor, on plasma lipids in patients with primary hypercholesterolemia. *Eur Heart J* 2003;24(8):729–741.
34. Brown G, Albers JJ, Fisher LD, et al. Regression of coronary artery disease as a result of intensive lipid-lowering therapy in men with high levels of apolipoprotein B. *N Engl J Med* 1990;323(19):1289–1298.
35. Graham DJ, Staffa JA, Shatin D, et al. Incidence of hospitalized rhabdomyolysis in patients treated with lipid-lowering drugs. *JAMA* 2004;292(21):2585–2590.
36. Harris WS, Connor WE, Illingworth DR, et al. Effects of fish oil on VLDL triglyceride kinetics in humans. *J Lipid Res* 1990;31(9):1549–1558.

Chapter 65

Heart Failure

Robert E. Hobbs

POINTS TO REMEMBER:

- The most common cause of heart failure in the United States is end-stage coronary artery disease (CAD), accounting for more than half of cases.

- *Systolic heart failure* refers to contractile impairment manifested by low left ventricular ejection fraction (LVEF).

- *Diastolic heart failure* occurs in the setting of preserved LVEF and is associated with abnormal left ventricular relaxation and filling, left ventricular hypertrophy, and elevated intracardiac pressures.

- The degree of functional impairment usually is stated in terms of the New York Heart Association (NYHA) classification:

  - *Class I* refers to no limitation of physical activity and no dyspnea or fatigue with ordinary physical activities.
  - *Class II* indicates mild limitation of physical activity and dyspnea or fatigue occurring with ordinary physical activities. The patient has no symptoms at rest.
  - *Class III* implies marked limitation of activity. Less than ordinary physical activities cause symptoms. The patient is asymptomatic at rest.
  - *Class IV* refers to symptoms at rest and with any physical exertion.

- The B-type natriuretic peptide (BNP) assay is a useful test for determining whether dyspnea is due to heart failure. Elevated levels of BNP correlate with the severity and prognosis of heart failure.

- Echocardiography is the most useful diagnostic test in heart failure.

Heart failure is a complex clinical syndrome characterized by structural, functional, and biological alterations leading to impaired cardiac function and circulatory congestion. In this syndrome, impaired cardiac function is inadequate to meet the metabolic needs of the body, resulting in decreased perfusion of organs and tissues as well as fluid retention. Half the cases of heart failure result from systolic dysfunction, in which the contractility of the left ventricle is impaired. An equal number of cases involve impaired relaxation of the ventricles during diastole (i.e., diastolic failure or heart failure with preserved systolic function).

ETIOLOGY

The most common cause of heart failure in the United States is end-stage CAD, accounting for more than half the cases. Other causes include cardiomyopathies, hypertensive heart disease, valvular heart disease, and congenital heart disease.

Heart failure may be characterized in several ways: acute versus chronic, systolic versus diastolic, left versus right sided, forward versus backward, low versus high output. *Acute heart failure* refers to a rapid decompensation leading to dyspnea, acute pulmonary edema, or fluid retention. *Chronic heart failure* refers to prolonged impairment due to dyspnea, effort intolerance, and fluid retention. Chronic heart failure with acute exacerbations is the most common clinical presentation. *Systolic heart failure* refers to contractile impairment manifested by a low LVEF. *Diastolic heart failure* occurs in the setting of preserved LVEF and is associated with abnormal left ventricular relaxation and filling, left ventricular hypertrophy, and elevated intracardiac pressures. Diastolic heart failure occurs with hypertensive heart disease, CAD, hypertrophic cardiomyopathy, restrictive cardiomyopathy, and aortic valve disease with or without valve replacement. Left-sided failure is manifested by effort intolerance and dyspnea. Right-sided failure is characterized by fluid retention, edema, and ascites. The causes of right-sided failure include left-sided failure, mitral stenosis, pulmonary hypertension (primary or secondary), cor pulmonale from chronic obstructive pulmonary disease, pulmonic valve disease, tricuspid valve disease, right ventricular infarction, and arrhythmogenic right ventricular dysplasia. Low cardiac output failure is common, but high-output failure is rare. The causes of high-output heart failure include thyrotoxicosis, arteriovenous fistula, pregnancy, Paget's disease, anemia, and beriberi.

EPIDEMIOLOGY

Heart failure affects 1% to 2% of the population (approximately 5 million Americans), with 550,000 new cases diagnosed each year. It is the only cardiovascular disease that is increasing in prevalence. During the last decade, hospitalizations for heart failure have increased 159% and now account for more than 1 million hospital admissions each year. The prevalence of heart failure increases with age and approaches 10 cases per 1,000 population after age 65 years. Seventy-five percent of patients have antecedent hypertension. In the Medicare population, heart failure is the leading diagnosis-related group, accounting for 20% of all hospitalizations. It the largest expense for the Center for Medicare and Medicaid Services, accounting for at least $29.6 billion in health care expenditures annually. Heart failure has the highest readmission rate of any medical condition, with half the patients readmitted for cardiac decompensation within 6 months. Heart failure is more common in men than in women until late in life. It is estimated that 10% of the population older than age 75 years has experienced heart failure.

The annual mortality for heart failure exceeds that of most malignancies, approaching 20% for all cases. The high annual mortality gives rise to a 70% all-cause mortality rate at 5 years. Sudden death occurs in half these patients and is six to nine times more common than in the general population. Heart failure deaths have increased 35% during the last decade, whereas mortality from myocardial infarction (MI) has declined. The prognosis of heart failure is related to a number of factors: exercise impairment, low LVEF, elevated neurohormones (BNP, norepinephrine, etc.), cachexia, wide QRS complex, renal impairment, hyponatremia, and hypocholesterolemia.

PATHOPHYSIOLOGY

Factors contributing to the syndrome of heart failure include structural cardiac abnormalities, hemodynamic derangements, and neurohormonal activation. Hemodynamic derangements characteristic of heart failure are low cardiac output and high intracardiac pressures. Low cardiac output accounts for fatigue and exercise intolerance, whereas high intracardiac pressures lead to exertional dyspnea and peripheral edema. Heart failure patients have poor exercise capacity because of low cardiac output and an exercise-induced pulmonary hypertension. Hemodynamic abnormalities contribute to symptoms, whereas neurohumoral abnormalities lead to progression and eventually death. Neurohormonal abnormalities consist of sympathetic nervous system activation, renin-angiotensin-aldosterone stimulation, release of vasopressin, elevation

of endothelin, activation of proinflammatory cytokines, and secretion of natriuretic peptides. In general, neurohormonal abnormalities lead to vasoconstriction and sodium and water retention as well as cardiovascular growth and remodeling. Although the immediate neurohormonal actions are beneficial, long-term effects are deleterious. Neurohormones are elevated in heart failure and correlate with severity and prognosis. Baroreceptor dysfunction contributes to sympathetic nervous system activation and inhibits the parasympathetic nervous system. Circulating catecholamines cause resting tachycardia, arrhythmias, myocyte toxicity, β-receptor dysfunction, and renin-angiotensin stimulation.

The renin-angiotensin system is activated when renin is released from the juxtaglomerular apparatus of the kidney by a variety of stimuli. Renin acts as a substrate for the conversion of angiotensinogen to angiotensin I. After passage through the pulmonary circulation, angiotensin I is converted to angiotensin II. Angiotensin II is a potent vasoconstrictor that stimulates thirst, releases aldosterone, and promotes sodium and water retention. It is a growth factor that may lead to progressive cardiac deterioration. Vasopressin is released from the hypothalamus secondary to baroreceptor or osmotic stimuli, and it causes vasoconstriction as well as sodium and water retention. The actions of the sympathetic nervous system, renin-angiotensin system, and vasopressin are balanced by the natriuretic peptides. These hormones are released from the cardiac myocytes and exert their physiological actions on the vasculature and kidneys. The physiological effects of natriuretic peptides include vasodilation, sodium and water excretion, vasodilation, and neurohormonal modulation. Endothelin is derived from a variety of sources from within the cardiovascular system. It is both a vasoconstrictor and a growth factor. The proinflammatory cytokine—tumor necrosis factor—is released from macrophages and may cause cardiac cachexia, exercise intolerance, and apoptosis in the failing heart. As a consequence of myocardial injury, the heart undergoes remodeling to compensate for low stroke volume. Remodeling consists of hypertrophy, dilatation, and spherical reshaping of the left ventricular chamber, which leads to increased wall stress, mitral regurgitation, and decreased inotropic reserve. In chronic heart failure, the skeletal muscles undergo biochemical and physiological deterioration. These abnormalities account for some of the exercise intolerance seen in these patients.

HEART FAILURE WITH PRESERVED SYSTOLIC FUNCTION (DIASTOLIC FAILURE)

Systolic dysfunction is characterized by impaired contractility, whereas diastolic dysfunction is characterized by impaired relaxation. In patients with diastolic dysfunction, the LVEF is normal but the ventricular filling is impaired (i.e., "stiff heart syndrome"). The left ventricle often is hypertrophied, left ventricular cavity size is small, and overall heart size is not grossly enlarged. Diastolic dysfunction occurs with hypertensive heart disease, ischemic heart disease, hypertrophic cardiomyopathy, restrictive cardiomyopathy (including infiltrative diseases), and aortic valve disease. Echocardiography is the most important test for assessing LVEF and diastolic filling patterns. Hemodynamically, diastolic dysfunction is characterized by elevated intracardiac pressures. Treatment is directed at the underlying cause. Therapeutic goals include relieving congestion, improving relaxation, decreasing hypertrophy, and reducing ischemia.

CLINICAL PRESENTATION

The symptoms of congestive heart failure (CHF) are caused by low cardiac output or high intracardiac pressures. The general manifestations of heart failure include breathlessness, fatigue, effort intolerance, and fluid retention. Respiratory symptoms are common: dyspnea, orthopnea, paroxysmal nocturnal dyspnea, cough, wheezing, or respiratory distress. Abdominal manifestations are indicative of right-sided heart failure: weight gain, fluid retention, bloating, early satiety, anorexia, weight loss, right upper quadrant pain, nausea, and vomiting. The degree of functional impairment usually is stated in terms of the NYHA classification:

- *Class I* refers to no limitation of physical activity and no dyspnea or fatigue with ordinary physical activities.
- *Class II* indicates mild limitation of physical activity and dyspnea or fatigue occurring with ordinary physical activities. The patient has no symptoms at rest.
- *Class III* implies marked limitation of activity. Less than ordinary physical activities cause symptoms. The patient is asymptomatic at rest.
- *Class IV* refers to symptoms at rest and with any physical exertion.

Physical Examination

Patients with severe, acute decompensated CHF and pulmonary edema have respiratory distress, tachypnea, diaphoresis, pallor, cyanosis, cool extremities, jugular venous distension, rales, rapid heart rate, and S_3 and S_4 gallops. Most patients with chronic heart failure have fluid retention, but are comfortable at rest. Those with end-stage heart failure may have cardiac cachexia and muscle wasting. The blood pressure may be low, normal, or high. The resting heart rate frequently is increased, and pulsus alternans (a beat-to-beat variation in the intensity of the pulse) may be present. Jugular venous distension is an important finding in patients with decompensated failure, indicating fluid overload. A prominent V wave is seen with tricuspid regurgitation. The lungs usually are clear in chronic heart failure, but rales indicate decompensation. Decreased breath sounds and dullness at the lung base reflect an underlying pleural effusion. Wheezing may occur because of bronchospasm (cardiac asthma). Cheyne-Stokes respirations, which are a manifestation of central sleep apnea, occur with advanced heart failure. Examination of the heart reveals a diffuse apical impulse that is displaced downward and to the left. A left ventricular heave and occasionally a right ventricular heave may be palpable. If the heart rate is rapid, the first heart sound will be accentuated. The second heart sound may be paradoxically split because of delayed electric activation or mechanical ejection of the left ventricle. A third heart sound is characteristic of left ventricular failure, whereas a fourth heart sound suggests a noncompliant left ventricle. Murmurs of mitral and tricuspid regurgitation are common. Abdominal examination may reveal hepatomegaly, right upper quadrant tenderness, and ascites. Pressing on the liver may further distend the jugular veins (positive hepatojugular reflux). An examination of the extremities may reveal edema, muscle wasting, or cyanosis.

Diagnostic Studies

The BNP assay is a useful test for determining whether dyspnea is due to heart failure. Elevated levels of BNP correlate with the severity and prognosis of heart failure. Electrocardiography may reveal normal sinus rhythm or atrial fibrillation. Left ventricular hypertrophy and left bundle-branch block are common patterns, and Q waves reflect previous MI. Chest radiography often shows cardiomegaly, increased pulmonary vascularity, redistribution of blood flow to the upper lobes, prominent pulmonary arteries, Kerley B lines, interstitial and alveolar edema, and pleural effusions.

Echocardiography is the most useful diagnostic test in heart failure. Imaging usually reveals a dilated left ventricle with decreased LVEF. The right ventricle may be normal or dysfunctional. Mitral and tricuspid regurgitation often is detected through Doppler imaging. Pulmonary artery pressures may be estimated indirectly and frequently are elevated. Echocardiography also excludes tamponade or pericardial diseases as possible causes of heart failure. Doppler measurements provide information about diastolic dysfunction.

Metabolic stress testing using respiratory gas measurement provides an objective assessment of functional capacity. Normal middle-aged adults achieve a peak oxygen consumption of ≥ 25 mL/kg per minute. Values < 14 mL/kg per minute indicate severe functional impairment.

Cardiac catheterization provides hemodynamic data that may guide therapy. Coronary angiography is the most accurate means of diagnosing CAD. The status of the cardiac valves and left ventricle also may be assessed by catheterization. Although right ventricular endomyocardial biopsy is no longer performed routinely in heart failure patients, myocardial tissue diagnosis may be helpful in assessing patients with giant cell myocarditis, restrictive cardiomyopathy, or infiltrative diseases.

TREATMENT PRINCIPLES

The management of heart failure consists of identifying the underlying cause of heart failure, determining precipitating factors for decompensation, initiating clinically proven therapies, and providing patient education. The etiology of heart failure should be determined if possible: CAD, cardiomyopathy, valvular heart disease, hypertensive heart disease, or congenital heart disease. Precipitating factors for decompensation include excessive salt or fluid intake; noncompliance with diet, fluids, medications, or follow-up; arrhythmias; infection; renal failure; ischemia or MI; drugs; pulmonary embolism; anemia; and thyrotoxicosis. Patient education is an important aspect of management, because noncompliance is the most frequent cause of rehospitalization. The management of heart failure has evolved during the last 40 years. Initially, bed rest, fluid removal, and oxygen were used for treatment. Later efforts were directed at increasing contractility and improving hemodynamics. Newer therapies for heart failure attempt to modulate neurohormonal factors. Sympathetic nervous system excess may be modulated through the use of β-blockers and possibly digoxin. The renin-angiotensin system may be inhibited by angiotensin-converting enzyme (ACE) inhibitors, angiotensin II receptor blockers (ARB), and aldosterone antagonists. Novel therapies that target other neurohormones are under investigation.

Stages of Heart Failure and Treatment

Heart failure may be divided into four stages, A through D. *Stage A* includes patients at risk for developing heart failure, such as those with hypertension, diabetes mellitus, CAD, metabolic syndrome, or obesity; those who use cardiotoxins; or those with a familial history of cardiomyopathy. Management involves risk factor modification as well as ACE inhibitors or ARBs for vascular disease or diabetes. *Stage B* patients are those with asymptomatic left ventricular dysfunction or hypertrophy. Management involves risk factor modification as well as ACE inhibitors or ARBs plus β-blockers to prevent adverse remodeling. *Stage C* includes patients with structural heart disease and current or past symptoms of heart failure. Treatment involves all measures used in stages A and B, plus diuretics, digoxin, aldosterone antagonists, hydralazine/nitrates, and electronic devices in selected patients. *Stage D* designates patients with refractory heart failure who might be candidates for cardiac transplantation, mechanical circulatory support, advanced surgical therapies, or hospice care.

OUTPATIENT THERAPIES

Angiotensin-converting Enzyme Inhibitors

ACE inhibitors are important drugs for treating patients with all levels of heart failure, including those with asymptomatic left ventricular dysfunction. These drugs inhibit the formation of angiotensin II by blocking converting enzyme (ACE). They enhance the action of kinins and augment prostaglandin synthesis. In addition to prolonging survival, ACE inhibitors improve symptoms, hemodynamics, neurohormones, quality of life, and exercise tolerance. The beneficial actions of ACE inhibitors appear to be a class effect. ACE inhibitors should be started at low dose and titrated to target doses to achieve optimal clinical benefit. ACE inhibitors may be limited by side effects including azotemia, hyperkalemia, cough, angioedema, dysgeusia, and agranulocytosis. ARBs may be substituted for ACE intolerance due to cough or angioedema. The combination of hydralazine and nitrates may be used when ACE inhibitors are not tolerated due to azotemia or hyperkalemia. Hydralazine is an arterial vasodilator that prevents nitrate tachyphylaxis and has antioxidant properties. Nitrates are venous dilators that inhibit cardiovascular growth and remodeling.

Beta-Blockers

Numerous studies have shown that β-blockers improve ejection fraction, symptoms, exercise capacity, quality of life, and survival. β-Blockers are as important as ACE inhibitors in the long-term management of heart failure. β-Blockers modulate catecholamine excess, which has numerous adverse effects on the failing heart, and they improve or prevent remodeling, apoptosis, β-receptor pathway dysfunction, wall stress, myocardial oxygen demand, and arrhythmias. These agents should be started in euvolemic patients at low doses and titrated slowly upward over a period of weeks to target levels. The initiation of a β-blocker decreases adrenergic stimulation of the failing heart and may be associated with a temporary decrease in LVEF, increased left ventricular volume, and worsening hemodynamics. Thus, patients may feel worse initially, but most patients improve clinically after several months of therapy. The risks of β-blocker use in heart failure include hypotension, lightheadedness, fluid retention, worsening heart failure, bradycardia, and heart block.

Angiotensin Receptor Blockers

ARBs modulate the peripheral effects of angiotensin II by blocking angiotensin II receptors at the tissue level. Clinical trials have shown that these agents are similar to ACE inhibitors in their beneficial effects. ARBs are better tolerated than ACE inhibitors, although they can cause hypotension, worsening renal function, and hyperkalemia. ARBs are still considered second-line drugs for heart failure in patients who are ACE intolerant due to cough or angioedema. ARBs may be added to an ACE inhibitor and a β-blocker for additional morbidity benefit.

Diuretics

Most patients with heart failure benefit from diuretics. These agents produce rapid symptomatic improvement and control fluid retention. Many diuretics are available; each group or class of diuretic has different sites of action in the kidney, different potencies, and different metabolic effects. Diuretics are useful in systolic or diastolic failure and are the key to success when used in conjunction with other drug therapies. These drugs are available at relatively low cost and may be administered once daily. Diuretics may cause electrolyte depletion, hypotension, and azotemia. They activate neurohormones and for this reason should not be prescribed as monotherapy for heart failure. It is important to achieve an euvolemic state without overdiuresis; a patient-directed flexible diuretic regimen helps to facilitate this goal.

Aldosterone Antagonists

Angiotensin II stimulates the release of aldosterone from the adrenal cortex. Aldosterone promotes the sodium and water retention associated with potassium and magnesium loss. It activates the sympathetic nervous system and inhibits parasympathetic outflow. Aldosterone may cause fibrosis of myocardial, vascular, renal, and cerebral tissue as well as cardiac and vascular remodeling. Spironolactone, an aldosterone antagonist, reduces mortality and heart failure hospitalizations in patients with severe heart failure. It has not shown the same benefit in patients with mild to moderate heart failure or in patients with asymptomatic left ventricular dysfunction. Therefore, an aldosterone antagonist is indicated in patients with NYHA functional class III and IV heart failure along with an ACE inhibitor, β-blocker, and diuretic. Hyperkalemia may occur, especially when the serum creatinine level is >2 mg/dL, and an aldosterone antagonist is best avoided in this group of patients. Potassium levels should be determined during the first week of therapy and regularly thereafter. Potassium supplementation may not be necessary when these drugs are administered. Ten percent of men taking spironolactone develop gynecomastia. Eplerenone, a selective aldosterone antagonist, improved survival in patients with MI complicated by left ventricular dysfunction or heart failure. It is associated with a lower incidence of side effects, especially gynecomastia, compared with spironolactone but may still cause hyperkalemia in 5% of patients.

Digoxin

Digoxin, a centrally acting neurohormonal modulating agent, has several direct and indirect actions on the myocardium and conducting system. It exerts its actions through the binding and inhibition of the enzyme sodium-potassium ATPase. In the heart, this leads to increased intracellular calcium, which enhances contractility. In the central nervous system, it reduces sympathetic excess; within the kidney, it decreases the release of renin. Clinically, digoxin improves exercise capacity, LVEF, and hemodynamics. Although it decreases the frequency of hospitalizations, digoxin has a neutral effect on mortality. Digoxin has a relatively low therapeutic–toxic range, and a low dose should be prescribed in women, the elderly, and patients with renal dysfunction or when combined with amiodarone. Serum digoxin levels should be maintained at <0.9 ng/mL.

Calcium Channel Blockers

Standard calcium channel blockers should not be used in patients with CHF, as these agents depress left ventricular function, activate neurohormones, worsen symptoms, and increase the risk of death. Amlodipine has a neutral effect on cardiac function and may be added to an ACE inhibitor and a β-blocker to treat patients with angina pectoris or hypertension associated with heart failure.

INPATIENT THERAPIES

Nitroprusside

Sodium nitroprusside is an intravenous vasodilator that dilates arteries and veins, thereby lowering systemic arterial blood pressure and intracardiac pressures. It is used to treat acute pulmonary edema, decompensated heart failure, or hypertensive emergencies in an intensive care unit using invasive hemodynamic monitoring. Nitroprusside is metabolized to nitric oxide and cyanide by the liver. Nitric oxide activates guanylate cyclase in smooth muscle and epithelial cells, increasing the intracellular concentration of cyclic guanosine-5' monophosphate (cGMP), a second messenger, and resulting in smooth muscle relaxation and vasodilation. The drug is administered by continuous intravenous infusion. Hypotension is a common side effect, mandating frequent blood pressure measurements. It rarely may cause coronary steal syndrome and should be avoided in acute ischemic syndromes. Prolonged infusions, especially in patients with hepatic or renal dysfunction, have been associated with thiocyanate toxicity.

Nitroglycerin

Intravenous nitroglycerin is a venous vasodilator at low doses and an arterial vasodilator at high doses. It is biotransformed into nitric oxide, which activates guanylate cyclase, increases cGMP, relaxes smooth muscle cells, and causes vasodilation. Intravenous nitroglycerin lowers intracardiac pressures and improves pulmonary congestion. It relieves myocardial ischemia through coronary artery dilation and increased collateral flow. Its long-term use is limited by tachyphylaxis (loss of effect) occurring within 24 hours as a result of sulfhydryl-group depletion. Headache occurs in 20% of patients and hypotension in 5%.

Nesiritide

Nesiritide, synthetic BNP, is a systemic and pulmonary vasodilator with modest diuretic and natriuretic properties. It is administered as a weight-based intravenous bolus followed by a continuous intravenous infusion in patients with decompensated heart failure. This vasodilator improves heart failure symptoms by lowering intracardiac pressures and increasing cardiac index. Nesiritide has no inotropic properties and no proarrhythmic effects. It is does not require frequent titrations and is not associated with tachyphylaxis.

Dopamine

Dopamine, an intravenous inotropic agent, is the immediate precursor of norepinephrine. It has distinct physiological properties (mesenteric vasodilation, positive inotropic effects, and peripheral vasoconstriction), depending on the infusion rate. When used at low doses, dopamine activates dopaminergic receptors in the mesenteric and renal arteries, causing vasodilation. At moderate doses, dopamine stimulates cardiac β-receptors and increases cardiac output. At high doses, it activates peripheral α-receptors, causing vasoconstriction.

Dobutamine

Dobutamine is a direct-acting positive inotropic agent. It is useful for treating hospitalized patients with decompensated heart failure who have hypotension or shock. Routine infusions of dobutamine for decompensated heart failure (without hypotension) are not recommended, and intermittent outpatient dobutamine infusions are discouraged. Continuous home dobutamine may be considered as palliative therapy to improve quality of life and prevent recurrent hospitalizations in patients with end-stage heart failure.

Milrinone

Milrinone, a phosphodiesterase III inhibitor, is a positive inotropic agent and a vasodilator. It may be used as a primary agent or combined with dobutamine or dopamine. It is more potent as a pulmonary vasodilator than dobutamine, and it is less likely to increase heart rate and myocardial oxygen consumption. It is the preferred inotrope for use in patients treated with β-blockers.

ELECTRONIC DEVICE THERAPIES

Defibrillator Therapy

Half of heart failure deaths occur suddenly and without warning. These deaths probably are caused by ventricular tachyarrhythmias or bradyarrhythmias. Sudden death is six to nine times more common in heart failure patients than in the general population. The most important risk factor for sudden cardiac death is the presence of heart failure. Current indications for implantable cardiac defibrillator placement include survivors of a cardiac arrest, sustained ventricular tachycardia, inducible ventricular tachycardia, and dilated or ischemic cardiomyopathy with ejection fraction ≤35%.

Resynchronization Therapy

Conduction abnormalities occur in approximately 50% of heart failure patients, usually left bundle-branch block, and are associated with poorer survival. Conduction abnormalities delay the electrical activation of the left ventricle and cause ventricular dyssynchrony (inefficient contractility), prolonged mitral regurgitation, and impaired diastolic filling. Resynchronization therapy involves the placement of a right atrial lead, right ventricular lead, and a third pacing lead in a left cardiac vein. Atrial contractility and biventricular contractility are synchronized by echocardiography. Resynchronization therapy improves ventricular contractility, cardiac output, mitral regurgitation, heart failure symptoms, functional class, exercise capacity, and survival. Indications include dilated or ischemic cardiomyopathy with ejection fraction ≤35% and NYHA functional class III and IV symptoms. Approximately 70% of patients experience immediate benefit through the use of resynchronization therapy, although symptomatic improvement may decline with time.

MECHANICAL CIRCULATORY SUPPORT

Intra-aortic balloon pumping (IABP) temporarily improves hemodynamics in patients with severe heart failure. A balloon pump may increase cardiac output by 20% as a result of improved forward flow and diastolic augmentation. Device complications, such as limb ischemia, bleeding, thrombosis, neurologic injury, and infection, occur at a rate of 10% per day and limit the usefulness of a balloon pump to a period of 1 week.

Currently available left ventricular assist devices (LVAD) include the HeartMate, Novacor, Thoratec, and Abiomed pumps. Small continuous flow devices (DeBakey, Jarvik 2000, HeartMate II, etc.) are undergoing clinical trials. The major indication for LVAD placement is cardiogenic shock that persists despite inotropes and IABP. Patients should be suitable candidates for cardiac transplantation, because most of these devices are used as a bridge to cardiac transplantation. More frequently, LVADs may be implanted as permanent mechanical support or "destination therapy." LVAD support occasionally functions as a "bridge to recovery" after acute myocardial failure.

Following LVAD placement, patients are weaned from respiratory and inotropic support. Renal and hepatic dysfunction improve with normalization of cardiac output. The LVAD allows patients to become physically rehabilitated, making them better candidates for cardiac transplantation. Complications from these devices are frequent and serious. Perioperative bleeding is common, resulting from coagulopathies and liver dysfunction. Most patients receive blood products at the time of device implantation, which may lead to antibody formation against potential organ donors. Infections are the limiting factor to long-term success. Thromboembolic and mechanical complications are less common with improved devices. Deaths after LVAD implantation usually result from irreversible organ dysfunction, stroke, or infection.

SURGICAL THERAPIES

Ventricular Reconstruction

Ventricular reconstruction surgery may be performed in patients with ischemic cardiomyopathy who have evidence of ischemic or hibernating myocardium. The procedure involves a combination of techniques, including coronary artery bypass grafting, mitral and tricuspid valve repair, left ventricular scar or aneurysm resection, left ventricular reconstruction, and epicardial left ventricular pacing lead placement. Postoperatively, the reconstructed elliptically shaped left ventricle becomes a smaller, more efficient pumping chamber. Candidates include patients with CAD, NYHA functional class III or IV symptoms, severe left ventricular dysfunction with scar/aneurysm plus hibernating or ischemic myocardium, and mitral and/or tricuspid regurgitation.

Cardiac Transplantation

Approximately 2,100 heart transplants are performed annually in the United States. This therapy is limited by inadequate numbers of donor hearts and serves only a small fraction of patients with severe heart failure who remain functionally impaired despite medical therapy. The criteria for transplant listing include end-stage heart disease refractory to medical or surgical therapy, disabling symptoms despite maximal medications, and anticipated poor survival. Contraindications include irreversible pulmonary hypertension, other serious illnesses limiting survival or rehabilitation, drug or alcohol abuse, and medical noncompliance. After transplantation, patients are treated with a multidrug immunosuppressive regimen. Complications often are related to immunosuppression and include infection, rejection, malignancy, and allograft CAD. Other problems occur frequently in the transplant population, including hypertension, renal insufficiency, weight gain, hyperlipidemia, diabetes mellitus, and osteoporosis. Mortality averages 10% to 15% during the first year and 4% annually thereafter.

OTHER THERAPIES

Antiarrhythmic Drugs

Antiarrhythmic drug prophylaxis in heart failure is controversial. Amiodarone is the preferred agent for treating atrial fibrillation or ventricular tachycardia in heart failure, but its use is limited by multiple toxicities. Defibrillator therapy is more effective than amiodarone in preventing sudden death. Amiodarone is not a substitute for β-blocker therapy in heart failure. Dofetilide, a restricted class III antiarrhythmic agent, is effective in maintaining sinus rhythm but does not improve overall survival in heart failure.

Anticoagulation

The routine use of warfarin in heart failure is controversial, as the risk of thromboembolic events and hemorrhagic complications from the drug is 1% to 3% annually. Specific indications for warfarin include mechanical heart valve, atrial fibrillation, intracardiac thrombus (especially mobile), left ventricular aneurysm, hypercoagulable state, history of thromboembolism, and patent foramen ovale. Aspirin is indicated in patients with ischemic cardiomyopathy. There is no evidence to support the routine use of aspirin in patients with normal coronary arteries. At present, the risk–benefit ratio does not justify the routine use of either aspirin or warfarin in heart failure patients as a group.

Treatment of Sleep Apnea

Sleep-related breathing disorders occur commonly in heart failure. Forty percent of patients have central sleep apnea (Cheyne-Stokes respirations), and 10% have obstructive sleep apnea. Sleep apnea is associated with nocturnal catecholamine surges, hypertension, cardiac arrhythmias, and increased mortality in heart failure. Patients suspected of having sleep apnea should undergo polysomnography. Central sleep apnea improves with the intensification of heart failure therapy and nocturnal oxygen. Persistent central sleep apnea should be treated with continuous positive airway pressure (CPAP) ventilation, whereas overdrive atrial pacing requires further study. Obstructive sleep apnea improves with weight loss and avoidance of alcohol and sedatives but not with heart failure therapy. CPAP ventilation is indicated for moderately severe obstructive sleep apnea associated with daytime somnolence. Surgical procedures and mandibular advancement devices have not been studied in heart failure populations.

Treatment of Anemia

Anemia occurs in 10% to 20% of patients with heart failure. The presence of anemia correlates directly with the severity of heart failure. Anemia is associated with worsening symptoms, impaired exercise tolerance, increased risk of hospitalizations, and poor survival. The causes of anemia in heart failure are multifactorial, with anemia of chronic disease the most common diagnosis. Low cardiac output impairs bone marrow production, whereas renal dysfunction and ACE inhibitors decrease erythropoietin production. Proinflammatory cytokines suppress bone marrow function and inhibit erythropoietin effects. Poor nutrition, gastrointestinal blood loss, and iron deficiency may contribute to low hemoglobin. The treatment of anemia using erythropoietin alone or in combination with iron therapy may improve the natural history of heart failure, quality of life, functional class, and exercise capacity. The threshold level for initiating therapy and the target level of hemoglobin as a therapeutic endpoint are unresolved at this time.

Ultrafiltration

The standard treatment for severe fluid retention from advanced heart failure consists of high-dose intravenous diuretics, combined loop and thiazide diuretics, or continuous diuretic infusion. Occasionally, diuretic resistance occurs in the setting of cardiorenal syndrome (persistent fluid overload, rising creatinine levels, and hyponatremia). In this setting, ultrafiltration may be utilized to remove water from the blood and extravascular spaces. The balanced diuresis from ultrafiltration maintains plasma volume and avoids hypotension. Ultrafiltration has been shown to relieve pulmonary edema, decrease ascites/edema, correct electrolyte abnormalities, improve hemodynamics, restore diuretic responsiveness, and reduce the length of stay in the hospital.

MISCELLANEOUS THERAPIES

Statins are recommended for patients with ischemic cardiomyopathy. Supplements such as coenzyme Q10, carnitine, antioxidants, growth hormone, and thyroid hormone are not recommended. Exercise training, especially cardiac rehabilitation, improves clinical status in heart failure patients. Disease management programs with multidisciplinary staff have been shown to decrease readmissions for cardiac decompensation.

REVIEW EXERCISES

QUESTIONS

1. Which of the following is not associated with poor prognosis in heart failure?

a) Obesity (body mass index 34)
b) QRS complex 170 msec
c) BNP level 800 pg/mL
d) Serum cholesterol 79 mg/dL
e) Serum sodium 119 mmol/L

Answer and Discussion
The answer is a. Heart failure is associated with reversed epidemiology. Better prognosis correlates with body mass index, level of blood pressure, and cholesterol level.

2. Which statement about angiotensin II is true?
a) It is a vasodilator.
b) It promotes sodium excretion.
c) It inhibits growth and remodeling.
d) It causes release of aldosterone.
e) It inhibits thirst.

Answer and Discussion
The answer is d. Angiotensin II is a potent vasoconstrictor that promotes sodium and water retention, releases aldosterone, stimulates thirst, and causes cardiovascular growth and remodeling.

3. Heart failure with preserved systolic function is not characteristic of
a) Hypertensive heart disease
b) Ischemic heart disease
c) Hypertrophic cardiomyopathy
d) Restrictive cardiomyopathy
e) Dilated cardiomyopathy

Answer and Discussion
The answer is e. Dilated cardiomyopathy is characterized by left ventricular enlargement and systolic dysfunction.

4. Which statement about ACE inhibitors is false?
a) They prevent degradation of bradykinin.
b) They cause gynecomastia in 8% of men.
c) They may improve cough due to heart failure.
d) They cause hyperkalemia in some patients.
e) Dysgeusia is a known side effect.

Answer and Discussion
The answer is b. Gynecomastia is a side effect of spironolactone and digoxin.

SUGGESTED READINGS

Adams KF, Lindenfeld J, Arnold JMO, et al. Executive summary: HFSA 2006 comprehensive heart failure practice guideline. *J Cardiac Fail* 2006;12:10–38.

American Heart Association. Heart disease and stroke statistics-2007 update. Dallas, TX: Author, 2007.

Bhatia RS, Tu JV, Lee DS, et al. Outcome of heart failure with preserved ejection fraction in a population-based study. *N Engl J Med* 2006;355:260–269.

Bonow RO, Bennett S, Casey DE Jr, et al. ACC/AHA clinical performance measures for adults with chronic heart failure: a report of the American College of Cardiology/American Heart Association Task Force on Performance Measures (Writing Committee to Develop Heart Failure Clinical Performance Measures). *J Am Coll Cardiol* 2005;46:1145–1178.

Bradley TD, Floras JS. Sleep apnea and heart failure. Part I: Obstructive sleep apnea. *Circulation* 2003;107:1671–1678.

Bradley TD, Floras JS. Sleep apnea and heart failure. Part II: Central sleep apnea. *Circulation* 2003;107:1822–1826.

Butler J, Young JB, Abraham WT, et al. Beta-blocker use and outcomes among hospitalized heart failure patients. *J Am Coll Cardiol* 2006;47:2462–2469.

Cesario DA, Dec GW. Implantable cardioverter-defibrillator therapy in clinical practice. *J Am Coll Cardiol* 2006;47:1507–1517.

Cleland JGF, Coletta A, Witte K. Practical applications of intravenous diuretic therapy in decompensated heart failure. *Am J Med* 2006;119:S26–S36.

Cleland JGF, Daubert JC, Erdmann E, et al. the effect of cardiac resynchronization on morbidity and mortality in heart failure. *N Engl J Med* 2005;352:1539–1549.

Costanzo MR, Guglin ME, Saltzberg MT, et al. Ultrafiltration versus intravenous diuretics for patients hospitalized for acute decompensated heart failure. *J Am Coll Cardiol* 2007;49;675–683.

Digitalis Investigation Group. The effect of digoxin on mortality and morbidity in patients with heart failure. *N Engl J Med* 1997;336:525–533.

Felker GM, O'Connor CM. Inotropic therapy for heart failure: an evidence-based approach. *Am Heart J* 2001;142:393–401.

Gheorghiade M, Filippatos G. Reassessing treatment of acute heart failure syndromes: the ADHERE Registry. *Eur Heart J* 2005;7(Suppl B):B13–B19.

Gring CN, Francis GS. A hard look at angiotensin receptor blockers in heart failure. *J Am Coll Cardiol* 2004;44:1841–1846.

Hogg K, Swedberg K, McMurray J. Heart failure with preserved left ventricular systolic function: epidemiology, clinical characteristics, and prognosis. *J Am Coll Cardiol* 2004;43:317–327.

Hunt SA, Abraham WT, Chin MH, et al. ACC/AHA 2005 guideline update for the diagnosis and management of chronic heart failure in the adult: a report of the American College of Cardiology/American Heart Association Task Force on Practice Guidelines (Writing Committee to Update the 2001 Guidelines for the Evaluation and Management of Heart Failure). *J Am Coll Cardiol* 2005;46:1116–1143.

Inglis SC, Pearson S, Treen S, et al. Extending the horizon in chronic heart failure: effects of multidisciplinary, home-based intervention relative to usual care. *Circulation* 2006;114:2466–2473.

Jessup M, Brozena S. Heart failure. *N Engl J Med* 2003;348:2007–2018.

Krum H, Cameron P. Diuretics in the treatment of heart failure: mainstay or therapy of potential hazard. *J Cardiac Fail* 2006;12:333–335.

Leclercq C, Hare JM. Ventricular resynchronization. *Circulation* 2004;109:296–299.

Levine TB, Levine AB. Clinical update: the role of angiotensin II receptor blockers in patients with left ventricular dysfunction. Part I. *Clin Cardiol* 2005;28:215–218.

Levine TB, Levine AB. Clinical update: the role of angiotensin II receptor blockers in patients with left ventricular dysfunction. Part II. *Clin Cardiol* 2005;28:277–280.

Lindenfeld J, Feldman AM, Saxon L, et al. Effects of cardiac resynchronization therapy with or without a defibrillator on survival and hospitalizations in patients with New York Heart Association Class IV heart failure. *Circulation* 2007;115:204–212.

Maggioni AP, Opasich C, Anand I, et al. Anemia in patients with heart failure: prevalence and prognostic role in a controlled trial and in clinical practice. *J Cardiac Fail* 2005;11:91–98.

McCarthy PM, Starling RC, Young JB, et al. Left ventricular reduction surgery with mitral valve repair. *J Heart Lung Transplant* 2000;19:S64–S67.

Metra M, Dei Cas L, Cleland JGF. Pharmacokinetic and pharmacodynamic characteristics of β-blockers: when differences may matter. *J Cardiac Fail* 2006;12(3):177–181.

Miller, LW, Lietz K. Candidate selection for long-term left ventricular assist device therapy for refractory heart failure. *J Heart Lung Transplant* 2006;25:756–764.

Mills RM, Hobbs RE. Nesiritide in perspective: evolving approaches to the management of acute decompensated heart failure. *Drugs Today* 2003;39:767–774.

Nieman MS, Bohm M, Cowie MR, et al.; Task Force on Acute Heart Failure of the European Society of Cardiology. Executive summary of the guidelines on the diagnosis and treatment of acute heart failure. *Eur Heart J* 2005;26:384–416.

O'Connor CM, Gattis Stough W, Gallup DS, et al. Demographics, clinical characteristics and outcomes of patients hospitalized for decompensated heart failure: observations from the IMPACT-HF Registry. *J Cardiac Fail* 2005;11:200–205.

Pervaiz MH, Dickinson MG, Yamani M. Is digoxin a drug of the past? *Cleve Clin J Med* 2006;73:821–833.

Pitt B, Rajagopalan S. Aldosterone receptor antagonists for heart failure: current status, future indications. *Cleve Clin J Med* 2006;73:257–268.

Rathore SS, Curtis JP, Wang Y, et al. Association of serum digoxin concentration and outcomes in patients with heart failure. *JAMA* 2003;289:871–878.

Schoenfeld MH. Contemporary pacemaker and defibrillator device therapy: challenges confronting the general cardiologist. *Circulation* 2007;115:638–653.

Shin DD, Brandimarte F, De Luca L, et al. Review of current and investigational pharmacologic agents for acute heart failure syndromes. *Am J Cardiol* 2007;99(suppl):4A–23A.

Strickberger SA, Conti J, Daoud EG, et al. Patient selection for cardiac resynchronization therapy. *Circulation* 2005;111:2146–2150.

Swedberg K, Cleland J, Dargie H, et al.; Task Force for the Diagnosis and Treatment of Chronic Heart Failure of the European Society of Cardiology. Guidelines for the diagnosis and treatment of chronic heart failure: executive summary (update 2005). *Eur Heart J* 2005;26:1115–1140.

Tang WHW, Parameswaran AC, Maroo AP, et al. Aldosterone receptor antagonists in the medical management of chronic heart failure. *Mayo Clin Proc* 2005;80:1623–1630.

Tang YD, Katz SD. Anemia in chronic heart failure: prevalence, etiology, clinical correlates, and treatment options. *Circulation* 2006;113:2454–2461.

Ware LB, Matthay MA. Acute pulmonary edema. *N Engl J Med* 2005;353:2788–2796.

Chapter 66

Cardiovascular Emergencies

Vidyasagar Kalahasti   *Samir R. Kapadia*

POINTS TO REMEMBER:

- Characteristic physical signs of cardiac tamponade are pulsus paradoxus, increased jugular venous pressure (JVP), and low blood pressure.

- Transthoracic echocardiogram (TTE) is helpful in making the diagnosis of tamponade.

- Volume resuscitation and immediate drainage of the fluid are essential in the treatment of tamponade.

- Acute pulmonary edema is the most common clinical presentation of papillary muscle rupture.

- A new holosystolic murmur may be an early clue in papillary muscle rupture.

- Echocardiography is the diagnostic imaging modality of choice for papillary muscle rupture.

- Free wall rupture is a catastrophic complication after large transmural myocardial infarction (MI).

- Surgery remains a treatment option for free wall rupture but has significant limitations.

- A contained left ventricular (LV) free wall rupture is known as a pseudoaneurysm.

- Surgical repair is the definitive treatment for LV pseudoaneurysm.

- The clinical presentation of ventricular septal defect (VSD) can be acute pulmonary edema, biventricular failure, or shock.

- A new holosystolic murmur with thrill is the important physical sign of VSD.

- Echocardiography with color and Doppler and right heart catheterization with oxygen step-up are confirmatory tests.

- Sharp or tearing chest pain radiating to the back in a hypertensive patient should alert the clinician to the possibility of aortic dissection.

- Aggressive blood pressure control is essential in ascending and descending aortic dissection.

- Emergent surgery is needed for the best outcome after ascending aortic dissection, while conservative management is preferred for descending aortic dissection.

Cardiovascular emergencies occur from hemodynamic compromise of the system resulting from mechanical or electrical dysfunction. In this chapter, we will focus on understanding the pathophysiology, modes of diagnosis, and appropriate management of mechanical problems of the cardiovascular system resulting in life-threatening emergencies. A prototypical case is presented for each condition, and salient features are discussed in a case-based approach.

Cardiac Tamponade

A 50-year-old man with history of lung cancer presents with shortness of breath and dizziness. On examination, his blood pressure is 90/60 mm Hg, and pulse rate is 110 beats per minute. He is breathing at a rate of 20 per minute. JVP is elevated. Heart sounds are distant. Lung examination reveals normal breath sounds bilaterally. There is no peripheral edema. Cardiac tamponade is suspected.

Which of the following is true?
a) Malignancy is the most common cause for pericardial effusion.
b) Pulsus paradoxus is pathognomonic of cardiac tamponade.
c) JVP will increase with inspiration.
d) Tachycardia, hypotension, and increased JVP constitutes Beck's triad for cardiac tamponade.
e) None of the above

DEFINITION

Cardiac tamponade is a clinical syndrome that is characterized by cardiac decompensation due to compression of cardiac chambers from increased intrapericardial pressure. It is important to recognize that this is a clinical diagnosis. Although imaging modalities help to visualize compression of different chambers of the heart, clinical decompensation has to be present for the diagnosis of cardiac tamponade. Hemodynamic compromise is determined by intrapericardial pressure, volume status, and peripheral vascular tone.

ETIOLOGY

Cardiac tamponade results from increasing intrapericardial pressure from increasing pericardial effusions. The intrapericardial pressure increases rapidly with even a small increase in pericardial fluid if the process is acute (Fig. 66.1). This typically is seen in patients with traumatic effusion where there is bleeding in the pericardium. Therefore, in acute trauma patients, any effusion is considered serious and warrants immediate attention. Table 66.1 lists common causes of pericardial effusion. Note that the most common cause of pericardial effusion in current practice is malignancy. Tuberculosis is a common cause of effusion in third world countries. Although autoimmune and infectious diseases are important causes of pericardial effusion, tamponade is not common in these disease processes because intrapericardial pressure is not greatly elevated (due to relatively small effusions that develop slowly in these diseases).

CLINICAL FEATURES

Cardiac tamponade is suspected based on history and physical examination. The symptoms of tamponade are reflective of a low cardiac output state and include dyspnea on exertion, restlessness, dizziness, drowsiness, and fatigue. The physical signs are increased JVP, tachypnea, tachycardia, hypotension, and decreased heart sounds. Low blood pressure, increased JVP, and distant cardiac sounds constitute Beck's triad.

The most characteristic physical sign is pulsus paradoxus, defined as decline in systolic blood pressure >10 mm Hg with inspiration (Fig. 66.2). With inspiration, *normally* there is some decrease in systolic blood pressure from the decrease in LV stroke volume. However, with normal breathing, the decrease in blood pressure is minimal. With pericardial tamponade, this normal response is exaggerated due to even further decrease in LV filling from the bowing of interventricular septum toward the left ventricle during inspiration (Fig. 66.3). It is important to note that patients should be asked to breathe normally while checking for pulsus paradoxus, because deep breaths can exaggerate the inspiratory pressure drop.

Pulsus paradoxus is not specific for cardiac tamponade. It is seen in other pericardial diseases like constrictive pericarditis (~50% of patients) or in situations where there are marked intrathoracic pressure changes as in emphysema, bronchial asthma, hypovolemic shock, pulmonary embolism, pregnancy, and extreme obesity. Pulsus paradoxus may be absent in severe LV dysfunction, positive pressure breathing, atrial septal defect, localized tamponade in postoperative cardiac surgery patients, and severe aortic regurgitation.

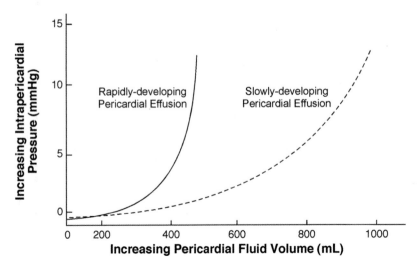

Figure 66.1 Relationship between pericardial fluid volume and intrapericardial pressure in acute and chronic pericardial effusion.

TABLE 66.1

CAUSES OF PERICARDIAL EFFUSION

Malignancy (~30%)
Secondary (metastatic):
- Lung
- Breast
- Hematologic cancers
- Adenocarcinoma (ovarian, GI, GU, unknown, thymoma, osteogenic sarcoma, mesothelioma)

Primary:
- Mesothelioma,
- Sarcoma

Infectious (~25%)
Viral (most common):
- Coxsackie, influenza, HIV, hepatitis A, EBV

Bacterial:
- TB (4%–7%)
- Sepsis, any organism
- Rickettsiae
- *Mycoplasma pneumoniae*

Parasitic:
- Hydatid cyst

Autoimmune Diseases (~20%)
Rheumatoid arthritis
SLE
MCTD
Scleroderma

Postoperative (~5%)
Post cardiac surgery

Others (~20%)
Metabolic diseases:
- Uremia
- Myxedema

Pleural/pulmonary diseases
Trauma
Iatrogenic:
- Pacemaker placement
- Extraction of pacemaker leads
- Coronary artery perforation

Radiation pericarditis
Post MI:
- <10% in postthrombolytic era

EBV, Epstein-Barr virus; GI, gastrointestinal; GU, genitourinary; MCTD, mixed connective tissue disease; MI, myocardial infarction; SLE, systemic lupus erythematosus; TB, tuberculosis.

Increase in jugular venous distension during inspiration, known as Kussmaul's sign, is seen in constrictive pericarditis. In inspiration, there is increased intra-abdominal pressure, which leads to increased venous return, which in turn leads to an increase in right atrial (RA) pressure. The increase in RA pressure is seen as distended jugular veins. Since the abdominal veins typically are not engorged in cardiac tamponade, this sign is not present in the majority of patients with cardiac tamponade.

The patient undergoes further diagnostic testing, including a chest x-ray (CXR), ECG, echocardiogram, and right heart catheterization.

Which of the following is *not* true?

a) "Water bottle heart" on CXR or "pulsus alternans" on the ECG is suggestive of a large pericardial effusion.

b) Early diastolic collapse of the right ventricle or right atrium, increased respiratory variation in mitral inflow, and a distended inferior vena cava indicate the presence of cardiac tamponade.

c) Equalization of pressures of the right and left atrium (pulmonary capillary wedge pressure [PCWP]) is pathognomonic of cardiac tamponade.

d) Echocardiography is useful in determining the approach for draining the effusion.

e) Cardiac tamponade can occur with small pericardial effusion.

The answer is c.

DIAGNOSIS

An ECG and CXR are performed routinely when a patient presents with symptoms of shortness of breath.

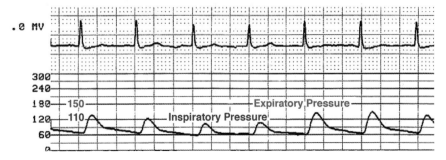

Figure 66.2 Arterial pressure tracing showing a significant decrease in arterial pressure during inspiration and an increase during expiration (pulsus paradoxus).

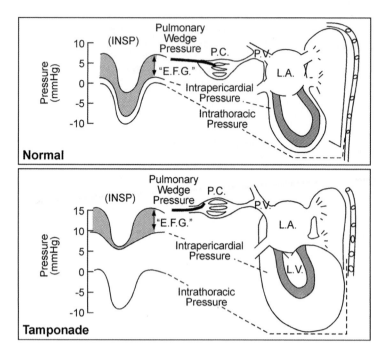

Figure 66.3 Interrelationships between pulmonary capillary wedge pressure, intra thoracic pressure, and intrapericardial pressure during inspiration (*INSP*) in normal patients and in patients with cardiac tamponade. Note that the intrapericardial pressure remains elevated in tamponade despite the decrease in intrathoracic pressure. (PC, pulmonary capillary; PV, pulmonary veins; LA, left atrium; LV, left ventricle; EFG, effective filling gradient.)

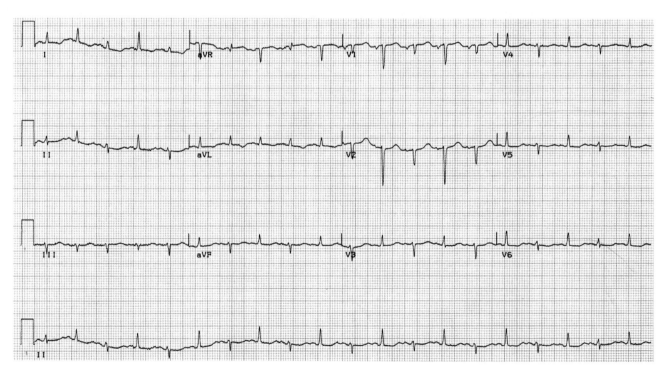

Figure 66.4 ECG in a patient with a large pericardial effusion demonstrating a classic "electrical alternans" pattern.

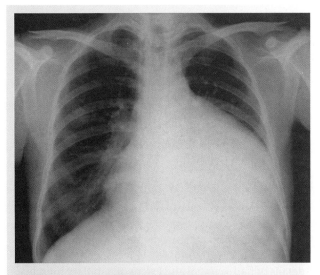

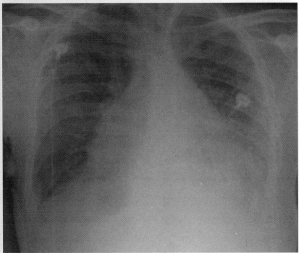

Figure 66.5   Chest x-rays in patients with large pericardial effusion and "water bottle heart" with enlarged cardiac silhouette.

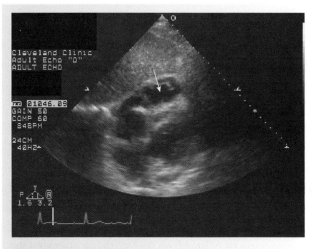

Figure 66.6   Subcostal image on transthoracic echocardiogram showing right ventricular collapse in a patient with cardiac tamponade. The *arrow* shows a large pericardial effusion with collapse of the right ventricle.

In patients with pericardial effusion, the ECG may be normal or may show pulsus alternans in patients with a large effusion (Fig. 66.4). The classic appearance of a large pericardial effusion on CXR is a "water bottle heart," with the small base of the heart and enlarged cardiac silhouette different from that seen with chamber enlargements (Fig. 66.5). TTE is the imaging modality of choice to confirm the diagnosis of cardiac tamponade when clinically suspected.

The signs of cardiac tamponade on TTE are collapse of the right atrium and right ventricle in early diastole (Fig. 66.6). Prominent respiratory variation in flows across all cardiac valves is seen in patients with hemodynamic compromise. This is analogous to the change in systolic pressures seen with pulsus paradoxus. A distended inferior vena cava corroborates the clinically observed elevated JVP. Transesophageal echocardio-graphy (TEE) may be needed in postoperative patients with clinical signs of tamponade, as the TTE images are not optimal. TEE is very useful to evaluate for hematoma, which is common in post-operative patients.

Hemodynamic pressure measurements can help to determine the functional significance of a pericardial effusion in difficult cases. The increased intrapericardial pressure is transmitted to all cardiac chambers; therefore, when the chambers are not actively contracting (diastole), pressures in all chambers are equal and reflect intrapericardial pressure. Although equalization of diastolic pressures (RA, left atrial [LA] [or PCWP], LV, and right ventricular [RV]) is typical for cardiac tamponade, it can be seen in other diseases affecting the pericardium, such as constrictive pericarditis.

TREATMENT

Volume resuscitation is the most important and useful medical intervention in patients with cardiac tamponade. Diuretics and vasodilators should not be used when tamponade is suspected. The definitive therapy for tamponade is drainage of pericardial fluid. In most situations, percutaneous drainage is the best approach. If the pericardial fluid is loculated and not approachable percutaneously, surgical drainage is necessary. In trauma patients, surgical exploration is required because pericardial hemorrhage is a sign for chamber rupture and percutaneous drainage is contraindicated. Pericardial fluid can be percutaneously drained using a subcostal, apical, or parasternal approach. The specific approach is dependent on the location of fluid and operator preferences. Echocardiographic guidance is extremely helpful for the drainage procedure.

KEY POINTS

- Cardiac tamponade is a clinical diagnosis.
- Characteristic physical signs are pulsus paradoxus, increased JVP, and low blood pressure.
- TTE is helpful in making the diagnosis of tamponade.
- Volume resuscitation and immediate drainage of the fluid are essential.
- Even a small amount of fluid (typically blood) can lead to tamponade if the accumulation is rapid.

PAPILLARY MUSCLE RUPTURE

An 80-year-old woman with inferior MI develops severe shortness of breath on the fourth day after MI. On examination, she has a systolic murmur. An echocardiogram was performed, which shows severe mitral regurgitation (MR).

Which of the following is least likely to be the cause of her MR?
a) Papillary muscle dysfunction
b) Papillary muscle rupture
c) Restricted mitral valve leaflet
d) Myxomatous degeneration of the mitral valve
e) All of the above

The answer is d.

ETIOLOGY

MR occurs in almost one-fourth (13%–45%) of patients suffering MI. Post-MI MR can result from various mechanisms. The most common mechanism is the restriction of the posterior mitral leaflet secondary to an akinetic inferior-posterior wall. The akinetic wall pulls the papillary muscle, restricting the movement of the posterior leaflet, and leading to incomplete coaptation with the anterior leaflet and MR. The ischemic papillary muscle can cause MR from a similar mechanism. The most serious cause of MR after MI is papillary muscle rupture, which rapidly can be fatal if not recognized and treated immediately. Papillary muscle rupture typically occurs 1 to 7 days after MI. Papillary muscle rupture occurs most commonly after inferior MI, as the blood supply of the posteromedial papillary muscle is from a single coronary artery, usually the posterior descending artery branch of the right coronary artery. The anterolateral papillary muscle derives its blood supply from dual coronaries (left anterior descending [LAD] and left circumflex), making it less vulnerable to an ischemic insult.

CLINICAL FEATURES

Patients with complete papillary muscle rupture may die of cardiogenic shock from severe acute MR. Patients with rupture of one of the heads of a papillary muscle may present with sudden onset of shortness of breath and hypotension. Notably, the MI leading to this complication is usually small in the vast majority of patients.

Signs of papillary muscle rupture include a new holosystolic murmur that is best heard at the apex and radiates to the axilla or to the base of the heart. The murmur may be soft and relatively short due to rapid increase in LA pressure from acute, severe MR in a noncompliant left atrium.

DIAGNOSIS

An ECG shows evidence of recent inferior or posterior MI, and CXR reveals pulmonary edema. Echocardiography is the diagnostic modality of choice to assess papillary muscle rupture. TEE may be needed to see the details of flail segment and extent of papillary muscle involvement (Figs. 66.7 and 66.8).

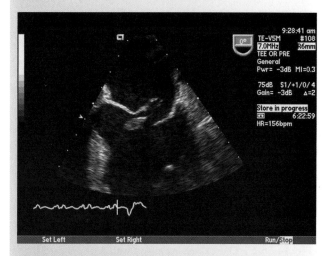

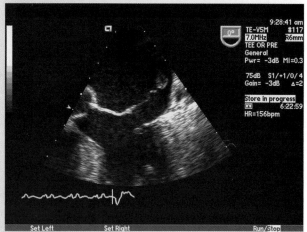

Figure 66.7   Transesophageal echocardiogram of a patient with a ruptured head of the papillary muscle. **Upper panel:** A flail anterior mitral valve leaflet attached to the ruptured papillary muscle head in early systole. **Lower panel:** The flail mitral valve leaflet prolapsing into the left atrium during systole. In this view, the top and bottom chambers are the left atrium and left ventricle, respectively.

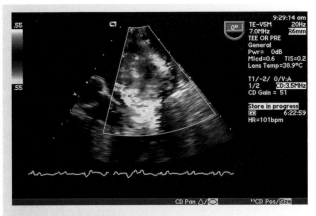

Figure 66.8 Transesophageal echocardiogram showing severe mitral regurgitation by color Doppler due to flail anterior mitral valve leaflet from a ruptured papillary muscle.

Hemodynamic monitoring with pulmonary artery catheterization shows large V waves on the PCWP tracing (Fig. 66.9). The large V wave represents the increase in sudden LA pressure from severe MR and a noncompliant small left atrium, which did not have time to dilate as in chronic causes of MR. It is important to note that large V waves are also seen with acute VSD after MI and therefore are not pathognomonic of acute MR.

TREATMENT

Acute MR should be recognized early, as 24-hour mortality is as high as 70% without immediate surgical repair. A high index of suspicion is required to diagnose this condition. Medical therapy with vasodilators to decrease afterload can be attempted after recognition of MR, but hypotension may limit the use of such therapy. In patients with hypotension and shock, an intra-aortic balloon pump (IABP) should be placed. An IABP decreases afterload, improves coronary blood flow, and augments forward cardiac output. Urgent surgery is needed for definitive repair of papillary muscle rupture.

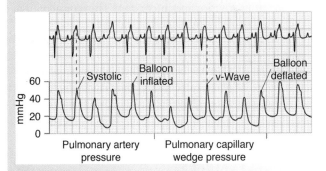

Figure 66.9 Prominent V waves on a pulmonary capillary wedge pressure tracing reflective of an increase in left atrial pressure from severe mitral regurgitation.

KEY POINTS

- Papillary muscle rupture causing acute MR is more common after inferior MI.
- Acute pulmonary edema is the most common clinical presentation.
- A new holosystolic murmur may be an early clue in papillary muscle rupture.
- Echocardiography is the diagnostic imaging modality of choice.
- Immediate surgical repair can be lifesaving in these patients.

FREE WALL RUPTURE

An 80-year-old woman presents to the hospital with severe chest pain for 4 hours and is found to have an acute anterior wall MI. She is taken to the cardiac catheterization laboratory emergently, and the LAD artery is stented. There is partial resolution of ST segments, and the final flow in the LAD is TIMI II. She does well for 3 days and starts having sharp substernal chest pain. The likely cause for chest pain is

a) Pericarditis
b) Recurrent MI
c) Pulmonary embolism
d) Myocardial rupture
e) All of the above

The answer is a.

ETIOLOGY

LV free wall rupture is a catastrophic complication that can occur after transmural MI. It is seen in 1% to 8% of patients after an acute MI. Free wall rupture accounts for approximately 10% of the mortality occurring after MI. This complication typically is encountered 1 to 4 days after MI, although early (within 24 hours) or delayed (3 weeks) presentations have been reported.

Unlike papillary muscle rupture, free wall rupture more frequently is seen with anterior wall MI. As well, free wall rupture is seen more commonly in elderly women with a history of hypertension and prior use of steroids and nonsteroidal anti-inflammatory drugs. It is more common with first MI, late thrombolytic therapy, and a large transmural MI involving ≥20% of the myocardium.

CLINICAL FEATURES

Patients with acute free wall rupture die suddenly due to electromechanical dissociation. Patients with subacute rupture may present with chest pain and hypotension suggestive of pericarditis and tamponade. Signs of tamponade and a to-and-fro murmur have been described in subacute rupture, although this is uncommon.

DIAGNOSIS

A high index of clinical suspicion is necessary to make a timely diagnosis. Any patient with a complaint of sharp pain within the first few days after a large anterior MI should have echocardiographic assessment. Intramural hematoma, partial rupture, subacute rupture, or any other mechanical complications of MI should be carefully excluded. Computed tomography (CT) or magnetic resonance imaging (MRI) may have a role in the evaluation of some stable patients.

TREATMENT

Anticoagulants should be discontinued immediately. Immediate surgical repair is the only treatment option if the patient is to survive. However, surgical mortality is high and secondary failure (i.e., dehiscence of patch) is common because the suturing may be difficult with a recent acute MI.

KEY POINTS

- Free wall rupture is a catastrophic complication after large transmural MI.
- It is seen more commonly after anterior MI.
- Surgery remains a treatment option but has significant limitations.

LEFT VENTRICULAR PSEUDOANEURYSM

ETIOLOGY

LV rupture contained by pericardial adhesions and thrombus is known as a pseudoaneurysm. A pseudoaneurysm has a narrow neck, which is characterized by having <50% of the size of the fundus of the aneurysm.

CLINICAL FEATURES

Patient typically presents with pleuritic pain. The presentation may be clinically silent and detected only on routine investigations. Alternatively, patients may present with heart failure symptoms and recurrent tachyarrhythmias. Examination may reveal a continuous murmur across the pseudoaneurysm.

DIAGNOSIS

CXR may reveal cardiomegaly with an abnormal bulge of the cardiac shadow. The ECG may show persistent ST segment elevation, as in a true LV aneurysm.

A variety of imaging modalities can be used to define the pseudoaneurysm. Echocardiography, cardiac CT, and cardiac MRI are used to confirm the diagnosis (Fig. 66.10).

TREATMENT

Patients with LV pseudoaneurysm need to be referred for definitive surgical repair, as there is a risk for sudden rupture and death. This is irrespective of the size or symptoms.

KEY POINTS

- A contained LV free wall rupture is known as a pseudoaneurysm.
- Surgical repair is the definitive treatment.

VENTRICULAR SEPTAL DEFECT

A 79-year-old woman with no history of coronary artery disease presents with an inferior wall MI. The patient develops severe shortness of breath and hypotension. On examination, a loud holosystolic murmur with a thrill is detected. A Swan-Ganz catheter is placed. Oxygen saturation in the right atrium was 50% and in the pulmonary artery was 75%. A large V wave was noted on the pulmonary capillary wedge tracing.

All of the following are true, *except*

a) Acute VSD explains the systolic murmur, a step-up in saturation but not a large V wave.
b) VSD can happen with a relatively small MI.
c) Surgical repair is the best treatment option for this patient.
d) An IABP prior to surgery may be helpful to stabilize the patient.
e) Recurrence of VSDs after surgical repair is relatively common.

The answer is a.

ETIOLOGY

VSD occurs as a result of necrosis of the interventricular septum following a transmural MI. It occurs in up to 2% of acute MI patients and accounts for 1% to 5% of all hospital deaths due to MI. VSD usually is seen within 3 to 7 days after MI but can occur in as early as 24 hours. The early presentation is seen after inferior MI and after thrombolytic therapy. The incidence of acute VSD is similar after anterior and inferior MI. The typical patient with VSD is an elderly, hypertensive woman with multivessel disease who presents late after a first MI and has not undergone revascularization.

An acute VSD is located apically in anterior MI and posterior-basally in inferior MI. The defect may be a through-and-through hole or a serpiginous meshwork of channels. Right ventricular involvement is common with posterior-basal defects.

CLINICAL FEATURES

Patients with acute VSD may present insidiously with few symptoms or may present precipitously with

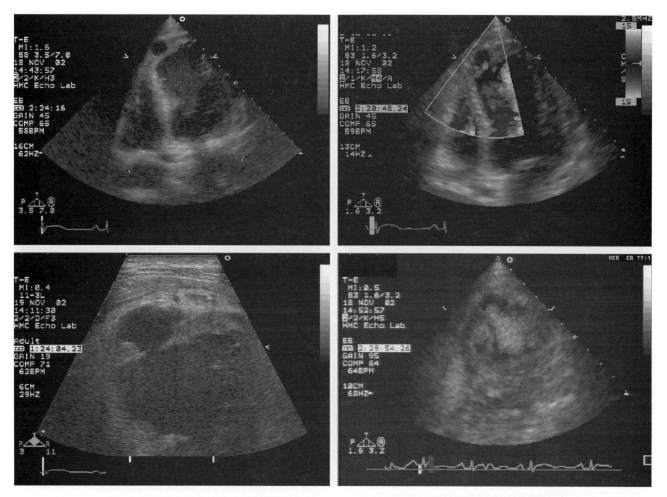

Figure 66.10 Echocardiographic images of a left ventricular pseudoaneurysm. **Upper left panel:** An apical pseudoaneurysm. **Upper right panel:** Flow through the neck of a pseudoaneurysm. **Lower left panel:** The classic appearance of a pseudoaneurysm with a narrow neck. **Lower right panel:** Echocardiographic contrast is used to delineate the pseudoaneurysm more clearly.

pulmonary edema, biventricular failure, and shock. A loud holosystolic murmur, best heard over the lower left sternal border, associated with systolic thrill is present in 50% of patients. The intensity of the murmur is inversely related to defect size.

DIAGNOSIS

Echocardiography with color flow Doppler is very useful in detecting a VSD. As well, it is useful in assessing the location and extent of defect and in the assessment of left and right ventricular function. Doppler flow helps in quantifying the magnitude of the left-to-right shunt (Fig. 66.11). Right heart catheterization with oximetry is helpful in the diagnosis of an acute VSD by demonstrating an oxygen step-up between the right atrium and pulmonary artery. The step-up allows the clinician to calculate the shuntfraction. V waves on the PCWP tracing may be seen in acute

VSD due to increased flow in the left atrium from the shunt.

TREATMENT

Medical therapy has a limited role but may be helpful in stabilizing the patient prior to surgical treatment. Intravenous vasodilators, such as sodium nitroprusside, are the treatment of choice, as they help decrease the left-to-right shunt and increase systemic flow. An IABP is helpful to decrease systemic vascular resistance and therefore decrease left-to-right shunting. Surgical repair is the treatment of choice for all but the smallest VSDs and should be performed early. Small VSDs have the best survival, and posterior-basal VSDs have the worst prognosis. Percutaneous closure of a VSD with various closure devices has been reported, but this approach still has technical limitations depending on anatomical location and the nature of the defect.

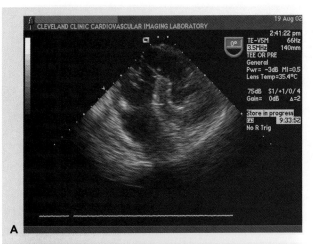

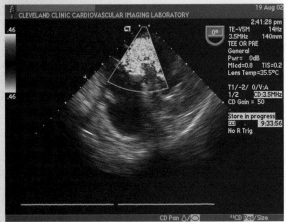

Figure 66.11 Echocardiographic images of a ventricular septal defect in the inferior septum of the left ventricle (*arrow*, **panel A**) with color Doppler depicting the blood flow from the left ventricle to the right ventricle (*arrow*, **panel B**). (See Color Fig. 66.11B.)

KEY POINTS

- VSD occurs equally after anterior and inferior MI.
- The clinical presentation of VSD can be acute pulmonary edema, biventricular failure, or shock.
- A new holosystolic murmur with thrill is the important physical sign.
- Echocardiography with color and Doppler and right heart catheterization with oxygen step-up are confirmatory tests.
- Surgical correction is the standard treatment, but percutaneous closure is emerging as a treatment option in some patients.

AORTIC DISSECTION

A 40-year-old man presents with acute onset of chest pain radiating to back, described as sharp and tearing. His blood pressure is 180/100 mm of Hg. Cardiac ex-amination is remarkable for tachycardia with normal first and second heart sounds and a soft 3/6 early diastolic murmur at the left lower sternal border. The lungs are clear. Distal pulses are equal bilaterally in both upper and lower extremities. Aortic dissection is suspected.

Which of the following is true about aortic dissection?

a) Thoracic aortic dissection is less common than abdominal aortic aneurysm rupture.

b) Marfan's syndrome is the most frequent cause of aortic dissection.

c) Blood pressure control is very important in ascending and descending aortic dissection.

d) Surgery is the treatment of choice for descending aortic dissection.

e) None of the above

The answer is c.

ETIOLOGY

Aortic dissection is the most common aortic emergency. The incidence is twice that of ruptured abdominal aortic aneurysm. Aortic dissection is rare in patients younger than 40 years of age and most commonly is seen between 50 and 70 years. The male-to-female ratio is 2:1. Aortic dissection is seen in patients with hypertension, Marfan's syndrome, Ehlers-Danlos syndrome, Turner's syndrome, giant cell arteritis, bicuspid aortic valve, and in any condition that leads to medial degeneration of the aortic wall. The other causes for aortic dissection are blunt trauma and iatrogenic trauma, such as following cardiac catheterization, IABP placement, and cardiac surgery.

PATHOLOGY

Intimal tear results in blood splitting the aortic media and leading to a false lumen that can progress in an antegrade or retrograde direction. Aortic rupture can occur back into the lumen or externally into the pericardium or mediastinum. External rupture often results in fatal cardiac tamponade. The most common site of intimal tear is within 2 to 3 cm of the aortic valve. The other common site is in the descending aorta distal to the left subclavian artery. The dissection can result in occlusion of aortic branches such as the renal, spinal, coronary, or iliac arteries, resulting in acute end-organ ischemia.

CLASSIFICATION

Two classifications that utilize anatomic location for dissection are commonly used: Stanford (types A and B) and DeBakey (types I, II, and III) (Fig. 66.12).

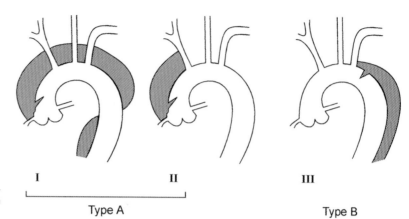

Figure 66.12 Stanford and DeBakey classification of aortic dissection by the anatomical location of the intimal tear.

I   II   III

Type A   Type B

CLINICAL FEATURES

Aortic dissection usually presents with severe chest or back pain that starts when patients are doing physical exertion. The pain usually is sudden in onset and is described as sharp, tearing, or stabbing. Other less common presentations include heart failure with acute aortic regurgitation or end-organ compromise (acute renal failure, paraplegia, acute limb ischemia, cerebrovascular accident, inferior MI, etc.) or syncope and collapse in the case of tamponade. Examination may show either hyper- or hypotension (depending on presentation), a soft early diastolic murmur of aortic regurgitation, and reduced or absent peripheral pulses.

DIAGNOSIS

CXR may show a widened mediastinum. The ECG may be normal or may show evidence of acute MI if the coronary arteries are involved. The diagnosis can be confirmed by a variety of imaging modalities. The choice of test depends on the availability and stability of the patient. TEE and CT are useful in emergency situations (Fig. 66.13). CT and MRI are useful in serial follow-up of chronic dissections.

TREATMENT

Aggressive control of blood pressure is important in the initial management of ascending and descending aortic dissection. The primary aim is to reduce blood pressure and the rate in rise of blood pressure (dP/dT). The agents commonly used are intravenous combined α- and β-blockers (e.g., labetalol) followed by sodium nitroprusside. Ascending aortic dissections require early surgical intervention. Surgery should be coordinated urgently, because there is approximately a 1% rate of mortality per hour with ascending aortic dissection. Type B dissections typically may be managed medically with aggressive blood pressure control. Percutaneous fenestrations can be considered if there is end-organ compromise from branches coming out of the

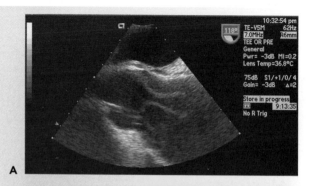

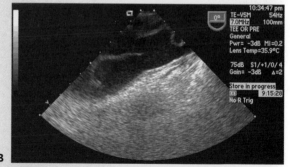

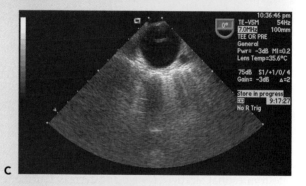

Figure 66.13 Transesophageal echocardiographic images of acute aortic dissection. **Panel A:** A dissection flap in a severely dilated ascending aorta with extension into the aortic valve. **Panel B:** A dissection flap extending into the arch of aorta. **Panel C:** A dissection flap extending into the descending aorta.

false lumen. Surgery is reserved for situations when there is threat of aortic rupture.

KEY POINTS

- Aortic dissection is the most common aortic emergency.
- Sharp or tearing chest pain radiating to the back in a hypertensive patient should alert the clinician to the possibility of aortic dissection.
- Aggressive blood pressure control is essential in ascending and descending aortic dissection.
- Emergent surgery is needed for the best outcome after ascending aortic dissection.

- Conservative management is preferred for descending aortic dissection.
- Stenting of the aortic dissection is emerging as a promising new therapy for some patients with aortic dissection.

SUGGESTED READINGS

Braunwald EG, ed. *Heart Disease. A Textbook of Cardiovascular Medicine*, 7th ed. WB Saunders Company, 2004.
Shabetai R. Diseases of the pericardium. *Cardiol Clin* 1990;8:627–639.
Topol EJ, ed. *Textbook of Cardiovascular Medicine*, 3rd ed. Philadelphia: Lippincott Williams & Wilkins, 2006.

Chapter 67

Mock Board Simulation

Anitha Rajamanickam

QUESTIONS

1. A 72-year-old man with a history of cirrhosis complicated by recurrent ascites is awaiting liver transplantation. He presents to the emergency department with a recent episode of upper gastrointestinal bleed 5 days ago and decreased urine output for the past 3 days. His white blood cell count is 10,000/mm^3, hemoglobin is 9.7 g/dL, and serum creatinine is 3.0 mg/dL. Baseline serum creatine is 0.6 mg/dL. Which of the following factors would *not* support the diagnosis of hepatorenal syndrome?
a) Acute onset of the renal failure
b) Oliguria

c) Benign urinary sediment
d) Fractional excretion of sodium <1%
e) History of primary biliary cirrhosis

Answer and Discussion

The answer is e. The development of acute renal failure in advanced cirrhotic liver disease, severe alcoholic hepatitis, metastatic tumor, or fulminant hepatic failure from any cause is called the hepatorenal syndrome. In patients with cirrhosis and ascites, the hepatorenal syndrome has been shown to occur in about 19% of patients at 1 year and in 39% of patients at 5 years. It is characterized by oliguria, benign urine sediment, a very low fractional excretion of sodium, and a progressive rise in the plasma creatinine concentration. Onset is typically insidious, but it can be acute following an insult, such as gastrointestinal bleeding, infection, or rapid diuresis. Patients with hyponatremia or those with hyperreninemia or pre-existing renal failure are at high risk for the hepatorenal syndrome. Strangely enough, patients with primary biliary cirrhosis are comparatively protected against the development of the hepatorenal syndrome. The best treatment is an improvement in hepatic function due to improvement of the primary disease or due to successful liver transplantation. Growing data suggest that combination therapy with midodrine and octreotide may be effective.

2. A 55-year-old man undergoing hemodialysis three times a week missed his previous dialysis 2 days ago and presents to the emergency department, concerned about his missed dialysis. He is without specific complaints, except stating that he is several pounds over his dry weight. His vitals signs reveal that he is afebrile at 36.5°C, heart rate is 80 beats/minute, respiratory rate is 14 breaths/minute, and blood pressure is 130/80 mm Hg. He has no jugular venous distension. His lungs are clear, and his heart sounds are regular with no S_3 gallop or murmur. He has 1+ peripheral edema. His chemistry profile shows Na^+ 138 mEq/L, K^+ 5.8 mEq/L, Cl^- 104 mEq/L, HCO_3^- 22 mEq/L, blood urea nitrogen 120 mg/dL, creatinine 7.0 mg/dL, and glucose 125 mg/dL. An ECG performed because of hyperkalemia is normal. Which of the following is an indication for emergent hemodialysis in this patient?
a) Hyperkalemia
b) Elevated blood urea nitrogen
c) Elevated creatinine
d) Metabolic acidosis
e) None of the above

Answer and Discussion
The answer is e. Indications for emergent hemodialysis should not be based on the value of blood urea nitrogen or creatinine levels. Indications for emergent hemodialysis include symptomatic uremia (including pericarditis, neuropathy, or unexplained alterations in mental status), significant fluid overload, refractory hyperkalemia, or refractory metabolic acidosis. This man is neither symptomatic from uremia nor significantly fluid overloaded. Furthermore, his ECG does not demonstrate changes typically seen with significant hyperkalemia (he may have a baseline K^+ of 5.5 mEq/L). His metabolic acidosis is probably also near his baseline. He may need hemodialysis in the very near future, but not emergently.

3. An 88-year-old woman is admitted to the hospital after a fall that resulted in a fractured hip. She previously lived alone and cared for most of her daily needs. She had recently employed a helper to do the weekly shopping and the heavier housework because the arthritis in her knees was limiting her efficiency in performing this heavier work. She had hip surgery yesterday, and today you are asked by the orthopedic surgeon to see her as a medical consult because she is combative and trying to get out of bed. The history and examination are difficult to perform because she fluctuates between falling asleep and shouting that she needs to go to the shops because the cupboards are empty and she has no food. She will listen to you and follow simple commands, but she is easily distracted by the noises of the hospital, is unable to concentrate, and wants to leave the bed to go shopping. All the following are true about the most likely cause of her confusion, *except*
a) It is a common condition in the hospitalized elderly.
b) Common causes include medications.
c) The best plan for her safety is to restrain her with soft restraints until the confusion resolves.
d) A reduced level of consciousness and inability to focus or sustain concentration are key characteristics.
e) Perceptual disturbances such as illusions, hallucinations, and delusions help establish the diagnosis.

Answer and Discussion
The answer is c. Delirium is a common condition in elderly hospitalized patients. Physical restraints are not the best plan in this case. The use of physical restraints has associated morbidity and mortality, and they should be used only when other management possibilities, such as environmental changes or nursing and family support, cannot be established. As well as immediate safety, evaluation and determination of the underlying cause of delirium is important to enable treatment of the underlying cause, and, consequently, the confusion.

4. A 60-year-old Asian man is referred to you for evaluation of a heart murmur. He speaks no English and is not accompanied by any family member able to translate. As you wait for the translator to arrive, you are able to communicate sufficiently to obtain permission for a physical examination. His pulse is regular, with a rate of 80 beats/minute, and his blood pressure is 100/85 mm Hg. Carotid pulse has a slow upstroke. No jugular venous distension is present. The apex is slightly displaced laterally. A systolic thrill is palpable over the aortic area and carotids. Auscultation reveals a harsh ejection systolic murmur. Valsalva's maneuver does not accentuate the murmur. The second aortic sound is soft. With which of the following are these findings most consistent?
a) Mitral regurgitation
b) Mitral valve prolapse
c) Aortic stenosis

d) Hypertrophic obstructive cardiomyopathy

e) Mitral stenosis

Answer and Discussion

The answer is c. It is important to know the clinical findings associated with all valvular abnormalities. All the signs and symptoms in this case point to aortic stenosis. This is a systolic murmur, which eliminates mitral stenosis. The murmur of hypertrophic obstructive cardiomyopathy is increased with Valsalva's maneuver. Neither mitral regurgitation nor mitral valve prolapse is associated with narrowed pulse pressure or slow upstroke.

5. A 42-year-old man presents with intermittent chest pain. Further history reveals that the character of the pain is typical of angina. He also has had episodes of dyspnea, dizziness, and syncope. He is a nonsmoker and denies illicit drug use. His past medical history is significant for tonsillectomy in childhood. Family history includes the sudden death of his brother of unknown cause at age 33 years. On examination of the cardiovascular system, the pulse is regular, with a rate of 68 beats/minute, and no jugular venous distension is present. The apical impulse is forceful and displaced laterally. A double apical impulse and a palpable systolic thrill are present. On auscultation of the heart, an S_4 and an ejection systolic murmur are heard. ECG shows left ventricular hypertrophy and Q waves in the inferior and lateral precordial leads. Chest radiograph reveals a mild increase in the cardiac silhouette. Echocardiographic findings include left ventricular hypertrophy with asymmetric septal hypertrophy and a small left ventricular cavity. This murmur may be increased by all of the following, *except*

a) Dopamine

b) Amyl nitrite

c) Diuretics

d) Valsalva's maneuver

e) Handgrip

Answer and Discussion

The answer is e. Features of hypertrophic obstructive cardiomyopathy include left ventricular hypertrophy with asymmetric septal hypertrophy, causing a dynamic left ventricular outflow tract pressure gradient and diastolic dysfunction from stiffness of the hypertrophied muscle. Interventions that increase the murmur include those that decrease preload (diuretics, nitrates, Valsalva's maneuver, standing from squatting), decrease afterload (vasodilators, amyl nitrite, angiotensin-converting enzyme inhibitor), or increase contractility (digoxin, dopamine, and premature ventricular contractions). Interventions that decrease the murmur include those that increase preload (intravenous fluids, passive leg raising, squatting), increase afterload

(handgrip), or decrease contractility (beta-blockers, disopyramide, verapamil).

6. A 45-year-old white woman with no significant past medical history presents with fatigue developing over the past few weeks. She does not take any medications or over-the-counter supplements. She is afebrile with a heart rate of 90 beats/minute and a blood pressure of 100/70 mm Hg. Physical exam is unremarkable, and the patient appears euvolemic. Laboratory workup reveals the following: white blood cell count 9,250/mm³, hemoglobin 12.1 g/dL, platelets 400,000 μL, sodium 146 mmol/L, potassium 4.0 mmol/L, chloride 110 mmol/L, blood urea nitrogen 54 mg/dL, creatinine 2.7 mg/dL, calcium 12.9 mg/dL, phosphorous 3 mg/dL, magnesium 2.2 mg/dL, albumin 2.0 g/dL, and uric acid 3.2 mg/dL. Urine dipstick is trace positive for protein. Urine sediment is bland. The sulphosalysylic acid test is markedly positive. Urine and plasma protein electrophoresis reveals elevated quantities of monoclonal free light chains. All the following should be instituted immediately in this patient *except*

a) Dexamethasone-based chemotherapy

b) Intravenous fluids

c) Avoidance of all nephrotoxins

d) Intravenous bisphosphonates

e) Plasmapheresis

Answer and Discussion

The answer is e. Renal failure is a fairly common problem in patients with multiple myeloma, with approximately 20% presenting with a plasma creatinine ≥2 mg/dL (176 μmol/L) at presentation. The diagnosis can be made clinically in a patient older than 40 years who has unexplained renal failure and elevated quantities of monoclonal free light chains in both the plasma and urine. However, definitive diagnosis is by a kidney biopsy. Biopsy is recommended when the history or clinical features are atypical for myeloma cast nephropathy (e.g., significant proteinuria, active urinary sediment, nephrotoxic drugs). Common causes of acute renal failure in multiple myeloma are cast myeloma kidney, hypercalcemia, and volume depletion. Patients with myeloma kidney should receive dexamethasone-based chemotherapy as rapidly as possible to decrease light chain formation. Intravenous fluids are given to treat volume depletion, hypercalcemia, and hyperuricemia, and to produce a high urine flow rate to minimize light chain precipitation. Loop diuretics should be used cautiously as they may promote cast formation. If the initial corrected serum calcium concentration is <14 mg/dL (4 mmol/L), fluid therapy is instituted for up to 12 hours, and then intravenous bisphosphonate is administered if there is no response. If the corrected serum calcium concentration is ≥ 14 mg/dL (4 mmol/L), bisphosphonates should be administered immediately, along with intravenous fluids. The evidence evaluating the effectiveness of plasmapheresis is conflicting and is not advocated as the first line of therapy.

7. A previously healthy 25-year-old man presents to his internist after referral from the emergency department for microhematuria. His vital signs and physical examination are normal. His urine dipstick is positive for both 1+ protein and 3+ hemoglobin, and the urine sediment, examined under the microscope, reveals red and white blood cells with granular and red cell casts. On further questioning, he denies a history of cough, hemoptysis, chest pain, sinus infections, or dyspnea. The chemistry profile reveals a blood urea nitrogen level of 40 mg/dL and a creatinine level of 4.0 mg/dL. He is sent for further testing, including a chest radiograph, which is reportedly normal. Anti–glomerular basement membrane antibody testing is positive, as is testing for perinuclear pattern antineutrophil cytoplasmic antibodies. A complete blood count is normal. Which of the following statements is false?

a) He has Goodpasture's syndrome.
b) He has anti–glomerular basement membrane antibody disease.
c) He has antibodies directed against myeloperoxidase.
d) He has antibodies directed against a chain of the type IV collagen found in basement membranes.
e) He has a more treatable disease than he would if perinuclear pattern antineutrophil cytoplasmic antibody tests were negative.

Answer and Discussion
The answer is a. With his positive anti–glomerular basement membrane (GBM) antibody status, this man has evidence of glomerulonephritis. These antibodies are directed to a target on the NC1 domain of the $\alpha 3$ chain of type IV collagen found in the basement membrane. Goodpasture's syndrome requires the presence of glomerulonephritis, pulmonary hemorrhage, and anti-GBM antibodies. This man does not have evidence of pulmonary hemorrhage. He also is positive for perinuclear pattern antineutrophil cytoplasmic antibodies (P-ANCAs), which can be seen in 10% to 38% of patients with anti-GBM antibody disease. P-ANCAs are directed against myeloperoxidase. Thus, overlap with Wegener's granulomatosis or a related disease may exist, with occasional evidence of a systemic vasculitis. Treatment for these patients has a more favorable outcome than for P-ANCA–negative individuals.

8. A 38-year-old woman presents to your clinic for a routine health examination. She questions whether she needs a Pap smear. "I have had Pap smears every year since I was 16 years old. When can I stop?" Which of the following statements regarding cervical cancer screening is false?

a) Initiate screening by 3 years after onset of sexual intercourse or by age 21 years, whichever comes first.
b) Annual screening every year for women younger than 30 years.
c) Discontinue screening in women ages 60 years and older.
d) Discontinue screening in women who have undergone total hysterectomy, including removal of the cervix for benign causes.
e) Women exposed in utero to diethylstilbestrol may warrant continued and more frequent screening.

Answer and Discussion
The answer is c. The U.S. Preventive Services Task Force (USPSTF), the American Cancer Society (ACS), and the American College of Obstetrics and Gynecology (ACOG) all recommend initiating cervical cancer screening at age 21 years or 3 years after the onset of sexual activity, whichever comes first. Low-risk women who have had three consecutive negative Pap smears in the past 10 years can stop screening at age 65 years, according to USPSTF recommendations, and at age 70, according to ACS recommendations. The ACOG advises that the determination of when an older woman may stop screening should be made on a case-by-case basis. The USPSTF recommends screening at least every 3 years; ACS and ACOG advise screening for women younger than age 30 every year and every 2 to 3 years for women ages 30 and older who have had three consecutive normal Pap smears. ACS and ACOG specify certain risk groups that may require more frequent screening: HIV infection, in utero diethylstilbestrol exposure, immunosuppression, or prior history of cervical cancer. All three organizations agree that women who have undergone total hysterectomy with removal of cervix for benign disease may discontinue screening for cervical cancer.

9. A 48-year-old man presents with his wife, who complains of her husband's snoring. Further history reveals snoring for at least 20 years, with restless sleep observed by the wife. The patient denies any problem sleeping, but on direct questioning, he admits to dry mouth and headaches in the morning and sleepiness throughout the day. He confesses that he almost fell asleep at the wheel of the car several times, but he ascribes this to long hours and overwork. Physical examination reveals a stocky man, somewhat overweight, but the examination is otherwise normal. Which would be the most appropriate next step?

a) Sedative medication for the patient to ensure that he gets a better night's sleep

b) Sedative medication for the wife so that she can sleep through his snoring

c) Sending the patient for sleep studies

d) Advising a weight loss program and following up in 6 months

e) Advising stopping smoking because doing so has been proven to stop snoring in more than 50% of patients

Answer and Discussion

The answer is c. This man's clinical picture suggests obstructive sleep apnea. Patients with unexplained excessive daytime sleepiness deserve further evaluation, and the diagnosis of obstructive sleep apnea requires examining a patient during sleep.

10. A 21-year-old male patient comes to the emergency room with itching and jaundice. He has a long history of recurrent pulmonary infections, chronic sinusitis, a recent diagnosis of diabetes, and two prior admissions for pancreatitis. Liver biopsy confirms cirrhosis. In regard to this patient's diagnosis, which of the following is the most accurate statement?

a) The disease is autosomal dominant in inheritance.

b) Alcohol abuse is a common cause for this disease.

c) The most common cause of death is liver failure.

d) A sweat chloride test result of <70 mEq/L is highly sensitive for diagnosis.

e) Digital clubbing is often seen in patients.

Answer and Discussion

The answer is e. Cystic fibrosis (CF) is a fatal autosomal recessive, multisystem disease that usually presents with persistent pulmonary infection, pancreatic insufficiency, and sinusitis. Additional features include pancreatitis, infertility, diabetes, deep vein thrombosis, and, rarely, biliary cirrhosis. Although CF is generally diagnosed in infants and children, patients may present later in life with atypical symptoms. One large retrospective cohort study of 1,051 patients with CF found that 7% received a diagnosis at age 18 years or older. Progressive lung disease and eventual respiratory failure continue to be the major causes of morbidity and mortality. The sweat chloride test is the gold standard for CF diagnosis, and a result of >70 mEq/L distinguishes CF from other lung diseases. More than 95% of men with CF are infertile, mostly due to incomplete development of the wolffian structures, particularly the vas deferens. Digital clubbing is often seen in patients with moderate to severe disease.

11. A 32-year-old woman presents with double vision. The significant findings on examination include ptosis, diplopia, and facial weakness, causing her to appear to snarl when she attempts to smile. During counting aloud, her speech becomes progressively less distinct and more nasal. Proximal muscle weakness is present, which increases with repetitive movements and improves with rest. All the following statements are true about this disease, *except*

a) It is more common in women.

b) The most common ages at presentation are the 20s and 30s for women and the 60s for men.

c) Pupils are small and irregular and react to accommodation but not to light.

d) The diagnostic test involves intravenous injection of an anticholinesterase inhibitor.

e) A pathophysiologically similar syndrome that affects proximal muscles but improves with brief exercise is associated with malignancy, most commonly, small cell carcinoma of the lung.

Answer and Discussion

The answer is c. Myasthenia gravis is the diagnosis suggested by the findings in this woman. The disease is more common in women than men (3:1). Pupillary reactions are always spared in myasthenia gravis. Small, irregular pupils that react to accommodation but not to light are described as Argyll Robertson pupils and are found in patients with neurosyphilis and, occasionally, in those with diabetes mellitus. The diagnostic test for myasthenia gravis involves intravenous injection of the anticholinesterase inhibitor edrophonium chloride.

12. A 55-year-old white man was recently diagnosed with colon cancer. He asks you what the average survival at 5 years is for people with his type of cancer. You obtain the surgical pathology report that indicates that the cancer extends into the perirectal fat. In addition, the report indicates that regional nodes are also involved. You report to him that the average 5-year survival is

a) 70% to 80%

b) 80% to 90%

c) 60% to 70%

d) 40% to 60%

e) Less than 40%

Answer and Discussion

The answer is d. According to Astler and Coller's modification of the Dukes' staging system (Table 67.1), this patient has stage C2 cancer. Penetration into the perirectal fat makes it stage B2, but lymph node involvement makes it stage C2. Furthermore, this staging system is helpful in predicting prognosis, which is directly related to cancer penetration and nodal involvement at the time of resection.

13. You are seated in the hospital cafeteria in the middle of a busy call day when the medical student with whom you are having dinner complains of pruritus and appears flushed. He states that he has felt like this previously, is allergic to peanuts, and thinks that there may have been nuts in the cake that he just ate. He states that he does not feel too bad and that this is nothing like the last time,

TABLE 67.1

STAGING OF COLORECTAL CANCER

Stage	Penetration	5-Year Survival (%)
A	Mucosal, above muscularis propria, no involvement of lymph nodes	97
B1	Into muscularis propria but above pericolic fat, no involvement of lymph nodes	78
B2	Into pericolic or perirectal fat, no involvement of lymph nodes	78
C1	Same penetration as B1 with nodal metastases	74
C2	Same penetration as B2 with nodal metastases	48
D	Distant metastases	4

when he had some difficulty with breathing; he says that he will go lie down in the call room for awhile and he should be fine. You assess his airway and breathing, and they are normal. What would be the most appropriate next step?

a) Let him go and rest; you will go and see a patient who has just arrived and then check on the medical student in an hour or so.

b) Keep him with you so that you can take him to the emergency department if he starts to feel any worse or has any pulmonary symptoms.

c) Take him to the emergency department, and administer 1 mL of 1:10,000 epinephrine intravenously with cardiac monitoring.

d) Take him to the emergency department, recruit assistance from the medical team there, have his airway and cardiopulmonary status assessed and monitored, obtain intravenous access, and administer 0.5 mL of 1:1,000 epinephrine subcutaneously or intramuscularly as soon as possible.

e) Give him an antihistamine that you happen to have in your pocket, and keep him with you so that you can take him to the emergency department if he starts to feel any worse or has any pulmonary symptoms.

Answer and Discussion

The answer is d. Anaphylaxis can occur within 5 to 60 minutes after exposure to an allergen. This medical student is at risk of anaphylaxis and death. He needs a controlled and monitored environment. Epinephrine is the drug of choice; fatality rates are highest in patients in whom epinephrine administration is delayed. Severe airway edema, severe bronchospasm, or hypotension requires intravenous administration of 0.5 to 1.0 mL of epinephrine. Mild or moderate symptoms without laryngeal edema, bronchospasm, or hypotension

should be treated with 0.3 to 0.5 mL of 1:1,000 epinephrine subcutaneously or intramuscularly.

14. A solitary pulmonary nodule is seen in the right upper lobe on the chest radiograph and CT scan of a 60-year-old woman with a history of stage IB breast cancer. She underwent right lumpectomy 20 years ago without any further treatment. Regularly scheduled follow-up mammograms have been negative to date. She has a 20 pack-year history of tobacco use and quit smoking 7 years ago. The chest CT scan shows a 1.2-cm mass with smooth borders, popcorn calcification, and a density of 214 Hounsfield units. What is the next step in management?

a) Follow up with serial CTs to evaluate change in size of the nodule.

b) Excise the mass for pathological diagnosis.

c) Obtain a fluoro-2-deoxyglucose–positron emission tomography scan.

d) Perform percutaneous needle aspiration and biopsy.

e) Order an MRI of the chest.

Answer and Discussion

The answer is a. A solitary pulmonary nodule is a lesion that is usually <3 cm and surrounded by pulmonary parenchyma. Larger lesions are more likely to be malignant than smaller lesions. Malignant lesions tend to have more irregular and spiculated borders as compared to the smooth and discrete border of benign lesions. Increased density on CT argues against malignancy with the cut off of >164 Hounsfield units for benign and <164 Hounsfield units for malignant lesions. Certain patterns of calcification such as "popcorn" calcification, laminated (concentric) calcification, central calcification, and diffuse homogeneous calcification suggest that a lesion is benign, whereas reticular, punctate, amorphous, or eccentric calcifications raise the concern for malignancy. A nodule with a low probability of being malignant may be followed with serial chest CT scans. A nodule that is ≥1 cm and has an intermediate probability of being malignant should be evaluated by fluoro-2-deoxyglucose–positron emission tomography (PET). If the nodule is negative by PET, they too can be followed with serial chest CT scans; if the PET is positive, the nodule should be excised. A nodule that is <1 cm and has an intermediate probability of being malignant can be followed by serial chest CT scans. Any nodule that has a high probability of being malignant should be excised. For nodules ≥4 mm, serial CT scans are not required if the patient is low risk. Patients who are high risk or have nodules >4 mm should have follow-up chest CT scanning.

15. A 55-year-old man with a history of polycythemia vera sees his family physician for routine follow-up. A hematocrit drawn at the visit is 48%. Which of the following is most likely?

a) The iron stores in his bone marrow would be increased.
b) He has decreased cerebral blood flow and is at increased risk of thrombotic complications.
c) His bone marrow will be hypocellular, except for hyperplasia of red cell progenitors.
d) An increased level of circulating erythropoietin is present in his plasma.
e) He does not have an increased bleeding tendency due to preservation of platelet function.

Answer and Discussion

The answer is b. Patients with polycythemia vera who have a hematocrit >45% usually have decreased cerebral blood flow and an increased thrombotic tendency. The bone marrow is usually hypercellular, with hyperplasia of all bone marrow elements. Iron stores are not increased, and patients may actually be iron deficient due to an increased tendency for gastrointestinal blood loss because of dysfunctional platelets. Finally, a characteristic finding in polycythemia vera is a decreased erythropoietin level due to feedback inhibition (i.e., the proliferation of marrow elements occurs independently of erythropoietin stimulation).

16. A 30-year-old man, who has been your patient for several years, presents for his regular checkup. He is known to have dextrocardia. He suffers from recurrent sinusitis and, for years, has had mucopurulent sputum and episodic hemoptysis. He has digital clubbing and bilateral crackles on auscultation of the lungs. With which of the following conditions are this patient's symptoms most consistent?

a) α_1-Antitrypsin deficiency
b) Kartagener's syndrome
c) Young's syndrome
d) Williams-Campbell syndrome
e) Yellow nail syndrome

Answer and Discussion

The answer is b. The pulmonary symptoms and signs are suggestive of bronchiectasis. Kartagener's syndrome consists of dextrocardia, sinusitis, and bronchiectasis. Young's syndrome is defined as obstructive azoospermia; approximately 20% to 30% of patients have bronchiectasis. Early panacinar emphysema, as well as bronchiectasis, may develop in patients with α_1-antitrypsin deficiency. Yellow nail syndrome is characterized by the triad of lymphedema, pleural effusion, and yellow discoloration of the nails; 40% of patients have bronchiectasis. Patients with Williams-Campbell syndrome have a deficiency of the bronchial cartilage of medium-size airways, which dilate and can be complicated by bronchiectasis.

17. A 38-year-old man with a history of hepatitis B virus infection and significant alcohol abuse, who has not seen a physician in 7 years, presents to the emergency department with fever and altered sensorium. On examination, he is febrile, tachycardic, hypotensive, and somnolent. He is markedly jaundiced, with a distended abdomen. Initial blood work reveals a Na^+ level of 130 mg/dL, creatinine level of 1.6 mg/dL, hemoglobin of 10 mg/dL, and platelet count of 90,000/mm^3. Which of the following diagnoses is most consistent with these findings?

a) Splenic sequestration
b) Idiopathic thrombocytopenic purpura
c) Thrombotic thrombocytopenic purpura
d) Heparin-induced thrombocytopenia
e) Systemic lupus erythematosus

Answer and Discussion

The answer is a. This man most likely has portal hypertension and ascites. Splenic sequestration of platelets secondary to portal hypertension often leads to a decrease in the platelet count. Alcohol also has a direct cytotoxic effect on megakaryocytes. Furthermore, inadequate thrombopoietin production may be present in the failing liver, also leading to the decreased production of platelets. Nevertheless, the platelet count rarely falls to <10,000/mm^3.

18. A 32-year-old woman is referred to you from her obstetrician. She has had mild hypertension for several years but has been hesitant to start any medications. She is now attempting to have a baby and is concerned that her elevated blood pressure may pose a risk to her baby. She is also concerned that any medications that she takes not be harmful to the fetus. At a preconception visit, her obstetrician recommended consultation with you. She denies any complaints. Her blood pressure during this visit is 160/90 mm Hg, and her heart rate is 85 beats/minute. She has a normal physical examination. Urinalysis is negative. You tell her all the following, *except*

a) Methyldopa and hydralazine have been shown to be safe to the developing fetus.
b) Reducing her blood pressure will reduce the chances of pre-eclampsia or eclampsia developing.
c) Eighty-five percent of hypertensive women have uncomplicated pregnancies.
d) Some women with mild hypertension can stop antihypertensive medications in the second trimester.
e) Drug treatment would be indicated if hypertensive end-organ damage were found on evaluation.

Answer and Discussion

The answer is b. Eighty-five percent of women with pre-existing mild hypertension do well through pregnancy. Of those taking medication, some may be able to reduce the dose or stop the antihypertensive agent during the second trimester because of the usual drop in blood pressure. Studies have shown that treatment of mild hypertension before and during pregnancy does not reduce the risk for pre-eclampsia or eclampsia and does not improve maternal or fetal health. Indications for drug treatment usually include a diastolic blood pressure (DBP) of >100 mm Hg or evidence of end-organ damage from the hypertension. Methyldopa and hydralazine have been shown to be safe for the fetus, as opposed to angiotensin-converting enzyme inhibitors, which have been associated with poor fetal outcome, perhaps related to dysregulation of uteroplacental blood flow.

19. A 60-year-old man reports generalized fatigue. He has been having red urine for the past few days and tarry stools for the past month. He has a history of severe arthritis for which he has been taking over-the-counter ibuprofen. Vital signs and physical examination are normal, but an initial complete blood count revealed a leukocyte count of 7,000/mm^3, hemoglobin of 7 mg/dL, hematocrit of 20%, and platelet count of 600,000 μL. The mean cell volume (MCV) is 62 fL, and MCH is 29 pG. He is hemodynamically stable. His stool for occult blood is positive. The most appropriate next step in this patient's management is which of the following?

a) Serum haptoglobin
b) Esophagogastroduodenoscopy
c) Colonoscopy
d) Cystoscopy
e) Iron tablets

Answer and Discussion

The answer is b. The low MCV and guaiac-positive stools point toward iron deficiency anemia. The red-colored urine is due to beeturia, which is an infrequent manifestation of iron deficiency in which the eating of beets leads to the formation of red urine. This is due to increased intestinal absorption and excretion in the urine of the reddish pigment betalaine. Betalaine is decolorized by ferric ions. This most likely explains the predisposition in iron deficiency to beeturia. The laboratory values in iron deficiency are microcytosis, hypochromia, a low serum iron, an increased total iron binding capacity (transferrin), a reduced transferrin saturation, and a reduced ferritin. The test with the highest sensitivity and specificity for the diagnosis of iron deficiency is serum ferritin. Iron-deficiency anemia is most often associated with blood loss. To find the cause, the first step is esophagogastroduodenoscopy (EGD) followed by a colonoscopy if the EGD is nondiagnostic. In this patient, iron deficiency anemia is most likely secondary to peptic ulcer disease caused by excessive use of nonsteroidal anti-inflammatory drugs for his severe arthritis.

20. A 26-year-old man has had recurrent episodes of mild, crampy abdominal pain accompanied by bloody diarrhea over the past year. He has no other significant past medical history and does not smoke or drink alcohol. He has undergone colonoscopy as part of his evaluation. The colon appears to be continuously inflamed from the anal verge to the more proximal colon. Shallow ulcers were noted, and there were no hemorrhoids. Biopsy is consistent with ulcerative colitis. He now presents with a 5-day history of bloody diarrhea and mild abdominal pain with a rather abrupt onset. Stool studies are negative for *Clostridium difficile* or a microbiological cause of colitis. All the following are true about this patient's condition, *except*

a) Total parenteral nutrition is not effective as primary therapy.
b) Sulfasalazine can be effective in maintaining remission, as well as in acute disease.
c) If he responds to a corticosteroid, he should be maintained on it indefinitely once in remission.
d) Sclerosing cholangitis may be an associated condition.
e) Oral anticholinergics for control of symptoms are contraindicated.

Answer and Discussion

The answer is c. This man most likely has ulcerative colitis. Corticosteroids are used in the treatment of ulcerative colitis and Crohn's disease, but controlled trials have shown no benefit in maintaining remission. In patients with a severe exacerbation of colitis, oral intake can promote colonic activity and intravenous alimentation serves as a component of therapy, although no evidence suggests that it alone is effective as primary therapy. Sulfasalazine is a well-established agent for use in remission, but can also be used in therapy of an acute flare. Drugs such as codeine, diphenoxylate, or anticholinergics are contraindicated because they can promote colonic dilatation and toxic megacolon.

21. A 50-year-old woman presents for a routine annual examination. She feels well. Past medical history is notable for peptic ulcer disease. Examination reveals a healthy-appearing, middle-age woman. Results of a chemistry panel are as follows:

Na$^+$	136 mEq/L
K$^+$	3.9 mEq/L
Cl	102 mEq/L
HCO$_3$	26 mEq/L
Blood urea nitrogen	18 mg/dL
Creatinine	1.0 mg/dL
Mg^{2+}	2.1 mg/dL
Ca^{2+}	11 mg/dL
P	2.0 mg/dL
Albumin	4.0 g/dL

Her parathyroid hormone level is 90 pg/mL. All the following statements about the diagnosis are true, *except*

a) An increased level of urinary excretion of cyclic adenosine monophosphate is present.

b) The majority of patients are symptomatic at presentation.

c) This condition occurs in multiple endocrine neoplasia types 1 and 2a.

d) Peptic ulceration and pancreatitis may be associated.

e) A single abnormal gland is the cause in approximately 80% of patients.

Answer and Discussion

The answer is b. The most likely diagnosis is primary hyperparathyroidism. Elevated circulating parathyroid hormone in the presence of elevated calcium is highly suggestive of primary hyperparathyroidism. Serum phosphorus is usually low but can be normal in patients with renal insufficiency. In the majority of cases, the diagnosis is made by routine blood samples when a chemistry panel is ordered. Peptic ulcer disease, pancreatitis, mental status changes, nephrolithiasis, and osteoporosis are all potential presentations.

22. A 19-year-old man is seen in an urgent care center. He reports dysuria for the past 2 days and admits to two sexual partners in the past 3 weeks. Physical examination reveals an otherwise healthy man with a purulent urethral discharge. A Gram-stained smear of the discharge reveals intracellular gram-negative diplococci. Along with appropriate counseling and serologic testing, which of the following would be the most appropriate treatment?

a) Intramuscular dose of a long-acting antimicrobial, such as benzathine penicillin G combined with a 7-day course of doxycycline

b) Single intramuscular dose of ceftriaxone, 125 mg

c) Single oral dose of azithromycin, 2 g

d) Single oral dose of ciprofloxacin, 500 mg

e) Intramuscular dose of cefazolin, 0.5 g, with a 7-day course of doxycycline

Answer and Discussion

The answer is c. This man most likely has gonorrhea. First-generation cephalosporins and long-acting penicillins have no place in the treatment of gonorrhea. Ceftriaxone or ciprofloxacin alone would be inadequate because a high incidence of chlamydial infection is present in patients with gonorrhea. Dual antimicrobial coverage is therefore necessary, and a single dose of azithromycin would be appropriate treatment.

23. A 64-year-old man schedules an urgent visit for severe pain in his right great toe. The pain was sudden in onset and has prevented him from bearing weight on the right foot. He was recently hospitalized for elective coronary angioplasty and is also known to have

moderate renal sufficiency as a result of long-standing diabetes mellitus. His medications consist of aspirin, lisinopril, and glyburide. He does not drink alcohol and is an ex-smoker. Physical examination shows him to be in moderate distress, and the right first metatarsophalangeal joint is inflamed. A polarizing light microscope is used to examine an aspirate from the joint, and needle-shaped crystals with negative birefringence are seen. A Gram stain of the fluid is negative for bacteria. What would be the *least* appropriate next step in management?

a) Single intramuscular dose of adrenocorticotropic hormone

b) Intravenous colchicine given through a carefully placed intravenous catheter

c) High dose of indomethacin

d) Allopurinol given orally for at least 2 weeks

e) Stopping aspirin and commencing naproxen

Answer and Discussion

The answer is d. This question relates to the acute management of gout. Intravenous radiocontrast dye can serve as a precipitant of gouty arthritis. Adrenocorticotropic hormone, 40 U in a single intramuscular injection, can be used in acute gouty arthritis. Intravenous colchicine is frequently given when a good intravenous site can be used; however, it is contraindicated in patients with renal insufficiency, as is high-dose indomethacin. Allopurinol should not be started while signs of acute inflammation are present. Stopping aspirin would not be appropriate because it is being used for prophylaxis against myocardial infarction.

24. A 28-year-old woman reports palpitations for the past 6 months. They are accompanied by lightheadedness, chest pressure, and nausea. Initially, they tended to occur only two or three times a day; however, they have now become more frequent, and she has missed work on several occasions and has stopped socializing with friends except at her own home. She has no psychiatric history and does not drink alcohol or abuse drugs. Her caffeine intake is limited. Her family history is notable for maternal hypertension; her father suffered a stroke 7 months ago. The workup reveals no evidence of thyroid disease. Ambulatory ECG monitoring shows that her symptoms are accompanied by sinus tachycardia. All the following statements about her condition are true, *except*

a) She may benefit from a short-acting benzodiazepine, such as alprazolam.

b) She may benefit from a serotonin reuptake inhibitor, such as paroxetine, in a dose similar to that used for depression.

c) First-degree relatives have an increased incidence of the same condition.

d) Behavioral exposure techniques may be helpful.

e) Patients using alcohol to relax in social situations have a lower incidence of this condition.

Answer and Discussion

The answer is e. Symptoms of panic disorder are characterized by discrete attacks of anxiety associated with a sensation of chest pain, palpitations, or nausea. Patients may have multiple emergency department visits before they are diagnosed. The embarrassment or fear of having panic attacks in public without an easy escape often disrupts social interactions. Alcohol can actually intensify symptoms.

25. A 69-year-old businessman is assessed for halitosis and a sensation of fullness in his throat. On being questioned, he explains that he is embarrassed by this and has started to avoid social situations. He has also found that he has some difficulty in swallowing that seems to be relieved by bringing up foul-smelling food particles. He has tried over-the-counter famotidine without relief. Which of the following is the single, most likely diagnosis?

a) Dental abscess
b) Gastroesophageal reflux disease
c) Zenker's diverticulum
d) Globus pharyngeus
e) Progressive systemic sclerosis

Answer and Discussion

The answer is c. The symptoms are most likely to be explained by the presence of a Zenker's diverticulum, which is an outpouching of the esophageal wall. This condition usually presents in older individuals complaining of cervical dysphagia, gurgling in the throat, halitosis, and regurgitation of foul food. Regurgitation of old food is unlikely with a dental abscess or gastroesophageal reflux disease. Symptoms of globus pharyngeus do not include dysphagia. Scleroderma of the esophagus can cause gastroesophageal reflux disease, but if dysphagia occurs, it is progressive.

26. A 17-year-old woman reports aching in the groin area. She is athletic, jogs several miles a day, and is a member of a cheerleading team. She describes an abnormal sensation over the anterolateral thigh. On occasion, she has noticed an "electric jab"–type sensation on extending the knee and has curtailed her running. Her past medical history is noncontributory, and she feels well otherwise. You observed her gait to be normal when she entered the office. A normal range of movement is present on examination, and reflexes in the lower extremities are symmetric. Tenderness is not elicited. What is the most likely diagnosis?

a) Early-onset hip arthritis (limited internal rotation)
b) Multiple sclerosis
c) Lumbar disc herniation (decreased knee reflex, posterior quadriceps weakness)

d) Lateral cutaneous nerve syndrome
e) Trochanteric bursitis

Answer and Discussion

The answer is d. Entrapment of the lateral cutaneous nerve is characterized by pain, dysesthesia, or hypesthesia at the lateral thigh. Repetitive exercise, particularly extending the hips while doing the splits, could be a factor in this woman. Tight clothing, obesity, and trauma have also been implicated in causing irritation to the lateral cutaneous nerve, particularly in its path adjacent to the anterosuperior iliac spine. Hip arthritis would be expected to demonstrate limited internal rotation. The diagnosis of multiple sclerosis requires documentation of neurologic events over time at different sites of the neuraxis. Normal knee reflexes are less likely with lumbar disc herniation, which can also affect quadriceps strength. Tenderness would be expected on physical examination in trochanteric bursitis.

27. A 40-year-old man undergoing treatment for lymphoma presents with new-onset vertigo. On further questioning, he also admits to a change in his sense of taste. Along with his prescribed medications, he is also self-medicating with *Echinacea*. On physical examination, he has a vesicular rash in the right external auditory canal and right-sided facial palsy. Which is the most likely etiology of his new symptoms?

a) Side effect of herbal medication
b) Disseminated malignancy
c) A virus often identified by Tzanck smear
d) Parvovirus infection
e) A virus often identified by heterophile antibody testing

Answer and Discussion

The answer is c. Immunocompromised individuals are particularly susceptible to symptomatic herpes zoster, which can result in Ramsay Hunt syndrome. Pain and vesicles appear in the external auditory canal, and there may be loss of taste sensation in the anterior two-thirds of the tongue. The geniculate ganglion of the sensory branch of the facial nerve is involved.

28. A 21-year-old woman is seen in the outpatient department with a 3-month history of watery diarrhea. She has had similar episodes on three prior occasions, with negative stool cultures. Past medical history is notable for knee surgery 2 years ago. Her medications include an oral contraceptive. She has not traveled out of state in the recent past and is a nonsmoker. Examination reveals a slender woman in no acute distress. Office proctoscopy shows black mucosa but an otherwise normal examination. Which of the following statements is correct?

a) Colonoscopy with multiple biopsies should be the next step in management.
b) Fecal smears should be examined using fluorescent techniques.
c) The patient's condition is highly infectious.
d) The patient's condition could be explained by surreptitious laxative abuse.
e) All first-degree relatives should undergo genetic testing.

Answer and Discussion

The answer is d. The appearance of black rectal mucosa is consistent with a diagnosis of melanosis coli, which results from laxative abuse.

29. A 41-year-old man reports dull pain over the maxillary areas for the past 10 days and a yellow nasal discharge. He has tried over-the-counter nasal decongestants without relief. Physical examination shows that percussion of the teeth causes pain. You recommend the use of oxymetazoline 0.05% spray and a 10-day course of trimethoprim-sulfamethoxazole. He is seen in routine follow-up 4 months later when he explains that his symptoms did improve for a few days but soon returned. His symptoms are much the same as they were 4 months ago, but he now has a postnasal drip associated with cough. Which of the following statements relating to this patient's condition is incorrect?
a) Oral amoxicillin for 1 month would be an acceptable next step in management.
b) CT is more sensitive than plain radiography.
c) Up to one-third of patients may respond to treatment with an antihistamine and decongestant preparation.
d) A topical corticosteroid is contraindicated.
e) For patients who do not respond to empiric medical therapy, surgical drainage should be considered.

Answer and Discussion

The answer is d. Symptoms of sinusitis of more than 3 months are termed *chronic*. Obstructed sinus drainage is implicated, leading to persistent infection. Diagnosis can be made, based on clinical history, although CT is particularly helpful if there is doubt. Oral amoxicillin for 1 month is appropriate, and an antihistamine/decongestant may help relieve the cough. A topical corticosteroid may actually accelerate resolution of symptoms.

30. A 64-year-old diabetic woman is hospitalized with a diagnosis of myocardial infarction. During hospitalization, she undergoes coronary angiography and is discharged on the sixth day. You see her in follow-up 8 weeks later, and she explains that she has right-sided shoulder discomfort. She also reports some stiffness in the fingers of her right hand. She explains the pain has come on gradually and is not related to ambulation. Use of the upper extremity on her dominant left side is without pain. She explains that after her hospitalization, she felt low in her mood, and a psychiatrist told her that she was depressed. Physical examination reveals significant reduction in both active and passive range of motion of the right shoulder compared with the left side. Movement of the right shoulder is painful. Tenderness to palpation is also present. Plain radiographs of the shoulder are reported as normal. Which is the most likely cause of her shoulder pain?
a) Adhesive capsulitis
b) Impingement syndrome
c) Angina
d) Rotator cuff tear
e) Fibromyalgia

Answer and Discussion

The answer is a. Adhesive capsulitis is characterized by gradual onset of symptoms, with pain and progressive reduction in active and passive range of motion. Patients often have a recent history of immobilization in a hospital bed. Diabetic patients are known to have an increased risk of capsulitis that is particularly resistant to treatment. Hypothyroidism and Parkinson's disease are also associated. Patients with impingement syndrome usually have good range of motion, and osteoarthritis would be seen on radiography. Examination in rotator cuff tear would show normal passive range of movement. Fibromyalgia is associated with depression, but this patient does not meet other criteria for the diagnosis. The symptoms of tenderness in this patient are not consistent with angina.

31–35. From the following list, match the characteristic clinical and laboratory feature with the appropriate vasculitis in questions 31 to 35:
a) Arterial bruits are present, and there are no peripheral pulses.
b) Pulmonary involvement is manifested as asthma.
c) Angiographic evidence of aneurysms is present in the small- and medium-size arteries of the kidneys.
d) Nonsyphilitic interstitial keratitis is present with vestibuloauditory symptoms.
e) Positive antineutrophil cytoplasmic antibody test is highly specific.

31. Wegener's granulomatosis
32. Churg-Strauss disease
33. Polyarteritis nodosa
34. Takayasu's arteritis
35. Cogan's syndrome

Answers
31. The answer is e.
32. The answer is b.
33. The answer is c.
34. The answer is a.
35. The answer is d.

36. A 29-year-old woman is seen in the outpatient department with a dry cough, dyspnea, and headache for 2 weeks. A physician in employee health gave her a 5-day course of clarithromycin without improvement. She had previously been well, except for recurrent sinus infections from which she is presently asymptomatic. She is not taking any medications at the moment, does not smoke, and has not traveled outside the country. Symptoms of fatigue since she returned from a field trip to Arizona 3 weeks ago have caused her to miss several days from work. On examination, a nonspecific maculopapular erythematous rash is noted. A chest radiograph demonstrates a focal upper lobe infiltrate and hilar adenopathy. Biopsy of the rash shows eosinophilic infiltrates. Which is the most likely cause of this presentation?
a) Mycoplasma pneumonia
b) Lyme borreliosis
c) Varicella pneumonia
d) Coccidioidal pneumonia (valley fever)
e) Streptococcal pneumonia

Answer and Discussion

The answer is d. The presentation is typical for coccidioidal infection. Coccidioidomycosis is a fungal infection acquired by the inhalation of fungal arthrospores. The disease is endemic in south central California, southern Arizona, Nevada, New Mexico, and parts of Texas. Many cases elude diagnosis because symptoms may be mild and nonspecific. Cutaneous lesions may be present in as many as 25% of patients. Chest radiology most commonly shows a single focal infiltrate. Laboratory studies typically show eosinophilia, and mild elevation of alanine transaminase may also be present. A common clue to the diagnosis is nonresolution of symptoms when treatment is directed toward bacterial pneumonia.

37. Which of the following statements regarding hepatitis C is false?
a) In patients with chronic infection with hepatitis C virus, hepatitis A virus immunization is indicated if patients have not previously been exposed.
b) Chronic infection develops in approximately 20% of patients.
c) Cirrhosis develops in 20% of infected patients.
d) Cryoglobulinemia is associated.
e) Of patients with hepatitis C, 30% to 40% have no identifiable risk factors for acquiring the infection.

Answer and Discussion

The answer is b. The most common presentation of hepatitis C is a chronic asymptomatic elevation of hepatic transaminases. A state of chronic infection occurs in at least 50% of patients, and in those in whom cirrhosis develops, an increased risk of hepatic malignancy is present.

38. A 42-year-old man is found to be anemic on workup for fatigue. He has been taking multivitamins and oral iron supplements for the past 20 years. He is a nonsmoker and seldom drinks alcohol. On direct questioning, he explains that he has frequent bowel movements with stools that are difficult to flush away. Physical examination is notable for a blistering rash at the elbows and knees. On testing, he is found to be anemic, with a mean corpuscular volume of 65. Review of his peripheral blood smear demonstrates Howell-Jolly bodies. Endomysial antibody test result is positive, and antinuclear antibody test is negative. He is instructed to eat a glutenfree diet, and his symptoms improve. All the following statements about this patient's condition are true, *except*
a) A positive endomysial antibody test is consistent with the clinical picture.
b) Small bowel biopsy shows periodic acid–Schiff-positive granules in macrophages.
c) Lymphoma is a late complication.
d) Osteomalacia is an association.
e) Response to the glutenfree diet is diagnostic.

Answer and Discussion

The answer is b. This man has a history suggestive of celiac sprue, a gluten-sensitive enteropathy. Iron-deficiency anemia unresponsive to oral supplements is often seen. Dermatitis herpetiformis and Howell-Jolly bodies are clues to the diagnosis. Although a positive endomysial antibody test is not specific, it is sensitive, and the response to the glutenfree diet is virtually diagnostic. If a patient becomes unresponsive to dietary therapy after many years, lymphoma should be a consideration. Periodic acid–Schiff-positive granules on small bowel biopsy are seen in Whipple's disease, not in celiac sprue.

39. A 27-year-old man, a concert pianist, reports gradually worsening back pain and stiffness for 6 months. He describes the pain as being worst on waking and located in the lumbar and gluteal region. He recalls being awakened by the pain on a number of occasions, and he has arisen and stretched his back to relieve the discomfort. Taking a warm shower helps alleviate the stiffness, and sitting for prolonged periods exacerbates it. The Schober's test demonstrates a separation of 3 cm. Which of the following is most compatible with this patient's illness?
a) Occupation-related illness
b) Finding of an early diastolic murmur
c) Positive antinuclear antibody test
d) Disease moderately responsive to systemic glucocorticoids
e) Dry mouth and eyes

Answer and Discussion
The answer is b. Insidious onset, morning stiffness, and symptom duration of longer than 3 months suggest that the most likely cause of the man's back pain is inflammatory. Limitation of spinal movement demonstrated by the Schober's test suggests the diagnosis of ankylosing spondylitis. Aortic insufficiency is an association, as are inflammatory bowel disease and iritis. A positive antinuclear antibody test is not a feature of the illness, although up to 90% of patients carry the *HLA-B27* gene. Glucocorticoids have not been found to be helpful in management. Sitting with a poor posture for prolonged periods may be implicated in back pain, as could be suspected in a pianist, but it would not explain morning stiffness. Dry mouth and eyes are features of Sjögren's syndrome.

40. A new ultrasound technique is available to screen for ovarian cancer. The sensitivity is said to be 80% and the specificity 95%. The prevalence of ovarian cancer is believed to be 2% in a sample population of adult women. If the entire sample population undergoes imaging with the new technique, what will be the predictive value of a positive test?
a) 10%
b) 49%
c) 24%
d) 80%
e) 95%

Answer and Discussion
The answer is c. Suppose a sample population of 1,000: The reader should construct a 2 × 2 table. A prevalence of 2% would mean 20 patients have the disease (a + c = 20). The sensitivity is 80%, and of the 20 patients with the disease, 16 would test positive (a = 20 × 0.8). Of the 980 patients without disease, 931 would test negative (d 980 × 0.95 [specificity]). This now means 49 patients (b − 931) would test positive despite the absence of disease. The positive predictive value is calculated as a/(a + b).

41. A 25-year-old woman reports rectal bleeding. She is admitted for further investigation. Physical examination reveals pigmented lesions of the mouth, hands, and feet. Radiologic investigation shows multiple polypoid tumors of the small bowel, which are also found on endoscopic evaluation of the ascending colon. Biopsy demonstrates findings consistent with hamartomas. Which of the following statements about this woman's condition is correct?
a) An increased incidence of ovarian sex cord tumors is present in patients with this condition.
b) A high risk of colonic malignancy is present.
c) Total colectomy is absolutely indicated.
d) First-line treatment is a corticosteroid.

e) The inheritance pattern of this condition is autosomal recessive.

Answer and Discussion
The answer is a. This woman most likely has Peutz-Jeghers syndrome of hamartomas and pigmented lesions. This condition is associated with an increased risk of ovarian sex cord tumors. The risk of colonic malignancy is close to that of the general population, and the inheritance pattern is autosomal dominant. Corticosteroids do not play a role in management. Total colectomy is not mandatory.

42. A 28-year-old woman reports not being able to sleep. On questioning, she admits to having lost 8 lb over the past 4 weeks despite an increased appetite. She also feels weak and has noticed difficulty in climbing stairs. Her menstrual cycle has become irregular over the past few months. On examination, she appears restless, and a starelike gaze is particularly noticeable. Her pulse is 96 beats/minute, and she appears diaphoretic. Diffuse enlargement of the thyroid gland is present. The dorsa of the legs show thickening of the dermis. Thyroid function tests are reported as follows:

Serum thyroid-stimulating hormone	Undetectable
Serum T4	22 μg/dL
Serum T3	690 μg/dL
Free T4 index	35
Radioactive iodine uptake	40%

Methimazole is started. Which of the following statements about this patient's condition is false?
a) Once a euthyroid state is achieved, the dose of methimazole can be reduced.
b) Once a euthyroid state is achieved, methimazole can be continued at the original dose and levothyroxine supplementation started.
c) Leukopenia is a potential complication.
d) Hypertrophic pulmonary osteoarthropathy may be seen.
e) Thyroglobulin levels will be low at the time of diagnosis.

Answer and Discussion
The answer is e. This case is typical of a patient with Graves' disease. The symptoms described are those of hyperthyroidism in general. Older patients may have apathy. Ophthalmopathy with exophthalmos and dermatopathy, also termed *pretibial myxedema*, are often seen and are characteristic of Graves' disease. Clubbing may be seen. Treatment is an oral antithyroid agent, and the dose can be lowered when euthyroidism is achieved, or levothyroxine can be added. After 12 to 24 months of treatment, the drug can be discontinued, and up to 50% of patients remain well for an extended time. Thyroglobulin levels are typically low in patients with thyrotoxicosis factitia; levels are usually elevated in Graves' disease.

43–47. Match the following drugs with the mechanism by which they can raise blood pressure in hypertensive patients in questions 43 to 47:
a) Alcohol
b) Prednisone
c) Nonsteroidal anti-inflammatory drugs
d) Monoamine oxidase inhibitors
e) Cold formulas

43. Prevention of metabolism of norepinephrine

44. Increased cortisol levels

45. Promotion of sodium retention

46. Increased peripheral resistance and activation of the sympathetic nervous system

47. Iatrogenic Cushing's disease

Answers
43. The answer is d.
44. The answer is a.
45. The answer is c.
46. The answer is e.
47. The answer is b.

48. Which of the following statements relating to colorectal cancer is false?
a) High-fat diet increases the risk of colorectal cancer.
b) High-fiber diet has a protective effect.
c) Personal history of female genital or breast cancer increases the risk for colorectal cancer.
d) Fecal occult blood testing is highly specific.
e) Hereditary nonpolyposis colon cancer is an autosomal dominant disease.

Answer and Discussion
The answer is d. Fecal occult blood testing has a low specificity and a positive predictive value of approximately 5% for colorectal malignancy.

49. A 45-year-old man has recently moved into the area and has been renovating his home. He reports severe pain over the right elbow and back of the upper forearm. Examination reveals pain to pressure over the wrist extensor muscles 1 cm below the lateral epicondyle. Strength is preserved. Which of the following is the most likely cause of his pain?
a) Tennis elbow
b) Radial nerve entrapment
c) Olecranon bursitis
d) Ruptured biceps tendon
e) Golfer's elbow

Answer and Discussion
The answer is a. Repetitive overuse of the forearm muscles can result in lateral epicondylitis, or tennis elbow. The description given is most suggestive of this process. Golfer's elbow is also associated with overuse of the forearm but involves the medial epicondyle. Ruptured

biceps tendon results in weakness, and olecranon bursitis most often manifests with posterior elbow pain. Radial nerve entrapment is rare and, therefore, not the most likely cause of pain.

50. All the following statements about the cough associated with angiotensin-converting enzyme inhibitors are true, *except*
a) Dry and hacking
b) More frequent in asthmatics
c) Women affected more often than men
d) Generally occurring on rechallenge
e) Usually beginning within 1 to 2 weeks of institution of therapy

Answer and Discussion
The answer is b. The cough associated with angiotensin-converting enzyme inhibitors does *not* occur more frequently in asthmatics than in nonasthmatics, although it may be accompanied by bronchospasm.

51. The following statements about influenza therapy are true, *except*
a) In recommended populations, frequency of immunization is annual because of the changing strains, as well as immunity declining over the year.
b) Concurrent administration of influenza and pneumococcal vaccines is safe and does not affect the effectiveness of either vaccine.
c) In a known outbreak of influenza B in a nursing home, amantadine or rimantadine should be prescribed with the vaccination because these drugs have been shown to reduce the development of influenza B.
d) Amantadine and rimantadine have been shown to be beneficial as prophylaxis in some situations.
e) Vaccination for pregnant women of at least 14 weeks' gestation is indicated because they are at risk for influenza-related complications.

Answer and Discussion
The answer is c. Amantadine or rimantadine is effective in the prophylaxis and treatment of influenza A but not influenza B. Amantadine and rimantadine have been shown to be beneficial as prophylaxis when taken daily during the period of highest risk, particularly in the nonimmunized and during institutional outbreaks of influenza A.

52. The following statements regarding uremic pericarditis are true, *except*
a) Pericarditis in patients with advanced renal failure is an indication for dialysis.
b) The ECG shows diffuse ST-segment–T-wave elevations.
c) Symptoms include pleuritic chest pain, which is worse in the recumbent position.

d) If dialysis is performed, it should be heparin free due to risks of pericardial hemorrhage.

e) It occurs in approximately 13% of patients on maintenance hemodialysis.

Answer and Discussion

The answer is b. Renal failure is a common cause of pericardial disease. Uremic pericarditis is observed in approximately 10% of patients with advanced renal failure and approximately 13% of patients on hemodialysis. Presenting signs and symptoms include fever and pleuritic chest pain. The pain increases with the recumbent position. Uremic pericarditis may be associated with worsening anemia. A strange feature of uremic pericarditis is that the typical diffuse ST- and T-wave elevations seen with other causes of acute pericarditis are absent on an ECG. This is secondary to the lack of penetration of the inflammatory cells into the myocardium. Systemic corticosteroids and indomethacin have had limited success in the treatment of uremic pericarditis. Unexplained pericarditis in a patient with advanced renal failure is an indication to institute dialysis provided the patient is hemodynamically stable. The response to dialysis is usually dramatic. Because heparin increases the risk of hemorrhage into the pericardial space, heparinfree hemodialysis should be performed. Pericardial effusion drainage may be required if intensive dialysis is ineffective.

53–55. You are considering the options for antianginal medications for a patient with stable angina. Select the major side effect associated with the medications in questions 53 to 55:

a) Constipation
b) Bronchospasm
c) Hypercalcemia
d) Headache
e) Hypertension

53. Verapamil

54. Nitroglycerin

55. Propranolol

Answers and Discussions

53. The answer is a.
54. The answer is d.
55. The answer is b.

In the prescription of medications, it is important to consider the side effect profile as it relates to the patient. Verapamil is associated with peripheral edema. Nitroglycerin is associated with headache, lightheadedness, and flushing due to vasodilation. Propranolol is associated with bronchospasm and, consequently, is contraindicated in asthma.

56. A 30-year-old woman is brought to the emergency department by ambulance after her boyfriend found her in her garage. He says that she may have ingested antifreeze. She is comatose. Which of the following sets of laboratory studies is most consistent with her diagnosis?

a) Na^+ 141 mEq/L, K^+ 2.6 mEq/L, Cl^- 115 mEq/L, HCO_3^- 14 mEq/L, creatinine 3.0 mg/dL, arterial pH 7.31, urine pH 6.1

b) Na^+ 138 mEq/L, K^+ 6.2 mEq/L, Cl^- 107 mEq/L, HCO_3^- 18 mEq/L, creatinine 3.0 mg/dL, arterial pH 7.34, urine pH 5.2

c) Na^+ 144 mEq/L, K^+ 4.7 mEq/L, Cl^- 100 mEq/L, HCO_3^- 10 mEq/L, creatinine 3.0 mg/dL, arterial pH 7.25, urine pH 5.0

d) Na^+ 136 mEq/L, K^+ 4.4 mEq/L, Cl^- 108 mEq/L, HCO_3^- 20 mEq/L, creatinine 3.0 mg/dL, arterial pH 7.38, urine pH 5.0

e) Na^+ 140 mEq/L, K^+ 5.2 mEq/L, Cl^- 105 mEq/L, HCO_3^- 22 mEq/L, creatinine 3.0 mg/dL, arterial pH 7.36, urine pH 5.2

Answer and Discussion

The answer is c. The anion gap is defined as the measured cations minus the measured anions or sodium concentration minus the combination of the chloride and bicarbonate concentrations. Traditionally, the normal range has been between 7 and 13 mEq/L, but because of newer analyzers, the normal range may fall to 3 to 11 mEq/L due to higher reported chloride concentrations.

Ethylene glycol ingestion causes acute renal failure in addition to a metabolic acidosis. In addition, the metabolic acidosis is characterized by a high anion gap; thus, choice c is correct. In choice c, the anion gap is 34 (144 – 100 – 10), whereas in choice a, the anion gap is 12 (141 – 115 – 14), and in choice b, it is 13 (138 – 107 – 18). Choice a may refer to a patient with a distal or type I renal tubular acidosis. These patients have hyperchloremic or non–anion gap metabolic acidosis and are unable to lower urinary pH. Choice b may refer to a patient with a type IV RTA. Choice d refers to a patient with a low anion gap, as seen in multiple myeloma due to the positive charge of paraproteins. Finally, choice e may refer to a patient with mild renal insufficiency who has a mild metabolic acidosis with a normal or mildly elevated anion gap and mildly elevated potassium.

57–60. For the clinical scenarios in questions 57 to 60, select the best treatment option.

57. A 45-year-old woman who recently immigrated from India exhibits a 6-mm reaction on a Mantoux skin test during an immigration physical. She is well, with a normal physical examination and chest radiograph. She denies any history of a bacille Calmette-Guérin vaccination. What is the best approach?

a) No treatment
b) Isoniazid daily
c) Isoniazid plus rifampin
d) Ethambutol and pyrazinamide

Answer
The answer is a.

58. A 30-year-old man diagnosed with HIV infection 5 years ago shows a 6-mm reaction on the Mantoux skin test. He is well, with a normal physical examination and chest radiograph. A friend recently died while undergoing treatment for multiple drug-resistant tuberculosis. What is the best approach?

a) No treatment
b) Isoniazid daily
c) Isoniazid plus rifampin
d) Ethambutol and pyrazinamide

Answer
The answer is d.

59. A 27-year-old medical resident 9 months into his training at a rural community hospital shows a 10-mm reaction on the Mantoux skin test. Testing 9 months ago revealed no reaction. He is well, with a normal physical examination and chest radiograph. He does not recall caring for a patient with tuberculosis. What is the best approach?

a) No treatment
b) Isoniazid daily
c) Isoniazid plus rifampin
d) Ethambutol and pyrazinamide

Answer
The answer is b.

60. A 55-year-old woman who denies any exposure to tuberculosis is found to have a 10-mm reaction on the Mantoux skin test. She was negative at a pre-employment physical 2 years ago. She is well, with a normal physical examination and chest radiograph. She is currently living at home with her husband. What is the best approach?

a) No treatment
b) Isoniazid daily
c) Isoniazid plus rifampin
d) Ethambutol and pyrazinamide

Answer
The answer is b.

Discussion for Answers 57–60
Each individual must be stratified in terms of his or her risk of progressing on to tuberculosis. The benefit of prevention then needs to be weighed with the risk of drug therapy for each patient.

61. A 67-year-old man reports "lethargy." History and physical examination suggest no physical disease, but he is not sleeping well, has lost his appetite, is not enjoying his retirement, and is staying in bed for much of the day. He states that his wife has been trying to get him to play golf and bridge with his friends, which he used to enjoy doing, but he feels too lethargic and is not interested in socializing. You are concerned that he may be depressed, and you consider his suicidal risk. All the following statements about suicide are true, *except*

a) His age puts him in a high-risk group.
b) Women are more likely to attempt suicide and successfully complete it than men.
c) Family history of suicide is a risk factor for suicide.
d) History of recent loss, such as retirement, is a risk factor for suicide.
e) Being single puts one at greater risk of suicide than being divorced.

Answer and Discussion
The answer is b. Suicide among men peaks at age 75 years and among women at 55 years. The predominant age groups for suicide are the elderly (older than 65 years) and adolescents (15–24 years). Women are more likely to attempt suicide (3:1), but men are more likely to complete it (3:1). History of recent loss, such as retirement or bereavement, is a risk factor for suicide. Marital status is important in assessing suicide risk. Single individuals have a higher suicide risk than those who are divorced. Widowed individuals are at higher risk than those who are married.

62. Which of the following statements regarding complications of mechanical ventilation in patients with acute respiratory distress syndrome (ARDS) is false?

a) Barotrauma is often a significant direct cause of death in ARDS patients.
b) Tissue breakdown, excessive tidal volumes, and low airway pressures predispose to barotrauma.
c) Although often accompanied by nonspecific findings, nosocomial pneumonia is an important cause of morbidity and mortality in ARDS patients, with a prevalence of approximately 55%.
d) The combination of a corticosteroid and a neuromuscular blocking agent used for paralysis in these patients can lead to a reversible myopathy.
e) Decreased radiolucency at the lung bases and the presence of the deep sulcus sign on a chest radiography are clues to the diagnosis of pneumothorax.

Answer and Discussion
The answer is a. ARDS patients who are mechanically ventilated have an intensive care unit course complicated by barotrauma, nosocomial pneumonia, and multiple organ failure. Additional complications

include deep vein thromboses, gastrointestinal bleeding, malnutrition, and side effects from sedatives and paralytics. Barotrauma occurs in a minority of ventilated patients (13% in one study), with barotrauma rarely directly causing death. The tissue breakdown seen in ARDS, high airway pressures, and high tidal volumes predisposes to barotrauma. Barotrauma is evidenced by the development of pneumothorax, subcutaneous emphysema, pneumomediastinum, and interstitial emphysema. Increased radiolucency at the lung bases and the presence of the deep sulcus sign on a chest radiograph are clues to barotrauma and pneumothorax. Nosocomial pneumonia is present in 55% of patients with ARDS and is accompanied by nonspecific findings. The combination of a corticosteroid and a neuromuscular blocking agent has been associated with a reversible myopathy that takes several months to resolve.

63. A 29-year-old woman presents to the emergency department with shortness of breath and palpitations. The triage nurse finds that she has a heart rate of 170 beats/minute and establishes an intravenous line, starts oxygen therapy, and attaches a cardiac monitor. You assess her airway, breathing, and circulation. Her respiratory rate is 24 breaths/minute and blood pressure 70/40 mm Hg. She starts to complain of chest tightness. What should your next step be?
a) Drawing blood for a metabolic profile and cardiac enzymes
b) Synchronized cardioversion
c) Defibrillation
d) Lidocaine
e) Verapamil

Answer and Discussion
The answer is b. This woman has unstable tachycardia with serious signs and symptoms, including hypotension, heart rate >150 beats/minute, shortness of breath, and chest tightness. According to the American Heart Association this should be treated with immediate synchronized cardioversion.

64. A 55-year-old man with a history of hypertension and renal artery stenosis is brought to the emergency department by his wife because of confusion. His blood pressure is 220/120 mm Hg. Head CT is negative for ischemia or hemorrhage. Which of the following additional findings would be *least* consistent with malignant hypertension?
a) Retinal hemorrhages and exudates
b) Hematuria
c) Proteinuria
d) Abrupt onset of confusion
e) Bilateral papilledema

Answer and Discussion
The answer is d. Malignant hypertension is characterized by elevated blood pressure. Retinal involvement may include hemorrhages, exudates, and bilateral papilledema. Malignant nephrosclerosis leads to hematuria, proteinuria, and acute renal failure. Renal injury is due to fibrinoid necrosis in arterioles and capillaries, the same pathology as in hemolytic-uremic syndrome and scleroderma. Neurologic symptoms may be due to intracerebral or subarachnoid bleeding, lacunar infarction, or hypertensive encephalopathy. The encephalopathy seen in malignant hypertension is insidious in onset, unlike the abrupt onset of encephalopathy seen in strokes or hemorrhage.

65. A 35-year-old woman reports dysuria. Other than minor back pain, for which she is taking ibuprofen, she has generally been healthy. Her vital signs and physical examination are normal. A urine dipstick test reveals 2+ leukocyte esterase. Urine is immediately sent to the laboratory for culture and sensitivity. She is told that she has a urinary tract infection and is given a prescription for trimethoprim-sulfamethoxazole. Two days later, the urine culture report indicates no bacterial growth. In interpreting this report, you consider all the following, *except*
a) Sterile pyuria may occur in the presence of urinary tract infection if this patient had been self-medicating with an antibiotic.
b) Sterile pyuria may be caused by an atypical organism such as *Chlamydia trachomatis, Ureaplasma urealyticum,* or *Mycobacterium tuberculosis.*
c) Obtain further history regarding her analgesic intake and consider chronic interstitial nephritis in the differential.
d) Repeat the urine dipstick because vaginal leukocytes may have contaminated the original urine sample.
e) You consider all of the above.

Answer and Discussion
The answer is e. True infection without pyuria is rare, but pyuria in the absence of infection does occur. This woman may have had a urinary tract infection that has been partially treated with an antibiotic. In addition, vaginal leukocytes may have contaminated the original urine specimen. Atypical organisms, such as *C. trachomatis, U. urealyticum,* or *M. tuberculosis,* may not grow in standard cultures, and thus patients who have symptoms of a urinary tract infection with a negative culture result should be tested for these organisms. Other important causes of sterile pyuria include chronic interstitial nephritis (hence the questioning regarding analgesic use), urothelial tumors, and nephrolithiasis. Nevertheless, the presence of leukocyte esterase and nitrite on urine dipstick has a 95% sensitivity and a 75%

specificity for the diagnosis of bacterial urinary tract infection.

66. All the following statements concerning acne vulgaris are true, *except*

a) It is the most common cutaneous disorder in the United States.
b) Inflammation results from the proliferation of the organism *Propionibacterium acnes* within follicles.
c) Typical areas affected include the face, neck, upper back, and upper arms.
d) A topical antibiotic may help eliminate *P. acnes* and thus help suppress the inflammation, but it may produce resistant strains.
e) Tetracyclines are effective only through inhibition of growth of *P. acnes*.

Answer and Discussion

The answer is e. Tetracyclines have direct anti-inflammatory properties, as well as inhibiting growth of *P. acnes*.

67. A 70-year-old man with a 10-year history of chronic obstructive pulmonary disease (COPD) comes to your outpatient office for routine follow-up. He is a current smoker with a 20 pack-year tobacco history. He has had two COPD exacerbations in the past year requiring hospitalization. His last episode was 1 month prior to this visit. He is currently on Advair 500/50 one puff twice a day, and Albuterol aerosols as needed. His laboratory values show white blood cell count of 6.7/mm^3, hematocrit 50%, platelets 350,000 μL, a normal basic metabolic profile, and a normal echocardiogram. Vitals signs were normal with SaO$_2$ of 92% at rest. SaO$_2$ drops to 89% on walking up two flights of stairs. His forced expiratory volume in 1 second (FEV$_1$)/forced vital capacity (FVC) is <70% predicted, and his FEV$_1$ is >50% but <80% predicted. All the following are indicated, *except*

a) Oxygen
b) Advise patient to quit smoking
c) Tiotropium
d) Pneumococcal vaccination
e) Influenza vaccination

Answer and Discussion

The answer is a. Infection is a frequent cause of COPD exacerbation. All patients with stable COPD should be offered pneumococcal vaccine, especially if they are 65 years or older, or with FEV$_1$ <40%. An influenza vaccine should be offered to all patients with COPD annually. All patients should be strongly encouraged to quit smoking because this can minimize exacerbations and retard the rate of FEV$_1$ decline. For all patients with COPD, a short-acting bronchodilator must be used on an as-needed basis and if that is insufficient to control

symptoms, a regularly scheduled long-acting inhaled bronchodilator or a long-acting inhaled anticholinergic should be added. Patients that continue to have exacerbations despite being on optimal long-acting inhaled bronchodilators may require inhaled corticosteroids. Indications for continuous long-term oxygen therapy in COPD patients include an arterial partial pressure of oxygen (PaO$_2$) of ≤55 mm Hg or arterial oxygen saturation (SaO$_2$) of ≤88%. If patients have cor pulmonale, right heart failure, or hematocrit >55%, oxygen is also warranted. Long-term oxygen therapy improves quality of life and increases survival in these patients.

68. All the following statements regarding coccidioidomycosis are true, *except*

a) Endemic areas include south central California, southern Arizona, Nevada, and New Mexico.
b) Sixty percent of infections are asymptomatic.
c) Cutaneous manifestations, such as a nonspecific maculopapular or erythematous rash, are seen in 25% of patients, indicate disseminated disease, and portend a poor prognosis.
d) A focal bronchopneumonic infiltrate in a single lobe is the most common finding on chest radiography.
e) Eosinophilia may be seen in up to 25% of patients with coccidioidomycosis.

Answer and Discussion

The answer is c. Coccidioidomycosis is a fungal infection caused by the inhalation of the spore form of *Coccidioides immitis*. In the United States, endemic areas include south central California, southern Arizona, Nevada, New Mexico, and the western half of Texas. Most (60%) of patients are asymptomatic; however, the vast majority of symptomatic patients usually have a self-limited pneumonic process, and a minority progress to disseminated disease. Most symptoms are nonspecific; they include fatigue, nonproductive cough, chest pain, dyspnea, headaches, myalgia, and arthralgia. Cutaneous manifestations, such as a nonspecific maculopapular or erythematous rash, are seen in 25% of patients and do *not* indicate disseminated disease, nor does their presence portend a poor prognosis. On skin biopsy, a nonspecific vasculitic process with variable eosinophilic infiltration is usually seen. A focal bronchopneumonic infiltrate in a single lobe is the most common finding on chest radiography. Occasionally, two or more lobes may be involved. In addition, pleural effusion of clinically insignificant sizes may occur. Laboratory abnormalities include the presence of eosinophilia in 25% of patients and mild elevations of aspartate aminotransferase and alanine transaminase. Diagnosis is made by serologic means. A new enzyme-linked immunosorbent assay has a sensitivity of 98.5% and a specificity of 94.8%. Treatment usually consists of antifungal azoles in mild cases and amphotericin B in severe cases and in patients with concomitant HIV infection.

69. Emergency medical services brings a 55-year-old man with a previous history of coronary artery disease and prior myocardial infarction (MI) to the emergency department with severe substernal chest pain radiating to the left shoulder and jaw. Pain has been persistent for approximately 20 minutes. On questioning, he has experienced similar pain intermittently throughout the previous 48 hours. In addition to the pain, he has experienced shortness of breath, diaphoresis, and nausea. His pain improves somewhat after he is given two nitroglycerin tablets sublingually. His vital signs are stable, and his ECG reveals changes consistent with an anterior MI. He is admitted to the coronary intensive care unit. While there, severe systemic hypotension (blood pressure 80/30 mm Hg) and dyspnea develop. He is given vasopressor and inotrope support. A pulmonary artery catheter is placed. The pulmonary artery wedge pressure is 18 mm Hg, and the cardiac index is calculated to be 2.0 L/minute/m^2. All the following statements regarding this man's diagnosis are true, *except*

a) It is unusual for cardiogenic shock to develop in this man because in most patients it develops before presentation to the hospital.
b) The hemodynamic measurements obtained for this patient are consistent with those for classic cardiogenic shock.
c) Severe mitral regurgitation from a ruptured chordae tendineae or papillary muscle, cardiac tamponade, or rupture of the intraventricular septum may also lead to cardiogenic shock in the setting of an acute MI.
d) Urgent echocardiography with Doppler flow is indicated and would be helpful in narrowing the differential for this man's hypotension.
e) All the above statements are true.

Answer and Discussion

The answer is a. Cardiogenic shock, clinically described as severe systemic hypotension, cool extremities, and respiratory distress, occurs in approximately 6% to 7% of patients with acute MI. These patients are often older and of the female gender, and have an anterior or large infarction, previous MI, or diabetes mellitus. In the Global Utilization of Streptokinase and t-PA for Occluded Coronary Arteries I trial, however, only 0.8% of patients had shock on presentation to the hospital, with shock developing either suddenly (as in this patient) or gradually in the remaining 5.3% after admission. Most cases occur within 24 hours to days afterward, with cases occurring 1 week afterward being rare. Severe left ventricular dysfunction is the most common cause of cardiogenic shock, most commonly from an anterior MI. Right ventricular dysfunction does not usually lead to respiratory distress unless the left ventricle is

also involved. Acute mitral regurgitation from ruptured chordae tendineae or papillary muscle, ruptured intraventricular septum, or cardiac tamponade may all lead to cardiogenic shock from mechanical means. As with any patient who is in "shock" (hypoperfusion), other causes and types of shock must be ruled out. Echocardiography (either transthoracic or transesophageal) is essential in the initial evaluation of patients with cardiogenic shock. Not only is left and right ventricular function assessed, but also mechanical complications of MI can be ruled in or out. Finally, the insertion of a balloon-tipped pulmonary artery catheter can confirm the hemodynamic criteria for cardiogenic shock. The American College of Cardiology and the American Heart Association Task Force guidelines define cardiogenic shock as two subsets:

1. Pulmonary capillary wedge pressure >15 mm Hg, systolic blood pressure (SBP) <100 mm Hg, and CI <2.5 L/minute/m^2
2. Pulmonary capillary wedge pressure >15 mm Hg, SBP <90 mm Hg, and cardiac index (CI) <2.5 L/minute/m^2

Subset 2 has a worse prognosis.

70. An 87-year-old woman presents for a checkup. She has no complaints and considers herself healthy. On direct questioning, she confesses to falling in her home a few weeks ago but states that she was in no way injured. She is taking no medications. She remains in the family home where she raised her seven children and had lived with her husband for 65 years until he died there 5 years ago. Her children live nearby and visit her frequently. You perform a full history and physical examination and assess her with respect to her risk for falls. All the following are risk factors for falls, *except*

a) Increasing age
b) Female sex
c) A history of falls
d) Arthritis
e) Hypertension

Answer and Discussion

The answer is e. Postural hypotension, rather than hypertension, has been associated with falls. In the elderly, it is important to assess the risk factors for falls and to address them to prevent falls because falls are one of the most common problems that threaten the independence of the elderly and are associated with significant morbidity and mortality.

71. A 48-year-old man reports drooping of the face and difficulty in speaking for 48 hours. On examination, a paralysis of the upper and lower face is present on the right side. He cannot raise his eyebrows or close his eye tightly. Drooping of the right side of the mouth is present, and the nasolabial fold is smoothed out. Which of the following is true about the most likely cause of this man's symptoms?

a) This is an upper motor lesion.

b) The most common cause is herpes zoster of the external auditory meatus and geniculate ganglion, called *Ramsay Hunt syndrome*.

c) This is a rare condition occurring in approximately 1 in 10,000 persons in a lifetime.

d) This is permanent in 60% of patients.

e) There may be associated loss of taste sensation from the ipsilateral anterior two-thirds of the tongue.

Answer and Discussion

The answer is e. These clinical findings are consistent with Bell's palsy, in which there may be associated loss of taste sensation from the ipsilateral anterior two-thirds of the tongue. Clinically, this is a lower motor lesion. In an upper motor lesion of the facial nerve, there would be sparing of the frontalis muscle and an ability to raise his eyebrows. Ramsay Hunt syndrome is a lower seventh cranial nerve lesion associated with herpes zoster of the external auditory meatus and geniculate ganglion, but it is not the most common cause of this facial nerve lesion; the most common cause is idiopathic. This is a common condition occurring in approximately 1 in 60 or 70 persons in a lifetime. Bell's palsy is usually a self-limiting disease; most patients recover in a few weeks.

72. All the following signs are associated with diffuse toxic goiter (Graves' disease), *except*

a) Lid retraction

b) Ectropion

c) Lid lag

d) Exophthalmos

e) Ophthalmoplegia

Answer and Discussion

The answer is b. Ectropion is not associated with Graves' disease; it is common in the elderly and may be seen in chronic facial nerve palsy.

73. Your patient reports a history of penicillin allergy and requests desensitization. All the following statements are true, *except*

a) It is important to verify the history because the patient may incorrectly assume that a nonallergic side effect, such as a gastrointestinal side effect, is allergic in origin.

b) Fatal reactions to penicillin skin tests have been reported.

c) Skin testing should not be performed in patients with a high risk for an anaphylactic reaction, unless no alternative drug to a beta-lactam is available.

d) Patients with a positive skin test to penicillin are at a fourfold increased risk for an allergic reaction to cephalosporins.

e) Desensitization helps reduce the incidence of Stevens-Johnson syndrome, hemolytic anemia, and serum sickness associated with penicillin.

Answer and Discussion

The answer is e. Desensitization has no effect on the incidence of Stevens-Johnson syndrome, hemolytic anemia, or serum sickness associated with penicillin because these are all non–IgE-mediated reactions. Fatal reactions to penicillin skin tests have been reported, but they occur in <1% of those tested.

74. A 30-year-old fit man presents with deep vein thrombosis (DVT). He has a history of allergic rhinitis each summer. He has had no recent trauma or surgery and has not traveled in the past 6 months. He is adopted and does not have any medical family history. What is the most common underlying cause of DVT?

a) Factor V Leiden, activated protein C resistance

b) Protein C deficiency

c) Protein S deficiency

d) Antithrombin III deficiency

e) Dysfibrinogenemia

Answer and Discussion

The answer is a. Inherited thrombophilia is associated with a genetically increased risk for venous thromboembolism. Factor V Leiden mutation accounts for 40% to 50% of cases. Protein C, protein S, and antithrombin III deficiencies and dysfibrinogenemia are all causes of inherited thrombophilia, but they are less common.

75. Which of the following is not a correctly matched drug and side effect?

a) Enalapril and hyperkalemia

b) Hydrochlorothiazide and hypouricemia

c) Metoprolol and heart block

d) Nifedipine and peripheral edema

e) Prazosin and orthostatic hypotension

Answer and Discussion

The answer is b. Hyperuricemia, not hypouricemia, is a side effect of hydrochlorothiazide.

76. A 42-year-old woman presents with a pruritic erythematous rash around her neck after wearing a new necklace. In the past, she experienced a similar reaction to a cheap pair of earrings. All the following statements are true, *except*

a) Perfumes and cosmetics can produce the same type of response.

b) Diagnosis can be confirmed with a patch test read in 48 hours.

c) This type of reaction can be caused by topical medications, including antibiotics.

d) Poison ivy produces the same type of response.

e) This is a type II cell-mediated response.

Answer and Discussion

The answer is e. Contact dermatitis is a type IV cell-mediated response.

77. Occupational exposure is associated with lung cancer in all the following, *except*
a) Asbestos
b) Silica
c) Inorganic arsenic
d) Chromium compounds
e) Polycyclic hydrocarbons (coal by-products)

Answer and Discussion

The answer is b. Silica exposure is associated with the lung disease silicosis but not associated with lung cancer. Silicosis has several different clinical manifestations, including chronic simple nodules or progressive pulmonary fibrosis. The calcification of hilar lymph nodes produces a characteristic "eggshell" pattern. Patients with silicosis are at increased risk for the development of *Mycobacterium tuberculosis* infections—silicotuberculosis.

78. A 25-year-old man presents to the emergency department with fever, chills, cough, shortness of breath, and dyspnea on exertion. He is reluctant to give any further history. On examination, he is febrile, tachypneic, tachycardic, and normotensive. He appears to have significant muscle wasting. The physical examination is notable for the presence of oral thrush, poor dentition, normal lung examination, and rapid but regular heart sounds without evidence of murmur. Further laboratory testing and radiologic examinations are done. Meanwhile, a friend mentions that he was diagnosed with HIV infection 9 years ago and last saw his physician 3 months ago. Which of the following findings or additional history would be *least* supportive of the diagnosis of *Pneumocystis carinii* pneumonia?
a) CD4 count is 600/mm^3.
b) He has been on aerosolized pentamidine monthly.
c) Arterial blood gas readings taken while breathing room air are pH 7.43, PCO$_2$ 36 mm Hg, PO$_2$ 64 mm Hg, HCO$_3^-$ 28 mEq/L, and SaO$_2$ 93%.
d) Chest plain film reveals a right lower lobe consolidation.
e) Lactate dehydrogenase level is 550 U/L.

Answer and Discussion

The answer is a. The two most common laboratory abnormalities in HIV patients with *Pneumocystis carinii* pneumonia is a CD4 cell count <200/mm^3 and an elevated lactate dehydrogenase level. Although it is possible, *P. carinii* pneumonia is unlikely to develop in patients with CD4 counts >200/mm^3.

79. The following are true in regard to screening for sexually transmitted diseases (STDs) *except*

a) All patients being evaluated for STDs should be offered counseling and testing for HIV.
b) Asymptomatic women with risk factors for STDs should be screened for gonococcal or chlamydial infection during their annual pelvic examination.
c) HIV-infected patients should be screened annually for *Neisseria gonorrhoeae*.
d) Pregnant women should be screened for *Chlamydia*.
e) All sexually active women and pregnant women need to be screened for herpes infection.

Answer and Discussion

The answer is e. According to the 2006 Centers for Disease Control and Prevention treatment guidelines for STDs, all patients being evaluated for STDs should be offered testing for HIV. All women with risk factors for STDs should be screened for gonococcal or chlamydial infection annually and offered human papillomavirus vaccination if cervical cytology is normal. Hepatitis B screening should be offered to men who have sex with men (MSM), patients with a history of multiple sex partners or intravenous drug abuse. Sexually active MSM are recommended to undergo annual testing for *N. gonorrhoeae*, *Chlamydia trachomatis*, HIV, and syphilis. Pregnant women should be screened for *C. trachomatis*, HIV, hepatitis B, and syphilis infections. Patients with HIV should be screened annually for *N. gonorrhoeae*, *C. trachomatis*, syphilis, hepatitis B, and hepatitis C. Local and state public health departments should be kept informed of chancroid, *C. trachomatis*, *N. gonorrhoeae*, acute hepatitis B and C, HIV, and syphilis. The U.S. Preventive Services Task Force (USPSTF) recommends against routine serologic screening for herpes simplex virus (HSV) in asymptomatic pregnant women at any time during pregnancy to prevent neonatal HSV infection and routine serologic screening for HSV in asymptomatic adolescents and adults.

80–82. The following hemodynamic indices are obtained: CI, systemic vascular resistance (SVR), pulmonary vascular resistance (PVR), mixed venous oxygen saturation (SvO$_2$), and pulmonary artery occlusion pressure (PAOP). Which of the following diagnoses is most consistent with the parameters in questions 80 to 82?

80. CI ↓; SVR ↑; PVR Normal; SvO$_2$ ↓; PAOP ↑
a) Neurogenic shock
b) Hypovolemic shock
c) Cardiogenic shock
d) Septic shock
e) None of the above

Answer

The answer is b.

81. CI ↑; SVR ↓; PVR Normal; SvO$_2$ Normal ↓; PAOP Normal ↓

a) Neurogenic shock
b) Hypovolemic shock
c) Cardiogenic shock
d) Septic shock
e) None of the above

Answer
The answer is d.

82. CI ↓; SVR ↑; PVR Normal; SvO$_2$ ↓; PAOP ↑

a) Neurogenic shock
b) Hypovolemic shock
c) Cardiogenic shock
d) Septic shock
e) None of the above

Answer
The answer is c.

Discussion for Answers 80–82
In hypovolemic and cardiogenic shock, the CI is low, SVR is high, and SvO$_2$ is low, whereas the PAOP is low in hypovolemic shock and high in cardiogenic shock. Finally, in septic shock, an increased CI is present due to a drop in SVR, the SvO$_2$ may be either normal or elevated (reflecting the increased cardiac output), and the PAOP is either normal or depressed.

83. A 25-year-old heterosexual man with a single sex partner presents to his primary care physician requesting an HIV test. Which of the following would be the most correct statement?

a) Testing should not be done because he has no risk factors.
b) A positive enzyme immunoassay test would need confirmation with a Western blot to lessen the likelihood of a false-positive test result.
c) The false-positive and false-negative rates of the enzyme immunoassay and Western blot tests are related to the prevalence of HIV in the population being tested.
d) b and c.
e) None of the above.

Answer and Discussion
The answer is d. This man should be tested because he is requesting it. To diminish the chances of a false-positive result, a Western blot should be performed to confirm a positive enzyme immunoassay. Unlike sensitivity and specificity, the false-positive and false-negative rates are directly related to the prevalence of disease in the population. For example, the higher the prevalence of disease, the higher the false-negative rate will be; the lower the prevalence of disease, the higher the false-positive rate will be.

84. Which of the following is the leading cause of cancer deaths in the United States?

a) Lung cancer
b) Breast cancer
c) Colorectal cancer
d) Prostate cancer
e) Ovarian cancer

Answer and Discussion
The answer is a. Lung cancer is the leading cause of cancer death in the United States.

85. Which of the following statements regarding the amniotic fluid embolism syndrome (AFES) is true?

a) Disseminated intravascular coagulation with resultant hemorrhage develops in <20% of women with AFES.
b) Maternal mortality is reported to be approximately 20% with supportive therapy and surpasses pulmonary embolism as a cause of maternal mortality.
c) The majority of women diagnosed with AFES die from cardiogenic shock or its complications.
d) Noncardiogenic pulmonary edema develops in approximately 70% of patients who survive the first hours of AFES. The resultant damage of the alveolar capillary membrane produces a clinical pattern typical of adult respiratory distress syndrome.
e) None of the above.

Answer and Discussion
The answer is e. AFES occurs in 1 in 20,000 to 30,000 births in the United States and is associated with an 80% to 90% mortality in affected women. It is second only to pulmonary embolism as an aggregate source of maternal mortality. Of patients diagnosed with AFES, 86% die from cardiogenic shock or its complications. Left-sided heart failure is more common than right-sided heart failure. Disseminated intravascular coagulation develops in approximately 40% of patients. Of the patients surviving the first hours, noncardiogenic pulmonary edema develops in 70%. Although damage to the alveolar-capillary membrane occurs, the clinical pattern seen in these survivors is *not* typical of adult respiratory distress syndrome (ARDS). In contrast to the protracted course often seen with ARDS, these patients' conditions improve rapidly. Diagnosis and anticipation of the complications of AFES are crucial in affording patients the best chances for survival.

86. A 50-year-old cirrhotic male patient with a past medical history of smoking, substance abuse, and alcohol abuse presents with acute hemoptysis, wheezing, and fever. His examination shows a cachetic individual with diffuse wheezing and thermal burns on his fingers and thumbs. Chest radiograph show diffuse alveolar infiltrates. Complete blood count shows a white count of

14,000/mm^3 with eosinophilia. In regard to this patient's diagnosis, all the following are true *except*

a) Expectoration of black sputum is frequently seen.
b) He is at an increased risk for pulmonary infections.
c) Fresh-frozen plasma is indicated.
d) He is at higher risk for acquiring HIV.
e) Pneumothorax may be frequently encountered.

Answer and Discussion

The answer is c. Crack lung may occur within 48 hours of smoking of cocaine, which presents as diffuse alveolar infiltrates, eosinophilia, and fever. Patients may present with pleuritic chest pain, dyspnea with even mild exertion, dry or productive cough, wheezing, and hemoptysis. Melanoptysis or expectoration of black sputum is seen from inhalation of black carbonaceous residue from inflammable substances that are typically used to set fire to crack. Finger burns are seen from handling crack pipes. Cocaine users are at increased risk for pulmonary infections, malnutrition, HIV, and tuberculosis. Crack smokers often perform Valsalva maneuver after inhalation or exhale vigorously into each other's mouths to augment the uptake of the drug, which may lead to the development of pneumothorax, pneumomediastinum, and pneumopericardium.

87. A 76-year-old man admitted to the hospital 2 weeks ago for pneumonia and transferred to the intensive care unit (ICU) 1 week ago has been deteriorating for the past 3 days, requiring mechanical ventilation with full support and 100% oxygen. He has a history of coronary artery disease and chronic obstructive pulmonary disease. Given the poor prognosis, the ICU team meets with his wife. Which of the following statements is most valid?

a) Instruct the wife that the patient's prognosis is poor and that she will need to make a decision regarding her husband's thoughts on end-of-life issues.
b) Instruct the wife that because there is no "do not resuscitate" order on the chart, even if her husband's physicians believe that cardiopulmonary resuscitation is futile, it will have to be performed in the event of cardiopulmonary arrest.
c) If a durable power of attorney for health care is appointed, that person should be making decisions, but only in the absence of the patient's wife.
d) Because the prognosis is poor, the ICU team should be instructed to only run "slow" codes on this patient.
e) Use of pain medications can be construed as a form of physician-assisted suicide because these medications can hasten the patient's death.

Answer and Discussion

The answer is a. Because this man cannot make decisions about end-of-life issues, the responsibility falls on his wife to make the decision on his behalf.

Essentially, she is being asked to decide what he would want done, not what she would want done. In addition, if a durable power of attorney for health care has been appointed, this individual would be the surrogate decision maker, even if the wife were involved in the patient's hospitalization or illness. The individual with the power of attorney must also act on behalf of the patient and not merely project his or her own view. Finally, "slow" codes have no role in the care of a terminally ill patient because there is also no requirement that cardiopulmonary resuscitation be performed in the event that it has been deemed futile. Competent physicians who use standard pain medications in terminally ill patients who suffer from chronic pain are not engaging in physician-assisted suicide.

88. A 35-year-old woman traveling to Africa in 2 weeks presents to her local physician. She takes no medications and has been healthy. Which of the following statements is most accurate?

a) Malaria prophylaxis with chloroquine is recommended because travel to sub-Saharan Africa does not increase her chance of chloroquine-resistant *Plasmodium falciparum* exposure.
b) Mefloquine is the drug of choice in most chloroquine-resistant areas and is effective against all strains of *P. falciparum*.
c) Mefloquine should not be prescribed for individuals with cardiac conduction abnormalities because of the association with sinus bradycardia and a prolonged QT interval.
d) If this patient is pregnant and travel cannot be deferred, she should be given doxycycline because chloroquine and mefloquine have been shown to be teratogenic.
e) None of the above.

Answer and Discussion

The answer is c. Malaria leads to 1 million deaths out of 200 million cases worldwide each year. Of *P. falciparum*, *Plasmodium vivax*, *Plasmodium ovale*, and *Plasmodium malariae*, *P. falciparum* can lead rapidly to coma and death. Travel to sub-Saharan Africa poses the greatest risk for acquisition of *P. falciparum* for American travelers. Strains of *P. falciparum* are becoming more and more resistant to chloroquine; thus, mefloquine is the chemoprophylactic agent of choice in areas where chloroquine resistance prevails (Fig. 67.1). Adverse effects associated with mefloquine include nausea, dizziness, and vertigo. Mefloquine has been associated with neuropsychiatric effects, including inability to concentrate, bad dreams, paranoid ideation, seizures, and psychosis, as well as cardiac conduction abnormalities leading to sinus bradycardia and a prolonged QT interval. Pregnancy should not be a

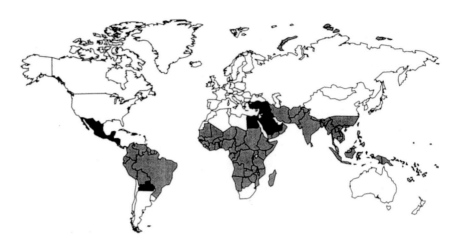

Figure 67.1 Distribution of malaria and chloroquine-resistant *Plasmodium falciparum*, 1997. (Reproduced with permission from Centers for Disease Control and Prevention Web site: www.cdc.gov.)

⬤ Chloroquine-resistant *P. falciparum*

⬤ Chloroquine-sensitive malaria

contraindication to chemoprophylaxis if travel cannot be postponed. Chloroquine is without any established teratogenicity, and mefloquine also seems to be safe. However, a tetracycline such as doxycycline should not be prescribed because of harmful effects on the fetus (dental discoloration and dysplasia and inhibition of bone growth).

89. A 65-year-old diabetic woman presents to the hospital with fever. On examination, her temperature is 38.5°C, heart rate 100 beats/minute, blood pressure 120/70 mm Hg, and respiratory rate 24 breaths/minute. On physical examination, she does not have a focus for infection. Laboratory studies reveal a white blood cell count of 12,500 cells/mm^3, and urinalysis is positive for leukocyte esterase and nitrites. Urine culture and blood cultures are ordered. Which of the following terms most accurately describes her present condition?
a) Septic shock
b) Systemic inflammatory response syndrome
c) Sepsis
d) Infection
e) Bacteremia

Answer and Discussion

The answer is c. The American College of Chest Physicians and the Society of Critical Care Medicine have defined this series of terms. This patient meets criteria for having systemic inflammatory response syndrome, as well as clinical evidence of urinary tract infection; thus, the most accurate term for her condition would be *sepsis*. The terms *infection* or *systemic inflammatory response syndrome* would not completely describe her condition. *Infection* is a microbial phenomenon characterized by an inflammatory response to the presence of organisms or to invasion of normally sterile host tissue by these organisms. *Bacteremia* is defined by the presence of viable bacteria in the blood. *Systemic inflammatory response syndrome* is a widespread inflammatory response defined by the presence of two or more of the following:

■ Temperature >38°C or <36°C
■ Heart rate >90 beats/minute
■ Respiratory rate >20 breaths/minute or PaCO$_2$ <32 mm Hg
■ White blood cell count >12,000/mm^3 or <4,000/mm^3 or >10% bandemia

Sepsis is the presence of systemic inflammatory response syndrome together with evidence of infection. *Severe sepsis* is the presence of sepsis associated with organ dysfunction, hypotension, or hypoperfusion. *Septic shock* is sepsis with hypotension despite adequate fluid resuscitation and the presence of lactic acidosis, oliguria, or acute mental status changes. *Hypotension* is defined as a systolic blood pressure of <90 mm Hg or a ≥40 mm Hg decrease from baseline (in the absence of other causes for the decrease).

90. A 32-year-old woman reports increasing shortness of breath. On examination, pulse is regular, and a parasternal heave is noted. On auscultation, a continuous, machinery-type murmur is present, with systolic accentuation that is best heard at the second intercostal space and left sternal border; it is also heard posteriorly. Clubbing and cyanosis of the toes is present, but not of the fingers. All the following are true of this condition, *except*
a) It is more common in men.
b) Endocarditis prophylaxis should be given before dental procedures.

c) Cyanosis of the lower extremities is associated with the development of Eisenmenger's syndrome.
d) Maternal rubella is associated.
e) It is normal anatomy before birth.

Answer and Discussion

The answer is a. Patent ductus arteriosus is more common in women than in men (3:1). It is associated with maternal rubella. Complications include infective endocarditis and Eisenmenger's syndrome. Prophylaxis for endocarditis is indicated, unless treatment by surgical ligation has been performed. Severe pulmonary vascular disease leads to a reversal of flow and shunting of deoxygenated blood to the lower extremities, resulting in differential cyanosis. Once Eisenmenger's syndrome has developed, corrective surgical intervention is no longer an option. The ductus is patent in the fetus but normally closes immediately after birth.

91. A 55-year-old woman reports gradually increasing shortness of breath. On examination, respiratory rate is 24 breaths/minute, and she appears in mild distress, with difficulty breathing. Blood pressure is 138/89 mm Hg. Expansion appears to be normal. Percussion is stony-dull in the right base and halfway up the right lung field, with diminished tactile fremitus, vocal resonance, and breath sounds in the same areas. Chest radiograph is consistent with the clinical suspicion of a pleural effusion. Which of the following statements about pleural effusion is true?
a) An exudative effusion is suggested by pleural fluid lactate dehydrogenase (LDH) more than one-third of the normal upper limit for serum.
b) A transudative pleural effusion is suggested by a ratio of pleural fluid LDH to serum LDH of >0.6.
c) Pulmonary emboli may be associated with both transudates and exudates.
d) The pleural effusion associated with neoplastic disease is usually transudative.
e) In a patient with a parapneumonic effusion, an indication for thoracostomy tube placement is a pleural fluid glucose level >50 mg/dL.

Answer and Discussion

The answer is c. An exudative effusion is suggested by at least one of the following three criteria, whereas a transudate has none of these criteria:

- Pleural fluid LDH more than two-thirds of the normal upper limit for serum
- A ratio of pleural fluid LDH to serum LDH of >0.6
- A ratio of pleural fluid protein to serum protein of >0.5

The pleural effusion associated with neoplastic disease is usually exudative. Pulmonary emboli are associated with both transudates and exudates. In a patient with a parapneumonic effusion, any of the following is an indication for thoracostomy tube placement:

- Pleural fluid glucose level <50 mg/dL
- Presence of gross pus in the pleural space
- Organisms visible on Gram stain of the pleural fluid
- Pleural fluid pH <7.0 and 0.15 U lower than arterial blood pH

92. Which of the following statements regarding renovascular hypertension is false?
a) Renovascular hypertension is less common in African Americans.
b) Renovascular hypertension should be suspected when an abrupt rise in plasma creatinine levels occur after the institution of an angiotensin-converting enzyme inhibitor.
c) Patients with moderate to severe hypertension who have recurrent episodes of acute "flash" pulmonary edema should be screened for renovascular hypertension.
d) The gold standard for diagnosing renal artery stenosis is the renal arteriogram.
e) The baseline plasma renin level is elevated in virtually all patients with renovascular hypertension.

Answer and Discussion

The answer is e. Renovascular hypertension is less common in African Americans. Moderately or severely hypertensive individuals with atherosclerosis, recurrent "flash" pulmonary edema, or asymmetric kidney sizes should be screened. In addition, patients who have a rise in serum creatinine levels after the initiation of an angiotensin-converting enzyme (ACE) inhibitor should also be screened. The gold standard for diagnosing renal artery stenosis is renal arteriography; however, intravenous pyelography can demonstrate delayed calyceal appearance of contrast and diminished kidney size in the presence of unilateral stenosis. In bilateral stenosis, the differences between the two kidneys may be difficult to see. Other methods for noninvasive screening are available; these include renogram, duplex Doppler ultrasound, magnetic resonance angiography, and spiral CT with angiography. The baseline plasma renin level is elevated in only 50% to 80% of patients with renovascular hypertension, but the administration of an ACE inhibitor can increase the predictive value of obtaining an elevated plasma renin level.

93. Which of the following features suggests a lower motor neuron lesion rather than an upper motor lesion?
a) Extensor plantar response
b) Hyperreflexia of the tendon reflexes
c) Increased tone (spasticity)

d) Fasciculation

e) Weakness

Answer and Discussion

The answer is d. Fasciculation suggests a lower motor neuron lesion rather than an upper motor lesion. Extensor plantar response, hyperreflexia of the tendon reflexes, and increased tone (spasticity) are all suggestive of an upper motor lesion. Weakness is a feature of both upper and lower motor lesions.

94. A 35-year-old man presents to the emergency department with abdominal cramping, tenesmus, and sudden onset of bloody diarrhea. On examination, he is toxic appearing with a temperature of 40°C. His blood pressure and respiratory rate are normal. He is slightly tachycardic. He is slightly tender in the right lower quadrant. A presumptive diagnosis is made after examination of the stool for fecal leukocytes and is confirmed by culture of rectal swab. All the following regarding this diagnosis are true, *except*

a) Stool examination would reveal polymorphonuclear leukocytes on methylene blue stain.

b) Blood cultures would likely reveal the causative organism.

c) In general, antibiotics are not essential in the treatment because this illness is generally self-limited in duration, averaging approximately 7 days.

d) Antibiotic treatment in infected patients can reduce the transmission of this organism to other individuals.

e) The development of bacteremia in this condition is more common in children than adults.

Answer and Discussion

The answer is b. Acute-onset bloody diarrhea, high fever, and crampy abdominal pain with tenesmus typically characterize *Shigella* gastroenteritis. Initial diagnostic tests may include an examination of stool stained with methylene blue to look for polymorphonuclear leukocytes. Fecal leukocytes may occur in other bacterial diarrheas and are not specific for *Shigella*. The presence of fecal leukocytes suggests a bacterial etiology. Culture of stool or rectal swab can confirm the diagnosis. Blood cultures are rarely helpful, as bacteremia is rare, occurring in approximately 7% of children but few adults. Patients at risk for bacteremia include those who are elderly, HIV infected, or malnourished, or those who have underlying diseases, such as diabetes mellitus. Untreated, shigellosis is highly contagious and is generally a self-limited illness with an average duration of 7 days. The organism can be shed in the stool for up to 6 weeks. For this reason, food handlers, day care workers and children, and health care workers should be treated, along with anyone with bacteremia. Treatment in the United States should start

with trimethoprim-sulfamethoxazole. Healthy adults with mild disease can alternatively be treated with norfloxacin. Ampicillin should not be used because of developing resistance. Treatment outside the United States generally consists of a quinolone.

95. A 65-year-old man reports back pain. In review of his chart, you note a hemoglobin level of 10 mg/dL and an elevated total protein. You entertain the diagnosis of multiple myeloma. Which of the following statements is true?

a) Among neurologic manifestations of myeloma, 5% to 10% of patients have extramedullary plasmacytomas leading to cord compression, although peripheral neuropathy is more common.

b) The anemia is most likely microcytic and hypochromic and occurs in a majority of patients with multiple myeloma.

c) Hypercalcemia is common, occurring in more than 50% of patients with multiple myeloma.

d) The two major causes of renal failure in these patients include cast nephropathy and hypercalcemia.

e) In myeloma kidney, casts accumulate in the loop of Henle. These casts are composed of precipitated monoclonal light chains that interact with Tamm-Horsfall mucoprotein synthesized by the tubular cells in the ascending limb of the loop of Henle.

Answer and Discussion

The answer is d. More than two-thirds of patients with multiple myeloma have a normocytic and normochromic anemia during their illnesses; 50% have rouleaux formation, and only approximately 15% have hypercalcemia. The most common neurologic manifestations are thoracic or lumbosacral radiculopathy, with a cord compression secondary to extramedullary plasmacytomas developing in 5% to 10% of patients. Peripheral neuropathy is rare. The major causes of renal failure in these patients are cast nephropathy and hypercalcemia. In myeloma kidney, casts formed by precipitating monoclonal light chains that interact with the Tamm-Horsfall mucoprotein (synthesized by the tubular cells in the ascending limb of the loop of Henle) accumulate in the distal and collecting tubules.

96. All the following statements concerning rhinitis are true, *except*

a) An increased risk of allergic rhinitis exists if there is a family history of allergic rhinitis.

b) Eosinophils can be seen on Wright's-stained nasal secretions.

c) Over-the-counter oral sympathomimetic agents may provide some relief of congestive symptoms, but they can cause elevation of blood pressure and can be dangerous in patients with hypertension or in those at risk for cardiac events.

d) Nasal sympathomimetic agents are an excellent choice for long-term symptom relief.

e) Hot and spicy foods may produce an episodic rhinitis termed *gustatory rhinitis*, which is a vagally mediated reflex.

Answer and Discussion

The answer is d. Nasal sympathomimetic agents are not to be used for long-term symptom relief. Their use is limited to 2 to 3 days to avoid the development of rhinitis medicamentosa. In rhinitis medicamentosa, rebound nasal congestion occurs after the discontinuation of a strong nasal decongestant, creating a vicious cycle, with the patient restarting the nasal spray to treat the congestion, which is directly caused by the nasal spray itself.

97. A 56-year-old man asks for advice concerning a nodule seen on a chest radiograph obtained during a physical examination for a new job. Which of the following statements concerning a solitary pulmonary nodule is true?

a) It is a single, radiologically visible lesion that must be surrounded on all sides by pulmonary parenchyma.

b) The upper limit in size is 2 cm.

c) The type of malignancy most commonly presenting as a solitary pulmonary nodule is small cell carcinoma.

d) It may present with associated pleural effusion.

e) It may present with associated mediastinal lymphadenopathy.

Answer and Discussion

The answer is a. The definition of a solitary pulmonary nodule is a single radiologically visible lesion that is within and surrounded on all sides by pulmonary parenchyma. It is not associated with potentially related pathology, such as pleural effusion or mediastinal lymphadenopathy. The upper limit of the size of a nodule may be 3 or 4 cm; larger lesions are considered masses. Adenocarcinoma most commonly presents as a solitary pulmonary nodule; small cell carcinoma usually presents as a central endobronchial lesion.

98. A 21-year-old woman with a history of sickle cell disease is admitted to the hospital with a pain crisis. This is her sixth admission in the past 4 years. She has been on folate and hydroxyurea therapy as an outpatient. On the day of admission, her temperature is 39°C, blood pressure 130/90 mm Hg, pulse 120 beats/minute, and respiratory rate 12 breaths/minute. Her physical examination reveals that she is in moderate distress. Her head, eyes, ears, nose, and throat examination is

unremarkable, as are her pulmonary and cardiovascular examinations, except for tachycardia. The abdomen is soft and nontender, with normal bowel sounds. Examination of her extremities does not demonstrate any edema. Initial laboratory tests show a normal chemistry profile. Complete blood count (CBC) shows that her white cell count is 15,000/mm^3, hemoglobin level is 7.5 mg/dL, and hematocrit is 20%. Which of the following is *least* appropriate in the initial management of this patient?

a) Continuous intravenous fluids: dextrose water with potassium chloride at 200 mL/hour

b) A narcotic analgesic given for adequate pain control

c) Packed red blood cell transfusion, 2 U, each over 4 hours

d) Cultures of blood and urine, chest radiograph, and careful examination of the skin for a potential source of fever and infection

e) Reticulocyte count

Answer and Discussion

The answer is c. Packed red blood cell transfusions are the least appropriate choice for a patient with sickle cell anemia. The reticulocyte count is essential in ruling out the possibility of an aplastic crisis. Cultures of the blood and urine, along with chest radiography, help rule out infection. Pain control and intravenous hydration are the mainstays of therapy for patients with a sickle cell crisis.

99. A 76-year-old man admitted to a general medicine ward for pneumonia is found by a nurse to be unresponsive and without a palpable pulse or spontaneous breathing. As the first physician to the scene, you confirm the absence of pulse and respiration. You then ask the respiratory therapist to establish an airway and begin mask-bag ventilation. Meanwhile, leads are placed for cardiac monitoring. A subclavian central access line had already been placed 2 hours before the arrest. The initial rhythm seen is pulseless electrical activity at 70 complexes/minute. A Doppler ultrasound, operated by the nurse, is unable to detect a blood pressure. Cardiopulmonary resuscitation is initiated. According to the American Heart Association guidelines on the advanced cardiac life support protocol, all the following steps are appropriate in the initial management of this patient, *except*

a) Give epinephrine, 1 mg intravenously.

b) Order a draw of arterial blood for blood gas and chemistry.

c) Begin synchronized direct-current cardioversion.

d) Start intravenous fluid infusion after bolus.

e) Order (but do not wait for) a portable chest radiograph and examine the patient for equal breath sounds bilaterally.

Answer and Discussion

The answer is c. This man is in cardiopulmonary arrest. Specifically, his electrical cardiac activity is pulseless electrical activity. All the choices are appropriate in the initial management of pulseless electrical activity, except synchronized direct-current cardioversion. In addition to pneumothorax, hypoxia, and hypotension, other causes of pulseless electrical activity that must be investigated in the initial management of these patients include cardiac tamponade, hypothermia, massive pulmonary embolism, drug overdose, hyperkalemia, severe acidosis, and massive myocardial infarction. Atropine may also be given in the event of bradycardia or relative bradycardia.

100. In the patient from question 99, the cardiac monitor now reveals a wide complex tachycardia; heart rate is 120 beats/minute. Blood pressure is now 80/50 mmHg. In the interpretation and treatment of this patient's rhythm, which of the following statements is incorrect?
a) If a wide complex tachycardia cannot be differentiated between supraventricular tachycardia (SVT) and ventricular tachycardia (VT), the patient should be treated initially with low-dose verapamil intravenously.
b) The presence of coronary artery disease in this patient would make the diagnosis of VT more likely than SVT.
c) The recurrence of a wide complex tachycardia over the past few years in the same patient would make it more likely that this is SVT.
d) The observation of cannon "a" waves would make the diagnosis of VT more likely.
e) None of the above.

Answer and Discussion

The answer is a. In the treatment of wide-complex tachycardia (heart rate > 100 beats/minute, QRS duration 120 milliseconds or more), if one cannot diagnose it as SVT, verapamil, adenosine, or a beta-blocker should not be given because they can lead to rapid deterioration in the presence of VT and hypotension. The presence of coronary artery disease is a strong predictor of VT rather than SVT. Multiple recurrences of the tachycardia over more than 3 years suggest SVT, and the development of the tachycardia after the recent diagnosis of myocardial infarction suggests VT. Finally, the observation of cannon "a" waves indicates atrioventricular disassociation and thus VT.

101. A 32-year-old woman presents with slurred speech and ataxia. You have seen her previously with two episodes of blurred vision, 10 and 6 months ago. On examination of her lower extremities, she has increased tone and bilateral spasticity and weakness. Bilateral ankle clonus is present, and the plantar reflexes are extensor. You consider the possibility of multiple sclerosis (MS). Which of the following statements about MS is true?
a) It is more common in men.
b) The predominant age at presentation is 50 to 65 years.
c) Northern European descent or living in a temperate climate are risk factors for MS.
d) CT and MRI are equally sensitive in the diagnosis of MS.
e) Cerebrospinal fluid examination that suggests the diagnosis of MS includes a normal or slightly low protein level, a low level of γ-globulin immunoglobulin G, and negative serology for syphilis.

Answer and Discussion

The answer is c. Northern European descent or living in a temperate climate are risk factors for MS. MS is more common in women. The predominant age at presentation is 16 to 40 years. MRI is more sensitive than CT in the diagnosis of MS. Cerebrospinal fluid examination that suggests the diagnosis of MS includes a normal or slightly *high* protein level (50–100 mg/dL), a *high* level of γ-globulin IgG, and negative serology forsyphilis.

102. All the following statements regarding renal tubular acidosis (RTA) are true, *except*
a) All forms of RTA are characterized by a normal anion gap (hyperchloremic) metabolic acidosis.
b) Proximal (type 2) RTA originates from the inability to reabsorb bicarbonate normally in the proximal tubule and is marked by a urine pH > 7.5 and the appearance of filtered bicarbonate during bicarbonate infusion. This is often associated with Fanconi's syndrome.
c) The most common causes of distal (type 1) RTA in adults are autoimmune disorders, such as Sjögren's syndrome and other hyperglobulinemic states.
d) Distal RTA is associated with hyperkalemia, unless decreased tubular sodium reabsorption occurs, in which case hypokalemia is present.
e) Type 4 RTA is due to aldosterone deficiency or resistance of the tubular cells to aldosterone; typically, urinary pH is acidic, and serum bicarbonate is > 17 mEq/L.

Answer and Discussion

The answer is d. All forms of RTA lead to a normal anion gap metabolic acidosis. Fanconi's syndrome is a generalized proximal tubular dysfunction and is most often associated with proximal or type 2 RTA. In Fanconi's syndrome, glucose, phosphate, uric acid, and amino acids are also spilled inappropriately, in addition to bicarbonate. The most common causes of Fanconi's syndrome in adults include the excretion of light chains in multiple myeloma and the use of a carbonic anhydrase inhibitor. Multiple myeloma should be excluded in all patients with a proximal RTA unless another cause is identified. Urinary pH is variable in proximal RTA. Distal RTA results from defects in hydrogen ion secretion: decreased proton pump (H^+-adenosine triphosphatase) activity, hydrogen back-leak due to increased luminal membrane permeability, and reduction of the electrical gradient necessary for proton secretion due to decreased distal tubular sodium reabsorption. Distal RTA is often associated with hyperglobulinemic states. The urinary pH is inappropriately high (>5.5) and is often associated with hypercalciuria due to bone loss from the chronic metabolic acidosis. In addition, hypokalemia is often seen, unless it is caused by decreased tubular sodium reabsorption. In this case, hyperkalemia is seen. Type 4 RTA is due to either aldosterone deficiency or resistance by the tubular cells. The most common cause of aldosterone deficiency in adults is hyporeninemic hypoaldosteronism, seen in mild to moderate renal insufficiency (especially diabetic nephropathy). Finally, aldosterone resistance is commonly seen with potassium-sparing diuretics and chronic tubulointerstitial disease. It is associated with a mild metabolic acidosis due to the suppression of ammonia excretion due to hyperkalemia and an appropriately low urinary pH (<5.3) and serum bicarbonate >17 mEq/L.

103. The following are all risk factors for the development of carcinoma of the bladder, *except*
a) Cyclophosphamide use
b) Family history
c) Tobacco smoke exposure
d) *Schistosoma haematobium* infestation
e) Recurrent stones

Answer and Discussion
The answer is b. Transitional cell carcinoma of the bladder is more common than either squamous cell carcinoma or adenocarcinoma and has a more favorable prognosis. A risk factor for the squamous subtype includes schistosomal infestations. Other risk factors include aromatic amines present in the products of chemical dyes and cigarette smoke, recurrent stones or infection, and use of cyclophosphamide. Family history is not a risk factor for bladder carcinoma; it is a risk factor for renal cell carcinoma.

104. A 65-year-old man with a history of chronic renal insufficiency is now progressing to end-stage renal disease. In preparation for hemodialysis, you counsel him about the possible complications of chronic hemodialysis. Which of the following do you *not* discuss as a possible complication?
a) Gastrointestinal bleeding
b) Hepatitis
c) Dementia
d) Osteoporosis
e) Cerebrovascular accidents

Answer and Discussion
The answer is d. Osteomalacia, not osteoporosis, is a complication of dialysis. In addition to osteomalacia, aluminum toxicity is also associated with dialysis dementia. Hepatitis is a potential complication arising from the increased need for blood product transfusions. Liver failure arising from hepatitis can lead to portal hypertension that can lead to gastrointestinal (GI) bleeding. In addition, heparin used during dialysis can also increase the risk of GI bleeding. Cerebrovascular accidents and cardiovascular disease are seen with increased frequency in uremic patients, accounting for 50% of deaths of hemodialysis patients.

105. A 35-year-old woman who was diagnosed with HIV infection 9 years ago and has been reluctant to start treatment now presents to you for advice. You obtain her CD4 cell count, which is 200/mm^3, and her viral load (RNA-polymerase chain reaction), which is 30,000 copies/mL. In addition, a pregnancy test is negative. Of the following options, which would you recommend as the most appropriate initial therapy for this patient?
a) No treatment because she does not meet criteria for drug therapy
b) Didanosine, zalcitabine, and indinavir
c) Zidovudine
d) Zidovudine, didanosine, and nevirapine
e) Zidovudine and didanosine

Answer and Discussion
The answer is d. The criteria for the initiation of therapy in HIV-infected patients include acute HIV infection or, within the first 6 months of seroconversion, symptomatic HIV infection, or asymptomatic infection with a CD4 cell count <500/mm^3 or viral load (RNA-polymerase chain reaction) >20,000 copies/mL. Recommended initial therapy in these patients includes the combination of two nucleoside reverse transcriptase inhibitors (zidovudine, lamivudine, zalcitabine, or didanosine) and a protease inhibitor (indinavir, saquinavir, ritonavir, or nelfinavir). Therefore, choice b would be correct, except that the combination of zalcitabine and didanosine should be avoided because of possible toxicity. Alternately, one can use two nucleoside reverse transcriptase inhibitors and a nonnucleoside reverse transcriptase inhibitor (nevirapine, delavirdine, or efavirenz). Therefore, choice d would be the best choice. Combination therapy with two nucleoside reverse transcriptase inhibitors or monotherapy is not recommended. In the case of a pregnant woman, however, in the absence of the indications mentioned previously, monotherapy with zidovudine is indicated

in the second and third trimesters to reduce the risk of fetal transmission.

106. A 60-year-old man on your inpatient service for 3 days presented with melenic stools. He has been doing well; his hemoglobin has been stable at 13 mg/dL, and his vital signs have also been stable and normal. He arrived on the Friday of a holiday weekend, and you have been unable to schedule an esophagogastroduodenoscopy until tomorrow. You are paged by his nurse, who reports that he has been restless all afternoon, and now he is demanding and threatening to leave and go home. You immediately go to see the patient, surprised at the behavior described to you by the nurse because he had been very pleasant the previous 3 days. You look at his vital signs chart outside his room. His blood pressure has been rising over the past 24 hours and is now 170/98 mm Hg; on admission, it had been 128/76 mm Hg. He has also developed a sinus tachycardia of 118 beats/minute and a temperature of 37.8°C. When you enter the room, he appears agitated and tremulous and is pacing around the room. On seeing you, he states that he must leave. He appears to be watching something in the room and, on inquiry, states that he is watching the little angels who are flying around the room. Which of the following is most likely to cause this presentation?
a) Alcohol withdrawal
b) Alcohol intoxication
c) Opiate withdrawal
d) Schizophrenia
e) Personality disorder

Answer and Discussion
The answer is a. Restlessness, tachycardia, fever, hypertension, and visual hallucinations after 3 days in the hospital are most suggestive of withdrawal from alcohol. Similar presentations may occur with withdrawal from sedative hypnotics. Withdrawal from either alcohol or sedative hypnotics can cause seizures and may be life threatening. Alcohol intoxication is suggested by slow or slurred speech, confusion, gait disturbance, and nystagmus. Opiate withdrawal may present with agitation, but other features include dilated pupils, rhinorrhea, nausea, cramps, and restlessness. Schizophrenia does disturb thoughts and behavior and may have features of tactile, auditory, olfactory, and visual hallucinations, but it does not usually present with restlessness, tachycardia, fever, and hypertension. Personality disorder can present with agitated, aggressive, or violent behavior, but it is not usually associated with restlessness, tachycardia, fever, and hypertension.

107. All the following statements about the medication adenosine are true, *except*

a) The American Heart Association subcommittee on advanced cardiac life support protocol recommends adenosine as the initial drug of choice for hemodynamically stable paroxysmal supraventricular tachycardia (PSVT).
b) It should be administered as a rapid intravenous push followed by a fluid flush.
c) Patients frequently experience a few seconds of chest discomfort similar to ischemic chest pain.
d) In the treatment of PSVT, the rhythm can recur in up to 50% to 60% of patients.
e) The highest dose recommended for use in PSVT is 6 mg.

Answer and Discussion
The answer is e. The highest dose recommended for use in PSVT is not 6 mg. If 6 mg fails to convert the rhythm after 1 to 2 minutes, a dose of 12 mg should be administered. A 12-mg bolus may be repeated if needed, but the maximum single dose is 12 mg. Adenosine should be administered as a rapid intravenous push followed by a fluid flush because of its very short half-life.

108. In a confused elderly patient, which feature suggests a diagnosis of delirium rather than dementia?
a) Onset over months to years rather than hours to days
b) Postural tremor, myoclonus, and asterixis
c) Normal rather than slurred speech
d) Impaired recent memory and preserved distant past memory
e) Normal electroencephalogram

Answer and Discussion
The answer is b. The differentiation between dementia and delirium is important because of the many reversible underlying causes that require treatment in patients with delirium. Motor signs of postural tremor, myoclonus, and asterixis are suggestive of delirium rather than dementia. Dementia rather than delirium is suggested by onset over months to years rather than hours to days, normal rather than slurred speech, and impaired recent memory and preserved distant past memory. A normal or mildly slow electroencephalogram is found in dementia, whereas in delirium pronounced diffuse slowing is typically seen.

109. All the following statements regarding aspirin intoxication are true, *except*
a) Toxicity can result with plasma levels of 400 to 500 mg/L.
b) Respiratory alkalosis can occur due to stimulation of the respiratory center by salicylates.
c) A nonanion gap metabolic acidosis develops soon after the respiratory alkalosis.
d) Sodium bicarbonate should be given to alkalinize the plasma.
e) All the above are true.

Answer and Discussion

The answer is c. Aspirin is rapidly converted to salicylic acid in the body. Toxicity is seen in most patients with plasma levels of 400 to 500 mg/L. Therapeutic levels are 200 to 350 mg/L. Fatal overdose can occur with 10 to 30 g in adults. Salicylates directly stimulate the respiratory centers, promoting respiratory alkalosis. In addition, the accumulation of organic acids, including lactic acid and ketoacids, leads to a high anion gap metabolic acidosis. The lactic acidosis may be a response to the respiratory alkalosis. Most patients have either a combined respiratory alkalosis with metabolic acidosis or just a respiratory alkalosis. Finding just metabolic acidosis in these patients is rare. Treatment consists of minimizing absorption of the aspirin with the use of charcoal and preventing accumulation by alkalinizing the plasma with sodium bicarbonate. Urinary alkalinization may also aid in removal of salicylic acid from the body.

110. A 30-year-old man is evaluated for dyspepsia. His history is remarkable for an 11-lb weight loss in the past month, and he also complains of diarrhea. He denies any nonsteroidal anti-inflammatory drug use. On endoscopic examination, duodenal bulb ulceration is noted. Biopsy of the involved area is negative for *Helicobacter pylori*. What would be the most appropriate next step in managing this patient?
a) Culture of the biopsy specimen for *H. pylori*
b) A 4-week trial of oral famotidine with follow-up endoscopy
c) Breath test for *H. pylori*
d) CT of the abdomen
e) Serum gastrin level

Answer and Discussion

The answer is e. The coexistence of duodenal bulb ulceration with diarrhea is suspicious for Zollinger-Ellison syndrome. This patient also lacks risk factors for *H. pylori* or nonsteroidal anti-inflammatory drug use. Histologic evaluation for *H. pylori* is 98% sensitive, and workup with culture and breath test is redundant here. CT can be used to localize a gastrinoma, but the first step would be to evaluate the serum gastrin level.

111. A 26-year-old woman is undergoing autologous bone marrow transplantation for non-Hodgkin's lymphoma. On the third day of her admission, she is found to have a temperature of 39°C. She feels well, and the examination does not reveal any localizing signs of infection. Laboratory studies show an absolute neutrophil count of 420/mm³. What would now be the most appropriate management for this patient?
a) Close observation only
b) Blood cultures
c) Blood cultures and empiric treatment with an aminoglycoside and piperacillin
d) Blood cultures and empiric treatment with an aminoglycoside only
e) Blood cultures and empiric treatment with vancomycin and an aminoglycoside

Answer and Discussion

The answer is c. This woman has neutropenic fever. Neutropenia is defined as an absolute neutrophil count $<500/mm^3$. Patients with an absolute neutrophil count $<500/mm^3$ due to chemotherapy or marrow failure are at high risk for overwhelming bacterial infection. Blood cultures are indicated, and antibiotics should be commenced as soon as possible. Most antibiotic regimens target gram-negative bacilli. The choice of a beta-lactam and an aminoglycoside is appropriate. Vancomycin should be added only if the patient has signs of cardiovascular compromise, positive blood cultures for gram-positive cocci before final identification of the organism, recent quinolone prophylaxis, patients receiving intensive chemotherapy causing substantial mucosal damage or if methicillin-resistant *Staphylococcus aureus* or penicillin resistance is suspected.

112. A 27-year-old obese female patient with history of hypertension presents with complaints of burning pain, numbness, and tingling over the upper outer thigh. The pain worsens with walking and standing and is relieved with sitting. The patient rubs the outer thigh when describing the symptoms. Which of the following statements regarding her condition is *not true*?
a) Sensory loss is seen in a discrete area in the anterolateral thigh.
b) The straight leg raise is positive.
c) The deep tendon reflexes and motor strength are normal.
d) Avoiding tight garments is helpful.
e) Weight loss will benefit patient.

Answer and Discussion

The answer is b. Meralgia paresthetica or painful mononeuropathy of the lateral femoral cutaneous nerve occurs when the nerve is trapped as it passes through the inguinal ligament. It is a purely sensory nerve and has no motor component. Hence, neurologic symptoms are limited to sensory changes only, and the neurologic exam is otherwise normal. The straight leg raising test is negative. The deep tendon reflexes are normal, and muscle strength is preserved. There is no evidence of bone or joint abnormality, and treatment is reassurance and education. Pregnancy, diabetes, and obesity can predispose to the previous syndrome. Patients are advised to avoid tight-fitting garments. Physical therapy has not proven to be of any benefit.

If symptoms persist, carbamazepine, phenytoin, or gabapentin may be useful.

113. A 51-year-old man consults you because he is concerned about his risk of cardiovascular disease. His father died at 52 years of age from myocardial infarction. For exercise, he runs for 30 minutes five times per week. In discussing his diet, you find that he typically eats eggs for breakfast and usually has some sort of fast food for lunch on working days. He does not smoke or drink alcohol and is normotensive on examination. Results of fasting cholesterol and glucose testing are as follows:

Total cholesterol	231 mg/dL
Low-density lipoprotein cholesterol	161 mg/dL
High-density lipoprotein cholesterol	56 mg/dL
Triglycerides	72 mg/dL
Glucose	107 mg/dL

Liver function tests are normal. He is concerned that he may die of a heart attack and urges you to treat him with "some of the pills" that he has seen advertised. What would be the most appropriate response?
a) Explain that he should be treated with active diet therapy, and there is no need to start medication at this time.
b) Repeat his laboratory work in 3 to 6 months and discuss the matter further at that time if the lipid profile has not improved.
c) Evaluate for primary and secondary causes of hypercholesterolemia and institute drug therapy.
d) Reassure him, explaining that he is not at increased risk and that he should continue exercising.
e) Suggest that he take a glass of red wine four to five times per week.

Answer and Discussion

The answer is c. This man has two risk factors for coronary artery disease: being a man older than 45 years and a significant family history. The National Cholesterol Education Program suggests that with a low-density lipoprotein cholesterol level > 160 mg/dL, active drug therapy should be instituted. Although epidemiologic studies suggest that a lowered risk of coronary events is present in those consuming certain types of alcohol, the recommendation that someone who does not otherwise drink starts taking red wine is controversial.

114. A 52-year-old man reports bilateral ear pain. He describes no change in his hearing or any febrile episodes. His past medical history is notable for a history of episcleritis, and he has stiffness and pain in both upper extremities, which have been bothering him intermittently over the past 6 months. He had some epistaxis after taking ibuprofen for the stiffness and was advised to discontinue it by a pharmacist. On examination, tenderness and swelling of the cartilaginous portion of the ears is present. You have to talk loudly to be understood, and you note that the patient's voice is hoarse. What is the most appropriate initial management for this patient?
a) Start oral prednisone, 40 mg daily.
b) Prescribe a mild topical corticosteroid to be applied to the ears twice daily.
c) Prescribe a nasal decongestant for 2 weeks.
d) Request antinuclear antibody studies.
e) Restart ibuprofen.

Answer and Discussion

The answer is a. This man has the typical features of relapsing polychondritis. Disease activity can be suppressed with oral glucocorticoids. Nonsteroidal anti-inflammatory drugs, topical steroids, and decongestants are unlikely to affect the disease course. Anemia of chronic disease and an elevated erythrocyte sedimentation rate can be seen. Although rheumatoid factor and antinuclear antibody may be positive, they do not contribute to the diagnosis in this case.

115. You have encouraged a 42-year-old patient to exercise more. He has recently started to play soccer and now comes to you, complaining of back pain. The pain is worse on standing or bending and eased by sitting or lying down. The pain does not radiate. Pain is not reproducible on straight leg raising, and neurologic examination is intact. All the following statements concerning this patient's condition are true, *except*
a) Spinal manipulation can be helpful, if used in the first month of symptoms.
b) Biofeedback has proved to be helpful in reducing recovery time.
c) Controlled physical activity, nonsteroidal anti-inflammatory drugs, and muscle relaxants have a role in the initial management.
d) Bed rest for more than 4 days may lead to debilitation.
e) Lumbosacral strain is the most likely diagnosis.

Answer and Discussion

The answer is b. The most likely diagnosis is lumbosacral strain. Biofeedback has not been proven to reduce recovery time.

116. A 21-year-old woman reports a thin, malodorous vaginal discharge with vulvar itch. She is sexually active with more than one partner and does not use condoms. She thinks her last menstrual period was 3 weeks ago. Examination of the discharge reveals a pH of 5.0 and a fishy odor on addition of 20% potassium hydroxide solution. The saline wet preparation is significant for squamous cells covered by adherent bacteria. Which of the following statements relating to this patient is the most accurate?

a) Treatment of choice is oral metronidazole, 2 g.

b) Treatment of choice is oral metronidazole, 500 mg twice daily for 7 days.

c) There is no need for pregnancy testing at this time.

d) There are no findings indicating an increased risk of cervical carcinoma.

e) Treatment with ketoconazole is effective.

Answer and Discussion

The answer is b. Bacterial vaginosis is characterized by the appearance of clue cells on a saline wet preparation, as described. The vaginal pH is usually >4.5, and a fishy odor may be present on addition of 20% potassium hydroxide solution. The treatment of choice is metronidazole, 500 mg twice daily for 7 days. Intravaginal clindamycin cream may also be used in the first trimester of pregnancy, when metronidazole is contraindicated. Human papillomavirus has been implicated in the etiology of cervical cancer. Multiple sex partners, smoking, and HIV infection are considered to be risk factors for cervical cancer. Ketoconazole is an antifungal agent and is not effective for bacterial vaginosis.

117. A 46-year-old overweight postal worker has had multiple emergency department visits for chest pain. Cardiac catheterization done 1 month ago was significant for mild atherosclerotic disease. His past medical history is notable for hypercholesterolemia. Exercise stress testing was negative for ischemia. He is worried that he should not continue working and seeks further evaluation. Which of the following tests would be the most appropriate for this patient?

a) Bernstein test

b) Ambulatory ECG monitoring

c) 24-Hour pH monitoring

d) Endoscopy

e) Esophageal manometry

Answer and Discussion

The answer is a. This man has chest pain that is unlikely to be of cardiac origin. Reflux disease may mimic cardiac chest pain. A positive Bernstein test would imply that the symptoms are due to reflux and should be treated as such. With convincing evidence that the cause is noncardiac, further evaluation for atherosclerotic disease is redundant. The use of pH monitoring helps establish whether reflux is present, but it may not explain symptoms. Similarly, endoscopy and manometry evaluate for esophagitis and the mechanism of reflux, respectively.

118. A 38-year-old nurse is seen for symptoms consistent with recurrent hypoglycemia. On occasion, she has collapsed at work. Her plasma glucose has been noted as 48 mg/dL on one occasion when she felt faint at work. Her past medical history is notable for irritable bowel syndrome, and her mother is known to be an

insulin-requiring diabetic. Fasting laboratory values are as follows:

Plasma insulin	468 μU/mL (normal, 626 μU/mL)
C-peptide	8.0 ng/mL (normal, 1.02.0 ng/mL)
Proinsulin-to-insulin ratio	15%

What would be the most appropriate next step in management?

a) Angiography with selective venous sampling for insulin levels

b) Two-phase contrast CT

c) Trial of octreotide and two-phase contrast CT

d) Search for needlestick marks

e) Urinary drug testing

Answer and Discussion

The answer is e. This woman has a laboratory picture consistent with factitious hypoglycemia. The most likely cause is sulfonylurea abuse. Patients with access to drugs are at higher potential for abuse. An elevated C-peptide level makes surreptitious insulin use an unlikely cause. Angiography and CT may be used to search for an insulinoma. An insulin-producing tumor can cause hypoglycemia; however, the proinsulin-to-insulin ratio is usually >20%. Urinary testing is the most effective way to search for evidence of sulfonylurea intake.

119. A 28-year-old male medical assistant is seen in occupational health for pre-employment screening. He is asymptomatic, and his physical examination is normal. He undergoes drug screening and is offered a hepatitis immunization. He explains that a physician at his previous place of employment told him that he does not need hepatitis B immunization. You take samples for hepatitis B virus serology and ask him to return in 2 days when you will have the results. The following results are reported:

HbsAg	Negative
Anti-HBs	Positive
HBc	Negative
HbeAg	Negative
Anti-Hbe	Negative

What would be the most accurate advice for this patient?

a) He has a high level of infectivity and should not be employed under federal guidelines.

b) He has low-level infectivity and can be employed as long as universal precautions are followed.

c) He most likely has chronic hepatitis B virus infection and should have liver function testing.

d) All his sexual partners must be advised to undergo testing.

e) None of the above.

Answer and Discussion

The answer is e. It is important to be aware of common serologic patterns relating to hepatitis B. This patient is positive only for surface antibody, which is consistent with prior immunization or past exposure. Hepatitis E virus antigen is correlated with high infectivity, and its disappearance (appearance of anti-HBe) in infected patients heralds lower infectivity. Patients with chronic infection would be positive for hepatitis B virus surface antigen.

120. A 59-year-old diabetic man is seen in the outpatient clinic. He reports left-sided ear pain for the past 2 weeks. His wife describes a greenish exudate. His diabetes is well controlled, and he is known to be compliant with your recommendations. His medications include an oral hypoglycemic agent, and he does not have any allergies. However, to help himself get to sleep without discomfort, he has self-medicated with tramadol that was prescribed for his wife. He appears comfortable but is noted to have a temperature of 39.1°C. On examination, the external auditory meatus is exquisitely tender, and you note some friable reddish tissue. What would be the most appropriate next step in management?

a) Recommend instillation of a suspension of polymyxin B/neomycin/hydrocortisone four times daily for 7 days, with a scheduled return outpatient visit every 7 days until cure is achieved.

b) Prescribe clotrimazole 1% solution, three drops twice daily for 14 days.

c) Prescribe clotrimazole 1% solution, three drops twice daily for 14 days in combination with a topical steroid cream.

d) Prescribe clotrimazole 1% solution applied to a wick left in the ear canal and recommend avoidance of moisture entering the ear canal when he is bathing by use of cotton wool for plugging.

e) Admit him for intravenous antibiotics and possible debridement.

Answer and Discussion
The answer is e. Otitis externa is also termed *swimmer's ear*. Maceration of the skin of the external auditory canal is present, and there may be impairment of hearing as debris obstructs the canal. A greenish exudate suggests *Pseudomonas* infection. In uncomplicated cases, debris should be removed and a topical antibiotic applied. If bacterial infection is suspected, an antibacterial steroid solution is appropriate. A fungal infection is treated with clotrimazole solution applied locally for 14 days. Malignant otitis externa is more common in diabetics and is characterized by severe pain and fever. In this situation, there may be rapid spread of infection to local skin and bone, and immediate hospital admission for intravenous antibiotics is indicated.

121. A 45-year-old woman reports a neck mass. On examination, she is found to have a goiter with a rubbery consistency. A review of systems is positive for weight gain, fatigue, and cold intolerance. High titers of antithyroid peroxidase antibody are present on laboratory studies. All the following statements about this patient's diagnosis are true, *except*

a) Some patients present with symptoms of hyperthyroidism.

b) The prognosis is poor despite appropriate hormone replacement treatment.

c) A small increased risk of lymphoma exists.

d) An association with autoimmune diseases exists.

e) It is a common cause of hypothyroidism in the United States.

Answer and Discussion
The answer is b. This woman almost certainly has Hashimoto's thyroiditis, which is most common in middle-age women. On histopathological examination, lymphocytic infiltration of the thyroid gland is present. Antithyroid peroxidase antibodies are invariably present. The disease is associated with a number of other autoimmune disorders, such as chronic active hepatitis, pernicious anemia, and diabetes mellitus. The goitrous form is associated with HLA-DR5 antigen. The prevalence of Hashimoto's thyroiditis is believed to be increasing due to increased iodine intake. A goiter is the usual presentation. High titers of antithyroid peroxidase in pregnant women suggest an increased risk of miscarriage. Elevated thyroid-stimulating hormone is a marker for replacement therapy, and prognosis is usually good. Long-standing disease is associated with an increased risk of lymphoma.

122. A 28-year-old visiting student from India is seen in an urgent care facility. He reports that his friend's dog bit his hand 1 hour ago. The dog is apparently in good health. Examination of the affected hand reveals small, superficial puncture wounds. He does not have any allergies. He does not recall any childhood immunizations. What is the most appropriate management for this patient?

a) Thorough cleansing of the wound with soap and water only

b) Wound irrigation and a 7-day course of antibiotics, with observation of the dog for 10 days

c) Wound irrigation and tetanus and diphtheria toxoid immunization, with destruction of the dog

d) Irrigation, 7 days of antibiotics, tetanus and diphtheria toxoid immunization, tetanus immunoglobulin, and observation of the dog for 10 days, with repeat tetanus and diphtheria immunizations in 1 and 6 months

e) Irrigation, tetanus and diphtheria toxoid immunization, tetanus immunoglobulin, and observation of the dog for 10 days, with repeat tetanus and diphtheria immunizations in 1 and 6 months

Answer and Discussion
The answer is d. The appropriate treatment of animal bites before the appearance of local infection is of paramount importance. Appropriate prophylaxis for tetanus is necessary. It is uncertain whether this patient previously received tetanus immunization, and he should therefore receive tetanus immunoglobulin and a primary series of immunizations. Dog bites can cause local infection with multiple organisms and always raise a concern about rabies. Precautions for rabies involve observing the dog for 10 days by quarantine, if necessary. If the dog cannot be observed, then human rabies immune globulin and diploid vaccine should be administered to the patient. Minor abrasions should be cleaned thoroughly and puncture wounds irrigated. Antibiotic use is necessary if bites involve the hand or face, or if there is any sign of infection.

123–127. Match the following antihypertensive agents with the most appropriate association.

123. Drug of choice in severe pre-eclampsia

124. First-line therapy in all patients who have history of myocardial infarction or left ventricular dysfunction

125. Avoidance in patients with coronary artery disease and ongoing cocaine abuse

126. Initial choice for secondary prevention of stroke

127. Avoidance in a patient who is noncompliant with medications
a) Hydrochlorothiazide
b) Lisinopril
c) Labetolol
d) Atenolol
e) Clonidine

Answer and Discussion
123. The answer is c. The definitive treatment of preeclampsia is delivery. However, if the baby is preterm, labetalol is the first drug of choice for intravenous use in patients with pre-eclampsia.

124. The answer is b. Angiotensin-converting enzyme inhibitors (ACE-Is) are considered first-line therapy in all patients that have had an ST elevation myocardial infarction (MI), non-ST elevation MI with anterior infarct, diabetes (especially with microalbuminuria or proteinuria), and left ventricular systolic dysfunction. Angiotensin receptor blockers are used if the patient is intolerant to ACE-I.

125. The answer is d. Beta-blockers and drugs with mixed alpha- and beta-adrenergic blocking properties should probably be avoided in cocaine abusers because they may intensify cocaine-induced vasoconstriction and increase the risk of cardiovascular complications.

126. The answer is a. Current guidelines suggest that a diuretic or the combination of a diuretic and ACE-I may prevent recurrences of stroke.

127. The answer is e. Clonidine should be avoided in a noncompliant patient because missed doses lead to severe rebound hypertension.

128. A 69-year-old man is seen in the emergency department, complaining of substernal chest pain at rest. He is admitted to the hospital for further evaluation. He is known to have hypercholesterolemia and is a long-time smoker. No other past medical history is noted as being significant. On the morning of the second hospital day, he undergoes cardiac catheterization and is found to have single-vessel coronary artery disease. He undergoes what appears to be a successful angioplasty. He is started on aspirin and a beta-blocker. On the evening of the second hospital day, he complains of new-onset abdominal pain that is not relieved by morphine administered by the house officer. Physical examination of the abdomen is noted to be normal. His respiratory rate is 24 breaths/minute. ECG done during the pain is unchanged from his postprocedure tracing. Which of the following statements about this patient's condition is correct?
a) A thrombolytic should be administered as soon as possible.
b) The pain that he is experiencing could be explained by a condition that would manifest itself on abdominal radiography with the appearance of thumbprinting.
c) The ECG should not have been done because it is not useful in this context.
d) Beta-blockers are contraindicated in this heavy smoker.
e) The normal physical examination rules out bowel pathology as the cause of his abdominal pain.

Answer and Discussion
The answer is b. This man exhibits a clinical syndrome consistent with mesenteric ischemia.

129. A 22-year-old woman, a nurse, has mild discomfort and tearing of her right eye. She is afebrile. On examination, no purulent drainage is present, but there is hyperemia of the conjunctiva. Preauricular adenopathy is also noted. Which of the following is the most important recommendation?
a) Topical vasoconstrictive drops and cold compress alone
b) Oral tetracycline, 250 mg four times daily for 21 days
c) No specific medication, but a request for her to use thorough hand washing, not to share towels, and to remain away from work until her tearing has settled down
d) Cold compress for symptomatic relief alone

e) Gentamicin solution, one or two drops every 4 hours

Answer and Discussion

The answer is c. This woman has viral conjunctivitis. Preauricular adenopathy is a characteristic feature, but it is not always found. The infection is highly contagious, and patients should be cautioned to use strict hygiene. If the patient is in an occupation that may pose the risk of spread, time off work may be prudent. Symptomatic treatment can be helpful, but hygiene advice takes priority. Oral tetracycline is used in inclusion conjunctivitis to treat chlamydial infection. Gentamicin drops are indicated in chronic bacterial conjunctivitis.

130. A 56-year-old woman reports urinary incontinence. She explains that she has leakage of urine associated with laughing or making sudden movements. Her past medical history is notable for migraines and two uncomplicated pregnancies. A postvoid residual volume is recorded as 30 mL. Urinalysis is unremarkable. What would be the most appropriate management at this time?
a) Prompted voiding
b) Intermittent catheter drainage
c) Environmental manipulation
d) Fluid intake modification
e) Pelvic muscle exercises

Answer and Discussion

The answer is e. This postmenopausal woman has stress incontinence. The history shows leakage associated with increased intra-abdominal pressure. Instruction in pelvic muscle exercises can be effective, as can bladder training. Prompted voiding, fluid-intake modification, and environmental manipulation are strategies used in functional incontinence. Intermittent catheter drainage can be used in overflow incontinence.

131. All the following statements regarding chronic myelogenous leukemia (CML) are true, *except*
a) It is genetically characterized by the Philadelphia chromosome, a reciprocal translocation between chromosomes 9 and 22, t(9;22).
b) The translocation that accounts for the Philadelphia chromosome is most commonly found in all hematopoietic cell lines but not nonhematopoietic cell lines.
c) The translocation seen in CML is also seen in other myeloproliferative disorders, such as polycythemia vera and idiopathic myelofibrosis.
d) The propensity of CML to progress to acute transformation is approximately 90%, much higher than that seen for other myeloproliferative disorders.
e) Patients often present with a palpable spleen and have an elevated leukocyte count, often >200,000/mm³.

Answer and Discussion

The answer is c. CML is the only myeloproliferative disorder characterized by the Philadelphia chromosome, a reciprocal translocation between chromosomes 9 and 22. This translocation is commonly found in all hematopoietic cell lines, but not in nonhematopoietic cell lines. The propensity of the myeloproliferative disorders to progress to acute transformation is highest in CML (approximately 90%) and lowest for essential thrombocytopenia (<5%).

132. All the following statements are true, *except*
a) Chronic use of long-acting beta-agonists has been associated with loss of potency of bronchodilation and decreased duration of effect.
b) Zafirlukast is an orally administered leukotriene receptor antagonist.
c) Cromolyn is a mast cell stabilizer that has no known serious side effects.
d) Long-term use of high-dose inhaled steroids (>1,000 μg daily) has been associated with cataracts.
e) Oral candidiasis is a side effect associated with inhaled corticosteroids.

Answer and Discussion

The answer is a. The chronic use of long-acting beta-agonists has *not* been associated with loss of potency or decreased duration of effect in bronchodilation.

133. All the following are features of a third (oculomotor) cranial nerve palsy, *except*
a) Loss of taste in the posterior one-third of the tongue
b) Ptosis
c) Dilatation of the pupil
d) Outward and downward deviation of the affected eye
e) Absent pupillary reflexes

Answer and Discussion

The answer is a. Taste sensation in the posterior one-third of the tongue is transmitted via the glossopharyngeal nerve.

134. After an appendectomy, a 2-year-old boy has significant bleeding. His parents deny any bleeding tendencies in the family. Results of laboratory studies are as follows:

Platelet count	250,000/mm³
Bleeding time	<4 minutes
Prothrombin time (PT)	12 seconds (same as control)
Partial thromboplastin time (PTT)	28 seconds (same as control)

Which of the following is the most likely diagnosis for this patient?
a) Thrombasthenia
b) Protein S deficiency
c) Factor XIII deficiency
d) Prekallikrein deficiency
e) Factor XII deficiency

The answer is c. Acquired or inherited factor XIII deficiency frequently leads to significant bleeding. An assay for clot solubility in urea screens for this disorder because the bleeding time, platelet count, PT, and PTT are all normal. PTT is prolonged in patients with factor XII deficiency or prekallikrein deficiency, although no associated increase in bleeding tendency is present. Patients with thrombasthenia do not have normal bleeding times because defective platelet aggregation is present. Finally, patients with protein S deficiency often have a thrombotic rather than a bleeding tendency.

135. All the following are common presenting symptoms of depression and *Diagnostic and Statistical Manual of Mental Disorders*, Fourth Edition, criteria for major depression, *except*

a) Fatigue or loss of energy
b) Beliefs of worthlessness or guilt
c) Recurring thoughts of death or suicide
d) Auditory hallucinations
e) Significant weight loss or weight gain

The answer is d. Auditory hallucinations are not common symptoms of depression and are not included among the nine *Diagnostic and Statistical Manual of Mental Disorders*, Fourth Edition criteria, of which at least five are required for the diagnosis of major depression.

136. All the following are true of Horner's syndrome, *except*

a) Ptosis
b) Dilatation of the pupil
c) Anhidrosis
d) Interruption of sympathetic nerve fibers
e) Occasional association with apical bronchogenic carcinoma

The answer is b. Horner's syndrome is associated with constriction (miosis) rather than dilatation of the pupil.

137. A 45-year-old man was admitted to the intensive care unit 5 days ago for acute respiratory failure. Which of the following statements about this man's risk of catheter-related infection is *not* true?

a) Peripheral catheters placed in the lower extremity in comparison with those placed in the upper extremity increase the risk of subsequent catheter-related infection.
b) Central venous catheters placed into the internal jugular vein increase the risk, compared with those placed into the subclavian vein.
c) The duration of catheterization has been established as a significant risk factor for catheter-related infection.

d) Heparin-bonded central venous catheters reduce the risk of infections.
e) Catheters placed under emergency conditions are associated with higher rates of infection.

The answer is c. The duration of catheter placement has not been firmly established as a risk factor for catheter-related infection. Several studies demonstrated an increased risk with increased duration, whereas others demonstrated no increased risk.

138. Which of the following statements regarding the mortality of intensive care unit patients is *not* true?

a) The in-hospital mortality of mechanically ventilated patients presenting with status asthmaticus ranges from 10% to 38%.
b) The in-hospital mortality of mechanically ventilated patients with a history of chronic obstructive pulmonary disease who present with acute respiratory failure ranges from 20% to 60%.
c) Patients with adult respiratory distress syndrome who present without multiple organ failure have a mortality of approximately 35%.
d) Patients who have systemic inflammatory response syndrome have a mortality of <10%, but patients who progress to septic shock have a mortality of >40%.
e) Cancer patients who require mechanical ventilation have an average in-hospital mortality of >70%; however, patients presenting after bone marrow transplantation have only a 50% in-hospital mortality.

The answer is e. In general, cancer patients have a mortality of 50%. If they are ventilated, mortality rises to >70%. Furthermore, bone marrow transplantation patients who require mechanical ventilation have a mortality that exceeds 95%.

139. A 78-year-old African American man is brought to the emergency department by his family. He is known to have a mild baseline dementia but still lives alone and has been able to carry out the basic activities of daily living. The family states that over the past 24 hours, he has become more confused. He has been unable to tolerate anything to eat or drink for the past 2 days and has been incontinent of very loose feces, with nausea, vomiting, and a low-grade fever. On examination, he appears frail and is oriented to person but not to place or time. Skin turgor is decreased. Lying blood pressure and pulse are 128/68 mm Hg and 80 beats/minute, and standing readings are 86/50 mm Hg and 118 beats/minute. Examination of the respiratory, cardiovascular, and abdominal systems is normal. Which of the following statements concerning this man's condition is true?

a) You expect a urinary Na$^+$ level <25 mEq daily.
b) You expect a urinary Na$^+$ level >25 mEq daily.
c) If the serum Na$^+$ level is >150 mEq/L, vasopressin therapy should be considered.
d) Because of the high risk of seizures in this case, prophylactic phenytoin should be started.
e) You expect a urinary K$^+$ level >20 mEq daily.

Answer and Discussion

The answer is a. This man is hypovolemic from gastrointestinal fluid loss. The serum sodium is likely to be raised and the urinary sodium low (<25 mEq daily) because the kidneys are attempting to retain sodium to compensate for the lost volume. In the same way, potassium is lost in vomiting and diarrhea, and the kidney attempts to compensate for this with a reduced urinary loss of potassium. Vasopressin may be used in the syndrome of central diabetes insipidus, but not in this case. Phenytoin is not indicated in this patient.

140. Which of the following statements regarding the diagnosis of minimal change disease (MCD) is incorrect?
a) It accounts for 90% of nephrotic syndrome cases in children younger than 10 years, 50% in older children, and approximately 15% to 25% in adults.
b) On electron microscopy, diffuse fusion of the epithelial cell foot processes is seen.
c) A renal biopsy is necessary in both children and adults to confirm the diagnosis before the start of treatment.
d) Corticosteroids are the mainstay of therapy in MCD.
e) Nonsteroidal anti-inflammatory drugs are the most common cause of secondary MCD, and most affected patients concurrently have an acute interstitial nephritis.

Answer and Discussion

The answer is c. MCD is the most common cause of nephrotic syndrome in children (age younger than 10 years, 90%; older than 10 years, 50%), but accounts for only 15% to 25% in adults. Immunofluorescence and light microscopy do not show immune complex disease, but electron microscopy reveals diffuse fusion of the epithelial cell foot processes. Corticosteroid therapy is the mainstay of empiric treatment in children without biopsy because of the high frequency of MCD in this nephrotic population. Even in young adults (20–30 years), corticosteroids treat both MCD and focal glomerulosclerosis, the second most common cause of nephrotic syndrome. In older adults, other causes (e.g., primary amyloid, membranous nephropathy) of nephrotic syndrome must be ruled out with a renal biopsy before treatment. Nonsteroidal anti-inflammatory drugs, ampicillin, rifampin, and interferon all have been reported to cause secondary

MCD. MCD may be associated with an underlying hematologic malignancy (Hodgkin's disease and, less commonly, other lymphomas or leukemias), whereas solid tumors usually produce an immune complex–mediated disease such as membranous nephropathy.

141. All the following statements about cholesterol screening are true, *except*
a) Cholesterol lowering and, therefore, cholesterol screening are more effective in primary prevention than in secondary prevention.
b) Measuring blood cholesterol levels is widely accepted as a convenient, safe, and inexpensive screening test.
c) Elevated blood cholesterol levels increase the risk for coronary heart disease (CHD).
d) The effects on CHD from lowering cholesterol depend on the magnitude of the cholesterol reduction.
e) In men and women with CHD, cholesterol reduction retards or reverses the progression of atherosclerotic plaques and reduces mortality from CHD.

Answer and Discussion

The answer is a. Smith et al. pooled primary and secondary prevention studies, and their meta-analysis shows that the net benefit of cholesterol lowering depends on the underlying risk for death from CHD. The risks for developing and dying of CHD are much lower in primary prevention settings than in secondary prevention settings. Hence, cholesterol lowering is more effective in secondary prevention (patients who have had a myocardial infarction) than in primary prevention. The effects of lowering cholesterol on CHD depend on the magnitude of cholesterol reduction. Each 10% reduction in cholesterol levels is associated with roughly a 20% to 30% reduction in the incidence of CHD.

142. A 45-year-old African American woman presents to the emergency department with fever, cough productive of reddish sputum, shortness of breath, and dyspnea on exertion. She was well until approximately 5 days ago. She denies any chest pain, palpitations, abdominal pain, diarrhea, or neurologic symptoms. Her vital signs reveal that she is febrile, normotensive, and tachycardic. On examination, she appears in mild respiratory distress. She has a normal head, eyes, ears, nose, and throat examination. Her neck is supple without any lymphadenopathy. On examination of her lungs, decreased breath sounds and egophony are heard in the left lower base, and dullness to percussion is present in the same region. Cardiovascular, abdominal, and neurologic examinations are unremarkable. All the following regarding the diagnosis of community-acquired pneumonia in this patient are true, *except*
a) The clinical presentation of an abrupt illness with fever, chills, cough, and pleuritic pain is compatible with *Streptococcus pneumoniae* infection.

b) *S. pneumoniae* is the most common pathogen responsible for community-acquired pneumonia in all age groups.

c) *S. pneumoniae* is acquired through the nasopharynx and is carried asymptomatically by 50% of people at some point in their lives.

d) If this patient has *S. pneumoniae* infection, sputum culture will grow the organism in more than 80% of cases.

e) Mortality of patients with *S. pneumoniae* infection is low, even among intensive care unit patients, who experience a 25% mortality.

Answer and Discussion

The answer is d. *S. pneumoniae* is the most common pathogen associated with community-acquired pneumonia and accounts for up to 66% of bacterial pneumonia in some series in which serologic techniques were used. Nevertheless, the organism is isolated in only 5% to 18% of the cases. In fact, the sputum culture is negative in 50% of patients with bacteremic pneumococcal pneumonia. Fever, chills, cough with rusty-colored sputum, and abrupt-onset pleuritic pain are the symptoms often ascribed to pneumococcal pneumonia. Rales and tubular sounds are often heard over the affected lobe. Most cases are uncomplicated, and even among patients in the ICU, mortality is only 25%. Risk factors for the development of complications include age, pre-existent lung disease, AIDS or other forms of immunodeficiency, or nosocomial acquisition. Abscesses are usually culture positive and respond rapidly to drainage. Parapneumonic effusions are associated with concurrent bacteremia with penicillin–nonsusceptible pneumococci. Finally, the most serious complication, bacteremia, occurs in 25% of patients. This complication is increased in splenectomized patients. The use of the sputum Gram stain and sputum culture in the diagnosis of *S. pneumoniae* infection is debated, but these tests may sometimes aid in choosing the optimal antimicrobial regimen. Penicillin covers the majority of cases, but increasing resistance to penicillin is occurring, thus necessitating use of a cephalosporin or, in some cases with significant resistance, vancomycin.

143. A 40-year-old woman presents to you after reading an article in the newspaper about screening for ovarian cancer. She is concerned because although she comes for annual physical examinations and has her regular pelvic examinations, Pap tests, and all the tests that are recommended to her, nobody has told her that she needs to have screening tests for ovarian cancer. She feels very well and wants to remain so. She has no family history of ovarian cancer, but a friend was recently diagnosed with it. Her history and physical examination reveal nothing that suggests any increased risk of ovarian cancer. What would be the most appropriate next step for this patient?

a) Call your lawyer in case she has ovarian cancer and you missed it.

b) Test for the tumor marker CA125.

c) Perform transvaginal ultrasonography.

d) Test for the tumor marker CA125, and perform transabdominal ultrasound.

e) Explain to her why no screening is indicated.

Answer and Discussion

The answer is e. No expert group in the United States recommends screening for ovarian cancer in asymptomatic women. A National Institutes of Health consensus conference on ovarian cancer recommends a family history and annual pelvic examination for all women. Screening for CA125 and vaginal ultrasound are recommended only for those with presumed hereditary cancer syndrome.

144. A 34-year-old woman reports shooting pain between the third and fourth toes of her left foot that has progressively worsened over the past 5 months. The pain occurs with walking and is relieved by stopping and massaging the affected area. On examination, compression of the forefoot causes the patient to wince in pain. Which of the following is the most accurate statement relating to this patient's condition?

a) Elevating the heel of her shoe will help alleviate her pain.

b) Nonsteroidal anti-inflammatory drugs are effective.

c) Men and women are affected in equal numbers.

d) The condition is caused by the compression of interdigital nerves.

e) Surgical treatment is never indicated.

Answer and Discussion

The answer is d. This is a description of Morton's neuroma, a common cause of metatarsalgia. The condition is not caused by a true neuroma, but is due to an interdigital nerve fibrosis caused by irritation. Women are affected approximately five times more often than men, and wearing high-heeled or restrictive shoes aggravates symptoms. Patients should be instructed to wear low-heeled shoes with a wide toe box. Local injection with lidocaine can be helpful in avoiding surgery, which may be necessary.

145. All the following statements concerning asbestos-induced lung disease are true, *except*

a) Most patients are asymptomatic for at least 20 to 30 years.

b) Cough, sputum production, and wheezing are the most common presenting symptoms.

c) Antinuclear antibody and rheumatoid factor may be present.

d) Cigarette exposure increases the risk of lung cancer associated with asbestos exposure.

e) Asbestos exposure increases the risk of lung cancer associated with cigarette smoke exposure.

Answer and Discussion

The answer is b. Dyspnea is the most common presenting symptom of asbestos-induced lung disease. Cough, sputum production, and wheezing are unusual presenting symptoms and, if present, tend to be due to cigarette smoke rather than asbestos exposure. It is true that antinuclear antibody and rheumatoid factor may be present, as may a raised erythrocyte sedimentation rate, but these are not clinically useful, being nonspecific and not related to disease severity. The risk of lung cancer associated with exposure to both asbestos and cigarette smoke appears to be multiplicative. A 1979 report in the *Annals of the New York Academy of Science* showed that asbestos is associated with a 6-fold increase, cigarette smoking with an 11-fold increase, and both cigarette smoke and asbestos exposure with a 59-fold increase in risk of lung cancer.

146. A 35-year-old woman presents with "recurrent chest infections." She has a long history of asthma, but no other past medical history. She is a nonsmoker. In the past year, she has had several episodes of fever, malaise, and increased sputum production; twice, she had chest radiographs that showed infiltrates consistent with pneumonia. She now has recurrence of her symptoms. Chest radiography shows a parenchymal infiltrate in the left upper lobe and some atelectasis in the right base. Immediate skin test reactivity is positive for *Aspergillus* antigens, and she has serum antibodies to *A. fumigatus*. All the following statements concerning this woman's condition are true, *except*

a) Proximal bronchiectasis is a feature of this disease.

b) Peripheral blood eosinophilia >55/mm^3 is a feature of this disease.

c) Treatment should be an antimicrobial effective against *Aspergillus*.

d) Treatment should be a corticosteroid.

e) Serum IgE concentration >1,000 ng/mL is a feature of this disease.

Answer and Discussion

The answer is c. Allergic bronchopulmonary aspergillosis is a hypersensitivity reaction in patients with asthma. Colonization with aspergilli occurs, rather than infection, and an antimicrobial is not indicated. Treatment with a corticosteroid is very effective.

147. A 65-year-old man with a history of coronary artery disease and hypertension is admitted for unstable angina. He has been taking ticlopidine since his last angioplasty with stent placement. Vital signs reveal a temperature of 37.5°C, heart rate of 90 beats/minute,

blood pressure of 130/90 mm Hg, and respiratory rate of 12 breaths/minute. His lungs are clear, and his heart examination reveals a regular rate and rhythm, without an S$_3$ gallop or murmur. He has no peripheral edema. He is started on aspirin, metoprolol, nitroglycerin, heparin, and simvastatin. He is also given haloperidol for the "mental confusion" experienced in the coronary intensive care unit. One day later, a platelet count is obtained, showing 25,000 cells/mm^3. His creatinine level is 2.5 mg/dL. Review of medical records from 6 months ago reveals a normal platelet count and creatinine. Heparin is stopped, and a hematology consultation is obtained. The peripheral smear reveals a few fragmented red blood cells. Which of the following diagnoses is most consistent with these findings?

a) Splenic sequestration

b) Idiopathic thrombocytopenic purpura

c) Thrombocytopenia purpura

d) Heparin-induced thrombocytopenia

e) Systemic lupus erythematous

Answer and Discussion

The answer is c. Although this man has been on heparin, abnormal mental status, abnormal renal function, and the presence of fragmented red blood cells should raise the suspicion of thrombocytopenia purpura (TTP). In addition, ticlopidine has been associated with TTP.

148. According to the 2007 American Heart Association guidelines for the prevention of infective endocarditis (IE), prophylaxis is indicated in all the following *except*

a) Prosthetic heart valves, including bioprosthetic and homograft valves

b) A prior history of IE

c) Unrepaired cyanotic congenital heart disease, including palliative shunts and conduits

d) Hypertrophic cardiomyopathy with latent or resting obstruction

e) Cardiac valvulopathy in a transplanted heart

Answer and Discussion

The answer is d. According to the 2007 American Heart Association guidelines for the prevention of IE, prophylaxis is indicated in prosthetic heart valves, patients with a prior history of IE, "valvulopathy" in a transplanted heart, unrepaired cyanotic congenital heart disease, completely repaired congenital heart defects within the first 6 months after the procedure, or repaired congenital heart disease with residual defects at the site or adjacent to the site of the prosthetic device. Prophylaxis is no longer indicated in common valvular lesions such as bicuspid aortic valve, acquired aortic or mitral valve disease, mitral valve prolapse with regurgitation, and hypertrophic cardiomyopathy. High-risk procedures that warrant antibiotic prophylaxis include all dental procedures that involve manipulation of gingival tissue or the periapical region, or that involve perforation of the oral mucosa; all respiratory procedures that involve incision of the respiratory mucosa; all procedures in patients with ongoing gastrointestinal or genitourinary tract infection; all procedures on infected skin or musculoskeletal tissue; and surgery to place prosthetic heart valves or prosthetic intravascular or intracardiac materials.

149. A 46-year-old man with a past history of coronary artery disease and diabetes mellitus presents to your office for a routine checkup. He denies angina since undergoing coronary artery bypass graft 3 years ago. His activity is limited by osteoarthritis of the knees and hips. Medications include an angiotensin-converting enzyme inhibitor (ACE-I), a beta-blocker, aspirin, digoxin, insulin, and ibuprofen. Routine laboratory studies reveal a K^+ level of 5.8 mEq/L. All the following medications can cause an increase in potassium levels, *except*
a) ACE-I inhibitors
b) Insulin
c) Beta-blockers
d) Digoxin
e) Ibuprofen

Answer and Discussion
The answer is b. Beta-blocker and digoxin toxicity can produce hyperkalemia through the redistribution of potassium. ACE-I and nonsteroidal anti-inflammatory drugs, as well as trimethoprim, cyclosporine, and pentamidine, can produce hyperkalemia through renal mechanisms. Insulin, along with beta-agonists, causes redistribution and may produce hypokalemia.

150. A 25-year-old woman is noted on preoperative laboratory testing to have an abnormal complete blood count. She is otherwise well and awaiting a laparoscopy for chronic abdominal pain. Leukocyte count is 5,000/mm³, hemoglobin level is 12 mg/dL, hematocrit is 36%, and platelet count is 14,000/mm³; chemistry profile and serum creatinine are normal. On further questioning, she admits to easy bruising and heavy menses. Further testing is done. An antinuclear antibody test result is negative. Which of the following diagnoses is most consistent with these findings?
a) Splenic sequestration
b) Idiopathic thrombocytopenic purpura
c) Thrombocytopenia purpura
d) Heparin-induced thrombocytopenia
e) Systemic lupus erythematous

Answer and Discussion
The answer is b. Idiopathic thrombocytopenic purpura in adults normally presents as chronic idiopathic thrombocytopenic purpura, a more indolent form. Patients are more often women (3:1) 20 to 40 years

of age and have a history of easy bruising and menometrorrhagia. Because a low platelet count may be seen in systemic lupus erythematous, antinuclear antibody testing and bone marrow biopsies are often required to rule out other causes.

151. A 39-year-old man presents with a nonproductive cough for 6 to 8 months. He states that the cough is very irritating because he frequently has to speak in public. Six months ago, he saw your colleague who he reports told him that it was a "postviral cough" and gave him an albuterol inhaler, which he used twice a day for 4 months. He discontinued it 2 months ago because it did not help the cough. Further history reveals nasal discharge, frequent throat clearing, and no wheezing or shortness of breath. The cough is worse in the morning but does not wake him from sleep; it is not associated with exercise. On examination, he appears generally well; his respiratory rate is 12 breaths/minute, and his pulse is 72 beats/minute. Nasopharyngeal mucosa has a cobblestone appearance, and the presence of secretions is noted. Auscultation of the lung fields is clear with no wheeze. Cardiovascular and abdominal examinations are normal. You observe his inhaler technique, and it is good. What would be the most appropriate next step in his treatment?
a) Obtain spirometry to investigate for asthma.
b) Recommend restarting the albuterol in addition to an inhaled steroid.
c) Start a trial of an H_2 blocker.
d) Reassure him that the cough is probably postviral, and have him return in 3 months if the cough has not resolved.
e) Start a trial of a nasal steroid spray.

Answer and Discussion
The answer is e. Chronic cough is defined as a cough persisting for 3 weeks or longer. Postnasal drip, asthma, and gastroesophageal reflux represent approximately 90% of the causes found for chronic cough (and an even higher percentage in nonsmokers with a normal chest radiograph). The approach to such patients should include a detailed history, including a drug history to evaluate for the use of an angiotensin-converting enzyme inhibitor (associated with cough in 3% to 20% of patients taking one), and an appropriate physical examination. This man has a history of nasal discharge and frequent throat clearing, and examination revealed nasopharyngeal mucosa with a cobblestone appearance and the presence of secretions, all of which suggest postnasal drip. Hence, a trial of a nasal steroid spray is the most appropriate next step. No clues are suggestive of gastroesophageal reflux, but if there were such clues, a trial of an H_2 blocker would have been a possible option. Postviral cough can persist for up to 8 weeks after the acute syndrome but should resolve after 6 months

in this case. The diagnosis of asthma is not suggested as the most likely diagnosis here because no night-time or exercise-related symptoms are present, and 4 months of twice daily albuterol with a good technique had no effect on the symptoms. Therefore, persisting with albuterol and adding an inhaled steroid are not indicated, and at this point, spirometry would not be the best choice.

152. A 45-year-old man undergoing rehabilitation after hip surgery as a result of a motor vehicle accident is noted on a routine complete blood count to have a platelet count of 55,000/mm^3; at hospital discharge 3 weeks ago, it was 200,000/mm^3. He has been taking a narcotic analgesic and lorazepam, as well as subcutaneous heparin injections, since admission to the rehabilitation center. Heparin has been stopped. Peripheral blood smear is unremarkable, except for thrombocytopenia. Which of the following diagnoses is most consistent with these findings?
a) Splenic sequestration
b) Idiopathic thrombocytopenic purpura
c) Thrombocytopenia purpura
d) Heparin-induced thrombocytopenia
e) Systemic lupus erythematous

Answer and Discussion
The answer is d. This man has been receiving heparin subcutaneously since his surgery. The development of heparin-induced thrombocytopenia may occur from 5 to 10 days after the initiation of therapy. A nonimmunogenic thrombocytopenia (type 1) may occur in 10% to 20% of patients on heparin. It is characterized by a decrease in the platelet count in the initial days of therapy, with a return to normal range with continued therapy, and poses no clinical risk. Immunogenic thrombocytopenia (type 2) may occur in 2% to 3% of patients on heparin; however, it is characterized by a progressive decrease in platelet count, along with an increased risk of both venous and arterial thrombosis. The antigen is believed to be a heparin–platelet factor IV complex in most patients. Treatment is immediate discontinuation of heparin therapy. The diagnosis of heparin-induced thrombocytopenia must be made clinically, although better assays are becoming available to detect the presence of heparin-induced platelet antibodies.

153. A 39-year-old woman presents to the emergency department with shortness of breath and chest pain. She reluctantly confesses to smoking two packs of cigarettes per day, although she had told her primary care doctor that she had stopped smoking. The only medication she is taking is an oral contraceptive. The chest pain is sharp and "catches" when she takes a deep breath. She has no fever, cough, or sputum production. She had a history of deep vein thrombosis (DVT) approximately 6 months ago, for which she was treated with warfarin for 3 months. Her left calf has remained a little swollen since the incident of DVT. On physical examination, she is breathing uncomfortably and rapidly at a rate of 28 breaths/minute; pulse is regular at 110 beats/minute. The trachea is central, percussion is resonant, and breath sounds are normal in all areas. The chest pain is not reproduced on palpation, although it occurs on deep inspiration. You highly suspect that she may have a pulmonary embolus. All the following statements concerning the diagnosis of pulmonary embolus are true, *except*
a) In this case, a high-probability perfusion scan would indicate a high likelihood of pulmonary embolus.
b) In this case, a low-probability lung scan does not exclude the diagnosis of pulmonary embolus.
c) A raised D-dimer (>500 ng/mL) is highly specific for the diagnosis of pulmonary embolus.
d) Pulmonary angiography is the gold standard.
e) Echocardiography has a low sensitivity.

Answer and Discussion
The answer is c. An elevated D-dimer level (>500 ng/mL) is present in the majority of patients with pulmonary embolus, but raised levels are also found in malignancy and postsurgery. Therefore, a raised D-dimer level is not specific for pulmonary embolus. A D-dimer value <200 ng/mL contributes to excluding the diagnosis of pulmonary embolus, with a negative predictive value of 97% when combined with a nondiagnostic lung scan.

154. A 38-year-old woman comes in with a history of nightly insomnia for the past 5 years. She has "weird" sensations in her legs at night when she tries to sleep. This feeling is relieved when she moves her legs or gets up and walks. Her husband complains that she kicks during her sleep. All the following are true regarding her condition, *except*
a) The prevalence is twice as high for women compared with men.
b) A trial of oral iron therapy is indicated in premenopausal women.
c) Pregnancy causes temporary relief of symptoms in patients.
d) It is associated with diabetes.
e) Dopaminergic agents are considered the first line of treatment.

Answer and Discussion
The answer is c. Restless leg syndrome (RLS) refers to an upsetting and overwhelming urge to move the legs, or sometimes even the arms or trunk, when the patient lies down to sleep. Dramatic relief is provided by movement. The prevalence of RLS increases with

age up to 80 years and is twice as high in women as in men. Primary (or idiopathic) RLS may show a dominant inheritance pattern in 40% of the cases. Secondary causes include iron deficiency, dialysis, diabetes mellitus, venous insufficiency, vitamin deficiencies, lumbosacral radiculopathy, spinal stenosis, hypoglycemia, Parkinson's disease, and hypothyroidism. Pregnancy can cause or worsen RLS. Dopaminergic agents (levodopa, bromocriptine, pergolide, and pramipexole) are considered the first line of treatment in idiopathic RLS. Opiates (propoxyphene, oxycodone, and methadone), benzodiazepines (clonazepam), and anticonvulsant agents (carbamazepine and gabapentin) have been shown to improve the symptoms of RLS. Among patients with RLS, a high prevalence of iron deficiency is seen, and treatment of the iron deficiency has been reported to improve symptoms. A trial of oral iron therapy is indicated for all patients with RLS.

155. While on call in the hospital, you are walking through a ward when a nurse comes running to you, requesting your help with a patient whose doctor she is unable to locate. The patient is a 62-year-old man who has a heart rate of 38 beats/minute and is feeling lightheaded and short of breath. Which of the following statements concerning this situation is true?
a) Atropine, 1 mg intravenously, is an appropriate treatment if the patient is recovering from heart transplantation.
b) High-dose isoproterenol is an appropriate treatment for this bradycardia.
c) Adenosine is a first-line choice of drug therapy.
d) Transcutaneous pacing can be effective treatment, but it is often painful.
e) If the patient is unstable with a falling blood pressure, then synchronized direct-current cardioversion is the appropriate therapy.

Answer and Discussion
The answer is d. Atropine, 1 mg intravenously, is not an appropriate treatment if the patient is recovering from heart transplantation because denervated hearts do not respond to atropine; transcutaneous pacing or catecholamine infusion would be an appropriate therapy in this situation. Low-dose isoproterenol may be used with caution after other therapeutic options have failed, but at high doses, it is a class III drug, has been shown to be harmful, and is thus never an appropriate treatment for bradycardia. Adenosine is an appropriate first-line choice of drug therapy for some tachycardias, but not bradycardia. If a patient is unstable with tachycardia and a falling blood pressure, then synchronized direct-current cardioversion is appropriate therapy; however, if a patient with bradycardia is unstable, then transcutaneous pacing is indicated.

156. A 55-year-old man presents with confusion and fever. He presented with an acute inferoposterior myocardial infarction 1 week prior and underwent coronary angioplasty with stent placement to the right coronary artery. He has been receiving aspirin, metoprolol, and clopidogrel since the procedure. On physical examination, he is febrile (38.4°C), disoriented to place and time, his heart rate is 85 beats/minute, and his blood pressure is 95/73 mm Hg. The medical resident witnesses a short-lived tonic-clonic seizure while examining the patient. Although his postictal state lasts an hour, no focal neurologic abnormalities are detected on repeated neurologic examinations. A brain CT is unremarkable. Laboratory studies reveal the following:

Hematocrit	24%
White blood cells	7,100/mm^3
Platelets	11,000/mm^3
Prothrombin time	12 seconds
Partial thromboplastin time	31 seconds
Blood urea nitrogen	21 mg/dL
Serum creatinine	2.9 mg/dL
Lactate dehydrogenase	900 U/L
Direct Coombs' test	Negative

The next step in the management of this patient at this time is
a) Pulmonary artery catheterization placement for hemodynamic guided management
b) Intravenous fluid resuscitation and positive inotropic agents
c) Broad-spectrum intravenous antibiotics and cerebrospinal fluid analysis
d) Transthoracic echocardiography
e) Peripheral blood smear review

Answer and Discussion
The answer is e. Thrombocytopenia purpura (TTP) is an acute syndrome that affects myriad systems. The classic pentad of clinical features includes thrombocytopenia, microangiopathic hemolytic anemia, neurologic changes, renal function abnormalities, and fever. Because of the association between ticlopidine use and TTP, clopidogrel, a newer thienopyridine derivative whose mechanism of action and chemical structure are similar to those of ticlopidine, has largely replaced ticlopidine in clinical practice. Several reports showed, however, that TTP could also occur after the initiation of clopidogrel therapy, often within the first 2 weeks of treatment. Although TTP remains an extremely rare complication of clopidogrel, physicians should be aware of the possibility of this potentially life-threatening syndrome when initiating clopidogrel treatment.

157–159. Match the host defense defect with the clinical presentation in questions 157 to 159:
a) Common variable immunodeficiency

b) Selective IgA deficiency

c) Reduced activity of the late components of serum complement pathway: C6, C7, or C8

d) Complement deficiency factors H and I (alternate pathways)

e) Job's syndrome

157. A 19-year-old white woman with history of recurrent sinus and lung infections presents with weight loss, anemia, night sweats, and mediastinal lymph node enlargement by chest radiograph

158. Recurrent *Neisseria meningitidis* and *Neisseria gonorrhoeae*

159. Recurrent "cold" staphylococcal abscesses, failure to shed primary teeth, eczema, hyperimmunoglobulinemia E, and impaired neutrophil chemotactic responses

Answers and Discussion

157. The answer is a.

158. The answer is c.

159. The answer is e.

Common variable immunodeficiency is a primary immunodeficiency characterized by defective antibody formation. Among populations of European origin, common variable immunodeficiency is the most frequent of the primary specific immunodeficiency diseases. It affects men and women equally. The usual age at presentation is the second or third decade of life. The clinical presentation of common variable immunodeficiency disease is generally that of recurrent pyogenic sinopulmonary infections. Recurrent attacks of herpes simplex are common, and herpes zoster develops in approximately one-fifth of patients. An unusually high incidence of malignant lymphoreticular and gastrointestinal conditions is present in common variable immunodeficiency. A 50-fold increase in gastric carcinoma has been observed. Lymphoma, which seems to be the presenting illness in this patient, is approximately 300 times more frequent in women with common variable immunodeficiency than in affected men.

Deficiencies in both the late and early components of the complement system can lead to increased susceptibility to meningococcal infection. The risk of meningococcal disease for a person with a complement deficiency is estimated to be 0.5% per year. This represents a relative risk of 5,000, as compared with the incidence of meningococcal disease among persons without a complement deficiency.

Job's syndrome is an autosomal recessive disorder characterized by a defective neutrophil chemotactic response, with the development of recurrent cold staphylococcal abscesses and eczema. Patients also have elevated levels of immunoglobin E in the serum.

Questions 160–165. Match the disease with the laboratory findings in questions 160 to 165:

	Alkaline Phosphatase	Serum Serum Calcium	Parathyroid Hormone	Urine Calcium
a)	–	– or		–
b)				
c)	–	–	–	–
d)	–			or –
e)	–	–	– or	– or
f)	–	–	–	–

160. Osteoporosis

161. Metastatic neoplasm to the bones

162. Osteomalacia

163. Paget's disease

164. Primary hyperparathyroidism

165. Vitamin D excess

Answers and Discussion

160. The answer is b.

161. The answer is e.

162. The answer is a.

163. The answer is d.

164. The answer is c.

165. The answer is f.

Osteoporosis, the most common bone disease, is characterized by low bone mass and a disruption of the normal bony architecture, which undermines the structural integrity of the bone and leads to skeletal fragility and an increase in fracture risk. The chemistry panel of patients with osteoporosis is nonspecific. The diagnosis of osteoporosis is established by measuring bone mineral density. Ten percent to 20% of cancer patients are hypercalcemic. Hypercalcemia can occur through three major mechanisms in cancer patients: osteolytic metastases, tumor secretion of parathyroid hormone–related protein, and tumor production of calcitriol. Osteomalacia is a disease of decreased bone mineralization. The diagnosis of Paget's disease is usually made incidentally through a routine chemistry screen showing an elevated serum alkaline phosphatase concentration or through a plain radiograph obtained for some other reason. Serum calcium and phosphorus concentrations are normal in most patients with Paget's disease. The diagnosis of primary hyperparathyroidism is made by the demonstration of an inappropriate parathyroid hormone (PTH) value in the face of hypercalcemia. The serum phosphorus concentration may be decreased but is typically in the lower range of normal. Approximately 40% of patients with primary hyperparathyroidism are hypercalciuric. Vitamin D excess can cause hypercalcemia by increasing calcium absorption and bone resorption. PTH is usually suppressed by negative feedback of the high calcium levels.

166. A 75-year-old man presents with fatigue and decreased energy. He has lived alone since his wife died 2 years ago. His last physical examination was in 1978, when he changed jobs. He is edentulous, and he cooks for himself. On examination, temperature is 36.5°C, respiratory rate is 18 breaths/minute, heart rate is 83 beats/minute, and blood pressure is 142/87 mm Hg. His lung, heart, and abdominal examinations are unremarkable. Perifollicular hyperkeratotic papules containing hemorrhages and purpuric rash are noted on the backs of his thighs. Laboratory tests reveal the following:

White blood cells	4,239/mm^3 (normal differential)
Hemoglobin	9.8 g/dL
Platelets	145,000/μL
Mean corpuscular volume	101
Blood smear	Hypersegmented neutrophils and macrocytic red blood cells
Blood urea nitrogen	32 mg/dL
Serum creatinine	1.3 mg/dL
Antinuclear antibody	Positive

The most likely diagnosis is
a) Vitamin A deficiency
b) Vitamin B$_{12}$ deficiency
c) Folic acid deficiency
d) Vitamin C deficiency
e) Lead poisoning

Answer and Discussion

The answer is d. Although rare in the United States, ascorbic acid deficiency (vitamin C deficiency, scurvy) occurs mostly in severely malnourished individuals, drug and alcohol abusers, or those living in poverty. One group at particularly increased risk comprises adults living alone, most commonly men ("bachelor" or "widower" scurvy) but sometimes women, who have deficient dietary intake because of such factors as poverty, poor access to groceries, dementia, or nutritional ignorance. They mostly prepare their own meals.

The clinical syndrome seen in vitamin C deficiency is due to impaired collagen synthesis. The most distinctive cutaneous finding in scurvy is hemorrhagic skin lesions that usually occur in a perifollicular distribution, especially on the legs, where the hydrostatic pressure is highest. Besides fatigue and decreased exercise tolerance, symptoms of scurvy include ecchymoses, bleeding gums, petechiae, hyperkeratosis, Sjögren's syndrome, arthralgias, and impaired wound healing.

167. A 45-year-old woman reports being "off-balance" for the past several weeks. She has sustained several falls and was treated at the local urgent care clinic for skin lacerations and mild bruises. She reports no head injury but states that she consumed five cans of beer and enjoyed two to three martinis with dinner daily for the past 9 years. On review of systems, she complains of chronic abdominal pain. Her past medical history is remarkable for hypertension and weekly marijuana use. On examination, she is mildly delirious, her temperature is 35.4°C, blood pressure is 187/110 mm Hg, and pulse is 78 beats/minute. She has poor dental hygiene, horizontal nystagmus, diplopia, ataxia, and a distended abdomen. A kidney, ureter, and bladder examination reveals calcifications in the midepigastric area. A brain CT reveals cerebral atrophy without evidence of intracranial bleed or masses. Laboratory tests indicate the following:

Hemoglobin	11.6 g/dL
White blood cells	8,323/mm^3 (normal differential)
Platelets	138,000/μL
Mean corpuscular volume	107

The most likely explanation of her neurologic symptoms is which of the following?
a) Acute alcohol intoxication
b) Cocaine overdose
c) Wernicke's encephalopathy
d) Cerebellar degeneration
e) Korsakoff's psychosis

Answer and Discussion

The answer is c. Wernicke's encephalopathy is caused by thiamine deficiency. Alcoholics are the most commonly affected population in the United States. Patients with significant malnutrition are also at risk. The classic triad is ophthalmoplegia, ataxia, and confusion. Cardiovascular beriberi may coexist. The treatment of choice is parenteral thiamine (50 mg daily until the patient resumes a normal diet, which should begin before starting intravenous glucose infusion). Korsakoff's psychosis is a part of Wernicke's disease and may occur together with the other components of the illness. Cocaine inhibits catecholamine reuptake at adrenergic nerve endings, thus potentiating sympathetic nervous system activity. Tachycardia, hypertension, pyrexia, and mood stimulation are seen in cocaine overdose.

168. An 82-year-old white man with past medical history of hypertension, coronary artery disease, cerebrovascular accident, T12 compression fracture, and asthma presents with malaise; anorexia; hip and shoulder pain and stiffness; and an inability to arise from chair, walk, and care for himself. On further questioning, he reports a 3-month history of fatigue, weight loss, and bilateral shoulder and hip stiffness. He recalls feeling relief from his symptoms after self-administration of tapered corticosteroid doses taken during episodes of asthma exacerbation. On examination, he is afebrile, has limited range of motion of the hips and shoulders, and is unable to raise the right arm laterally above 30 degrees. Point tenderness at the subacromial bursa is noted. His examination is otherwise unremarkable. A brain CT shows no evidence of intracranial hemorrhage or recent infarct. Laboratory tests indicate the following:

Na^+	135 mEq/dL
K^+	4.1 mEq/dL
Blood urea nitrogen	21 mg/dL
Creatinine	1.1 mg/dL
HCO_3^-	23 mEq/dL
White blood cells	5,300/mm^3
Hemoglobin	10.0 g/dL
Platelets	389,000/μL
Westergren sedimentation rate	99 mm/hour
C-reactive protein	6.6
Creatine phosphokinase	241 U/L

He receives prednisone (20 mg/day) and exhibits dramatic subjective and objective improvement after 24 hours. Ten days after the initiation of prednisone, he has no further complaints, and his Westergren sedimentation rate and C-reactive protein levels have decreased to 22 mm/hour and 0.3, respectively; his Hgb level has increased to 12.3 g/dL. The most likely cause of this patient's musculoskeletal symptoms is

a) Inflammatory polymyositis
b) Fibromyalgia
c) Pseudo-osteoarthritis
d) Inclusion body myositis
e) Polymyalgia rheumatica

Answer and Discussion

The answer is e. Although this patient has several medical problems, note that the examiner is interested in the most likely cause of his musculoskeletal problems. Polymyalgia rheumatica is the leading diagnosis when an elderly patient presents with girdle pain and stiffness, increased acute-phase reactants, and anemia, especially when the symptoms improve with systemic glucocorticoids.

Polymyositis is less likely in the absence of elevated creatine phosphokinase and with the presence of muscle pain. Fibromyalgia does not cause the laboratory abnormalities described in this case. Pseudo-osteoarthritis is a condition that describes the progression of calcium pyrophosphate dihydrate crystal deposition disease to joint degeneration. Multiple joints are usually involved, but the most commonly affected joints are the knees, followed by the wrists and metacarpophalangeal joints. Inclusion body myositis is an idiopathic inflammatory myopathy that presents with the insidious onset of weakness over several years. Symmetric proximal lower extremity weakness is usually the first sign. Myalgias are encountered in approximately 40% of cases.

169. A 79-year-old African American man presents to the office for follow-up of hypertension and hyperkalemia. His past medical history is remarkable for long-standing diabetes mellitus and congestive heart failure. His medications include enalapril (5 mg/day), hydrochlorothiazide (25 mg/day), insulin (70/30, 20 U in am and 14 U in pm), digoxin (1.25 mg/day), metoprolol (25 mg/day), and aspirin (81 mg/day). He reports medical and dietary compliance and denies using any over-the-counter medications. On examination, he is afebrile, heart rate is 74 beats/minute, and blood pressure is 173/102 mm Hg. His weight is 73 kg, and his height is 5 ft, 10 in. A nonradiating systolic murmur, best heard at the apex, is auscultated. Abdominal examination reveals no bruits. Trace pitting pedal edema and decreased distal pulses are evident on lower extremity examination. His funduscopic examination reveals grade II arteriolosclerotic retinopathy on the Keith-Wagener-Barker classification scale. Laboratory studies obtained the morning of the visit were as follows:

Na^+	132 mEq/dL
K^+	5.9 mEq/dL
Blood urea nitrogen	58 mg/dL
Creatinine	1.8 mg/dL
HCO_3^-	21 mEq/L
Chloride	115 mEq/L
Calcium	8.4 mg/dL
Glucose	Fasting 198 mg/dL
Arterial blood gases (room air)	
PO_2	94 mm Hg
PCO_2	41 mm Hg
pH	7.31
O_2 saturation	77%

His aldosterone and renin activity shows low normal values, which do rise with postural changes and diuretics. The most likely cause of this patient's abnormalities is

a) Addison's disease
b) Conn's syndrome
c) Secondary aldosteronism
d) Hyporeninemic hypoaldosteronism
e) Iatrogenic Cushing's syndrome

Answer and Discussion

The answer is d. Hyporeninemic hypoaldosteronism is seen in elderly patients with diabetes mellitus or renal disease. Patients usually have mild renal insufficiency, hyperchloremic metabolic acidosis, and hyperkalemia. Coexisting hypertension and congestive heart failure are common in this patient population. The acidosis is best corrected by treating the hyperkalemia with cation exchange resins and, in the absence of contraindications, mineralocorticoid replacement.

170–172. Match the laboratory findings of a 72-hour fast with the most likely underlying cause of fasting hypoglycemia in questions 170 to 172:

	Insulin	C-Peptide	Urine Drug Screen
a)	–	–	
b)	–	–	
c)	–	–	Positive
d)	–	–	

170. Exogenous insulin use

171. Sulfonylurea use

172. Insulinoma

Answers and Discussion

170. The answer is b.

171. The answer is c.

172. The answer is a.

Plasma C-peptide distinguishes endogenous from exogenous hyperinsulinemia. C-peptide is high in patients with insulinomas and sulfonylurea-induced hypoglycemia. Plasma insulin values are high in patients with exogenous insulin administration, whereas plasma C-peptide values are appropriately low.

173–181. Correctly match the vitamin or mineral deficiency with their symptoms.

173. Bleeding gums, easy bruising, impaired wound healing, joint pains, loose teeth, malaise, tiredness

Answer and Discussion

The answer is g. Vitamin C deficiency causes bleeding gums, easy bruising, dental cavities, low infection resistance, nosebleeds, poor digestion, stress, weakened cartilages, blood clots, and impaired healing.

174. Acne, dry hair, fatigue, growth impairment, insomnia, hyperkeratosis, immune impairment, night blindness

Answer and Discussion

The answer is e. Vitamin A deficiency causes acne, allergies, colds, dry hair and skin, eye sties, hyperkeratosis, fatigue, insomnia, impaired growth, loss of smell, and night blindness.

175. Loss of vibration sensation, low stomach acid, mental disturbances, numbness, spinal cord degeneration

Answer and Discussion

The answer is f. Vitamin B_{12} deficiency causes appetite loss, diminished reflexes, fatigue, irritability, memory impairment, mental depression and confusion, pernicious anemia, and spinal cord degeneration.

176. Myocardial infarction, hyperactivity, insomnia, muscular irritability, restlessness, weakness

Answer and Discussion

The answer is d. Magnesium deficiency causes hypotension, hypothermia, tachycardia, confusion, disorientation, hair loss, hyperactivity, muscle tremors, nervousness, noise sensitivity, depression, muscle weakness, twitching, heart disease, and disruption in proper pH balance.

177. Anxiety, fatigue, glucose intolerance, adult-onset diabetes

Answer and Discussion

The answer is a. Chromium deficiency causes disturbed amino acid metabolism, increased serum cholesterol, impaired glucose tolerance, lack of energy, myopia, and protein/calorie malnutrition.

178. Delayed sexual maturation, impotence, alopecia, dysgeusia, delayed wound healing, and decubitus ulcers

Answer and Discussion

The answer is b. Zinc deficiency causes acne, brittle nails, decreased learning ability, delayed sexual maturity, eczema, fatigue, loss of taste and smell, poor appetite, poor circulation, poor memory, prolonged wound healing, and decubitus ulcers.

179. Cardiomyopathy and skeletal muscle dysfunction
a) Chromium
b) Zinc
c) Selenium
d) Magnesium
e) Vitamin A
f) Vitamin B_{12}
g) Vitamin C

Answer and Discussion

The answer is c. Selenium deficiency causes cardiomyopathy and skeletal muscle dysfunction.

180. A 63-year-old man with severe chronic obstructive pulmonary disease presents to the emergency department with severe respiratory distress. Arterial blood gas measurement is obtained as follows:

	Current	1 Month Ago (Office Visit)
PaO_2	51 mm Hg	59 mm Hg
PCO_2	73 mm Hg	51 mm Hg
pH	7.25	7.38

He continues to deteriorate despite maximal therapy, and mechanical ventilation is instituted.
Which of the following arterial blood gas values would be most desirable for this patient?

	PaO_2	$PaCO_2$	pH	FiO_2	SaO_2
a)	91	62	7.31	40%	94%
b)	55	42	7.43	50%	86%
c)	65	50	7.37	40%	93%
d)	65	40	7.47	40%	93%

Answer and Discussion

The answer is c. The goal of mechanical ventilation in patients with chronic obstructive pulmonary disease exacerbation is to achieve an arterial oxygen tension (PaO_2) of 60 mm Hg. Although higher levels increase the risk of oxygen toxicity, they do not increase tissue oxygenation. PaCO$_2$ should be brought as close to the baseline value (i.e., the value recorded when the patient was compensated) but not necessarily normalized. For this patient, choice c meets these criteria.

181. A 33-year-old woman at 34 weeks' gestation presents with petechial rash and epistaxis. Laboratory tests reveal the following:

White blood cell	6,000/mm^3 (normal differential)
Hemoglobin	14.8 g/dL
Platelets	18,000/μL
Chemistry profile	Normal
Bone marrow aspirate	Normal with abundant megakaryocytes

She is started on prednisone (60 mg/day). Four days later, she begins to have contractions, and delivery is expected within the next 12 hours. Repeat complete blood count reveals a platelet count of 31,000/μL. Your next step in management is which of the following?

a) Pulse glucocorticoid (Solu-Medrol, 1 g/day for 3 days)
b) Danazol, orally
c) Continuous platelet transfusion until 6 hours after delivery
d) Emergent plasma exchange
e) Intravenous gamma globulin

Answer and Discussion

The answer is e. The management of idiopathic thrombocytopenic purpura in the early stages of pregnancy is similar to the management of the disease in non-pregnant patients. Prednisone is the drug of choice for patients whose platelet counts are between 30,000 and 50,000/μL. Although splenectomy remains the most effective treatment for severe idiopathic thrombocytopenic purpura, splenectomy should be reserved for refractory cases that fail medical therapy. Intravenous immunoglobulin is a temporary therapy, especially useful for patients with severe thrombocytopenia who have to undergo urgent surgical procedures or those who go into labor.

182–187. For each patient listed, select the most likely set of liver function test findings.

182. A 23-year-old man develops mild icterus 48 hours after fasting. His examination is otherwise unremarkable.

183. A 28-year-old college student presents with right upper quadrant pain, diarrhea, anorexia, and fever 2 weeks after returning from a trip to Mexico.

184. A 55-year-old woman with 10-year history of progressive pruritus develops increasing abdominal girth and dark urine.

185. A 51-year-old farmer develops increasing abdominal girth over the preceding month. He presents with fever, abdominal pain, and vomiting. He drinks four to six beers every day and two glasses of wine with dinner.

186. A 35-year-old African American woman presents with progressive shortness of breath on exertion. Her chest radiograph reveals hilar lymphadenopathy and interstitial infiltrates. She is found to be anergic on skin testing.

187. A 49-year-old woman with history of hepatitis C and bipolar disorder was found unconscious. An empty bottle of acetaminophen was found on the floor.

Answers and Discussion

182. The answer is e.
183. The answer is a.
184. The answer is b.
185. The answer is d.
186. The answer is f.
187. The answer is c.

Gilbert's syndrome is the most common inherited disorder of bilirubin glucuronidation. Routine laboratory tests are usually normal, except for hyperbilirubinemia. Baseline bilirubin levels are usually <3 mg/dL. Certain stressors such as fasting (or receiving a lipidfree diet), febrile illnesses, and physical exertion cause further elevation in serum bilirubin levels, but the level usually stays <6 mg/dL. The bilirubin level returns to normal 12 to 24 hours after resuming normal diet, removal of the stressor, or both.

Hepatitis A infection is common in areas in which food and water hygiene and sanitation are suboptimal.

	Alanine Aminotransferase (ALT) (U/L)	Aspartate Aminotransferase (AST) (U/L)	Alkaline Phosphatase (U/L)	Total Bilirubin (mg/dL)	Albumin (g/dL)	PT/Control (Seconds)
a)	994	518	110	2.2	4.1	11.8/11
b)	87	81	902	6.1	3.1	14.8/11
c)	18,900	17,230	269	7.1	3.1	20/11
d)	63	273	121	3.7	2.2	16/11
e)	21	23	70	2.6	4.1	11.2/11
f)	44	46	444	0.9	4.5	12.2/11

The incubation period averages 30 days. Patients experience prodromal symptoms, including malaise, nausea, vomiting, anorexia, fever, and right upper quadrant pain. Jaundice and hepatomegaly are the most common physical findings in symptomatic patients. Serum aminotransferases are markedly elevated (usually >1,000 IU/dL); serum bilirubin (total and direct) and alkaline phosphatase are also elevated. Alanine transaminase (ALT) is commonly higher than aspartate aminotransferase (AST).

Ninety-five percent of primary biliary cirrhosis patients are women. Although fatigue and pruritus were once the most common presenting symptoms of primary biliary cirrhosis, presently up to half the patients are asymptomatic at diagnosis. Significantly elevated serum alkaline phosphatase is characteristic of primary biliary cirrhosis. The aminotransferases may be normal, and, when elevated, they rarely increase more than five-fold above normal. The serum bilirubin concentration becomes elevated in most patients as the disease progresses. Antimitochondrial antibodies are the serologic hallmark of primary biliary cirrhosis.

A disproportionate elevation of serum AST compared with ALT is the most common biochemical abnormality in alcoholic liver disease. Although the absolute values of serum AST and ALT are almost always <500 IU/L, the AST-to-ALT ratio is usually <2.0.

Although hepatic granulomas are present in almost all patients who have sarcoidosis with involvement of their gastrointestinal tract, clinically apparent liver disease is uncommon even in patients who have numerous hepatic granulomas. Mild elevation in alkaline phosphatase and γ-glutamyltransferase is the usual laboratory finding.

Liver function abnormalities peak from 72 to 96 hours after ingestion in patients with acetaminophen overdose. The plasma ALT and AST levels often exceed 10,000 IU/L. Total bilirubin concentration generally does not exceed 4.0 mg/dL, which is primarily indirect.

188. A 19-year-old man presents with dysuria and penile discharge for 5 days. He reports having unprotected sexual encounters with multiple prostitutes over the past 3 weeks. On examination, an indurated 2- to 4-cm warm, tender inguinal mass is palpated. An ultrasound examination of the groin suggests that the mass represents enlarged inguinal lymph nodes. A Gram stain of the discharge shows numerous neutrophils and gram-negative intracellular diplococci. Rapid plasma reagin is nonreactive, and HIV serology is negative. The next most appropriate step in management is
a) Give a single dose of ceftriaxone intravenously, 250 mg.

b) Give a single dose of ceftriaxone intravenously, 250 mg, and doxycycline for 7 days.
c) Give a single dose of ceftriaxone orally, 2 g, and doxycycline for 14 days.
d) Give a single dose of ceftriaxone (125 mg intramuscularly) and doxycycline (100 mg two times a day for 7 days), until *Chlamydia trachomatis* serology is back.
e) Await the results of culture and sensitivity testing, and counsel him regarding safe sex practices.

Answer and Discussion
The answer is d. Penile discharge should be treated aggressively, and the physician should look carefully for clinical and laboratory clues for coinfections with sexually transmitted diseases. The Centers for Disease Control and Prevention recommend concomitant chlamydia treatment for cases of presumed or confirmed gonorrheal infection at any site. Choice d represents the preferred recommended therapy.

Conversely, the history of exposure to several prostitutes and presence of inguinal lymph node enlargement in this patient is suspicious for concomitant lymphogranuloma venereum (LGV) infection. The diagnosis of LGV is difficult because there is no characteristic clinical presentation. Sexual partners of patients diagnosed with *Neisseria gonorrhoeae* who have had sexual contact with the infected patient within the past 60 days should be evaluated and treated, even if they were asymptomatic.

189. A 53-year-old man with a history of chronic pancreatitis and chronic hepatitis secondary to alcoholism presents to the emergency department complaining of worsening epigastric pain and dizziness. Recently, his chronic pain has been hard to control despite adequate pain medications. On examination, he is afebrile, orthostatic, and has heme-positive stool. Laboratory evaluation reveals the following:

Hemoglobin	5.0 g/dL
Platelets	402,000/μL
Mean corpuscular volume	86.4
White blood cell	9,800/mm^3
Prothrombin time	11.2 seconds
International normalized ratio	0.98
Partial thromboplastin time	31.1 seconds
Albumin	3.0 g/dL
Aspartate aminotransferase	81 U/L
Alanine transaminase	56 U/L
Alkaline phosphatase	377 U/L
Bilirubin	0.8 mg/dL
Amylase	55 U/L
Lipase	12 U/L

Fresh blood is apparent on gastric lavage, and an urgent esophagogastroduodenoscopy confirms the presence of fresh blood clots in the fundus, with multiple gastric varices and one bleeding varix. The bleeding site is successfully injected with epinephrine. Blood transfusion, octreotide, and propranolol therapy are initiated. The bleeding does not recur, and his hospital course is uncomplicated. Before discharge, which of the following diagnostic tests is indicated to further explore the cause of this patient's gastric varices?

a) Endoscopic retrograde cholangiopancreatography
b) Percutaneous transhepatic cholangiography
c) Visceral angiography
d) Transjugular hepatic biopsy
e) Radionuclide (hepatobiliary iminodiacetic acid) biliary scan

Answer and Discussion

The answer is c. Splenic and portal vein thrombosis is a relatively common complication of chronic pancreatitis. In patients with the disorder, studies have estimated a splenic vein thrombosis prevalence rate of between 5% and 24%. In a surgical series, a surprising 10% prevalence of portal or superior mesenteric vein thrombosis has been noted. Besides the fact that many cases are silent, splenic and portal vein thrombosis symptoms in chronic pancreatitis patients may be indistinguishable from the patients' chronic symptoms. Hence, it is not uncommon that many cases go undetected until patients present with complications of portal hypertension. Worsening of the chronic abdominal pain in chronic pancreatitis patients warrants further evaluation to rule out splenic and portal vein thrombosis. Visceral angiography is the diagnostic test of choice for splenic and portal vein thrombosis.

190. A 59-year-old man with a history of hypertension and end-stage renal disease develops refractory hypotension during dialysis. He has missed two dialysis sessions, and his blood urea nitrogen level on presentation is 109 mg/dL. He reports constant chest discomfort, dyspnea on exertion, and easy fatigability over the past week. On examination, he is alert and oriented, heart rate is 112 beats/minute and regular, and blood pressure is 88/57 mm Hg. On inspiration, his systolic blood pressure falls to 62 mm Hg. His jugular veins are distended and elevated to the jaw angle. Chest radiography shows cardiomegaly and mild interstitial edema, and the ECG reveals diffuse low voltage. The most appropriate next step in management is which of the following?

a) Start heparin infusion, aim for a prothrombin time of 55 to 75 seconds, and obtain lung perfusion scan.
b) Start dobutamine and place pulmonary artery catheter to guide management.
c) Infuse 1 L of normal saline followed by dextrose 5% in water and observe.

d) Admit to the telemetry unit and obtain a set of cardiac enzymes.
e) Admit to the ICU and obtain an urgent echocardiogram.

Answer and Discussion

The answer is e. Pericardial tamponade is a well-recognized complication in patients with chronic renal failure and uremic pericarditis. Pericardial tamponade is a medical emergency. The management of patients suspected of having pericardial tamponade includes aggressive fluid resuscitation and immediate echocardiography by a cardiologist trained to perform pericardiocentesis.

191–194. For each patient described with dysphagia, select the most likely diagnosis.

a) Esophageal carcinoma
b) Esophageal web
c) Achalasia
d) Gastroesophageal reflux disease
e) Scleroderma

191. A 42-year-old woman with a history of episodes of digital pallor

192. A 49-year-old man with recurrent chest pain and negative recent stress test presents with nocturnal cough

193. A 56-year-old man with a history of progressive dysphagia and constant retrosternal discomfort over the past 2 months who requests a prescription for a nicotine patch

194. A 48-year-old woman with long-standing menorrhagia and glossitis

Answers and Discussion

191. The answer is e.
192. The answer is d.
193. The answer is a.
194. The answer is b.

Raynaud's phenomenon is an early manifestation of scleroderma. Esophageal involvement in scleroderma is present in up to 50% of patients and includes burning pain in the retrosternal region. Gastroesophageal reflux disease and the subsequent esophagitis and esophageal spasm can cause retrosternal chest pain that mimics angina. It is not uncommon for these patients to undergo full cardiac evaluation before the attention is directed to the esophagus. Smoking is a risk factor for esophageal carcinoma. Plummer-Vinson syndrome is a combination of iron-deficiency anemia and a hypopharyngeal web in middle-age women.

195. A 42-year-old Boy Scouts scoutmaster presents with a painful violet pustule on the dorsum of his right hand that appeared 2 weeks after returning from a fishing trip. A crusted ulcer is seen in the midportion of the pustule. He denies any constitutional symptoms. The most likely cause of this infection is

a) *Mycobacterium leprae*
b) *Pseudomonas aeruginosa*
c) *Sporothrix schenckii*
d) *Rickettsia rickettsii*
e) *Mycobacterium marinum*

Answer and Discussion

The answer is e. Swimming pool and fish tank granuloma is caused by *Mycobacterium marinum*. A small violet nodule or pustule appears at a skin surface exposed to contaminated water. A crusted ulcer or a small abscess evolves thereafter. The incubation period is 1 to 8 weeks after exposure. *Mycobacterium leprae* is the causative agent of leprosy. The incidence of leprosy in the United States has fallen to an average of 150 cases/year. The incubation period ranges between 3 and 5 years. *Pseudomonas aeruginosa* bacteremia may be associated with ecthyma gangrenosum, which is characterized by central necrosis surrounded by violaceous ecchymotic areas. Lymphangitic sporotrichosis is the most common manifestation of *Sporothrix schenckii* infection. A painless, red nodule forms at the site of inoculation, followed by several nodules along the lymphatic channels over the next few weeks. *Rickettsia rickettsii* causes Rocky Mountain spotted fever, a tickborne disease. This is a systemic disease with skin rash that manifests as macules, up to 5 mm in diameter, on the wrists and ankles.

196. Paradoxical splitting of the second heart sound may be heard with which of the following?
a) Right bundle branch block
b) Restrictive cardiomyopathy
c) Pulmonic stenosis
d) Aortic dissection with new diastolic murmur
e) Aortic stenosis

Answer and Discussion

The answer is e. Because the left ventricular systole may become prolonged in severe aortic stenosis, the aortic valve closure may no longer precede the pulmonic valve closure. This phenomenon causes paradoxical splitting in the second heart sound. Left bundle branch block is another common cause of paradoxical splitting in S_2. In right bundle branch block, however, the delayed activation of the right ventricle causes the S_2 splitting, which normally occurs during inspiration, to persist during expiration.

197. A 23-year-old man with a history of nephrotic syndrome presents with the acute onset of severe right flank pain, gross hematuria, and left testicular pain. On examination, he is afebrile, heart rate is 87 beats/

minute, and blood pressure is 158/94 mm Hg. A left-sided varicocele is palpated, and severe left flank tenderness is evident. He has 2+ pitting pedal edema. His medications include prednisone (20 mg/day) and cyclophosphamide (2 mg/kg/day). Laboratory tests reveal the following:

	Currently	3 Weeks Ago
Blood urea nitrogen	76 mg/dL	34 mg/dL
Serum creatinine	4.3 mg/dL	1.9 mg/dL
Serum albumin	2.4 g/dL	3.2 g/dL
Serum uric acid	6.9 mg/dL	7.1 mg/dL
Serum calcium	7.1 mg/dL	7.9 mg/dL
Urinalysis		
Red blood cell	Too numerous to count	510/high-power field
White blood cell	05/high-power field	03/high-power field
Protein	4+	1+
Casts	Occasional granular	Occasional granular

Renal ultrasound shows an increased size of the left kidney with no collecting system dilatation or nephrolithiasis. The most likely diagnosis is which of the following?
a) Renal cell carcinoma
b) Obstructive uropathy secondary to retroperitoneal hematoma
c) Emphysematous pyelonephritis
d) Perinephric abscess
e) Renal vein thrombosis

Answer and Discussion

The answer is e. Nephrotic syndrome leads to a reduction in antithrombin III and free protein S levels and an elevation in total protein S and protein C levels. These abnormalities predispose to thrombosis, especially renal vein thrombosis. An abrupt deterioration in renal function or exacerbation of baseline proteinuria and hematuria in a patient with known nephrotic syndrome warrants investigation to rule out renal vein thrombosis.

198. A 21-year-old college student who was found confused and disruptive by the dorm security staff is brought to the emergency department. He states that he has no complaints, is not tired, and is "getting ready to party for 8 more hours." On examination, he is agitated, heart rate is 113 beats/minute, blood pressure is 155/96 mm Hg, respiratory rate is 19 breaths/minute, and temperature is 37.1°C. His pupils are dilated. Heart examination reveals regular tachycardia, and an ECG confirms sinus tachycardia. A urine drug screen is most likely to be positive for which of the following?
a) Nicotine
b) Cocaine

c) Opiates
d) Amphetamines
e) Hallucinogens

Answer and Discussion

The answer is d. The use of amphetamines as drugs of abuse has increased markedly since 1975. This use affects myriad systems, resulting in a wide range of symptoms that may make it a difficult addiction to recognize. The drug is known to cause a massive release of dopamine in the brain, resulting in agitation, anxiety, delirium, hallucinations, and death. In addition, it causes a decrease in *N*-acetylaspartate in the frontal lobes and basal ganglia that may explain the chronic central nervous system side effects, such as lasting psychosis after its use is stopped and choreoathetoid movements. A high index of suspicion is necessary to make an early diagnosis.

199. A 56-year-old diabetic woman presents with new-onset diplopia and headache. On examination, she has left eye ptosis, and her left pupil is dilated and fixed to light. The left eye is deviated laterally and slightly downward. The etiology of these abnormalities is which of the following?
a) Diabetic third nerve palsy on the left
b) Diabetic sixth nerve palsy on the right
c) Left pontine lacunar infarct
d) Surgical third nerve palsy secondary to aneurysm of the posterior communicating artery
e) Migraine attack

Answer and Discussion

The answer is d. Total palsy of the third nerve causes ptosis, a dilated pupil, and diplopia. Typically, the eye looks down and out. This occurs when all the nerve fibers are affected, which is the case when a circle of Willis aneurysm causes nerve compression and subsequent injury, especially when such an aneurysm ruptures. Most cases of pupil-sparing oculomotor (third cranial nerve) palsy result from microvascular infarction of the nerve. This occurs in patients with long-standing diabetes mellitus and hypertension. Spontaneous recovery over a period of months is the rule.

200–207. For the following periodic fever syndromes, correctly match the appropriate description.

200. Familial Mediterranean Fever

Answer and Discussion

The answer is e. Familial Mediterranean Fever is the most common of the hereditary recurrent inflammatory disorders. It affects people of Mediterranean descent such as Arabs, Armenians, Turks, Jews, Lebanese, Italians, and Greeks. It is caused by muta-

tions in the *MEFV* gene, which encodes for the protein pyrin (marenostrin). Inheritance is autosomal recessive, but secondary to its high prevalence, it has a pseudodominant mode of inheritance. It presents as persistent fever with peritonitis, scrotitis, pericarditis, arthritis, and erysipelaslike erythema of the lower limbs. Length of the attack varies from hours to 3 or 4 days. The attacks stop spontaneously and recur irregularly.

201. Muckle-Wells syndrome

Answer and Discussion

The answer is f. The three cryopyrin-associated periodic syndromes are familial cold autoinflammatory syndrome, Muckle-Wells syndrome (MWS), and neonatal onset multisystem inflammatory disorder. They are all secondary to mutations in a single gene, *CIAS1* on chromosome 1, which encodes a protein called cryopyrin. MWS is characterized by a triad of intermittent fever, urticarial rash, and joint pain with progressive sensorineural deafness and amyloidosis with nephropathy.

202. Pyogenic sterile arthritis, pyoderma gangrenosum, and acne

Answer and Discussion

The answer is c. Pyogenic sterile Arthritis, Pyoderma gangrenosum, and Acne (PAPA) occurs secondary to recently identified mutations in the gene *PSTPIP1* that encodes for a protein that interacts with pyrin. Inheritance is autosomal dominant. It presents in the first decade of life with pauciarticular, destructive arthritis involving the elbow, knee, or ankle and severe cystic acne. PAPA may also include pyoderma gangrenosum and pathergy (sterile abscesses at sites of injections).

203. Blau syndrome

Answer and Discussion

The answer is g. Blau syndrome has been associated with *NOD2* mutation, the same gene that has been associated with granulomatous Crohn's disease. Inheritance is autosomal dominant. It is characterized by granulomatous inflammation of the skin, eye, and joints and with progressive flexion contractures of the fingers (camptodactyly). Biopsy usually reveals synovial granulomas.

204. Familial cold autoinflammatory syndrome

Answer and Discussion

The answer is h. In familial cold autoinflammatory syndrome, exposure to cold usually causes a classical response, which usually resolves within 24 hours. This includes fever, an urticarial rash, conjunctivitis, and arthralgias. Patients may also have daily symptoms even in the absence of cold exposure, especially toward the afternoons and evenings.

205. Neonatal onset multisystem inflammatory disease

Answer and Discussion

The answer is d. Neonatal onset multisystem inflammatory disease is also called chronic infantile neurologic cutaneous and articular syndrome. It causes impaired growth with frontal bossing, protruding eyes, and saddle-shaped nose. Limb and joint pain is common, and there is "tumorlike" proliferation of cartilage at growth plates and epiphyses.

206. Hyper-IgD syndrome

Answer and Discussion

The answer is a. Hyperimmunoglobin D syndrome (HIDS) results from mutations in the *MVK* gene that encodes mevalonate kinase. It is seen in patients of Dutch, French, or Italian origin. HIDS presents as unremitting fever lasting about a week, palpable tender lymphadenopathy, splenomegaly, arthralgias, abdominal pain, and rash. Elevated levels of age-specific serum immunoglobin (Ig) D and/or IgA levels, elevation of acute-phase reactants, and urinary excretion of mevalonic acid during, but not between, attacks are characteristic.

207. Tumor necrosis factor receptor-1–associated periodic syndrome
a) Caused by mutations in the *MVK* gene
b) Most patients are of Irish (Hibernian) or Scottish descent and inheritance is autosomal dominant
c) Pathergy or development of sterile abscesses at the sites of injection
d) Clinical features include frontal bossing, protruding eyes, and saddle-shaped nose
e) Mutations of *MEFV* gene
f) Triad of intermittent fever and rash with progressive sensorineural deafness and amyloidosis with nephropathy
g) Causes granulomatous inflammation of the skin, eyes, and joints
h) Exposure to cold results in fever, urticarial rash, conjunctivitis, and arthralgias

Answer and Discussion

The answer is b. Tumor necrosis factor (TNF) receptor-1–associated periodic syndrome results from mutations in the TNF receptor *TNFR1* gene. Inheritance is autosomal dominant. Penetrance is variable. Many patients are of Irish (Hibernian) or Scottish descent. It presents usually with prolonged periods of fever, myalgias, rash, conjunctivitis, and periorbital edema. Persistent inflammation may result in secondary amyloidosis.

SUGGESTED READINGS

Question 1

Gines A, Escorsell A, Gines P, et al. Incidence, predictive factors, and prognosis of the hepatorenal syndrome in cirrhosis with ascites. *Gastroenterology* 1993;105(1):229–236.

Question 2

Blumberg A, Weidmann P, Shaw S, et al. Effect of various therapeutic approaches on plasma potassium and major regulating factors in terminal renal failure. *Am J Med* 1988;85:507–512.

Conger JD. Interventions in clinical acute renal failure: what are the data? *Am J Kidney Dis* 1995;26:565–576.

Rutsky EA, Rostand SG. Treatment of uremic pericarditis and pericardial effusion. *Am J Kidney Dis* 1987;10:2–8.

Question 3

Rummans TA, Evans JM, Krahn LE, et al. Delirium in elderly patients: evaluation and management. *Mayo Clin Proc* 1995;70:989–998.

Question 6

Johnson WJ, Kyle RA, Pineda AA, et al. Treatment of renal failure associated with multiple myeloma: plasmapheresis, hemodialysis, and chemotherapy. *Arch Intern Med* 1990;150(4):863.

Sanders PW. Pathogenesis and treatment of myeloma kidney. *J Lab Clin Med* 1994;124(4):484–488.

Question 7

Hellmark T, Johansson C, Wieslander J. Characterization of anti-GBM antibodies involved in Goodpasture's syndrome. *Kidney Int* 1994;46:823–829.

Hoffman GS, Specks U. Antineutrophil cytoplasmic antibodies. *Arthritis Rheum* 1998;41:1521–1537.

Jayne DR, Marshall PD, Jones SJ, et al. Autoantibodies to GBM and neutrophil cytoplasm in rapidly progressive glomerulonephritis. *Kidney Int* 1990;37:965–970.

Kalluri R, Meyers KM, Mogyorosi A, et al. Goodpasture syndrome involving overlap with Wegener's granulomatosis and anti-glomerular basement membrane disease. *J Am Soc Nephrol* 1997;8:1795–1800.

Question 8

ACOG Practice Bulletin: clinical management guidelines for obstetrician-gynecologists. Number 45, August 2003. Cervical cytology screening (replaces committee opinion 152, March 1995). *Obstet Gynecol* 2003;102(2):417–427.

Saslow D, Runowicz CD, Solomon D, et al. American Cancer Society guideline for the early detection of cervical neoplasia and cancer. *CA Cancer J Clin* 2002;52(6):342–362.

U.S. Preventive Services Task Force. *Screening for Cervical Cancer: Recommendations and Rationale.* Rockville, MD: Agency for Healthcare Research and Quality, 2003. Available at: www.ahrq.gov/clinic/3rduspstf/cervcan/cervcanrr.pdf.

Question 10

Ramsey B, Richardson MA. Impact of sinusitis in cystic fibrosis. *J Allergy Clin Immunol* 1992;90:547–552.

Question 11

Phillips LH II, Melnick PA. Diagnosis of myasthenia gravis in the 1990s. *Semin Neurol* 1990;10:62–69.

Ryder REJ, Mir MA, Freeman EA. *Myasthenia Gravis: An Aid to the MRCP Short Cases.* Oxford: Blackwell Scientific, 1991:246–247.

Question 12

Cohen AM, Tremiterra S, Candela F, et al. Prognosis of node-positive colon cancer. *Cancer* 1991;67:1859–1861.

Eisenberg B, Decosse JJ, Harford F, et al. Carcinoma of the colon and rectum: the natural history reviewed in 1,704 patients. *Cancer* 1982;49:1131–1134.

Question 13

Sampson HA, Mendelson L, Rosen JP. Fatal and near-fatal anaphylactic reactions to food in children and adolescents. *N Engl J Med* 1992;327:380–384.

Question 14

MacMahon, Austin JH, Gamsu G, et al. Guidelines for management of small pulmonary nodules detected on CT scans: a statement from the Fleischner Society. *Radiology* 2005;237(2):395–400.

Question 15

Adamson JW. The myeloproliferative diseases. In: Wilson JD, Braunwald E, Isselbacher KJ, et al., eds. *Harrison's Principles of Internal Medicine*, 12th ed. New York: McGraw-Hill, 1991:1563–1565.

Dickstein JI, Vardiman JW. Hematopathologic findings in the myeloproliferative disorders. *Semin Oncol* 1995;22:355–373.

Question 17

Girard DE, Kumar KL, McAfee JH. Hematologic effects of acute alcohol abuse. *Hematol Oncol Clin North Am* 1987;1:321–324.

Peck-Radosavljevic M, Zacherl J, Meng YG, et al. Is inadequate thrombopoietin production a major cause of thrombocytopenia in cirrhosis of the liver? *J Hepatol* 1997;27:127–131.

Question 18

Cunningham FG, Lindheimer MD. Hypertension in pregnancy. *N Engl J Med* 1992;326:927–932.

Redman CW. Controlled trials of antihypertensive drugs in pregnancy. *Am J Kidney Dis* 1991;17:149–153.

Remuzzi G, Ruggenenti P. Prevention and treatment of pregnancy-associated hypertension: what have we learned in the last 10 years? *Am J Kidney Dis* 1991;18:285–305.

Shotan A, Widerhorn J, Hurst A, et al. Risk of angiotensin-converting enzyme inhibition during pregnancy: experimental and clinical evidence, potential mechanisms, and recommendations for use. *Am J Med* 1994;96:451–456.

Sibai BM. Treatment of hypertension in pregnant women. *N Engl J Med* 1996;335:257–265.

Sibai BM, Mabie WC, Shamsa F, et al. A comparison of no medication versus methyldopa or labetalol in chronic hypertension during pregnancy. *Am J Obstet Gynecol* 1990;162:960–966.

Question 19

Killip S, Bennett JM, Chambers MD. Iron deficiency anemia. *Am Fam Physician* 2007;75(5):671.

Rockey DC. Occult gastrointestinal bleeding. *N Engl J Med* 1999;341:38

Question 20

Kirsner JB, Shorter RG, eds. *Inflammatory Bowel Disease*, 3rd ed. Philadelphia: Lea & Febiger, 1988.

Podolsky DK. Inflammatory bowel disease (1). *N Engl J Med* 1991;325:928–937.

Question 21

Silverberg SJ, Bilezikian JP. Evaluation and management of primary hyperparathyroidism. *J Clin Endocrinol Metab* 1996;81:2036–2040.

Question 22

1998 Guidelines for treatment of sexually transmitted diseases. Centers for Disease Control and Prevention. *MMWR Morb Mortal Wkly Rep* 1998;47(RR-1):1–111.

Question 23

Pascual E. The diagnosis of gout and CPPD crystal arthropathy. *Br J Rheumatol* 1996;35:306–308.

Terkeltaub RA. What stops a gouty attack? *J Rheumatol* 1992;19:8–10.

Question 24

Anderson DJ, Noyes R Jr, Crowe RR. A comparison of panic disorder and generalized anxiety disorder. *Am J Psychiatry* 1984;141:572–575.

Lydiard RB, Ballenger JC. Antidepressants in panic disorder and agoraphobia. *J Affect Disord* 1987;13:153–168.

Question 25

Koch W. Swallowing disorders: diagnosis and therapy. *Med Clin North Am* 1993;77:571–582.

Zenker FA, Von Ziemssen H. Krankheiten des Oesophagus. In: Von Ziemssen H, ed. *Handbuch der Specielen Pathologie und Therapie*. Leipzig: FC Vogel, 1877.

Question 26

Lieberman JR, Berry DJ, Bono JV, et al. The hip and thigh. In: Snider RK, ed. *Essentials of Musculoskeletal Care*. Rosemont, IL: American Academy of Orthopaedic Surgeons, 1997:265–303.

Question 27

Locksley RM, Flournoy N, Sullivan KM, et al. Infection with varicella-zoster virus after marrow transplantation. *J Infect Dis* 1985;152:1172–1181.

Question 28

Donowitz M, Kokke FT, Saidi R. Evaluation of patients with chronic diarrhea. *N Engl J Med* 1995;332:725–729.

Ewe K, Karbach U. Factitious diarrhea. *Clin Gastroenterol* 1986;15:723–740.

Question 29

Fairbanks DN. Inflammatory diseases of the sinuses: bacteriology and antibiotics. *Otolaryngol Clin North Am* 1993;26:549–559.

Question 30

Johnson TR. The shoulder. In: Snider RK, ed. *Essentials of Musculoskeletal Care*. Rosemont, IL: American Academy of Orthopaedic Surgeons, 1997:72–121.

Lequesne M, Dang N, Bensasson M, et al. Increased association of diabetes mellitus with capsulitis of the shoulder and shoulder-hand syndrome. *Scand J Rheumatol* 1977;6:53–56.

Pal B, Anderson J, Dick WC, et al. Limitation of joint mobility and shoulder capsulitis in insulin- and non-insulin-dependent diabetes mellitus. *Br J Rheumatol* 1986;25:147–151.

Question 35

Hunder GG, Arend WP, Block DA, et al. American College of Rheumatology 1990 criteria for the classification of vasculitis: introduction. *Arthritis Rheum* 1990;33:1065–1067.

Question 36

Galgiani JN. Coccidioidomycosis. *West J Med* 1993;159:153–171.

Stevens DA. Coccidioidomycosis. *N Engl J Med* 1995;332:1077–1082.

Question 37

Alter MJ, Mast EE. The epidemiology of viral hepatitis in the United States. *Gastroenterol Clin North Am* 1994;23:437–455.

Takahashi M, Yamada G, Miyamoto R, et al. Natural course of chronic hepatitis C. *Am J Gastroenterol* 1993;88:240–243.

Question 38

Kagnoff M. Celiac disease: a gastrointestinal disease with environmental, genetic, and immunologic components. *Gastroenterol Clin North Am* 1992;21:405–425.

Trier JS. Celiac sprue. *N Engl J Med* 1991;325:1709–1719.

Question 39

Mau W, Zeidler H, Mau R, et al. Clinical features and prognosis of patients with possible ankylosing spondylitis: results of a 10-year follow-up. *J Rheumatol* 1988;15:1109–1114.

O'Neill TW, King G, Graham IM, et al. Echocardiographic abnormalities in ankylosing spondylitis. *Ann Rheum Dis* 1992;51:652–654.

Question 40

Goldman L. Quantitative aspects of clinical reasoning. In: Isselbacher KJ, Braunwald E, Wilson JD, et al., eds. *Harrison's Principles of Internal Medicine*, 13th ed. New York: McGraw-Hill, 1994:43–48.

Question 41

Utsunomiya J, Gocho H, Miyanaga T, et al. Peutz-Jeghers syndrome: its natural course and management. *Johns Hopkins Med J* 1975;136:71–82.

Young RH, Welch WR, Dickersin GR, et al. Ovarian sex cord tumor with annular tubules: review of 74 cases including 27 with Peutz-Jeghers syndrome and four with adenoma malignum of the cervix. *Cancer* 1982;50:1384–1402.

Question 42

Singer PA, Cooper DS, Levy EG, et al. Treatment guidelines for patients with hyperthyroidism and hypothyroidism. Standards of Care Committee, American Thyroid Association. *JAMA* 1995;273:808–812.

Torring O, Tallstedt L, Wallin G, et al. Graves' hyperthyroidism: treatment with antithyroid drugs, surgery, or radioiodine—a prospective, randomized study. Thyroid Study Group. *J Clin Endocrinol Metab* 1996;81:2986–2993.

Question 48

Hardcastle JD, Thomas WM, Chamberlain J, et al. Randomised, controlled trial of faecal occult blood screening for colorectal cancer: results for first 107,349 subjects. *Lancet* 1989;1:1160–1164.

Question 49

Johnson TR. The elbow and forearm. In: Snider RK, ed. *Essentials of Musculoskeletal Care*. Rosemont, IL: American Academy of Orthopaedic Surgeons, 1997:125–129.

Question 50

Israili ZH, Hall WD. Cough and angioneurotic edema associated with angiotensin-converting enzyme inhibitor therapy: a review of the literature and pathophysiology. *Ann Intern Med* 1992;117:234–242.

Lunde H, Hedner T, Samuelsson O, et al. Dyspnoea, asthma, and bronchospasm in relation to treatment with angiotensin converting enzyme inhibitors. *BMJ* 1994;308:18–21.

Question 51

Prevention and control of influenza: recommendations of the Advisory Committee on Immunization Practices (ACIP). Centers for Disease Control and Prevention. *MMWR Morb Mortal Wkly Rep* 1998;47(RR-6):1–26.

Question 52

Maisch B, Seferovic PM, Ristic AD, et al. Guidelines on the diagnosis and management of pericardial diseases executive summary: the task force on the diagnosis and management of pericardial diseases of the European Society of Cardiology. *Eur Heart J* 2004;25(7):587–610.

Question 56

Gabow PA. Disorders associated with an altered anion gap. *Kidney Int* 1985;27:472–483.

Gabow PA, Kaehny WD, Fennessey PV, et al. Diagnostic importance of an increased anion gap. *N Engl J Med* 1980;303:854–858.

Winter SD, Pearson R, Gabow PA, et al. The fall of the serum anion gap. *Arch Intern Med* 1990;150:311–313.

Question 60

Management of persons exposed to multidrug-resistant tuberculosis. *MMWR Morb Mortal Wkly Rep* 1992;41(RR-11):61–71.

Prevention and control of tuberculosis in U.S. communities with at-risk minority populations. Recommendations of the Advisory Council for the Elimination of Tuberculosis. *MMWR Morb Mortal Wkly Rep* 1992;41(RR-5):1–11.

Prevention and treatment of tuberculosis among patients infected with human immunodeficiency virus: principles of therapy and revised recommendations. Centers for Disease Control and Prevention. *MMWR Morb Mortal Wkly Rep* 1998;47(RR-20):1–58.

Question 61

Currier MB, Olsen EJ. Suicide. In: *Griffith's 5-Minute Clinical Consult*. Baltimore: Lippincott Williams & Wilkins, 1999:1030–1031.

Question 62

Chastre J, Trouillet JL, Vuagnat A, et al. Nosocomial pneumonia in patients with acute respiratory distress syndrome. *Am J Respir Crit Care Med* 1998;157:1165–1172.

Gammon RB, Shin MS, Buchalter SE. Pulmonary barotrauma in mechanical ventilation: patterns and risk factors. *Chest* 1992;102:568–572.

Gammon RB, Shin MS, Groves RH Jr, et al. Clinical risk factors for pulmonary barotrauma: a multivariate analysis. *Am J Respir Crit Care Med* 1995;152:1235–1240.

Schnapp LM, Chin DP, Szaflarski N, et al. Frequency and importance of barotrauma in 100 patients with acute lung injury. *Crit Care Med* 1995;23:272–278.

Question 64

Kaplan NM. Management of hypertensive emergencies. *Lancet* 1994;344:1335–1338.

McGregor E, Isles CG, Jay JL, et al. Retinal changes in malignant hypertension. *BMJ* 1986;292:233–234.

Phillips SJ, Whisnant JP. Hypertension and the brain. The National High Blood Pressure Education Program. *Arch Intern Med* 1992;152:938–945.

The sixth report of the Joint National Committee on prevention, detection, evaluation, and treatment of high blood pressure. *Arch Intern Med* 1997;157:2413–2446. [Erratum: *Arch Intern Med* 1998;158:573.]

Strandgaard S, Paulson OB. Cerebral blood flow and its pathophysiology in hypertension. *Am J Hypertens* 1989;2:486–492.

Question 65

Michel DM, Kelly CJ. Acute interstitial nephritis. *J Am Soc Nephrol* 1998;9:506–515.

Pappas PG. Laboratory in the diagnosis and management of urinary tract infections. *Med Clin North Am* 1991;75:313–325.

Stamm WE, Wagner KF, Amsel R, et al. Causes of the acute urethral syndrome in women. *N Engl J Med* 1980;303:409–415.

Question 66

Hurwitz S. Acne vulgaris: pathogenesis and management. *Pediatr Rev* 1994;15:47–52.

Kaminer MS, Gilchrest BA. The many faces of acne. *J Am Acad Dermatol* 1995;32:S6–S14.

Webster GF, Toso SM, Hegemann L. Inhibition of a model of in vitro granuloma formation by tetracyclines and ciprofloxacin: involvement of protein kinase C. *Arch Dermatol* 1994;130:748–752.

Question 67

Niewoehner DE, Rice K, Cote C, et al. Prevention of exacerbations of chronic obstructive pulmonary disease with tiotropium, a once-daily inhaled anticholinergic bronchodilator: a randomized trial. *Ann Intern Med* 2005;143:317.

American Thoracic Society/European Respiratory Society Task Force. *Standards for the Diagnosis and Management of Patients with COPD* (Internet), Version 1.2. New York: American Thoracic Society, 2004 (updated 2005 September 8). Available at: www.test.thoracic.org/go/copd/.

Question 68

Drugs for AIDS and associated infections. *Med Lett Drugs Ther* 1995;37:87.

Martins TB, Jaskowski TD, Mouritsen CL, et al. Comparison of commercially available enzyme immunoassay with traditional serological tests for detection of antibodies to *Coccidioides immitis*. *J Clin Microbiol* 1995;33:940–943.

Sarosi GA, Davies SF. Therapy for fungal infections. *Mayo Clin Proc* 1994;69:1111–1117.

Stevens DA. Coccidioidomycosis. *N Engl J Med* 1995;332:1077–1082.

Question 69

Califf RM, Bengtson JR. Cardiogenic shock. *N Engl J Med* 1994;330:1724–1730.

Goldberg RJ, Gore JM, Alpert JS, et al. Cardiogenic shock after myocardial infarction: incidence and mortality from a community wide perspective, 1975 to 1988. *N Engl J Med* 1991;325:1117–1122.

Guidelines for the early management of patients with acute myocardial infarction. A report of the American College of Cardiology/American Heart Association Task Force on Assessment of Diagnostic and Therapeutic Cardiovascular Procedures (Subcommittee to Develop Guidelines for the Early Management of Patients with Acute Myocardial Infarction). *J Am Coll Cardiol* 1990;16:249–292.

Hands ME, Rutherford JD, Muller JE, et al. The in-hospital development of cardiogenic shock after myocardial infarction: incidence, predictors of occurrence, outcome and prognostic factors. *J Am Coll Cardiol* 1989;14:40–46.

Holmes DR Jr, Califf RM, Van de Werf F. Differences in countries' use of resources and clinical outcome for patients with cardiogenic shock after myocardial infarction: results from the GUSTO trial. *Lancet* 1997;349:75–78.

Question 70

Tinetti ME, Speechley M, Ginter SF, et al. Risk factors for falls among elderly persons living in the community. *N Engl J Med* 1988;319:1701–1707.

Question 71

Ryder REJ, Mir MA, Freeman EA. *Lower Motor Neurone VIIth Nerve Palsy: An Aid to the MRCP Short Cases.* Oxford: Blackwell Scientific, 1991:192–193.

Question 73

Lin RY. A perspective on penicillin allergy. *Arch Intern Med* 1992;152:930–937.

Question 74

Mateo J, Oliver A, Borrell M, et al. Laboratory evaluation and clinical characteristics of 2,132 consecutive unselected patients with venous thromboembolism: results of the Spanish Multicentric Study on Thrombophilia (EMET-Study). *Thromb Haemost* 1997;77:444–451.

Ridker PM, Hennekensch, Lindpainter K, et al. Mutation in the gene coding for coagulation factor V and the risk of myocardial infarction, stroke, and venous thrombosis in apparently healthy men. *N Engl J Med* 1995;332:912–917.

Question 75

Kostis JB, Shelton B, Gosselin G, et al. Adverse effects of enalapril in the Studies of Left Ventricular Dysfunction (SOLVD). SOLVD Investigators. *Am Heart J* 1996;131:350–355.

Langford HG, Blaufox MD, Borhani NO, et al. Is thiazide-produced uric acid elevation harmful? Analysis of data from the Hypertension Detection and Follow-up Program. *Arch Intern Med* 1987;147:645–649.

Materson BJ, Reda DJ, Cushman WC, et al. Single-drug therapy for hypertension in men: a comparison of six antihypertensive agents with placebo. The Department of Veterans Affairs Cooperative Study Group on Antihypertensive Agents. *N Engl J Med* 1993;328:914–921. [Erratum: *N Engl J Med* 1994;330:1689.]

Oren S, Gossman E, Frohlich ED. Effects of calcium entry blockers on distribution of blood volume. *Am J Hypertens* 1996;9:628–632.

Question 78

DeLorenzo LJ, Huang CT, Maguire GP, et al. Roentgenographic patterns of *Pneumocystis carinii* pneumonia in 104 patients with AIDS. *Chest* 1987;91:323–327.

Hoover DR, Saah AJ, Bacellar H, et al. Clinical manifestations of AIDS in the era of *Pneumocystis* prophylaxis. Multicenter AIDS Cohort Study. *N Engl J Med* 1993;329:1922–1926.

Jules-Elysee K, Stover DE, Zaman MB, et al. Aerosolized pentamidine: effect on diagnosis and presentation of *Pneumocystis carinii* pneumonia. *Ann Intern Med* 1990;112:750–757.

Stansell JD, Osmond DH, Charlebois E, et al. Predictors of *Pneumocystis carinii* pneumonia in HIV-infected persons. Pulmonary Complications of HIV Infection Study Group. *Am J Respir Crit Care Med* 1997;155:60–66.

Zaman MK, White DA. Serum lactate dehydrogenase levels and *Pneumocystis carinii* pneumonia: diagnostic and prognostic significance. *Am Rev Respir Dis* 1988;137:796–800.

Question 79

Centers for Disease Control and Prevention. Sexually transmitted diseases: treatment guidelines 2006. *MMWR Recomm Rep* 2006; (RR-11) 55:1–95. Available at: www.cdc.gov/STD/treatment/2006/toc.htm.

U.S. Preventive Services Task Force. Screening for genital herpes. Rockville, MD: Agency for Healthcare Research and Quality, March 2005. Available at: www.ahrq.gov/clinic/uspstf/uspsherp.htm.

Question 82

Rodgers KG. Cardiovascular shock. *Emerg Med Clin North Am* 1995;13:793–810.

Shoemaker WC. Temporal physiologic patterns of shock and circulatory dysfunction based on early descriptions by invasive and noninvasive monitoring. *New Horiz* 1996;4:300–318.

Question 83

Public Health Service guidelines for counseling and antibody testing to prevent HIV infection and AIDS. *MMWR Morb Mortal Wkly Rep* 1987;36:509–515.

Recommendations for HIV testing services for inpatients and outpatients in acute-care hospital settings. Centers for Disease Control and Prevention. *MMWR Morb Mortal Wkly Rep* 1993;42(RR-2):1–6.

Update: serologic testing for HIV-1 antibody—United States, 1988 and 1989. *MMWR Morb Mortal Wkly Rep* 1990;39:380–383.

Question 85

Clark SL. Amniotic fluid embolism. *Crit Care Clin* 1991;7:877–882.

Dashow EE, Cotterill R, Benedetti TJ, et al. Amniotic fluid embolism. *J Reprod Med* 1989;34:660–666.

Question 86

Tashkin DP. Airway effects of marijuana, cocaine, and other inhaled illicit agents. *Curr Opin Pulm Med* 2001;7(2):43–61.

Question 87

Consensus report on the ethics of foregoing [sic] life-sustaining treatments in the critically ill. Task Force on Ethics of the Society of Critical Care Medicine. *Crit Care Med* 1990;18:1435–1439.

Consensus statement of the Society of Critical Care Medicine's Ethics Committee regarding futile and other possibly inadvisable treatments. *Crit Care Med* 1997;25:887–891.

Guidelines for the appropriate use of do-not-resuscitate orders. Council on Ethical and Judicial Affairs, American Medical Association. *JAMA* 1991;265:1868–1871.

Quill TE, Cassel CK, Meier DE. Care of the hopelessly ill: proposed clinical criteria for physician-assisted suicide. *N Engl J Med* 1992;327:1380–1384.

Schneiderman LJ, Jecker NS, Jonsen AR. Medical futility: response to critiques. *Ann Intern Med* 1996;125:669–674.

Question 88

Centers for Disease Control and Prevention Web site: www.cdc.gov.

Davis TM, Dembo LG, Kaye-Eddie SA, et al. Neurological, cardiovascular and metabolic effects of mefloquine in healthy volunteers: a double-blind, placebo-controlled trial. *Br J Clin Pharmacol* 1996;42:415–421.

U.S. Department of Health and Human Services, Public Health Service, Centers for Disease Control and Prevention, National Center for Infectious Diseases, Division of Quarantine. *Health Information for International Travel, 1996–97.* Washington, DC: U.S. Government Printing Office, December 1, 1996.

Question 89

American College of Chest Physicians/Society of Critical Care Medicine consensus conference: definitions for sepsis and organ failure and guidelines for the use of innovative therapies in sepsis. *Crit Care Med* 1992;20:864–874.

Question 90

Ryder REJ, Mir MA, Freeman EA. *Eisenmenger's Syndrome: An Aid to the MRCP Short Cases.* Oxford: Blackwell Scientific, 1991:192–193.

Question 92

Detection, evaluation, and treatment of renovascular hypertension: final report. Working Group on Renovascular Hypertension. *Arch Intern Med* 1987;147:820–829.

Mann SJ, Pickering TG. Detection of renovascular hypertension: state of the art: 1992. *Ann Intern Med* 1992;117:845–853.

Olin JW, Piedmonte MR, Young JR, et al. The utility of duplex ultrasound scanning of the renal arteries for diagnosing significant renal artery stenosis. *Ann Intern Med* 1995;122:833–838.

Setaro JF, Saddler MC, Chen CC, et al. Simplified captopril renography in diagnosis and treatment of renal artery stenosis. *Hypertension* 1991;18:289–298.

Van de Ven PJ, Beutler JJ, Kaatee R, et al. Angiotensin converting enzyme inhibitor-induced dysfunction in atherosclerotic renovascular disease. *Kidney Int* 1998;53:986–993.

Question 94

Dupont HL. *Shigella* species. In: Mandell GL, Douglas RG Jr, Bennett JE, eds. *Principles and Practice of Infectious Diseases,* 4th ed. New York: Churchill Livingstone, 1995:203.

Gotuzzo E, Oberhelman RA, Maguina C, et al. Comparison of single-dose treatment with norfloxacin and standard 5-day treatment with trimethoprim-sulfamethoxazole for acute shigellosis in adults. *Antimicrob Agents Chemother* 1989;33:1101–1104.

Struelens MJ, Patte D, Kabir I, et al. Shigella septicemia: prevalence, presentation, risk factors, and outcome. *J Infect Dis* 1985;152:784–790.

Question 95

Blade J, Kyle RA. Multiple myeloma in young patients: clinical presentation and treatment approach. *Leuk Lymphoma* 1998;30:493–501.

Cohen DJ, Sherman WH, Osserman EF, et al. Acute renal failure in patients with multiple myeloma. *Am J Med* 1984;76:247–256.

Winearls CG. Acute myeloma kidney. *Kidney Int* 1995;48:1347–1361.

Question 96

Lundback B. Epidemiology of rhinitis and asthma. *Clin Exp Allergy* 1998;28(Suppl 2):3–10.

Raphael GD, Raphael MH, Kaliner M. Gustatory rhinitis: a syndrome of food-induced rhinorrhea. *J Allergy Clin Immunol* 1989;83:110–115.

Question 97

Lillington GA, Caskey CI. Evaluation and management of solitary and multiple pulmonary nodules. *Clin Chest Med* 1993;14:111–119.

Midthun DE, Swensen SJ, Jett JR. Approach to the solitary pulmonary nodule. *Mayo Clin Proc* 1993;68:378–385.

Quoix E, Fraser R, Wolkove N, et al. Small cell lung cancer presenting as a solitary pulmonary nodule. *Cancer* 1990;66:577–582.

Question 98

Bunn HF. Disorders of hemoglobin. In: Wilson JD, Braunwald E, Isselbacher IL, et al., eds. *Harrison's Principles of Internal Medicine*, 12th ed. New York: McGraw-Hill, 1991:1544–1548.

Platt OS, Thorington BD, Brambilla DJ, et al. Pain in sickle cell disease: rates and risk factors. *N Engl J Med* 1991;325:11–16.

Question 99

Guidelines for cardiopulmonary resuscitation and emergency cardiac care. Emergency Cardiac Care Committee and Subcommittees, American Heart Association. Part III. Adult advanced cardiac life support. *JAMA* 1992;268:2199–2241.

Question 100

Akhtar M, Shenasa M, Jazayeri M, et al. Wide QRS complex tachycardia: reappraisal of a common clinical problem. *Ann Intern Med* 1988;109:905–912.

Buxton AE, Marchlinski FE, Doherty JU, et al. Hazards of intravenous verapamil for sustained ventricular tachycardia. *Am J Cardiol* 1987;59:1107–1110.

Stewart RB, Bardy GH, Greene HL. Wide complex tachycardia: misdiagnosis and outcome after emergency therapy. *Ann Intern Med* 1986;104:766–771.

Tchou P, Young P, Mahmud R, et al. Useful clinical criteria for the diagnosis of ventricular tachycardia. *Am J Med* 1988;84:53–56.

Question 101

Ryder REJ, Mir MA, Freeman EA. *Multiple Sclerosis: An Aid to the MRCP Short Cases*. Oxford: Blackwell Scientific, 1991:316.

Smith SG. Multiple sclerosis. In: Dambro MR, ed. *Griffith's 5-Minute Clinical Consult*. Baltimore: Lippincott Williams & Wilkins, 1999:700–701.

Question 102

Gluck SL. Acid–base. *Lancet* 1988;352:474–479.

Rose BD. *Clinical Physiology of Acid–Base and Electrolyte Disorders*, 4th ed. New York: McGraw-Hill, 1994:572–586.

Question 103

Garnick MB, Brenner BM. Tumors of the urinary tract. In: Wilson JD, Braunwald E, Isselbacher KJ, et al., eds. *Harrison's Principles of Internal Medicine*, 12th ed. New York: McGraw-Hill, 1991:1211–1212.

Question 104

Delmez JA, Slatopolsky E. Hyperphosphatemia: its consequences and treatment in patients with chronic renal failure. *Am J Kidney Dis* 1992;19:303–317.

Farias MA, McClellan W, Soucie JM, et al. A prospective comparison of methods for determining if cardiovascular disease is a predictor of mortality in dialysis patients. *Am J Kidney Dis* 1994;23:382–388.

Henrich WL. Dialysis considerations in the elderly patient. *Am J Kidney Dis* 1990;16:339–341.

Sherrard DJ, Hercz G, Pei Y, et al. The spectrum of bone disease in end-stage renal failure: an evolving disorder. *Kidney Int* 1993;43:436–442.

Zuckerman GR, Cornette GL, Clouse RE, et al. Upper gastrointestinal bleeding in patients with chronic renal failure. *Ann Intern Med* 1985;102:588–592.

Question 105

Carpenter CC, Fischl MA, Hammer SM, et al. Antiretroviral therapy for HIV infection in 1998: updated recommendations of the International AIDS Society–USA Panel. *JAMA* 1998;280:78–86.

Drugs for HIV infection. *Med Lett Drugs Ther* 1997;39:111–116.

Guidelines for the use of antiretroviral agents in HIV-infected adults and adolescents. Department of Health and Human Services and the Henry J. Kaiser Family Foundation. *Ann Intern Med* 1998; 128:1079–1100.

Montaner JS, Reiss P, Cooper D, et al. A randomized, double-blind trial comparing combinations of nevirapine, didanosine, and zidovudine for HIV-infected patients. The INCAS trial. Italy, the Netherlands, Canada and Australia Study. *JAMA* 1998;279:930–937.

Question 106

Turner RC, Lichstein PR, Peden JG Jr, et al. Alcohol withdrawal syndromes: a review of pathophysiology, clinical presentation and treatment. *J Gen Intern Med* 1989;4:432–444.

Question 108

Rummans TA, Evans JM, Krahn LE, et al. Delirium in elderly patients: evaluation and management. *Mayo Clin Proc* 1995;70:989–998.

Question 109

Gabow PA, Anderson RJ, Potts DE, et al. Acid–base disturbances in the salicylate-intoxicated adult. *Arch Intern Med* 1978;138:1481–1484.

Hill JB. Salicylate intoxication. *N Engl J Med* 1973;288:1110–1113.

Prescott LF, Balali-Mood M, Critchley JA, et al. Diuresis or urinary alkalinisation for salicylate poisoning? *BMJ (Clin Res Ed)* 1982;285:1383–1386.

Question 110

Deveney CW, Deveney KE. Zollinger-Ellison syndrome (gastrinoma): current diagnosis and treatment. *Surg Clin North Am* 1987;67:411–422.

Question 111

Elting LS, Rubenstein EB, Rolston KV, et al. Outcomes of bacteremia in patients with cancer and neutropenia: observations from two decades of epidemiological and clinical trials. *Clin Infect Dis* 1997;25:247–259.

Question 112

Entrapment syndrome of peripheral nerve injuries. Lee, CC. In: Winn HR, ed. *Youman's Neurological Surgery*, 5th ed. Elsevier: Philadelphia, 2004:3923.

Question 113

Summary of the second report of the National Cholesterol Education Program (NCEP) Expert Panel on Detection, Evaluation, and Treatment of High Blood Cholesterol in Adults. *JAMA* 1993;269:3015–3023.

Question 114

Michet CJ. Vasculitis and relapsing polychondritis. *Rheum Dis Clin North Am* 1990;16:441–444.

Question 115

Bigos S, Bowyer O, Braen G, et al. *Acute low back pain problems in adults: clinical practice guideline.* Rockville, MD: U.S. Department of Health and Human Services, Public Health Service, 1994. Agency for Health Care Policy and Research Publication No. 95-0643.

Lahad A, Malter AD, Berg AO, et al. The effectiveness of four interventions for the prevention of low back pain. *JAMA* 1994;272:1286–1291.

Question 117

Richter JE. Typical and atypical manifestations of gastroesophageal reflux disease: the role of esophageal testing in diagnosis and management. *Gastroenterol Clin North Am* 1996;25:75–102.

Question 118

Bauman WA, Yalow RS. Hyperinsulinemic hypoglycemia: differential diagnosis by determination of the species of circulating insulin. *JAMA* 1984;252:2730–2734.

Service FJ. Hypoglycemic disorders. *N Engl J Med* 1995;332:1144–1152.

Question 119

Maddrey WC. Chronic viral hepatitis: diagnosis and management. *Hosp Pract (Off Ed)* 1994;29:117–120.

Question 120

Bojrab DL, Bruderly T, Abdulrazzak Y. Otitis externa. *Otolaryngol Clin North Am* 1996;29:761–782.

Question 121

Mariotti S, Caturegli P, Piccolo P, et al. Antithyroid peroxidase autoantibodies in thyroid diseases. *J Clin Endocrinol Metab* 1990;71:661–669.

Question 122

Dire DJ. Emergency management of dog and cat bite wounds. *Emerg Med Clin North Am* 1992;10:719–736.

Goldstein EJ. Bite wounds and infection. *Clin Infect Dis* 1992;14:633–638.

Question 123–127

Sacco RL, Adams R, Albers G, et al. Guidelines for prevention of stroke in patients with ischemic stroke or transient ischemic attack: a statement for healthcare professionals from the American Heart Association/American Stroke Association Council on Stroke. *Stroke* 2006;37:577.

Lange RA, Cigarroa RG, Yancy CW Jr, et al. Cocaine-induced coronary-artery vasoconstriction. *N Engl J Med* 1989;321:1557.

Mancia G, De Backer G, Dominiczak A, et al. Guidelines for the management of arterial hypertension: the task force for the management of arterial hypertension of the European Society of Hypertension (ESH) and of the European Society of Cardiology (ESC). *J Hypertens* 2007;25:1105.

Question 128

Schneider TA, Longo WE, Ure T, et al. Mesenteric ischemia: acute arterial syndromes. *Dis Colon Rectum* 1994;37:1163–1174.

Silen W. *Cope's Early Diagnosis of the Acute Abdomen.* Oxford: Oxford University Press, 1990.

Question 129

Newell FW. *Ophthalmology: Principles and Concepts,* 8th ed. St. Louis, MO: Mosby, 1996.

Schachat AP, Cruess AF. *Ophthalmology.* Baltimore: Williams & Wilkins, 1984.

Question 130

Fantl JA, Newman DK, Colling J, et al. Urinary incontinence in adults: acute and chronic management. Urinary Incontinence in Adults Guideline Panel. Clinical practice guideline update. Rockville, MD: U.S. Department of Health and Human Services, 1996. Agency for Health Care Policy and Research Publication No. 96-0682.

Question 131

Gaidano G, Guerrasio A, Serra A, et al. Molecular mechanisms of tumor progression in chronic myeloproliferative disorders. *Leukemia* 1994;8:S27–S29.

Najean Y, Rain JD. The very long-term evolution of polycythemia vera: an analysis of 318 patients initially treated by phlebotomy or ^{32}P between 1969 and 1981. *Semin Hematol* 1997;34:6–16.

Tefferi A, Litzow MR, Noel P, et al. Chronic granulocytic leukemia: recent information on pathogenesis, diagnosis, and disease monitoring. *Mayo Clin Proc* 1997;72:445–452.

Question 132

Drazen JM, Israel E, Boushey HA, et al. Comparison of regularly scheduled with as-needed use of albuterol in mild asthma. Asthma Clinical Research Network. *N Engl J Med* 1996;335:841–847.

Question 134

Girolami A, Sartori MT, Simioni P. An updated classification of factor XIII defect. *Br J Haematol* 1991;77:565–566.

Suchman AL, Griner PF. Diagnostic uses of the activated partial thromboplastin time and prothrombin time. *Ann Intern Med* 1986;104:810–816.

Question 135

American Psychiatric Association. *Diagnostic and Statistical Manual of Mental Disorders,* 4th ed. Primary Care Version (DSM-IV-PC). Washington, DC: American Psychiatric Association Press, 1995.

Question 136

Smith SG. Horner's syndrome. In: Dambro MR, ed. *Griffith's 5-Minute Consult.* Baltimore: Lippincott Williams & Wilkins, 1999:502–503.

Question 137

Appelgren P, Ranjso U, Bindslev L, et al. Surface heparinization of central venous catheters reduces microbial colonization in vitro and in vivo: results from a prospective, randomized trial. *Crit Care Med* 1996;24:1482–1489.

Cobb DK, High KP, Sawyer RG, et al. A controlled trial of scheduled replacement of central venous and pulmonary-artery catheters. *N Engl J Med* 1992;327:1062–1068.

Eyer S, Brummitt C, Crossley K, et al. Catheter-related sepsis: prospective, randomized study of three different methods of long-term catheter maintenance. *Crit Care Med* 1990;18:1073–1079.

Maki DG, Ringer M. Risk factors for infusion-related phlebitis with small peripheral venous catheters: a randomized, controlled trial. *Ann Intern Med* 1991;114:845–854.

Question 138

Abel SJ, Finney SJ, Brett SJ, et al. Reduced mortality in association with acute respiratory distress syndrome (ARDS). *Thorax* 1998;53:292–294.

Crawford SW, Petersen FB. Long-term survival from respiratory failure after marrow transplantation for malignancy. *Am Rev Respir Dis* 1992;145:510–514.

Mansel JK, Stogner SW, Petrini MF, et al. Mechanical ventilation in patients with acute severe asthma. *Am J Med* 1990;89:42–48.

Marquette CH, Saulnier F, Leroy O, et al. Long-term prognosis of near-fatal asthma: a 6-year follow-up study of 145 asthmatic patients who underwent mechanical ventilation for a near-fatal attack of asthma. *Am Rev Respir Dis* 1992;146:76–81.

Milberg JA, Davis DR, Steinberg KP, et al. Improved survival of patients with acute respiratory distress syndrome (ARDS): 1983–1993. *JAMA* 1995;273:306–309.

Rangel-Frausto MS, Pittet D, Costigan M, et al. The natural history of the systemic inflammatory response syndrome (SIRS): a prospective study. *JAMA* 1995;273:117–123.

Schapira DV, Studnicki J, Bradham DD, et al. Intensive care, survival, and expense of treating critically ill cancer patients. *JAMA* 1993;269:783–786.

Weiss SM, Hudson LD. Outcome from respiratory failure: predicting intensive care unit outcome. *Crit Care Clin* 1994;10:197–215.

Westerman DE, Benatar SR, Potgieter PD, et al. Identification of the high-risk asthmatic patient: experience with 39 patients undergoing ventilation for status asthmaticus. *Am J Med* 1979;66:565–572.

Question 140

Dabbs DJ, Striker LM, Mignon F, et al. Glomerular lesions in lymphomas and leukemias. *Am J Med* 1986;80:63–70.

Nolasco F, Cameron JS, Heywood EF, et al. Adult-onset minimal change nephrotic syndrome: a long-term follow-up. *Kidney Int* 1986;29:1215–1223.

Warren GV, Korbet SM, Schwartz MM, et al. Minimal change glomerulopathy associated with nonsteroidal antiinflammatory drugs. *Am J Kidney Dis* 1989;13:127–130.

Question 141

Garber AM, Browner WS, Hulley SB. Cholesterol screening in asymptomatic adults, revisited. Part 2. *Ann Intern Med* 1996;124:518–531.

Guidelines for using serum cholesterol, high-density lipoprotein cholesterol, and triglyceride levels as screening tests for preventing coronary heart disease in adults. American College of Physicians. Part 1. *Ann Intern Med* 1996;124:515–517.

Screening for high blood cholesterol and other lipid abnormalities. In: *Guide to Clinical Preventive Services: Report of the U.S. Preventive Services Task Force*, 2nd ed. Baltimore: Williams & Wilkins, 1996:15–38.

Smith GD, Song F, Sheldon TA. Cholesterol lowering and mortality: the importance of considering initial level of risk. *BMJ* 1993;306:1367–1373.

Summary of the second report of the National Cholesterol Education Program (NCEP) Expert Panel on Detection, Evaluation, and Treatment of High Blood Cholesterol in Adults. *JAMA* 1993;269:3015–3023.

Question 142

Fine MJ, Smith MA, Carson CA, et al. Prognosis and outcome of patients with community-acquired pneumonia: a meta-analysis. *JAMA* 1996;275:134–141.

Potgieter PD, Hammond JM. The intensive care management, mortality and prognostic indicators in severe community-acquired pneumococcal pneumonia. *Intensive Care Med* 1996;22:1301–1306.

Tuomanen EI, Austrian R, Masure H. Pathogenesis of pneumococcal infection. *N Engl J Med* 1995;332:1280–1284.

Question 143

NIH consensus conference. Ovarian cancer: screening, treatment, and follow-up. NIH Consensus Development Panel on Ovarian Cancer. *JAMA* 1995;273:491–497.

Question 144

Wu KK. Morton's interdigital neuroma: a clinical review of its etiology, treatment, and results. *J Ankle Foot Surg* 1996;35:112–119.

Question 146

Greenberger PA, Patterson R. Diagnosis and management of allergic bronchopulmonary aspergillosis. *Ann Allergy* 1986;56:444–448.

Question 147

Bennett CL, Weinberg PD, Rozenberg-Ben-Dror K, et al. Thrombotic thrombocytopenic purpura associated with ticlopidine: a review of 60 cases. *Ann Intern Med* 1998;128:541–544.

George JN, Gilcher RO, Smith JW, et al. Thrombotic thrombocytopenic purpura–hemolytic uremic syndrome: diagnosis and management. *J Clin Apheresis* 1998;13:120–125.

Leavey SF, Weinberg J. Thrombotic thrombocytopenic purpura associated with ticlopidine therapy. *J Am Soc Nephrol* 1997;8:689–693.

Question 148

Wilson W, Taubert KA, Gewitz M, et al. Prevention of infective endocarditis: guidelines from the American Heart Association: a guideline from the American Heart Association Rheumatic Fever, Endocarditis, and Kawasaki Disease Committee, Council on Cardiovascular Disease in the Young, and the Council on Clinical Cardiology, Council on Cardiovascular Surgery and Anesthesia, and the Quality of Care and Outcomes Research Interdisciplinary Working Group. *Circulation* 2007;116:1736.

Question 150

George JN, el-Harake MA, Raskob GE. Chronic idiopathic thrombocytopenic purpura. *N Engl J Med* 1994;331:1207–1211.

Stasi R, Stipa E, Masi M, et al. Long-term observation of 208 adults with chronic idiopathic thrombocytopenic purpura. *Am J Med* 1995;98:436–442.

Question 151

Irwin RS, Curley FJ, French CL. Chronic cough: the spectrum and frequency of causes, key components of the diagnostic evaluation, and outcome of specific therapy. *Am Rev Respir Dis* 1990;141:640–647.

Israili ZH, Hall WD. Cough and angioneurotic edema associated with angiotensin-converting enzyme inhibitor therapy: a review of the literature and pathophysiology. *Ann Intern Med* 1992;117:234–242.

Mello CJ, Irwin RS, Curley FJ. Predictive values of the character, timing, and complications of chronic cough in diagnosing its cause. *Arch Intern Med* 1996;156:997–1003.

Pratter MR, Bartter T, Akers S, et al. An algorithmic approach to chronic cough. *Ann Intern Med* 1993;119:977–983.

Question 152

Brieger DB, Mak KH, Kottke-Marchant K, et al. Heparin-induced thrombocytopenia. *J Am Coll Cardiol* 1998;31:1449–1459.

Warkentin TE, Levine MN, Hirsh J, et al. Heparin-induced thrombocytopenia in patients treated with low-molecular-weight heparin or unfractionated heparin. *N Engl J Med* 1995;332:1330–1335.

Question 153

Ginsberg JS, Wells PS, Kearon C, et al. Sensitivity and specificity of a rapid whole-blood assay for D-dimer in the diagnosis of pulmonary embolism. *Ann Intern Med* 1998;129:1006–1111.

Question 154

Earley CJ. Restless legs syndrome. *N Engl J Med* 2003;348:2103.

Silber MH, Ehrenberg BL, Allen RP, et al. An algorithm for the management of restless legs syndrome. *Mayo Clin Proc* 2004;79:916.

Question 155

Austrian R, Gold J. Pneumococcal bacteremia with especial reference to bacteremic pneumococcal pneumonia. *Ann Intern Med* 1964;60:759.

Barrett-Conner E. The non-value of sputum culture in the diagnosis of pneumococcal pneumonia. *Am Rev Respir Dis* 1970;103:845.

Question 156

Amorosi E, Utmann J. Thrombotic thrombocytopenic purpura: report of 16 cases and review of the literature. *Medicine (Baltimore)* 1966;45:139.

Bennett CL, Connors JM, Carwile JM, et al. Thrombotic thrombocytopenic purpura associated with clopidogrel. *N Engl J Med* 2000;342:1773–1777.

CAPRIE Steering Committee. A randomised, blinded, trial of clopidogrel versus aspirin in patients at risk of ischemic events (CAPRIE). *Lancet* 1996;348:1329–1339.

Connors JM, Gopfert C, Robson S, et al. Clopidogrel associated TTP. *Transfusion* 1999;39(Suppl):56S.

Questions 157–159

Cunningham-Rundles C, Siegal FP, Cunningham-Rundles S, et al. Incidence of cancer in 98 patients with common varied immunodeficiency. *J Clin Immunol* 1987;7:294–299.

Densen P. Complement deficiencies and meningococcal disease. *Clin Exp Immunol* 1991;86(Suppl 1):57.

Ellison RT III, Kohler PF, Curd JG, et al. Prevalence of congenital or acquired complement deficiency in patients with sporadic meningococcal disease. *N Engl J Med* 1983;308:913.

Kinlen LJ, Webster AD, Bird AG, et al. Prospective study of cancer in patients with hypogammaglobulinaemia. *Lancet* 1985;1:263–266.

Questions 160–165

Consensus Development Conference. Consensus development conference: diagnosis, prophylaxis, and treatment of osteoporosis. *Am J Med* 1993;94:646.

Gardsell P, Johnell O, Nilsson BE. The predictive value of forearm bone mineral content measurements in men. *Bone* 1990;11:229–232.

Kanis JA, Melton LJ III, Christiansen C, et al. The diagnosis of osteoporosis. *J Bone Miner Res* 1994;9:1137.

Rosen FS, Cooper MD, Wedgwood RJP. Medical progress: the primary immunodeficiencies. *N Engl J Med* 1995;333:431–440.

Rosol TJ, Capen CC. Mechanisms of cancer-induced hypercalcemia. *Lab Invest* 1992;67:680.

Seymour JF, Gagel RF. Calcitriol: the major humoral mediator of hypercalcemia in Hodgkin's disease and non-Hodgkin's lymphomas. *Blood* 1993;82:1383.

Silverberg SJ, Shane E, Jacobs TP, et al. Nephrolithiasis and bone involvement in primary hyperparathyroidism. *Am J Med* 1990;89:327.

Silverberg SJ, Bilezikian JP. Evaluation and management of primary hyperparathyroidism. *J Clin Endocrinol Metab* 1996;81:2036.

Sneller MC, Strober W, Eisenstein E, et al. NIH conference: new insights into common variable immunodeficiency. *Ann Intern Med* 1993;188:720–730.

Walport MJ. Advances in immunology: complement—first of two parts. *N Engl J Med* 2001;344:1058–1066.

Question 166

Connelly TJ, Becker A, McDonald JW. Bachelor scurvy. *Int J Dermatol* 1982;21:209–211.

Hirschmann JV, Raugi GJ. Adult scurvy. *J Am Acad Dermatol* 1999;41:95–906.

Hodges RE, Baker EM, Hood J, et al. Experimental scurvy in man. *Am J Clin Nutr* 1969;22:535–548.

Reddy AV, Chan K, Jones JIW, et al. Spontaneous bruising in an elderly woman. *Postgrad Med J* 1998;74:273–275.

Reuler JB, Broudy VC, Cooney TG. Adult scurvy. *JAMA* 1985;253:805–807.

Stewart CP, Guthrie D. *Lind's treatise on scurvy*. Edinburgh: Edinburgh University Press, 1953:113–126.

Question 167

Lieber CS. Medical disorders of alcoholism. *N Engl J Med* 1995;333:1058.

Victor M, Adams RD, Collins GH. *The Wernicke-Korsakoff Syndrome and Related Disorders due to alcoholism and Malnutrition*. Philadelphia: Davis, 1989.

Question 168

Beyenburg S, Zierz S, Jerusalem F. Inclusion body myositis: clinical and histopathological features of 36 patients. *Clin Invest* 1993;71:351.

Gerster JC, Vischer TL, Fallet GH. Destructive arthropathy in generalized osteoarthritis with articular chondrocalcinosis. *J Rheumatol* 1975;2:265.

Hamilton EBD, Richards AJ. Destructive arthropathy in chondrocalcinosis articularis. *Ann Rheum Dis* 1974;33:196.

Kula RW, Sawchak JA, Sher JH. Inclusion body myositis. *Curr Opin Rheumatol* 1989;1:460.

Questions 170–172

Service FJ, O'Brien PC, McMahon MM, et al. C-peptide during the prolonged fast in insulinoma. *J Clin Endocrinol Metab* 1993;76:655–659.

Question 181

George JN, Woolf SH, Raskob GE, et al. Idiopathic thrombocytopenic purpura: a practice guideline developed by explicit methods for the American Society of Hematology. *Blood* 1996;88:3–40.

Moise KJ Jr. Autoimmune thrombocytopenic purpura in pregnancy. *Clin Obstet Gynecol* 1991;34:51–63.

Questions 182–187

Balasubramaniam K, Grambsch PM, Wiesner RH, et al. Diminished survival in asymptomatic primary biliary cirrhosis: a prospective study. *Gastroenterology* 1990;98:1567–1571.

Gollan JL, Bateman C, Billing BH. Effect of dietary composition on the unconjugated hyperbilirubinaemia of Gilbert's syndrome. *Gut* 1976;17:335–340.

Kaplan MM. Primary biliary cirrhosis. *N Engl J Med* 1996;335:1570–1580.

Lednar WM, Lemon SM, Kirkpatrick JW, et al. Frequency of illness associated with epidemic hepatitis A virus infections in adults. *Am J Epidemiol* 1985;122:226–233.

Question 197

Llach F. *Renal Vein Thrombosis*. New York: Futura, 1983.

Questions 200–207

Grateau G. Clinical and genetic aspects of the hereditary periodic fever syndromes. *Rheumatology* 2004;43(4):410–415.

Simon A, Van der Meer JW, Vzsely R, et al. Approach to genetic analysis in the diagnosis of hereditary autoinflammatory syndromes. *Rheumatology (Oxford)* 2006;45(3):269–273.

Index